# Meat Hygiene

Commissioning Editor: *Catriona Byres*
Project Editor: *Deborah Russell*
Project Controller: *Mark Sanderson*
Production Editor: *Tim Kimber*

# Meat Hygiene

J. F. GRACEY

PhD, BAgr, FRCVS, DVSM, FRSH
(formerly City Veterinarian, Belfast)

D. S. COLLINS

MVB, DVPH (MH), CBiol, MIBiol, MBIAC, MRCVS
Consultant in Veterinary Public Health
(formerly City Veterinarian, Belfast)

R. J. HUEY

MVB, DVPH (MH), MRCVS
(currently) Divisional Veterinary Officer, Veterinary Service,
Department of Agriculture for Northern Ireland, Belfast

TENTH EDITION

W. B. SAUNDERS COMPANY LTD
London • Edinburgh • New York • Philadelphia • Sydney • Toronto

WB SAUNDERS
An imprint of Harcourt Brace and Company Limited



First published 1949 as *Textbook of Meat Inspection* by H. Thornton
Seventh edition published 1981 as *Thornton's Meat Hygiene* by J. F. Gracey
Eighth edition 1986 *Meat Hygiene* by J. F. Gracey
Ninth edition 1992 by J. F. Gracey and D. S. Collins

English Language Book Society edition of eighth edition 1986
Italian edition of seventh edition (Ermes, Milan) 1984

ISBN 0 7020 2258 6

**British Library Cataloguing in Publication Data**
A catalogue record for this book is available from the British Library

**Library of Congress Cataloging in Publication Data**
A catalog record for this book is available from the Library of Congress

**Note**
Medical knowledge is constantly changing. As new information becomes available, changes in treatment, procedures, equipment and the use of drugs become necessary. The editors/authors/contributors and the publishers have, as far as it is possible, taken care to ensure that the information given in this text is accurate and up-to-date. However, readers are strongly advised to confirm that the information, especially with regard to drug usage, complies with the latest legislation and standards of practice.

Typeset by IMH (Cartrif), Loanhead, Scotland

Printed in China

The publisher's policy is to use **paper manufactured from sustainable forests**

# Contents


| | | |
|---|---|---|
| | List of Colour Plates | vi |
| | Preface | vii |
| | Acknowledgements | ix |
| 1 | The Food Animals | 1 |
| 2 | Anatomy, Meat Composition and Quality | 19 |
| 3 | Meat Plant Construction and Equipment | 77 |
| 4 | Preservation of Meat | 101 |
| 5 | By-products Treatment | 129 |
| 6 | Plant Sanitation | 143 |
| 7 | From Farm to Slaughter | 163 |
| 8 | Humane Slaughter | 197 |
| 9 | Meat Hygiene Practice | 223 |
| 10 | Red Meat Inspection | 243 |
| 11 | Poultry Production, Slaughter and Inspection | 261 |
| 12 | Exotic Meat Production | 289 |
| 13 | Chemical Residues in Meat | 299 |
| 14 | Food Poisoning and Meat Microbiology | |
| | Part 1 – Food Poisoning | 321 |
| | Part 2 – Meat Microbiology | 339 |
| | Part 3 – The Meat Plant Laboratory | 355 |
| 15 | Occupational Injuries and Infections | 409 |
| 16 | Pathology | 421 |
| 17 | Infectious Diseases | 505 |
| 18 | Diseases Caused by Helminth and Arthropod Parasites | 635 |
| 19 | Metabolic Diseases and Nutritional Deficiencies | 699 |
| 20 | Diseases Caused by Environmental Pollutants | 709 |
| 21 | Disease Data Retrieval and Feedback | 725 |
| | Appendix I: By-products of the UK Meat Industry | 741 |
| | Index | 743 |

# List of Colour Plates


**Plate 1**

Fig. 1 Lumpy skin disease. Bovine.
Fig. 2 Scrapie. Ram.
Fig. 3 Scrapie. Lesions in vestibular nucleus of brain.
Fig. 4 Melanosis. Liver, lungs, kidney and heart. Sheep.
Fig. 5 Endocarditis. Heart. Bovine.
Fig. 6 Contagious bovine pleuropneumonia. Lung. Bovine.

**Plate 2**

Fig. 7 Lymphosarcoma. Peritoneum. Bovine.
Fig. 8 Epizootic lymphangitis. Leg. Horse.
Fig. 9 Haematoma. Spleen. Bovine.
Fig. 10 Goitre. Thyroid. Calf.
Fig. 11 Goat pox. Tail. Goat.
Fig. 12 Vitamin D deficiency. Sheep.

**Plate 3**

Fig. 13 Deep pectoral myopathy. Fowl.
Fig. 14 Haemorrhagic septicaemia. Lungs. Bovine.
Fig. 15 Coenurus *serialis*. Rabbit.
Fig. 16 Coenurus *cerebralis*. Sheep.
Fig. 17 Anaplocephala magna. Small intestine. Horse (1 year old).
Fig. 18 Hydatid cyst. Liver. Sheep.

**Plate 4**

Fig. 19 *Onchocerca gibsoni*. Oesophagus. Bovine.
Fig. 20 *T. saginata*. Scolex and proglottids.
Fig. 21 *Cysticercus cellulosae*. Diaphragm. Pig.
Fig. 22 Blackhead. Liver. Turkey.
Fig. 23 Cholangiohepatitis. Broiler.
Fig. 24 Marek's disease. Proventriculus. Broiler.


**Plates 1–4**


Grateful thanks for loan of transparencies are accorded to the following: Central Veterinary Laboratory (Fig. 3); D. E. Counter (Figs 5, 10, 12); R. M. Edelsten (Figs 6, 8, 11, 14, 19); M. Fussey (Figs 4, 7, 9); M. Jeffrey (Fig. 13); J. A. Kendrick (Fig. 1); Dr K. A. Linklater (Fig. 2); C. J. Randall (Figs 22, 23, 24); Professor A. J. Trees (Figs 15 to 18, 20, 21).



**Between pages 342–343 and 406–407.**

# Preface

This tenth edition of *Meat Hygiene* has been largely rewritten and enlarged to take account of the many developments in the last decade, to further emphasise the importance of microbiology and to make the book more international in character.

Bovine spongiform encephalopathy and *E. coli* O157 H7 in particular, along with the introduction of some genetically-modified food, have served to undermine the confidence of the consumer in the safety of food in Britain and elsewhere, despite the reassurances issued by authorities. It is difficult to place reliance on oft-repeated pronouncements about food safety, especially when these emerge suddenly, are later contradicted, are sometimes associated with vested interests or are suddenly imposed on the population without evidence of adequate and competent research findings.

The concept of 'Plough to Plate', 'Stable to Table' is at last being recognised since accountability cannot be laid solely at the door of meat inspection. Livestock producers have the chief responsibility to ensure that clean, healthy livestock, free from potentially harmful residues, are presented for slaughter with close attention being paid to welfare on the farm, through transport and in the meat plant. It is depressing to reflect, however, that the classic work of Empey and Scott on carcase contamination was carried out in Australia in 1939.

To cater for this ever-increasing task, it has been necessary to enlist the help of other experts. Robert Huey is an officer in charge of meat hygiene in the Department of Agriculture for Northern Ireland where he is in touch with developments in the European Union and further afield, in addition to his extensive experience in livestock husbandry. Along with other text material, he has been responsible for updating the important chapter on Farm to Slaughter.

Professor W.J. Reilly, BVMS, BSc, MRCVS, DVSM, of the Scottish Centre for Infection and Environmental Health, Glasgow, has been involved in public health matters, especially foodborne disease, for many years and has made a significant contribution to our knowledge of this vital area. Such is the importance of this sector that we have also seen fit to introduce a section on the function of the meat plant laboratory, this especially in view of the fact that little is known of the intangible potential pathogens passing through many abattoirs making final judgement based solely on visual inspection at best a doubtful procedure. Indeed, such is the load of bacteria currently entering meat plants that reliance in the future may well have to be based on carcase pasteurisation with subsequent microbiological testing of meat samples.

The oft-neglected, yet vital subject of sanitation has been revised and expanded by Stan R. Brown, BSc, (Hons), Dip. MGMT MSIM, Marketing Director, Kleencare, Europe, and that of the other intangibles (chemical residues) by Dr. W.J. McCaughey, MVB, MA, MSc (Ohio), PhD, FRAgS, late Deputy Director of Veterinary Sciences Division, Department of Agriculture, Northern Ireland.

J. F. Gracey

# Acknowledgements

The cooperation we received from the many associates and firms listed in the ninth edition of *Meat Hygiene* continued for the most part.

In particular, we have to pay tribute to the United States Department of Agriculture's Food Safety and Inspection Service for their generous assistance. Their 'MEAT and POULTRY HOTLINE – We are just a phone call away', which gives valuable advice to consumers, business people, health professionals, teachers, Members of Congress, etc., on safe food handling, storage, temperature control, cooking, foodborne illness, etc., is a service which could with advantage be copied by other authorities. Staffed by a team of qualified food technologists, registered dieticians and home economists it also provides excellent publications.

We are grateful to Dr. David Sainsbury, Cambridge Centre for Animal Health & Welfare, Cambridge for information on livestock housing.

Dr Anne-Marie Farmer, BVSc. (Qu), MRCVS, Brian Kennedy, MRCVS, Dr Alaistair F. Carson and Dr George McElroy, MRCVS, wrote and commented on the 'Food Animals' chapter.

The UK Ministry of Agriculture, Fisheries and Food was unstinting in providing up-to-date legislation, information bulletins and, through the Meat Hygiene Agency, material for their Operations Manual and our thanks are accorded to them, especially the Chief Executive, Johnston McNeill and the Head of Operations, Peter Soul. The Ministry of Agriculture and Scottish Environment Protection Agency (MAFF/SEPA) provided us with their much-appreciated regular copies of their reports (Radioactivity in Food and the Environment). We are indebted to the Northern Ireland Department of Agriculture through its veterinary officials (C.D. Hart, R.H.S. Moore, J.A. Ross, M.B. Geddis, J.H. O'Neill, Dr S.W.J. McDowell, K.A. Elliott (now with the European Commission) and meat inspector A. Rice for information on pathology and carcase dressing and related items. Peter I. Hewson, Veterinary Head, Joint Food Safety and Standards Group, Dr J.A. Storrar and F.A. Eames, MRCVS, gave advice on exotic meat production. Dr Raymond Cooper, C.Eng., F.Inst.R., gave valuable information on refrigeration.

The assistance of Dr. I. Blair of the University of Ulster on matters microbiological is gratefully acknowledged as is that of his colleagues, J.V. Kyle and O. Hetherington, Environmental Health Department, on processing and meat plant construction, respectively, and Alan McBride and Derek Boucher on by-product processing.

Valuable information on meat hygiene was available from the British Veterinary Association, London via their summaries of EU legislation and events of veterinary interest for which we would like to thank Helena Cotton. Miss B.A. Horder and Miss Jenny Harris of the Royal College of Veterinary Surgeons Wellcome Library were always to hand for photocopies of articles and deserve our thanks.

We would like to thank the Leatherhead Research Association, Leatherhead, Surrey, UK, especially P.N. Church, David Pimbley and J.M. Wood for supplying data on microbiology and quality assurance in general. We have utilised their splendid Manual of Manufacturing Meat Quality, produced under the chairmanship of Dr. Tom Toomey of Ventress Technical Services, Cambridge, that doyen of the food industry to whom one of us (JFG) is forever appreciative for a constant supply of food industry information.

## *Acknowledgements*

We are indebted to Dr. G. Georghiev, Head, Joint FAO/WHO Food Standards Programme, Rome and Dr. K. Stohr, Division of Communicable Diseases, Veterinary Public Health, World Health Organization, Geneva, Switzerland for help with Codex Alimentarius reports.

Our knowledge of the Australian system of meat inspection was augmented by Drs B. Biddle, P. Hickey and P.J. Corrigan of the Australian Quarantine and Inspection Service, Department of Primary Industries, Canberra and acknowledged with thanks.

New Zealand made its much appreciated contribution to our task mainly through advice on meat hygiene practice and humane slaughter, the latter via the publication by the late Professor D.K Blackmore and M.W. Delany.

It has been a pleasure over the years to collaborate with the Danish Meat Research Institute at Roskilde. Developments in lairage construction and carcase data retrieval and feedback are kindly acknowledged to its Director, Dr. Nielsen and to Dr. R. Zachrau.

Copies of transparencies/photographs were provided by D.E. Counter, J. Lucas, F.T.W. Jordan, J.A. Kendrick, Profs C. Mahon and G. Manuselis, M. Jeffrey, Prof. K.A. Linklater, M. Fussey, R.M. Edelston, D.W. Sainsbury, C.J. Randall, Prof. A.J. Trees, G.H. Wells, Prof. Diane Newell, S.E. Gold, P. Hawtin, T.Y. Fletcher, P.G.G. Jackson, R.W. Blowey and B.E.C. Shreuder. All are acknowledged with thanks.

We are grateful to the UK Meat and Livestock Commission who provided valuable information on the British livestock industry through its Director, C.W. Maclean and Head of Veterinary Services, J.H. Pratt who has always been a source of encouragement.

The UK Humane Slaughter Association, The Old School, Brewhouse Hill, Wheathampstead, Hertfordshire AL4 8AN collaborated in the field of livestock handling and humane slaughter. Our thanks are accorded to Sir Michael Simmons, Miss Miriam Parker and Charles Mason.

Dr Steve Watton and Dr Mohan Raz, University of Bristol, also advised on humane slaughter and handling.

As longstanding members of the UK Veterinary Public Health Association, we have profited from their various meetings and also from discussions with colleagues, a large number of whom are involved in active meat inspection duties. To VPHA and the members we express our thanks. A special thanks is accorded to Dr. R.A. Jones, Maun, Botswana whose encouragement and advice have always been available.

We are grateful to Professors J. Hannan, J.D. Collins and P.J. Quinn of the National University of Ireland Faculty of Veterinary Medicine, Dublin whose excellent Laboratory Handbook on Food Hygiene (Hannan & Collins) and Veterinary Microbiology and Parasitology (Quinn) we have been pleased to consult.

Cooperating private firms supplying advice and photographs include Accles & Shelvoke, Witton, Birmingham, England; Biotrace Ltd., Bridgend, Glamorgan, Wales; Stork PMV B.V. of Boxmeer, Holland; Alfa-Laval Meat By-products, Soborg, Denmark; Anglia Airflow, Diss, Norfolk, England; Oxoid Ltd., Basingstoke, Hampshire, England; Sovereign Food Group, Eye, Suffolk, England; Rentokil Environmental Services, East Grinstead, West Sussex, England; Metal Box Ltd.; North West Water, Warrington, England; Merck Ltd., Laboratory Supplies, Poole, Dorset, England: Kleencare Hygiene, Cheadle, Cheshire, England; bioMerieux Vitek Inc. Missouri, USA; Scan Farmek, Skara, Sweden; SFK Meat Systems of Kolding, Denmark; Nijhuis, Lichtenvoorde, The Netherlands and Idexx Laboratories, Maine, USA. Our thanks are accorded to them.

Paul Fforde Gracey, HND, Food Technologist, supplied valuable advice on meat plant operations and food industry quality assurance for which we are duly thankful.

An enlarged *Meat Hygiene* required expert copyediting. We are indebted to Richard Cook of Keyword Publishing Services, Barking, Essex, England and to Len Cegielka, Farington, Preston, Lancashire, England who corrected our numerous errata.

Finally, we would like to show our appreciation for the guidance and patience of the staff of Harcourt Brace & Company; Sean Duggan, Editor-in-chief, Catriona Byres, Deborah Russell, Tim Kimber, Jonathan Price and Mark Sanderson.

J. F. Gracey

# Chapter 1
# The Food Animals

'HEALTH is a state of complete physical, mental and social well-being and not merely the absence of disease or infirmity.' *World Health Organization Chronicle*, 1978.

Meat is normally regarded as the edible parts (muscle and offal) of the food animals which consume mainly grass and other arable crops, *viz.* cattle, sheep, goats, pigs, horses, deer, reindeer, buffalo, musk oxen, moose, caribou, yak, camel, alpaca, llama, guanaco, vicuna, etc. In addition, poultry have become a major meat-producing species while rabbits, guinea pigs, capybara and various game animals and birds provide a substantial amount of protein, particularly in localised areas. Fish and other seafood have also been an important part of man's diet since earliest times.

Although, theoretically, hundreds of animals could supply meat for human consumption, in practice only a relatively small number of species is used today. This is all the more remarkable since it represents in general the instruction of the Levitical Law of the Old Testament, most of which is in accord with modern sanitary science. The animals suitable for the food of man had to part the hoof and chew the cud. Only those fish with fins and scales were wholesome. It is true that today we eat pig, rabbit and hare, but it is recognised that they are subject to parasitic infestation. There appears to be little doubt that the dangers of trichinosis and of *Cysticercus cellulosae* were recognised 1400 years before the birth of Christ. In many parts of the world, horse flesh forms an important article of human diet. The Danes reintroduced the consumption of horse flesh into Europe during the siege of Copenhagen in 1807; slaughter of horses for human consumption is now well established in Denmark, Belgium, Holland and Germany.

All the above animals, including fish, are *converters*, i.e. they utilise green vegetable material with varying efficiency to produce protein. Even microorganisms can be classified as converters in that they use carbohydrates from plants to make protein from simple nitrogenous compounds. Especially when an animal eats something which is inedible for man or could not easily be made into food for man, it is considered valuable as a source of food; so when pigs and poultry, and even other animal species, are used as scavengers to eat scraps, by-products, etc., they are very useful indeed. However, when food which could be utilised by human beings is fed to livestock, the question of efficiency becomes more problematic. Nevertheless, other factors, such as the production of manure for fertiliser usage, variety in the human diet, etc., have to be borne in mind.

Not only did the Creator command the earth to 'bring forth grass, the herb yielding seed and the fruit tree yielding fruit after his kind' (Genesis 1:11), He also 'made the beast of the earth after his kind, and cattle after their kind, and everything that creepeth upon the earth after his kind' (Genesis 1:25). For both plant and beast, 'God saw that it was good' (Genesis 1:12 & 25). They were *both* to be used for the food of man.

In more recent times efforts have been made to domesticate certain *wild animals*, although many of these have been used as food since ancient times. In Africa and Russia, elands are being domesticated, as well as antelope in the latter country. Kangaroos are being kept for meat in Australia and, in South America, the large rodent capybara, which is a semi-aquatic vegetarian, is being used as a source of meat, although it is not especially palatable. There are probably many other wild species which could be utilised in meat production and would have some advantages over the domesticated animals since they exist on less valuable land, need only rough grazing, are more disease-resistant and act as a tourist attraction. Some problems, however, arise in connection with feeding, protection from predators, slaughter and meat inspection.

Recent innovations have included the breeding of *wild boar* in England and *buffalo* in Germany, France and Poland. Wild boars introduced from Germany and Denmark into England are used to produce purebreds as well as crosses with established breeds of pigs. Differences in quality and flavour are said to exist between the wild variety and the various crosses. Litter sizes average six piglets and only one litter is produced yearly. Slaughtered at 12–14 months, wild boar has a liveweight of about 59 kg and a deadweight of around 45 kg. The meat is very lean with an acceptable flavour but stress is sometimes associated with abattoir slaughter, which may necessitate on-farm handling. In Great Britain the keeping of wild boar is subject to the Dangerous Wild Animals Act.

*Buffalo* meat is said to be more tender, leaner and gamier than beef, with lower levels of cholesterol. Although expensive in France, it is cheaper than beef in Canada. The name buffalo is often applied to the bison (*Bison bison*) of North America, a different species of the order Bovidae. There are several species, the Indian buffalo (*Bubalus bubalis*), sometimes called the water buffalo or arna, is the only one to be domesticated. It is found in many parts of the Old World, with significant numbers in Hungary, Italy and France.

The future for meat and meat products will depend mainly on consumer demand and the prices at which they can be profitably produced. As living standards rise, so also does the consumption of meat. Factors such as the cost of production, feed conversion efficiency, land use and availability, consumer taste, price to consumers, diet, attitudes of people to meat production methods, use of protein from non-animal sources, etc., will all play a part in determining future demands.

Procedures such as genetic engineering, embryo transfer, cross-breeding and twinning will continue to be utilised in attempts to produce more productive livestock with improved milk and meat quality. But if close attention is not paid to the vital importance of *disease resistance*, we may well see the development of stock susceptible to existing and novel conditions, some of which may have serious public health implications. Consumer attitudes must always be borne in mind by research workers and those engaged in the agriculture and food industries, which will only prosper in a climate of real consumer confidence in the quality and safety of food.

In order to address this point, much food from animals is produced under 'Farm Quality Assured Schemes'. These provide customers with some assurance that the animals have been reared in a manner which involves animal welfare and environmental issues and are fit to produce wholesome, safe, food products. This complements the 'plough-to-plate' approach to meat production with control over all the nutritional, welfare, housing and other management factors, as well as ensuring the traceability of the food product. Veterinarians have a pivotal role in this discipline, both on the farm and at the meat plant.

## DIETARY FACTORS

Concern about the amount of fat, especially saturated fat, in the diet, has been given prominence in the USA and the UK. In the former country the incidence of ischaemic heart disease (IHD) has decreased owing to the reduction of fat intake. In the UK a report on *Diet and Cardiovascular Disease* was produced by the Committee on the Medical Aspects of Food and Nutrition Policy (COMA) in 1984. This recommended that saturated fat consumption should be reduced by 25% but that some increase in polyunsaturated fat would be acceptable, in which case the total fat intake need only be reduced by 15%.

Since the COMA Report is an official document which has been accepted as government policy, it means that government agencies including the Ministry of Agriculture, Fisheries and Food are obliged to put its recommendations into effect. Already steps are being taken to have legislation which will require total fat and saturated fatty acid content labelling on a wide variety of foodstuffs. While much of the intake of fat is derived from milk and dairy products, meat and meat products, margarine, cooking fat and salad oils, some comes from vegetable sources, where it is either produced in a saturated form, e.g. coconut oil, or converted into such during manufacture.

The sources of fat in the average British diet are given in Table 1.1.

If people respond to the COMA recommendations, and there are indications that this is already the case, there will be major

**Table 1.1** Average British diet – sources of fat (1981).

| Food groups | % Total fat |
|---|---|
| Milk and dairy products, excluding butter | 18.9 |
| Total meat | 27.0 |
| Total fish | 1.1 |
| Eggs | 2.7 |
| Total fats, i.e. butter, margarine, cooking fats, salad oils, etc. | 36.6 |
| Total vegetables | 2.0 |
| Total fruit | 0.9 |
| Total cereals | 9.6 |
| Total beverages | 0.1 |
| Other foods | 1.1 |
| Total, all foods | 100.00 |

Source: National Food Survey.

changes in food consumption which will inevitably have an impact on production methods in agriculture, especially in milk and livestock production, despite the fact that not all is known about the aetiology of the commonest cause of death in most industrialised countries. (In the UK, in 1995, 27% of all deaths in men and 18% of all deaths in women, under 75 were ascribed to IHD.) Factors such as heredity, blood pressure, obesity, blood haemostasis, physical inactivity, water hardness, smoking and alcohol consumption are also involved in the causation of this serious condition.

In 1997 COMA reported on diet and cancer. It recommended:

1. Maintain a healthy body weight and do not increase it during adult life.
2. Increase intake of a wide variety of fruits and vegetables.
3. Increase intake of dietary fibre from a variety of food sources.
4. Eat average amounts of red meat (UK average is 90 g cooked per day).

Over the last 20 years, the amount of red meat eaten in the UK has fallen by 25%, yet the incidence of colon cancer has increased by 20% over the same period. The consumption of meat per head of the population in the UK is among the lowest of all the EU countries, as Table 1.2 shows.

Consumer demand is now for leaner meat in smaller, waste-free cuts, easy and quick to prepare. On the livestock breeding and rearing side, changes have taken place with the emphasis on animals which produce leaner carcases. Appropriate grading and certification standards are applied in meat plants. Quite apart from the health aspect, overfat stock are

**Table 1.2** Annual consumption of meat (kg/head) (EC 1996).

| | Beef and veal | Sheep and goat meat | Pig meat | Poultry meat | Total meat |
|---|---|---|---|---|---|
| Bel/Lux | 20.7 | 2.1 | 48.1 | 24.6 | 95.5 |
| DK | 19 | 1.2 | 58.6 | 15.9 | 94.7 |
| D | 15.2 | 1.2 | 54.9 | 13.6 | 84.9 |
| GR | 20.9 | 13.9 | 22.9 | 19 | 76.7 |
| SP | 12.2 | 6.4 | 56.6 | 26.6 | 101.8 |
| FR | 26.5 | 5.2 | 36 | 23.2 | 90.9 |
| IR | 19.2 | 5 | 33.9 | 30 | 88.1 |
| IT | 23.5 | 1.8 | 33.8 | 20 | 79.1 |
| NL | 21.8 | 1.4 | 50.1 | 21.5 | 94.8 |
| AUS | 16.5 | 1.2 | 58.6 | 14.5 | 90.8 |
| PO | 14.4 | 4 | 36.2 | 25.2 | 79.8 |
| FIN | 19.4 | 0.2 | 30.9 | 7.4 | 57.9 |
| SWE | 18.7 | 0.6 | 37.3 | 7 | 63.6 |
| UK | 14 | 6.3 | 23.6 | 28.1 | 72 |
| EU | 18.6 | 3.7 | 41.3 | 20.8 | 84.4 |

too costly to produce, and farmers will have to realise that energetic competition will have to be faced from vegetarians (sincere and insincere), 'animal welfarists' and a wide range of branded convenience and 'health foods', many not based on a meat content.

There have been attempts to increase the use of potentially cheaper non-meat proteins in human foods, i.e. vegetable protein derived mainly from soya beans, cottonseed, groundnuts, sunflower, rape and sesame. The three main classes of vegetable protein products, usually based on soya, are meat analogue, textured vegetable protein and extended meat, which all vary in composition and production cost. Analogue is soya protein spun into filaments and bound with more protein such as egg albumin. Textured vegetable protein may be meals, concentrates or protein isolates combined with carbohydrate in the form of starch or carageenan by extrusion, i.e. forcing the protein mass through extrusion dies under high pressure at 115–117°C. Extended meat is a mixture of vegetable and meat protein which is subjected to normal heat processing. Various flavours, colours and even fat can be added.

Many technical problems still have to be overcome before vegetable protein products can be regarded as acceptable commercial entities. A survey in England showed that they could be much improved in flavour, texture and formulation.

In the UK the annual consumption of meat and meat products, which represent about 22.4% of the total household expenditure on food, amounted to approximately £15 200 million in 1996 at retail prices.

It is estimated that only 60% of the world's population eats 18 kg or more of meat per year, which is regarded as the nutritional minimum. The remaining 40% represents some 1500 million people who consume less than this amount. This stark fact is exemplified by countries in equatorial Africa and OPEC where the average annual consumption is only 10 kg per head and in the underdeveloped countries of Asia where it is as low as 3 kg.

## WORLD LIVESTOCK PRODUCTION

In general, those countries with the highest meat consumption rates are also the major producers. Some parts of the world such as Argentina, Australia, New Zealand and Denmark are large exporters of meat and meat products, while the United States, Britain and Germany import large quantities, although the former also have a considerable export trade as have many other countries.

Many factors operate to determine levels of food animal populations, economics playing the principal role, but disease outbreaks, weather conditions, overproduction, consumer preference, feed availability, etc. are also important reasons, along with trade barriers imposed by individual states, often on ill-defined, even unjustified, grounds.

In 1996 *beef* and *veal* production was similar to that in 1995 and is not expected to alter much for the following two years. Sheepmeat production on a global basis is rising slowly, primarily as a result of rising production in China. Expected improved world prospects for the wool trade had encouraged extra production in Australia. In eastern Europe and countries of the former Soviet Union, production continues to contract. Pig production in most of the major world producing countries is forecast to be stable or declining in 1999. The exception is China.

Poultry production continues to expand throughout the world.

## UK MEAT PLANTS AND THROUGHPUTS

Each year some 93 million animals (excluding poultry) are slaughtered in around 480 meat plants. There has been a great reduction in the number of plants, from 2062 in Great Britain in 1968 to 444 in 1999. At the same time the total number of animals slaughtered has increased from over 11 million cattle units in 1968 to over 29 million cattle units in 1998. The trend, as far as size of plant is concerned, is for the smaller ones to close, although this is not always a result of lower efficiency (Tables 1.3, 1.4 and 1.5).

## CATTLE

The 1996 FAO Production Yearbook gives the world cattle population as 1320 million with 145.7 million buffaloes. The numbers in the main countries are as follows (in millions):

**Table 1.3** Abattoirs and total throughputs (1996/97) in Great Britain.

| Abattoir number (April–March) | Total cattle units* (1000s) | Average no. of cattle units* per year |
|---|---|---|
| 453 | 13 138 | 29 002 |

* 1 cattle unit = 1 beast/2 pigs/3 calves/5 lambs.
Courtesy of MLC Information Service.

**Table 1.4** Throughputs by species (1996/97) in Great Britain.

| Species | Average annual throughput (1000s) |
|---|---|
| Cattle | 7 470 |
| Pigs | 43 400 |
| Sheep | 42 240 |

Courtesy of MLC Information Service.

**Table 1.5** Meat plant numbers and throughputs per size of operation (1996/97) in Great Britain.

| Cattle units per year | No. of plants | % |
|---|---|---|
| 1–1000 | 159 | 0.4 |
| 1001–5000 | 71 | 1.2 |
| 5001–10 000 | 35 | 2 |
| 10 001–20 000 | 56 | 6.3 |
| 20 001–30 000 | 32 | 5.8 |
| 30 001–50 000 | 28 | 8.5 |
| 50 001–1000 000 | 72 | 75.6 |
| Total | 453 | 99.9 |

Courtesy of MLC Information Service.

India 276.1 (inc. 80.1 buffalo); Brazil 166.7 (inc. 1.7 buffalo); China 127.3 (inc. 22.8 buffalo); USSR for 1989–91 118.3 (inc. 0.412 buffalo); USA 103.5; Argentina 54; Pakistan 38.1 (inc. 20 buffalo); Ethiopia 29.9; Mexico 28; Australia 27; Columbia 26; Bangladesh 25.2 (inc. 0.8 buffalo); Sudan 23.5; France 20.7; Nigeria 18.1; Germany 15.9; Indonesia 15; Venezuela 14.6; Tanzania 13.4; Canada 13.2; S. Africa 13.0; Turkey 12 (inc. 0.25 buffalo); UK 11.6; Madagascar 10.3; New Zealand 9.2.

In the United Kingdom, beef and milk account for about one-third of the total agricultural output. Britain now produces almost 80% of its beef requirement, compared with about 50% just before the Second World War. The remaining 20% is imported mainly from Ireland and Argentina. About 52% of the home-produced beef is derived from the dairy herd, i.e. from calves reared for beef. Specialised beef cattle and their crosses provide 48% of the home kill.

## Breeds

In Britain's dairy herd the Friesian (British Friesian/Holstein) is the dominant breed, representing in England 80% of all dairy cows and in Scotland 25%. About one-third of the dairy cows and almost half of the dairy heifers are mated with beef bulls, mostly Belgian Blue, Limousin and Charolais, in order to increase the beef potential of calves not required as dairy herd replacements.

Exotic breeds have been introduced into the United Kingdom in an attempt to improve beef production. The first of these (in 1961) was the French Charolais, which is typical of the large cattle breeds of western Europe with their mature body size, rapid growth rate and lean carcases. Charolais and Belgian Blue, are, however, liable to some difficulty in calving, often necessitating caesarian section, but this is apparently regarded as an acceptable risk by many farmers. British Charolais, through selective breeding, have easier calvings.

Other breeds which have been imported include: Blonde d'Aquitaine, Brown Swiss, Limousin, Murray-Grey (which was developed in Australia but has been in the UK for decades and is now widely considered to be British), Piedmontese, Romagnola, French Salers and Simmental. The Luing was evolved from Beef Shorthorn and Highland cattle on the island off the west coast of Scotland.

British breeds have been exported to many other countries to improve local strains, as live animals, frozen embryos or semen.

Throughout the world there are numerous breeds of domestic cattle used for meat and milk production and also in some cases as draught animals. Most are humped Zebu cattle or cross-breeds of these with cattle of European origin. In addition, the domestic buffalo, the water buffalo of Asia (*Bubalus bubalis*), is an animal of great importance mainly in the Far East (India and China) but is also found in the Caribbean, Middle East and the former USSR. (It has to be distinguished from the buffalo of North America, which is not a buffalo at all but a bison, and from the African wild buffalo, which has never been domesticated.) Many consider that the full potential of the water buffalo as a meat and milk producer has not yet been realised. A breed of Droughtmaster cattle (*Bos taurindicus*) has been developed by cross-breeding the Zebu or Brahman (*Bos indicus*) of the tropics with British beef breeds, notably Shorthorn and Hereford (*Bos taurus*). The Droughtmaster is said to combine the hardiness and disease resistance of the Zebu with the productivity and early maturity of the British breeds. Since 1974, Droughtmasters have been exported from Australia to many tropical countries including Nigeria, Ghana, Pakistan, New Guinea, Solomon Islands and Taiwan.

## Systems of beef production

Beef production systems vary from almost range conditions to semi-intensive and intensive units. The efficiency of animal production is the ratio of output to input: the main outputs are meat, milk, power and transport, hides, fur and by-products; and the principal inputs are feed, land, labour, capital, energy and water.

In the United Kingdom, consumer demand has dictated that meat be lean with a minimum of fat cover, tender, nutritious, palatable and, not least, relatively inexpensive. Accordingly, it is now the custom to slaughter not only cattle but all animals and poultry at much earlier ages. The economically important beef production systems in Britain usually involve slaughter of cattle at between 15 and 24 months of age. Even lower slaughter ages are adopted for certain specialist beef systems; for example, in the so-called barley-beef system calves are weaned early and fed concentrates ad lib to slaughter at 11 months of age and 400 kg, with an overall feed conversion ratio of 5.5:1. At the other extreme, there may be a high utilisation of grass with a lower overall liveweight gain, with animals slaughtered at 2 or more years of age at weights of 499 kg and over. A popular intermediate system is 18-month beef in which autumn-born calves are fed through the winter, kept on grass from 6 to 12 months of age and then finished during their second winter on hay, silage and feed grains.

In Britain the term 'fatstock' used to mean exactly what it said. The meat industry was traditionally based on well-finished animals with substantial fat depots. However, the term *fatstock* is no longer appropriate; '*leanstock*' or '*meatstock*' is more suitable. Changes in the grades of fatness of livestock will probably be promoted by the production of intact males, use of bulls for larger, leaner, late-maturing breeds on the dairy herd and genetic selection of types with efficient feed conversion rates, rapid growth rates and less fat.

Most male cattle in Britain today are reared as castrates (steers or bullocks), although the production of *young bulls* may become more important. The practice of castration was adopted to prevent indiscriminate breeding, to make animals more docile and less dangerous to man and to facilitate fattening. Only the latter factor can be regarded as significant today, since modern husbandry methods for the most part eliminate the breeding problem and present consumer demand is for lean meat. While bulls are more dangerous to handle than steers, experience has shown that the problem has been overemphasised. It has also been well demonstrated under experimental and practical farm conditions that bulls grow faster (by 12%), convert food more efficiently (by 8%) and produce heavier (by 10%) and leaner carcases than steers. Bull beef production is much more important in Europe, especially in Italy, Germany and eastern Europe, than it is currently in Britain.

In Europe, *bulls* are reared in intensive feedlot systems largely based on maize silage, and also in grass-finishing systems with slaughter ages of 24–30 months. The main breeds are Simmentals and Friesians. In New Zealand grass-finishing systems have been used over the last 25 years.

Although the production of bull beef in Britain was initially slow, the rearing of young bulls doubled during the 1980s and will undoubtedly expand further. Some sections of the meat trade have considered bull beef to be of inferior conformation and tenderness as well as being subject to dark cutting (DFD) development. However, recent trials have shown most of these objections to be ill-judged.

In fact, young bull carcases are heavier and leaner than steers of the same age. Careful handling of young bulls will obviate the DFD problem (which is not confined to bulls), and chilling efficiency will offset any tendency to meat toughness, bull beef being inclined to cool more rapidly than steer beef.

Young bull beef must be distinguished from the inferior product supplied by old cull bulls, which is much darker in colour. Investigations by the UK Meat and Livestock Commission on groups of young bulls and steers transported and slaughtered under comparable commercial conditions have shown that bull flesh is only marginally darker than that of the steers, and there are only a few dark cutters among the bulls. The solution is to avoid pre-slaughter stress by gentle, efficient handling, keeping social groups intact and providing for immediate slaughter. Some of the other meat trade criticisms can be ascribed to pure conservatism. In the UK full use is made of grassland and grass products in cattle rearing systems, unlike in certain EU countries, e.g. Germany, where bulls are housed for beef production (51% bulls and 2% steers as against 40% steers and 17% bulls in the UK).

Calves range from the 'bobby' calves, slaughtered within a few days of birth, to specially fed veal calves producing carcases of 115–135 kg at slaughter. A great variation in quality exists in the various age groups, only the heavier carcases being of real value. The typical 'bobby' calf not only has a low muscle/bone ratio but is also very oedematous, rendering it of little value from a consumer standpoint.

## Growth promoters

Many different factors are associated with growth and the muscle/bone ratio in animals, including nutrition, hereditary factors and certain hormones. *Growth hormone* (GH) is probably the most important regulator of growth before puberty is reached, and androgenic and oestrogenic hormones are not active.

*Androgens* stimulate the growth of all body tissues, as well as the organs specific to the male. They are responsible for the characteristic development of the male with his well developed forequarter and neck and greater size. *Oestrogens* also appear to exhibit anabolic effects, causing early maturation of muscles and bones.

The main purpose of using *growth-promoting compounds* is to replace the metabolic growth action lost at castration. Much controversy, however, surrounded the use of these compounds, a lot of it in response to the illegal use of *diethylstilboestrol* in veal calf production in certain EC countries with the occurrence of carcinogenesis in human beings. Widespread consumer concern finally resulted in the introduction of EC Directive 81/602/EU, as amended by Directives 85/358/EU and 88/146/EU, which prohibited the use in livestock farming of certain substances having a hormonal action. These directives were supplemented by Council Directive 86/469/EU, which established controls for the examination of animals and fresh meat for the presence of residues, and Council Directive 88/299/EU, which dealt with trade in animals treated with certain substances having a hormonal action. There was no scientific evidence to show that the use of the licensed substances, with a hormonal action, was harmful and these are still used legally in some countries.

*Probiotics* are benign bacteria which are administered by mouth to animals (calves, lambs and piglets) sometimes at birth and/or after disease. The introduction of a probiotic into the digestive tract is claimed to ensure more efficient feed conversion, earlier slaughter and a healthier animal. Unlike antibiotics, which often kill useful intestinal microorganisms and create undesirable residues, probiotics are said to be natural products without any side effects.

*Beta-agonists* ($\beta$-adrenergic blocking agents) are drugs normally used in human medicine (sometimes also in small-animal practice) to block the effects of adrenaline (epinephrine) and noradrenaline (norepinephrine) in, for example, peripheral vascular disease, cardiac arrhythmias and hypertension. There have been reports of the alleged misuse of these compounds, for example, propanolol, chlorpromazine and clenbuterol, in livestock farming to produce lean meat. These products act as a partitioning agent and produce lean meat at the expense of fat. The meat is said to be tougher than in non-treated animals. While approved for therapeutic purposes, they are not authorised as growth promoters.

### Definitions

*Bull*

An uncastrated bovine.

*Heifer*

A female up to its first calf.

*Cow*

A female which has had one or more calves.

*Steer or bullock*

A castrated male (usually castrated at 6–12 weeks old).

*Stag*

A male bovine castrated late in life, and therefore presenting a more masculine conformation than the bullock.

## SHEEP

The principal sheep-producing countries in the world are (in millions): China 127.2; Australia 126.3; Iran 51.5; New Zealand 48.8; India 45.4; Turkey 33.8; Pakistan 29.8; South Africa 29; UK 28.8; Sudan 23.4; Ethiopia 21.7; Spain 21.3 (FAO Production Yearbook 1996).

Sheep were probably among the first animals to be domesticated by man. They can be found under a wide range of environments throughout the world and, just like goats, their system of husbandry has changed very little over the centuries in most countries. In the main this can be classed as an extensive grazing system, the most natural for the three main species of meat animals: cattle, sheep and pigs. This system probably explains why sheep have the fewest lesions and condemnations at post-mortem compared with cattle and pigs, at least under UK conditions.

Various breeds are adapted to living in areas of high altitude where wind, rainfall, low temperatures and snow are common. The hill ewe lives a very hazardous life exposed to these adverse elements and with low food intake, especially during pregnancy. It is little wonder that up to one-third of body weight can be lost and that neonatal mortality is high. Indeed, of all the farm animals, the relative mortality rate is highest in sheep. Other breeds can be found in desert or semi-desert regions where high temperatures or fluctuating high and low temperatures predominate, with arid conditions and sparse vegetation. With some breeds, such as those kept under lowland conditions in Britain, stocking rates can be as high as 20 ewes and their lambs per hectare; under hill and other extensive systems the rate may be as low as one sheep to 20 hectares.

The quality of forage consumed by sheep varies from good grass under semi-intensive husbandry to low-quality (high-cellulose) plants, such as thorn scrub, rushes and heather, where the stock are relatively few in number. The ability of sheep to eat plants of little use to man and to survive in places which cannot easily be cultivated is very much in their favour. On the other hand, except for specialised breeds like the Finnish Landrace and Russian Romanov, which can produce over three lambs per ewe a year, low reproductive rates, difficulties with husbandry (e.g. fencing and labour) and the disposition towards carcases of fairly high fat content are definite drawbacks. It has been shown that with housing of ewes and subjecting them to artificial photoperiods and hormone treatment they can produce a lamb crop every 8 months and an average of 2.2 lambs per ewe yearly. Unless fecundity can be improved by suitable breeding methods, and leaner carcases ensured, it is possible that in many hill areas sheep may be replaced by goats or deer.

In addition to meat, sheep produce wool and, in some countries, milk, which is used in the making of cheese.

In the United Kingdom there are some 50 breeds of sheep classified by habitat and type of wool. They are kept mainly for meat production, with wool as an important secondary product. Two major systems of sheep farming exist: hill sheep farming, by far the larger of the two, where the sheep are hardy and thrifty, small in size, long of wool, late in maturity and low in fecundity; and lowland sheep farming, in which short-woolled breeds predominate, possessing characteristics of early maturing, higher carcase weights and superior lambing percentages.

True *hill* breeds include the North Country Cheviot, South Country Cheviot, Scottish

Blackface, Swaledale, Welsh Mountain, Exmoor Horn, Herdwick, Rough Fell, Derbyshire Gritstone and Lonk. Hill flocks provide store stock for fattening on lowland farms along with cast ewes which are retained for a year or two for further breeding. The famous Half-Bred, which is the product of the Border-Leicester ram and the Cheviot ewe, is one of the foremost utility sheep in Britain. Although the flesh of the Border-Leicester carries an excessive amount of fat, its prolificacy and milk yield potential when blended with the hardiness of the Cheviot make the resulting cross an excellent animal, the dams bred to Down rams being very popular for fat lamb production in lowland areas. Another example of this close association between hill and lowland breeds is the use of the Border-Leicester ram on Scottish Blackface ewes, the cross being known as the Greyface, which is second only in importance to the Half Bred. Another Half-Bred, the Welsh Half-Bred, results from the crossing of the Border-Leicester with Welsh Mountain ewes. The Mule is a cross-bred ewe which has grown in popularity in the UK; it now makes up 20% of the UK ewe flock. The term Mule covers a number of Blue-faced × hill breed ewe crosses. The most common of these are the Blue-Faced Leicester × Scottish Blackface cross and the Blue-Faced Leicester × (Welsh) Hardy Speckled Face. Reported prolificacy levels are higher in Mules than Greyfaces. Where certain hill sheep, e.g. Scottish Blackface ewes, are grazed on lowland pastures, the good feeding can result in up to 200% lamb crops.

*Lowland* breeds are represented by the short-woolled Downland types, the Suffolk, Dorset Horn and Dorset Down, Southdown, Oxford Down, Ryeland, Shropshire, and the long-woolled breeds of Leicester, Lincoln Longwool, Kent or Romney Marsh, Wensleydale and the Blue-faced or Hexham Leicester. The three most common terminal sires used in the industry at present are Suffolk, Texel and Charolais.

The Dorset Horn, a white-faced short-wool, has a much-extended mating season and can produce three crops of lambs in 2 years. In this way it resembles the Merino. Breeds like these along with Finnish Landrace (high prolificacy), East Friesland (good milking potential) and the Ile de France (excellent carcase quality) could feature in cross-breeding programmes. It is possible that many of the present British breeds may disappear with the development of new hybrids: it is certain that some 50 breeds are unnecessary for successful sheep production. Indeed, this has already taken place with the appearance of the Colbred sheep, named after Oscar Colborn, a Cotswold farmer who crossed Cluns, Dorset Horns, Suffolks and East Frieslands in order to increase fecundity, mothering ability and carcase quality. More recently, French Texels, Beltex, Berrichon du Cher, Rouge de l'Ouest and Charolais have been imported for crossing purposes. The Cambridge breed of sheep is another recently developed breed which is very prolific.

British breeds of sheep are not found extensively in Europe, although Cheviots and some lowland types occur in Scandinavia, but many have found their way to other parts of the world. In Australia, about 75% of the 126 million sheep are Merinos, the remainder being crosses with certain British breeds. In New Zealand, the Romney Marsh predominates, followed by Corriedales, Merinos and South-Downs and their crosses. In the United States, the Rambouillet is the main representative of the Merino and a lot of cross-breeding occurs, with larger sheep units under confined systems of management becoming more important. However, it is doubtful whether sheep grazing in the United States will expand very much. In South Africa and the USSR, the most important breed is the Merino. Fat-tailed and fat-rumped sheep are found in the Middle and Far East; the Awassi breed is an important coarse-wool type in the eastern Mediterranean and Iraq, where the wool is used mainly for making carpets.

In some parts of Europe, milk or dairy sheep are of significance: the common breeds are East Friesland (Holland), Cochurro, Lancha and Mancha (Portugal and Spain).

In recent years more attention is being given to the production of fine wools, cashmere and mohair which the textile industry needs and presently has to import. In addition to sheep, angora goats and rabbits, alpacas and llamas also produce quality fibres. Judicious crossing of British sheep with Merinos, e.g. Merino de l'Ouest from France, produces sheep capable of high lambing percentages, good growth rates and carcase quality as well as fine fleeces.

In addition to better feeding methods, improvements in sheep production are currently centred on the use of hormones to increase the number of lambs born and out-of-season lambing, hybridisation to produce a superior stock of leaner types, oestrous synchronisation, early weaning and artificial rearing of lambs. Intensification on grass and fodder is possible as long as farmers are aware of the problems involved.

In the United Kingdom the demand for young and small carcases means that lamb is the more important product. Lambs are usually slaughtered at between 36 and 45 kg liveweight giving a dressed carcase of 17–23 kg. 'Mutton' is derived from lambs not attaining a finished condition before weaning and from ewes, wethers, hoggets and rams.

As in the case of cattle and pigs, use has been made of *entire ram lambs* to produce leaner carcases. Work carried out at the Meat Research Institute, Bristol and in New Zealand has shown that carcases from entire ram lambs grade about one fat class lower than those from ewes at the same weight without deterioration in eating quality. The entire ram lambs had lower values of subcutaneous and intermuscular fat and a higher proportion of the total fat in the rams was deposited subcutaneously where it can be removed by trimming – an important commercial consideration. Some 30% of the New Zealand kill is now composed of entire ram lambs, non-castration being encouraged.

Research work on carcase and meat composition and tenderness of meat from ram, wether and ewe Dorset-Down-cross and Suffolk-cross lambs slaughtered at 20 weeks of age showed that differences in meat quality were very small, tenderness of ram meat being ensured by efficient refrigeration control. The fact that the rams, especially the Suffolk crosses, grew faster, yielded larger joints and had good carcase conformation in addition to meat tenderness would indicate potential for ram lamb production in the UK (Dransfield *et al.* 1990). When the adverse aspects of castration, *viz.* sepsis, which often leads to pyaemia and sometimes death, the improvement in welfare, and labour and equipment costs are considered, the lead given by New Zealand would seem a good one to follow.

The desirable features required by the butcher in both lamb and mutton carcases of any breed are short stocky plump legs, thick full loin, broad full back, thick fleshy ribs with a wide breast and shoulder, a good depth of chest cavity, a short plump neck, and overall lean content.

### Definitions

*Lamb*

A sheep from birth to weaning time (generally at 3½–4½ months old). Butchers apply a more generous interpretation to the term 'lamb' and use it to denote a sheep from birth until shearing time the following year; by this interpretation a sheep 13 months old is still classed as lamb.

*Tup or Ram*

The uncastrated male.

*Hogg or Wether*

The castrated male sheep (usually castrated before 1 week of age with a rubber ring or at 3 weeks to 3 months old by other methods).

*Gimmer*

A female which has not yet borne a lamb.

*Ewe*

A female which has borne lambs.

*Cast Ewe*

One which has been removed from the breeding flock.

## PIGS

According to the most recent world census data, the leading 12 pig-producing countries in order of production are: Republic of China 452.2; USA 58.2; Brazil 36.6; Germany 23.7; Russian Federation 22.6; Poland 18.7; Mexico 18; Spain 18; Vietnam 16.9; France 14.8; Netherlands 14; Ukraine 13.1 (FAO Yearbook 1996). However, since these data were published, pig production in the USA has grown significantly while in the Netherlands a severe outbreak of Classical Swine Fever during 1997 led to a major culling programme which removed 40% of the Dutch annual production (6% EU total annual output) during that year. Since then the Dutch government has decided to introduce stringent new legislation which will in future limit the size of the national herd to 80% of the 1996 herd size.

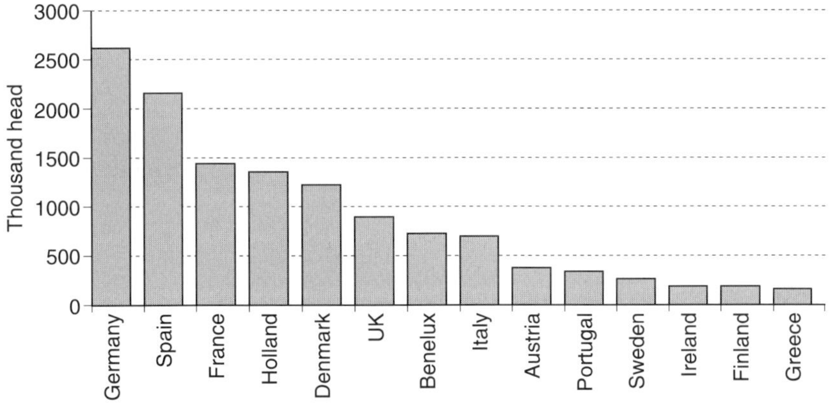


**Fig. 1.1** Breeding sow herd sizes by country (1997). (Source: SOEC)

## Pig breeds

A pig breed is defined as 'A group of animals that has been selected by man to possess a uniform appearance that is inheritable and distinguishes it from other groups of animals within the same species.' In essence a breed relies on being recognisable because it possesses a number or combination of features, e.g. coat colour, body conformation, head shape, etc.

When viewed from a worldwide perspective, the domesticated pig appears to have converged from the breeding of what was essentially two divergent extremes: (a) the European 'Wild Boar' type, a flighty muscular animal with an arched back, coarse body shape and coarse coat type and with body fat deposited mainly within the muscle mass; and (b) the Asian type, a more docile pig whose body is lighter in shape with a low back and whose fat deposition tends to lie predominantly below the skin.

As the pig was domesticated it was selected for a variety of different characteristics such as fertility, mothering ability, muscle and fat deposition, durability and amenability to handling under a variety of husbandry systems. This process continues today on two distinct levels. There are those who breed *pedigree* pigs with the aim of preserving the 'purity' of their breed and the *commercial* pig-producing companies and pig farmers who use cross-bred varieties to utilise hybrid pigs to optimise production traits. Through selection there are now estimated to be some 300 different breeds of pigs.

Unlike some species, the pig has suffered little from man's selection to maximise production and appearance. The most noted exception was the introduction of the *halothane gene* following the introduction of the Piétrain breed. This breed was chosen with the aim of increasing muscle production via the double muscle gene carried naturally by the Piétrain breed. However, pigs which carry the double recessive gene known as the halothane gene tend to drop dead if stressed and those that do survive and are slaughtered express a high frequency of pale, soft, exudative (PSE) muscle tissue such that the meat appears pale and suffers from high drip-loss, making it less suitable for processing and sale. For many years after this gene was introduced, the commercial breeding companies tested breeding stock by exposing all potential breeding pigs to the anaesthetic gas halothane because it was found that if 10-week-old pigs which were double recessive for this gene were exposed to this gas they would become rigid; pigs not carrying the gene retained a relaxed posture. Recently a gene probe has been developed which is cheaper and more welfare-acceptable. This new test has also made it possible for the breeding companies to retain some of the benefits of this gene in terms of muscle production without the risk of pigs being stress-susceptible and producing PSE meat (see also p. 64).

More recently breeding companies in the UK and France have imported and experimented with genes introduced by crossing European breeds with the Meisham breed which originates in China. The Meisham is a highly prolific breed with the potential of producing up to 30 piglets per litter. The aim is to introduce the genes for prolificacy while retaining the leaner carcase characteristics of the European breeds.

## Pig breeds in the United Kingdom

In the UK pedigree pig breeding is carefully recorded by the British Pig Association (BPA), which began keeping breeding records in 1884 when the association was known as the National Pig Breeders Association (NPBA). The aim of the NPBA was to 'maintain the purity and improve the breeds of swine in the United Kingdom of Great Britain and Ireland by the means of livestock inspection and herdbook recording all pedigree pure-bred pigs'.

Today the BPA recognises three major pedigree pig breeds: Large White, Landrace and Welsh and eight minor breeds: Berkshire, British Hampshire, British Saddleback, Duroc, Gloucester Old Spot, Large Black, Middle White and Tamworth.

*Commercial* breeding companies in the UK supply approximately three-quarters of all the replacement gilts bought by commercial pig farmers. These companies use pedigree pigs at the top of their breeding pyramids to produce cross-bred grand-parent and parent pigs.

Increasingly, the force which has been driving the selection made by the breeding companies is coming from the retail sector where the demand is for a leaner, 'healthier' carcase which produces a tender, succulent meat not showing signs of PSE or excessive drip loss and which has sufficient intramuscular fat to provide flavour. Added to this is a new demand which places emphasis on the production system used, with the requirement being for what are termed 'high-welfare' production systems but which equate to loose housing systems. These demands influenced the choice of breed used by the breeding companies in their breeding programmes. For example, although the traditional crosses of the White breeds still account for 84% of all commercial indoor production, sales of Duroc crosses to produce hardier pigs, more suited to the more demanding outdoor environment, are on the increase.

## Pig production

The UK, with some 23% of its pigs outdoors, has the highest percentage of *outdoor production* in Europe. The availability of suitable outdoor sites will probably limit further development since pig welfare can be severely compromised if pigs are put on to sites where the rainfall exceeds 750 mm per year and the land is not free-draining or relatively flat. In fact, much of the outdoor rearing of pigs has now ceased in the UK since farmers have discovered that the environmental conditions were too severe and too difficult to manage.

European Council Directive 91/630 EEC set out the 'Minimum Standards for the Protection of Pigs'. This legislation was incorporated into UK law by SI 2126 'The Welfare of Livestock Regulations 1994'. However, the UK legislation not only implemented the European Directive but added the abolition of stalls and tethers by 1 January 1999. Some of the other European countries decided to address other aspects of production; for example, in the Netherlands fully slatted flooring systems have to be phased out by 2006.

The imposition of legislation on production inevitably affects the way pigs are produced. Pig production in the future is likely to be even more tightly controlled by legislation as pressure from welfare and other lobbying bodies mounts on governments. This, plus the change in the way world trade is changing, will inevitably affect the economics of pig production and accordingly the size and structure of the UK pig industry. The breeds of pigs used and the husbandry procedures adopted, will continue to evolve.

## Pigmeat production

By 1997 the EU was about 105% self-sufficient for pigmeat based on a total consumption figure of 15.4 million tonnes or 41.3 kg per person. The UK industry produced in the region of 871 000 tonnes of pork and 236 000 tonnes of bacon. When compared with other European countries, the UK consumer eats less pigmeat, with the total consumption figures being 839 000 tonnes for pork and 453 000 tonnes for bacon. The UK pig industry is about 104% self-sufficient for pork but only 52% for bacon. The balance of bacon production comes from Denmark, Holland and France. The UK industry is unusual in that it produces pigmeat from uncastrated males, which means that in order to avoid *boar taint*, pigs are slaughtered at lighter weights in that country. The average slaughter weight, at 69 kg deadweight (90 kg liveweight), is lower than in most other countries.

Historically, pigs in the UK were sold as pork pigs, cutters, bacon pigs and heavy hogs. This classification has largely disappeared and been replaced by three weight bands. According to the MLC Year Book 1998, in 1997 these weight bands, P2 measurements and distribution of kill were:

| Liveweight | Average carcase weight | P2 | % of GB kill |
|---|---|---|---|
| Less than 60 kg | 54.6 kg | 9.4 | 9.2 |
| 60–80 kg | 70.2 kg | 11.2 | 83.3 |
| Greater than 80 kg | 83.7 kg | 13.2 | 7.6 |

In recent years the trend in the UK has been to allow pigs to grow to heavier carcase weights because it has been more economically advantageous to do so. However, as a result, fat content as measured by P2 has also increased. This has had a negative influence on grading, which in the UK is now done using the EU grades as follows:

| Grade | Lean meat% |
|---|---|
| S | 60% or more |
| E | 55–59% |
| U | 50–54% |
| R | 45–49% |
| O | 40–44% |
| P | less than 40% |
| Z | partially condemned or with soft fat or pale muscle |
| C | poor conformation |

Carcase dressing can be different in the UK when compared with the rest of Europe; in the UK if the tongue, flare fat, kidneys and diaphragm remain with the carcase, adjustments to payment are made to take this into account.

### Glossary of terms

The following definitions are those used in EU legislation:

*Pig:* an animal of the porcine species of any age, kept for breeding or fattening

*Boar:* a male pig after puberty, intended for breeding

*Gilt:* a female pig intended for breeding, after puberty and before farrowing

*Sow:* a female pig after the first farrowing

*Piglet:* a pig from birth to weaning

*Weaner:* a pig from weaning to the age of ten weeks

*Rearing pig:* a pig from ten weeks to slaughter or service

### Additional facts

In Europe piglets must not be weaned from the sow at an age of less than 3 weeks unless the welfare or health of the sow or piglets would otherwise be adversely affected. This is not the case in the United States where it is not unusual to find piglets weaned between 16 and 19 days of age.

On average, UK producers weaning between 24 and 28 days will achieve between 2.3 and 2.44 litters per sow per year, and expect to produce between 22 and 25 piglets per sow per year born and sell in the region of 18 to 22 slaughter pigs per sow per year. Feed conversion is around 2.5:1. Producers using outdoor systems tend now to produce only one pig less per sow per year than those using indoor systems.

## GOATS

The principal goat-producing countries of the world are (in millions): China 88.2; India 49; Pakistan 24.8; Bangladesh 15; Nigeria 10.2 (FAO Yearbook 1996).

Consumer demand for meat with a low saturated fat content has seen an increase in the numbers of those species which are naturally lean, e.g. goats and deer. In Britain there are now over 100 000 goats producing milk, which is also utilised for making hard and soft cheeses and yoghurt. Allergy to cow's milk has also been a factor in the increased goat population. Meat is a by-product, as are skins and goat hair. Steps were recently taken in Britain to produce home-bred mohair and cashmere from imported Angora goats.

Domesticated goats, descended from native breeds in the East, probably Iran, are found throughout the world, even in torrid and frigid zones where they are superior to cows for milk production. Besides milk, some breeds are kept for their wool, e.g. Angora and Cashmere, while young goats are a source of kid leather. They are especially useful for small-scale milk production and can be maintained in buildings and on pasture where it would not be possible to keep cattle or sheep.

Breeds can be roughly classified into two main groups: Swiss, which are prick-eared and include Alpine and Toggenburg; and Nubian, which are African in origin, chiefly Egyptian, and have long drooping ears and roman noses, e.g. Angora, Cashmere, Maltese.

While the market for goat meat in Britain has not yet assumed much importance, in France there are now some 121 000 goat farmers. Many of these have developed broiler goat units in which 3–7-day-old kids are reared on high-vitamin milk powder to a liveweight of 10 kg at 1 month of age, when they are slaughtered. The average carcase deadweight is 6.3 kg. The carcases are split and the meat is exported, mainly to Italy, skins being utilised for shoemaking.

## POULTRY

The main poultry-producing regions of the world include (in 1000 metric tonnes ready to cook equivalent, 1998 forecast): USA 15 435; China 12 500; Brazil 4650; France 2350; Mexico 1749; UK 1509; Japan 1235; Italy 1170 (Foreign Agricultural Services USDA).

It is probably true to say that no other farm enterprise is as widespread throughout the world as is that of poultry farming. Certainly no other farming activity has made such vast strides in recent years as the production of meat and eggs for table use. In many countries it is regarded as the most important sector of the agricultural industry. While many farmers keep a few poultry for their own use to provide meat and eggs, the other extreme is represented by large commercial organisations in which thousands of birds are kept under the most modern systems of management. The major part of the poultry industry consists of domestic fowls, but turkeys, ducks, geese and guinea fowl are also reared, turkeys being especially common in the United States and Britain. While it is still not unusual for meat and egg production to go hand-in-hand on small enterprises, they are mostly separate activities with the larger concerns. Indeed, the early 1950s saw the commencement of the broiler industry, which in the UK now has an annual production of 750 million broilers and combines in most instances breeding, hatching, rearing, slaughter, processing, packing and marketing; efficiency and competition are the motivating forces. This operation is said to be 'vertically integrated'.

The rapid trend towards larger enterprises is exemplified by the broiler industry in the UK, where some 75% of the whole industry is controlled by six companies. While in the early years only a few hundred birds were reared on one holding, nowadays it is not uncommon for one million birds to be housed on a single poultry farm, as many as 40 000 birds being kept in one house. In the UK, house size generally varies from 12 000 to 35 000 birds and there may be one to ten houses on each individual site rather than in huge integrated units, this trend being dictated by disease control and welfare considerations.

Concentrated efforts have been put into the breeding of poultry for both egg and meat production, not only to enhance productivity but also to control disease, which could be devastating to the industry. Instead of pure breeds, commercial poultry are now represented by hybrids.

Poultry meat production in the United Kingdom is provided in the main by broilers, turkeys and ducks, together with geese, poussins and end-of-lay hens, guinea fowl and some game species such as grouse, partridges, pheasants and quail. Ostrich farming for meat production and leather is a significant enterprise in South Africa and has recently been introduced into Britain and other areas of Europe.

## Definitions

### *Broilers*

Slaughtered normally at around 42 days at liveweight of about 2.3 kg. Food conversion rate is 1.75:1 with a kill-out of 69%. Broilers are housed in environmentally-controlled buildings.

### *Poussins*

Young birds, 23–28 days old, with an average liveweight of 0.5 kg. Oven-ready they weigh 0.25–5 kg. Poussins are mainly sold to the retail trade.

### *End-of-lay hens*

Birds at the end of their laying life, sometimes called boiling fowl, and weighing around 2 kg, form a substantial trade in meat for processing. Some live, fat hens are required for Halal slaughter in Britain.

Nearly all the *broilers* in the major production areas in the world are reared on deep litter on the floor. Using modern strains of fast-growing birds, the majority are raised until they are approximately 6 weeks of age, when they are harvested, i.e. caught, crated, loaded and transported to the processing plant. Nowhere is intensivism more evident than in broiler production, where the health of the breeding stock and the growing birds is essential for economic and welfare reasons. Breeding flocks have a detailed vaccination programme which gives protection against respiratory diseases such as infectious bronchitis and Newcastle disease as well as Marek's disease, egg drop syndrome, avian epidemic tremor and infectious bursal disease (IBD). The broilers themselves may be vaccinated against Gumboro disease and other infections and in addition will have a coccidiostat in the ration to prevent coccidiosis.

The keeping of large numbers of birds together makes it essential that nutrition, ventilation and temperature, stocking densities and management are optimal. Very close supervision of the birds is essential and correct treatment/management changes must be prompt. It is vital that detailed records are kept since it is usually from these that early signs of disease are detected, e.g. water consumption, reduced food intake, weight gain, egg production in layers.

Two aspects of management help birds keep free from disease. *Biosecurity* – safety from transmissible infectious diseases, parasites and pests – is a term that embodies all the measures that can or should be taken to prevent viruses, bacteria, fungi, protozoa, parasites, insects, rodents and wild birds from entering or surviving and infecting or endangering the well-being of the poultry flock. An *'all in-all out'* policy operates where the birds on a unit are approximately the same age and all are slaughtered, the unit then thoroughly cleaned and disinfected prior to the arrival of a new batch of birds.

*Turkeys* are nowadays not confined to the Christmas period. A wide range of weights is produced, depending on the particular trade, and these may be as low as 4 kg and as high as 9 kg or more. Some large cocks can be as heavy as 18 kg. The popular weight of bird for the average family in Britain is between 5 and 6 kg.

*Ducks* are produced both oven-ready frozen – used mainly in the catering trade – and oven-ready fresh chilled – sold mainly retail – and are available in weights from 2 kg upwards. Table ducks can make very fast liveweight gains, attaining 3.6 kg in 49 days at a food conversion of 2.3:1. The kill-out percentage is 72%. In the UK, 90% of ducks are Pekin. Small specialist producers use other breeds such as Barberi. Generally Pekin ducks are considered a cold weather duck and are predominant in northern Europe, and Barbari are predominant in southern Europe and warmer countries.

Compared with domestic fowls and turkeys, geese and ducks are of minor importance. Sales of *geese* are usually confined to the Christmas period. They are generally regarded as being a specialised product in that they have a high feed conversion ratio, 5:1, and are expensive to produce. A female can produce 50–60 offspring which are killed normally at 18–22 weeks weighing around 10 kg liveweight with a kill-out of about 75%. Nowadays, owing to hybridisation, the meat content of the carcase is much higher. In Denmark, Germany, Austria, Poland and parts of France, commercial geese production is an important enterprise; in some instances force-feeding with noodles or other foods is carried out to produce enlargement of the liver, from which the delicacy *paté de fois gras* is prepared.

In the UK the keeping of geese and ducks is subject to the terms of the Agriculture (Miscellaneous Provisions) Act of 1968, and other legislation, as is all livestock farming, so that geese and ducks have the same welfare protection as other animals. Their force-feeding might, therefore, be regarded as causing unnecessary stress, depending on the professional assessment of the inspecting veterinary officer, and would not be allowed in the UK.

*Guinea fowl* can be reared intensively and kept indoors, the first part of their life under brooders. They are killed at 8–9 weeks of age and have a food conversion ratio of 3:1. France and Italy produce large numbers.

There is no doubt that poultry is Britain's favourite meat at the moment, its market continuing to grow at the expense of red meat. Chicken has a 78% share of the retail market, while turkey now stands at 19%. The major growth sector in the poultry industry in recent years has been that of value-added products, now estimated to be worth over £600 million for chicken. Altogether, poultry are worth some £2000 million. Most of the retail sales of chicken (87%) go to the multiples, only 6% going to butchers. The trade is divided into fresh chilled and frozen birds and portions.

## RABBITS

Under commercial rabbit-rearing conditions in the UK, only two of the 40 breeds of rabbit, are used for meat production. These are the Commercial White and Californian.

Rabbits have high fertility rates (some breeds can produce 60 offspring per year), fast growth rates (1.75 kg at 8 weeks of age) and a food conversion efficiency of 2.5:1. A killing-out percentage of around 50 head-off, hot carcase weight can be achieved. A measure of the potential of the rabbit as a meat-producing animal can be gauged by comparing it with a breeding ewe. A 70 kg ewe is capable of producing 20 kg of lamb carcase per year, whereas a 4.5 kg doe is able to produce 75 kg of rabbit meat in the same time.

Rabbit meat is low in fat (3.8%) and high in protein (20.7%), which compares favourably with chicken (2.5% fat and 21.5% protein), beef forequarter (18.9% fat and 18.3% protein), lamb leg (17.5% fat and 18.7% protein) and pork ham (19.6% fat and 19.7% protein).

Rearing is often a large-scale enterprise in Europe, where farms of several thousand does can be found, but rabbits are mainly kept on small farms where labour costs are low. The average size of a rabbit farm in the UK is a 40–50 doe unit. For the industry to be successful it must develop on the same lines as the poultry industry, i.e. highly organised with specialist attention to the cost of labour, food, equipment, breeding, nutrition, disease prevention and housing.

The optimum weight for slaughter lies around 2.7 kg, which is achieved at about 12–14 weeks of age, although this depends on factors such as breed, feeding systems and management, but mainly the environment.

Rabbit-processing plants have to conform to EC standards. Integrated premises have facilities for rearing, slaughter, refrigeration and packing, the end products consisting of whole fresh rabbits, sausages and burgers, stewpacks and cooked and coated portions as in the poultry industry.

Stunning is by electricity, as opposed to home killing where animals are stunned by a blow to the head, which is immediately removed, or the spinal cord is broken in a manner similar to that for poultry.

Imports of Chinese rabbits have been a serious source of competition for the British industry, but they are not of the same standard as British supplies.

While the rabbit is an animal which can utilise many types of feedingstuffs unsuitable for human consumption, it is susceptible to certain conditions such as the enteritis complex, which may be a form of nutritional deficiency allied to an infection caused by microorganisms. Respiratory diseases are also common and these, along with the above, represent important areas for research as well as good husbandry. Labour input is very high for rabbit breeding and one person can only manage a maximum of 250–300 does.

## DEER

The farming of red deer has now become firmly established in the UK and other European countries and on a much larger scale in New Zealand. In the latter country the emphasis is on the production of antler in velvet for the lucrative oriental trade, a practice prohibited by law in the UK.

There are three different kinds of pasture land which, taken together with the system of livestock production practised, provide a basis for the classifying of farm units into hill farms, upland farms and lowland farms. *Hill* deer farms produce weaned calves which are sold to upland and lowland farms, where they grow much faster to breeding or slaughter liveweights. *Upland* farms breed stags which may be suitable for use on hill farms, and sell breeding stock and store calves to lowland farms; they can also produce prime venison. Some upland farms will also export breeding stock and import new blood lines from abroad. *Lowland* farms sell breeding stags to the upland farmer and can import and export livestock as well as being a major producer of prime venison.

It was estimated by the British Deer Society Farmers' Association in 1997 that some 10 000–15 000 carcases were being handled from 200 deer farms containing 10 000 deer. Park deer are also increasingly being used for venison production. Estimates made in 1993 show that Scotland had at least 300 000 wild red deer as well as between 150 000 and 200 000 roe deer, in comparison with a total of about 10 000 red deer and 200 000 roe deer in the rest of Britain.

While most of the deer farmed in Britain are red deer, smaller numbers of fallow, roe, sika and wapiti are also kept.

New Zealand's 1.5 million farmed deer graze on approximately 4000 farms. Average herd size is about 375, although the largest herds comprise several thousand. Deer are processed in specialist plants. Revenue from New Zealand venison exports (14 186 tonnes) was around £61 million in 1995. The major market group was Europe, with Germany the main importer, followed by Scandinavia and France.

Consumer demand for lean meat is fully met in venison, which has a low fat content (5–10%), the polyunsaturate content is 50–55%, compared with levels of 4–5% in beef and lamb.

*Husbandry* mainly centres round the red deer *(Cervus elaphus)* because of its ease of handling compared with the other species, some of which can be aggressive, e.g. wapita *(Cervus canadensis).*

The calves are weaned in September. Housed calves appear to thrive much better than those outwintered unless very good shelter is available. The principal problem in housing deer is bullying and it is important to separate deer into groups of similar size and to quickly identify and remove either aggressive deer or those being bullied. Where there is abundant fenced rough pasture and forest to provide shelter, adult deer are best outwintered because of bullying indoors.

The most suitable areas for deer farming are good, well-sheltered grassland with good fencing and shelter because of the lower subcutaneous fat content than in cattle and sheep and the consequent poorer insulation.

Rutting (the annual sexual display in the male) occurs in the autumn and is accompanied by increased aggression, vocalisation, testicular activity, shedding of velvet and a strong urine odour. The rut lasts for 2–5 weeks (late September–October).

Single calves are born in the Spring (late May–June) after a gestation of 231 days. At birth they weigh an average 8.5 kg and reach sexual maturity at 16 months. Farmed deer are slaughtered at various ages (8–30 months) and produce dressed carcase weights of 53–60% liveweight. Some 56% of the carcase is regarded as first-class meat.

Stocking rates vary according to the type of land and pasture utilised, from 0.66/hectare on heather-dominant hills to 12–16 hinds with their calves, per hectare, on good lowland pasture.

## Handling of Deer

Because of their relatively sensitive nature, aggression at times and powers of agility, it is essential that they are handled efficiently and with care. Housing has been shown to be of value, especially for calves, but care has to be taken with dominant types (which must be removed) and to allow sufficient trough space.

Good handling systems are necessary for collection of deer for tuberculin testing, blood sampling, weighing, anthelmintic and other treatments, etc. Drugs such as etorphine hydrochloride (Immobilon) and diprenorphine (Revivon) are frequently used to immobilise animals humanely, projectile syringes being fired from rifles or blowpipes into the hindquarter or shoulder.

## REFERENCE

Dransfield, E., Nute, G. R., Hogg, B. W. and Walters, B. R. (1990) *Animal Production* **50**, 291.

## FURTHER READING

Universities Federation for Animal Welfare (1988) *The Management of Farm Animals*. London: Baillière-Tindall.

Alexander, T. L. and Buxton, D. (eds) (1994) *Management and Diseases of Deer*. A Veterinary Deer Society Publication. London: B.V.A.

*Farm Animal Welfare Council*

*Report on the Welfare of Broiler Chickens*, 1992.

*Report on the Welfare of Sheep*, 1994.

*Report on the Welfare of Turkeys*, 1995.

*Report of the Welfare of Pigs Kept Outdoors*, 1996.

MAFF Codes of Practice.

MLC Year Books Cattle, Pigs and Sheep.

# Chapter 2
# Anatomy, Meat Composition and Quality

## ANATOMY

*Cells* are the basic building blocks of all living matter. Billions of different types of cells form the tissues of the body; each type is distinct in shape and function.

Each cell is a tiny, microscopic unit, surrounded by a cell membrane, which contains a jelly-like material called protoplasm, and a nucleus. The cell membrane acts as a filter, allowing certain substances to enter the cell and others to leave.

The chemical processes which sustain life occur in the protoplasm. The nucleus governs cell structure and function. Bounded by a nucleus membrane, it contains: nucleoproteins, particularly chromatin; deoxyribonucleic acid (DNA), the molecule governing hereditary characteristics; ribonucleic acid (RNA), which is involved with protein synthesis; and nucleoli, which contain RNA and protein.

About 80% of any cell is water. The next most important substance is protein, composed of numerous amino acids, followed by the carbohydrates, such as sucrose, glucose, maltose and fructose, and the lipids or fats, which can be combined with, for example, carbohydrates or phosphates (phospholipids). Steroids are complex lipids of great biological significance, e.g. cholesterol, bile salts, cortisol and oestradiol. Cells also contain a number of inorganic salts such as potassium, sodium, calcium and magnesium salts, as well as nitrogenous compounds, enzymes, organic acids, gases and vitamins, all the numerous substances taking part in the complex metabolic processes of the animal body.

In complex organisms, cells are specialised in form and function. There is also differentiation of cells between different types of organism in the animal kingdom, which acts as a basis for their classification. There are four main types of *tissues* in animal bodies:

1. *Epithelial tissues* are found on external and internal surfaces and also form specialised structures such as the liver.
2. *Muscular tissues*, constituting the flesh of animals, are of three main types: voluntary (striped, striated), involuntary (unstriped, unstriated, smooth) and cardiac (a special form of striated muscle found in the heart).
3. *Connective tissues* include the skeleton, which gives rigidity to the body. Blood is a specialised form of connective tissue although it is sometimes classified alone.
4. *Nervous tissue* is the most specialised of all the tissues. It transmits the nerve impulses of both sensation and movement.

The animal body is a highly developed multicellular organism, consisting of billions of cells specialised to form tissues. Each tissue has a special function; the tissues are further grouped together to form organs. An *organ* is a group of tissues arranged in a special manner to carry out a special task; for example, the heart, stomach, kidney, bone. Organs are again grouped to form *systems*, each of which performs essential body functions.

The systems of the body are 11 in number, as follows: osteology and arthrology (bones and joints), digestive, respiratory, circulatory, lymphatic, urogenital, nervous, endocrine, myology (muscles), sense organs (ear, eye, organ of smell and organ of taste) and common integument (skin and appendages).

### Descriptive terms

Certain terms are used to describe the exact position and direction of the different body parts, it being assumed that the animal is in the standing position.

*Dorsal*, superior or upper structures or positions lie towards the back or dorsum of the body, head or tail.

*Ventral*, inferior or lower positions are directed towards the belly or venter.

The longitudinal *median plane* divides the body into two similar halves. Structures that are nearer than others to the median plane are said to be *medial* or *internal* while those farther away from it are *lateral* or *external*. Planes parallel to the median plane are *sagittal* to it. Parts which lie towards the head are *cranial* or *anterior* while those towards the tail are *caudal* or *posterior*.

In relation to the *limbs* the terms proximal and distal are used, those lying towards the junction with the body being *proximal* and those at a greater distance away from the body being *distal*. Above the knee and hock the terms cranial and caudal are used for front and rear positions, those below the knee and hock being dorsal and *palmar* and dorsal and *plantar* respectively.

The terms *superficial* and *deep* denote relationships from the surface of the body, e.g. superficial and deep flexor tendons of the legs.

## OSTEOLOGY AND ARTHROLOGY

(See Appendix I for use of parts.)

### Bones

The skeleton, composed of some 200 bones, acts as a support and protection for the soft tissues of the body and provides a system of levers for locomotion and body movement (Fig. 2.1). It also acts as a blood-forming organ, producing red and white cells, haemoglobin and platelets.

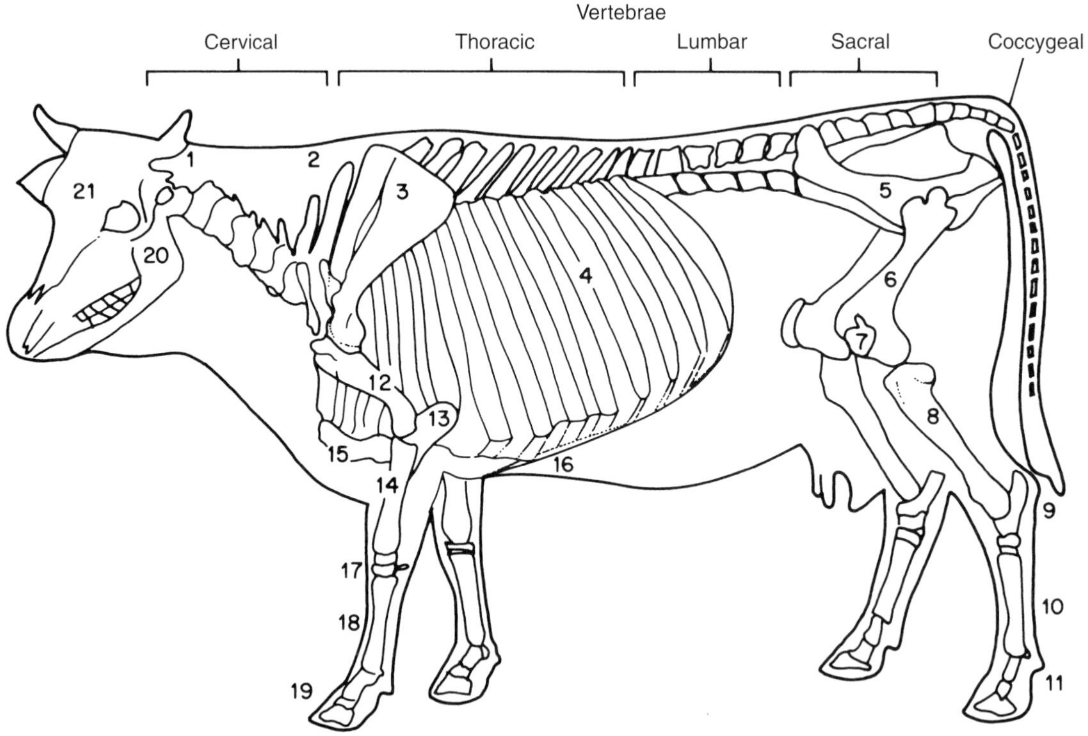


**Fig. 2.1** Skeleton of ox. 1, Atlas; 2, 7th Cervical vertebra; 3, Scapula; 4, Ribs; 5, Pelvic girdle; 6, Femur; 7, Patella; 8, Tibia; 9, Tarsus; 10, Metatarsus; 11, Phalanges; 12, Humerus; 13, Ulna; 14, Radius; 15, Sternum; 16, Xiphiod process; 17, Carpus; 18, Metacarpus; 19, Phalanges; 20, Mandible; 21, Cranium. (By courtesy of Sisson and Grossman, 1975)

The long bones of the very young animal are very long, slender and smooth, with their prominences less pronounced. With age, ossification of cartilage takes place and the bone becomes more rigid. In the very old animal there is a decrease in bone organic matter, making the bone more brittle and liable to fracture. Though a proportion of the carcase bone is often sold with the retail joints, the head bones, thigh bones, etc., are retained by the butcher and are collected for processing.

The proportion of bone in the dressed carcase of beef, i.e. the two sides, varies between 12% and 28%, according to breed and bodily condition, being about 15% in a good beef carcase and increasing with the age and weight of the animal. It is lowest in Aberdeen Angus cattle, but is as high as 28% in second-quality cows. The average percentage of bone in lamb is 17–35%, in bobby calves 50%, in veal calves 25%, in pork 12–20%, in poultry 8–17%. Ox bone is composed of the following constituents:

| | | % |
|---|---|---|
| Organic matter: | Ossein or bone collagen | 33.3 |
| Inorganic matter: | Calcium phosphate | 57.7 |
| | Calcium carbonate | 3.5 |
| | Sodium carbonate and chloride | 3.5 |
| | Magnesium phosphate | 2.0 |
| | | 100.0 |

The organic matter is the only edible constituent of bone and forms gelatin when boiled.

Bone also contains blood vessels, lymphatics and nerves, and a typical long bone is composed of a hard, compact substance within which is a cancellated spongy substance. The shaft of the long bone has a medullary cavity lined by a fibrous membrane, the *endosteum*, and containing *marrow*. Covering the outside of bone, except where cartilage occurs, is the *periosteum*, another specialised membrane capable of producing bone in certain circumstances.

Two types of bone marrow may be distinguished: the red marrow and the white, which is fatty and gelatinous. In the fetus and newborn animal the marrow has an important blood-forming function and is red in colour. Later, in the adult, the marrow in the medullary cavity of long bones becomes white bone marrow, which is rich in fat, is yellowish in colour and may represent 15% of the weight of the bone; the marrow in the epiphyses of long bones usually remains red. Another important position of red bone marrow in the adult is in those bones which possess no medullary cavity, such as the bodies of the vertebrae, the scapula and pedal bones.

Two or more bones form a *joint* or *articulation*, which may be:

1 fibrous, where there is no movement, e.g. bones of the skull;
2 cartilaginous, in which cartilage unites the bones, e.g. vertebral joints, pelvic symphysis; or
3 synovial, in which a joint capsule is formed with the operation of tendons and ligaments to make a movable joint.

Bones are classified according to their overall shape and function as follows:

*Long bones* Elongated with enlarged extremities, acting as levers and supports, e.g. humerus, radius, femur.

*Flat bones* Expanded to furnish large areas for muscle attachment, e.g. scapula or shoulder blade.

*Short bones* Cuboidal in shape, e.g. small bones in the carpus (knee) and tarsus (hock).

*Irregular bones* Vertebrae forming the axial skeleton, for example.

The *skeleton* of the meat animals is divided into two parts: the *axial skeleton* comprising the vertebral column or the spine, ribs, sternum and skull; and the *appendicular skeleton* representing the bones of the limbs. The *foreleg* contains the scapula, humerus, radius and ulna, carpus, metacarpus and digits which are composed of phalanges. The *hindleg* is made up of the pelvic girdle (ilium, pubis and ischium), femur, tibia and fibula, tarsus, metatarsus and digits.

The *vertebral column* or spine is divided into five regions—cervical (C), thoracic (T), lumbar (L), sacral (S) and coccygeal (Cy), representing the neck, chest or thorax, loins, sacrum (fused sacral vertebrae) and tail, respectively. In meat animals it consists of the number of individual vertebrae shown in Table 2.1.

**Table 2.1** Vertebrae of the spine.

| | | | | | |
|---|---|---|---|---|---|
| Ox | C7 | T13 | L6 | S5 | Cy 18–20 |
| Sheep and goat | C7 | T13 | L6 | S4 | Cy 16–18 |
| Horse | C7 | T18 | L6 | S5 | Cy 15–21 |
| Pig | C7 | T14–T15 | L6–7 | S4 | Cy 20–23 |
| Rabbit | C7 | T12 | L7–8 | S3–4 | Cy 14–20 |
| Chicken | C15–17 | T7 | L + S14 (fused synsacrum) | | Cy 5–6 + pygostyle (fused caudal vertebrae) |

The *sacrum* is in the shape of a pyramid and formed of three to five fused sacral vertebrae, except in the fowl in which 14 fused lumbar and sacral vertebrae form the synsacrum. The *sternum* or breast bone in mammals is composed of six to eight fused segments. In the fowl the sacrum is a very large bone covering almost all of the ventral part of the body.

There are generally the same number of *ribs* as thoracic vertebrae; they are divided into sternal or asternal ribs depending on whether or not they articulate with the sternum.

Carcase bones are valuable means of *identification* of the different species of food animals, e.g. where substitution is suspected. Where the teeth of a bovine animal are unavailable for examination, the *age* can be estimated with reasonable accuracy by examination of the carcase bones. This estimation is based on the degree of ossification of certain parts of the skeletal system, the most valuable of which are the cartilaginous extensions of the spines of the first five dorsal vertebrae. Ossification in these spines develops as shown in Table 2.2.

In *cows* these changes take place more rapidly and the cartilage has ossified after 3 years.

A further useful guide as to *age* can also be obtained from the ischiopubic symphysis. In cattle up to 3 years of age this can be cut with a knife, but after this age a saw is necessary. Similarly, the red bone marrow of the vertebrae is gradually replaced by yellow bone marrow and distinction can be drawn between the soft vascular bones of the young animal with cartilage discernible at the joints, and the hard, white, bleached appearance of bones in old cows. In young bovines, cartilage is discernible between the individual segments of the sternum, but after 5 years of age begins to be replaced by bone; at 8 years two or three cartilaginous divisions are still apparent, but at 10 years the cut surface of the sternum presents a uniform bony structure.

In *sheep* the break at the carpus, or knee joint, is a valuable guide as to age. In *lambs* the joint breaks in four well-marked ridges resembling the teeth of a saw, the ridges being smooth, moist and somewhat pink or congested. In older sheep the surface of the joint is rough, porous, dry and lacks redness. The determination by X-ray of the amount of cartilage present at the epiphysis of a long bone in a joint of meat provides unassailable evidence in cases where there is dispute as to the age of the animal from

**Table 2.2** Ossification of the cartilaginous extensions of the spines of the first five dorsal vertebrae. (Bovines.)

| Age (years) | Ossification |
|---|---|
| 1 | The extension is entirely cartilaginous, soft, pearly white and sharply delineated from the bone, which is soft and red. |
| 2 | Small red islets of bone appear in the cartilage. |
| 3 | The cartilage is greyish, and red areas are more numerous. |
| 4–5 | The area of ossification within the cartilage extends until the proportion of bone is greater than that of cartilage. |
| 6 | The cartilage has ossified into compact bony tissue, though the line of junction between cartilage and bone can still be defined. |

which the meat was derived. The degree of ossification, determined by X-ray, in the ischial portion of the pubic symphysis enables a leg of lamb to be differentiated with certainty from that of an old sheep.

### *Poultry*

In the *domestic fowl* the bones of the skeleton are very light in weight and contain air sacs. The skeleton also differs from that of other animals. There is a *pectoral girdle* which consists of a clavicle or wishbone, scapula and coracoid (Raven's beak), and a fused *pelvic girdle* comprising an ilium, ischium and pubis, which does not meet ventrally as in mammals.

The *wings*, comparable with the forelimbs of mammals, are composed of a large humerus, a smaller radius and ulna and a manus or wing tip consisting of a carpus (two bones), metacarpus (two fused segments) and three digits. The legs are formed by a large femur (thigh bone), a very large tibiotarsus with a slender fibula forming the drumstick, a tarsometatarsus or shank bone and digits (four).

## DIGESTIVE SYSTEM

### Tongue

#### *Ox*

In the ox tongue the filiform papillae are horny and directed backwards; they have a rasp-like roughness which aids in the prehension of food. The posterior part of the dorsum, i.e. the upper surface, is prominent and defined anteriorly by a transverse depression which is frequently the seat of erosions due to actinobacillosis. On either side of the midline on the prominent dorsum are 10–14 circumvallate papillae; the epiglottis, if left on the tongue, is oval in shape. Black pigmentation of the skin of the tongue is frequently observed but is quite normal and of no pathological significance.

#### *Sheep and goat*

The tongue is similar to that of cattle, but the centre of the tip is slightly grooved and the papillae are not horny. The sheep tongue may be differentiated from that of the calf by the fact that it is narrower, the dorsal eminence is more marked, the surface is smoother and the tip more rounded. Black pigmentation of the surface of the tongue is common in black-skinned sheep.

#### *Pig*

The tongue is long and narrow and there is no dorsal ridge. One, or possibly two, circumvallate papillae are present on each side of the midline near the base of the tongue and the surface is studded with fungiform papillae.

#### *Horse*

The tongue is long and flat with a spatulate end. There is no dorsal ridge and only one circumvallate papilla is present on each side. The epiglottis is pointed. Pigmentation is never seen.

### Stomach

#### *Ox* (Figs 2.2, 2.3, 2.4)

The *oesophagus* is comparatively short and wide, measuring about 1 m long and 5 cm wide. The voluntary muscle, which performs the reverse peristaltic action in rumination, weighs about 340 g and is used for sausage meat. After removal of this muscle, the serous covering of the oesophagus is used for sausage casings.

The *stomach* (*paunch*) consists of four compartments: the rumen, the reticulum, the omasum and the abomasum, which is the true digestive stomach and secretes gastric juice. The *rumen* occupies 75% of the abdominal cavity; it is bounded on the left side by the abdominal wall, on the anterior extremity by the reticulum and part of the omasum, and on the right side by the remainder of the omasum, the abomasum and intestine. The *reticulum*, which is placed transversely between the anterior extremity of the rumen and the posterior surface of the diaphragm to which it is adherent, causes a depression on the posterior aspect of the thin, left lobe of the liver (Fig. 2.2). The omasum and abomasum are attached to the posterior surface of the liver by means of the *omentum* or *caul fat*, the root of this membrane being apparent on the posterior aspect of the liver to the left of the portal lymph nodes when the liver is removed from the carcase. The omentum, after connecting the

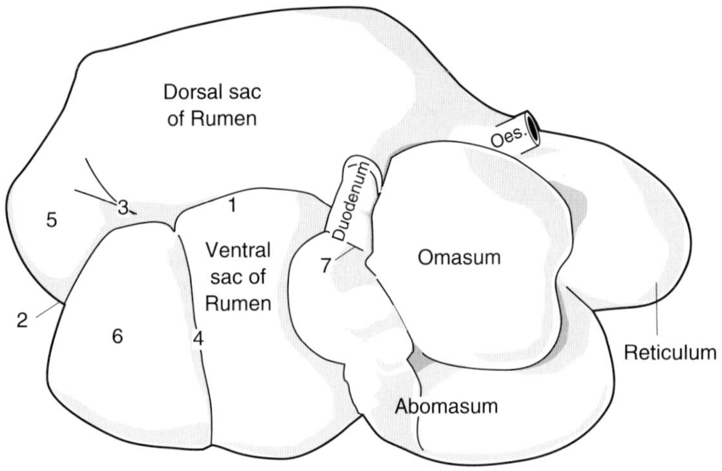


**Fig. 2.2** Stomach of ox; right side. Oes, oesophagus; 1, insula between right longitudinal groove below, and accessory groove above; 2, caudal groove of rumen; 3, 4, right dorsal and ventral coronary grooves; 5, 6, caudodorsal and caudoventral blind sacs; 7, pylorus. The positions of the reticulum, omasum and abomasum have been altered by removal of the stomach from the abdominal cavity and inflation.

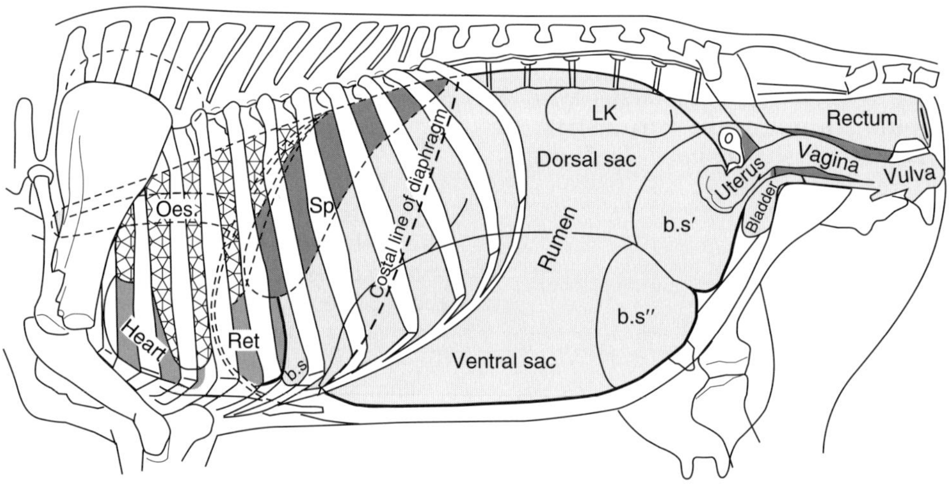


**Fig. 2.3** Projection of viscera of cow on body wall; left side. b.s., atrium of rumen; b.s.′, b.s.″, blind sacs of rumen; O, ovary; Oes, oesophagus; Ret., reticulum; Sp, spleen. The left kidney (LK) is concealed by the dorsal sac of the rumen, is indicated by dotted lines. The median line of the diaphragm is dotted.

liver and omasum, is continued to the lesser curvature of the abomasum and thence to the duodenum. The anatomical relations of the bovine stomach play an important part in the aetiology of traumatic pericarditis. The average capacity of the stomach is 150 litres.

### *Mucous membranes*

*Rumen* Brown or black in colour except on pillars or folds where it is pale. Studded with large papillae.

*Reticulum* Honeycomb-like appearance with four, five or six-sided cells.

*Omasum* Prominent longitudinal folds, about 100 in number. Sometimes called the 'Bible'.

*Abomasum* Some 30 prominent oblique folds in the body of the abomasum, but absent in the pyloric portion.

A feature of the calf stomach is the relatively large size of the abomasum as compared with the small size of the rumen, which remains small until the animal is weaned. As the calf

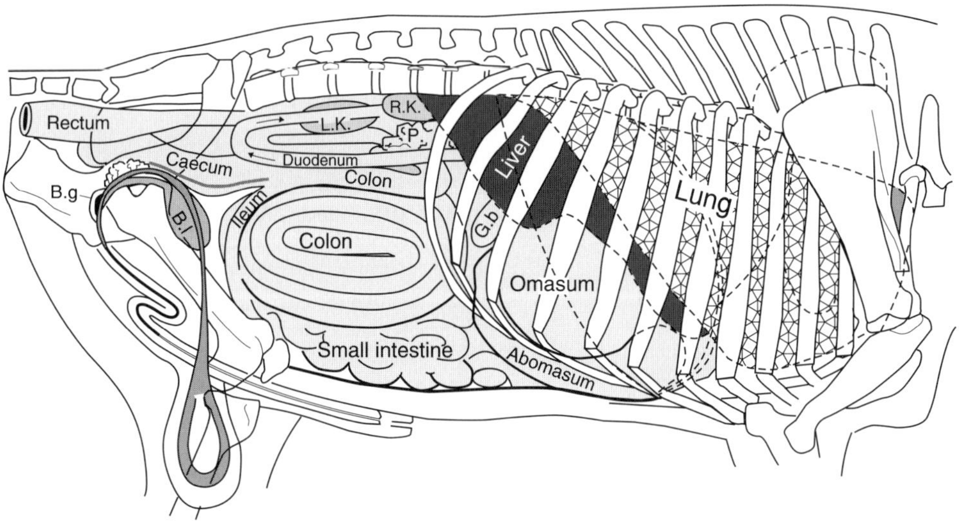


**Fig. 2.4** Projection of viscera of bull on body wall; right side. B.g., bulbourethral gland; Bl., urinary bladder; G.b., gallbladder; L.K., left kidney; P (above duodenum), pancreas; P (below G.b.), pylorus; R.K. right kidney; V.s., vesicular gland. Costal attachment and median line of diaphragm are indicated by dotted lines.

commences to take solid foods, the size of the rumen increases until in the adult animal it represents 80% of the total stomach capacity and the abomasum 7–8%.

*Sheep and goat* (Fig. 2.5)

The stomach is similar in structure to that of the ox and has an average capacity of 18 litres. The first and second stomachs together yield 0.9 kg of tripe; the fourth stomach is also sometimes used, but the third is often discarded. The sheep rumen is also used in Scotland as a container for haggis (cooked minced heart, liver and lungs, seasoned with salt, pepper, cayenne, nutmeg and grated onion mixed with oatmeal and shredded beef suet). Mechanical methods for the cleaning of both ox and sheep stomachs are now operating satisfactorily in modern triperies.

*Pig*

The pig stomach is a simple one, semilunar in shape, with a small pocket or diverticulum at the cardiac (i.e. oesophageal) end. The mucous membrane of the cardiac end is pale grey, while the central fundic region is reddish brown, becoming paler and corrugated towards the pyloric end. The average capacity of the stomach is 6.5 litres.

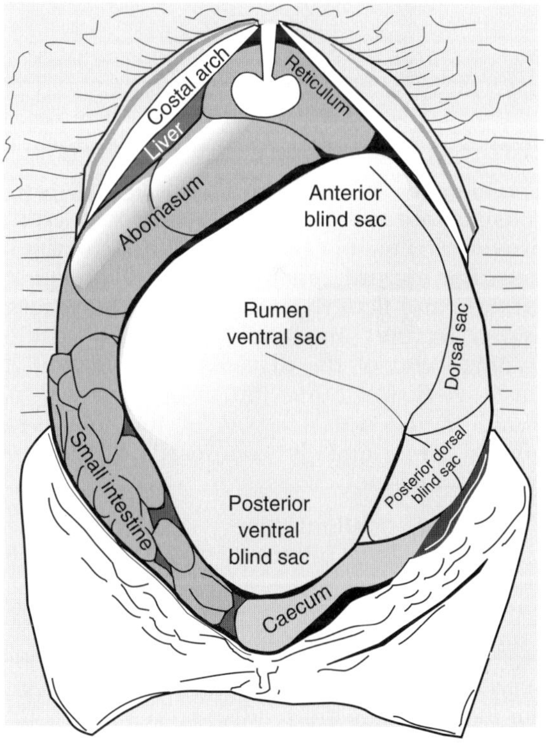


**Fig. 2.5** Abdominal viscera of sheep; ventral aspect. For 'Anterior blind sac' read cranial end of ventral sac; for 'Posterior ventral blind sac' read caudoventral blind sac; for 'Posterior dorsal blind sac' read caudodorsal blind sac.

*Horse*

The horse stomach is a simple one; the mucous membrane of the whitish oesophageal portion is clearly distinguishable from the reddish, soft and vascular fundic and pyloric portions. The average capacity is 12 litres.

## Intestines

*Small* Duodenum, jejunum, ileum.
*Large* Caecum, colon, rectum.

The average length of the intestines is shown in Table 2.3. Thus, for practical purposes, the ratio of the length of the small intestine to the large intestine is 4 to 1.

**Table 2.3** Length of intestines (m).

| | Small intestine | Large intestine |
|---|---|---|
| Cattle | 36.5 | 9 |
| Horse | 24.3 | 6 |
| Sheep | 25.6 | 6 |
| Pig | 17.1 | 4.8 |

*Fowl*

The alimentary tract of the domestic fowl consists of an oesophagus, fusiform crop, proventriculus or glandular stomach, thick muscular gizzard, small intestine (duodenum, jejunum and ileum), large intestine (two caeca and a rectum) and a cloaca, which is the common end of the digestive and urogenital tracts. A cloacal bursa (bursa of Fabricius) is found in the dorsal aspect of the cloaca in young birds and is composed mainly of lymphoid tissue.

Length of small intestine: 120–170 cm.
Length of large intestine: 22–35 cm.

## Liver

With the exception of the horse, the livers of all the food animals are reddish-brown in colour. The liver, the largest gland in the body, lies mainly to the right of the midline in all animals, its convex anterior surface conforming to the hollow of the diaphragm to which it is attached on its dorsal surface and its concave visceral surface (with portal vein, hepatic lymph nodes, gall bladder, common hepatic duct and hepatic artery) in contact with the pancreas, reticulum, omasum and abomasum with the caudal vena cava prominent on its dorsal border.

*Functions:*

1 Concerned with the formation and destruction of red blood cells (RBCs). (It is a site of RBC formation in the fetus.)
2 Removes bilirubin from the blood and excretes it via the bile duct into the duodenum.
3 Manufactures plasma proteins except for some of the globulin fraction.
4 Manufactures blood-clotting factors (prothrombin and fibrinogen) and heparin.
5 Manufactures glycogen from protein and fat and stores it along with the fat and protein.
6 Maintains the normal blood sugar level (100 mg%) and converts galactose into glucose.
7 Detoxifies certain foreign substances in the blood.
8 Deaminates surplus amino acids.
9 Produces bile salts for the digestion of fats. Forms and stores bile, vitamins A, D and $B_{12}$, copper and iron.

*Ox* (Fig. 2.6)

The liver is poorly divided into three lobes: a thin left, a thicker right, and a caudate lobe or thumb piece. The left and right lobes are divided by a slight notch, the umbilical fissure, which indicates the point of entry of the umbilical vein while the calf is *in utero*. In the cow the left lobe of the liver is thin, elongated and often markedly cirrhotic. Running transversely across the upper border of the liver is the posterior vena cava and on its posterior aspect the liver shows the root of the omentum, the gall bladder, portal vein and portal lymph nodes, the vein and lymph nodes being partly concealed by the pancreas.

The weight of the ox liver is about 5.4 kg, i.e. about 1% of the liveweight, although in feedlot cattle and heavier animals the liver may weigh up to 6.3 kg. The calf liver, which is relatively larger than in the adult, weighs 0.9–1.1 kg; its tenderness, its usual freedom from parasitic and other pathological conditions and its therapeutic value in the treatment of anaemia ensures the highest price.

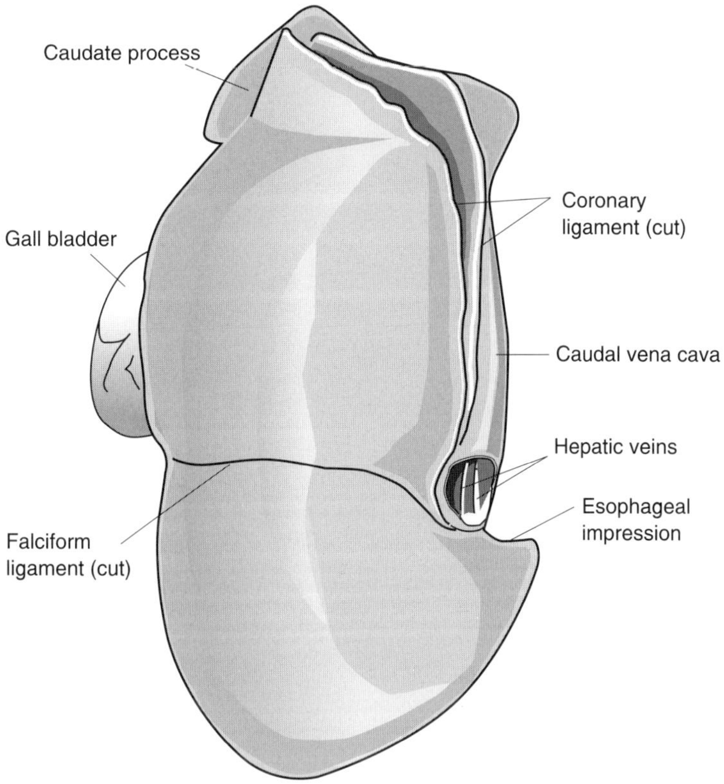


**Fig. 2.6** Liver of ox; diaphragmatic surface, hardened *in situ*.

*Sheep* (Fig. 2.7)

The liver is similar in shape to that of the ox, but the caudate lobe is more pointed and its edges are well defined. This is a useful distinguishing feature between sheep and calf liver. The caudate lobe in the latter is more rounded and has a blunter extremity which frequently extends beyond the lower edge of the liver. When the calf liver is laid on the table, anterior surface uppermost, the caudate lobe fits neatly into the liver like a carpenter's joint.

An adult sheep's liver weighs 453–680 g but undergoes a marked hypertrophy in ewes approaching parturition.

*Pig* (Fig. 2.8)

Pig liver has five lobes, two smaller inner, two smaller outer and a caudate lobe. The oesophageal notch is prominent but the identifying feature is the large amount of visible interlobular tissue which gives the surface of the organ its classical 'morocco leather' appearance. The lobules are mapped out sharply and are polyhedral, and the organ, because of the amount of interlobular tissue, is less friable than in the other food animals.

Its weight varies from 0.9 kg in pork pigs to 2 kg in sows.

*Horse* (Fig. 2.9)

Horse liver has three distinct lobes and a thumb piece which terminates in a point. A notable feature is the absence of a gall bladder. The horse liver is purplish and weighs about 4.5 kg.

*Fowl*

The liver consists of right (larger) and left lobes with fusiform gall bladder.

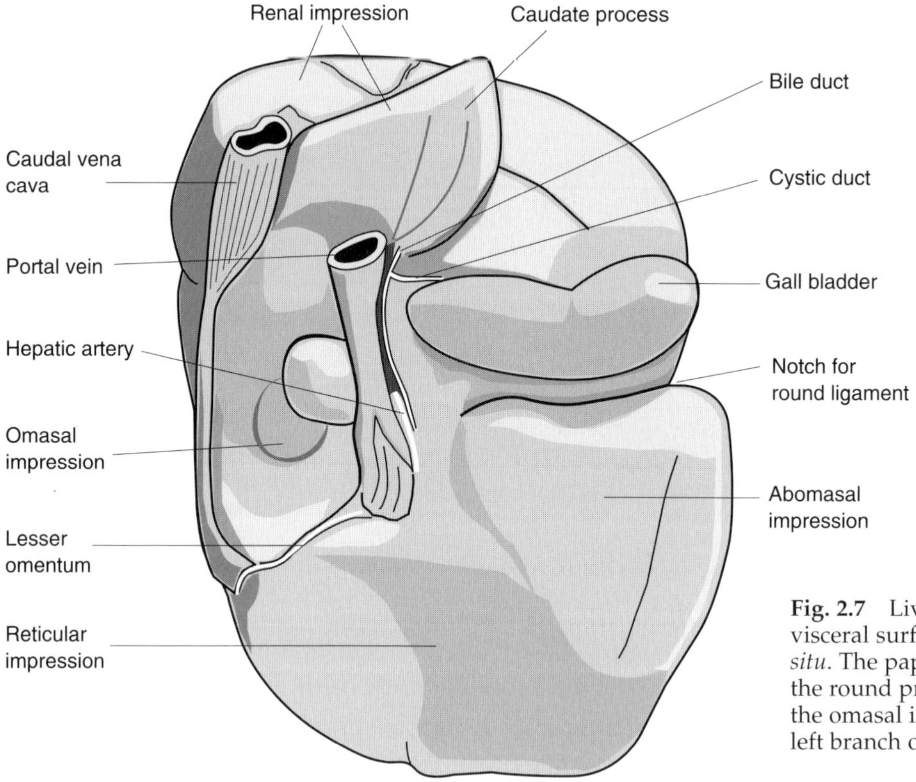


**Fig. 2.7** Liver of sheep; visceral surface; hardened *in situ*. The papilliary process is the round projection between the omasal impression and the left branch of the portal vein.

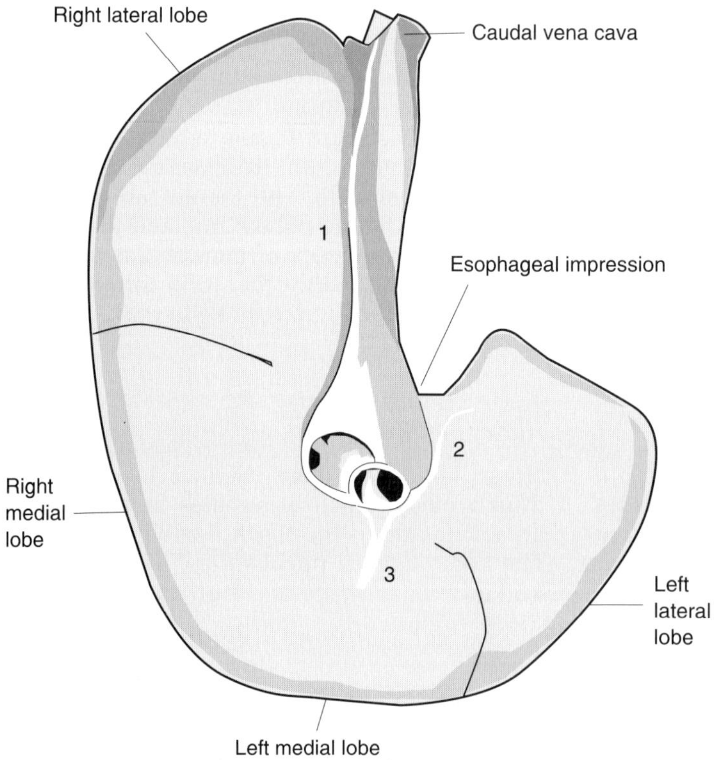


**Fig. 2.8** Liver of pig; parietal surface. 1, Large hepatic veins opening into caudal vena cava; 2, coronary ligament; 3, falciform ligament .

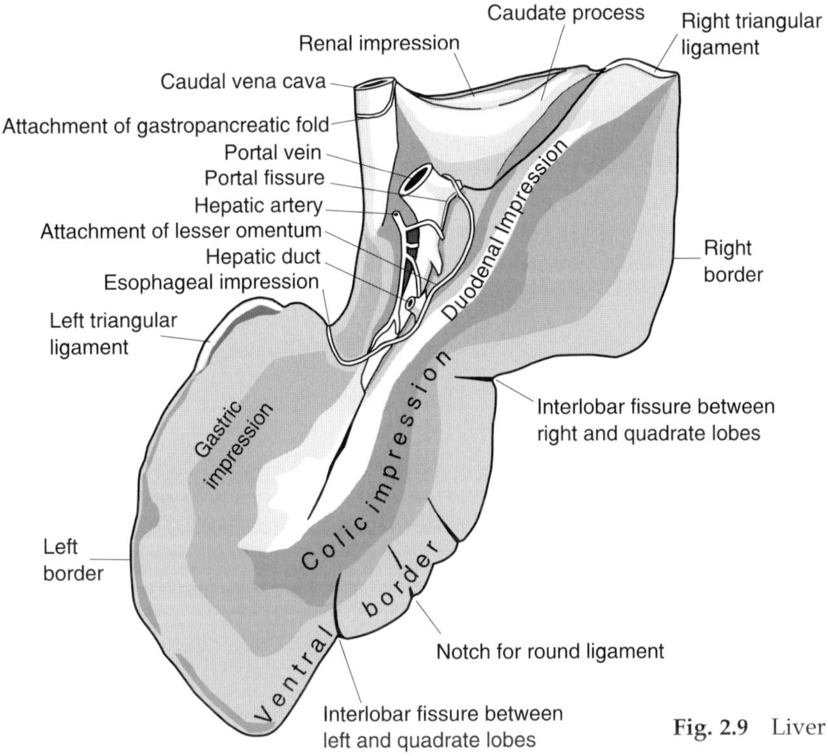


**Fig. 2.9** Liver of horse; visceral surface.

### Pancreas (gut sweetbread)

Two hormones, insulin and glucagon, are produced by the islet cells of Langerhans in the pancreas. These substances control the levels of blood sugars: an excess of insulin causes the blood sugar to drop, while excess glucagon raises it. Lack of insulin causes diabetes mellitus, in which there are high blood levels and reduced fat and protein formation in the body.

The ox pancreas is reddish brown, loosely lobulated and roughly the shape of an oak leaf. It is attached to the back of the liver and is deeply notched to accommodate the portal vein. The average weights of the pancreas are: cattle, 226–340 g; horse, 340 g; sheep, 85–142 g; pig, 28–56 g.

In the fowl the pancreas has dorsal, ventral and splenic lobes. It is yellow or reddish in colour.

## RESPIRATORY SYSTEM

The much smaller thoracic cavity (containing lungs, heart and associated large vessels) is separated from the abdominal cavity (in which all the other body organs are situated) by the strong musculomembranous *diaphragm* (convex in front and concave posteriorly).

The respiratory system comprises the nose, nasal cavity, part of the pharynx, larynx, trachea and lungs. Respiration allows an adequate intake of oxygen and the removal of carbon dioxide by bringing blood in the lungs into close proximity with the alveolar air.

The pleura lines the chest cavity and in the healthy animal is a smooth, glistening membrane divided into a right and left sac. Each sac covers the chest wall (the parietal pleura) and the lung (the visceral pleura). The two sacs (pleurae) join in the central mediastinal space in which are situated the mediastinal lymph nodes and which is traversed by the aorta, oesophagus and trachea.

### Lungs

*Ox* (Fig. 2.10)

The cartilaginous rings of the ox trachea meet at an angle and form a distinct ridge along the

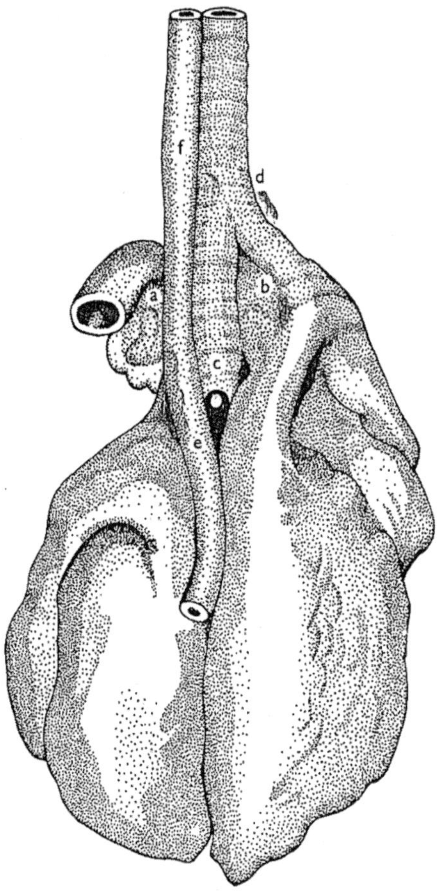


**Fig. 2.10** Lymph nodes of the bovine lungs. a, left bronchial partly covered by the aorta; b, right bronchial; c, middle bronchial; d, apical; e, posterior mediastinal; f, anterior mediastinal, related inferiorly to the oesophagus and trachea.

dorsal aspect. The *left lung* has three lobes named, from before backwards, the apical, cardiac and diaphragmatic. The *right lung* has four or five lobes, its apical lobe receiving an accessory bronchus from the trachea. The lung lobulation is well marked by the large amount of interlobular tissue and is particularly evident in old cows. The pair of ox lungs weighs 2.2–3.0 kg.

*Sheep*

Sheep lungs resemble those of the ox in the division of the lobes, but their consistency is more dense and leathery, they are duller in colour, and the lobulation is less distinct. They weigh 340–907 g.

*Pig*

The number of lobes varies, with two to three on the left and three to four on the right, because the apical and cardiac lobes can be subdivided. The tissue is very spongy and compressible, and the surface lobulation is particularly well marked. Of all the food animals, pig lungs show the greatest variations in colour, varying from red to a light pink, but these variations are due to slight variations in the amount of blood left in the lungs after bleeding and are of no pathological significance. Pig lungs weigh 340–453 g.

*Horse*

The lobar divisions are very indistinct in the horse; only two left lobes and three right lobes can be clearly distinguished. The horse lungs are long and may be further differentiated from those of the ox by the absence of surface lobulation and the absence of an accessory bronchus, while the ends of the cartilaginous rings of the trachea overlap like a piston ring. Horse lungs weigh 2.2–3.0 kg.

*Domestic fowl*

The respiratory system of the fowl is distinguished by the presence of an anterior or cranial larynx, which opens into the floor of the pharynx, and a posterior larynx or *syrinx*, located at the terminal part of the trachea and partly formed by the bronchi. Associated with the respiratory system are 10 paired air sacs and one single (clavicular) air sac. These form a communication between a bronchus and the interior of some of the pneumatic bones. The sacs are lined with a mucous membrane covered with a serous coat and play an active part in respiration. The walls are very thin and, while not easy to see in the healthy bird, are often involved in respiratory disease with thickening of the walls and cheesy or purulent exudation.

**Pluck**

In the pig, sheep and calf the internal organs comprising the larynx, trachea, lungs, heart and liver constitute the *pluck*. In the pig pluck the oesophagus remains attached and is related to the trachea, which is short and consists of 32 cartilaginous rings. In the sheep the oesophagus is removed with the stomachs in the dressing of the carcase. The trachea is long and composed of about 50 rings.

## CIRCULATORY SYSTEM (heart, arteries, capillaries and veins)

### Heart

The heart, a hollow muscular organ acting as a pump, lies in the pericardial sac in the mid-mediastinal region of the thorax between the lungs. Its muscular portion, the *myocardium*, has a smooth lining, the *endocardium*, to its four cavities (left ventricle and atrium, right ventricle and atrium). Covering the cardiac muscle is the *epicardium*, the visceral layer of the pericardium.

In reality the *circulation* consists of two pumps, the left and right sides, the former being involved with the systemic circulation and the latter the pulmonary circulation.

*Systemic circulation:*

1. Left atrium and ventricle (LA and LV) via aorta, arteries, arterioles and capillaries to tissues (oxygenated blood).
2. Return via venae cavae and veins to right side of heart (RV and RA) (carbonated blood).

*Pulmonary circulation:*

1. RV and RA via pulmonary artery (two branches) to lungs (carbonated blood).
2. Return via pulmonary veins to left side of heart (LA and LV) (oxygenated blood).

The heart itself receives blood from the right and left coronary arteries and is drained by several veins which pass into the coronary sinus and the right atrium.

The heart is reddish-brown in colour in all the food animals; the myocardium has a firm consistency and the epicardium and endocardium are smooth and glistening. The right and left ventricles may be readily distinguished by palpation, the wall of the left ventricle being three times as thick as that of the right, while the mitral valve and its chordae tendineae are stronger than the tricuspid valve of the right side. A certain amount of blood clot is found normally in each of the ventricles after death.

*Ox*

The ox heart shows three ventricular furrows on its surface. Two *ossa cordis*, which are cartilaginous until 4 weeks after birth, develop at the base of the heart in the aortic wall. The ox heart weighs 1.8–2.2 kg. In pregnant cows and in those with a septic infection it is frequently pale, flabby and friable.

*Sheep*

There are three ventricular furrows, while in later years a small *os cordis* may develop on the right side. The heart weighs 85–113 g.

*Pig*

Only two ventricular furrows are normally present in the pig heart although a rudimentary posterior furrow may be present. The apex is more rounded than in sheep, and the heart cartilage ossified in older animals. The weight is 170–198 g.

*Horse*

The heart has two ventricular furrows, the aortic cartilage becoming partly ossified in older animals. The average weight is 2.7 kg although much greater in racehorses; in the thoroughbred horse Eclipse the heart weighed 6.3 kg.

*Domestic fowl*

The heart possesses a very pointed apex which in round-heart disease becomes distorted, dimpled at the apex and brownish.

### Portal circulation

The portal circulation is important in the study of the spread of certain parasitic and bacterial infections throughout the body.

The portal vein is formed by two main branches, the gastrosplenic and mesenteric veins which drain the stomach and intestines. The veins also drain blood from the pancreas. Venous blood from these organs is conveyed by the portal vein to the liver. The liver is drained by the hepatic veins which enter the posterior vena cava, wherein the blood is conveyed to the heart.

Bacteria or parasites which gain entry to the portal vein may be arrested within the sinusoids of the liver, but this organ is an imperfect filter and organisms may pass through to the heart and thence to the lungs. For example, hydatid cysts may be found in the lungs and occasionally immature liver flukes in the lungs of cattle and older sheep but not in pigs.

## Fetal circulation

The fetal circulation plays an important role in the occurrence of congenital tuberculosis in the calf and in the distribution of lesions.

Although the fetus *in utero* receives oxygen and nutrient material from the mother there is no actual passage of blood from mother to fetus. Transference of essential materials is rendered possible by the intimate contact of the mucous membrane of the maternal uterus with the fetal membrane, this contact being attained by means of the *cotyledons* of the *placenta*. Corresponding to each maternal cotyledon is a fetal cotyledon containing fine branches of the umbilical vein. These branches are received into the sponge-like structure of the maternal cotyledon and close contiguity of the two blood supplies is thus assured. Fetal blood is conveyed from the placenta by the umbilical veins (two in the ox and sheep) to the umbilicus, where they join to form a single vein. This main umbilical vein then passes forward along the floor of the abdominal wall and enters the liver at the umbilical fissure. The umbilical vein is the only fetal vessel which carries unmixed arterial blood.

In the *fetal* calf a portion of the blood borne by the umbilical vein, having entered the liver, passes into the *ductus venosus* and thus discharges directly into the posterior vena cava. The amount of blood side-tracked in this way is insignificant compared with the amount which passes through the liver substance, but by whichever route the blood passes through the liver its destination is the right auricle of the heart and then the lungs.

The lungs do not function in the *fetus*, as oxygen is supplied to it by the placenta, and the blood requirements of the fetal lungs are accordingly small. Blood which reaches the right auricle is therefore largely directed from the right to the left auricle by way of the *foramen ovale*, an orifice situated in the interauricular wall. A certain amount of blood, mostly draining from the head, does pass from the right auricle to the right ventricle and into the pulmonary artery, but a large portion of this blood passes from the pulmonary artery into the *ductus arteriosus*, a connecting vessel to the posterior aorta, and consequently does not reach the lungs. The blood supply to the fetal lungs, then, is the minimum amount necessary for the growth of these organs.

Blood which supplies the fetal structures through the aorta and its branches is eventually collected by two umbilical arteries which arise from the two iliac arteries in the pelvic cavity. These pass back to the umbilicus and thence to the placenta where the blood receives fresh oxygen and nutriment. After birth, the umbilical arteries retract and, like the umbilical vein, ductus venosus and ductus arteriosus, become cord-like and cease to function, while the foramen ovale becomes occluded. Although the elastic umbilical arteries retract within the abdomen of the calf immediately after birth, the umbilical vein remains open for a day or so. This is filled with liquid blood which coagulates to form a physiological thrombus; it is by this channel that the organisms causing navel ill gain entry to the body.

Although the placenta acts as an excellent filter, normally preventing the passage of bacteria into the umbilical veins and thence into the body of the fetus, certain foreign invaders do, at times, enter the umbilical vein from the placenta. Where bacteria or parasites gain entry to this vein, the place where these organisms are most likely to be arrested is the fetal liver.

### *The umbilical cord*

In the cow this cord from fetal membranes to umbilicus is 33–46 cm long, the fetal calf being born free of its membranes. In both cow and ewe the umbilical cord is embraced in a jelly-like tissue which contains the following vessels: two umbilical veins, two umbilical arteries and the *urachus*, the tube which drains the fetal bladder.

## Blood

Blood consists of a suspension of cells or corpuscles (red and white) and platelets in a straw-coloured fluid called plasma. It constitutes about one-thirteenth of the body weight of the animal. At any one time, about 20% of the blood volume is in the lungs, 20% in the heart and arterial system and 60% in the veins of the body.

The *red blood cells* are small biconcave discs about 7.2 µm thick. There are about six million red blood cells in every millilitre. The red cells give the blood its colour, although under the microscope they appear pale orange. They are manufactured in the red bone marrow, especially of the sternum, vertebrae, ribs and, in early life, the long bones. In fetal life, red cells are also formed in the liver, kidneys, spleen and muscles. Each red cell has a life of about 120 days, after which time it is broken down and replaced by a new cell.

Unlike mammalian blood, the avian red blood cells are nucleated.

*White blood cells* or *leukocytes* are much fewer in number than the red cells, there being only one in every 600 of the latter, and between 7000 and 14 000 white cells per millilitre. In certain diseases leukocytes are greatly increased in number, and young animals possess more than older stock. Leukocytes are manufactured in the bone marrow, spleen and lymph nodes (especially the lymphocytes). They play vital parts in the defensive mechanism of the body, destroying bacteria, dead cells and foreign material, and producing antibodies, heparin, histamine and antihistamine substances.

*Blood platelets* or *thrombocytes* are very minute bodies, measuring 2.4 µm in diameter. There are some 160 000–250 000 per millilitre. Their exact origin is not fully known, but some are thought to be produced in the lungs. Platelets aggregate and break down at sites of injury and when they come into contact with a foreign surface. They can arrest bleeding by forming a plug, especially in capillaries.

Blood obtained from the food animals at slaughter contains 77–82% of water and 18–23% of solids, of which 18–19% is protein. It therefore forms an article of food, though it is an essential preliminary process to whip or defibrinate it to prevent clotting. If any suppurative lesion, however slight, or other gross lesion of infection is found, the blood should not be used for food purposes. Further, the blood of animals slaughtered by the Jewish method is contaminated by stomach contents and should be rejected.

*Fetal blood*

This is an important biological substance, its serum being used for cell or tissue culture, following collection at slaughter via the umbilical cord or by direct heart cannulation and subsequent chilling.

## Spleen (melt)

The spleen is not essential to life. In the fetus it forms red and white cells, lymphocytes being produced during the life of the animal. It also acts as a store for RBCs and for the destruction of old red cells and platelets. Antibodies are formed in the spleen, which, in certain diseases, e.g. anthrax or trypanosomiasis, becomes very enlarged.

*Ox* (Fig. 2.11)

The spleen of the ox is related to the left dorsal side of the rumen and also to the diaphragm. In

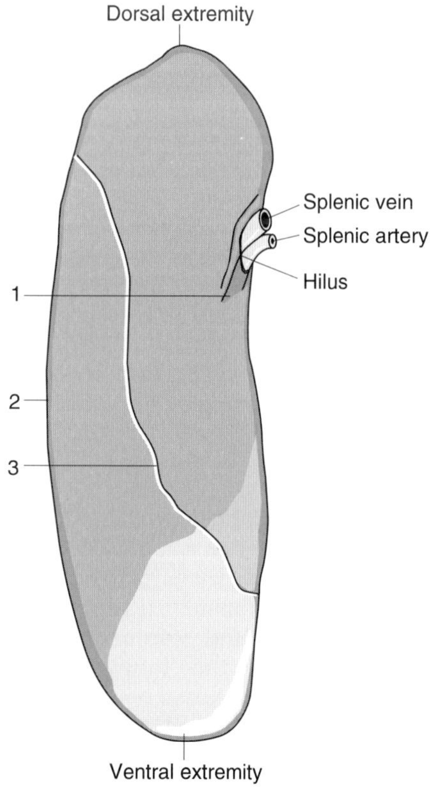


**Fig. 2.11** Spleen of ox; visceral surface. 1, Area of attachment to rumen (non-peritoneal); 2, caudal border; 3, line of peritoneal reflection.

the young bovine, it is reddish-brown, elongated and slightly convex with rounded edges; lymph follicles are apparent on the cut surface. In the cow the organ is bluish and flat with sharp edges and rounded extremities; it weighs 0.9–1.3 kg.

*Sheep*

The spleen is usually found attached to the pluck, being removed with it in the dressing of the carcase. It is oyster-shaped, soft or elastic to the touch and weighs 56–85 g. In both ox and sheep the spleen is adherent to the rumen.

*Pig*

The pig spleen is connected to the greater curvature of the stomach by the serous membrane known as the gastrosplenic omentum. The organ is elongated, tongue-shaped and triangular in cross-section, while its under surface shows well-marked longitudinal ridge to which the omentum is attached; it weighs 113–425 g. The relatively loose attachment of the pig spleen to the stomach often leads to splenic rotation, resulting in torsion and acute swelling of the organ.

*Horse*

The equine spleen is flat, sickle-shaped and bluish and weighs 453–907 g.

*Fowl*

In fowl the spleen is reddish-brown, small and spherical (1.5 cm in diameter.); it weighs 3–5 g.

## LYMPHATIC SYSTEM (Figs 2.10, 2.12)

*Lymph* is the medium by which oxygen and nutritive matter are transferred from the blood to the body tissues and waste products are removed. Although the blood capillaries approximate to the individual body cells, actual contact is through the lymph. The presence of lymph around the tissue cells is maintained by a slow exudation of fluid through the capillary walls and into the surrounding tissue; this fluid is similar to the plasma of the blood but is thinner, more watery and poorer in protein, which cannot pass readily through the capillary walls.

After lymph has fulfilled its function of feeding the tissue cells it is forced by the animal's muscular movements into the fine-walled *lymphatics*, which arise as blind-ended vessels in the tissues. These are similar to veins, but have thinner walls and more valves; when distended with lymph they have a characteristic beaded appearance.

Practically all lymph vessels discharge their contents into *lymph nodes* and, with rare exceptions, all the lymph throughout the system passes through at least one lymph node before it returns into the blood circulatory system. In every case the direction of flow of lymph in an organ is from the centre of the organ towards its surface. Lymph nodes consist of a reticular framework of elastic and smooth muscle fibres enclosing lymphatic tissue which contains lymphocytes. The intestinal lymphatics are the route of absorption of fat from the digestive tract.

Lymphatic vessels conveying lymph to a lymph node are known as *afferent* lymphatics and the area drained by the particular lymph node is known as its drainage area. An appreciation of the drainage system of lymph nodes is of particular value in the judgement of septic infections and of the tuberculous carcase (Fig. 2.12).

After passing through one or more lymph nodes, where some impurities are removed, lymph is conveyed by *efferent* lymphatics to discharge eventually into larger lymph-collecting vessels, which all flow towards the heart. The largest of these lymph-collecting vessels is the *thoracic duct*, which commences as a thin-walled dilation about 19 mm in width and known as the *receptaculum chyli*. This dilation is situated in the abdomen, lying above the aorta at the level of the last dorsal vertebra, and receives lymph from the lumbar and intestinal trunks; it is the main receptacle for lymph from the posterior part of the body. The thoracic duct is about 6.3 mm in width, passes forward through the diaphragm, traverses the thorax and opens into the anterior vena cava in the anterior thorax. Lymph from the anterior part of the body is carried towards the heart by two tracheal lymph ducts, which commence at the lateral retropharyngeal lymph nodes and pass down the neck on each side of the trachea and oesophagus; each duct discharges into the jugular vein of its own side.

The size of lymph nodes varies from that of a pinhead to that of a walnut, though the posterior mediastinal lymph node of the ox may reach a length of 20 cm. Lymph nodes are generally round or oval and somewhat compressed; in the ruminant they are large and few in number, but in the horse they occur in large numbers and in clusters. The size of lymph nodes is relatively greater in the young growing animal than in the adult.

The colour of lymph nodes shows considerable variation, and may be white, greyish-blue or almost black. The mesenteric lymph nodes of the ox are invariably black but in the pig the lymph nodes are lobulated and almost white, with the exception of those of the head and neck which are reddish.

The consistency of lymph nodes varies in different parts of the body, the nodes of the abdomen being generally softer than those of the thorax. A physiological oedema of the supramammary and iliac lymph nodes will invariably be encountered in the lactating animal.

The response of a lymph node to an irritant is normally rapid, involving enlargement, congestion and possibly tissue breakdown; thus *the size, colour and consistency of lymph nodes form a valuable guide in the estimation of disease processes in the animal body.*

Lymph nodes are absent in most poultry, although lymphatics are present.

## Haemal lymph nodes

These are deep red or almost black in colour, oval in shape and up to the size of a pea, but differ from lymph nodes in their anatomical

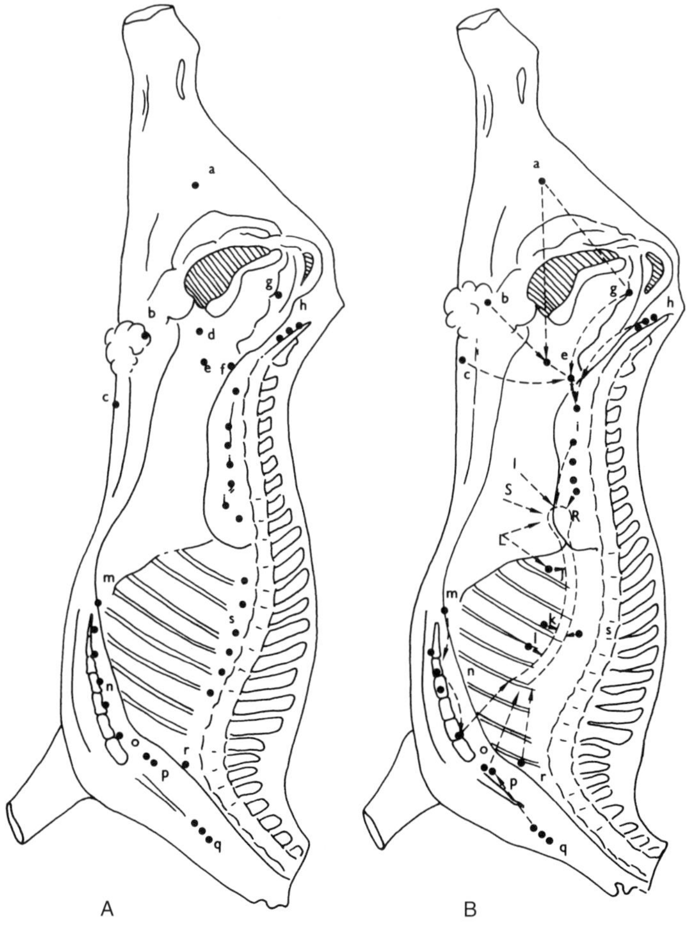


**Fig. 2.12** Carcase of bullock. A, Position of lymph nodes: a, popliteal; b, superficial inguinal; c, precrural; d, deep inguinal; e, external iliac; f, internal iliac; g, ischiatic; h, sacral; i, lumbar, i″, renal; m, xyphoid; n, suprasternal; o, presternal; p, prepectoral; q, middle cervical; r, costocervical; s, intercostal. B, Direction of the lymph flow: I lymph from intestine; S, lymph from stomach; L, lymph from liver; R, receptaculum chyli; j, lymph from posterior mediastinal lymph node discharging into thoracic duct; k, lymph from bronchial lymph nodes; l, lymph from anterior mediastinal lymph nodes.

structure and in the absence of afferent and efferent lymphatics. Haemal lymph nodes are supplied by arteries which break up in the gland substance and discharge their blood into tissue spaces; in this respect these nodes bear a resemblance to the spleen and may, in fact, be described as accessory spleens. Like the spleen, they contain numerous white blood corpuscles together with red blood corpuscles in various stages of disintegration, hence the red coloration of the nodes.

Haemal lymph nodes are numerous in the ox and sheep but are not found in the horse or pig. In cattle they occur especially along the course of the aorta and in the subcutaneous fat, while in sheep and lambs they are commonest beneath the peritoneum in the sublumbar region, being larger and more numerous in animals suffering from anaemic and cachectic conditions. The red lymph nodes of the head and neck of the pig are frequently mistaken for haemal lymph nodes.

In poultry, mural lymph nodules are present on the lymphatic vessels.

## LYMPH NODES OF THE OX

**P**: Position. **D**: Drainage area. **E**: Destination of efferent lymph vessels of node. (Nomenclature varies in different texts, countries, etc.)

### Nodes of the head and neck

*Submaxillary*

**P**: One on each side, just inside the angle of the jaw and embedded in fat. **D**: Head, nose and mouth. **E**: Lateral retropharyngeal nodes.

*Parotid*

**P**: One on each side, on the edge of the masseter muscle and covered by the parotid salivary gland which must be incised to expose it. It is a flat node 7.5 cm long by 2.5 cm wide, and should always be examined in old cows. **D**: Muscles of head, eye and ear, tongue and cranial cavity. **E**: Lateral retropharyngeal nodes.

*Retropharyngeal*

These are divided into two groups:

1. The *internal retropharyngeal nodes*, two to four in number and situated between the hyoid bones. **D**: Pharynx, tongue and larynx. **E**: Lateral retropharyngeal nodes.
2. The *lateral retropharyngeal nodes* situated beneath each wing of the atlas and therefore usually located at the neck end of the dressed carcase. **D**: Tongue, and receive efferents from submaxillary, parotid, and internal retropharyngeal nodes. **E**: Tracheal lymph duct.

*Middle cervical*

**P**: Situated in the middle of the neck on each side of the trachea and often absent in cattle. They vary in number from one to seven and also in position and size. **D**: Lateral retropharyngeal nodes. **E**: Prepectoral nodes.

### Nodes of the chest and forequarter (Figs 2.10 and 2.12)

*Prepectoral*

These are known also as the *lower cervicals* and may be considered anatomically as a continuation of the upper and middle cervical chain. The middle cervical group may, in fact, extend to the upper group or may reach back almost to the prepectorals. **P**: The prepectorals are two to four in number on each side, and are embedded in fat along the anterior border of the first rib. The main node of this group is superficially situated about the middle of the first rib and just anterior to it; haemal lymph nodes are usually present in the fat around this group. The second node of this group is on the same level and just anterior to the main node but is deep-seated and is exposed by making an incision 10 cm long and 5 cm deep through the triangular-shaped *scalenus* muscle. **D**: Efferents from upper and middle cervical nodes, together with efferents from the prescapular; thus all lymph from the head and neck passes through the prepectoral lymph nodes. **E**: Thoracic duct.

*Costocervical*

**P**: This may be found on the inner side or just anterior to the first rib and close to its junction with the first dorsal vertebra. It lies adjacent to the oesophagus and trachea and is frequently removed with these in the dressing of the carcase, being then found anterior to the heart and lungs. **D**: Neck, shoulder, parietal pleura and first few intercostal nodes. **E**: Thoracic duct.

*Prescapular*

**P**: This node is elongated, commonly 7.5–10 cm long and 2.5 cm or more in width. It lies about 10 cm in front of the point of the shoulder and a deep incision 15 cm long and 5 cm deep must be made to expose it. The node is embedded in fat and its exposure is greatly facilitated if the carcase is examined before the onset of rigor mortis. **D**: Head, neck, shoulder and forelimb. **E**: Thoracic duct.

The importance of the prescapular lymph node in relation to bovine tuberculosis lies in the fact that it drains not only the head, neck, shoulder and forelimb, but also muscle and bone. When lesions of tuberculosis, therefore, are found in the prescapular node without lesions being present in the head or its lymph nodes, it is strongly suggestive that the infection of the node is the result of either local inoculation or haematogenous dissemination.

*Intercostal*

**P**: Known also as the *dorso-costal*, these are situated in the intercostal spaces at the junction of the ribs with their vertebrae, and are deep-seated, being covered by the intercostal muscle. Most of these nodes are small, and not all of the spaces may contain nodes. **D**: Muscles of dorsal region, intercostal muscles, ribs, and parietal pleura. **E**: Mediastinal lymph nodes.

*Subdorsal*

**P**: This superficial group lies in the fat between the aorta and the dorsal vertebrae. The nodes are irregular in arrangement, varying in length from 12 to 25 mm, and are frequently removed with the lungs in the dressing of the carcase; they may then be found by incising the upper surface of the mediastinal fat between the lungs. In some areas the thoracic portion of the posterior aorta is left attached and the subdorsal lymph nodes, which run down each side of the vessel wall, will then be found on the carcase. The more posterior nodes of the group, no matter how the carcase is dressed, usually remain on the forequarter and can be found by incising the fat below the dorsal vertebrae just anterior to the diaphragm. **D**: The same structures as the intercostals and also the mediastinum, pericardium, diaphragm and efferents from the intercostal lymph nodes. **E**: Thoracic duct.

*Suprasternal*

**P**: Known also as the *sternocostal*, these nodes lie between the costal cartilages and are covered by muscle. They may be exposed by an incision 7.5 cm from and parallel to the cut surface of the sternum, and are found at the junction of the internal thoracic vein with a line continuing the posterior border of each rib. The node in the fourth intercostal space is large and readily exposed, but nodes are not present in every intercostal space. The largest of this group, known as the *presternal* or anterior sternal node, is superficially placed and embedded in fat on the first segment of the sternum. **D**: Diaphragm, abdominal muscles, intercostal muscles, parietal and visceral pleura and peritoneum. **E**: Thoracic duct and prepectoral nodes.

*Bronchial* (Fig. 2.10)

**P**: There are two main bronchial nodes, the right and left, together with two smaller nodes. The left bronchial is 4 cm × 2.5 cm in size, often irregular in shape, and found close to the left bronchus, being embedded deeply in fat and partly covered by the aorta. The right bronchial is related to the right bronchus, is usually smaller than the left and partly hidden by the right lung; it is absent in 25% of cases, while in others two nodes may be found. The middle bronchial node is situated in the middle line above the bifurcation of the trachea but is absent in 50% of cases; a further node, the *apical*, is placed on the accessory bronchus where it enters the apical lobe of the right lung. **D**: Lungs. **E**: The left bronchial node discharges into the thoracic duct, the right bronchial node into the posterior mediastinal node or thoracic duct, the middle bronchial or apical into the anterior mediastinal nodes. When the right bronchial node is absent, the lymphatics of the diaphragmatic lobe of the right lung discharge into the posterior mediastinal and left bronchial node. A node known as the *inspector's node* is present in 75% of cases and is situated at the junction of the two cardiac lobes of the right lung.

*Anterior mediastinal* (Fig. 2.10)

**P**: These are numerous, lying in the mediastinal space anterior to the heart, and are related anatomically to the oesophagus, trachea and anterior aorta. **D**: Heart, pericardium, mediastinum and thoracic wall, and receive efferents from apical and middle bronchial lymph nodes. **E**: Thoracic duct.

*Posterior mediastinal* (Fig. 2.10)

These nodes are 8 to 12 in number and situated in the fat along the dorsal wall of the oesophagus. The largest and most posterior of these nodes lies posterior to the heart, being up to 20 cm long and extending almost to the diaphragm; in some cases this large node is replaced by two smaller ones. **D**: Lungs, diaphragm and, via the diaphragm, the peritoneum, surface of the liver and spleen. They receive efferents from the right bronchial node. **E**: Thoracic duct.

*Axillary*

**P**: Known also as the *brachial*, this node is about 2.5 cm long, covered by the scapula and situated in the muscle external to and about midway along the second rib. **D**: Muscles of shoulder and forelimb. **E**: Prepectoral node.

*Xiphoid (ventral mediastinal)*

**P**: Found in the loose fat at the junction of the sternum and diaphragm at the level of the sixth rib, and related anatomically to the apex of the heart. This node is absent in 50% of cases. **D**: Pleura, diaphragm and ribs. **E**: Suprasternal lymph nodes.

### Nodes of the abdomen and hindquarter (Fig. 2.12)

The position of these nodes is described as if the hindquarters were suspended by the hock in the normal manner.

*Lumbar*

**P**: These are situated in the fat covering the lumbar muscles and are related anatomically to the aorta and posterior vena cava. Some of these nodes are superficial, others being embedded in the loin fat; haemal lymph nodes are common in this region. **D**: Lumbar region and peritoneum. They receive efferent vessels from the internal and external iliacs, sacral and popliteal nodes. **E**: Receptaculum chyli.

*Portal*

**P**: Known also as the *hepatic*, these form a group around the portal vein, hepatic artery and bile duct, and are covered by the pancreas. Another group, which includes the lymph node draining the pancreas, lies between the edge of the pancreas and the caudate lobe of the liver. The portal nodes vary from 10 to 15 in number. **D**: Liver, pancreas and duodenum. **E**: Receptaculum chyli.

*Renal*

**P**: This node belongs in reality to the lumbar group, and is found in the fat at the entrance to the kidney. In this position a split blood vessel is found and the node can be exposed by making an incision lengthwise through this vessel and continuing the incision 2.5 cm deep into the lumbar suet. **D**: Kidneys and adrenal body. **E**: Receptaculum chyli. The renal lymph nodes vary in size and number.

*Mesenteric*

**P**: These comprise a large number of elongated nodes which lie between the peritoneal folds of the mesentery and receive lymph from the intestines. These nodes may be divided into a small duodenal group which drains the duodenum, the efferent lymphatics passing to the portal nodes of the liver, and a jejuno-ileal group ranging in number from 10 to 50, and 0.5–12 cm in length. The long nodes form the main chain parallel to and some 5 cm from the intestine, while the small nodes are scattered throughout the mesentery between the small intestine and the colon. **D**: The small intestine (jejunum and ilium). **E**: Receptaculum chyli.

*Splenic*

Splenic lymph nodes are absent in the ox and sheep. Lymph drained from the spleen passes to the gastric chain of lymph nodes. Several splenic lymph nodes are present in the horse and pig.

*Gastric*

**P**: These are numerous and difficult to group satisfactorily; a number form a chain along the right and left longitudinal grooves of the rumen. **D**: Walls of stomach and spleen. **E**: Receptaculum chyli. The gastric group are rarely incised in meat inspection.

*Iliacs*

These are situated near the terminal branches of the aorta and are embedded in fat.

**Internal iliac** **P**: This may be exposed by an incision level with the junction of the sacrum and the last lumbar vertebrae. Several nodes are present, lying some 18 cm from the vertebrae and 1–5 cm in length. **D**: This node drains muscle and pelvic viscera, including muscles of the sublumbar region, pelvis and thigh, the femur, tibia, patella, tarsus and metatarsus, the male and female genital organs and kidneys. It receives efferent vessels from the external iliac, precrural, ischiatic and superficial inguinal nodes. **E**: Lumbar lymph nodes and receptaculum chyli.

**External iliac** **P**: A single or double node 1–2.5 cm in length and situated laterally to the internal iliac. It lies beneath the external angle of the ilium at the bifurcation of the circumflex iliac artery, but is sometimes absent on one or both sides. **D**: Abdominal muscles, sublumbar area, posterior part of the peritoneum, and some efferents from the popliteal node. **E**: Internal iliac and lumbar lymph nodes.

*Superficial inguinal (male)*

**P**: These lie in the mass of fat about the neck of the scrotum and behind the spermatic cord. **D**: External genitals and adjoining skin area. **E**: Deep inguinal when present, or failing this, the internal iliac.

*Supramammary (female)*

**P**: These lie above and behind the udder; there are usually two present on each side, one large and one small, the larger pair, about 7.5 cm in size, approximating to each other, the small pair being found above or in front of the larger pair and 0.5–1.5 cm in size. In the heifer these nodes may be found on a straight line level with the cut pubic tubercle. **D**: Udder and external genitals. **E**: Deep inguinal when present, or internal iliac.

*Deep inguinal*

**P**: In the inguinal canal and frequently absent; when absent, the internal iliac functions in its place. **D**: Hind limb and abdominal wall. **E**: Internal iliac. According to some authors the deep inguinals are part of the external iliacs.

*Ischiatic*

**P**: This lies on the outer aspect of the sacrosciatic ligament, and is exposed by a deep incision on a vertical line midway between the posterior part of the ischium and the sacrum. **D**: Posterior pelvic organs and also receives efferents from popliteal node. **E**: Internal iliac.

In many countries in Africa the ischiatic node is incised on routine post-mortem examination of beef carcases because the bites of the tick *Hyalomma rufipes*, which attaches itself to the perianal region, frequently cause abscess formation.

*Sacral*

**P**: These are not constantly present and are unimportant. If present they are difficult to distinguish from the medial iliac lymph nodes.

*Precrural (Sub-iliac)*

**P**: This node is known also as the *prefemoral* and is embedded in fat; it may be exposed by an incision at the edge of the tensor fascia lata, the incision being made about 18 cm down from the apex of this muscle. **D**: Skin, prepuce and superficial muscles. **E**: Internal iliac nodes.

The precrural nodes, draining the umbilicus, should always be palpated in calves, and if necessary incised.

*Popliteal*

**P**: This is deeply seated in the round of beef and is exposed by a deep incision along the superficial seam or division which connects the ischium and *os calcis*, the node lying midway between these and 15 cm deep. **D**: Lower part of the leg and foot. **E**: Lumbar and iliac nodes and also ischiatic node.

## LYMPH NODES OF THE PIG (Fig. 2.13)

### Head and neck

The nodes of the head and neck are numerous and somewhat difficult to group satisfactorily. They include the following.

*Submaxillary (mandibular)*

These lie anterior to the submaxillary salivary gland near to the angle of the jaw, and are covered by the lower part of the parotid salivary gland. There are commonly two nodes on each side, one large and one small.

*Anterior or upper cervical*

Known also as the *accessory submaxillary* or submandibular these lie a short distance behind and above the preceding nodes, being separated from them by the submaxillary salivary gland.

*Parotid*

There are several nodes on each side, which are red in colour, one of the largest being situated just posterior to the masseter muscle of the lower jaw and partly covered by the parotid salivary gland. One or two nodes may be left on the inner side of the jaw after the head is removed.

*Prescapular (superficial cervical)*

On account of the short neck of the pig these nodes lie close to the parotid salivary gland, being partly covered by its posterior border. They form an oblique chain which is directed downwards and backwards to the shoulder joint. This chain really includes all the superficial cervical nodes and is best exposed by a long incision, made on the inside of the carcase, from the nape of the neck to the lower border of the neck and just anterior to the shoulder joint. The prescapular lymph nodes in the pig receive lymph from the submaxillary, parotid and upper cervical nodes and thus may become tuberculous as a result of primary infection of the lymph nodes of the head. Enlargement of the prepectoral node in pigs may occur as a result of arthritic changes in the forelimbs.

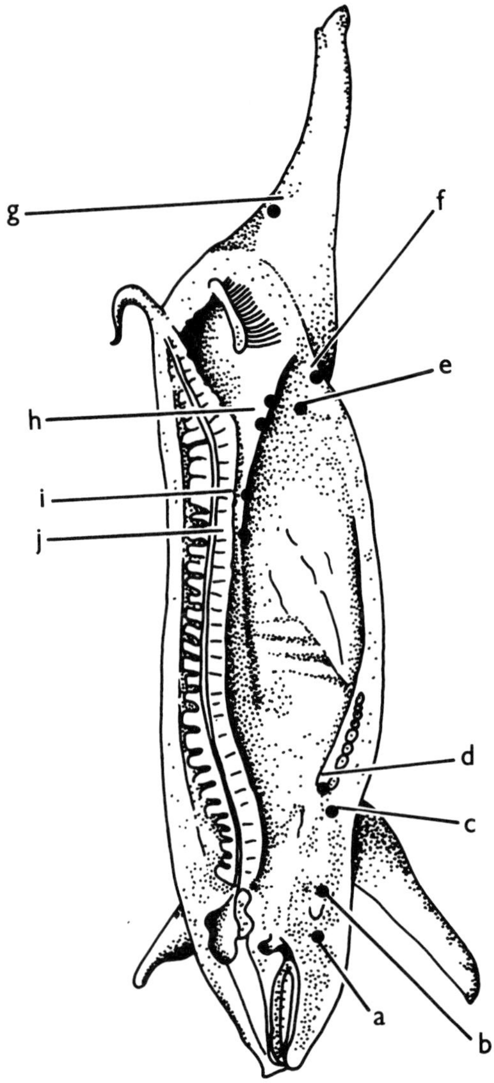


**Fig. 2.13** Side of pork showing position of lymph nodes: a, submaxillary; b, anterior or upper cervical; c, prepectoral; d, presternal; e, precrural; f, superficial inguinal; g, hock node; h, iliac; i, lumbar; j, renal.

### Other nodes

*Precrural (sub-iliac)*

In adult pigs this is up to 5 cm in length by 2.5 cm wide, and is most easily exposed by an incision through the peritoneal aspect of the carcase deep into the fat and 2.5 cm in front of the stifle joint, the incision being made at right angles to the vertebral column.

*Popliteal*

When present these are superficial, but are absent in 50% of cases. A small subcutaneous node, known as the *hock node* or *Hartenstein's gland*, can constantly be found, and is superficially placed on the posterior aspect of the limb about a hand's breadth above the *tuber calcis*.

*Gastric*

These and the pancreatic nodes are situated on the lesser curvature of the stomach.

*Bronchial*

In addition to the right and left bronchial, this group includes one on the bifurcation of the trachea and another at the apical bronchus of the right lung. The posterior mediastinal nodes are rudimentary or absent.

*Portal*

Several nodes are present about the portal vein, the largest being about 2.5 cm long. The portal lymph nodes may be removed during evisceration of the carcase, and can then be found on the mesentery beneath the pancreas or in the fat attached to the lesser curvature of the stomach.

## UROGENITAL SYSTEM

### Urinary organs

Two kidneys, two ureters, bladder and urethra.

### Genital organs

*Female* two ovaries, two uterine (fallopian) tubes, uterus, vagina, vulva, clitoris and mammary glands.

*Male* two testes and epididymes, two vasa deferentia, seminal glands, prostate, bulbo-urethral (Cowper's) glands, urethra and penis.

### Kidney

In addition to their functions in the excretion of urine and in acid–base balance, the kidneys produce two hormones, *renin* and *erythropoietic factor*. Renin acts in the formation of a blood peptide which increases blood pressure and stimulates the secretion of aldosterone, a hormone controlling the reabsorption of sodium. The erythropoietic factor stimulates the formation of a protein which increases the red cell production in the bone marrow.

*Ox* (Fig. 2.14)

The kidneys are reddish-brown and composed of 15–25 lobes which are fused at their deeper portions; each lobe terminates in a blunt process or papilla, visible when the kidney is split. When the rumen is empty, the left kidney lies to the left of the vertebral column but, as the rumen becomes filled, it propels the kidney towards the right side of the body, though injury due to pressure on the ureter is usually

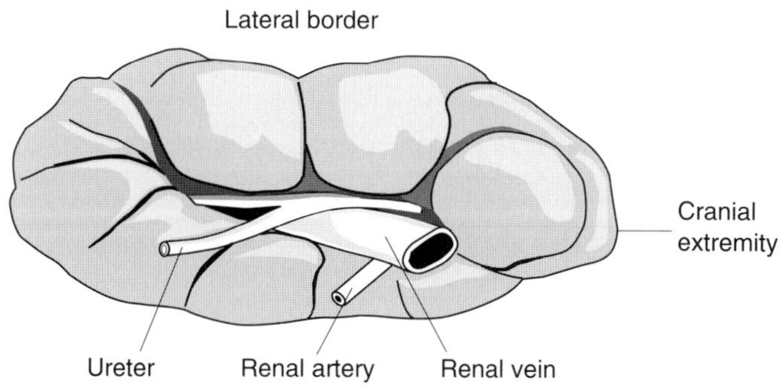


**Fig. 2.14** Right kidney of ox; ventral surface. Organ hardened *in situ*. Fat has been removed from fissures between lobes.

avoided. This orientation of the left kidney is rendered possible by its loose attachment to the lumbar region. The left kidney, by reason of its mobility, is roughly three-sided and of a somewhat twisted appearance, but the right kidney has a more regular, elliptical outline. The weight of each kidney is 283–340 g.

*Sheep and goat*

The kidneys are dark brown, bean-shaped and unlobulated and possess a single renal papilla. As in the ox, the left kidney of the sheep and goat is freely movable. Each kidney weighs 56–85 g.

*Pig* (Fig. 2.15)

The kidneys are smooth, bean-shaped and reddish-brown but thinner and flatter than in the other food animals; 10–12 renal papillae are present internally. The weight of each kidney is 85–170 g. In the pig the bladder is large with a long neck; the ureters enter posteriorly in the neck region. This predisposes the animal to bilateral hydronephrosis, because, when full, the bladder hangs down into the abdominal cavity and the long neck presses against the pubis, thus closing the ureter openings and interfering with urination.

*Horse*

The right kidney is triangular or heart-shaped, the left is bean-shaped and longer than broad. The weight of each kidney is 680 g.

*Domestic fowl*

The kidneys lie on either side of the vertebral column from the level of the sixth rib to the iliac fossa. They each consist of four dark red, friable lobes. The ureters empty into the cloaca medial to the ductus deferens of the male or the oviduct of the female. The end products of protein metabolism are excreted as uric acid which can be seen as whitish turbid crystals in the ureters.

## REPRODUCTIVE SYSTEM

**Uterus** (Fig. 2.16)

*Cow*

The *uterus* consists of a small *body*, less than 2.5 cm long, and two *cornua* or *horns* about 38 cm

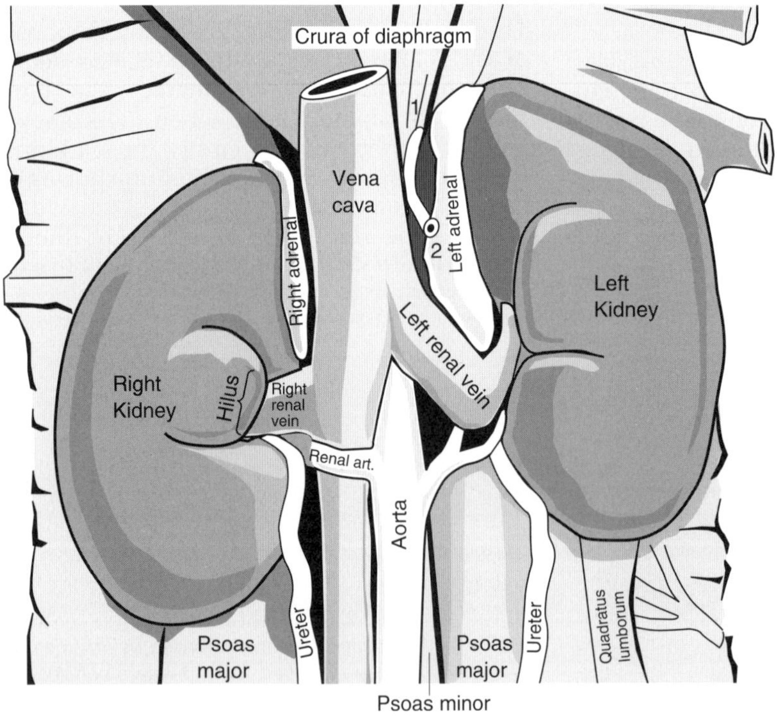


**Fig. 2.15** Kidneys of pig *in situ*; ventral view. 1, hepatic artery; 2, splenic artery.

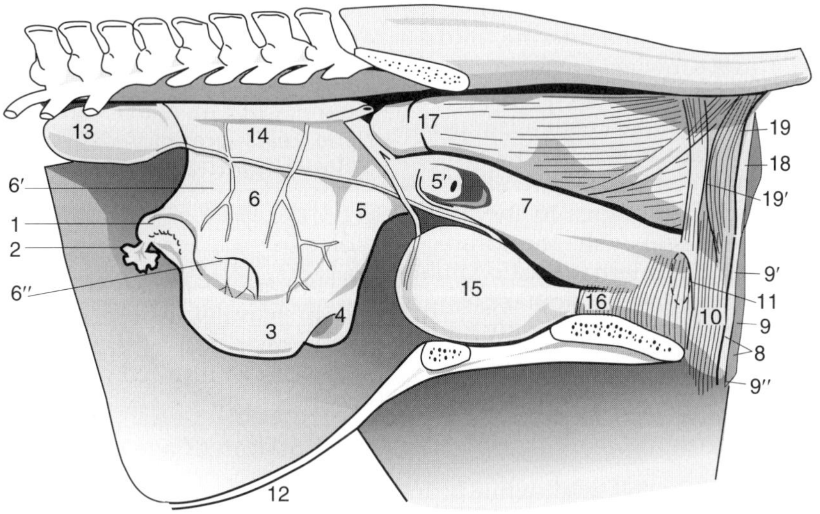


**Fig. 2.16** Lateral view of genital organs and adjacent structures of mare. 1. L. ovary. 2. Fallopian tube. 3. L. horn of uterus. 4. R. horn of uterus. 5. Body of uterus. [5′ Cervix] 6. Broad lig. of uterus. 7. Vagina. 8. Vulva. 9. Rim and commissures of vulva. 10. Constrictor muscle of vulva. 11. Vestibular bulb. 12. Abdominal wall. 13. L. kidney. 14. L. ureter. 15. Bladder. 16. Urethra. 17. Rectum. 18. Anus. 19. Anal sphincter muscle.

long. The uterus of the cow and ewe has characteristic cotyledons on the mucous membrane of the body and uterine horns; these are oval prominences, about 100 in all, and in the non-gravid bovine uterus are about 1.5 × 0.5 cm. During pregnancy, and as the fetus develops, the cotyledons hypertrophy, becoming pitted or sponge-like, and then measure up to 10–12.5 cm in length and 4 cm in width. Evidence as to whether a slaughtered female is a heifer or a cow may be established by opening each uterine horn and cutting transversely through the wall, including the diameter of a cotyledon. Generally, in the uterus of a heifer the cotyledons are surrounded by a shallow moat which usually disappears in the cow. The blood vessels in the exposed wall of the uterus of the cow are contorted and bulge from the surface. In the heifer the blood vessels can be seen clearly but do not bulge and show little contortion. The blood vessels in the cotyledon are the most valuable guide; in the heifer they are very fine and straight, whereas in the cow they are very distinct, contorted and bulge slightly from the cut surface. This method assumes that the cotyledons enlarge if the animal is in calf and regress in the non-pregnant uterus, i.e. that the animal must have been at least 3½ months or longer in calf.

### *Ewe*

The *uterine horns* are relatively long, the cotyledons being circular, pigmented and much smaller than in the cow, while in advanced pregnancy the centre of each is cupped or umbilicated.

### *Gilt and sow*

The *uterine horns* are very long and arranged in coils. The mucous membrane has no cotyledons but is arranged in numerous thin longitudinal folds. The *ovaries* are rounded with an irregularly lobulated surface. The sow and gilt carcase may be differentiated not only by the developmental condition of the udder and teats but also by examination of the uterine arteries. In the sow, the *udders* are enlarged and, in the broad ligaments of the uterine horns, the peripheral branches of the uterine middle arteries are torturous owing to pregnancy. In the gilt, these arterial vessels are less apparent and almost straight. Characteristic histological changes also take place in the uterine arteries during and after pregnancy; there is hyperplasia of the elastic fibres in the intima and media of the vessel wall, the intima is hypertrophied and the internal elastic lamina split into two or more layers. Similar changes can be observed in the arteries supplying the ovary.

### *Domestic fowl*

In the *male* there are two yellowish-white bean-shaped *testes* situated in the dorsal part of the abdomen and related to the right lobe of the liver (right testis) and the glandular stomach and intestine (left testis). The testes vary in size according to the size of the bird, breed and season. The vasa deferentia pass backwards to the cloaca, which they enter lateral to the ureters.

Although there are two *ovaries* in the embryo, the right one atrophies. The left ovary is situated in the dorsal abdomen opposite the last two ribs. The associated *oviduct* is a very flexuous organ and extends backwards to enter the cloaca lateral to the left ureter. Its mucosa produces the albumen, shell membrane and shell, while the yolk represents the ovum produced in the ovary.

## Udder

### *Cow*

The right and left sides of the udder are separated anatomically by a tendinous septum. Although a strong septum does not exist between the fore- and hindquarters of the same side, all four quarters are anatomically distinct and injection of differently coloured fluids into the four teats shows that they each drain separate and distinct areas.

The smooth udder of the heifer, which is composed almost entirely of fat, must be distinguished from the pendulous fleshy udder of the cow in which glandular tissue predominates and which is grey to yellowish-white in colour.

### *Ewe and goat*

The udder is composed of two halves, each with one small teat. In the goat the udder is similar but the halves are more pendulous and the teats are more strongly developed and directed forwards.

### *Sow*

There are 10–16 mammary glands, arranged in two parallel rows; each possesses a flat triangular teat and the glandular substance appears whitish-red on section.

## Estimation of age of the bovine fetus

By the end of the first month of pregnancy the bovine fetus is about 10 mm long. At the end of the second month the fetus is 5–6.5 cm long and digits and depressions for mouth and nose appear. After 3 months the fetus is 15 cm long, stomach divisions are present and hoofs and horns appear.

In the fourth month there is little change except growth, but towards the end of the fifth month hair appears and the testes descend into the scrotum. At the end of five months the fetus is 30 cm long.

During the next 3 months the fetus attains a length of 60 cm. By 8 months the eyes are open, the limbs are covered with hair, and the hoofs are hardened. At the end of the ninth month the fetus is full size, about 90 cm long, and weighs 36 kg, which is the average weight for a newborn calf, though variations occur according to the breed.

## Testis

(See Endocrine System.)

# NERVOUS SYSTEM

The nervous system, which forms a very delicate and complicated link between different parts of the body, consists of two main parts:

1 *Central nervous system* (CNS), comprising the brain and spinal cord.
2 *Peripheral nervous system*, consisting of 12 pairs of cranial nerves, approximately 40 pairs of spinal nerves, and the automatic

(involuntary) nervous system. Also associated with the peripheral nervous system are the specialised sense organs—eye, ear, olfactory (smell) organ, gustatory (taste) organ and tactile (touch) organs.

The nervous system is made up of numerous *nerve cells* or *neurons*, each consisting of a nucleated *cell body*, short cell processes called *dendrites*, and a single long process, the *axon*. The dendrites receive impulses from other axons and transmit them to the nerve cell, which conveys them onwards via the axon. A nerve fibre consists of the axon and a covering of sheath cells. In the peripheral nerves the sheath is composed of *Schwann cells*, forming a thick fatty (lipoidal) covering, the myelin sheath, which acts as an insulator and gives the white colour to nerves of the brain and spinal cord. In myelinated nerves, conduction of impulses takes place by means of jumps between notches (the nodes of Ranvier) in the myelin sheath. In unmyelinated nerve cells, conduction is a smooth continuous process. Bundles of nerve fibres are bound together by an extensive connective tissue sheath, the *perineurium*; the complete nerve trunk is covered by the *epineurium*.

Nerve cells may be sensory or motor. *Sensory* (afferent) fibres carry impulses to the brain from the sensory organs while *motor* (efferent) fibres carry impulses away from the brain to produce muscular movement and glandular secretion.

### Central nervous system

The *brain* is that part of the CNS situated in the cranial cavity and containing the vital centres. It consists of an upper main part, the *cerebrum*, and a lower smaller part, the *cerebellum*; the lowest portion of the brain, the *medulla oblongata*, is continuous through the *foramen magnum* with the spinal cord. The cerebrum is divided into two hemispheres by a longitudinal fissure.

The *spinal cord* is situated in the spinal or vertebral canal and extends from the foramen magnum at its juncture with the medulla oblongata to about the middle of the sacrum. It is approximately cylindrical in cross-section but somewhat flattened dorsoventrally. From it emerge a varying number of spinal nerves: in the *bovine* there are 40 pairs made up by 7 cervical, 14 thoracic, 6 lumbar, 5 sacral, and 8 coccygeal.

To the naked eye the central nervous system is composed chiefly of two kinds of tissue—*white* and *grey*. The outer white substance or matter is soft in consistency and consists of numerous nerve fibres, while the inner grey substance, even softer in make-up, is modified to form the gelatinous substance, which is a pale yellowish-grey and jelly-like. The grey matter is comprised of large numbers of nerve cells.

The brain and spinal cord are covered by three membranes known as the *meninges*. The *dura mater* is the tough, fibrous outer coat lining the cranial cavity and spinal canal, while the *arachnoid mater* (arachnoidea) is a delicate membrane loosely covering the brain and serving to contain the cerbrospinal fluid. The *pia mater* is another delicate membrane closely attached to the convoluted surface of the brain and spinal cord, to which it supplies blood.

The clear cerebrospinal fluid, which occurs in the subarachnoid space between the arachnoid and pia mater, serves to protect the brain and the spinal cord as well as to nourish and cleanse these structures.

### Peripheral nervous system

The 12 cranial nerves (motor and sensory) supply the head and neck and include the nerves involved in the sensations of sight, smell, taste and hearing in addition to the vagus nerve, an important entity of the parasympathetic division of the *autonomic nervous system*.

The 40 or so spinal nerves supply the muscles of the body and limbs. They are mixed nerves; the motor fibres give movement to these parts and the sensory fibres give sensation to the skin and to a lesser extent to body and limb muscles. Associated with some of the cranial nerves and all of the spinal nerves (on their ventral roots) are swellings (collections of nerves cells) called ganglia, which are part of the sympathetic nervous system.

### Autonomic (visceral, vegetative) nervous system

The *autonomic nervous system* is a set of nerves and ganglia supplying ennervation to all the internal organs, glands and blood vessels. It is so named because it acts independently of the conscious will, although it can be affected by the emotions.

Like the cerebrospinal system, it possesses conducting paths which transmit impulses to and away from the vital centres, but the nerves are mainly efferent. The efferent neurons are both motor, supplying the involuntary muscles of the walls of the stomach, lungs, intestines, heart, eye, bladder and blood vessels, and secretory, supplying glands such as the liver, salivary glands, pancreas as well as the external genitalia.

The autonomic nervous system consists of two subdivisions, the sympathetic and parasympathetic, both of which supply fibres to some organs (eye, bronchi, heart, digestive tract, sphincters, of digestive tract and bladder), although the *sympathetic system* mainly supplies the blood vessels and sweat glands and the *parasympathetic* the salivary, gastric and pancreatic glands and the external genitalia. The actions of these two systems are largely antagonistic to each other. Increased *sympathetic* activity dilates the pupil of the eye, the bronchi and the blood vessels, increases heart rate, inhibits motility of the digestive tract and allows the bladder to fill; the *parasympathetic* system produces the opposite effects and enhances the secretions from the salivary, gastric and pancreatic glands and produces vasodilation in the external genitalia.

## ENDOCRINE SYSTEM

The *endocrine* or *ductless glands* (thyroid, parathyroids, thymus, adrenals, and gonads-testes and ovaries) produce secretions or hormones which pass directly into the bloodstream to act on another organ or tissue. The liver and pancreas are both endocrine and exocrine glands, each possessing ducts, and are usually described with the digestive system. (*Exocrine* glands such as the sweat, mammary and lachrymal glands pass their secretions along ducts to the surface of the body.)

The *placenta*, formed from the outer chorionic membrane (the inner is the *amnion*) surrounding the developing fetus, is a ductless gland in addition to its function as a means of transferring nutrients from the mother to the embryo and conveying away waste material. It produces oestrogen, progesterone and chorionic gonadotrophin. The *corpus luteum* (yellow body), formed from the ovarian follicle of the ovary after the ovum has been expelled, produces the hormone progesterone, which prevents further ovulation.

*Hormones* are either peptides, containing two or more amino acids, or steroids, which are lipid substances. Insulin, produced by the islets of Langerhans in the pancreas, is a polypeptide composed of two amino acid chains, while the hormones of the adrenal glands, noradrenaline and adrenaline, are steroids, as are the hormones of the reproductive system (oestrogens and progestins in the female and androgens in the male). These organic substances are 'chemical messengers' responsible for regulating the physiological activities of the body; only minute amounts are necessary to evoke responses in target glands and tissues.

### Thyroid

In the *ox* the thyroid consists of two lateral lobes lying on either side of the trachea immediately posterior to the larynx. The lobes are flat, dark red, about 7.5 cm long, and are connected inferiorly by a narrow band-like isthmus about 13 mm wide.

In *sheep* the glands are dark red, resembling muscle, and are about 5 cm long and 1.5 cm wide. Each lateral lobe is long and elliptical and covers the first five rings of the trachea, but the isthmus is indistinct.

In the *pig* the lobes are large, dark red, about 5 cm long, and irregularly triangular in shape; they lie below the trachea and posterior to the larynx and are connected with each other inferiorly. The dark red colour of the thyroid gland is due to its rich blood supply.

The thyroid gland produces three hormones: thyroxine (tetraiodothyronine) and triiodothyronine, which contain iodine, are involved in the control of the general body metabolism; and thyrocalcitonin (calcitonin) which controls serum calcium levels.

Overactivity of the thyroid glands with excess secretion of the thyroid hormones in *man* causes toxic goitre (exophthalmic goitre, thyrotoxicosis, Graves' disease) with enlargement of the thyroid gland, excitability, irritability and loss of weight. Underactivity of the thyroid, on the other hand, results in myxoedema (hypothyroidism), which is characterised by slowness of physical and mental processes and an increase in body weight. Cretinism is hypothyroidism or myxoedema which begins before birth or early childhood and in which there is stunted growth and loss of intellectual ability. These syndromes occur infrequently in man and are rare in animals. However, goitre caused by iodine deficiency is seen occasionally in newborn animals of all species which show thyroid enlargement with loss of hair or wool and thickened skin. Hyperthyroidism occurs only in dogs and cats.

### Parathyroids

The position of the parathyroids relative to the thyroid gland varies, but they may sometimes be found near the posterior extremity or on the deep surface of the lateral lobes of the thyroid and are little larger than a grain of wheat in the *ox*. Their small size and similar colour to the thyroid makes them difficult to identify. One pair occurs in the *pig* in front of the thyroid gland.

The parathyroids produce a polypeptide hormone, which controls the levels of serum calcium and inorganic phosphorus and stimulates the removal of calcium from bone. Thyrocalcitonin, produced by the thyroid, has the opposite effect on calcium levels.

### Thymus

The thymus is pinkish-white and distinctly lobulated, and constitutes the *true sweetbread*. It consists of two portions; the thoracic portion (heart bread) is rich in fat, roughly the shape of the palm of the hand in the ox, and lies in the thoracic cavity, extending back to the third rib where it contacts the base of the heart; the second portion (neck bread) is poor in fat and consists of two lobes joined at their base and extending up the neck on either side of the trachea, diverging and diminishing in size as they pass up the neck and reaching almost to the thyroid gland.

In the *calf* the thymus is at its largest at 5–6 weeks, when it weighs 453–680 g, but gradually atrophies. By the onset of sexual maturity, little of the cervical portion remains. It is very small in 3-year-old cattle but a vestige of the thoracic portion may be seen in cows even after 8 or 9 years. In the *pig* the thymus is large, greyish-yellow, and reaches to the throat.

In early life, the thymus is necessary for the development of certain immune responses and antibodies. It is probably also associated with lymphocyte production. If this is removed shortly after birth, the production of lymphocytes, lymphoid tissue and plasma cells is much reduced, antibodies are not formed, and skin grafts, even from different species, are not rejected. Since no hormone has yet been isolated from the thymus, it should probably be classified as belonging to the circulatory system rather than the endocrine system. In animals certain autoimmune diseases such as haemolytic anaemia and systemic lupus erythematosus are associated with a defective thymus.

### Adrenal (suprarenal) bodies

In the *ox*, the adrenal glands are related to the two kidneys, and lie anterior to them. The left adrenal body is in contact with the dorsal sac of the rumen, though it does not rotate with the left kidney when the rumen is distended. After dressing of the carcase, portions of the right adrenal body may sometimes be found attached to the posterior aspect of the liver, or sometimes to the central muscular portion of the diaphragm.

In the *sheep* both the adrenals are bean-shaped, but the left is not in contact with its kidney. In the *pig* the adrenals are long and narrow, each lying on the inner aspect of the kidney.

The adrenals are reddish-brown in colour, and a section of them reveals a well-marked cortex and medulla.

The adrenal glands produce two completely different types of hormones. The medulla or central part of the gland produces hormones known as *catecholamines*, particularly *adrenaline* (epinephrine) and *noradrenaline* (norepinephrine). Being supplied by the preganglionic fibres of the sympathetic nervous system, the hormones of the adrenal medulla augment the action of this system, increasing blood pressure, constricting the sphincters of the alimentary tract, inhibiting the bladder musculature, mobilising liver glycogen to form glucose, relaxing the bronchioles of the lungs and constricting the arterioles and veins (except those of the heart and muscle). These effects are associated with excitement and emotions such as fear and anger. The adrenals are therefore sometimes referred to as the '*glands of fight and flight*' or the emergency glands.

The adrenal cortex, unlike the medulla, has no nerve supply. It is rich in vitamin C and cholesterol, which is the probable precursor of its hormones, the corticoids: glucocorticoids, mineralocorticoids and sex hormones.

The glucocorticoids (chiefly cortisol or hydrocortisone) regulate the metabolism of carbohydrates, fats and proteins on a long-term basis, decreasing the metabolism of carbohydrates, increasing the breakdown of protein to amino acids and mobilising fats. An excess of cortisol in the blood elevates blood glucose and causes ketosis, i.e. diabetes mellitus.

Mineralocorticoids, represented mainly by aldosterone, regulate the mineral salts in the body by stimulating the reabsorption of sodium in the kidney tubules and increasing the excretion of potassium. Aldosterone is also concerned with the control of blood and fluid volumes in the body.

The sex hormones (androgens, oestrogens and progesterone) are known to affect the development and function of the reproductive organs and secondary sexual characteristics, but are less important than the sex hormones produced by the gonads.

## Pituitary gland (Hypophysis)

The pituitary gland is situated on the lower aspect of the cerebrum, being connected to it by a short stalk, and rests in the pituitary fossa of the sphenoid bone formed by the base of the skull. Sometimes termed the master gland of the body, it exerts through its many hormones, an influence on almost all the other ductless glands. It consists of an anterior lobe (adenohypophysis) and a posterior lobe (neurohypophysis), each having very different activities (Table 2.4).

## Testicles (testes)

In the *bull* the testes have an elongated oval outline; they are about 12.5 cm long and weigh 283–340 g. The epididymis is narrow, but is closely attached to the testicle along its posterior border. In the *ram* the testicles are large, pear-shaped, and more rounded than in the ox, being 10 cm long and 255–283 g in weight. In the *boar* the testicles are very large and irregularly elliptical, while the epididymis is well developed and forms a blunt conical projection at both ends of the testicle.

The testes or male gonads have two functions; the production of spermatozoa and the production of *testosterone*, the main hormone responsible for the development of male secondary sexual characteristics.

## Ovaries

The ovaries, in addition to producing ova, secrete three hormones: *oestradiol*, *progesterone* and *relaxin*. Oestradiol, formed in the ovarian follicles, promotes female secondary sexual characteristics and sexual behaviour.

**Table 2.4** Pituitary gland hormones.

| Hormone | Action |
|---|---|
| *Adenohypophysis* | |
| Growth hormone | Growth promotion. |
| Thyrotrophin | Control of thyroid. |
| Corticotrophin/adrenocorticotrophic hormone (ACTH) | Control of adrenocorticoid hormones |
| Gonadotrophic hormones (follicle stimulating hormone, luteinising hormone, luteotrophic hormone) | Control of growth of gonads and their reproductive functions. |
| *Neurohypophysis* | |
| Oxytocin | Milk let-down, uterine contractions at parturition. |
| Antidiuretic hormone | Control of water secretion. |

Progesterone is formed in the corpus luteum and during pregnancy it prevents ovulation by inhibiting the secretion of luteinising hormone. Relaxin, also produced by the corpus luteum, relaxes the pelvic ligaments during parturition. The ovaries also control cyclical changes in the reproductive system which ensure development of breeding seasons when weather conditions, temperature, food, etc. are suitable.

## Pineal gland

The pineal gland is located in the brain posterior to the third ventricle. It is believed to be the source of the hormone *melatonin*.

Darkness and light are believed to affect the synthesis and release of melatonin, the former promoting and the latter inhibiting them. Melatonin in turn is thought to control the formation and release of gonadotrophic hormone-releasing factors from the brain.

## Collection and yield of glands (Table 2.5)

Although valuable pharmaceutical products are prepared from the ductless glands, it is only when there is a very large weekly kill that their collection becomes an economic proposition.

Successful utilisation of glands entails careful handling from the moment the animal is killed. The entire glands should be removed immediately, freed from surrounding fat or tissue and, according to the variety of gland, either frozen to a temperature of −10°C or placed in acetone. Cutting into the substance of a gland significantly reduces the hormone yield and it should not be soaked in water. In the case of the pancreas, care must be taken to leave the gland whole and not to remove adjoining portions of the duodenum whereby trypsin might be liberated and the insulin destroyed.

The occurrence of BSE in Britain has given more urgency to the need for extreme care in the collection of glands to be used for pharmaceutical purposes. Guidelines have been issued by the UK Committee on the Safety of Medicines and the Veterinary Products Committee for all products licensed under the Medicines Act of 1968 not only for material of bovine origin but also for material from sheep, goats, deer and other animals susceptible to scrapie-like agents. The main points of the guidelines are as follows.

1. Tissues to be excluded: all nerve tissue, spleen, thymus and other lymphoid tissue, placental tissue and cell cultures of bovine origin.
2. Bovine material should be taken from closed herds (since 1980), BSE-free and which have not received ruminant-derived feedstuff during this period.
3. Sterile equipment must always be used and needles, syringes, scalpel blades, etc. should be disposable items.
4. Whenever possible, source animals should be calves up to 6 months of age.
5. No tissue is to be used in relevant medicinal products when collected from an animal after brain penetrative stunning.
6. All cellular components must be removed from serum and fetal calf serum, care being

**Table 2.5** Yield of glands used in medicine.

| Gland | No. of animals required to produce 500 g of fresh material | No. of glands required per 500 g finished product |
|---|---|---|
| Pituitary, whole (cattle) | 199 | 1100 |
| Ovary (cow) | 39 | 210 |
| Ovary (sow) | 50 | 298 |
| Parathyroid (cattle) | 243 | 1990 |
| Suprarenal (cattle) | 22 | 127 |
| Pancreas (beef) | 2 | 26 500 |
| Pancreas (calf) | 18 | 8830 |
| Pancreas (pig) | 11 | 132 500 |
| Testis (bull) | 1.5 | 7 |
| Thyroid (cattle) | 22 | 100 110 |

taken to avoid contamination from placenta and fetal fluids.

7 Sterilisation of equipment must be capable of inactivating scrapie-like agents—autoclaving using a porous load cycle at 134–138°C for 18 min at 30 psi.

8 The final product must be sterilised adequately.

(See also Orders relating to SBM and Heads of Sheep and Goats.)

A European Commission Decision of 11 June 1996, 96/362/EC, amending 96/239/EC, prohibited the despatch to other Member States and to third countries, of materials destined for use as medicinal products, cosmetics or pharmaceutical products which had been obtained from bovines slaughtered in the United Kingdom.

## SKIN

The skin or common integument acts as a protective covering for the body and merges at the natural orifices with the mucous membranes of the digestive, respiratory and reproductive systems. With its covering of hair, wool, feathers, nails or horn it acts also as a temperature-regulating mechanism and, since it contains many sensory nerve endings, it protects the body against injury and is thus an important sense organ.

Sweat (sudoriferous) and sebaceous glands are found in the skin, the former involved in temperature and tissue fluid regulation and the latter secreting sebum which prevents loss of fluid and in some species playing an important part in the sexual life of the animal.

The *mammary glands* are modified skin glands associated in function with the reproductive system.

## HORNS

*Estimation of the age of cattle* by means of the horns entails counting the number of rings on the animal's horns, but these rings must not be confused with the small wrinkles situated at the root of the horn which are an indication that the animal has been ill-fed during its growth. The first ring appears at about two years and thereafter one ring is added annually so that the age in years in cattle equals the number of rings plus one. In cows it is not unusual for the rings to be removed by scraping, and greater accuracy as to age may be obtained by examination of the incisor teeth or carcase bones.

## MUSCULAR SYSTEM

The muscular system is composed of skeletal (voluntary, striated), cardiac (involuntary, striated) and smooth (involuntary, non-striated) muscle. Smooth muscle is found in certain organs, glands and blood vessels and responds to the demands of the autonomic nervous system.

Skeletal muscle along with associated connective tissue and intermuscular fat forms the flesh or butcher meat and represents 25–45% of the animal's liveweight.

There are some 300 muscles in the *animal* body which, despite vast differences in the size, shape, and function of each, all possess the same basic structure. Muscles are made up of numerous tiny spindle-shaped multinucleated *muscle cells* or *fibres*, each encased in a thin membrane, the *sarcolemma*. Groups of muscle cells joined by a loose connective tissue (*endomysium*) form bundles sheathed in connective tissue *perimysium* and fatty deposits. Connective tissue *epimysium* covers the complete muscle.

The muscles of *domestic birds* resemble in general those of mammals except that many are greatly enlarged and adapted for flight purposes, e.g. the pectoralis which lowers the wing and the supracoracoideus which raises it. Two forms of muscle occur: white muscle, and dark muscle which contains numerous myoglobin-containing cells. Specialised breeding of domestic poultry, and especially turkeys, has resulted in the enlargement of the pectoral muscles.

## CONNECTIVE TISSUE

Connective tissue is present in two forms in the animal body, white and yellow. A typical example of white connective tissue is the *fascia* connecting the muscular bundles. The main constituent of white connective tissue is *collagen*, which is converted into gelatin by boiling. Yellow connective tissue, as seen in the yellow fascia covering the abdominal muscles and in the *ligamentum nuchae*, consists of elastin, which cannot be softened by boiling.

## FAT

Fat develops in connection with connective tissue and has an important influence on both the odour and flavour of the different meats. It varies in consistency according to its composition, which is again controlled by the species, the feeding method and the site of the fat in the carcase.

The amount of fat in a carcase affects the rate of chilling, a greater amount slowing it down owing to its insulating property. So lean bull carcases chill more quickly than fatter steer carcases while trimming of subcutaneous fat from the hot carcase increases the chilling rate of the underlying muscle (Allen, 1990). But fat insulation also serves to prevent *cold shortening* in rapidly chilled carcases. Changes in refrigeration techniques have accordingly been recommended for leaner carcases in order to achieve tenderness combined with flavour. Work in Denmark has indicated that lean carcases should be conditioned at 4°C and chilled at 6°C, while in the USA even higher temperatures (up to 25°C) have been advocated, the implication being that slow early chilling shortens the conditioning time necessary for producing tenderness. (See *Conditioning of meat*.)

The deposition of fat between the muscle fibres is known as '*marbling*'. It occurs only in young, well-nourished cattle and not in older animals where fat tends to be deposited subcutaneously, e.g. on the hips and pin bones of fat cows. Marbling of fat does not occur in the horse. In the pig, fat cells between the individual muscle fibres prevent the gastric juice from reaching the fibres and thus render pork less digestible. The muscle fat is basically polyunsaturated, but as adipose tissue is laid down the saturated fat increases in amount. The eating of saturated fats has a bearing on the development of coronary heart disease in man, and the general tendency today is to reduce their level in the diet.

Marbling has a marked effect on eating quality. Studies at the USDA Meat Animal Research Center showed that a marbling rating of 'slight', which contained 3.7% fat, had a good eating quality, similar Danish work putting this figure at 2–3% of marbling fat. Leaner European breeds of cattle, e.g. Limousin, Simmental and Charolais, should therefore not be slaughtered at stages leaner than EEC fat class 3 in order to ensure minimal marbling. The Aberdeen-Angus has excellent marbling qualities. The amount of marbling in a given muscle can be reliably measured using the technique of magnetic resonance imaging.

Excess fat is expensive to produce since, weight for weight, it requires five to seven times as much energy to produce as meat. Much of the fat trimmed from carcases is used in manufactured meat products, which contribute some 9.4% of fat in the human diet.

The *edible fat* from the ox carcase, other than that intermixed with the muscle, is obtained from certain well-defined positions: the omentum, mesentery, stomach, mediastinum and kidney, which yield an average of 19 kg, varying between 11 kg in the lean cow and 29.5 kg in the well-finished bullock. Of the various by-products, edible fat has historically ranked second only to the hide in value. Abnormal amounts of kidney fat, sometimes up to 91 kg, are sometimes encountered; these are known as 'balloon kidneys', but the fat is marketable and edible. The butcher may render down his edible beef and mutton fat to produce dripping. On a commercial scale edible fat is converted into oleo oil and oleo stearin for margarine manufacture; oleo stearin is also used for soap and candle manufacture and is mixed with cooking fats to harden them. Inedible fat is used for the production of lubricants, soap, candles and glycerine, and as a binder for animal feed.

## DETERMINATION OF AGE BY DENTITION

Determination of age and sex is important in the keeping of records of disease found on routine examination, and also in the recognition of the carcase of the cow, ewe and sow, animals in which dangerous affections of a septic nature are most likely to occur. It is also of value where a system of mutual insurance of animals intended for slaughter exists and an inspector may be called upon to pass expert judgement as to the age and sex of any animal in dispute. Where meat is supplied to public institutions there is the possibility of the substitution of cow

**Table 2.6** Dental formula for the ox, sheep and goat.

| | |
|---|---|
| *Temporary (deciduous) teeth* Upper / Lower | $2\left(I\frac{0}{3}\ C\frac{0}{1}\ P\frac{3}{3}\right) = 20$ |
| *Permanent teeth* Upper / Lower | $2\left(I\frac{0}{3}\ C\frac{0}{1}\ P\frac{3}{3}\ M\frac{3}{3}\right) = 32$ |

I = Incisor, C = canine, P = premolar, M = molar.

**Table 2.7** Dental formula for the pig.

| | |
|---|---|
| *Temporary* | $2\left(I\frac{3}{3}\ C\frac{1}{1}\ P\frac{3}{3}\right) = 28$ |
| *Permanent* | $2\left(I\frac{3}{3}\ C\frac{1}{1}\ P\frac{4}{4}\ M\frac{3}{3}\right) = 44$ |

I = Incisor, C = canine, P = premolar, M = molar.

meat for that from bullocks or heifers, or for the substitution of ewe mutton for that of lambs or young sheep. Here again the judgement of the inspector will be of value.

In the food animals, age may be estimated with reasonable accuracy from the teeth (Tables 2.6–2.9), from the horns of cattle, or from the carcase bones.

## Teeth

### *Ox*

The age is estimated by the period at which the permanent incisor teeth erupt and come into wear; these periods are subject to variation, depending on sex, breed and method of feeding.

**Table 2.8** Dental formula for the horse.

| | |
|---|---|
| *Temporary* | $2\left(I\frac{3}{3}\ C\frac{0}{0}\ P\frac{3}{3}\right) = 24$ |
| *Permanent* | $2\left(I\frac{3}{3}\ C\frac{1}{1}\ P\frac{3(4)}{3}\ M\frac{3}{3}\right) = 40(42)$ |

I = Incisor, C = canine, P = premolar, M = molar.

The corner pair of permanent incisors are subject to the greatest variation in the time of eruption and well-bred cattle or animals that are well fed and well housed tend to erupt their teeth earlier than scrub animals or those that are poorly fed and poorly housed. In pedigree cattle the corner incisors may appear soon after completion of the third year, and in bulls they are not uncommonly present at 2 years 10 months.

The dental formulae for the temporary and permanent teeth are shown in Table 2.6. The upper and lower figures corresponding to the teeth of the upper and lower jaw. After the permanent incisor teeth have erupted, the degree of wear on their cutting surface and the amount of neck visible above the gums are a guide to the animal's age. The neck of the central pair of incisors is perceptible at the sixth year, that of the lateral centrals at 7 years, of the laterals at 8 years, and of the corner incisors at 9 years. Subsequent to this, the incisor teeth are small and much worn and it is then possible to confuse an animal 1½ years of age, and therefore possessing all its milk incisors, with an animal of about 10 years, but this can be avoided by recognition of the exposure of the roots of the teeth in the older animal due to shrinkage of the gums and projection of the roots from the alveolar sockets.

### *Sheep*

The milk incisors in sheep are all present at birth or shortly after and remain until the

**Table 2.9** Ages at which the permanent incisors appear.

| | 1st pair | 2nd pair | 3rd pair | 4th pair |
|---|---|---|---|---|
| Ox | 1½–2 years | 2–2½ years | 3 years | 3½–4 years |
| Sheep | 1–1½ years | 1½–2 years | 2½–3 years | 3½–4 years |
| Pig | 1 year | 16–20 months | 8–10 months | Canines 9–10 months |
| Horse | 2½ years | 3½ years | 4½ years | Canines 4–5 years |

animal is 1 year old. Where sheep are fed on turnips, however, a number of the temporary incisors may be broken off before the animal is 1 year old.

A notch develops between the central pair of incisors at 6 years of age. The formula for the temporary and permanent dentition in sheep is identical with that in cattle.

*Goat*

It is generally accepted that up to 4 years of age the goat is as many years old as it has pairs of permanent incisor teeth. Thus a goat in which the last pair of permanent incisors have erupted may be estimated as 4 years old.

*Pig*

The period of eruption of temporary and permanent teeth in pigs is subject to considerable variation, and dentition is not a really satisfactory or accurate guide to the animal's age. Estimation of the age in pigs is only likely to be necessary in the case of show animals in connection with their eligibility for particular age classes. There is variation in the figures quoted by various authorities as to the ages at which the permanent incisors appear in the various animals. Sisson & Grossman (1975) give the figures shown in Table 2.9.

## DETERMINATION OF SEX

### Cattle

Differentiation may be established between the carcase of the bull, stag, bullock, heifer and cow.

*Bull*

The outstanding characteristic in the bull carcase is the massive development of the muscles of the neck and the shoulder, with the forequarter, except in well-bred animals, being better fleshed than the hindquarter. This development of the crest is diagnostic in bulls, and in some American packing houses the funicular portion of the ligamentum nuchae is cut at its insertion to the dorsal vertebrae, the effect being to make the carcase approximate more in appearance to that of the bullock.

In the dressing of the bull carcase the testicles and spermatic cord are removed, leaving an open external inguinal ring partly covered by scanty scrotal fat. The pelvic cavity is narrow and can be spanned with the hand, while the pelvic floor (ischiopubic symphysis) is angular and the pelvic tubercle strongly developed. The bulbocavernosus muscle, often referred to as the erector and retractor penis muscle, is well developed and the cut adductor, or gracilis muscle, is triangular in shape; in young bulls, however, the posterior portion of this muscle is not covered with fat and the gracilis muscle therefore appears bean-shaped. The muscle of young bulls is light or brick red in colour and similar to that of the bullock, but in older bulls it is dark red, dry and poor in fat.

In some European countries and the northern countries of South America cattle are rarely castrated and it is the custom in dressing the carcase to leave the testicles attached to the hindquarters. These organs are much in demand by the population, many of whom regard them as an aphrodisiac.

*Stag*

If the male bovine is castrated later in life, at perhaps a year old, it will have developed certain bullish characteristics, the chief of which is the strong development of the muscles of the neck and shoulder. Such animals are known as stags and, except for the muscular development of the forequarter, differ little in appearance or quality from the normal bullock.

*Bullock (steer)*

The muscles of the neck and crest are not so strongly developed as in the bull, but fat is more evenly distributed over the carcase and is particularly abundant in the pelvic cavity; the scrotal fat is abundant and completely occludes the external inguinal ring. The pelvic cavity is narrow and can be spanned with the hand but although the pelvic floor is angular and the pubic tubercle is prominent, these characteristics are not so marked as in the bull carcase.

The posterior or ischial portion of the gracilis muscle, which presents a triangular appearance, is covered with fascia and fat, while there is a well-marked bulbocavernosus muscle, though this is less strongly developed than in the bull. Bullock flesh is lighter in colour than bull flesh and has a brick red colour with a shiny, marbled appearance due to the presence of intermuscular fat.

*Heifer*

In the dressing of the heifer carcase the udder remains on each side of beef and is characterised by its smooth, regular convexity and, on section, by the predominance of fat and lack of evidence of glandular tissue. The absence of bulbocavernosus muscle may be noted, and a useful feature in distinguishing the forequarter of the heifer or cow from that of the bullock is the enlargement at the end of the foreshank (radius). In the cow or heifer the bone is slim and rather straight, but in the bullock it is markedly enlarged. In the heifer or cow, remains of the broad ligament of the uterus are apparent on the inner abdominal wall, about a hand's breadth below the angle of the haunch.

*Cow*

The cow carcase is more slender and less symmetrical than that of the bull or bullock and shows a long tapering neck, a wide chest cavity, curved back and prominent hips. The pelvic cavity is wide and can scarcely be spanned with the hand, while the pelvic floor is thin, only slightly arched, and the pubic tubercle is only slightly developed. The exposed gracilis muscle is crescentic or bean-shaped, but no bulbocavernosus muscle is present. The udder, except occasionally in animals which have had only one calf, is removed, leaving a triangular ragged space on the outer aspect of the abdominal wall. In the cow both external and internal fat is irregularly distributed and yellowish in colour.

*Calf*

In the dressed bobby calf, the male may be recognised by the presence of testicles and the open external inguinal ring. A transverse cut with a knife just above the pubic tubercle will expose the root of the penis. In the heifer calf the rudimentary udder remains on the carcase.

## Sheep

*Ram*

The carcase has strong muscular development of the forequarter, the inguinal rings are open, and the scrotal or cod fat is sparse or absent.

*Wether*

The carcase is usually well proportioned with evenly distributed fat and abundant, lobulated cod fat. The root of the penis can be exposed by a transverse section with the knife above the pubic tubercle and in the wether is no thicker than an ordinary pencil.

*Gimmer*

The carcase is characterised by its symmetrical shape and the presence of a smooth convex udder.

*Ewe*

The carcase is angular in shape, with long thin neck and poor legs. The udder is brown, spongy and never sets; it is removed in dressing, leaving a roughened area on the outer abdominal wall, though portions of the supramammary lymph nodes frequently remain on the carcase.

Differentiating features of the carcases of the sheep and goat are shown in Table 2.10.

## Pigs

Differentiation must be established between the carcase of the boar, hog, gilt and sow.

*Boar*

The boar possesses an oval, strongly developed area of cartilage over the shoulder region which may become calcified in old boars, and is known as the *shield*. The scrotum is removed in the dressing of the carcase, the area of removal being apparent on the inside of the thigh. The cut gracilis muscle is triangular, while the root of the penis will be present on one of the sides when the carcase is split and a strongly developed bulbocavernosus muscle will then be apparent. Strong, curved canine teeth (the tusks) are present in the boar.

Castration of the adult boar produces an animal known as a *stag*, which is both heavier and fatter and commands a higher price than the boar carcase. Stag pigs show some reduction in the density of the shield as a result of castration, but as both boars and stags may be used only for manufacturing purposes, being skinned and boned out, this reduction of the

**Table 2.10** Differentiation of carcases of sheep and goat.

| Feature | Sheep | Goat |
|---|---|---|
| Back and withers | Round and well fleshed. | Sharp, little flesh. |
| Thorax | Barrel-shaped. | Flattened laterally. |
| Tail | Fairly broad. | Thin. |
| Radius | 1½ times length of metacarpus. | Twice as long as metacarpus. |
| Scapula | Short and broad. Superior spine, bent back and thickened. | Possesses distinct neck. Spine straight and narrow. |
| Sacrum | Lateral borders thickened in form of rolls. | Lateral borders thin and sharp. |
| Flesh | Pale red and fine in texture. | Dark red coarse with goaty odour. Sticky subcutaneous tissue which may have adherent goat hairs. |

shield is not of great importance and the chief advantage is the diminution of the boar odour.

*Hog*

The differentiation of the hog and gilt carcases frequently presents difficulty, as teats are present in both male and female pigs, though in the male they are small and underdeveloped. Evidence of castration in the hog is seen as two puckered, depressed scars and in both the hog and the boar there is evidence of the removal of the preputial sac. The belly fat on one side of the abdominal incision is grooved, and on the floor of this incision can be seen the retractor penis muscle, which is long, thin and pale red in colour. When the carcase is split, remains of the bulbocavernosus muscle can be seen, while the gracilis muscle is covered with connective and fatty tissue.

*Gilt*

In the gilt the space left below the tail after removal of the anus and vulva is greater than in the hog, the abdominal incision is straight and uninterrupted, and the cut surface of the gracilis muscle is bean-shaped. In sows there is greater development of the udders and teats, and though canine teeth are present in the female pig, they do not develop.

## HORSE AND OX DIFFERENTIATION

Carcases of the horse and ox may be differentiated by the following details.

1. In the horse, the unusual length of the sides is noticeable, together with the great muscular development of the hindquarters.
2. The thoracic cavity is longer in the horse; this animal possesses 18 pairs of ribs, whereas the ox has 13 pairs.
3. The ribs in the horse are narrower but more markedly curved.
4. The superior spinous processes of the first six dorsal vertebrae are more markedly developed in the horse and are less inclined posteriorly.
5. In the forequarter, the ulna of the horse extends only half the length of the radius; in the ox it is extended and articulates with the carpus.
6. In the hindquarter, the femur of the ox possesses no third trochanter; the fibula is only a small pointed projection, but in the horse it extends two-thirds the length of the tibia.
7. In the horse, the last three lumbar transverse processes articulate with each other, the sixth articulating in a similar manner with the sacrum. They do not articulate in the ox.
8. The horse carcase shows considerable development of soft, yellow fat beneath the peritoneum, especially in the gelding and mare, but in the stallion the fat is generally of a lighter colour and almost white. In the ox the kidney fat is always firmer, whiter and more abundant than in the horse.
9. Horse flesh is dark bluish-red, beef lacking the bluish tinge. Horse meat has a pronounced sweet taste and well-defined muscle fibres.

## CHEMICAL AND BIOLOGICAL DIFFERENTIATION OF MEATS

The differentiation of the muscle and fat of animals is of importance in connection with the possible substitution of inferior, and at times repugnant, meat for that of good quality.

There is little difficulty in differentiating the flesh and fat of these animals in carcase form or in joints, but recognition in mince or in sausage depends on chemical or biological tests and therefore comes properly within the province of the analytical chemist.

### Chemical tests

A number of differential chemical tests are based on the fact that horse flesh is richer in *glycogen* than the flesh of other food animals. Glycogen, however, starts to disappear from meat from the time of slaughter and, unless the examination is made soon after the carcase is cut up, very little may be found. Furthermore, the liver of all animals, particularly the pig, contains appreciable quantities of glycogen and if this organ is used as an ingredient of sausage a positive result to a glycogen test might occur from the presence of liver. Any deductions made from the presence of glycogen, particularly in sausage, should therefore be advanced with extreme caution.

A method of identifying horse fat when admixed with lard or beef and mutton fat is by demonstrating the presence of 1–2% of *linoleic acid*. In other animal fats this is not present in proportions higher than 0.1%.

A valuable test for horse fat depends on estimation of the *iodine value*. This test is based on the amount of iodine absorbed by the unsaturated fatty acids present in the fat, and varies in the different animals. In the horse the iodine value of fat is 71–86, in the ox 38–46, in the sheep 35–46, and in the pig 50–70; good lard has an iodine value of 66.

A further valuation test for fats which can be liquefied by heat and thus converted into oil is by the estimation of the *refractive index*. All liquids, including oils, possess a specific refractive index; that of horse fat is 53.5, of ox fat less than 40 and of pig fat not above 51.9.

### Biological tests

Three main biological methods are employed for the differentiation of the flesh of various animals: the precipitin test, the complement fixation test and the ELISA (enzyme-linked immunoabsorbent assay) test. The tests are particularly applicable to mince or sausage meat.

The *precipitin* test depends on the fact that specific antibodies develop in the blood of an animal which receives repeated injections of blood serum from another animal. If, for example, it is desired to test for horse flesh, a rabbit is injected periodically with blood serum from the horse. The rabbit, as a result, develops antibodies specific for horse serum, which possess the property of precipitating proteins of the horse but of no other animal. Therefore, when blood serum from the injected rabbit is mixed in a test tube with a filtered extract from the suspected meat, a turbidity of the solution occurs if horse meat is present, and this is followed by a definite precipitation.

*Complement fixation* utilises a normal component of serum complement, which is a thermolabile mixture of substances capable of reacting with any antigen–antibody system to lyse the antigen agglutinated by the antibody. Certain antigen–antibody reactions do not produce any visible result, e.g. precipitation or agglutination, and these can be detected by the fact that they use up or 'fix' complement, thus making it no longer available for other reactions. Complement is usually derived from guinea pig serum and the indicator system normally consists of sheep red cells and rabbit serum (heated to destroy its own complement before use in the test).

As with the previous biological tests, the *ELISA* technique relies on the ability of antibodies to bind with specific antigens. Used in blood grouping, tissue typing and bacteriological work, the ELISA test can be applied to meat identification because of the differences in protein composition in the food animals, slight though these generally are. In addition to the foregoing uses, ELISA is being applied in the detection of boar taint and soya in a variety of products.

The test is carried out by making an extract (containing antigens) from the meat sample under investigation, placing this in a Petri dish or test tube and then adding different specific sera (containing antibodies). The antibody that binds with the corresponding antigen forms a complex which is afterwards recognised and bound by a second antibody containing an enzyme which catalyses the reaction to produce a colour. If the sample under investigation was horse meat, a reaction would take place only in the presence of specific horse serum. Positive identification can be carried out in as short a time as six hours and the test is able to detect low levels of suspect meats, even as low as 3%. A diagnostic kit for routine use in commercial practice is available. This uses polystyrene tubes and gives a marked colour reaction in positive cases, and the colour can be more accurately measured using a spectrophotometer. The test can be adapted for use in cooked meats, meats which have been frozen and some canned products. Heating to the temperatures which are required for the manufacture of meat and bone meal, however, denatures the species specific protein. This fact allows the test to be carried out to ensure that this has been the case.

*Polymerase chain reaction* (PCR) analysis can be used to differentiate marinated or heat-treated meats from closely related species. The technique involves the identification of DNA fragments recovered from meat samples.

Other techniques used in species identification include microscopy, electrophoresis, various chemical procedures, agar gel diffusion and gas–liquid chromatography.

### Debasement of food (adulteration and substitution)

In the UK the composition and labelling of food is controlled by the Food Act 1984 (Sections 1–7):

- Section 1 Offences as to the preparation and sale of injurious foods.
- Section 2 General protection of purchasers of food.
- Section 3 Defences under Section 2.
- Section 4 Making of regulations relating to composition, etc.
- Section 5 Gives powers to Ministers to obtain particulars of ingredients of foods.
- Section 6 Refers to food falsely ascribed.
- Section 7 The making of regulations for the description of food.

The term *'wholesome'* is defined as "promoting or conducive to good health or well-being". It was recognised many centuries ago that food must be sound and entirely fit for human consumption. Meat must be derived from healthy animals reared and slaughtered under high standards of welfare and hygiene and their products processed with due attention to cleanliness.

*Continuous control of operations from livestock production to the consumer's home is essential if a safe quality product is to be created and enjoyed.* Regrettably, many opportunities exist from the farm to retail outlet for adulteration, accidental or malicious, and misrepresentation to occur.

The chief substitutions of inferior flesh for that which is more highly valued are those of horse for beef, goat for lamb, cat for rabbit and rabbit for poultry. Another form is the replacement of steer and heifer meat of high quality with lower-quality cow and bull beef. The use of *C. bovis*-infected meat which has been refrigerated to replace Grade A heifer and steer beef is not unknown and the perennial use of the word 'lamb', when in fact mutton is being sold, is yet another form of substitution and deception.

In recent times, kangaroo meat has been imported from Australia into Britain and the United States and has been used in the UK in the manufacture of meat pies, pasties and beefburgers, on occasions along with the inclusion of condemned meat. A widespread racket involving the use of unfit meat and the meat from animal species other than that specified has been in existence in the UK for some years, it being estimated that the annual trade in unfit meat may amount to some 10 000 tonnes internally with about 5000 tonnes imported.

While substitution can, and does, occur at the carcase and meat cut stage, it is when meat is in a comminuted form that adulteration most often takes place. Using modern technology, production techniques are used to create debasement at a very sophisticated level. This pernicious practice creates great problems for the food analyst and enforcement agencies, besides being a health threat for the consuming public.

That it is not a new practice is illustrated by the introduction to a standard text on food law, Bell and O'Keefe's *Sale of Food and Drugs*, which states 'The act of debasing a food or drug with the object of passing it off as genuine, of the substitution of an inferior article for a superior one to the detriment of the purchaser, whether done in fraud or negligence, appears to be as old as trade'.

In Great Britain, some basic laws are contravened by this practice, probably the main one being Section 8 of the Food Act 1984, which relates to the sale of unfit food. But legislation relating to the labelling, description and composition of food, whose provisions ensure that all food is not adulterated or misdescribed and is of a reasonable quality, is also contravened.

The high price of meat, the wide range of proteins of an inferior nature which can be used, the processed form of the product, the analytical difficulties presented and the economic considerations, all appeal to the unscrupulous manufacturer.

### *Ingredients used*

Many different types of non-meat proteins and animal-based proteins are used in an attempt to disguise the true meat content on analysis. These ingredients are often referred to in the trade as 'meat extenders' or 'meat substitutes', which can, of course, be used legitimately. It is their illegal use which results in fraud.

*Non-meat proteins* include vegetable protein, e.g. soya bean, which can be given a 'texture' simulating a meat appearance and cereal.

*Cereal* is an ingredient which is sometimes added to 'all-meat products' and has the ability to absorb water, giving the product a drier appearance more like its natural form, besides affecting the initial analytical determination, depending on the type of cereal used.

The consumption of certain forms of cereal adversely affects the health of persons suffering from coeliac disease, a condition in which the mucosa of the small intestine becomes abnormal owing to contact with dietary gluten, a reserve protein found in wheat, barley, rye and probably oats. The undeclared presence of cereal probably therefore has a serious relevance.

*Animal-based proteins* often include those parts of the carcase which are of low value and only some of which are legally defined as 'meat', e.g. pork rind, bone protein, urea, dried blood and plasma. While there can be no objection to their inclusion, it is the excessive extent of usage, in amounts far in excess of that naturally associated with the type of meat involved, which constitutes abuse and fraud. On occasions, pork rind is incorporated into a product in which there is no pork flesh present.

*Rind* may be cooked with water, emulsified with milk protein or vegetable proteins or dehydrated, ground and rehydrated (using as much as four times its own weight of water) before being incorporated into a sausage or 'meat' product.

*Bone protein* or *ossein* is extracted from animal bones. Like rind, it is an incomplete protein but, hydrated with four parts of water, is used to replace a similar weight of proper meat, yet another disguise to the true meat content of the product.

*Urea*, a natural nitrogenous waste product found in the urine of animals and man, can also be manufactured from ammonia and carbon dioxide by heating under pressure. It has no nutritional value at all and is normally used as a fertiliser and animal feed additive. Very soluble in water, its presence in a meat product for human consumption adds nitrogen and thereby increases the 'protein' calculation.

*Dried blood and plasma* are normally used for animal feed, petfood or fertiliser, or are discharged as effluent, only a small amount being consumed as black puddings. There can be no objection to the proper inclusion, after suitable treatment, of sterile blood and plasma in meat products, provided their presence is declared and they are not used in lieu of real meat. Rehydrated with water, blood and plasma have the effect of disguising the true meat content for the food analyst.

*Crushed bone and waste* have on occasions been used in a very fine form for incorporation into sausages. This must not be confused with accepted mechanically-recovered meat (MRM) systems. The Food Standards Committee have reported on this form of meat and considered that MRM is not meat as would be understood by the consumer, its essential structure compared with hand-trimmed meat being destroyed. This Committee also felt that, used in amounts exceeding 5%, its presence should be declared.

*Water* is a natural constituent of meat, varying in amount according to its age, method of handling, species, form of refrigeration, environmental factors, etc. In today's technology of curing, more pickle than is necessary to effect a proper cure is used. Increased water uptake of meat has been shown to be a property of the myofibrils (which are involved in muscle contraction), which make up about 70% of lean meat. In addition to excess cure, polyphosphate is also added to the curing solution and ensures that only minimal water loss occurs at the cooking stage. Tumbling or massaging of the cured meat enables the curing solution to be more thoroughly absorbed. The end result is a product (cooked ham or shoulder) which contains added water in the form of curing solution. While consumers probably on the whole prefer moist ham, there must obviously be a limit to the water content of cured meats. Accordingly, in the Ministry of Agriculture's Meat Products and Spreadable Fish Products Regulations the water content of cured meat must be expressed on the label in terms of 'added water' as opposed to 'additional curing solution' and that it should be banded at 10% levels.

There is a distinction between cooked and uncooked products in relation to water content labelling. Uncooked products are allowed a maximum of 10% added water without requiring label declaration, but cooked products require a label declaring the amount of added water in steps of 10%. Meat products which have the appearance of raw and unprocessed meat to which no ingredient has been added must be labelled with the maximum water content, this applying also to cuts, joints, slices, portions and carcases of cooked meat, although fresh and frozen poultry are not as yet included.

## MEAT COMPOSITION AND QUALITY

Butcher meat is a valuable part of the human diet because:

1. It is the most concentrated and easily assimilable of nitrogenous foods, and is a good source of first-class protein, i.e. it contains the amino acids essential for human life.
2. It is stimulating to metabolism because of its high protein content, i.e. it assists the body in the production of heat and energy.
3. It is satisfying, for the presence of fat in the diet delays emptying of the stomach (meat contains fat and therefore remains in the stomach for some hours and allays hunger).
4. After suitable treatment, which includes the processes of ripening and cooking, meat acquires a palatable flavour, acts as a stimulant to gastric secretion and is readily digested.

The term 'meat' may also refer to the edible offals such as liver, heart and tongue which are not parts of the skeletal muscular system.

A vegetable diet, compared with a meat diet, is usually incomplete in essential amino acids; the vegetable proteins are less easily digested and remain in the stomach for a shorter period than meat protein, with the result that hunger recurs more rapidly.

The approximate composition of lean bovine muscle (immediately after onset of rigor mortis) is given in Table 2.11.

### *Protein*

Protein is the most important muscle constituent and is made up of myofibrillar, sacroplasmic and connective tissue proteins.

*Myofibrillar protein* gives rigidity to the muscle and forms about two-thirds of the total protein, the most important types being *myosin* and *actin*.

*Sacroplasmic proteins* are the water-soluble proteins of the fluid cytoplasm of the muscle cells and include myoglobin muscle pigment, haemoglobin blood pigments and soluble glycolytic enzymes.

*Connective tissue proteins*, along with the bony segments of the body, form its supporting mechanism. They include *collagen*, which is insoluble in water and salt and can be converted into gelatin on heating; *elastin*, a tough yellow connective tissue; and *reticulin*, another form of connective tissue not converted to gelatin on heating.

### *Lipids*

The lipids are mostly composed of triglycerides, which are fats and oils, both of which are insoluble in water but soluble in

**Table 2.11** Composition of lean meat.

| | % net weight |
|---|---|
| Water | 75.0 |
| Protein | 19.0 |
| Lipids (fats and oils) | 2.5 |
| Carbohydrates (glycogen) | 1.2 |
| Non-protein nitrogen | 1.65 |
| Minerals | 0.65 |
| Vitamins | minute quantities |

ethyl ether. The lipids also include phospholipids, saturated, monounsaturated and polyunsaturated fatty acids and other fat-soluble substances, including cholesterol, the level of the latter in carcase meat being relatively low, although much higher in liver. Marked differences in intramuscular lipid levels occur in the different species of meat animals. The quantity of fat in all meat animals is very much lower than it used to be, because fat is an expensive tissue to produce and is not desired by the consumer. Differences in breed, sex, age and level of nutrition also vary the fat content in meat.

### *Carbohydrate*

Carbohydrate is present mainly as glycogen (animal starch), which has a major influence on muscle changes after death. Glycogen also occurs in the liver and is especially abundant in horse meat and in the fetus. Its level in the animal body does not vary as much as does fat, although older animals in general have lower reserves of glycogen.

### *Non-protein nitrogen*

Non-protein nitrogen is mainly represented by free amino acids, creatine, nucleotides, inosine monophosphate and carnosine (a dipetide), some of which, notably the free amino acids and nucleotides, give meat its *flavour* on cooking. Some sugars (e.g. glucose), lipids (e.g. certain lower fatty acids), nitrogen-containing compounds termed pyrazines, and oxygen- and sulphur-containing compounds also contribute to the flavour of meat. The production of flavour in meat is a very complex subject and not all the various compounds and interactions have yet been identified. Flavour can be influenced by many pre-slaughter factors. For example, it is more pronounced in the flesh of fully grown animals than in young immature ones, especially in muscles which are exercised and less tender. Veal has a very weak flavour compared with 18-month old beef. The flesh of animals which are properly rested prior to slaughter has a better flavour which is more readily released on cooking. Breed does not appear to exert much influence on the degree of flavour in a carcase, but sex can, especially in pigs, which on occasion have a boar-odour taint. As far as beef and lamb are concerned, there would appear to be little difference in flavour between the castrate and the entire animal. Recent work has shown that there is little or no correlation between the level of nutrition and flavour, although there are many who still hold that fatness is a guarantee of good flavour and tenderness.

The *extractives* of meat are the principal constituents of the commercial extracts and are obtained by concentrating liquors in which beef muscle and offal parts have been soaked and cooked, or by concentrating the liquor in which beef has been cooked prior to canning. It requires about 13.6 kg of lean meat to yield 453 g of extract. The food value of extractives is thought to be low, but they stimulate the flow of gastric juice and aid in the digestion of food.

### *Minerals*

The inorganic minerals or ash of muscle constitute a little less than 1% of the content, the main elements being, in order of importance, sulphur, potassium, phosphorus, sodium, chlorine, magnesium, calcium, iron, copper, chromium, selenium, cobalt (as vitamin $B_{12}$) and zinc.

### *Vitamins*

Vitamins occur in the form of the water-soluble B vitamins thiamin (vitamin $B_1$), riboflavin (vitamin $B_2$), nicotinic acid (niacin), pyridoxine (vitamin $B_6$), pantothenic acid, biotin, folic acid (pteroylmonoglutamic acid) and vitamin $B_{12}$ (cyanocobalamin), along with some vitamin A (lipid-soluble) and vitamin C (water-soluble ascorbic acid). Meat is our most important source of vitamin $B_{12}$, which is not found in vegetable foods. This vitamin is essential for cell division and nuclear maturation as well as the formation of red blood cells. Deficiencies of $B_{12}$ often occur in man and animals, causing pernicious anaemia in the former and anorexia (lack of appetite), loss of condition and growth, muscular weakness and fertility in the latter. Pork contains about ten times as much thiamin as beef and lamb, while beef has considerably more folic acid than either pork or lamb. Liver is another good source of B vitamins, especially thiamin, as well as vitamin A; 100 g of raw lamb's liver contains 25 times the recommended adult daily amount. The level of vitamins in meat is reduced by cooking, the amount depending on the temperature and time employed.

### *Other constituents*

Other important constituents of meat include the *pigments* myoglobin and haemoglobin. The redness of meat is largely due to its myoglobin content, which is greatest in beef (0.30–1.0%) and less in pork (0.06–0.40%) and poultry (0.02–0.18%). The myoglobin content is higher in male animals, old animals and certain muscles such as the heart and diaphragm which are in constant activity.

### *Reducing bodies*

Reducing bodies which possess an enzyme action with marked oxidising properties are present in meat; their action is manifested typically in carcases affected with icterus, for the yellow coloration of the tissues caused by the presence of the bile pigment bilirubin may often disappear if the icteric carcase is detained for 24 hours.

## QUALITY

### Physical and chemical changes

Considerable changes occur in the nature of meat within 1–2 days of slaughter. Shortly after death, the meat appears dark and is sticky and adherent when minced; water can only be squeezed from it with difficulty; it is resistant to the penetration of salt and sugar and its electrical resistance is high. A day or so later, the meat is lighter in colour and is moist but not sticky when minced; over 30% of fluid can be squeezed from it; and the electrical resistance drops to one-fifth of its initial value. The rate at which meat undergoes such changes depends on the atmospheric temperature, but the change cannot take place unless adequate amounts of glycogen are present and the pH falls to a satisfactory level. For this reason the meat of exhausted animals, in which the glycogen content is depleted, remains dark and fiery; there is little concrete evidence that this state is due to incomplete bleeding.

### **Rigor mortis** (See also Chapter 9, Stress and Meat Quality)

The first and most considerable post-mortem change which occurs in muscle is *rigor mortis*. The phenomenon is characterised by a hardening and contraction of all the voluntary muscles, by a loss in transparency of the surface of the muscle, which becomes dull, and by stiffening of the joints. It is accompanied by a slight rise in temperature of the carcase to 1.5°C or more above normal in the case of beef carcases, the temperature then gradually dropping to that of the surrounding atmosphere. Rigor mortis affects first the muscles that have been most active and best-nourished prior to death and commences at the head and neck, extending backwards to involve the body and limbs. The heart is affected very early, usually within an hour of slaughter. Rigor reaches its greatest intensity in the left ventricle and this cavity is therefore usually free of blood on post-mortem examination, although some blood may remain in the right ventricle. In a physiologically normal animal, rigor in the skeletal muscles does not appear for 9–12 hours after slaughter, and maximum rigidity is attained at 20–24 hours and then gradually declines.

The development of rigor mortis is influenced by:

1. The atmospheric temperature: a high temperature accelerates its onset whereas a low temperature retards it.
2. The health of the animal: where an animal is slaughtered while affected with a febrile condition, rigor mortis may be absent or scarcely apparent. Certain drugs are said to encourage the early onset of rigor mortis, including sodium salicylate, alcohol and ether.
3. The supply of energy stored as glycogen and adenosine triphosphate (ATP) in the muscle at the time of death. This is one of the most important factors controlling the production of rigor mortis.

Rigor mortis occurs when, after death, the muscles lose their extensibility owing to the supply of adenosine triphosphate and glycogen being used up. Energy is required to maintain muscle in a relaxed state. When the energy is used up, a bond forms between the myosin (in thick fibrils) and actin (in thin fibrils), the binding together of the protein forming *actomyosin*. The gradual disappearance of rigor is due, at least in part, to the action of proteolytic enzymes. Under certain conditions the onset of rigor mortis after slaughter may be very rapid and may pass off as rapidly, as for example, in hunted animals or excited young bulls. In this case the supply of energy in the muscle is low and is rapidly used up so that rigor mortis occurs rapidly. The pH of the muscle remains high in this case since there has been little conversion of glycogen into lactic acid. (See *DFD meat* below.)

In the meat trade the occurrence of an adequate degree of rigor mortis and a low ultimate pH of the flesh are desirable characteristics. The low pH inhibits bacterial growth and the lactic acid brings about the conversion of the connective tissue into gelatin so that the meat when cooked is more tender.

It is thus apparent that absence of rigor mortis may result from unfavourable ante-mortem treatment such as fatigue or the fear and excitement engendered during transport, or it may result from an illness. Although poor pre-slaughter treatment does not usually render carcases unfit for food, they are difficult to cut up, the joints lose their shape, there is more waste and the durability of the meat is lowered. These undesirable changes also occur where absence of rigor mortis is due to illness before slaughter, but these carcases, besides being less durable, may contain organisms or deleterious toxins harmful to man.

## EFFECTS OF BREEDING AND PRE-SLAUGHTER STRESS

The constant search for animals with a high meat-to-bone ratio and, more recently, the demand by the consumer for lean meat have on occasion resulted in meat which many claim lacks colour, flavour, succulence and tenderness.

Nowhere is this illustrated more frequently than in pig meat, where producers have played their part by reducing backfat by some 0.5 mm a year in the past 10 years but may at the same time have produced defects which affect the appearance, cutting, cooking and eating qualities of pork and bacon.

While breeding and breeding systems as well as the manner in which the animal is handled before slaughter are undoubtedly important, it is also likely that post-mortem factors, such as the length of time the meat is held before consumption are also of significance, as is the final method of cooking.

The use of specialised boar lines with the emphasis on leanness and the adoption of high-energy diets can affect the type and distribution of carcase fat. At the present time the grading of pigs is largely based on the use of the backfat probe, but this may soon prove to be inadequate in assessing carcase quality, giving way to the use of ultrasonic screening, fibre optics to measure colour and a fat firmness metre. With a decrease in fat thickness the fat itself becomes softer and there is a tendency for it to separate from the lean, this defect being exaggerated on diets high in unsaturated fatty acids. Lean meat separation, soft fat, drip loss, lack or excess of colour, flavour and tenderness all make the product less acceptable to the consumer.

### Dark, firm and dry meat (DFD), dark cutting meat

This is a troublesome condition in which the colour of the musculature of freshly killed animals, as a whole or in parts, is appreciably darker and drier than normal. The condition, which is most common in cattle, occurs most frequently where animals are subjected to pre-slaughter stress, including the mixing of stock 24–48 hours prior to slaughter. Young bulls are frequently affected because of their enhanced temperament and behaviour. In deer, stag carcases are more often affected than those from hinds.

In post-mortem glycolysis, glycogen reserves in the muscle are broken down into lactic acid and $CO_2$. The amount of lactic acid determines the ultimate pH of the meat. In normal animals the final pH is in the region of 5.5–5.8, but in some animals which are physically exhausted or otherwise stressed at the time of slaughter and have low glycogen reserves, the extent of post-mortem glycolysis is very limited and the pH fall is small, i.e. from 7.0 to, for example, 6.8. This results in very dark, firm and dry meat which has poor keeping quality. Thus the rate and extent of acidification taking place in muscle in the first few hours after slaughter greatly influences the quality of meat and is largely determined by the degree of stress to which the animal has been subjected in the last hours prior to slaughter. If this has been prolonged, with a consequent depletion of glycogen, DFD meat develops.

The presence of an attractive bright red hue on the exposed surface of meat is due to oxygenated myoglobin. The effect of a high pH in meat is to increase the activity of the muscle enzymes that utilise oxygen and to hinder the penetration of oxygen into the meat substance. The unpleasant purplish-red colour of DFD meat is therefore due to the fact that the myoglobin of muscle is only partly converted to oxymyoglobin. Dark, firm and dry meat, while perfectly fit for food, has a less desirable colour and flavour and a lower keeping quality. It is resisted by the meat trade for use as normal meat cuts.

## Pale, soft, exudative muscle (PSE, watery pork)

In healthy, rested pigs the amount of lactic acid produced shows a gradual increase after slaughter and the muscle pH falls from 7.0 to about 5.5 over a period of 4–8 hours. Watery pork is a direct result of a *rapid* fall in muscle pH after death. Muscle which is normal in appearance at the time of death can become affected, and this occurs when pH values of about 5.5 are attained within an hour or so of slaughter while the temperature of the muscle is still above 35°C. Under these conditions, changes occur in the properties of the muscle proteins and the flesh becomes watery, assumes a pale, unattractive colour and lacks flavour.

Many factors have been associated with this condition, e.g. high environmental temperature, rough ante-mortem handling, fighting, physiological differences between breeds and individual muscles, inefficient slaughtering techniques and handling of carcases.

Certain *breeds* are particularly susceptible to stress because of endocrinological imbalances induced by selective breeding. The modern bacon pig carries more muscle and less fat than earlier types, has relatively greater oxygen requirements, and certain breeds (Danish Landrace, Piétrain and Poland China) appear to be prone to rapid post-mortem glycolysis and the production of watery pork. Work has shown that crossing a pig of high PSE incidence with one having a low incidence of PSE results in an intermediate incidence. Since PSE and leanness are closely related, it has been suggested that steps should be taken to select against PSE or at least to maintain it at the current levels within breeds.

PSE muscle is a serious problem if pork is to be sold fresh because of the amount of drip, which causes weight loss (up to 10%) and may necessitate repackaging, and to a lesser extent its pale colour. Such meat is more likely to be tougher when cooked and to have higher cooking losses. In curing, PSE meat takes up more brine than normal pig meat but appears to cure fairly satisfactorily as Wiltshire sides, except for reduced weight gain due to diffusion of proteins and low-molecular-weight substances into the brine. Exudative hams lose 2.2% more weight than normal hams and pasteurised canned hams have 1% more gelatin than hams with normal water-holding properties. Large pig meat processors do not consider PSE to be a serious problem because their batch processing techniques and use of polyphosphates make the differences become less evident.

Watery pork generally affects the leg, loin and fillet. A condition termed *travel oedema*, which may be analogous to PSE meat, is occasionally encountered in New Zealand in lambs slaughtered after an arduous journey, in which the carcase, particularly the shoulders, is unduly watery. To alleviate the condition, the animal must be properly rested and the carcase, particularly in the summer months, transferred immediately to the chiller to ensure rapid reduction in temperature. Careful selection of breeding stock is necessary for the long-term control of this particular condition.

Besides pre-slaughter stress, there are indications that the actual slaughter procedure may influence the onset of DFD and PSE. The following procedures will help reduce the incidence of PSE and DFD meat.

1 Animals should be handled gently and quietly at the farm and the meat plant.
2 Loading ramps should be provided at the farm and efficient unloading facilities at the meat plant.
3 Stock should be kept in their original social groups as far as possible and there should be no mixing within the last vital 24–48 hour period before slaughter.
4 Lairage pen design and race arrangements should allow for easy and efficient movement of stock.
5 Water should be provided at all times in the lairage, and food when necessary.

6 The use of sticks and electric goads should be avoided.
7 Aggressive animals should be isolated in the lairage as should females in oestrus.
8 The use of overhead fine sprays of water in lairages has been shown to reduce the incidence of PSE. This is thought to be due to the cooling effect.
9 Careful selection of stock for slaughter is important so that the period of time animals spend in the lairage is the optimum for the particular species, sex and time of year.
10 Feeding of sugar in liquid form to pigs in the lairage is recommended to replace depleted liver glycogen reserves.

### Porcine stress syndrome (PSS)

Allied to the PSE condition are the porcine stress syndrome (fatal syncope, herztod, shock heart failure syndrome) and malignant hyperthermia. *Fatal syncope* is relatively common in the Piétrain and Landrace but not in the Large White. The condition is characterised by sudden death, preceded by elevated temperature, skin blanching, erythema and dyspnoea in fat pigs which have been subjected to stress. Post-mortem examination shows diffuse and severe degeneration of skeletal muscle with excess pericardial fluid.

The condition is similar to *malignant hyperthermia* in man occurring during inhalation anaesthesia, usually with halothane. Susceptible patients (about 1 in 20 000) are affected with a very high body temperature, muscular rigidity, tachycardia (very rapid heart rate) and other heart abnormalities, elevated metabolic rate, acidosis, increased creatine phosphokinase levels and profound shock which may lead to death. The condition appears to be associated with a halothane-induced calcium activity in skeletal muscle, especially in the sarcoplasmic reticulum, necessitating immediate cessation of anaesthesia and surgery and correction of the metabolic acidosis, etc. Halothane anaesthesia has been used as a test for pigs prone to PSS as there is a definite association between halothane sensitivity, liability to fatal syncope and the occurrence of PSE meat. Studies have shown that halothane sensitivity in pigs is caused by a single recessive gene, which suggests that selection using the halothane test would be an effective method of reducing the incidence of PSS and PSE. On a practical basis, 80–100 pigs from at least six and preferably eight or more sires are tested to obtain a reliable estimate of the status of the herd in relation to PSS and PSE.

Pigs aged 3–11 weeks are subjected to full halothane anaesthesia and their reactions determined as positive when extreme rigidity of the hind limb occurs. An obvious disadvantage of the test is the high mortality (which may reach over 8%) among the positive reactors. Study of the positive and negative reactors shows that the former have significantly shorter and leaner carcases, fewer pigs born alive in litter, poorer meat quality and higher mortality in general.

The halothane test is only capable, however, of detecting the homozygous recessive animals which have received the halothane gene from both parents. A DNA test which can identify the presence of the specific gene has been developed in Canada and should have the potential to eliminate the gene from a pig population.

## INFLUENCE OF FEEDING ON ANIMAL TISSUE

The effect of feeding on the colour and texture of animal tissue is much more evident in fat than in muscle. The fat in grass-fed cattle is a rich yellow colour, particularly noticeable in animals which have come off grass in early summer; in animals coming off grass later in the year and in stall-fed cattle, the fat is almost white.

The yellow colour of fat due to grass feeding is linked to the presence of *carotene*, a pigment converted in the animal body into vitamin A and abundantly present in fresh young grass, some varieties of maize, certain root crops such as carrots, and linseed and cotton cake. Mammalian fat consists of three substances—olein, stearin and palmitin—which are present in varying proportions. Palmitin acts as a solvent of carotene so that animals such as cattle, horses and, to a lesser extent pigs which have a large proportion of palmitin in their fat will accumulate carotene if fed on carotene-containing foods and produce fat of a yellow colour. However, where such animals are fed on foods such as grain, hay or straw, which contain little or no carotene, the fat remains white in colour.

In the case of sheep, goats and buffaloes very little palmitin is present in their fat, so that they assimilate only small quantities of carotene and the fat remains white in colour irrespective of the nature of the feed. If the body fat should be lost, however, as in under-nourishment or postnatally in cows, such carotene as is present in the body fat is either used up more slowly or completely left behind, so that it becomes more concentrated and the fat becomes yellow in colour.

In Jersey and Guernsey breeds of cattle *yellow fat* is, however, a normal breed characteristic, probably due to a genetic factor influencing the deposition of carotene or other pigments from grass, etc. In the young calves the fat is white, but it becomes yellow when the animals are taken from their mothers and fed on grass or other foods. The deep yellow coloration of the fat occasionally seen in sheep carcases is a condition well known in Iceland and Ireland; it is attributed to a recessive factor which prevents oxidation of the yellow pigments, the xanthophylls, in their foodstuffs. The coloration may be so marked as to render the carcase unmarketable.

Pigs fed too long on swill develop a fat which is soft and unattractive and possesses an insipid taste. The soft fat of swill-fed pigs renders the carcase difficult to cut up, causes heavy loss in frying and contains a high proportion of unsaturated fatty acids, leading to early rancidity. Feeding pigs on fish meal produces fat of a brownish yellow colour, a condition known as *brown fat disease* and attributable to an acid-fast pigment caused by the presence of excessive unsaturated fatty acids in the meal.

## ABNORMAL ODOURS AND TAINTS

Abnormal odours are commonly encountered in meat, and may often be acquired from outside sources, e.g. from the consumption of certain foodstuffs, from drugs administered as medicine or by the absorption of the odour of strong-smelling substances whilst the meat is stored. Abnormal odours may also be intrinsic, as in the odour of acetone in the carcase of cows affected with ketosis or in the sexual odour of certain male animals. The causes of abnormal odours in meat may be classified as follows.

### Feeding

The most common example of abnormal odour acquired as a result of feeding is that which occurs from excessive feeding on fish meal resulting in pork or bacon with a fishy odour and taste, while the carcase fat is soft and greyish-yellow. Fishiness in pork or bacon is attributed to the high percentage of fat in fish meal and it can be avoided if the fat content of the meal is lowered to between 3% and 7%. Although it is claimed that the fishy odour of pork can be obviated if the feeding of fish meal is discontinued 6 weeks prior to slaughter, it is questionable whether this period is sufficient. Feeding pigs cod-liver oil, particularly the cheaper brands, also produces pork or bacon with a fishy odour and brownish coloration of the fat. In Denmark the feeding of cod-liver oil is discontinued after the animal has reached 50 kg liveweight. Where pigs are fed on restaurant swill, the flesh may possess an odour and taste similar to that of pigs fed on fish meal.

In cattle, an abnormal flesh odour is observed when animals are slaughtered after being moved from grass in the autumn and feeding on turnips has commenced; this turnipy odour is present only during the first week of turnip feeding and the continuance of root feeding after that period produces no odour. A turnipy odour may also be present in bovine carcases slaughtered due to obstruction or rupture of the oesophagus by a portion of root and may be so marked as to render the carcase unmarketable.

The recently introduced practice of feeding cattle with ensiled poultry litter is said to be associated with an abnormal meat odour and also, on occasions, with the onset of disease, e.g. botulism. Various food factory wastes, e.g. orange skins, are sometimes used as feed for livestock, usually cattle and pigs, and can give rise to undesirable odours in meat. An abnormal and persistent *garlic* odour in meat, resulting in carcase condemnation, has followed the feeding of vegetable waste containing decomposing onions to cattle (M. Fussey 1990, private communication). A *leek* taint in beef carcases has been reported by Lund *et al.* (1991). Four intensively reared bulls had been fed on vegetable waste obtained from a wholesale market garden at an inclusion rate of 50–60% of the feed (barley straw, ensiled grass and maize). The final ration was estimated to contain 1–2% of leek waste. The genus *Allium* includes several species of onions (cultivated and wild), chives, garlic and leeks and all contain the toxic principle *n*-propyl disulphide, which has caused haemolytic anaemia, sometimes ending fatally, in cattle and horses (Humphreys, 1988). The feeding of waste materials, of whatever type, is clearly fraught with danger.

In sheep, the feeding of turnips rarely produces an abnormal odour of the flesh, but a rancid odour and soapy taste may occur in sheep fed on fermenting beet; this would appear to be due to the *beatine* present in beet, for the feeding to cows of sugar-beet tops in excessive quantities is known to produce an abnormal flavour of the milk. The carcases from lambs fattened intensively in houses and fed on a mixture of fish or soya bean meal and barley have sometimes shown an abnormal flavour. In some cases the fleeces of such lambs are very damp and possess a 'pig' odour, which may taint the hot meat during dressing operations. Intensively fed lambs receiving these diets have very soft fat in their carcases. The problem would appear to be nutritional in origin, the carcase fat containing many unsaturated fatty acids. The eating of young garlic leaves by rabbits and sometimes by cattle may give the carcases a strong odour resembling phosphorus.

A boiling test should be performed in all cases of suspect odours.

## Absorption of odours

Abnormal odours and taste of flesh due to the administration of *drugs* are commonly encountered in cattle, particularly dairy cows, and attention should be paid in emergency-slaughtered animals to the stomach contents; detection of a drug odour calls for an examination of whether the odour is also present in the flesh. The odour of drugs persists longest in the thickest parts of the carcase. Drugs which may affect the meat adversely in this way are linseed oil, turpentine, carbolic acid, ether, chloroform, asafoetida, nitrous spirits of ether, aromatic spirits of ammonia and aniseed. In addition, it is inadvisable to administer aloes, magnesium sulphate, treacle, chloral hydrate and bromides to animals which are likely to require emergency slaughter. Apart from abnormal odours caused by the administration of drugs shortly before slaughter, abnormal odours may occasionally occur owing to the inspiration of air containing the vapour of chlorine or carbolic acid used in the cleansing of transport vehicles. The drinking of water impregnated with tar may likewise render the flesh unmarketable, as may chlorine leaking from a refrigeration system.

Certain of the chlorinated hydrocarbons, including DDT, used externally on animals as insecticides and acaricides may accumulate in the fat as a result of spraying or by the animal consuming contaminated feeds. Organophosphorus compounds are also used externally for a similar purpose but do not create a hazard to the consumer when properly used on animals destined for slaughter, provided immediate slaughter is not carried out.

In the imported meat trade the absorption of abnormal odours by refrigerated meat during transport or storage is a common cause of depreciation and even of condemnation. Contamination by the odour of citrus fruit may occur during a sea voyage if the fruit becomes over-ripe or unsound and the excessively generated gas filters through to an accompanying meat cargo. Such odours are readily absorbed by meat, particularly by the fat; odours of oil or tar in meat may occur in a similar way.

## Products of abnormal metabolism

The existence of a peculiar odour, described as sweet but repugnant, is frequently observed in the flesh of cattle which have been affected with fever or which were close to parturition prior to slaughter; it is often apparent in cows suffering from milk fever which have been slaughtered owing to failure to respond to treatment by calcium injections. This odour is caused by appreciable amounts of *acetone* present in the flesh and is most readily detected in the large connective tissue sheets, in the kidney fat or in the muscular tissue. The odour, which does not disappear from the meat even when grilled, may be sufficient to render it unfit for sale and for this reason a *boiling test* should always be applied on the flesh of animals slaughtered while suffering from fever or in an advanced stage of gestation, especially where the liver shows evidence of fatty change.

**Sexual odour**

In male animals the meat may possess an abnormal odour and taste, which may be so marked as to lower its value and marketability. This sexual odour, which is specific for each animal and may be described as resembling stale urine, is markedly apparent in the boar and male goat, though of little or no significance in bulls or rams. The sexual odour in boars is caused by a steroid substance, *androstenone;* the odour becomes apparent in the flesh when the carcase exceeds 63 kg weight, though it can be prevented by treatment of the animal with oestrogens. Experiments immunising boars with luteinising hormone releasing-hormone (LHRH) at 30 kg and again at 90 kg has demonstrated that this technique is effective in reducing the level of androstenone in the carcase fat when the pigs were slaughtered at 105 kg (Bonneau *et al.* 1994). In castrated boars, i.e. stags, the degree of odour depends on the length of time between castration and slaughter, as well as on the age of the pig and the length of time it has been used for breeding; it is most marked in older, coarser animals. Boar odour persists in flesh for a considerable time after the animal is castrated and can be completely obviated only if the boar pig is castrated before it is 4 months; about 11 days after castration the meat is odourless, but the boar odour persists in the fat for 10 weeks before it finally disappears. A pronounced sexual odour may also be present in the flesh of cryptorchid pigs. The carcases of hermaphrodite pigs often possess an abnormal odour which, however, is distinguishable from the odour of boars.

Male sexual odour is most apparent in the meat immediately after slaughter, particularly in the fatty tissues and while the carcase is still warm. The odour largely disappears as the carcase cools but may reappear when the meat is boiled or fried, and for this reason animals exhibiting a marked sexual odour immediately after slaughter are detained for 24 hours in German, Danish and Dutch abattoirs and a boiling test is then applied to portions of the flesh.

A survey in Northern Ireland involving 525 households in which bacon was eaten at least once a week showed that less than 3% of eaters marked boar bacon much less pleasant and no more than 1% very much less pleasant than either their usual bacon or the previous week's supply. Of the 13% who classed the aroma of the boar bacon as much stronger than that of their usual bacon, only 0.6% of the total sample rated it as much or very much less appetising. Strangely, a strong aroma, far from being disagreeable, was positively liked by the consumers. The survey concluded that, assuming that the householders and the pigs selected for the test were representative samples, it was safe to market bacon from boars under current rearing and processing procedures (Ulster Curers Association, Technical Division).

It is commonly contended that the slaughtering of gilts and sows during oestrus is likely to result in taint of the bacon or ham subsequently prepared. In the case of the home-cured product, there is a possibility that the lowering of the glycogen content of the muscle due to the restlessness and excitement associated with oestrus may be a predisposing factor to the onset of adverse bacterial changes. Some support for the empirical objection against the slaughtering of gilts while in oestrus is provided by Dutch workers who have detected organoleptically what is described as 'boar odour' in the flesh of gilts and have suggested a relationship between oestrus and this abnormal odour. The odour is said to disappear in 3 weeks after slaughter but may persist in subcutaneous fat for 2½ months. The odour is most marked in the parotid salivary gland, and it is practice in Denmark to apply a boiling test to this gland, other samples of meat and fat being examined if the test is positive.

The alleged dark fat and lack of setting of the carcases of cows affected with cystic ovaries may conceivably be due to the depletion of glycogen resulting from the excitement associated with nymphomania in which there are short and irregular intervals between heat periods and the periods themselves often prolonged.

A taint in poultry meat, referred to as 'off-flavour' or 'musty taint', was reported in England by the Food Research Institute in 1972. It is caused by chloroanisoles released by microorganisms from the wood preservatives in certain types of wood shavings, which are used in deep litters. Very low levels of chloroanisoles can produce the taint: 4 mg tetrachloroanisole in $10^6$ litres of water can be detected by smell. Fortunately, incidents of this taint have been isolated ones, and the problem is not considered to be a risk to human health. The problem is considered to be essentially one of food quality by the UK Advisory Committee on Taint, which consists of representatives from the Agricultural Research Council, the Laboratory of the Government Chemist and the Ministry of Agriculture, Fisheries and Food.

## Judgement of abnormal odours

In Britain, the meat of boars, castrated boars and cryptorchid pigs (rigs) is of lower value than the flesh of sows because of the boar odour. The flesh of these animals and of sows is, however, used regularly as an ingredient of sausage, and the existence of a sexual odour cannot be regarded as a justification for seizure of the meat as unfit for human food. In addition, the low price paid for such meat is sufficient to ensure that the practice of slaughtering boars is not encouraged, while the boar odour is minimised if the carcase is expeditiously cooled after slaughter, and largely disappears during the mincing and preparation for sausage. It is, however, not advisable to add more than one part of boar meat to 20 parts of other meat ingredient. In Great Britain, the Fresh Meat (Hygiene and Inspection) Regulations 1995 (para. 13(2)) requires that fresh meat from breeding boars and cryptorchid or hermaphrodite swine should not be sold for human consumption unless it has undergone one of the treatments which would render it a 'product' under EU legislation and has been specially marked.

Flesh with a pronounced odour of drugs or disinfectants must be regarded as unfit if the abnormal taste and smell are still apparent by a boiling test after the carcase has been detained for 24 hours. A marked and persistent fishy odour in pork may be regarded as sufficient to render it unmarketable, and it should be condemned. In imported meat the odour caused by the absorption of gases from cargoes of fruit during storage, and also superficial taint in meat due to oil or tar, can be removed almost entirely by subjecting the meat to long periods of ozonisation.

## Other abnormal constituents

These are more likely to occur in comminuted meats and usually gain access through careless processing methods, although some may be malicious in origin. (See *Food tampering*.) The absence of or presence of faulty metal detectors is occasionally responsible for the inclusion of pieces of metal in minced meats. Recent detections have included portions of hypodermic needles and of wire from car tyres and chicken fencing which have been discovered in pig tongues. Some dangerous foreign bodies are displayed in Fig. 2.17.

Current meat inspection routines are concerned with a visual inspection of carcase meat, which fails to detect deep-seated lesions which include small abscesses that are only discovered by the consumer during the preparation of a meal. Research work is being conducted on sonar technology in an attempt to detect these lesions at meat inspection. While the presence of a few flukes in livers may cause no harm in terms of food poisoning they are, nevertheless, aesthetically unacceptable.

Most of these problems could be averted by responsible husbandry methods at the farm, during meat inspection and meat processing.

## Food tampering

Malicious tampering with food has become a major concern for food companies and authorities. The display of various kinds of products on supermarket and other shelves is an opportunity for the criminal to introduce deleterious materials on and into food, usually for purposes of extortion. Attacks have occurred on meat companies and butchers' shops, although the main forms of food product

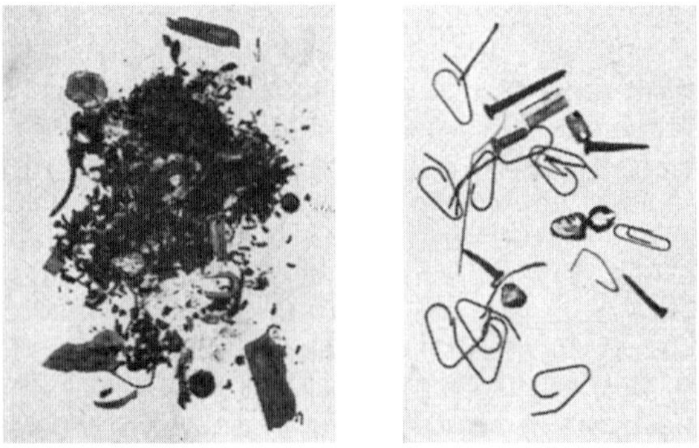

**Fig. 2.17** Metallic foreign bodies recovered from manufacturing meat imported into England from Europe. The objects include nails, needles, paper clips, pieces of wire and irregular lumps of metal. Some of the material on the left is solid purple dye.

involved have been packaged entities other than meat. Nevertheless, the threat to meat and meat products is very real, mainly because of the animal connection. Even though most of the threats are bogus, panic and fear are created, and with media publicity involvement there is a resulting loss of consumer confidence, institution of laboratory tests, and recall and destruction of product, all of which entail much monetary loss.

Control measures include close liaison with police authorities, the creation of an emergency management team and plan, the establishment of a security system, alerting of all staff to this menace, the appointment of a public relations officer to deal with the media, formulation of a recall plan, liaison with independent laboratories, and use of tamper-proof packaging where appropriate.

## CUTTING OF MEAT

Traditional methods of cutting up carcases of meat are based on their division into reasonably large wholesale or primal cuts convenient for the butchers to handle. The shape and size of these primal cuts depend to some extent on the anatomy of the animal, but they also have regard to the suitability of the final smaller cuts for cooking. The cutting involves sawing across bone and seaming along groups of muscles. In the past wholesale cuts were supplied to the retailer with the bone in, but it is more common now to trade in boneless primals. The final retail cuts, across the grain of the meat, are made as required.

In England, beef fore- and hindquarters are commonly separated between the 10th and 11th ribs, but the point of separation varies regionally. Within EEC countries there is also a demand for 'pistola' fores and hinds, which are officially recognised for the purpose of 'intervention buying'. The pistola hind has eight ribs attached, leaving a five-rib pistola forequarter with all the thin flank (normally part of the hind) attached. For intervention purposes the kidneys, kidney fat and channel (pelvic) fat (KKCF) are removed. The KKCF constitutes about one-third of the fat which has to be sold over the counter. Removal of the KKCF at the warm carcase stage means that there is less variability in carcases. None the less, there is no doubt that unless great care combined with hygiene is taken in its removal, the valuable fillet can be damaged by knife cuts, resulting in drying and deterioration. There is now general agreement that since the KKCF represents 3.75% of the carcase weight, weighings may be made with or without it present.

Although there are similarities between English and American methods of cutting beef, there are marked differences in the sub-primal and retail cuts. The American cuts reflect a consumer preference for grilling steaks, convenience foods and grinding beef for hamburgers.

### Hot boning of meat

The traditional method of cutting up meat has generally been carried out after the carcase has been cooled for 18 hours or more, although hot bull beef has been used for manufacturing purposes in Germany and the United States for many years. The integration of slaughtering and cutting operations on the one site makes hot boning, with direct preparation and vacuum packing of the primal cuts, a possibility.

EEC legislation stipulates that hot boning must be carried out in a room separate from the slaughterhall but within the same group of buildings and sufficiently close for the meat to be transferred in a single operation. Cutting must be carried out immediately after transfer and, following appropriate packaging, the meat must be chilled. The temperature of the cutting room, in all circumstances, must not exceed 12°C and the room must be equipped with a recording thermometer or recording telethermometer.

The hot deboning procedure removes meat from the bones as intact groups of muscles, although the traditional cutting method can be adopted. The former seaming method is preferred, however, because of the reduced bacterial levels (the cut surface of a muscle is much more susceptible to deterioration than a muscle with the connective tissue covering or epimysium intact). After removal, the muscles are vacuum packed, using different shapes and sizes of bag. The packs may be held at 10°C for 24 hours, then chilled to 0–1°C. Alternatively, a three-stage cooling system may be used in which the hot-boned joints are chilled at 15°C for 7 hours, 7°C for 24 hours and final holding at 2°C. With all chilling regimes after hot-boning, however, tenderisation of the carcase by electrical stimulation is considered to be a necessary prerequisite to avoid toughening of the meat due to *cold shortening* (q.v.).

The *advantages* claimed for this method are that:

1 More efficient and quicker chilling of the meat results in reduced refrigeration costs.
2 Since only the usable meat is chilled, approximately 65% of the carcase, less refrigeration, is needed.
3 Meat yield is higher owing to reduced evaporative weight loss of up to 1%.
4 Reduced amount of drip in the vacuum pack saves weight loss and avoids staining of the fat.
5 Colour uniformity is better.
6 Warm meat can be moulded.

The *disadvantages* include:

1 operational difficulties in the synchronisation of slaughter and boning lines;
2 fat being more difficult to trim;
3 the unconventional shapes of cuts;
4 the absolute need for high standards of hygiene throughout the whole operation;
5 the fact that hot boning virtually always requires tenderisation of the carcase by electrical stimulations;
6 need for very high standards of knife hygiene.

## Vacuum packing

In addition to the sale of wholesale cuts in a fresh or chilled form, a considerable trade has developed in vacuum-packed deboned primal cuts. This process started in the United States in the early 1950s and was introduced into Great Britain after the foot-and-mouth disease epidemic of 1967–68. When the United Kingdom refused to accept further shipments of bone-in-beef from South America, vacuum-packing was the only practical alternative to freezing. Two basic systems of vacuum packaging have been developed:

1 Drawing a low vacuum within a plastic film of copolymers with polyvinylidine chloride, sealing the bag with a metal clip, and then heat shrinking in hot water for 2 seconds.
2 Creating a much higher vacuum inside a nylon/polythene laminate film and then heat-sealing the bag. The package may then be passed through a heat tunnel which causes the bag to shrink tightly around the meat, forming a firm seal.

The secondary shrinking of the vac-pac produces a broad seal which reduces the incidence of 'leakers', and retains the drip around the meat, preventing it from spreading around the bag and appearing unsightly.

Because of the commercial success of vac-pac beef there is now a demand for the vacuum-packing of pork and lamb. Shelf-life is shorter (2–3 weeks) than with beef. Punctures from bone are said to be more common with lamb and pork, but this can be reduced by protecting the ends of bones with plastic caps or padding.

Whichever system is used it is essential to pay close attention to the following requirements:

1 Initial bacterial levels in the meat must be low.
2 Handling must be hygienic throughout the process.
3 Packs and boxed packs must be treated with care. For fresh chilled trade, the packs are usually transported in rigid baskets rather than cartons, so as to reduce rupturing of the pouch.
4 The meat must have a low pH, preferably below 5.8. At a high pH, hydrogen sulphide-producing bacteria can grow, leading to the development of putrid odours and the conversion of the muscle pigment at the meat surface to green sulphmyoglobin.
5 A temperature of 0–2°C must be maintained.
6 The film must not be punctured until the meat is ready to be used, and then the surplus fluid must be drained. Meat will normally take about 10 minutes to regain bloom. Once opened the meat will have the same shelf-life as fresh carcase meat.

## Modified-atmosphere retail packs

The fact that vacuum-packed meat retains the purple colour of myoglobin, rather than the bright red colour of oxymyoglobin associated with quality by the consumer, has limited the use of chilled vacuum-packed retail cuts. This requirement for colour has led to the widespread use of modified-atmosphere packaging (MAP) where the meat is contained within an impermeable plastic pack in an atmosphere of selected gases. Beef placed in an atmosphere of 60–80% $O_2$ and 20–40% $CO_2$ within a gas-impermeable pack can retain a bright red colour for at least a week. This is sufficient to allow for centralised cutting and distribution and a five-day 'best-before-date'. With cured meats and poultry, oxygen is not required to maintain the optimal colour, so an atmosphere of 75–80% nitrogen with 20–25% $CO_2$ is used. (Carbon dioxide is used for its bacteriostatic effect.)

The following problems may be encountered with MAP.

1 Drip from the meat can be unsightly when it accumulates within the MAP. Trays are therefore designed with patterned bases to disperse the liquid, but in most cases absorbent pads are also included.
2 Condensation can occur on the inside of the lid of the pack. This can be avoided by minimising temperature fluctuations in the display cabinet and by anti-fog coating on the inner surface of the lid.
3 Leakers can be difficult to identify until the meat has spoiled.
4 Where MAP is to be used strict attention must be paid to temperature control and hygienic production. The meat should be chilled to < 2°C prior to packing since the gas space around the meat makes further chilling difficult.
5 If MAP is to be used, it is usually necessary to utilise accelerated conditioning through, for example, electrical stimulation, since no more than 4 days of conditioning is recommended.

## Conditioning (tenderising) of meat

When meat is stored above freezing point at temperatures between 0°C and 3°C, all the changes that usually occur at higher temperatures take place but at a reduced rate. Atmospheric oxidation of fat, leading to rancidity, proceeds very slowly as meat is usually stored in the dark, and enzyme action in the fat which leads to the production of free fatty acids is also very slow. The action of bacteria is retarded but not arrested at these temperatures, while the proteolytic enzyme of the muscle fibres is active and brings about a desirable change known as *conditioning* or *ripening*, which is manifested by a marked increase in flavour, juiciness and tenderness of the meat. The action of enzymes is almost completely inhibited when the meat is stored at temperatures below freezing. Conditioning is not brought about by bacterial action.

Tenderness of meat is influenced by the breed, age, condition of nutrition and amount of muscular exercise of the animal from which it is obtained; it depends primarily on the amount of connective tissue present between the muscular fibres and, to a lesser extent, on the thickness of the muscle fibres themselves. The muscle of the thin flank, for example, is three times as rich in connective tissue as the muscle of the fillet or undercut.

Tenderness of meat post-mortem depends on changes which occur during the first 24 hours after slaughter within (1) the myofibrils and (2) the connective tissue surrounding the myofibrils which consists of collagen and a proteinaceous ground substance, *proteoglycan*. The changes which occur in the myofibrils are due to calcium-activated proteases, the calpins, and lysosomal cysteine proteases, the cathepsins. These cause a degradation of the Z-discs which separate the sarcomeres, the functional units within the myofibril. The loosening of the myofibrillar structure allows the myofibril, when stretched, to fracture along the Z-discs, resulting in the reduction in toughness. The actomyosin complex formed during the onset of rigor mortis remains intact.

Evidence available suggests that there is little post-mortem enzymatic breakdown in the connective tissue surrounding and supporting the myofibrils. The type of collagen present, however, and the extent of cross-linking within the structure of the molecule vary with the age of the animal and plays a significant role in meat tenderness. This helps to explain why older animals produce tougher meat.

A procedure recommended for the commercial ripening of beef is:

1 The dressed carcase should be cooled for 1–2 days at –0.5 to 3°C.
2 The sides or quarters should be held for 10–12 days at 2 to 3°C.
3 Before cutting up or removal for retail sale, the quarters should be held at ordinary room temperature or, if that is too high, at 4.5 to 7°C for 24 hours. In commercial practice, conditioning of meat is limited to from 2 to 6 weeks, and when beef is cut into small joints the greatest increase in palatability is ensured by a storage period of about 9 days.

Conditioning of lean meat is of value in the preparation of canned meats for, if properly matured, the muscle fibres are softened, the meat is more easily sliced and the pink colour is more vivid. Again, the hanging of venison and game for long periods need not be regarded as evidence of a perverted taste but as an appreciation of the fact that improved flavours will develop and that, unless these foods are allowed to hang, the abundant connective tissue which is developed as a result of exercise will not be broken down into more tender substances and the food may therefore be so tough and stringy as to be almost inedible. Tenderness of meat can also be improved by hammering and muscle stretching, which breaks down the muscle fibres; by 'quick' freezing before rigor mortis sets in (due probably to the mechanical effects of freezing); by the application of the enzymes *papain* and *bromelin* (obtained from the papaya and pineapple), which act on the structural components of muscle; and by electrical stimulation.

*Tenderstretch method of hanging beef sides*

While stretching of muscles tends to produce a tenderising effect (with little or no alteration in their appearance), shortening of muscles results in considerable toughening. The traditional system of hanging beef sides is by means of a hook inserted behind the Achilles tendon. Work carried out originally at the Texas A&M University showed that hanging beef sides from the aitch bone (by means of a hook inserted into the *obturator foramen or* 'pope's eye'), which allows the hind limb to assume a relaxed position, largely prevents the muscles from shortening and becoming tough. The hot beef side or quarter must be suspended by the aitch bone within 1½ hours of slaughter. After 24 hours in the chiller it can be hung by the Achilles tendon. Subsequent work at the UK Meat Research Institute showed that five important muscles from the hindquarter were more tender than muscles from carcases treated by the conventional method of hanging; although the psoas major muscle was tougher, it was still one of the most tender cuts. The improvement in tenderness of the rump, thick flank, striploin and scotch fillet is said to be equivalent to 3 weeks of ageing at 2°C. Similar improvements in sheep and lamb carcases can be achieved by the tenderstretch method. Although aitch-bone hanging slightly alters the appearance of various cuts, there was no difficulty in cutting, nor was there any reduction in the amount of saleable meat, juiciness or flavour. Hanging of beef carcases from the ischium bone may produce the same effect and is believed to be safer provided the proper long hook is used.

*Tendercut process*

Another method of altering the tension on individual muscles in the suspended carcase is to sever selected bones and ligaments. This method may be easier to implement than tenderstretch on commercial slaughterlines since it allows the carcase to be suspended normally by the Achilles tendon. The process has been carried out in both cattle and pigs and measurements indicate very significant improvements in tenderness over controls when the process is carried out within 45 minutes of slaughter.

*Tenderising by electrical stimulation*

Electrical stimulation (ES) was first introduced in New Zealand in an attempt to avoid the *cold shortening* of muscle resulting from too rapid cooling of lamb carcases. Its use however, was suggested by Harsham and Deatherage in the United States as far back as 1951. With appropriate stimulation it is claimed that beef is as tender at 4 days after slaughter as non-stimulated meat is at 10 days of normal ageing.

The effect of ES is to advance the process of rigor mortis by producing a pH of about 6.0 in 2–3 hours after slaughter. Pulses of electricity are passed through the carcase immediately after slaughter, the current causing the muscles to contract and thereby use up glycogen, ATP and creatine phosphate. A number of muscle contractions are made to occur in a short time, thereby accelerating the onset of rigor.

The operation is carried out using two electrodes, one live in contact with the carcase neck muscles or nose and the other earthed through the overhead conveyor rail and hook in the hock. It is important that good electrical contact be maintained between the electrode and the carcase.

The ES unit may be sited on the dressing line between the evisceration and carcase-splitting points or just before the weighing area. In the latter site it is claimed that a large proportion of the blood which would normally drip in the coolers is removed on the carcase dressing floor, a distinct advantage from a hygiene, neck cleanliness, labour and plant effluent standpoint.

A typical installation for beef carcases may use a voltage of 500–1000 V, 5–6 amps of current being pulsed at 25 pulses per second for 2 seconds about 30 minutes after slaughter. Lower voltages (< 100 V) can be used, which avoid expensive safety measures. Low voltage is effective only for a few minutes after death and is normally applied during bleeding. In all cases voltages must be adequate to overcome resistance at the electrodes and ensure enough flow of current through the carcase.

In addition to preventing cold shortening, ES will also avoid *thaw shortening*, a phenomenon which occurs in muscles that have been frozen at any stage up to almost the full rigor point and subsequently thawed. Both cold and thaw shortening occur more often in muscles that are severed at dressing, but can take place in muscles fixed at both ends.

The benefits of ES can be summarised as follows.

1 Accelerates tenderness and reduces ageing times.
2 Avoids cold and thaw shortening.
3 Allows rapid chilling.
4 Promotes better flavour and colour.
5 Allows for hot boning on the dressing line since cuts can be chilled rapidly.
6 Improves neck cleanliness in carcase.

### *Tenderising by infusion of calcium chloride*

Research has demonstrated that post-mortem, pre-rigor, infusion or injection of *calcium chloride* can accelerate the tenderisation process. Measurements suggest that after one day of ageing calcium chloride-infused bovine muscle was similar in tenderness to control cuts that had been aged for 7–14 days (3–7 days for lamb). The precise mechanism of action for this process is unknown, but it presumably involves the calcium-activated proteases, the calpins, which are involved in the breakdown of the myofibrillar proteins immediately post-mortem while the carcase is still warm and the pH is high (Marriott and Claus, 1994).

### *Pre-slaughter tenderising*

Since tenderness is generally regarded as being one of the desirable qualities of meat, it is not surprising that, in addition to normal ageing of meat by adequate hanging, attempts have been made to increase tenderness in meat by artificial means. Many different *enzymes* originating in certain fruits and in bacteria and fungi have been used in addition to trypsin from the pancreas. Proteolytic enzymes are used extensively in the baking industry, in cereal manufacture, in brewing and in meat products. Those most commonly utilised are: papain, a proteolytic enzyme of the *Carica papaya* or pawpaw fruit; ficin, a protease derived from figs; and bromelin, a proteolytic enzyme of the pineapple. These substances may be used separately or in combination.

Enzymes may be applied directly to meat cuts as a solution or a powder, being most effective with steaks or thin cuts of meat. Disadvantages are lack of uniform action, discoloration and surface mushiness or granulation.

Another method utilises the vascular system of the living animal to distribute the enzyme throughout the body tissues—the so-called Pro Ten Process of the Swift Company of Chicago, USA, developed in the late 1950s. In this way there is an even distribution of enzyme in the meat and the activity is controlled; the raw meat contains about four parts per million of the enzyme. This process comprises the introduction by gravity of a solution of papain into a jugular vein. The amount used varies between 300 and 500 ml, the dose being carefully controlled according to the breed, age, sex and weight of the animal. After the injection the animal must be slaughtered within 10–15 minutes, the optimum time range for maximum tenderness. The enzyme is activated and therefore tenderises when the meat is cooked, at an optimum temperature of 60–71°C. In the normal untreated animal the proportion of carcase meat which is suitable for grilling is no more than 35%. Pro Ten treatment increases this to 75%.

*Advantages* claimed over conventional methods of tenderising meat include:

1 Shorter time to achieve a uniform tenderness.
2 No loss of weight due to shrinkage or trimming.
3 Lower cost.

*Disadvantages* include the facts that:

1 The tongue, liver and kidneys of the treated animal become over-tender when cooked.
2 Some animals display an anaphylactic reaction to the process, resulting in very marked rigors and death in some cases, necessitating total condemnation of the carcase and organs.
3 The texture and flavour of the tenderised meat does not appeal to all palates.
4 There are animal welfare and ethical concerns. The UK Farm Animal Welfare Council in its report on the *Welfare of Livestock (Red Meat Animals) at the Time of Slaughter* described the process as 'an unnecessary interference to an animal for a non-veterinary purpose which can create additional stress and suffering for the animal at the time of slaughter', a conclusion with which we agree.

Where the process is used, regular tests must be carried out to ensure that moisture pick-up in the tenderised product does not exceed 3% and to determine the degree of proteolysis or tenderness. Any faults can result in product rejection.

## Mechanically recovered meat (MRM)

The need to recover as much meat as possible from bones has always been a part of good butchery practice. Carried out in the conventional manual way using knives, however, it is a laborious and time-consuming practice, and even when performed efficiently does not collect all the meat. Mechanical and other equipment employing wet extraction, screening and pressure systems can remove several extra pounds of meat per carcase, a great saving in a cost-conscious industry. As much as an additional 5% net yield has been reported.

The wet extraction methods involve cooking the bones or agitating them in cold brine in order to loosen the meat and produce bone stock. For those processors who are able to utilise the liquid extracts in meat products this is a useful method, but it is otherwise limited. Steam cooking with the use of ultrasonics is a newer variation.

In the screening methods the bones are crushed and then pressed against a fine screen which allows the soft bone to pass but not the solid bone.

Pressure methods employ a powerful press to compress a charge of uncrushed bones against a series of channels, meat being separated from a column of compressed bone.

Other methods, some of which are as yet only in the experimental stage, include the use of liquid or gas jets, brushes or flails, freezing followed by flotation in cryogenic liquids and digestion by proteolytic enzymes.

The composition of mechanically-recovered meat varies with different methods. Essentially it consists of comminuted red meat, bone marrow, collagen, bone and fat (this in addition to marrow fat). The marrow content can be reduced if long bones are excluded from the bones to be treated. The amount of actual bone is very important and must be kept to a minimum since large amounts, especially if they contain large particles, could be harmful to the consumer. In 1976 there was considerable consumer resistance to the use of MRM in the United States, but a subsequent investigation by the US Food Safety and Quality Service of the Department of Agriculture showed that there was no health hazard and that such meat might actually benefit the consumer by providing better nutrition. New regulations were brought into force which controlled bone particle size and fat content, although the panel concluded that existing particle sizes and lipid content were no worse than those in manually deboned meats. It was also arranged that mechanically-recovered meat should be labelled so that people on strictly limited calcium intakes could avoid it. EEC regulations stipulate that, in contrast to the American regulations, the calcium content should not be higher than 0.25%.

In addition to particle size and calcium content, the US panel concluded that fluoride content of MRM posed no threat to adult consumers but it advised caution in the case of young children. High amounts may cause mottling of the teeth and other changes in infants who normally ingest significant amounts. The levels of cadmium, selenium, strontium-90, copper, cobalt, iron, nickel, zinc, arsenic and mercury were not considered to be of importance. Arsenic has not been found in MRM in the United States and mercury does not accumulate in bone, while the zinc content is about the same as in manually-deboned meat. Chlorinated hydrocarbon residues have been detected only in minute quantities well below the established tolerance levels. Tetracyclines accumulate in the bones of young animals but these are below the tolerance levels.

Providing good and hygienic manufacturing and quality control practices are adopted, the bacterial content of MRM should be low. It is essential that the initial raw material is low in bacteria and that the bones are treated without undue delay and handled at low temperatures. It is recommended that the bones are stored at a temperature not exceeding +3°C and processed within 24 hours. If the procedure involves a method in which the temperature is raised, the resultant MRM must be cooled down quickly and held at freezer temperature, especially if it is not to be used immediately. Frozen MRM should be kept at a temperature not exceeding −18°C and processed within 3 months of production. All comminuted meats are liable to acquire microorganisms unless great care is taken over hygiene, method and temperature. They are also liable to oxidative colour changes.

The European Fresh Meat Directive 91/497/EEC defines mechanically-removed meat as 'meat obtained by mechanical means from flesh-bearing bones apart from the bones of the head, the extremities of the limbs below the carpel and tarsal joints and, in the case of swine, the coccygeal vertebrae, and intended for establishments approved in accordance with article 6 of Directive 77/99/EEC', i.e. EEC-approved products plants. MRM may not be used to make minced meat, but under some circumstances may be incorporated into meat preparations. In Great Britain the Minced Meat Preparations (Hygiene) Regulations 1995, which enacts the European Directives on minced meat and preparations, 88/657/EEC and 92/110/EC, adds to this definition a requirement for the meat to have 'been passed through a fine mesh such that its cellular structure has been broken down and that it flows in purée form'. There is no definition for poultry MRM.

The advent of bovine spongiform encephalopathy (BSE) has led to a prohibition on the use of the bovine vertebral column for the production of MRM. The definition of the vetebral column excludes the coccygeal vertebrae. The export of MRM from the UK to another Member State is at present banned.

## REFERENCES

Allen, D. (1990) *Meat Industry*, International Edn, November, 7.

Bonneau, M., Dufour, R., Chouvet, C., Roulet, C., Meadus, W. and Squires, E. J. (1994) *J. Anim. Sci.* **72**(1), 14–20.

Humphreys, D. J. (1988) *Veterinary Toxicology*, 3rd edn. London; Baillière-Tindall.

Lund, L. J. *et al.* (1991) *Vet. Rec.* **128**, 263.

Marriott, N. G. and Claus, J. R. (1994) *Meat Focus Int.*, 372–375

Sisson's & Grossman's (1975) *Anatomy of the Domestic Animals*, 5th edn. W. B. Saunders, Philadelphia.

Taylor, A. A. (1995) *Meat Focus Int.*, 280–285.

## FURTHER READING

Varman and Sutherland (1995) *Meat and Meat Products, Technology, Chemistry and Microbiology*. London: Chapman & Hall.

# Chapter 3
# Meat Plant Construction and Equipment

Since the cost of providing and maintaining an abattoir is very high, it is essential at the outset to ensure that there is a need for a new plant and that it will operate at maximum throughput. All too often, particularly in municipal abattoirs, vested interests have caused abattoirs to be built which have incurred, and are still incurring, serious financial losses due to inadequate business.

Inspection of efficient modern plants provides positive, as well as negative, *design information*. It is essential to appoint competent architects, engineers and other experts who have had experience in abattoir construction. The use of efficient and durable equipment, even if more expensive, cannot be overemphasised, nor can the need for future modifications. Equally important is the employment of a competent maintenance staff to ensure smooth mechanical operations.

Most basic legislation stipulates separate slaughter for horses and swine. Indeed, so specialised is the slaughter and dressing of pigs that separate abattoirs for handling them should be considered. At least special sections for pigs must be provided under EU legislation where two or more different species are slaughtered.

Pigs must be slaughtered at different times and scalding, depilation, scraping and singeing must be carried out in a place clearly separated from the other slaughter line by a 5-metre space or a 3-metre-high wall. Construction, layout and equipment must all be geared to promote efficient and hygienic operations.

The first step in planning an abattoir is to ascertain the ultimate maximum daily kill of each class of animal and the proposed disposal and treatment of the edible and inedible by-products. The actual system of operation must also be determined, bearing in mind local conditions. It may comprise a complete meat plant including full processing facilities on one or more floors or an abattoir adapted solely for slaughter and dressing. The factory abattoir requires regular full-time operatives to deal with all the livestock; it is a method that ensures economic handling of the by-products including hides, offals, glands, blood and condemned material. It also reduces overheads on buildings, equipment and labour.

The overall number and siting of abattoirs in any country should be geared closely to the demands of livestock production, due attention being paid to transport (journey to be as short as possible) as well as the need for casualty slaughter.

## Site

A suitable site for an abattoir should have the following facilities.

1. Mains water and electricity supply (daily usage of water can be in excess of 10 000 litres/tonne dressed carcase weight).
2. Mains sewerage.
3. Contiguity with uncongested road and rail systems.
4. Proximity with public transport.
5. Proximity to supply of varied labour.
6. Freedom from pollution from other industries' odours, dust, smoke, ash, etc.
7. Ability to separate 'clean' and 'dirty' areas and access.
8. Remoteness from local housing and other development to avoid complaints about noise and smell.
9. Good availability of stock nearby.
10. Ground suitable for good foundations including piling, and freedom from flooding.
11. Sufficient size for possible future expansion.

The actual site need not be a flat one. Indeed, slopes can provide suitable loading bays for stock and product and are of value when two or more floors are contemplated. In general, therefore, urban sites should be avoided; rural and nominated industrial sites are preferred.

### Environmental statement

It will be important at a very early stage in the planning and design of a meat plant to consider the possible effects of the operation of the plant on the local and wider environment. Planning authorities will often require the production of an *Environmental Statement* (ES) which will be used in determining the suitability or otherwise of the proposed plant in the particular location.

Before an environmental statement can be produced, an *Environmental Assessment* (EA) must be carried out. The EA will consider the outputs to the environment, not only from the plant in normal operation but during the construction phase. In the case of a meat plant it is likely that the following would be considered:

- Effect of increased traffic movements in the locality
- Noise and dust during construction phase
- Operational noise
- Odour
- Emission of combustion gases
- Waste water disposal.

The Environmental Statement will normally include the following elements:

- Justification of the need for the development
- Description of site and processes
- Identification of outputs to the environment
- Report of established baseline data (ambient air quality levels, traffic flows, etc.)
- Anticipated environmental impacts at both construction and operational stages
- Proposed measures to mitigate impacts.

The Environmental Statement is likely to be a substantial document and will normally be accompanied by a non-technical summary for use by lay persons. These documents will be available to all interested parties and will be used by the planning authority in determining a *planning application* and possibly by review bodies in the event of any appeal or public enquiry.

### Submission of plans

It is usual to submit two sets of *drawings* and four sets of *specifications* to the responsible authority for approval. The latter must include details of proposed throughput and capacity, number of employees, building construction, water supply, plumbing, drainage, sewage disposal, hot water supply, refrigeration capacity, lighting, ventilation, equipment and operations. Details for pest control, fly screening and the methods to be used for steam and vapour removal must also be supplied. Proposed flowlines for product, equipment, personnel and packaging must be indicated.

Guidance notes for prospective applicants and their consulting architects and engineers are normally available from government departments and these should be carefully studied beforehand.

The *site plan* (scale 1:500) must show the complete premises and the location in relation to roads, railways, waterways and adjoining properties and their function. Catch basins, water and sewer lines, storage tanks, etc. must also be shown. The *floor* plan (scale 1:50 or 1:100) relates to layout of walls, doorways, windows, partitions, rail systems, equipment, benches, platforms, toilets, chutes, conveyors, staircases, hot and cold water connections, ventilation fans, work positions of operatives, etc. The position of drainage gutters and floor gradients must also be included.

The *plumbing* plan gives details of the drainage system, which must ensure that toilet and floor soil lines are separated until outside the building and that the former do not connect with grease traps.

In addition to compliance with planning, hygiene, health and safety and EC regulations it is necessary in the UK to adhere to the *Building Regulations 1991*, which deal with good building standards and practices as well as Fire Regulation requirements.

Since specialised knowledge is required in the design and construction of a meat plant, it is vital that competent architects, veterinarians and engineers with years of experience are employed along with reputable contractors.

## Area size

Careful consideration must be given to the size of the site, with allowance for the various buildings and traffic circulation. Modern livestock and meat transport vehicles have very large turning circles: 14 m for a vehicle 15 m long. Completely separate routes for stock and meat vehicles should be provided. Approach roads should be at least 6 m wide. When all the various buildings are considered, it will be realised that a large area is necessary.

Generally, a small abattoir (up to 30 000 units/year) will occupy 1–2 acres, a medium plant (50 000+ units/year) 2–4 acres, and a large meat plant handling over 100000 units annually about 4–6 acres. (One adult bovine is equivalent to two pigs, three calves or five sheep.)

The 64/433 Directive of the EEC, as amended, states that there must be an adequate partition between the clean and dirty sections, ideally with completely separate entrances and exits for traffic involved. If only one entrance is possible, such vehicles must be routed in different directions after entry.

Lairage accommodation should be sited away from main roads or alternatively screened from them.

## Facilities

The European Council Directive No. 64/433/EEC, as amended, requires the following basic facilities for cattle, sheep, pigs, goats and solipeds:

1 Adequate lairage or, climate permitting, waiting pens for the animals.

2 Slaughter premises large enough for work to be carried out satisfactorily. Maximum slaughter rates for the different species must be specified.

3 A room for emptying and cleansing stomachs and intestines.

4 Rooms for dressing guts and tripe if this is carried out on the premises.

5 Separate rooms for the storage of fat and hides, pig bristles, horns and hooves which are not removed on the day of slaughter.

6 A separate room for preparing and cleaning offal, including a separate place for storing heads if these operations are carried out but do not take place on the slaughter line.

7 Lockable premises reserved respectively for the accommodation of sick or suspect animals, the slaughter of such animals, the storage of detained meat and the storage of seized meat.

8 Sufficiently large chilling or refrigerating rooms.

9 An adequately equipped, lockable room for the exclusive use of the veterinary service and a laboratory suitably equipped for microbiological and trichinoscopic tests when such tests are compulsory.

10 Changing rooms, wash basins, showers and flush lavatories which do not open directly on to the work rooms. The wash basins must be near the lavatories and must have hot and cold running water, materials for cleansing and disinfecting the hands and hand towels which can be used only once. There should be a receptacle for used towels.

11 Facilities enabling the required veterinary inspections to be carried out efficiently at any time.

12 Means of controlling access to and exit from the plant.

13 An adequate separation between the clean and the contaminated parts of the building.

14 In rooms where work on meat is undertaken: waterproof *flooring* which is easy to clean and disinfect, rat-proof, slightly sloping and which has a suitable *drainage* system for draining liquids to drains fitted with traps and gratings and smooth walls with light-coloured, washable coating or paint up to a height of at least 3 m with coved angles and corners with a radius of at least 75 mm.

15 Adequate *ventilation* and *steam extraction* in rooms where work on meat is undertaken.

16 In the same rooms, adequate natural or artificial *lighting* which does not distort colours or cause shadows. High-intensity lighting is now being demanded in many countries, e.g. 600 ux for pm, offal, boning + inspection rooms with 220 ux elsewhere (Australia).

17 An adequate supply, under pressure, of *potable water* only. *Non-potable water* may be used in exceptional cases for steam production, provided that the pipes installed for the purpose do not permit this water to be used for other purposes; in addition, non-potable water may be allowed in exceptional cases for cooling refrigeration equipment but these pipes must be painted red and must not pass through rooms containing meat.

18 An adequate supply of *hot potable water*.

19 A *waste water disposal system* which meets hygiene requirements.

20 In the work rooms, adequate *equipment for cleansing and disinfecting hands and tools*, and as near as possible to the work stations. Taps must not be hand-operable; there must be hot and cold running water, cleaning and disinfecting materials and hand towels which can be used only once. For cleaning of instruments the water must be not less than 82°C.

21 Equipment for dressing to be carried out as far as possible on the suspended carcase. Where flaying is carried out on metal cradles, these must be of non-corrodible materials and high enough for the carcase not to touch the floor.

22 An overhead system of rails for the further handling of the meat.

23 Appropriate *protection against pests*.

24 Instruments and working equipment of non-corrodible and easily cleaned material.

25 A special section for *manure*.

26 A place and adequate equipment for cleansing and disinfecting vehicles.

Similar provisions are made in the case of poultry by EEC Directive No. 71/118/EEC as amended.

### *Water*

Mains water supply usually provides an ample supply of potable water in the UK and most parts of the world. In many countries it must pass standard tests, such as the EEC Directive relating to the Quality of Water Intended for Human Consumption (80/778/EEC). In the UK mains water will meet the requirements of potable (drinking or wholesome) water. Water must be distributed to all parts of the plant under adequate pressure, which in the mains pipeline should be at least 20 psi. Hot and cold water are necessary; the hot from a central heating system, at not less than 82°C. On-site water storage tanks holding at least one day's consumption are usual. The recommended water requirement is 454 litres/day per pig, 272 litres/day per bovine, 45 litres/day per sheep, plus 25% at a reasonable pressure of 15 psi. Bacon factories and manufacturing operations require special assessment.

If non-potable water is used for steam production, refrigeration or fire control, it must be carried in separate lines and identified as such.

### *Electricity*

Industrial three-phase electricity should be supplied, and a stand-by generator installed. Central steam boilers may be fuelled by oil or gas, which require storage tanks of adequate size.

### *Drainage*

This most important function should have floors in wet areas that slope uniformly to drains, the gradient being 1:50. Good drainage also depends to a large extent on the type of floors provided. Floor drains should be fitted at the rate of one drain for each 40 $m^2$ of floor area.

Low places where water and blood could collect are to be guarded against. Where blood tends to collect, e.g. under dressing rails, special provision must be made to supply drainage valleys which should slope to drains in the valleys at a gradient of at least 1:25. The valleys themselves should be 60 cm wide and should continue under dressing lines for the collection of all blood and bone dust.

*Catch basins* for grease recovery and *traps* and *vents* on drains must also be provided, both to be properly sealed and easily cleanable and the latter to be effectively vented to outside the building.

Special arrangements have to be made for dealing with stomach and intestinal contents, the drains for bovine material to be at least 20 cm in diameter and for the smaller species 15 cm.

In the UK it is recommended that all drains in the slaughterhall be trapped with 4 mm screens, to prevent the possibility of contamination of the effluent with pieces of nervous tissue greater than 1 g—the possible infective dose of BSE.

Grids covering drains should be made of cast iron or other approved material.

Close attention to drainage is essential for hygienic operations besides assisting in cleaning procedures.

### *Lighting*

Adequate natural or artificial lighting must be provided throughout the meat plant. Natural lighting should take the form of efficient north lights. North-facing windows will largely preclude solar gain, but frosted glass or glass fitted with solar film will also reduce solar radiation.

The type of lighting must not distort colours. It is generally recommended that the overall intensity should not be less than:

540 lux (50 foot-candles) at all inspection points
220 lux (20 foot-candles) in work rooms
110 lux (10 foot-candles) in other areas.

These intensities of light are usually taken at levels of 0.9 m from the floor, except in inspection areas where the height is 1.5 m. Protective shields must be fitted to lights in areas where fresh meat and offal are exposed to prevent contamination from shattered glass.

### *Ventilation*

Adequate ventilation must be provided to prevent excessive heat, steam and condensation. Ventilation prevents the accumulation of odours, dust, etc., but it should not cause draughts and thus problems for staff. Particularly in multistorey plants, draughts arising from lift wells, stairways, chutes, etc. should be prevented. Opening ventilators and windows should be screened and internal window sills sloped.

### *Floor and wall finishes*

All parts of the meat plant must be capable of being easily cleaned. This means that all floors and walls should be non-toxic and non-absorbent, the floors also being non-slip. The floors of slaughter halls, lairage, work and chill rooms should be coved at wall junctions.

It is recommended that walls should be faced with a smooth, durable, impermeable material with a light-coloured washable finish up to a height of not less than 3 m from the floor and preferably reaching the ceiling, which should also be smooth, hard and impervious.

The types of operations encountered in abattoirs inevitably involve *impact damage*. Good design and layout can do much to prevent this, as can the employment of careful, skilful operatives. Surface materials should be capable of withstanding impact, doors should be wide enough to allow easy passage of personnel, carcases and offal on conveyorised lines and trucks, and their jambs should be protected with metal covers (they should be solid where necessary, self-closing or in the form of double-action doors). Hard-wearing materials are also essential.

High levels of humidity combined with low temperatures and the nature of the operations make for varying degrees of condensation, depending on the time of the year. Good ventilation, insulation and easily cleaned surfaces will do much to minimise this nuisance, but additional extractors may be necessary on occasion.

Abattoir operations entail wet floors on which are usually present quantities of fat and blood. While floor finishes should be easily cleaned, they should also be non-slip. Operatives are required to wear easily cleaned, safety (non-slip) footwear, and no one should be allowed on a slaughter hall floor, in particular, without proper footwear. In certain places it is wise to incorporate carborundum or aluminium oxide in order to provide a non-slip surface. Pin-rolling or tamping of the surface also assists in preventing slipping.

Walls and floors may be made of concrete, granolithic concrete or tiles (ceramic, quarry, steel-surfaced, cast iron or polymers). Wall sheets are often used in the form of plastic laminates, aluminium, polished asbestos, PVC-faced rustless metal or stainless steel. Although it is the most expensive, stainless steel is undoubtedly the most satisfactory; it is very strong, easily cleaned, completely non-corrosive, and does not flake, cause discoloration or affect the taste of meat and offal. Studies on the cleanability of various materials carried out at the University of Michigan, USA, showed that stainless steel ranks almost equal with glass and china.

### *Doors*

These should be wide enough to allow passage of product without contact with the doorway. A width of 1.37 m (4.5 ft) is usually adequate. Doors must be constructed of rust-resistant material. If made of wood, they should be covered with rust-resistant smooth impermeable material. Double-acting doors should have a glass (reinforced) panel at eye level. Plastic strip doors, because of difficulty of cleaning and their liability to scratch, crack or break, are unsuitable except where packaged product is moved.

## Equipment design

Since mechanical handling systems and other types of equipment used in meat plants usually form the major part of the overall cost, it is wise to consider design aspects as well as operating efficiency, durability, etc. Faults in construction and design include:

1. Use of wood for equipment and tools. Wood cannot be cleaned and disinfected with ease and is liable to deteriorate rapidly in moist surroundings.
2. Use of unsuitable fastenings which can work loose and contaminate the product.
3. Provision of ledges and corners where meat, fat, etc. can lodge and cause bacterial build-up.
4. Badly recessed nuts, bolts and screws can also gather scraps and hinder cleansing.
5. Use of expanded metal for decks, walkways and staircases especially near conveyors. All these should be constructed from non-slip solid plate.
6. Metal joints which are rough. Joints should be welded and then ground to a smooth finish.
7. Fixed covers for conveyors that make cleaning difficult.

The design and location of equipment should be such as to allow for ease and efficiency of cleaning and disinfection.

## Pest control

The ingress of birds, rats, mice and insects such as flies and cockroaches can cause serious problems since in addition to the dirt they create they may carry food-poisoning organisms, even those responsible for zoonoses. *Birds*, especially sparrows, starlings, feral pigeons and gulls inhabit areas where food and nesting material are available. They feed on meat scraps, dung, insects, grain and food scraps discarded or even on occasions purposely laid by personnel.

In some food factories sparrows have become an even greater problem than mice, defying air curtains and currents, netting, flashing lights, bird distress noises, anti-perch gel, etc.

While these measures may be useful in some instances, avoidance depends on a high level of hygiene and the discouragement of anthropomorphic attitudes to providing food. An effective final means of control is the use of narcotic baits (alphachloralose and pentobarbitone sodium baited on wheat with a sticker oil, e.g. risella oil).

*Rats and mice* are also attracted by the presence of food and may gain entrance from adjoining properties or be transported into the plant in fodder, etc. Mice have been known to be introduced into an abattoir in polystyrene insulation for use in chill rooms. Droppings and musk trails are indicators of their presence.

Control is effected by ensuring cleanliness, absence of food scraps and the use of specialist pest control firms. A sketch plan of the premises indicating numbered bait points should be produced and a record of usage of each point noted, as well as dates of inspection and any structural defects. These should be inspected regularly and if increased activity is seen further control measures must be taken.

*Insects* are drawn into food premises mainly by the presence of pre-digested food, such as excreta, and by warmth. Nearby breeding grounds such as waste tips, stagnant ponds and sewage works may be responsible for the advent of flies. Plant location and design are important factors in prevention of fly infestation, for example, the manure bay must be sited away from meat areas.

Scrupulous cleanliness, the avoidance of direct sunlight in rooms, the use of air curtains with horizontal air draughts, strip door curtains, ultraviolet light, electrocutors, mesh screens, etc. are of value, especially cleanliness. Insecticidal sprays should be used with discretion and confined to non-meat sectors.

## Small abattoir units

While larger meat plants are capable of greater throughputs per man, they have high fixed overheads which can be a problem for their operators. Under these circumstances the smaller plant has advantages, particularly in remote areas, by being sited close to production regions, thereby cutting transport costs.

The FPE plant (Food Processing Engineering Ltd, Thankerton, Biggar, Lanarkshire MLI2 6PA, UK) is a prefabricated unit 9.14 m (30 ft)

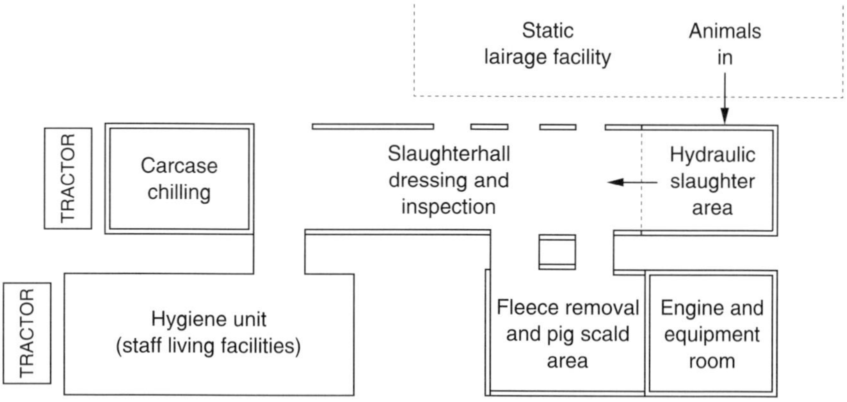


**DIMENSIONS**

| | |
|---|---|
| Main slaughterhall (including hydraulic extension) | 17.0 m |
| Trailer unit (scald area + engine room) | 7.5 m |
| Hygiene unit | 9.0 m |

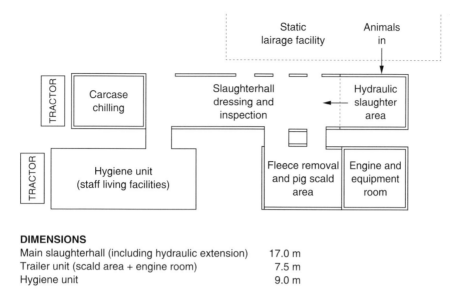

**Fig. 3.1** General layout of the mobile slaughterhall.

long, 3.7 m (12 ft) wide and 4.6 m (15 ft) high in the slaughter section combined with refrigeration, cutting and boning and by-products facilities, etc. It is capable of handling 10 cattle, 20 sheep and 10 pigs daily. Deer can also be catered for as well as casualty animals.

A recent innovation is the concept of a *mobile slaughter facility*, which has been developed by the Humane Slaughter Association (Humane Slaughter Association and Council of Justice of Animals, The Old School, Brewhouse Hill, Wheathampsteal, Herts AL4 8AN, UK (Fig. 3.1). This is based on a large trailer unit on an HGV tractor. Fitted with a stunning box, it includes hoists, bleeding area, dressing cradles, chill room and storage for by-products, detained and effluent material. The unit operates from a home base and visits farms on request, the farms providing basic facilities of water, electricity, lairage pens, toilet and changing rooms. While the advantages in animal welfare are obvious, the organisation of the important items of ante-mortem and post-mortem inspection must be given careful attention.

## LAIRAGE

A knowledge of animal behaviour is fundamental to lairage design. The importance of suitable lairage accommodation for animals awaiting slaughter cannot be overestimated, since a period of rest before slaughter can often have a markedly beneficial effect on the appearance and subsequent marketability of the carcase.

The *livestock reception area* should preferably be roofed to protect animals and staff, particularly during identification, handling and sorting of stock. If at all possible the off-loading dock should be about 1.2 m high to permit careful offloading, especially of stock carried on upper tiers of lorries. Although such vehicles should have a lowering device, all too often injuries and fractures are sustained. A suitable office for reception area staff is an essential, as are efficient cleansing facilities. Sufficient room should be allowed for manoeuvring and temporary parking. A weighbridge, suitably located, is a useful facility.

The entry point to the meat plant for livestock is a suitable place for the instruction of all and sundry in the careful handling of animals and disease control measures. A useful notice is *'All stock must be handled gently and quietly'*, which is a reminder for lorry drivers and lairage personnel. Irregularities in transporation can be noted at the reception area and the appropriate action taken.

In the handling of livestock it must be remembered that animals prefer walking up slopes rather than down steep gradients. Drain inlets in the centres of passageways should be avoided since stock will refuse to walk across them. Every effort must be made to avoid sharp corners and projections of any kind and gates should preferably be placed at the end, not in the middle, of the pen side. If tubular partitions are used, the horizontal bars should be correctly spaced to prevent strangulation. Lairage floor gradients should be at least 1:50.

Instead of straight *passageways* or lanes it is advantageous for them to be curved, especially the main passageway leading from the holding pens to the single-file chute prior to the stunning box. Associated with this curved lane is a series of elongated *pens*, each 3–3.7 m wide, and set at an angle of 60° to it. The pen gates are longer than the drive lane, eliminating sharp corners. The movement of stock is in one direction. The main curved holding lane has solid sides, gates to separate different lots and a catwalk for lairage personnel. There would appear to be no reason why cattle, sheep and pigs cannot be handled in this system, providing the species can be separated towards their respective slaughter areas.

Animal behaviour is an important consideration in lairage design and operation, particularly the reaction of animals to extreme change in environment. Strident voice and noises, dark objects (especially if these are moving), sudden movements of personnel, drain openings in the centres of passageways, sharp corners, etc., are contraindicated. The animal has good depth of vision in front of it but not laterally. Cattle, indeed all the herd animals, will follow a leader and use can be made of this in utilising trained goats or sheep to lead stock forward.

While durable tubular fencing has been found satisfactory for holding pens, final *drive races* should have solid sides, non-slip floor surfaces and lighting to encourage the animals to go forward. In larger plants it is necessary to have two single-line crushes for cattle to allow for stock movement should an animal fall in one race. Side gates should be installed to handle such emergencies and also to provide escape gates for personnel in the drive race when they are confronted with wild animals. The length of the final race is determined by the overall throughput of the meat plant. It is an important area for ensuring an even flow forward, checking slaughter sequence numbers and other forms of identification. In a large plant this race can be 36 m long, with stop gates to prevent the animals going backwards, 80 cm wide, and reach to about waist height. Catwalks must be provided alongside the race to enable handlers to control stock movement, check identification, etc.

All too often animals will baulk on approaching the stunning pen because of the noise generated by the pen doors. Equipment manufacturers must recognise the need for noise-free equipment. Gates located in the drive race and sliding or one-way gates in the single-file race should be made of expanded metal or closely-spaced bars to enable the animals to see through them.

Every effort must be made to avoid frightening the animals. Constant vigilance is required to ensure that there is no bullying by dominant individuals and these, in addition to females in oestrus and horned stock, must be kept separate.

In the United Kingdom the Ministry of Agriculture, Fisheries and Food recommend the following pen sizes for the housing of livestock in abattoirs:

| | |
|---|---|
| Cattle (loose) | 2.3–2.8 m$^2$ |
| Pigs (bacon and small porkers) | 0.6 m$^2$ |
| Heavy pigs, calves and sheep | 0.7 m$^2$ |

## Ante-mortem (AM) inspection facilities

The essential task of veterinary AM examination requires ample natural or artificial lighting, which should be even and diffuse, and an isolation pen with a *crush* where a suspect animal can be clinically examined.

## Cattle lairage

A suitable lairage has a series of pens with wall or tubular partitions and 2.4 m wide gates (at the end of each pen) which can be used for the pens and/or closing the adjoining passageway. For cattle, pens may be 7.6 m × 6 m, large enough to hold 20–25 cattle.

*Drinking water* must always be available to animals and each pen should be provided with a gravitational water supply; one cistern is sufficient to feed three troughs. Automatic water bowls, though satisfactory for cows, tend to frighten young cattle if they are not used to them. In a lairage of the tie-up type, long water troughs in front of the cattle are quite satisfactory and are more easily cleansed than individual troughs or bowls. Hayracks must be provided and regulations require that animals must be fed twice daily except on the morning of the day of intended slaughter or the afternoon preceding the morning of intended slaughter. Horses, however, must be fed on the afternoon preceding the day of intended slaughter.

Hydrant points should be placed conveniently, so that all parts of the lairage can be reached by a sufficient supply of water for cleansing; an adequate estimate is 680 litres per beast slaughtered. An important factor which facilitates cleansing is a lairage with a passage wide enough to admit entry of a vehicle for the removal of manure and dead animals. Whatever system of lairage is adopted, special emphasis must be placed on ease of cleansing, comfort for the animals and ease of handling them.

## Sheep lairage

Sheep pens should be 0.9 m high with passages 0.9 m wide between them. To prevent animals putting their heads through the lower rails of the pens, these rails should not be more than 15 cm apart. Double-hinged gates should be used in all sheep and pig pens, as they greatly facilitate entry and exit of stock; two adjoining pens can accommodate an overflow of animals if a sliding gate is provided between the pens. Since sheep drink quite freely, sheep pens must be provided with water troughs, placed some 50 cm from the floor to prevent fouling. Hayracks should also be provided above the level of the sheep's heads.

Straw should be provided for solid floors to help keep the sheep dry. Clean or expanded metal floors will achieve the same purpose.

There is no objection to cattle and sheep lairages being provided in the same building, but while pigs and sheep may be housed together without detrimental effect, cattle do not appear to rest well in the company of pigs.

## Pig lairage (Figs 3.2 and 3.3)

Pig pens are preferably constructed with solid walls. If rails are used they should be stronger than those required for the sheep lairage; the lower horizontal rails of the pen should not be more than 15 cm apart to prevent pigs putting their heads between the rails. The feeding troughs should be so designed that the pigs cannot gain access to them while the troughs are being cleansed and filled. The pens should be long and narrow to allow more pigs to rest against the walls.

In most Danish pig plants the handling of pigs in pens is carried out manually using gates mounted on side rollers for emptying the pens (Fig. 3.2). The driveway towards the race connected with the stunning area, however, is normally fitted with mechanical push gates.

A recent innovation in Danish pig plants is an *automatic lairage system* with pens divided into sections each holding a maximum of 15 pigs. Automatic filling and emptying of the pens is

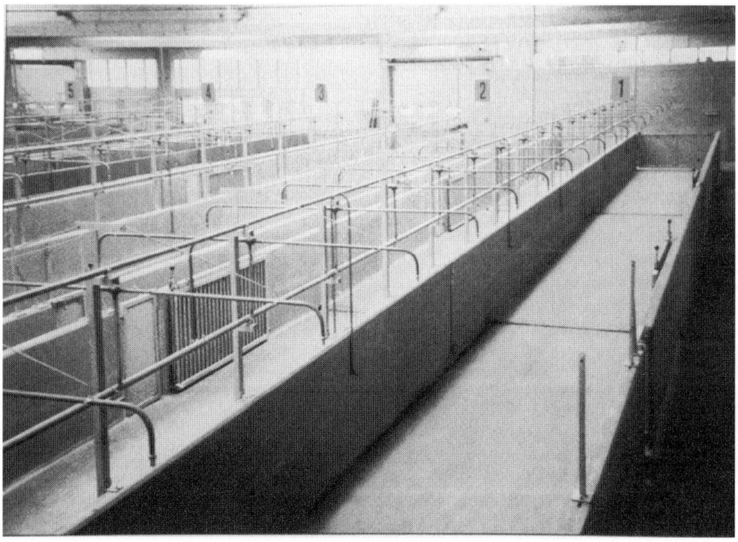

**Fig. 3.2** Danish pig lairage showing long pens with concrete wall and manually-pushed gates on rollers for forward emptying of the pens. (By courtesy of Danish Meat Research Institute, Roskilde, Denmark)

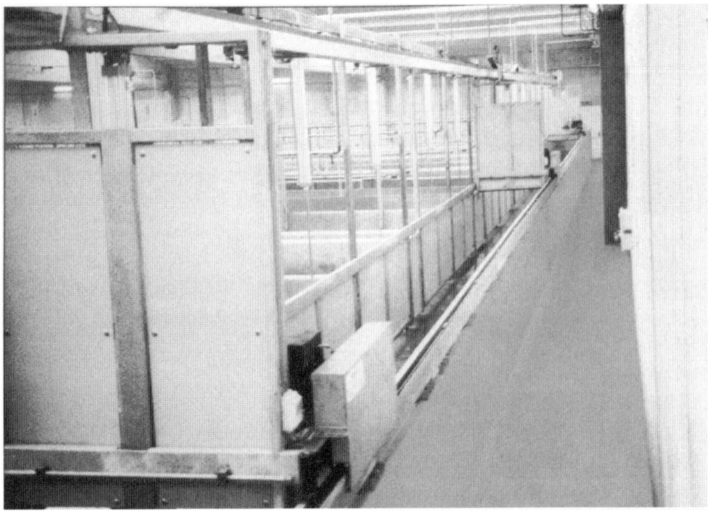

**Fig. 3.3** Danish automatic lairage system showing lifting/driving gates. (By courtesy of Danish Meat Research Institute, Roskilde, Denmark)

achieved using PLC-controlled lifting/driving gates. The system is said to improve welfare standards with reduction of damage due to fighting. Two single files are employed in the race section where some manual assistance is required.

A fine water spray and/or litter in the lairage pens are useful means of reducing fighting among pigs, cooling them and reducing the incidence of pale, soft, exudative (PSE) pork.

### Deer lairage (Figs 3.4 and 3.5)

Although the majority of farmed deer in Britain are still slaughtered by shooting in the field, some are handled in special farm abattoirs and others in larger abattoirs. Because of the nervous nature of these animals, which are very subject to stress, it is essential that good facilities for holding and slaughter are provided. It is also vital that expert handlers are on hand.

The UK Farm Animal Welfare Council (FAWC) has recommended that the slaughter of deer should take place only in specially licensed premises, and that deer should not be slaughtered while other species are being handled/slaughtered unless separated from those other activities by solid walls to exclude noise.

The Farmed Game Directive 94/495 implements their recommendations. Reception areas for unloading and lairage pens should

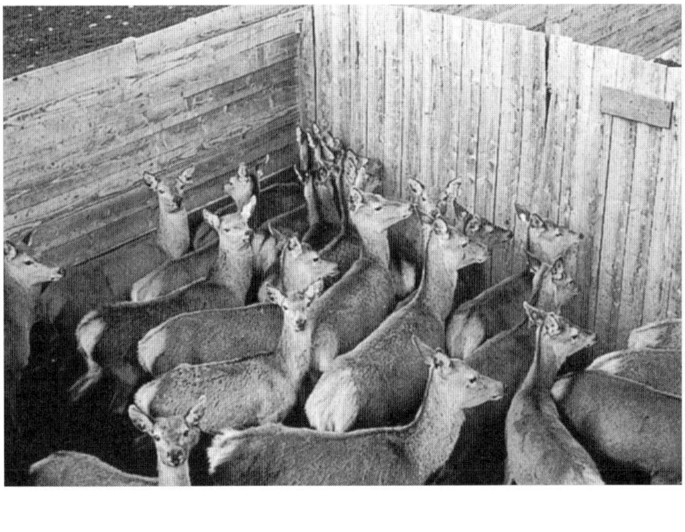

**Fig 3.4** Deer lairage showing pen with high partitions. (By courtesy of Dr T. J. Fletcher)

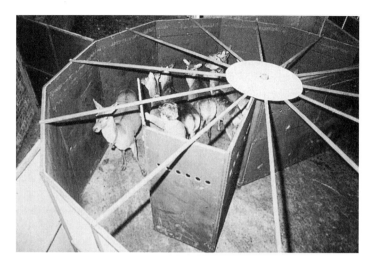

**Fig. 3.5** Deer lairage showing pen with revolving crush. (By courtesy of Dr T. J. Fletcher)

have smooth high-impact walls, and a circular crush gate of 5 m maximum diameter with two solid swing gates, centrally hung at least 1.83 m (6 ft) high. Unlike the requirements for cattle and sheep, lighting should be subdued throughout the lairage and stunning areas, which should interconnect (FAWC, 1985).

*Toilet* and *handwashing facilities* must be provided in the vicinity of the lairage. *Bootwashing equipment* is an essential component for lairage staff. *Electric goads* should be regulated to the lowest effective voltage – less than 50 v AC.

### Washing of livestock

Although washing of animals, e.g. cattle, bison, horses etc., is practised in tropical and subtropical countries, it is contraindicated in temperate regions, e.g. the United Kingdom, except possibly for pigs. Facilities usually consist of a foot bath spray system or bath and an adequate draining area prior to slaughter. A system for recovering solids and a final potable water wash must be included.

### Manure disposal

Considerable quantities of lairage waste in the form of bedding and dung require periodic removal, preferably to an elevated, covered site near the lairage, from which it can be conveniently reloaded for removal. It is convenient to load it directly on to a large trailer which can be removed as necessary. The manure obtained from the stomachs and intestines of slaughtered animals requires separate treatment. It is sometimes used as compost for horticultural purposes, and recently in the United States as cattle feed, after dehydration (see Chapter 4).

## SLAUGHTERHALL

The transfer of animals from lairage to slaughterhall is easy if the abattoir is well designed (see also Chapter 7). If an upper kill floor is used and the site is on a slope, the animals can be walked directly on the slaughter floor; alternatively, a ramp can be provided. Cattle and sheep can readily be driven up a ramp as steep as 1 in 6, though the ramp should be provided with battens and a catwalk. In some cases animals are stunned on the ground level then hoisted after bleeding for subsequent dressing on the top floor. This procedure is not recommended because of the problems of muscle splashing and poor bleeding brought about by delayed sticking.

The size and type of slaughterhall for cattle depends on which of the slaughtering systems is adopted, but in all cases it should be an open hall, with generous floor space, and well ventilated and lighted.

### Stunning area

(See also Chapter 7.)

The area in front of the stunning pen should be at least 3 m in width to the opposing wall or bleeding trough and be fitted with upright bars 5 cm in diameter and 1.2 m high, spaced at 40 cm intervals for safety purposes should improperly stunned animals regain their feet. The floor must be properly drained and possess high-impact and non-slip properties. A raised sturdy frame of expanded metal on to which the animal is ejected aids cleanliness and reduces wetness. Every effort must be made to reduce hide contamination.

### Bleeding area

No meat plant should be built without careful consideration being given to the full utilisation of by-products, edible and inedible. Blood is too valuable a commodity to be discarded, as in past customs. Edible is more valuable than inedible.

The *bleeding trough* should be at least 1.5 m wide, possess a good gradient, side walls of the same height, and two drains, one for blood only and the other for water when cleansing only. The length of the bleeding line will depend on the throughput and the system of conveying carcases, but should be generous, since the majority of blood flow requires 6–8 min. The bleeding trough has two points for the reception of blood: one at the actual point of sticking where the greater volume of blood will be handled; and thereafter a longer gradual slope that collects 'drip' blood classed as inedible. The overhead bleeding rail should be about 4.9 m above the floor of the dry landing area, dressing rails about 3.4 m high. The bleeding trough must have a smooth impervious surface, often a suitable grade of stainless steel.

Efficient arrangements for bleeding of stock will make for better-quality meat and cleaner conditions on the carcase dressing floor.

Various systems of hygienic bleeding of livestock, mostly cattle and pigs, are in use and these may or may not be combined with an in-plant blood processing department. The specialised nature of blood processing, as with inedible by-product processing, means that it may be more satisfactory to collect these items efficiently and then consign them to an outside central plant for final processing.

For hygienic bleeding for edible purposes, *the stainless hollow knife* combined with cleanliness and a sodium citrate/phosphate anticoagulant is used. The knife is held in the wound by hand, by a rotating endless screw, or by other means. For meat plants of small capacity, individual containers are used for holding the blood; with large throughputs and high rates of slaughter, several blood draining knives (as many as 14) can be used in a 'carousel' which rotates synchronously with the bleeding conveyor. Arrangements must be made for routine sterilisation of the knives and adequate staff to man this additional operation.

The hollow knife is made of stainless steel in two sizes, for cattle and pigs. Various designs are available, but they usually consist of a tubular handle with a deflector plate and two blades set at right-angles to each other. They are easy to strip for sharpening and cleaning and are combined with an anticoagulant dispensing tube. The broad blade should be directed in the longitudinal direction of the animal and, provided the animals have been properly stunned, it is not necessary to fix forelegs, still less to indulge in *pithing*, a totally unnecessary practice in modern meat plants. A suitable form of tubing, e.g. made of collagen, connects the knife to containers where the blood is cooled prior to collection.

A system which correlates each batch of blood to the carcase from which it originates must be operated so that if a carcase is subsequently condemned the blood from that animal may also be condemned.

The bleeding trough for sheep and pigs should preferably be enclosed on both sides as for cattle and have a width of 1.1–1.2 m with the overhead bleeding rail 2.7 m high, and dressing rails 2.3 m high for sheep and 3.4 m high in the case of pigs.

Subsequent leg, hide or fleece removal, evisceration, carcase splitting, inspection, kidney and channel fat (KKCF) removal, carcase washing and shrouding stations must have platforms at suitable positions and heights for operatives and inspectors to work efficiently and without unnecessary stooping and labour. Of particular importance is the position of the *viscera inspection table*, especially for adult cattle (see Fig. 3.6), where the top of the moving-top table should be about 2.7 m from the top of the conveyor rail and the vertical centre of the carcase positioned at the edge of the viscera inspection table (1.5 m wide).

### On-the-rail dressing

The development of *line dressing* of carcases originally emanated from Canada. Essentially,

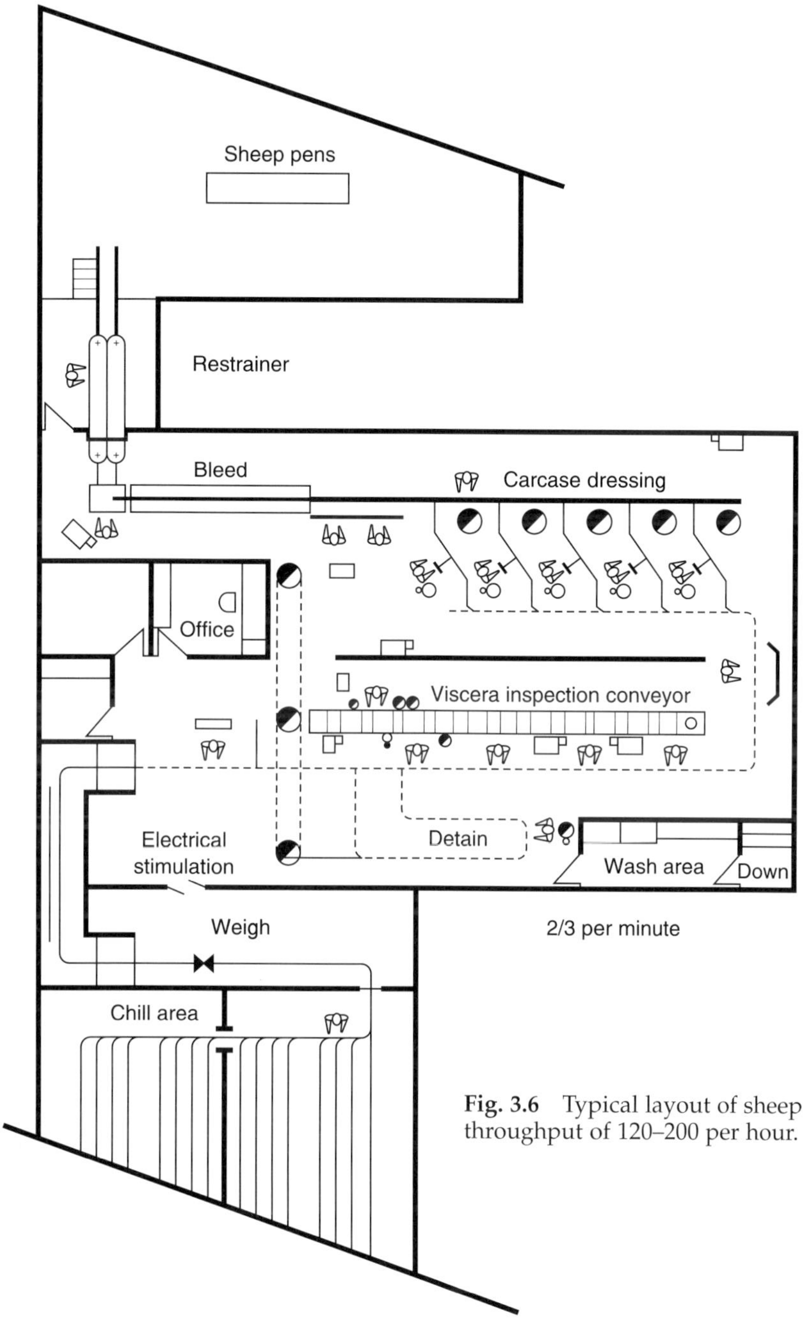


**Fig. 3.6** Typical layout of sheep facility for throughput of 120–200 per hour.

the carcase is conveyed by gravity or power along an overhead rail; after stunning and bleeding, the process of dressing is divided up into various stages, each undertaken by a separate operator as the carcase reaches him. Although most plants use the traditional one man–one job approach, a more modern method, currently in operation in New Zealand, is to allow one operative to follow the carcase through several operations. Besides reducing the labour load, this arrangement also makes for better job satisfaction. A combination of several machines, tools and correlated items of equipment (brisket saw, hock cutters, hide puller, aitch bone cutter, etc.) enables complete dressing to be carried out at high rates of slaughter.

Without the line method of slaughter it would be impossible to reach the production achieved in modern meat plants, which may be as high as 5000 cattle, 10 000 sheep and 3500 pigs every 10 hours.

Several systems of line dressing are in operation, the type depending mainly on the level of throughput, equipment design and species, being most complicated in cattle. Constant research is undertaken with a view to effecting more efficient methods of line dressing.

There are four main types of line dressing for cattle:

*Gravity rail system*

In this method the carcases, suspended from a spreader and single-wheel trolley or runner, are gravitated to each station and stopped by a manually-operated stop on the overhead rail.

The system is used for lower slaughter rates of 10–40 cattle/h. It is probably the most compact and economical of the systems. Being the simplest in design, there is less chance of serious breakdowns with consequent loss of production. Various items of equipment may be used with the gravity rail, e.g. a moving-top viscera inspection table or a paunch truck, but, because throughput is small, a mechanical hide-puller is rarely used. Adequate ceiling height is necessary because of the pitch of the rail to gravitate the carcases.

*Intermittent powered system*

This system can be used for rates of 10–75 cattle/h. It involves the mechanical moving of the carcases suspended on a spreader (gambrel) and trolley along a level rail at intervals by means of a variable timing device which can be pre-set to suit the slaughter rate.

*Continuous powered system*

In this method the dressing line is in continuous motion and is used for higher rates of kill, 40–120 cattle/h. More sophisticated equipment is associated with this slaughter line, e.g. mechanical hide-puller, moving top inspection table as with the 'Canpak' system.

The carcase can be revolved a full 360° while on the rail, allowing the operator to work all sides from one position. Associated with all line systems are platforms which can be varied in height and position, enabling the operator to carry out his task more efficiently.

*'Canpak' system*

This is a continuous conveyorised method in which the carcases are suspended by heavy beef trolleys or runners from the overhead rail; no spreader or gambrel is used. Developed and patented by Canada Packers Ltd, Toronto, Canada, it is probably the most common form of line system now used in large modern meat plants. Rates of slaughter from 50 to 150 cattle or more per hour can be achieved depending on the type and extent of associated equipment and the number of operators.

A typical sequence of operations on a modern line system is shown in the beef slaughter flow chart in Fig. 3.7.

In the UK a number of additional tasks are carried out to remove the bovine specified offals, and to check their removal.

*Advantages of line dressing*

1. Since carcases are conveyed to each dressing station, there is no need for operatives to be idle while carcases are being hoisted or positioned.
2. The line system is said to be safer for operatives than traditional slaughter systems.
3. Because carcases do not touch the floor and their dressing is more conveniently carried out, 'on the rail' dressing is hygienic.
4. Elimination of the handling of heavy shackles, trolleys and spreaders, the comfortable platform position for personnel and the use of mechanical tools reduce tedious labour.
5. The reduction of lost motion and unnecessary movement of the carcase saves space.
6. An efficient line system increases throughput and enhances the value of the carcase, hide and offal because of superior workmanship.

*Possible disadvantages*

The line system, however, being mechanically complex, demands a high standard of engineering maintenance, and when

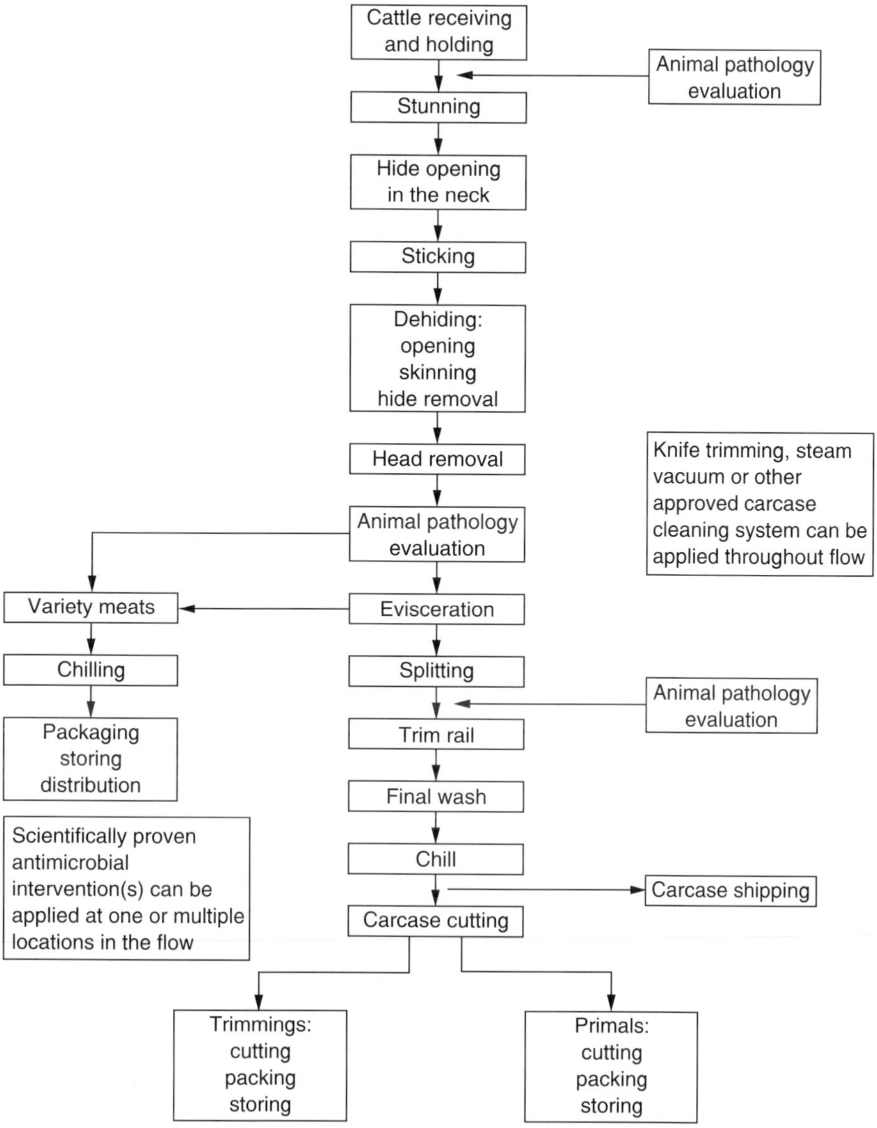


**Fig. 3.7** Beef slaughter, cutting and packing.

breakdowns do occur production ceases completely. The repetitive nature of the work can be largely offset by job rotation if personnel are so trained. Meat inspection is sometimes said to be made more difficult and possibly less efficient. An efficient system of meat inspection on a line system involves proper carcase and offal conveyor synchronisation, a good identification system, adequate, efficient and conscientious inspection staff, proper inspection points with ability to coordinate findings, an efficient recording setup and adequate *time* for the examination of each carcase. At the higher rates of slaughter, separate recording staff should be utilised, particularly for detailed information. A system of audio links can be used for communication between inspectors and recorders, one of whom is required for each line.

A line system of slaughter with a rate of 60–75 cattle/h needs approximately nine meat inspectors and one veterinarian for initial and final inspection. Correspondingly smaller numbers are necessary for pig and especially sheep inspection. Adequate space and facilities for inspection must always be provided. Indeed the all-too-common tendency to over-save on space when installing line slaughter systems must be resisted.

For new beef installations, consideration should be given to the performance of *hot boning* subsequent to the dressing line. This practice allows for the preparation and chilling of cuts without the problem of cold shortening.

*Sterilisers*

An adequate number of efficient sterilisers operating at 82°C for hand tools, shackles etc. must be provided on all slaughter/dressing floors, all conveniently placed for operator use.

*Bootwash/apronwash* facilities are necessary for operative cleanliness.

## **Sheep slaughterhall** (Fig. 3.6)

Though larger installations are best served by retaining the cattle slaughterhall for cattle only, in smaller establishments where cattle and sheep killing are not likely to take place at the same time a portion of the cattle hall can be adapted for slaughter and dressing of sheep. In the latter, sheep are driven to a passageway adjoining the slaughterhall, carried by hand into the slaughterhall and placed on crates (cradles, cratches, crutches) preparatory to stunning and dressing.

Line slaughter is frequently carried out on sheep and a line employing 17 operatives with a potential production of 150 sheep/h would have the following stations :

- **1** Pen sheep and stun
- **2** Shackle and hoist
- **3** Stick
- **4** De-elevate to crutch conveyor
- **5–9** Conveyor dressing (remove feet, commence fleece removal, saw brisket)
- **10** Elevate to overhead rail
- **11** Clear tail and commence backing
- **12** Back and chute fleece
- **13** Remove head
- **14** Eviscerate abdomen
- **15** Wash
- **16** Eviscerate thorax
- **17** Weigh and tag
- **18** Final wash.

The feet should be removed with a special instrument, avoiding the usual practice of individual removal with the skinning knife and the all-too frequent littering of the floor with these parts.

The New Zealand Meat Industry Research Institute (MIRINZ) have developed a superior method of *automatic pelt removal* to produce blemish-free and hygienic carcases with the minimum of labour. The valuable hindquarter is completely untouched and there is no stretching of the pelt. Termed the 'inverted' method, the carcase is suspended by the forelegs or in a near-horizontal position on twin conveyors. A 'Y' cut is made from forelegs to throat releasing the 'vee' flap, which is fed into the brisket skinner to clear the foreleg pockets. The two shoulder flaps are then pulled down and the 'vee' flap is split by hand. The head is removed and discarded under veterinary control. The pelt is further prepared for automatic removal by skinning the belly and groin. The carcase is now ready for the operation of two pelting machines – the shoulder puller and the final puller, the former drawing the shoulder flaps in a downward/backward direction while the latter (a hydraulically-operated arm and clamp) grips the fleece centrally and strips it downwards off the hindquarter and shanks. The fleece is then released through a floor chute to the pelt room.

## **Pig slaughterhall**

Pig slaughter is better carried out in a separate hall from that used for cattle and sheep, as the moist atmosphere, which is inseparable from the scalding of pigs, is not conducive to the good setting and drying of beef and mutton carcases. EEC regulations require that in slaughter premises where both pigs and other animal species are slaughtered a special place must be provided for slaughtering pigs. However, such special place shall not be compulsory if the slaughter of pigs and that of other animals takes place at different times; but in such cases scalding, depilation, scraping and singeing must be carried out in special places

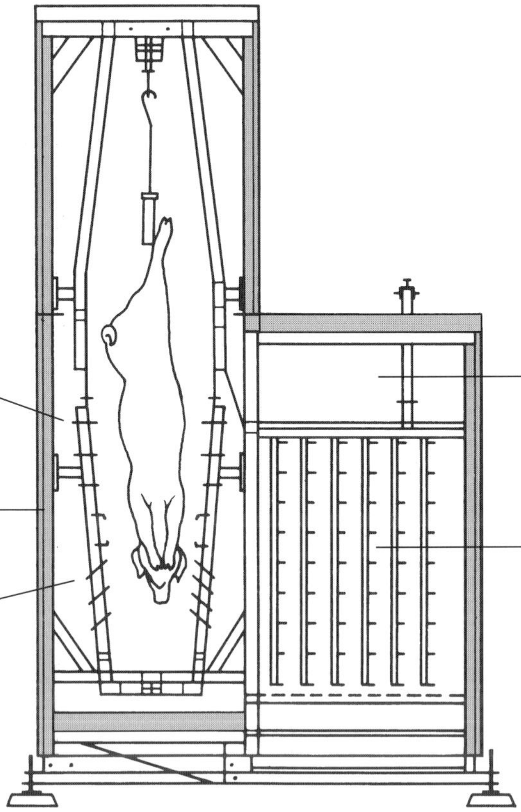


**Fig. 3.8** Vertical scalding of pigs showing cross-section of humidifying chamber, channel for recirculated air and humidifying zone. (By courtesy of SFK AmbA, Copenhagen, Denmark)

which are clearly separated from the slaughter line either by an open space of at least 5 m or by a partition of at least 3 m high.

After bleeding, pigs are scalded and then scraped to remove the hair. In the smaller abattoirs scraping is done by hand, but in large abattoirs and bacon factories a mechanical dehairing machine is used. It is estimated that if there is a regular throughput of some 200 pigs on 2–3 days per week, a dehairing plant is necessary. An extraction system, which removes steam from the canopies over the scalding tanks and keeps the temperature of the steam raised by heated air, serves to prevent condensation and fogginess. Provision must also be made so that the offals from each animal can be easily identified with the carcase.

A typical pig slaughter operation of up to 350 pigs/h would consist of the operations shown in the pork slaughter flow chart in Fig. 3.9.

*Scalding and dehairing*

The factors to be considered relating to scalding and dehairing are: hourly rate of slaughter; size of pig to be handled; ease of operation of the machines; efficiency of cleansing; and corrosion.

Because of the unhygienic circumstances associated with the typical scalding tank, it is likely in the future that other systems of removing hair and cleaning the surface of the skin will become commonplace. It has been shown in West Germany, for example, that before operations begin there can be as many as 39 400 bacteria per ml in the tank, rising to 45–800 million organisms per ml after the scalding of 600 pigs. Among these were aerobic and anaerobic spore-forming bacteria, cocci and organisms belonging to the coli-proteus groups; of 220 samples of scalding water, *Salmonella paratyphi* and *S. typhimurium* were isolated on

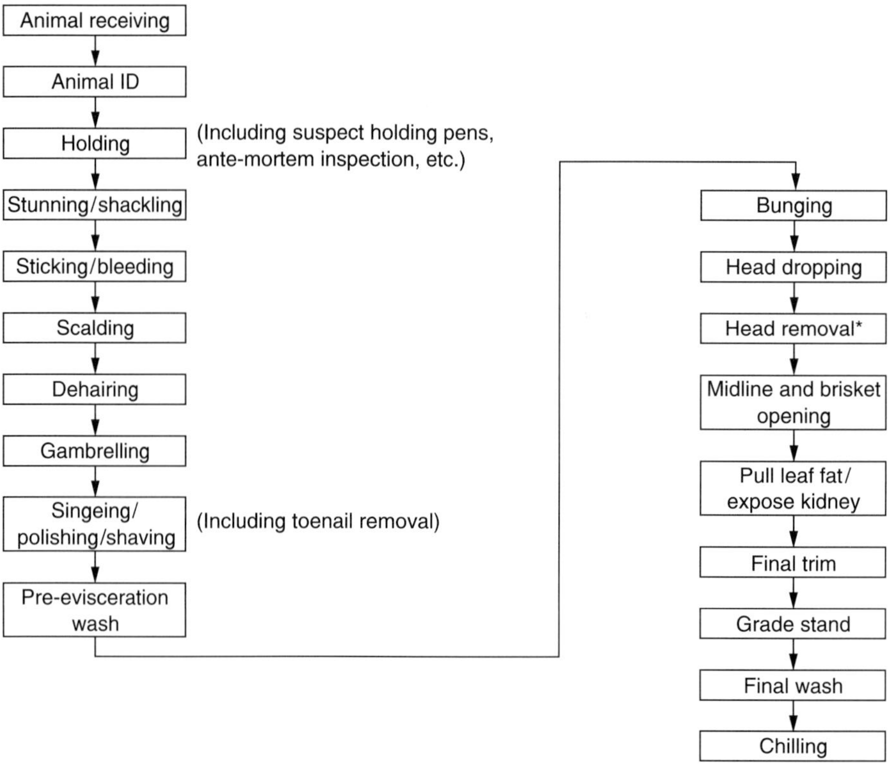


**Fig. 3.9** Pork slaughter flow chart (skin-on carcase). *The majority of industry operations remove the head following evisceration or splitting. In these situations the head removal step should be followed by an antibacterial intervention and the step be designated as a critical control point (CCP).

one occasion. In Holland, it has been discovered that developmental types of *Salmonella* could occur in the sludge of the scalding water and that a deep infection of the pig meat can arise from the bacterial flora on the surface. In addition to microorganisms, parasites such as *Ascaris suum* and whipworm *(Trichuris trichiura)*, hair, epithelial cells, *Balantidium coli*, and moulds such as *Aspergillus* and *Mucor* may be found. Many of these can gain entrance to the lungs and to the blood vessels in the stab wound (see also Chapter 9).

### *Vertical scalding*

Vertical scalding (Figs 3.8 and 3.10) of pig carcases involves the use of a double-walled tunnel in which steam, generated from a water bath in its bottom, is blown over the carcases and through a ventilator located over the condenser. The temperature in the tunnel is controlled by a thermostat at 61–64°C. The cooling water from the condenser in the tunnel is used to flush the pig carcases during the dehairing process. Before entry into the tunnel, the carcase should hang for 3 min and then lie on its side for 2 min. The pig carcases are then transported to the tunnel on a rising rail so that the head is lower than the other parts of the body during the whole scalding process, which lasts 6 min. Trimming and singeing take place afterwards. Vertical scalding is claimed to greatly improve the bacteriological standard of the pig meat, produce bacteria-free lungs and reduce muscular degeneration. This reduced incidence of PSE (pale, soft, exudative muscle) is said to be due to the fact that vertical scalding does not produce a rise in body temperature to above 41°C as in normal scalding operations. Dehairing is also said to be better with this method, and operating costs are also claimed to be reduced.

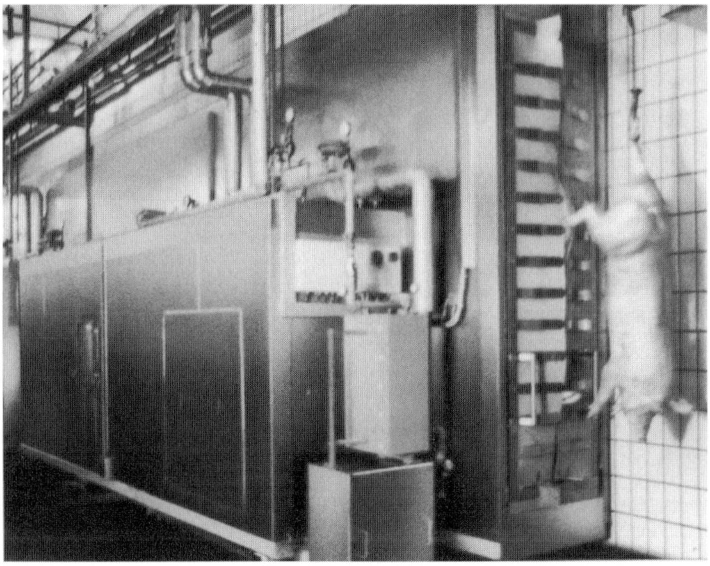

**Fig. 3.10** Vertical scalding of pigs. View of circulation chamber/humidifying zone with pig emerging. Cross-contamination is eliminated by humidified air at 61–64°C being blasted on to the carcase without immersion. (By courtesy of SFK AmbA, Copenhagen, Denmark)

## The isolation block (emergency slaughter unit)

This essential facility is actually a miniature abattoir, with a lairage for up to four cattle, a slaughter hall and hanging room. It should be situated near to the suspect meat detention room, and should also be in direct communication with the by-products department.

## Refrigeration accommodation

EEC Directive No. 64/433/EEC, as amended, provides that for the approval of slaughterhouses there must be sufficiently large *chilling* or refrigerating rooms. Fresh meat intended for intra-Community trade must be chilled immediately after the post-mortem inspection and kept at a constant temperature of not more than 7°C for carcases and cuts or 3°C for offal.

Except in the case of hot boning of meat after slaughter, it is essential that the specified temperatures be achieved quickly in order to offset bacterial spoilage, but not too quickly (see *Cold shortening*). Where hot boning is carried out, the resultant joints must be chilled before dispatch.

Since the Directive implies a continuous movement of carcases into chill following slaughter, it becomes necessary to provide a series of chilling units suited to the capacity of the meat plant and possessing a system of high rails for beef and low rails for sheep and pigs. In some smaller plants it may be possible to combine species, utilising the high rails for double-tiered pork and lamb carcases. A number of small rectangular chill rooms will reduce the time during which the chill room doors are open, speed up the chilling process and increase efficiency by reducing the mixing of hot and cold carcases.

The carcases must be hung in such a way as to allow free movement of cold air around them; rail spacing should be 0.9 m for beef, 0.7 m for pigs and 0.5 m for lambs. The minimum space between carcases on rails should be 0.3–0.4 m.

It is essential to record temperatures in order to control the chilling process, preferably on a continuous basis using charts or computer-generated records. The recording of relative humidity is also of value as is the occasional checking of air speed. *Temperature recording facilities* are required by the legislation of most countries.

EEC regulations forbid the use of exposed wood for chill doors; these should be made of durable, high-impact materials such as stainless steel, aluminium or reinforced plastics. They may be sliding or single- or double-hinged, and if hinged should open outwards.

Internal finishes should be durable and impervious, with good insulation and floor drainage. Areas of walls where contact with carcases occurs on loading should be protected with stainless steel or aluminium or plastic sheeting.

It is vital that chill and freezer doors be close-fitting and that they be provided with an internal opening device to avoid personnel being closed in the rooms.

The EEC requirements stated above present problems under commercial abattoir conditions. To begin with, the temperature of 7°C is too high a temperature for long-term storage of meat. Secondly, since many abattoirs wish to operate on a 24-hour schedule it is impossible to reduce the temperature of deep tissues to 7°C in this period without the onset of cold shortening. If a longer chilling period is possible, a pre-chilling period of 6–8 h will usually offset this undesirable result, which is more liable to occur in lamb.

As with chilling, different authorities specify different temperatures for *freezing*, which begins at temperatures below –2°C. In its regulations for 'intervention freezing' the EEC stipulates that beef quarters must be frozen to below –7°C, and pork to below –15°C, and stored at below –17°C for beef and below –20°C for pork; freezing times are not specified. These temperatures are considered to be low in comparison with current UK and USA practice.

### Detained meat room

Carcases detained for further examination should be routed by a special rail to the *detained meat room*, which should be located adjacent to the main slaughterhall inspection points in order to achieve close liaison over disease findings. All parts of the carcase must be identifiable pending the final decisions. From this detained meat room the overhead rail must reconnect with the main slaughter line for direction of carcases either to the chill rooms or to the condemned meat room. It is important that there should be ample space for the examination of carcases which, being hot at this stage, and prior to final inspection, should not be allowed to touch each other. If they are to be held for any period, for example, pending laboratory examination, chilling accommodation is necessary.

Good lighting which does not distort colours and is of an intensity of not less than 50 foot-candles (540 lux) is required. The normal facilities of good drainage, easily cleaned surfaces and adequate sterilisation and recording equipment are also necessary. A hydraulic lift stand is an advantage for detailed examination and trimming of beef carcases. If this particular department is situated adjacent to the meat plant laboratory, this is an added advantage, since microbiological, pathological, parasitological and biochemical examinations, as well as photography, can be more conveniently carried out. This room should be enclosed and entry restricted to authorised personnel. It must be lockable.

### Condemned meat room

All too often the condemned meat room does not receive the attention it deserves at the planning stage of the plant, especially with regard to space. In order to arrange for proper sorting and holding of materials unfit for human consumption prior to dispatch, adequate space, refrigeration and drainage along with the supply of durable and lockable containers and weighing facilities are essential. A suitable rail linkage with the detained meat room and other means of handling materials complete this important area, which must have lockable doors.

### Hide and skin store

Although primarily intended for the stacking and cooling of hides and sheep skins awaiting collection, the hide and skin store can conveniently be used for the reception of cattle and sheep feet.

Careful thought should be given at the planning stage to suitable arrangements for all areas where by-products are held pending dispatch, not only in relation to their position, size, layout, chute system with slaughterhall floor, etc., but also in connection with the facilities for easy loading on to vehicles. A system of handling hides and skins in palletised containers is of value, as is gravity feeding of vehicles which collect feet. As for by-product handling, gravity feeding of hides and skins is easier if the slaughterhall floor is on a higher level, and connected with the various by-products departments by stainless steel chutes.

### Gut and tripe room

The initial separation and emptying of stomachs and intestines is normally carried out in the gut and tripe room. Usually it is convenient to have this room associated with moving-top tables, with an arrangement for discharging to a macerator or holding pending collection for composting, etc. Heavy cattle stomachs should be handled either by mechanical equipment or by suitable gradients. The cattle-paunch emptying table should be at a convenient height in relation to the moving-top table or be provided with a power-operated hoist for elevating paunches to the higher level. The table must be fitted with an 'umbrella' of spray rods for cleaning the inside and the outside of the paunches.

Subsequent processing of stomachs and intestines should take place in a separate unit.

### Red offal room

Offal such as liver, lungs and kidneys should be trimmed and then placed in a chill or freezing room depending on the ultimate system of disposal. Offal for edible purposes must be held at a temperature not exceeding 3°C.

### The edible fat room

This is a completely separate holding room, usually situated near the gut room and where edible fat is held pending dispatch.

### Cutting rooms

The hygienic procedures undertaken with the initial carcase dressing are continued in the cutting rooms. So vital are these rooms and the techniques employed in them that legislation usually gives special consideration to them.

There are separate EEC conditions for the approval of cutting plants, whether or not they are an integral part of the abattoir. Building services, equipment and hygiene conditions are similar to those applying to abattoirs.

During the cutting process the temperature of the building must not exceed 12°C and the rooms must have sufficient refrigeration accommodation to keep meat at an internal temperature of not more than 7°C. There must also be a thermometer or telethermometer installed in the cutting room.

Adequate facilities are necessary in the form of suitable equipment, an adequate supply of hot, potable water to keep the whole area hygienic, and a waste disposal system that meets hygiene requirements.

### Inedible area

All materials unfit for human consumption, with the exception of hides and skins, should be sited away from edible areas. One of the difficulties associated with the inedible area is the arrangement for handling items such as omasa after separation from cattle paunches, since improper handling of these organs can result in unhygienic conditions.

### Equipment wash

A properly designed equipment wash adjacent to work rooms is essential to avoid buggies, bins, and other equipment being washed in work rooms, corridors or other inappropriate places. There should be a one-way system through the wash room, to avoid the mixing of clean and dirty equipment, good drainage and, most importantly, good steam extraction.

### Fresh meat dispatch area

The fresh meat dispatch area must be sited away from the dirty part and access to it restricted to vehicles associated with meat and offal for human consumption. If at all possible, the floor level of the loading bay should be at vehicle floor height and the whole area should be roofed so that personnel can work in inclement weather conditions. A system whereby the meat plant rails coordinate with those of the meat transport vehicles is of great value in efficiently and hygienically loading meat for delivery. There must be protection against pests of various kinds as well as stops to prevent damage to plant walls. This is best achieved by a docking system whereby there is no air movement from outside the premises into the dispatch area or vehicle. If quartering of carcases or any other butchering takes place in this area, it should be refrigerated to 12°C.

### Manure bay

This should be sited near the lairage on the dirty side of the plant. In some cases stomach and intestinal material is handled along with manure or it may be processed separately. Size and design depend mainly on throughput but in all cases ease of transfer to transport vehicles should be made a priority, which usually means having the bay in an elevated position. Its floor and sides should be impervious, with provision made for overflow liquors to be drained away.

In certain weather conditions there may be a need to treat the manure to prevent problems with flies.

Disposal of waste material must be carried out without creating objectionable conditions.

## Vehicle washing

An often neglected facility is that for the cleaning of meat transport and animal transport vehicles.

The former should be provided in the clean side of the plant and have adequate high-pressure hoses with hot water and detergent along with good drainage for vehicles and wash area. For animal lorries it is sufficient to provide a supply of cold water under pressure along with provision for disinfection. As for the meat vehicle wash area, suitable floor gradients are necessary in the plant dirty section. It is not unreasonable, in view of the great importance of having clean vehicles, to insist on the cleaning of all meat vehicles before loading and all stock lorries after unloading.

## Facilities for personnel

In addition to the full complement of locker rooms, a sufficient number of water closets, showers and wash-hand basins must be provided (one for every 15 employees). Alternatively, individual wash-hand basins may be replaced by suitable communal hand-washing facilities of an elongated or circular type which are more easily maintained. Separate units must be provided if both sexes are employed.

The dressing rooms should be properly separated from the toilets and these must not open directly on to working areas.

Lockers should be of metal construction with sloping tops and placed 40 cm above the floor in order to facilitate cleaning. A plastic, stainless steel or wooden bench along the front of the lockers at this level completes the furniture. Separate lockers should be provided for each employee's personal and work clothing, if alternative means of storing work clothing and equipment is not provided. Soiled working clothing should not be stored in lockers but be directed to the laundry.

Urinals should be installed in toilet rooms for male personnel.

It is well worthwhile giving close consideration to the layout and design of changing facilities for staff. Ventilation in these areas is of great importance, as is a code of practice for their use.

In addition to the changing areas, it is necessary to have mess rooms for the staff, access to which should be restricted to hygienically clad individuals. Separate welfare facilities may be provided for those employees working in inedible and other unwholesome areas.

The efficient operation of a meat plant depends greatly on the well-being of its personnel. Although a fully trained *industrial nurse and* a well appointed *first aid room* are considered beneficial, especially for the larger premises, not only to deal with the many cuts and other problems associated with slaughtering operations but also to assist materially in raising hygiene standards and preventing the onset of zoonoses, they have mostly been replaced by a trained first-aider.

A *laundry* and conveniently-sited *car park* are necessary departments of the modern meat plant and a comprehensive *system of communication* comprising internal telephones, a staff location system of the VHF-radio type and loudspeaker equipment should be installed along with adequate *security arrangements*.

In UK abattoirs, it has to be remembered that the Health and Safety at Work Act 1974 operates in addition to the Slaughter of Animals (Hygiene & Inspection Regulations 1995).

## Veterinary office

An adequately equipped lockable room for the exclusive use of the veterinary service is essential for intra-Community trade meat plants, and a larger one is necessary for the meat inspectors. The rooms should be provided with hand-washing and shower facilities, and lockers for clothing (work and personal) and meat inspection equipment. A convenient means of cleaning footwear before entry into changing rooms is an advantage.

### Veterinary laboratory

Under EEC regulations, a room equipped for carrying out a trichinoscopic test is compulsory where pigs or horses are slaughtered In the larger premises, a well-equipped laboratory is essential, not only for the preliminary diagnosis of animal disease and monitoring of potential pathogens but also to maintain the overall hygiene standards. These premises are very often also utilised for the training of meat inspectors and other employees.

## FURTHER READING

Food and Agriculture Organization (FAO) (1978) *Slaughterhouse and Slaughterslab Design and Construction*. FAO Animal Production and Health Paper No. 9. Rome: FAO.

UK Meat and Livestock Commission (1979) *Guidelines for Export Slaughterhouses.*

US Department of Agriculture, Food Safety and Inspection Service (1984) *A Guide to Construction, Equipment and Layout.* Agricultural Handbook No. 570.

## LEGISLATION

### EEC

Directive 89/778 concerning the quality of water intended for human consumption.

Document 7491/91 (19 July 1991) extends Directive 64/433 (with amendments).

Directives 71/118, 75/431, 78/50 and 86/642 are the main poultry Directives.

# Chapter 4
# Preservation of Meat

The primary purpose of food preservation is to prevent food spoilage. Whether food spoilage is mild or extreme, the primary cause is the action of microorganisms – bacteria, moulds or yeasts – aided by enzymes. As living organisms they can survive and develop only under particular environmental conditions; under unfavourable conditions they die or fail to develop.

The underlying principle of all food preserving methods, then, is the creation of conditions unfavourable to the growth or survival of spoilage organisms by, for example, extreme heat or cold, deprivation of water and sometimes oxygen, excess of saltiness or increased acidity. The methods by which meat foods may be preserved are drying, curing, cold, heat, chemicals, irradiation, and high pressure.

Preservation by *chemicals* may be achieved by artificial means, e.g. the addition of sulphur dioxide to foodstuffs, but this and the use of other chemicals is greatly restricted by food regulations in most countries, although research continues to find an acceptable chemical means of preservation.

Chemical preservation by natural means, as in the smoking of meat and fish, is employed as an adjuvant to commercial salting and pickling.

For preservation of food from meat animals to be successful it is essential that all livestock are correctly managed on the farm, in transport and in the lairage to ensure the supply of clean, healthy animals to the meat plant, and that the operations there are carried out in an exemplary manner (see Chapter 7). The meat from animals properly handled and processed will have a low pH value which will aid in the preservation process.

## Physical changes in stored meat

Meat undergoes certain superficial changes as a result of storage, chief of which are shrinkage, sweating and loss of bloom.

### *Shrinkage*

Shrinkage or loss of weight occurs as a result of *evaporation* of water from the meat surface; carcases cut into quarters dissipate water vapour rapidly and continuously and retail joints even more so. On the other hand, evaporation is inhibited by membranes such as the pleura and peritoneum and, in carcases of well-nourished animals, by the solidification of the superficial fat and drying of the connective tissue. A freshly-killed carcase dissipates body weight slowly, losing 1.5–2.0% of weight by evaporation during the first 24 h of hanging. Further loss of weight during storage depends on the humidity of the storage room: the drier the air the greater the amount of evaporation. The high-velocity cold air system (Turbo-Chill) reduces body heat of freshly killed animals by increasing the rate of heat removal from the surface of the carcase and hence reduces surface temperature quickly. Avoidance of all evaporative weight losses by high humidity facilitates the formation of moulds, so an accurate balance between temperature and humidity must be maintained; the dry, impervious film on the carcase surface is perhaps the best protection against the growth of spoilage organisms.

### *Sweating*

This denotes the *condensation* of water vapour on meat brought from a cold store into ordinary room temperature. The condensation occurs because the refrigerated carcase lowers the temperature of the air to below the dewpoint. In the winter months in Britain the dewpoint is generally below 4.5°C and sweating is unlikely to occur, but in the summer the dewpoint is always over 7°C and moisture will be deposited on the carcase. If the quarter or side is cut up immediately after removal from the chilling room, sweating will be extended to the individual joints.

*Loss of bloom*

*Bloom* is defined as the colour and general appearance of a carcase surface when viewed through the semitransparent layers of connective tissue, muscle and fat which form the carcase surface. If these tissues become moist, the collagen fibres in the connective tissue swell and become opaque and the meat surface assumes a dull, lifeless appearance. Loss of surface bloom in beef carcases may also be caused by dehydration or undue oxidation, but it may be prevented by avoiding temperature fluctuations that permit alternate drying and dampening of the carcase surface. It is also important to keep the relative humidity of cooling chambers high and ensure free circulation of air. Muscular tissue also tends to become brownish on exposure to air as myohaemoglobin changes to the brown pigment methaemoglobin, but the actual amount of exposed muscle in a side of beef is so small that this is of little or no consequence. Refrigeration has little effect on the carcase fat except in the case of frozen meat which has undergone a prolonged period of storage, in which case rancidity may develop.

## Chemical changes in stored meat

The chemical changes that take place after slaughter are indicative of a slight degree of breakdown in protein, due either to endogenous enzymes or to those of microorganisms. The odour of the meat becomes progressively more marked but never undesirable; the flavour may be described as stale, rendering the meat unpalatable but not repulsive.

The storage life of meat is more dependent on the chemical changes that take place in fat rather than in muscle, for fat rancidity, even if only slight, is objectionable. The condition of the fat therefore determines the length of storage, for whilst the lean muscle of a carcase may be still improving in flavour the changes in fat may render the meat repugnant and unmarketable.

*Drying*

Although drying as such plays only a minor role in preservation today, the whole vast process of refrigeration is largely based on the principle of drying, i.e. the removal of water available for microbial growth. Again, salting largely owes its preservation action to the extraction of water by osmosis.

It is essential that as little water as possible is put on sheep and cattle carcases during dressing.

## Water activity or water availability ($a_w$)

Water activity or water availability, $a_w$, is a measure of the partial vapour pressure of the foodstuffs compared to that of pure water at its surface. Water molecules are loosely orientated in pure liquid water and can easily rearrange. When solutes are introduced, these orient the water molecules around them and make them much less available for use by microorganisms. With the exception of *Staphylococcus aureus* and most moulds, microorganisms are poor at competing with solutes for the water molecules.

The $a_w$ varies little with temperature over the normal growth range of microorganisms. Pure water has the highest $a_w$ possible (1.0) and the $a_w$ decreases with the addition of solute (always <1).

Various NaCl solutions will give the following $a_w$.

| %NaCl (w/v) | $a_w$ |
|---|---|
| 0.9 | 0.995 |
| 3.5 | 0.98 |
| 7.0 | 0.96 |
| 16.0 | 0.90 |
| 22.0 | 0.86 |

The $a_w$ may greatly affect the ability of an organism to survive heat. The thermal death time ($D_{60}$) for *Salmonella typhimurium* at 60°C is 0.18 min at an $a_w$ of 0.94.

The $a_w$ stated for an organism is usually the minimum at which growth will take place, but growth will increase with increasing $a_w$. Lower than minimal $a_w$ will not necessarily kill the organisms, and they will remain infectious. It is difficult to standardise an $a_w$ for a specific food as this may vary depending on the source, the age of the food and even different parts of the food.

## MEAT CURING

While curing may be applied to all kinds of meat, it is best adapted to those with a high fat content, e.g. pork or fine-fibred beef intermixed with fat, and it is for this reason that brisket and flank of beef make high-quality pickled meat. On the other hand, lean beef, veal or mutton become dry and unpalatable on pickling.

### *Salt*

Salt is the principal preserving material used in curing on a commercial scale, though it appears to have little directly harmful effect on bacteria; large quantities of salt or sugar produce the same result as would be obtained by the extraction of water. Indeed, the osmotic pressure of the strong salt or sugar solution removes the water necessary for bacterial growth from the meat. Halophilic (salt-loving) bacteria require salt for optimum growth and are not affected; they are, however, slower growing than non-halophilic bacteria.

Distinction must be made between salted meats (beef, pork) and cured meats (bacon, ham, corned beef). In salted meats the dry salt first dissolves in the surface fluid and then passes slowly inwards until it is evenly distributed throughout the meat substance. A considerable amount of the moisture is removed when the salt draws to the surface some of the fluid in which it dissolves. Microscopically, salted meat, compared with fresh meat, shows a diminution in the size of the intercellular spaces as a result of loss of water.

*Curing* may be defined as the addition of *salt* (NaCl) and *nitrate/nitrite* or *nitric oxide* to the meat, which results in a conversion of the meat pigments, predominantly myoglobin, to the nitroso or cured form. Myoglobin in freshly cut uncured meat is in the reduced form (purple), which in contact with air is rapidly oxygenated to oxymyoglobin, which is bright red and responsible for the 'bloom' on meat. If oxidised, these pigments are converted to metamyoglobin, which is unattractive and gives a brown or grey colour. Under suitable conditions these pigments can be converted to the nitroso form (nitrosomyoglobin) by the addition of nitric oxide. During the curing process nitric oxide is formed by reduction of nitrites formed by bacteria from nitrates. Nitrosomyoglobin gives freshly-cut cured meat its bright red colour, but is unstable and rapidly oxidises to the brown and grey forms. However, on heating, the nitrosomyoglobin is converted to nitrosohaemochrome, a pink colour (e.g. of cooked ham or corned beef) as distinct from the grey and brown of the cooked uncured meat (e.g. roast beef).

### Ingredients used in curing

Basically to produce a cured meat only *sodium chloride* and a source of *nitric oxide (nitrate* or *nitrite)* are required. However, with a demand by consumers for a greater variety of cured meats in relation to saltiness and other flavour

**Table 4.1** Curing salts and additives.

| Ingredient | Level in curing brine | Function |
|---|---|---|
| Sodium chloride | 15-30% | Preservative; improves texture |
| Sodium nitrate* | 0.15–1.5% | A source of nitrite |
| Sodium nitrite* | 500–1000 ppm | Preservative; reduced by meat enzymes to NO, which combined with myoglobin (the uncured meat pigment) forms nitrosomyoglobin, the cured meat pigment |
| Polyphosphates | 2-4% | Reduce cooking losses, e.g. during smoking; improve texture |
| Sugars, e.g. sucrose, maple syrup | 1-4% | Improves flavour by masking the harshness of the salt |
| Liquid smoke † | ca. 1% | Flavouring agent |
| Sodium ascorbate | 0.2-1.0% | Reducing agent. Improves colour formation and stability by effecting rapid reduction of $NO_3$ to $NO_2$ in the meat |

* In the UK, levels must not exceed 500 ppm $NaNO_3$ and 200 ppm $NaNO_2$ in the final product.

† Varies considerably; refer to manufacturer's instructions.

components, a wide range of substances can be used (Table 4.1). Each ingredient has a specific function and is used accordingly.

## PRODUCTION OF BACON AND HAM

Pork may be cured by either salting or pickling. Dry salting gives a less consistent product and takes longer and is therefore more expensive.

The raw material, a 85–90 kg liveweight pig, is slaughtered and eviscerated to produce a 70 kg carcase. White-skinned pigs have traditionally been preferred as the bacon rind has a more attractive appearance. A pig with light shoulders, long, level back, deep and level flanks with broad hams is most likely to yield a carcase well-endowed in the region of the most valuable bacon cuts, for in a side of bacon the collar and foreleg together should not weigh more than 25% of the whole side.

After *stunning*, and *bleeding* for at least 6 minutes, most pig carcases in the British Isles are *scalded*, *dehaired*, *singed* and *scraped* in preparation for bacon production rather than being skinned. The scalding water may contain different types of bacteria originating from the pig's skin and gastrointestinal tract, including *Salmonella*. The temperature of the water in the drag-through scalding tank at 60°C is generally sufficient to reduce vegetative growth. The skins of scalded pigs have low numbers of both enteric pathogens and spoilage bacteria, but the subsequent dehairing process recontaminates the skin. The bacterial content of the muscle and viscera does, however, appear to be affected by the type of scalding equipment. Vertical scalding of pigs on the line in a 'steam cabinet' reduces the opportunity for contamination of the carcase via the stick wound. After dehairing, the carcase is hoisted on to a greased skid rail and transferred to a singeing plant, which consists of two vertical half-cylinders lined with heatproof bricks. The carcase is *singed* by a fired combination of oil and air at a temperature of 1371–1537°C. Singeing colours the skin brown, removes any hairs still remaining, hardens the subcutaneous fat, enhances the keeping quality of the meat and sterilises the external surface of the pig so that following singeing the bacterial load on the carcase surface is of the order of 10 bacteria/cm$^2$.

On leaving the furnace, the carcases are sprayed with cold water and scraped and polished in a tunnel containing banks of stainless steel scrapers and nylon brushes until the burnt brown epidermis has been removed and the pig appears white. These procedures, however, recontaminate the surface of the carcase to the order of 10$^4$ bacteria/cm$^2$. The majority of these are spoilage bacteria, predominantly *acinetobacteria*, *moraxellae* and *pseudomonads*; with enteric organisms such as *E. coli* and *Campylobacter* at single figures per cm$^2$.

The carcases are then ready for evisceration, inspection, weighing and grading followed by immediate transfer via overhead rails to the chills where they are chilled to <4°C within 24 hours.

### Cutting

Under modern systems very few Wiltshires (full sides of bacon) are produced, it being more common to reduce the side to individual primal cuts before curing. The butchery processes vary, but generally commence on removal from the chillers with the removal of the head and forelegs while the pig is still suspended on the overhead rail. This produces two sides which are dropped on to a moving steel conveyor, before the removal of the jaw flap from the fore. The hind leg is cut mid-way through the hock, and the fore-end is removed by a band saw at the level of the third and fourth rib. The fillet (also known as the tenderloin) runs from the third most posterior rib back along the dorsal surface of the abdominal cavity to the gammon. This is carefully removed and any loose pieces of meat, e.g. the diaphragm, are trimmed off the side. The gammon, the hind leg, is removed by a band saw, mid-way between the head of the femur and a part of the sacrum known as the oyster bone. The pelvic bones are removed and the gammon is trimmed.

The spinal column, or chine bones, are removed using a circular saw and the middle is slit into belly and back cuts. The ribs may be removed individually, by a process known as single ribbing, or in sheets. Finally, excess fat is trimmed off, and in most cases the rind is removed.

### Application of the pickle

Salt for the cure may be kept in a large silo through which water filters to produce a saturated salt solution. This is chilled to −2 or −3°C and *nitrite* added to a concentration, at an average of 160 ppm. Usually nitrate is not used as a constituent of the pickle. This is because nitrate is only effective in so far as it is converted into nitrite by bacteria present in the cover brine. *Sodium ascorbate* is added as a source of ascorbic acid, a reducing agent, which aids the formation of nitrosomyoglobin and hence ensures that the bacon or ham has good colour formation and stability. In a maple cure, sugar, maple crystals and seasoning give the bacon a unique flavour. *Polyphosphates* aid water retention in the cured meat during the cooking process, so reducing shrinkage during cooking, making the hams more succulent and improving the texture of smoked product.

In 1971 the amount of curing salts which could be used was restricted to 500 ppm of sodium nitrate and 200 ppm of sodium nitrite. This was in recognition that nitrites can react with secondary and tertiary amines to form nitrosamines, which are carcinogenic. Earlier methods of curing, by hand injection of pumping brine (called stitching) followed by immersion of the sides in cover brine for at least 4 days, have largely been superseded. The brine or pickle is now introduced into all sides of the prepared cuts by automatic pumping machines which introduce pickle under pressure through needles approximately 2 cm apart. The addition of pickle increases the weight of the piece by approximately 10%.

Immediately after pumping, the middle cuts, back and belly, are vac-packed and heat-sealed. They are held in cellars at a temperature below 4°C for at least 48 hours before going for blast freezing (−6°C for 5 h), slicing and packing. The freezing process suspends curing and assists high-speed slicing.

The gammons, after pumping, are immersed in traditional tiled or stainless steel tanks of cover brine for 3 days. The cover brine is used for approximately 3 weeks before it is discarded and is constantly monitored bacteriologically. In former times cover brine was used indefinitely and was thought to impart unique flavours to the product.

## Production of cooked hams

Re-formed cooked hams are produced from de-fatted lean cuts. Following pickle injection, these are tumbled in a machine that looks like a cement mixer with sharp stainless steel blades in a rotating drum, or massaged in a 'Bel Lagan' massager. In general, small pieces of meat are *tumbled* while large pieces are *massaged*. The machines rotate for 7 minutes in every hour for 18 hours, moving the meat around and ensuring that a uniform cure and colour are attained. The physical action also tenderises the muscle and aids fast penetration of the curing agent, thus saving on curing time. The process releases the albuminous protein myosin from the meat, leaving its surface in a gelatinous state. When cooked, the meat binds together, the myosin acting as a seal, aiding water retention.

When removed from the tumbling or massaging process, the product may be allowed to rest for up to 24 hours, or it may be immediately further processed.

Large pieces are manually packed into pots with pressure lids and cooked for 14 hours to a core temperature of 70°C. Smaller pieces are automatically fed into presses which extrude the pork into pre-soaked fibrous casings. These are semi-cooked for 4–5 hours to a core temperature of 42°C in preparation for slicing and vacuum packing.

To ensure consistently high quality, a mid-process analysis is carried out. A random sample of product, selected from different cuts, is analysed for levels of nitrite, salt and added water. There is a standard declaration of not more than 10% added water for middles, backs and streak. Massaged or tumbled product is allowed up to 20% added water.

## Traditional dry cure bacon

Although described as dry cure, some brine is injected by hand into the eye muscle of the back and deep into the gammon. Both cuts are then sprinkled with the dry cure mixture, which contains nitrite, before being covered in salt. The middles are stacked, cut surface up, for 5 days, after which excess salt is shaken off and the sides are turned rind up, and left for 2–3 weeks. The gammons are packed into tanks with salt for 4 weeks. On removal, all cuts are washed down to remove some of the salt. They are then hung on racks and singed with a blowtorch to remove any slime on the surface and dried over night, in a room with circulating air at 10–20°C. The bacon produced may then be smoked, if required, and prepared for dispatch by trimming the gammons, and rolling and placing the middles in stockinette.

### New dry cure

A new type of dry curing entails placing fresh rindless pork backs on racks, freezing, pressing into shape, allowing to temper and slicing. As it comes to the end of the slicing line, the product is sprayed on both sides with salt and nitrite solution and then packaged. Curing takes place in the bag, there being not more than 3½% salt in the final product.

### Smoking

Smoking of cured pork improves its keeping properties further, as well as imparting an appetising colour and flavour. Traditionally, smoking was carried out over several days in a brick oven with smouldering oak, hickory or hardwood sawdust and hot ash piled on the floor.

It is now more common to use an insulated steel cabinet enclosing a heat-exchanger system. The cuts to be smoked are hung on racks and placed in the cabinet and the temperature raised to approximately 32°C for 30 minutes. Smoke, produced by a smoke generator consisting of a hopper which automatically feeds dry hardwood sawdust on to a cast iron hotplate, is drawn into the cabinet for 1–2 hours. It is important to ensure that the temperature does not rise above 37°C or the fat may melt.

The chief bacteriostatic and bacteriocidal substances in wood smoke is formaldehyde. The combination of heat and smoke usually causes a significant reduction in the surface bacterial population. In addition, a physical barrier is provided by superficial dehydration, coagulation of protein and the absorption of resinous substances.

### Common defects in cured meat

1 *Fiery red areas* are caused by lack of available nitrite – miscure. This may occur in deep meat cuts.
2 *Jelly pockets* are caused by injection of brine into connective tissue, which it denatures.
3 *Areas of discoloration* may be caused by bruising or blood splashing. This can be very obvious in the cooked product.
4 *Rancidity in frozen bacon* may be identified by pronounced yellowing of the fat. Although all bacterial growth stops when bacon is frozen, certain chemical reactions can proceed at −8°C.
5 *Browning*. The cured meat pigment nitrosomyoglobin changes to the brown metamyoglobin owing to dehydration caused by low humidity, high temperature and oxidation caused by prolonged exposure to air, excessive nitrate and poor packaging.
6 *Greening* may be caused by excessive nitrate and by bacterial contamination.

### Bacteria on cured product

*Spoilage*

The most common form of spoilage found on cured meats is mouldiness, which may be due to *Aspergillus, Alternaria, Fusarium, Mucor, Rhizopus, Penicillin* and other moulds.

*Micrococci* are resistant to salt and consequently are most common where salt levels are high, especially the fat. *Lactobacilli* are less resistant to salt but more resistant to smoke. These, together with *Acinetobacter, Bacillus, Pseudomonas* and *Proteus* may result in the fermentation of sugars in the product to produce *sours* of various types. Pickling cannot be relied upon to destroy parasitic infections, e.g. *cysticerci* in beef or pork.

## REFRIGERATION

The modern meat industry is based on efficient refrigeration. Carcases of freshly slaughtered animals have surfaces that are warm and wet and thus provide a perfect substrate for the growth of pathogenic and spoilage organisms. Chilling immediately post-slaughter reduces the surface temperature to a value below the minimum growth temperature for many pathogens. The combination of low temperatures and surface drying inhibits the growth of spoilage bacteria. To provide a long, safe, high-quality shelf-life, the temperature of the meat needs to be kept at a temperature close to its initial freezing point. Combining a high standard of hygiene and packaging with a temperature of −1 to +0.5°C during storage, transport and display can routinely extend shelf-life to 12 weeks. If longer periods are required, then freezing the meat will extend the storage period into years. Scientific studies show that freezing has little if any affect on the eating quality of red meat. Overall the studies indicate that the meat may be slightly more tender after freezing. Freezing does increase the ultimate amount of drip from meat and this makes the meat less attractive. However, the increased drip does not influence the eating quality after cooking.

In the process of refrigeration, heat is extracted from the carcase in the chillrooms, two basic laws of physics being involved in this process. First, the boiling point of a liquid – the temperature at which it is turned into vapour – depends on the pressure. At normal atmospheric pressure (1 atmosphere = 760 mm Hg; 29.92 inches Hg; 14.7 lb in$^2$, 1013.25 Nm$^{-2}$ at sea level) water boils at 100°C but at a pressure of 0.1 atmosphere it boils at 46°C. Conversely, water vapour at 50°C and 0.1 atmosphere can be condensed back to water by increasing the pressure to 1 atmosphere. When a liquid passes into a vapour it absorbs heat which is given off again when it condenses.

Refrigerants are liquids or liquefied gases with low boiling points, e.g. ammonia or hydrofluorocarbons, which, in the refrigeration cycle, extract heat at low temperature when evaporated and give off this heat to the outside air when re-condensed.

The preservative action of refrigeration is based on the prevention of multiplication of harmful bacteria, yeasts and moulds by the artificial lowering of the temperature. The failure of bacteria to grow at or below freezing depends mainly on the removal of the available water as ice; about 70% is removed at −3.5°C and 94% at −10°C. A further factor is the inhibition of the life processes of spoilage organisms at low temperatures, though the actual lethal effect is small. At a temperature of −8°C the multiplication of all microorganisms stops and only resumes when the temperature is raised later to a suitable level. Neither fast (cryogenic) nor slow (blast) freezing completely destroys the bacteria commonly found in beef carcases; frozen meat which is thawed yields an abundant supply of water and forms an excellent medium for bacterial growth. In addition, the pH of muscle, which remains constant while the meat is frozen, falls rapidly after thawing, but then rises rapidly to create an environment which favours bacterial multiplication.

The surface growth of *mould* on meat is controlled not only by the temperature but by the relative humidity of the atmosphere. Some moulds are capable of growing on the surface of meat at several degrees below freezing point, but they require the presence of water in the surrounding atmosphere as otherwise they lose water by evaporation and wither. For the prevention of mould the temperature and relative humidity must therefore be kept as low as possible.

There is an obvious need to control the whole cold chain, not just in specific processes, to achieve truly effective refrigeration. This requires attention to the specification, design, commissioning, testing, monitoring and fault rectification at every stage.

## EU regulations on refrigeration

The regulations concerning the temperatures at which meat, offal and meat products are held vary in different countries.

The EEC Directive 64/433 (as amended) and Directive 69/349, in addition to requiring that abattoirs should have sufficiently large chilling or refrigerating rooms, lay down the following.

1. Meat must be chilled immediately after post-mortem inspection and kept at a constant temperature of not more than +7°C for carcases and cuts and +3°C for offal.
2. Cutting plants must have cooling equipment in the cutting rooms to keep meat at a constant internal temperature of not more than +7°C.
3. Cutting plants must have a thermometer or telethermometer in the cutting room.
4. During cutting the temperature of the building must not exceed +10°C.

In connection with *poultry*, EEC Directive 71/118 specifies that after inspection and evisceration poultry meat must be cleaned immediately and chilled in accordance with the hygiene requirements and afterwards kept at a temperature which may not at any time exceed +4°C.

*Transport of fresh meat* (red and white) in the European Union must be carried out under conditions which maintain the above temperatures. These standards apply to trade within the EU and also to imports from outside the EU.

Carcases of beef and veal which are destined for *freezing* for intervention purposes must be chilled immediately after slaughter and up to the time they have been taken over and, when taken over, must have an inner temperature not exceeding +7°C.

In *South Africa* detailed regulations prescribing temperature, relative humidity and air circulation rates are in operation as follows:

1 For *initial* chilling of 'warm' carcases, sides or quarters, the temperature must be maintained below 7°C and the mean air speed at a level above 0.75 m/s. In the *terminal* stages of chilling, the air temperature must be maintained at a level between –1°C and 2°C. For meat packed in cartons or on trays the temperature must be below 3°C and the air speed above 0.75 m/s.
2 For *storage* of chilled carcases, sides, quarters or portions, the temperature must be within the range – 1°C to 5°C and the mean air speed over the product above 0.5 m/s. The relative humidity (RH) must be maintained below 95% or, if the product is stored for longer than 72 h, below 90%.
3 For the storage of *offal*, the temperature must be maintained below – 2°C or, if stored for longer than 72 h, below – 10°C.

A very useful adjunct to the South African regulations is the requirement for a plate outside each refrigeration room which gives details of cubic capacity, type of product which may be chilled or stored within maximum permissible product loading in kg; for chillers, the mean product temperature reduction in °C and the minimum period in hours for this temperature reduction to take place; and for the storage of chilled meat, the maximum permissible mean temperature at which a product can be introduced into the storage room.

It is very evident that in different countries different temperatures, relative humidities and air speeds are utilised, reflecting differences in operating practices as well as opinions of refrigeration engineers and meat scientists.

The Codex Alimentarius Commission of the Joint FAO/WHO Food Standards Programme published in 1976 *Recommended International Codes of Hygienic Practice for Fresh Meat, for Ante-mortem and Post-Mortem Inspection of Slaughter Animals and for Processed Meat Products.* The Codes, which are advisory in nature, were sent to all Member Nations and Associate Members of FAO and/or WHO, the Commission expressing the view that they might provide useful checklists of requirements for national enforcement authorities. While not actually specifying temperatures, these excellent documents, in relation to refrigeration, make the following practical points:

1 Meat passed for human consumption should be removed from the dressing area without undue delay and placed into refrigeration under close supervision of the inspector. Pre-rigor cutting and boning is permitted in temperature-controlled rooms, but there should be no delay and immediately thereafter the meat should be transported to chilling or processing rooms.
2 The following provisions should apply where carcases, parts of carcases, or edible offals are placed in chilling rooms, freezing rooms or frozen storage as the case may be:
(a) Entry should be restricted to personnel necessary to carry out operations efficiently.
(b) Doors should not be left open for extended periods and should be closed immediately after use.
(c) No chilling room, freezing room or freezer store should be loaded beyond its designed capacity.
(d) Where refrigerating equipment is not manned, automatic temperature recorders should be installed.
(e) If no automatic device is installed, temperatures should be read at regular intervals and the readings recorded.
3 Where carcases, parts of carcases or edible offals are placed in a chilling room for chilling:
(a) There should be a reliable method of monitoring the chilling.
(b) Meat should be hung or placed in suitable corrosion-resistant trays with adequate air circulation.
(c) Drips from one piece of meat to another must be avoided.
(d) Temperature, relative humidity and air flow should be maintained at suitable level.
(e) Condensation should be prevented by the efficient operation of refrigerating facilities combined with, for example, the proper insulation of walls and ceilings and the application of heat near the ceilings. If overhead refrigeration coils are installed, insulated drip pans should be placed beneath them. All floor-type refrigerating units should be placed within curbed and separately

drained areas unless located adjacent to floor drains.

4 Where carcases, or parts of carcases, or edible offals are being frozen:

(a) Meat which is not in cartons should be hung or placed on suitable corrosion-resistant trays with adequate air circulation. Cartons should be stacked to permit adequate circulation.

(b) Drips on to uncartoned meat must be prevented.

(c) The base of any tray should not be in contact with the meat stored beneath.

(d) Refrigeration coils should be defrosted frequently to prevent loss of refrigerating efficiency. Provision should be made for the removal of water without affecting the product.

5 Where carcases, or parts of carcases, or edible offals are placed in any freezer store:

(a) No meat should be placed in a freezer store until its mean temperature is of an acceptable level.

(b) Meat should not be stacked directly on the floor but on pallets or dunnage with adequate air circulation around the stacks.

(c) The temperature of the freezer store should give adequate protection to the product. Temperature fluctuations should be kept to a minimum. Where unpackaged meat is stored, the temperature difference between the evaporator and the meat should be kept to a minimum.

(d) Refrigeration coils should be defrosted regularly to prevent loss of refrigeration efficiency. Provision should be made for the removal of water without affecting the product.

The Codex Alimentarius standard proposed for *beef chilling* calls for a temperature of 15°C or lower at the centre of the round within 20 h.

## Mechanical refrigeration

Carbon dioxide and sulphur dioxide were at one time commonly used as cooling liquids (refrigerants) but carbon dioxide is uneconomical and sulphur dioxide is corrosive and toxic.

*Ammonia*, first introduced in 1876, is still used extensively today, although it is somewhat corrosive and has a penetrating odour so that leaks can affect stored products. There is a revival of interest in ammonia as a refrigerant for larger plants because of the lesser effect on the ozone layer. Today the chloroflourocarbons (CFCs) – primarily the freons – are being replaced by hydroflourocarbons (HFS), again because of the absence of chlorine and hence lower ozone depletion potential.

The temperature utilised in refrigerating chambers falls into two main categories according to whether the meat is *chilled* or *frozen*, but whichever method is employed the important points are constant temperature, good air circulation and the right humidity.

## Chilling of meat

*Chilling* scarcely affects the flavour, appearance or nutritional value of meat and is particularly useful for short-term preserving. The meat is maintained at about +1°C and preferably in the dark, for light accelerates the oxidation of fat with the liberation of free fatty acids and the production of rancidity. The atmosphere is kept dry to hinder the formation of moulds, which are more likely to attack chilled meat than frozen.

In recent years, emphasis has been placed on shorter chilling cycles and lower temperatures – 'quick chilling' – for the following reasons:

1 Both time and building space are saved and higher rates of product handling are achieved. Overheads in labour are reduced and capital investment in buildings is minimised.

2 The meat is said to have a better keeping quality because lower air temperatures (usually below – 3°C initially) retard the rate of growth of bacteria on the surface of carcases where their concentration is most pronounced.

3 Shrinkage of meat is reduced substantially – an important economic factor.

4 The 'bloom' is said to be enhanced by quick chilling.

In order to achieve the above objectives, different time–temperature schedules exist for the different kinds of carcases. Surface discoloration and freezing of the carcase must be avoided.

In pre-war years it was customary to hang beef carcases at ambient temperatures for 24 h before placing them in chill rooms. (Indeed, in many abattoirs at that time refrigeration was non-existent.) Chilling times of 36–48 h for lowering the deep round temperature of beef carcases to 7°C are still common.

*Quick chilling* refers to a rapid lowering of carcase temperature starting not later than 1 h after slaughter and avoiding freezing.

Low temperatures and high air speeds incur a risk of cold shortening. Pig carcases, however, should be cooled as quickly as is economically feasible as they are less susceptible to cold shortening.

The phenomenon of *cold shortening* was first encountered in New Zealand when rapid cooling schedules for lamb freezing were first introduced. Toughness of the meat occurred owing to extreme contraction of muscles subjected to temperatures of around 10°C before the muscles were in normal rigor, i.e. while the pH was still above 6.2 and adenosine triphosphate (ATP) was still present. Cold shortening can also occur with beef carcases and even in parts of the carcase, e.g. the loin, with fairly slow chilling. It can be avoided by delaying the start of chilling, e.g. for 10–12 h when the pH will be below 6.2 and rigor will have taken place with the complete disappearance of ATP from the muscle, or not chilling to below 10°C in less than 10 h. Cold shortening can also be prevented by the use of electrical stimulation, which advances the onset of rigor (see Chapter 2).

Various schedules are in operation for the chilling of meat, but many of these pay little attention to the time required for heat to be extracted from the centre of heavy muscle and dispersed at the surface. Important issues are the velocity of air over the carcases, the uniform air flow throughout the chill room (although this depends also on the evenness of carcase hanging), temperature and relative humidity. Higher temperatures and air velocities and low relative humidity increase the weight loss due to drying out. The Meat Research Institute in Britain estimated that beef carcases stored in chill rooms can lose as much as 0.1% per day, while lambs can lose 0.5% in a relative humidity of 90%. Smaller items of meat lose relatively more because of their relatively larger surface area. On the other hand, high relative humidity increases spoilage. A relative humidity of about 90% appears to be suitable for commercial chilling and for retail purposes.

Hanging of carcases from the hole in the aitch bone (obturator foramen of the os coxae) and adequate maturation improves the eating quality of the meat.

### *EU legislation*

According to EEC Directive 64/433 as amended (81/476/EEC), fresh meat intended for intra-Community trade must be chilled immediately after the post-mortem inspection and kept at a constant temperature of not more than +7°C for carcases and cuts and +3°C for offal. Except for meat for immediate distribution, +7°C is too high for good keeping quality. This maximum temperature of +7°C applies also to meat in transit, but many operators aim at keeping the air temperature in vehicles below +2°C.

There is now a derogation from this requirement which, for technical reasons relating to maturation of the meat, may be granted by the competent authority on a case-by-case basis for the transportation of meat to cutting plants or butcher's shops in the immediate vicinity of the meat plant, provided that such transportation takes no more than 2 hours.

All chill rooms should have room air *temperature indicator-recorders*, and carcase temperature indicator-recorders should be fitted to the control panel so that proper adjustments to the chilling cycle can be easily carried out when necessary.

*Air circulation rates* are high in quick-chilling operations, often 70–110 times the room volume per hour. The carcase is initially warm and wet but evaporation from the surface is rapid. In order to minimise loss of carcase weight while maintaining a short chilling cycle, high air-circulation rates are necessary to lower the carcase temperature and carcase surface-water vapour pressure as quickly as possible. Later, when the carcase temperature has been sufficiently lowered, slower air circulation rates are more beneficial.

The Food Safety and Inspection Division of the United States Department of Agriculture advises that, for carcase-chilling coolers, rails should be placed at least 0.6 m from refrigerating equipment, walls and other fixed parts of the building and 0.9 m (especially for header and traffic rails) from walls in order to promote cleanliness and protect walls from damage. The top of the chill rails should be at least 3.3 vm (for beef sides) from the floor level;

**Table 4.2** Chilling shrinkage of pig carcase ca. 60 kg dressed weight.

| | Air temperature (°C) | Air speed (m/s) | Chilling shrinkage (%) A | B |
|---|---|---|---|---|
| Quick chilling | ½ | ¼ | 1.9 | 1.5 |
| Rapid chilling | −7 | 2 | 1.4 | 1.0 |

A: 24 h after slaughter. B: 1 h after slaughter.
Source: Cooper, R. (1970) *Proc. int. Inst. Refrig.*, Leningrad.

2.7 m for headless pigs and calves; 2.2 m for beef quarters; and 2 m for sheep and goats.

It is necessary to have several chill units, rather than one large chill room, with dimensions 18–30 m long (maximum), 7.6–15 m wide and 4.8 m high (minimum). Refrigeration requirements for the above cycle would be approximately 755–880 kcal/h per carcase of 290 kg weight (dry) with about 9.9–11.3 m$^3$/min of air circulated per carcase.

Pork carcases, because of their smaller size, the presence of a skin and relatively greater fat content, can tolerate much lower air temperatures and consequently shorter quick-chilling cycles, even as short as 4–7 h, but most British abattoirs produce pork, like beef and lamb, during a 24 h cycle, the carcases usually being chilled in air at 4°C and at an air speed of 0.5 m/s. Work at the British Meat Research Institute showed that *ultrarapid chilling of pork* in air at −30°C and 1 m/s for 4 h resulted in complete loss of heat in this short time with a 1% saving in evaporative weight loss compared with the control carcases handled in the traditional manner. But while early cutting and packing was possible and there was no difference in appearance and bacteriological quality, loins showed a marked increase in drip loss and were tougher than controls.

## Freezing of meat

The chief types of meat foods preserved by *freezing*, as distinct from chilling, are mutton, lamb, pork and rabbit, but there are rather wide differences of opinion as to the proper freezing temperature. In Germany the temperature is maintained at −6°C and in Australia −11°C. In South America much lower temperatures may be used in what are termed *sharp freezers*; for example, pork may be stored at −18°C, which prevents oxidation and resultant rancidity. During sea transport a temperature of −9°C to −8°C is maintained in the holds, while the air is kept dry and in circulation.

In the UK, it has been customary to hold meat in *cold stores* at temperatures of −20°C. It is now generally recognised that lower temperatures are more satisfactory since they reduce deterioration of carcase meat, and temperatures no higher than −18°C, even −30°C, are now being advocated. It was believed that very low temperatures resulted in excessive dehydration; this is now known to be incorrect.

Entry of the UK into the EEC led to more attention being paid to freezing rates and storage temperatures for frozen meat because of the requirements for intervention freezing, an essential part of the price-support system for beef and pig meat. These EEC regulations lay down that *beef* quarters shall be accepted for freezing at a temperature not above +7°C and frozen within 36 h to an internal temperature of −7°C or below. The acceptance temperature of *pig* sides is below +4°C; they must be frozen at −30°C and held in the freezer until all the meat is at −15°C or below. Frozen storage for beef must be at a temperature of −17°C and at −20°C for pig meat. The meat must be wrapped in polyethylene film at least 0.05 mm thick and in stockinette. Such low temperatures can be attained only in special *blast freezers* with air temperatures of around −34°C, air speeds of about 3–5 m/s and holding times of up to 25 h. The form of wrapping greatly affects the freezing time; if it is loose, the pockets of air or cartons act as insulation and thereby increase freezing times. Wrapping in moisture-proof packaging can offset water loss.

Cold stores are designed to hold frozen meat and other foods at a required temperature, although various temperatures and air speeds are used in different premises. While the meat trade in Britain is resistant to the use of very low temperatures for cold storage, work at the UK Meat Research Institute at Bristol has shown that at −10°C weight losses of meat are much greater than at −30°C because the amount of water vapour that air can hold before it becomes saturated increases as temperature rises.

The commonly held belief that frozen meat will keep indefinitely is not true. The practical

**Table 4.3** Practical storage life (PSL) (months) at different storage temperatures.

| | PSL (months) | | |
|---|---|---|---|
| | −12°C | −18°C | −24°C |
| Beef carcases | 8 | 15 | 24 |
| Lamb carcases | 18 | 24 | >24 |
| Pork carcases | 6 | 10 | 15 |
| Edible offals | 4 | 1–2 | 18 |

Source: Refrigeration and Process Engineering Research Centre, University of Bristol, Churchill Building, Langford, Bristol, UK.

storage life of frozen carcase meat is given in Table 4.3.

For *optimum results in chilling and freezing* and the prevention of growth of spoilage and food-poisoning bacteria, the following criteria should be adopted:

1 Initial design of refrigeration space must consider product tenderness, weight loss, possibility of spoilage, size of individual units, space required, rail height, and floor and wall surfaces.
2 Temperatures must be checked regularly.
3 Overloading must be avoided and carcases must not touch each other.
4 Door opening and closing must be kept to a minimum.
5 Adequate air flow around carcases is essential.
6 Carcases of different species must not occupy the same area.
7 Cold shortening must be avoided by not chilling below 10°C in less than 10 h.

### *Liquid nitrogen*

This refrigerant is increasingly being used in the food industry, especially for freezing and automated production lines. A moving belt carries the food through a tunnel and under a liquid nitrogen spray at the outlet. The food is frozen and the vaporised nitrogen is extracted by fans and discharged to the atmosphere. The liquid nitrogen is stored in vacuum-insulated tanks.

This form of *cryogenic freezing* is said to produce less dehydration (usually less than 0.3%) and better flavour, colour, aroma, texture and nutritive value in the food than the conventional types which utilise large volumes of cold air on the product. Higher operating efficiency and low running and maintenance costs are also claimed. Being constructed in stainless steel and capable of being quickly stripped down, the freezer tunnel can be rapidly and thoroughly cleaned.

Mobile meat containers are now nitrogen-cooled using either the gas, at −196°C from a tanker via a towed distribution unit, or the liquid as a coolant. The latter can reduce the temperature of the container more quickly but requires heavy storage vessels to be carried and is thus relatively expensive. There is also a tendency towards discoloration of the carcase and condensation on unloading; exposure to the air may restore the colour, while the use of loading hatches with an awning can reduce condensation. The cost, however, is some four times that of mechanical refrigeration.

## Refrigeration instrumentation

Good monitoring of refrigeration performance should always be insisted upon. Chill and freezer rooms should have *temperature indicators*, preferably with recording facilities, on the outside wall. There are a variety of portable instruments available for measuring temperature, air velocity and relative humidity. A *thermograph* is a chart recorder which can record temperatures for a period up to 7 days over a range of −25°C to 40°C. A *thermo-hygrograph* which can measure temperature and relative humidity (range 10–100% RH ±3% RH) is also available. 'Spear' thermometers may be inserted into carcases and cuts. Modern electronic and thermistor probe thermometers give accurate results and are durable. Instruments which can record temperature on charts may be obtained and an anemometer (records air velocity and some can also record temperature) is available.

Various types of relative humidity meters are available. These are electronic and instantaneous in measurement. A hair type thermohygrograph (using hair as a humidity sensor) is also a useful means of measuring and recording relative humidity (RH). This is the proportion of moisture to the value for saturation at the same temperature.

Temperatures measured can range from −40°C (in blast freezer) to +40°C for freshly slaughtered meat.

The relative humidity in chilled rooms after chilling is completed is around 85% RH, but when fresh carcases are first put into the chill room the air is supersaturated with moisture and in this case the humidity meter or thermohygrograph would read 100% RH. Infrared thermometry is now being more widely adopted.

## Freeze drying or lyophilisation

This is the process of removing water from frozen foods. The food products must be in comminuted form (sliced or diced) and packaging must be completely moisture-proof since the dried products are hygroscopic. At the present time beef, pork, chicken, shellfish and other foods such as mushrooms, fruits, peas, vegetables are preserved by this process. Since meat has a relatively high moisture content, it is relatively expensive to preserve by freeze-drying methods, which at this stage of development can be regarded only as a supplement to traditional methods of refrigeration.

## Vacuum packing

This is a process in which primal cuts of meat are placed in a gas-impermeable form of plastic (polythene, nylon/polythene, polyester/polythene) laminate bags at 2–4°C and a pH of 5.5–5.8. Two basic systems are used: (1) 'Cryovac', in which the air is sucked out and then the pack is passed through either a water dip or a hot air tunnel. (2) Drawing a vacuum without heat shrinkage. The advantage of (1) is that drip is reduced and there is less possibility of the package being torn. The packs are stored at between –18 and 1°C. The residual oxygen is consumed by tissue respiration and carbon dioxide accumulates. In the absence of water and air bacterial multiplication is significantly reduced and shelf-life can be maintained for up to 3 months, provided that the meat is of good microbiological standard. In the absence of air the meat assumes a bluish discoloration, but on re-exposure to air regains its normal red colour.

### *Carbon dioxide gas*

Great success in mould inhibition has been achieved by a process that depends on the ability of carbon dioxide gas, when present in high concentration, to prevent the growth of moulds. Facultative bacteria may or may not be suppressed by carbon dioxide, while lactic acid bacteria and anaerobes are virtually unaffected. On the other hand, the highly aerobic bacteria and yeasts and moulds are selectively inhibited by carbon dioxide, and the storage of meat in an appropriate concentration of this gas will therefore retard surface decomposition, though it will not prevent deep-seated anaerobic spoilage. Mould growth can be arrested completely at 0°C if 40% $CO_2$ is used, but any concentration over 20% rapidly produces methaemoglobin on the exposed muscle and fat, and the bloom is lost. Experiments have shown that in 10% $CO_2$ the storage life of meat at 0°C is double that of meat stored in ordinary air at a similar temperature, and in this way the storage life of chilled meat can be extended to 60–70 days.

## Refrigerated meat transport and storage

Depending on the type of trade and length of journey, meat may be transported by road in properly insulated and refrigerated (mechanical or liquid nitrogen) vehicles or insulated or non-insulated non-refrigerated vehicles. Only refrigerated transport can be considered adequate; all other modes are totally ineffective, especially the non-insulated type, particularly for chilled meat.

A well-designed *refrigerated road vehicle* should have the following qualities: high standard of insulation, good internal lining, air-tight door seals, water-tight flooring, rigidity of construction, efficient refrigeration unit, provision of temperature indicators in the driving cab and properly spaced overhead rails. In addition, it should be economical, lightweight and noiseless.

*Solid carbon dioxide* is sometimes used, either as solid blocks or crushed, and provides a temperature of 0–10°C. The van cooler is provided with a fan which blows the cool air over the carbon dioxide and load. A thermostat switches off the fan when the desired temperature is reached and a microswitch ensures that the unit does not operate when the vehicle doors are open.

The maintenance of the internal temperature is influenced by the difference between the inside and outside temperatures, insulation, the number of times the doors are opened and closed, loading temperature of the cargo, capacity rating of the refrigeration system, respiration rate of the product, etc. Vehicles left standing with doors wide open in high summer temperatures attract not only heat but also undesirable arthropods.

An efficient insulating medium is provided by urethane foam sprayed between inner and outer linings. This material expands to fill all crevices and has a low heat loss factor, a low water absorption rating and a density of 23–38 kg/cubic metre. Lining materials must be smooth, impermeable, durable, easily cleaned and able to withstand detergents and hot water. They must also be non-toxic and as far as possible free from seams. Typical lining materials are glass-fibre-reinforced panels, special non-marking aluminium (bare aluminium can mark fresh unwrapped hanging meat), plastic-coated and stainless steel sheeting.

Floors should be very durable, water-tight and easily cleaned. There should be no crevices or sharp corners throughout the inside of the vehicle which would hinder cleaning.

While construction of transport vehicles is normally suitable for hanging quarters of beef, lamb carcases, packaged meat, etc., the same does not hold for offal which is not in cartons. It is important that for the retail delivery of meat and offal there should be good handling facilities; it must not be placed in an unwrapped state on the floor. Loading should be effected into a previously chilled vehicle which has its own refrigeration unit and is well-insulated, should be direct from the cold store into the vehicle and, whenever possible, should be made using an enclosed loading bay. This prevents temperature increase during the loading operation. The vehicle temperature during transit should be monitored and recorded.

When the vehicle is unloaded, either into a transit cold store or at its final delivery point, product temperature should be checked before unloading, and transfer to the chilled storage should be immediate.

Over the last ten years, the market in chilled or refrigerated, as against frozen, foods has shown a marked increase in Europe, USA and Japan. The increase has been both in terms of value, including shelf space in the supermarkets and in the range of products available. These include those sold directly to the consumer and food service (catering) sales, where chilled products are sold in delicatessens, 'work place' cafeterias, restaurants or institutions for consumption on the premises.

These are appealing as 'convenience foods' for the consumer and as an added-value product for the manufacturer. Freshness is regarded as being healthier than, for example, in traditional heat processed foods and the sensory quality will be more 'natural'. Healthier foods, in the consumer's view, should not contain 'chemical' preservatives, and this has resulted in lower levels of salt and nitrates in preserved meats. Consumers often do not appreciate that added-value chilled foods are in fact processed.

## CHANGES IN FROZEN MEAT

Two outstanding and unfavourable changes take place as a result of the freezing of meat:

1 The physical state of the muscle plasm (globulin and albumen proteins) is considerably altered. When meat is frozen below −2°C the formation of ice crystals so raises the concentration of these proteins that they become insoluble and do not regain their solubility when the meat is thawed. A similar irreversible change may be observed if eggs are frozen.

2 The freezing point of meat lies between −1 and −1.5°C, when crystals begin to form: at −1.5°C, 35.5% of the muscle water is ice; at −5°C, 82% is ice; and at −10°C, 94% is ice. During freezing, the water present in the muscle fibres diffuses from the muscle plasm to form crystals of ice. In the past it has been believed that the speed of freezing has an important bearing on the size of the ice crystals and the future quality of the product. It has previously been postulated that when meat is frozen *slowly* the largest crystals are formed between the temperatures of −0.5°C and −4°C and are largely located outside the muscle fibres; this temperature range is known as the *zone of maximum ice formation*, and where meat is subsequently stored within this range the ice crystals continue to grow in size during storage. It has also been surmised that if meat is frozen *rapidly* to a temperature lower than −4°C, the ice crystals are small and lie mainly within the muscle fibres; if lowering of the temperature is sufficiently fast, many of the crystals are ultramicroscopic in size, and all of them are smaller than the cells in which they are formed. Doubt is now being cast on this theory as the *rate of freezing* appears to have minimal effect on thawing drip loss. *Quick freezing of meat* has made

rapid strides and is applied to lambs, calves, pigs, poultry, fish and various wholesale cuts, the latter being distributed wrapped in cellophane or a latex rubber container base. The temperature of a food may be reduced by quick freezing to as low as –46°C by contact with metal against which streams of brine at very low temperatures are directed; some methods use atomised sprays of cold brine, which produce no distortion of the muscle cells and practically no 'drip' on thawing. It is, however, unlikely that the quick freezing of whole quarters of beef will become a commercial proposition, for a temperature of –275°C would be required to quick-freeze a quarter of beef in 30 min.

## 'Weeping' or 'drip'

Weeping denotes the presence of a watery, blood-stained fluid which escapes from frozen meat when it is thawed and consists mainly of water, together with salts, extractives, protein and damaged blood corpuscles. The latter are responsible for the pink coloration of the fluid and are readily recognisable on microscopical examination. Weeping is an undesirable feature and is caused partly by the rupture of the muscle cells and tissues by crystals of ice, and partly by irreversible changes in the muscle plasm. The amount of drip is greater in beef than in mutton, lamb or pork, but the better the original quality of a beef carcase the less on average will be the drip from the meat after thawing. Quarters of frozen beef defrosted at 10°C for 3 days and cut into large wholesale joints lose about 1–2% of their weight during the following day, while smaller joints of the retail trade lose 1.5–2.5%.

It is claimed that drip is minimised if thawing is very slow. One method employed for beef is to subject the meat to a temperature of 0°C with 70% humidity, gradually increasing the temperature to 10°C and the humidity to 90%; the forequarter requires 65 h for complete thawing and the hindquarter 80 h. The major effect on drip is the final temperature on thawing.

It is known that the faster the rate of breakdown of ATP in muscle the more rapid is the onset of *rigor mortis* and the greater the release of fluid from the muscles. If the rate of breakdown of ATP could be slowed, i.e. rigor mortis delayed, less free fluid would be available for drip formation on subsequent freezing and thawing.

## Durability of frozen meat

Frozen meat stored too long becomes dry, rancid and less palatable, the most important change being the breaking down of the fat into glycerine and free fatty acids, with the production of *rancidity*. The better the quality of meat the less trouble one encounters in its storage. The storage temperature, the degree of fluctuation in the storage temperature and the type of wrapping (packaging) in which the meat is stored are generally thought to have the main influence on frozen storage life.

Temperature fluctuation is of limited importance when the product is left at a temperature below –18°C and the variation in temperature is only 1–2°C. Well-packed products and those that are tightly packed in palletised cartons are also less likely to show quality loss. However, poorly-packed items are severely affected by temperature changes.

### *Freezer burn*

This occurs on the outer surface of frozen offals, particularly liver, hearts and kidneys, and is caused by loss of moisture from the outer tissues. It may sometimes be seen where a carcase is stored, unwrapped, close to the opening of a cold air duct. The meat or offals have a brown, withered discoloration. This can be prevented by using suitable packaging or cryogenic freezing.

## Effect of freezing on pathogenic micro-organisms and parasites

Some bacteria are destroyed by freezing, but low temperatures merely inhibit the growth and multiplication of most until conditions favourable to their growth appear. Freezing is therefore of no great value in rendering a carcase affected with pathogenic bacteria safe for human consumption, nor are the bacteria commonly found on beef carcases destroyed by slow or sharp freezing. Anthrax bacilli can withstand a temperature of –130°C, while *Salmonella* can withstand exposure to –175°C for 3 days, and tubercle bacilli have been found alive after 2 years in carcases frozen at –10°C. The virus of foot-and-mouth disease can remain viable for 76 days if carcases of animals slaughtered during the incubative stage of the disease are chilled or frozen immediately afterwards. Under similar conditions the virus of swine fever may remain infective in bone marrow for at least 73 days, and has also been shown to be viable in frozen pork for 1500 days. Freezing is, however, a valuable method for the treatment of meat affected with certain *parasitic infections*. For example, pork affected with *Cysticercus cellulosae* can be rendered safe if held for 4 days at −10.5 to −8°C as can beef with *Cysticercus bovis* by holding for 3 weeks at a temperature not exceeding −6.5°C or for 2 weeks at a temperature not higher than −10.5°C. *Trichinella* cysts in pork are destroyed by holding the carcase for 10 days at −25°C, but this is unreliable if the pork is more than 15 cm thick.

### Storage of fresh meat

Meat cutting in supermarkets is labour-consuming and, as the cost of labour continues to increase, means to reduce these costs are being sought. Deboned and trimmed meat, in the unfrozen state offers cost savings in labour and transportation and requires less energy for storage than does frozen meat. This has resulted in a shift to more centralised meat cutting at packing plants where the carcase is reduced to smaller sections called *primal* and *subprimal cuts* which may represent one-fourth to one-eighth of a whole carcase. These cuts are vacuum-packed in high-barrier bags and paperboard boxes for shipment to retailers, where they are further reduced to retail-sized cuts. They are then repacked in the familiar tray and overwrap packages. Beef and pork may be vacuum-packed in a high-barrier film and stored at 0°C (unfrozen) for up to 3 weeks. Such meat acquires the purplish colour of myoglobin at its cut surfaces. When the film is removed, the myoglobin reoxygenates to oxymyoglobin and the meat reddens. Such meat is further cut into retail portions and wrapped in an oxygen-permeable film for consumer purchase. It also has been proposed that consumer cuts be centrally prepared and wrapped in oxygen-permeable film and then vacuum-packed as a group in an oxygen-impermeable overwrap. When the latter is removed, the individual units would redden and be ready for direct sale.

Most recently, new technologies have been developed which are designed to allow centralised processing and packaging of retail cuts, thus eliminating entirely the need for further processing in the retail store. The most successful technology is called *modified atmosphere packaging* (MAP). MAP utilises sealed high-barrier packages in which the air has been replaced with a mixture of gases which will reduce the rate of deterioration of the meat. Most often these gases include 10–50% carbon dioxide, which inhibits the growth of many microorganisms that cause spoilage of refrigerated meats. For fresh red meats the gas mixture often contains 20–50% oxygen so that the myoglobin will be in the oxygenated cherry-red form. The meats must be sealed in high-barrier films which will keep the air out and prevent the modified atmosphere from escaping.

## HEAT – THERMAL PROCESSING

The underlying principle of all food preserving methods is either the creation of unfavourable environmental conditions under which spoilage organisms cannot grow, or the destruction of such organisms. In commercial canning, carefully selected and prepared foods contained in a permanently sealed container are subjected to heat for a definite period of time and then cooled. In most canning processes, the heat destroys nearly all spoilage organisms and the permanent sealing of the container prevents reinfection.

Current canning practice, known as *aseptic canning*, involves the use of high temperatures for shorter periods. The food is sterilised at 120°C for 6 seconds to 6 minutes depending on the food, before it enters a sterilised can which is then closed with a sterilised lid. This method is said to improve the flavour and the vitamin content of the canned product.

Aluminium or coated aluminium may be used as alternatives to mild steel and tin in the fabrication of *cans*. While it has the advantage of lightness (and thereby lower transport costs), and freedom from sulphiding and rust, it buckles fairly easily. Efforts are being made to produce an alloy strong enough to withstand the stresses of processing, packing and transport.

Flexible *pouches* made from laminates of thermoplastic and aluminium foil are widely used in Japan and are now being adopted in Europe and the United States. They will not, however, withstand the high internal pressure developed during processing and must therefore be sterilised in media (water or steam and air) capable of providing an external pressure sufficient to balance the internal one.

For the thermal processing of the open or sanitary can, flame sterilisation, e.g. the Tarax flame steriliser developed in Australia, combined with rotation of the can, is now used for certain products. This system has the advantage of being relatively cheap and is capable of providing very efficient heat transfer in those products with some liquid.

Future forms of thermal processing may involve the use of microwave energy, hydrostatic sterilisers using high-efficiency steam and fluidised-bed systems.

When bacteria in a suspension are exposed to heat, the number remaining alive follows a logarithmic course (survivor or thermal death-rate curve) against the length of heating time at a constant temperature. The *D* value or *decimal reduction time* is the time taken at a constant temperature to reduce the *surviving* bacteria in a suspension to 10% of their original number. Total sterility is never achieved and the effect of any thermal processing is measured against the activity of the spores of *Clostridium botulinum*, the most heat-resistant pathogenic form known.

In modern canning operations there must be sufficient heat to reduce the population of *Cl. botulinum* spores by a factor of $10^{12}$, i.e. a heat process equal to 12 times the *D* (decimal reduction time) of *Cl. botulinum* spores. Foods with a pH of less than 4.5, in which *Cl. botulinum* spores do not germinate, may be subjected to milder heat treatments.

## Traditional canning methodology (Figs 4.1 and 4.2)

As a food container, the metal can – first developed by Nicholas Appert in France in 1795 – has certain virtues possessed by no other type of container for heat processed foods. It has a high conductivity, which is of importance during processing, it cannot easily be broken and, being opaque, any possible deleterious effects of light on the foodstuff are avoided.

There are currently three main methods of can manufacture, the most common being the traditional *three-piece food can*. Constant research and development are in operation to improve techniques and designs. Over the years the amount of metal in cans has been reduced and soldering, which involved the use of lead, has long been discarded. The process of can manufacture begins with sheets of tinplated steel (Fig. 4.2) (1). Some of these may be coated with lacquer and dried in ovens for 15–20 min. Lacquers are used to prevent contact between food and tinplate and vary in type according to the class of food to be canned – acid foods like fruit, high-protein foods such as meat, etc. The lacquer-coated sheets are cut into lengths and widths for specific can sizes (2, 3). Individual strips are then rolled into cylinders (4) and the two edges of the cylinder drawn together with an overlap which is *electrically welded* (5). At this stage the cylinders are given a further coat of lacquer on the seams and dried in an oven. A lip is next formed on each end of the cylinder (6). Separate ends (lids and bases) (7) are made in a different area and the rims of these ends are curled and a sealing compound is injected into the curl (8) (Fig 4.1). The base is next joined to the cylinder body, the sealing compound forming an airtight seal. The cans, with their separate lids, are now ready for use by the food processor.

The *two-piece drawn and wall-ironed can* (DWI) consists of two pieces of tinplate, the body and

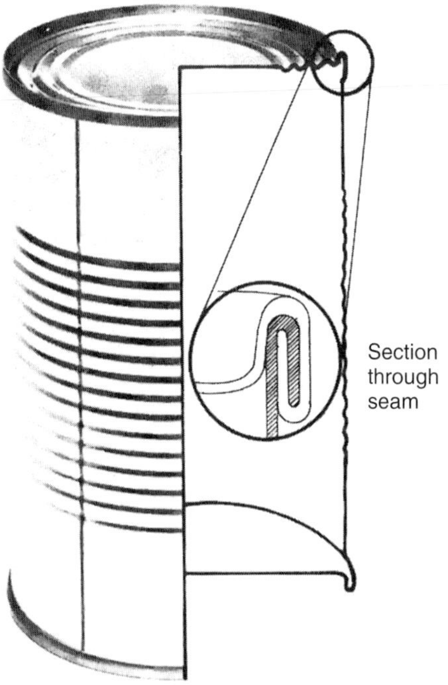


**Fig. 4.1** Modern food can showing section through seam. (By courtesy of Metal Box Ltd)

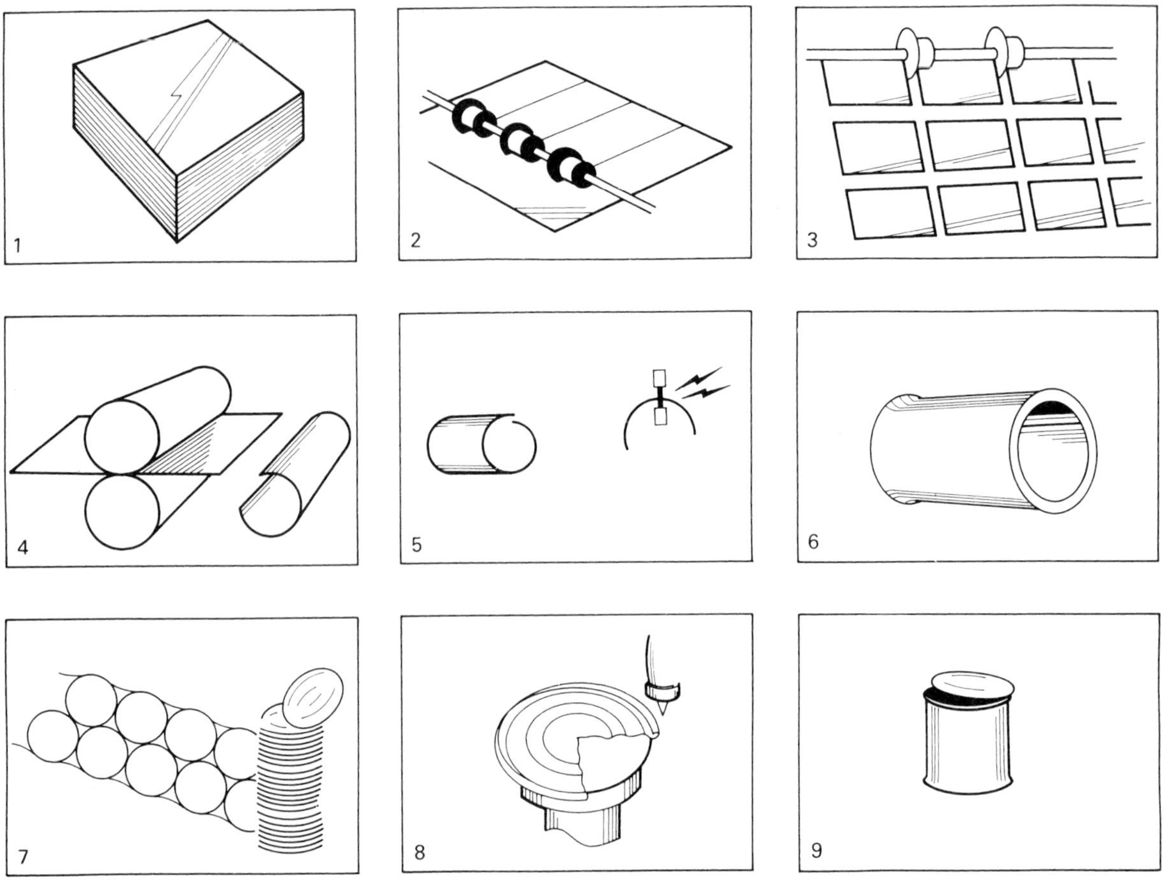


**Fig. 4.2** Stages of can manufacture. (By courtesy of Metal Box Ltd)

base being formed from one piece of metal and the lid from another. The body and base are shaped from a thick piece of tinplate which is drawn up, ironed and ridged for strength and then given a coat of lacquer.

The *drawn and redrawn* (DRD) can is manufactured from two pieces of tinplate, the body being made from a disc-shaped piece, lacquered on both sides, and drawn up to form a shallow cup and then redrawn a second and third time to make a deep cup.

Although the term *tin can* is applied to currently used containers, this is something of a misnomer as they are constructed of mild steel with a thin coating of pure tin representing about 1.5% of the can's weight. Coating of the steel plate is necessary to prevent corrosion, and in some foodstuffs, such as fish or fruit, a fish or fruit lacquer is used. Unsightly staining of the surface of certain foodstuff, known as *sulphiding*, may also occur and is avoided by use of a phenolic meat lacquer or a sulphur-resistant lacquer. An alternative method of avoiding sulphiding is now being extensively employed for meat packs and consists of chemical treatment of the inside of the can to form an invisible film, the solution used being a strong alkali bath containing phosphates and chromates.

## Treatment of food to be canned

The food to be canned must be clean and of good quality; the use of any material showing obvious signs of spoilage will result in deterioration in quality of the product. Many foods, particularly fruit and vegetables, are scalded or blanched before treatment, to cleanse the product, to produce shrinkage which permits adequate filling of the can, to remove gases, and to prevent oxidative changes which might cause deterioration. A firm, dry pack is required for meat foods without any excess of free liquor in the can; the moisture content of meat is therefore reduced by parboiling in steam-heated water, which produces up to 40% shrinkage in corned beef, 32% in ox tongues and 30% in pork tongues. Highly fattened animals are unsuitable for corned beef, as the meat is too fat and the finished product has an objectionable taste and appearance. The meat is therefore obtained from cattle which are older and leaner than those furnishing the supply of chilled or frozen beef.

After meats have been parboiled they are taken to the trimming table where inedible parts such as bones, cartilage and tendons, together with surplus fats, are removed.

## Canning operations

Cans may be filled either by hand or by automatic machinery, the next process being exhaustion or removal of air from the can before it is sealed. When meat with gravy is being canned it is important to put the gravy in first in order to ensure freedom from air bubbles, which could aid bacterial growth. It is essential to make sure the cans are not being overfilled.

### *Filling*

It is important that the correct weight is filled into each can. Overfilling can result in underprocessing and distortion of the can's seams. Underfilling may result in air pockets within the product which may interfere with the transfer of heat by conduction during processing. Any delay between filling and processing may allow bacterial growth with a resulting loss of quality.

### *Exhausting*

Exhaustion is necessary for the following reasons: to prevent expansion of the contents during processing, which may force the seams; to produce concave can ends so that any internal pressure may be readily detected and warrant rejection of the can; to lower the amount of oxygen in the can and prevent discoloration of the food surface; and, in fruit packs, to reduce chemical action between the food and container, and to avoid hydrogen swells. Although the production of a vacuum probably has little effect on microorganisms, experience has shown that tins containing a vacuum keep better than those with air in.

Exhaustion of a can may be carried out in two ways:

1. *Heat exhausting*, in which the contents are filled cold into the can, which is then passed through a steam-heated chamber before sealing. The ends of the can are loosely attached to permit the escape of air, sealing being completed when the cans leave the exhauster.
2. *Vacuumising*, in which the cold material is filled into the can, which is then closed in a vacuum-closing machine, the can being subjected to a high vacuum during the sealing operation.

Following closure, the cans are usually washed, before processing, in water at 80–85°C, containing a non-ionic detergent.

### *Processing*

With the exception of such foods as sweetened condensed milk or jam, all canned foods are processed, i.e. given final heating, after hermetic sealing. The term 'processing' is an exact one; it is not sterilisation since certain canned foods after processing may still contain living organisms. Although canned foods will keep with certainty if sterilised, they are then liable to alteration in colour and texture. Food to be canned is threatened on the one hand by bacterial spoilage and on the other by danger of overheating. The canner therefore chooses a middle course, the minimum heat employed in processing being controlled by the nature of the food in the can and the types and number of bacteria likely to be present.

During processing, heat penetrates to the centre of the can by conduction and by convection currents. In solid meat packs the heat diffuses by *conduction* only and the process is therefore slow; the *convection* currents in loosely packed foodstuffs transfer heat faster. Solids loosely packed in a liquid will, therefore, heat more rapidly than those that are tightly packed. Canned ham, being the largest and most solid pack of all the canned foods, requires very careful processing.

In non-acid foods, such as meat, the destruction of bacterial spores is slow; temperatures of about 115°C are required for adequate processing within a practical time limit. In commercial practice, the cans are placed in metal baskets in closed retorts and processed by pressurised steam.

The amount of heat used is based on that required to destroy the spores of *Cl. botulinum*, the so-called botulinum cook. It is quantified as the '*D-value*', which is a measure of the time taken to achieve a 10-fold reduction in the bacterial numbers at a given temperature. The accepted standard for a safe heat treatment is the time/temperature combination which will achieve a reduction in *Cl. botulinum* by a factor of 10, otherwise expressed as 10D. (Directive 92/5 refers to the *F* value. This is a measure of the LETHAL effect of the heat process to destroy spores or vegetative cells, and is expressed as minutes spent at 250°F – so an *F* value of 3.0 is the lethal heat equivalent of 3 minutes at 250°F. *Z Value* refers to the degrees *F* required for the destruction curve to traverse one log cycle.)

Monitoring of this CCPI must ensure that the time/temperature and pressure parameters are measured continuously and automatically to ensure all cans receive the correct 'cook'. The system must also ensure that processed and non-processed cans cannot be mixed.

### *Cooling*

Prompt cooling after processing is important, as it checks the action of heat and prevents undue change in texture and colour. In addition, cooling reduces the considerable internal pressure of the cans which builds up during processing. The cans may be placed under cold water showers, immersed in a cold water tank or pressure-cooled in the retort. The standard of the cooling water should be that acceptable for public drinking water supply, i.e. it should be clean and wholesome. Reliance cannot be placed on chlorination alone, which has little effect on any organisms if organic matter is present; river water will require sedimentation and filtration before final chlorination. The amount of chlorine added to cooling water should be enough to produce, after 30 min contact time, a free residual chlorine content of 0.5 ppm or more, and a chlorinated water supply should show no coliform bacteria in 100 ml water, a standard readily obtained by effective treatment. In commercial practice, cans are water-cooled to 38°C and the residual heat dries the exterior and prevents corrosion.

### *Can washing*

Cans that have just been cooled are dirty and greasy on the outside, and are therefore washed in a bath with soap or saturated with fatty alcohols and rinsed to facilitate subsequent handling, lacquering and labelling.

### *Outside lacquering*

Commercial lacquer or enamel is a colour varnish containing vegetable or synthetic resin. Lacquer may be applied to the outside of the tin to prevent external corrosion, particularly when the cans are destined for humid climates. Although external lacquering is not common in the canning of vegetables and fruits, it is almost universal in the salmon canning industry, not only because the UK market insists on shipments finished in this way, but also because the loss through rusting would otherwise be enormous.

### *Container handling*

The contents of hot, wet cans may be infected if the cans are subjected to mechanical abuse and exposed to excessive concentrations of microorganisms around the seam or seal areas, e.g. from operatives' hands. Thus, manual handling of hot wet cans must be avoided, and it is wise to discard cans manually handled while, for example, clearing run-way blockages. Surfaces coming into direct contact with cans must be checked for efficiency of cleaning ($<10\,cfu/cm^2$).

## Canning of meats

*Corned beef* is perhaps the best known of the canned meat products, although considerable quantities of canned ham, ox, sheep and pig tongues and spiced hams are now manufactured. The preparation of corned beef will illustrate the procedure normally adopted in the preparation of canned meats.

*Corned beef*

Corned beef is prepared from beef pickled in salt, nitrite and sugar, boiled for 1 h and then trimmed of soft fats, tendons, bones and cartilage. The texture and the fat content depend on the taste of the country for which it is intended, some countries preferring a lean corn beef, others a higher fat content; that for the UK market generally contains about 10% fat. Pickling is essential, for without it the meat after processing would be very much shrunken and dark in colour, while the can would contain liquid and dripping. The meat is machine-cut and packed automatically into cans. The shrinkage from original fresh boneless meat to its weight when finally packed is 40–45%. The cans are then capped with the vent open, and sealed under a vacuum. In some cases exhaustion is carried out, with the vent open, in a process retort for 45 min at 104.6°C; the can is then removed and the vent is closed as soon as it ceases blowing.

Subsequent processing varies in different plants. In some cases the cans are put into retorts and processed at a pressure of 0.632 $kgf/cm^2$ for 2½ h or more, depending on the size of the can. A 453 g tin of corned beef requires 21½ h at 104.6°C, a 2.7 kg tin 5 h at 105.5°C, and a 6.3 kg tin 6 h at 108.3°C. In other cases, the cans are immersed in boiling water for 3½–4 h. Processing is followed by cooling, degreasing and lacquering.

*Canned hams*

Hams are boned by hand and forced into a pressure mould to produce the required shape. The metal container for hams is double-seamed, though without a rubber gasket, sealing being done by hand-soldering followed by exhausting and soldering of the vent hole. The hams are finally cooked without pressure at 93.5°C for several hours Cooking at a higher temperature for a shorter time in a pressure retort is contraindicated, as it produces deleterious changes in the ham texture and heavy weight loss due to exudation of fat and gelatin. An increase of only 10 min in cooking at these higher temperatures can increase the overall cooking loss to 5%. Large hams 1.4 kg–7 kg, would be unpalatable if cooked at normal canning temperatures and should be subjected to 80°C for up to 60 min. This produces a 'pasteurised' ham which will have potentially a greater bacterial flora. The cans should be stored at 0°C.

## Foods packed in glass

A great variety of foods is packed in hermetically-sealed glass containers and, though the treatment of these differs somewhat from foods packed in cans, the principles of preservation are the same. The disadvantages of the glass container are that its greater weight, fragility, lessened output for the same amount of equipment and labour, together with the extra expense in packing, limit its use for the higher-grade products. On the other hand, it is less susceptible to attack by the product it contains and the contents may be readily inspected. The metal caps of glass containers are usually lacquered tin plate, with a paper liner inside to prevent discoloration resulting from corrosion of the metal. The cap is held firmly against a rubber gasket on the rim of the glass container and thus forms a hermetic seal.

Glass-packed foods are processed for a longer period than canned foods but at a lower temperature, as there is risk of fracture of the glass, and both heating and cooling must therefore be carried out more slowly. The modern method is to process in pressurised steam-heated water. At the conclusion of processing, the steam is shut off and cold water is slowly admitted to the retort but the air pressure is still maintained to prevent the cap from being blown off by the internal pressure which develops in the container.

## Spoilage in canned foods

It was at one time thought that the keeping qualities of canned goods depended upon the complete exclusion of air. Later it was suggested that the heating destroyed all microorganisms, while the sealing of the can prevented the entry of others, and that decomposition, when it occurred, was due to faulty sterilisation or to entry of bacteria through a fault in the can. Neither of these views expresses the whole truth because living bacteria can often be found in sound and wholesome food, and bacteriological methods show that any canned meats or meat products contain living organisms, even after modern processing methods. The mere presence of living organisms is of little or no significance in assessing the soundness of canned goods.

The organisms responsible for *spoilage* in canned goods may be spore-forming and therefore resistant to commercial processing, or they may be non-sporing organisms which gain access via leakages after processing. Aerobic spore-forming bacteria may be present in sound samples of canned goods. Spores probably remain dormant under the anaerobic conditions of a properly sealed can but, if supplied with air through faulty sealing, may develop and produce enzymes which decompose the foodstuff.

Non-sporing proteolytic or fermenting bacteria, e.g. *Proteus* and *E. coli*, may cause decomposition of canned foods; no single type of organism is responsible for microbial spoilage. The problem of spoilage in canned goods is not the simple one of the presence or absence of such bacteria, but why in some cans bacteria of this type decompose the contents, while in others they remain inactive. Though *yeasts* and *moulds* are of great importance as a cause of unsoundness in acid substances containing sugars, e.g. canned fruits, they are of less importance in canned meats and marine products. The presence of yeasts, moulds and non-sporing bacteria in canned meat foods is evidence of leakage after sealing and can make the food unsound. Canned goods which, on opening, show such evidence should be condemned.

## Types of spoilage

Canned goods are classified as spoiled when the food has undergone a deleterious change, or when the condition of the container renders such change possible. Spoiled cans may show obvious abnormalities such as distortion, blowing, concave ends or slightly constricted sides; or they may present a perfectly normal external appearance.

A can with its ends bulged by positive internal pressure due to gas generated by microbial or chemical activity is termed a *swell* or *blower*. A *flipper* has a normal appearance and though one end flips out when the can is struck against a solid object it snaps back to normal under light pressure. A *springer* is a can in which one end is bulged but can be forced back into normal position, whereupon the opposite end bulges. All blown cans pass successively through the *flipper* and *springer* stages and these two conditions must be regarded as suspicious of early spoilage of the can contents. A change in the appearance of the gelatin surrounding meat packs is usually associated with the formation of gas, the gelatin being discoloured and more liquid in consistency. It should be remembered however, that in hot weather the gelatin of meat packs is likely to be of a more fluid nature. These abnormal cans are brought about by imperfect canning operations such as inadequate exhaustion of air before sealing, overfilling and the so-called '*nitrate swell*' which arises during thermal processing and is recognised during subsequent cooling, but whose nature is not fully understood.

A *leaker* is a can with a hole through which air or infection may enter or its contents escape. An *overfilled can* is one in which the ends are convex due to overfilling, but filling by weight or accurate measurement has done much to obviate this condition and most tins classified as overfilled are actually in the early stage of blowing. Though an overfilled can cannot properly be regarded as a spoiled can, it must be differentiated from a blower, and it emits a dull sound when struck, whereas a blown tin emits a resonant note. The term *slack caps* denotes a can which has a movement of one of the ends similar to that of a can in the early stages of blowing but is now rarely, if ever, encountered, and the great majority of cans classed as slack caps are blown and should be treated as such.

Spoilage of canned goods may be of microbial origin or chemical origin due to deleterious influences such as rust or damage.

### *Microbial spoilage*

Bacteria of the decomposing or fermenting type are the most important as regards canned foods, while spore-forming bacteria are the most resistant. There are three main types of spore-forming organisms which can resist normal processing and may cause spoilage in canned foods; gas-producing anaerobic and aerobic organisms with an optimum growth temperature of 37°C; gas-producing anaerobic organisms growing at an optimum temperature of 55°C; and non-gas-producing aerobic or facultative anaerobic spore-forming organisms with an optimum growth temperature of about 55°C, which produce '*flat-sours*'.

Processing is not a substitute for cleanliness and will destroy a small number of bacteria rather more easily than a large number. Bacteria subjected to heat or other harmful influences are destroyed in accordance with a definite law which prescribes that where two different suspensions of the same organism are subjected to heat under uniform conditions, the number of bacteria will be reduced by the same *percentage* over equal periods of time.

*Insufficient processing* is a cause of unsoundness of canned goods, though not the all-important factor generally assumed.

The bacteria found in canned meat or fish are nearly always secondary invaders gaining access through a leak. Microbial spoilage may thus result from underprocessing or from *leakage* through the seam. Leakers may be detected by the disappearance of the vacuum from the sides and ends of the can, and bubbles appear if the can is held under water and squeezed. Another test for leakage is to heat the can to 38°C in the interior and allow it to cool slowly; if a leak is present, there will be no concavity of the sides or ends. The detection of leakers by striking the suspect can with a mallet has little value in industrial practice. The commonest form of leaking occurs at the seams, and may sometimes be detected by liquid or stain on the can surface. Mould formation on the surface of canned meats is also indicative of leakage, but cannot be detected until the can is opened.

*Flat-souring* in canned goods produces a sour odour of the foodstuff but the can is not blown. Canned foods susceptible to flat-souring are those containing sugar or starches, and meat products such as sausages or pastes containing cereal. True flat-sours are caused by thermophilic organisms (*B. coagulans, B. stearothermophilus, B. circulans*) which are exceptionally heat-resistant and attack carbohydrates, producing acid but not gas. Sourness in canned foods may also arise due to leaking cans, or it may have developed in the foodstuff before processing. This latter form of spoilage is most likely in packs cold-filled in warm weather, particularly if the cans are open for even short periods prior to processing.

Flat-souring of canned goods due to thermophilic spore-forming organisms cannot be detected until the can is opened and its contents are examined, but is unlikely to occur in temperate climates unless storage conditions have been exceptionally hot; it is, however, comparatively common in tropical and subtropical countries, or in cans imported from them.

Ham spoilage may be caused by faecal streptococci, e.g. *Streptococcus liquefaciens*, which may liquefy jelly and cause off-colour, off-flavour souring.

### *Chemical spoilage*

*Hydrogen swell* may occur quite independently of fermentation or bacterial decomposition, and is associated with the formation of hydrogen gas in the can following *internal corrosion*. Imperfections or scratches on the inner tin coating may expose small areas of steel, and, where the contents are acid, an electric couple may result, the reaction producing hydrogen gas. Electrolytic action is accelerated by oxygen and by the colouring matter (anthocyanins) of red fruit. Cracks in the inner lining of lacquer serve to concentrate electrolytic action on the areas of steel exposed and increase the rate of hydrogen release. Cans affected with hydrogen swell may show varying degrees of bulging from flipping to blowing. If the tin is punctured, there is emission of hydrogen gas, which is colourless and burns on the application of a flame. The condition is chiefly associated with foods containing organic acids such as *fruits*, particularly plums, cherries, raspberries, blackcurrants and loganberries.

The *range of acidity* most favourable to the production of hydrogen swell lies between pH 3.5 and 4.5, and the less acid fruits therefore give more trouble than those of higher acidity, but with proper precautions there should be very little trouble from hydrogen swells in commercially-packed English fruits for at least a year after canning. The condition is seldom encountered in canned vegetables and is practically unknown in canned meat foods, but it is sometimes seen in tinned sardines. Although the contents of a can in hydrogen swell may be quite harmless, the routine methods employed in the examination of canned goods render it impossible to distinguish between tins blown owing to hydrogen swell and those blown as a result of deleterious changes due to bacteria or yeasts. All blown tins, whether fruit, meat, vegetables or condensed milk, must be regarded as unfit for food, and leakers, springers and flat-sours, together with tins whose contents show evidence of mould, should likewise be condemned.

*Purple staining* on the inner surface of cans in which sulphur-containing foods are packed may occur with all fish and meat products, especially liver, kidneys and tongue. It is due to the breakdown of sulphur-containing proteins in high-temperature processing by the thermophilic *Clostridium nigrificans* ('sulphur stinker'); hydrogen sulphide is liberated and a thin layer of tin sulphide is formed on the inside of the can. This discoloration does not involve the foodstuff itself and varies from a light pink to a dark purple, but it may be accompanied by a blackening of both the inside of the can and surface of the foodstuff if the hydrogen sulphide attacks the steel base-forming iron sulphide. It is of more serious import than the deposition of tin sulphide, as it may lead to pitting of the steel and disfigurement of the surface of the meat pack. Discolorations of both types may be prevented by a sulphur-resisting lacquer, the basis of which is copal gum dissolved in a suitable solvent to which are added substances capable of uniting with the volatile sulphur gases released while the food is being processed.

### *Rust or damage*

Cans showing external *rust* require careful consideration. It is a condition particularly liable to occur beneath can labels when the adhesive contains hygroscopic substances. Cans in which the external surface is slightly rusted without noticeable pitting of the iron may be released for immediate sale and consumption, but if the rust is removed with a knife and inspection with a hand lens reveals the iron plate to be definitely pitted, there is danger of early perforation and the cans should be condemned. Minute perforations of the tin plate, known as *pinholing*, permit the entrance of air and lead to spoilage of the can contents. Pinholing may originate from the outside, but also from the inside of the can where the tin plating is imperfect or has been fractured during seaming, and in this case lacquer lining aggravates the trouble, as the cracks that occur in the lacquer aid in concentrating the chemical action on a small area. A can which is a leaker or pinholed may occasionally seal itself by blocking of the holes with the contained foodstuffs, and may then proceed to blow; such self-sealing cans may blow at any period of their storage life, whereas an underprocessed can will blow early in its life, generally within the first few months. Where unfilled cans are stored and allowed to rust internally before being filled, the can edges may become rusted, with the result that during processing a chemical action may take place between the rust and meat juices and give rise to an unsightly grey precipitate of iron phosphate in the meat jelly.

Considerable significance should be attached to cans *damaged* by rough handling, the important factor in their judgement being the extent and location of the damage. Marked deformation of the can seam is attended by considerable risk of leakage and such cans should be condemned. Slight indentations on the can body are permissible, but severe dents on the body may cause seam distortion and such cans should be rejected; any can having a dent at one end should also be rejected for it is possible to reduce a springer to normal, at any rate temporarily, by hitting it upon the corner of a box. Nail holes in cans caused during the closing of packing cases may also be encountered, and such cans should be rejected even if the contained foodstuff appears perfectly normal. It is important to reject any can which is in the least suspicious or which shows lack of concavity of the ends.

## The public health aspect of canned foods

Improvements in the canning industry during recent years, together with greater appreciation of its hygienic requirements, have done much to remove the public prejudice against canned foods, which were thought to cause food poisoning. Food poisoning is usually the result of improper handling of food during preparation or storage, and, with the exception of botulism, food poisoning outbreaks are nearly always caused by bacteria which would be destroyed during processing. *Salmonellae* are destroyed with certainty by the temperatures attained in commercial processing. The minimum standard of processing now universally recognised by reputable canners ensures the destruction of *Cl. botulinum* spores in low- and medium-acid foods (see *Botulism*). A lower processing temperature is, however, permissible in cases such as cured meats, in which the curing salts have an inhibitory effect on the growth of the organism and the production of toxin.

Staphylococci, and more rarely streptococci, are now recognised as a cause of food poisoning mainly in prepared or unheated foods, such as cheese, salad, milk or ice cream. These organisms are ubiquitous in nature but their main source is the human or animal body, where they are normally present on the skin, in the intestine and the respiratory tract. Staphylococci, however, are relatively susceptible to heat, and even the more resistant staphylococcal enterotoxin, which may withstand a temperature of 100°C for 30 min, is destroyed during commercial processing. Cans may occasionally become infected by these organisms through a leak, and in the absence of accompanying gas-forming bacteria, there will be no 'blow' and the can will appear normal. Most cases of food poisoning now associated with canned foods are the result of contamination after the can is opened, but a number of cases of typhoid fever associated with canned foods have occurred in Britain. The outbreak in Aberdeen in 1964, in which there were over 400 confirmed cases, was attributed to the post-processing entry of contaminated cooling water in a 2.7 kg tin of corned beef of South American origin.

Viewing the question as a whole, canned foods are considerably less likely to be a source of food poisoning than ordinary fresh foods. The possibility of secondary contamination of canned foods with pathogenic bacteria also raises the question of the wisdom of leaving food in a can after it has been opened. From the public health standpoint there is no reason why an open can, properly stored, should not be used as a food container; it should, however, be covered to prevent contamination and kept cool.

#### *Microbiological examination of canned meats*

Where suspected outbreaks of food poisoning attributed to canned food occur, the normal laboratory procedures for isolation of the responsible organism (*Salmonella, Staphylococcus, Clostridium*, etc.) are adopted, care being taken in the sampling, transport, identification, handling, etc. of the suspect food.

In order to ensure the safety and stability of large consignments of hermetically-sealed containers of meat products, attention should be directed at the standards of *methods used at the point of production* (quality assurance), *viz.* hygiene levels, temperatures for heat treatment, water supply, etc., which should supply more important information than the microbiological testing of numerous containers, which would not only be wasteful but would be unlikely to detect entities such as botulism.

Examination of the *quality of containers* is important to ensure that there are no damaged, rusty, blown, etc. cans. If there is reason to suspect that a consignment of meat products in hermetically-sealed containers is unsatisfactory, sampling and inspection procedures should be adopted anlong the lines recommended by the Codex Alimentarius Commission (1983). The number of samples to be taken is assessed according to the expected hazard and the laboratory facilities available in the case of shelf-stable canned products. For non-shelf-stable products, five containers are examined visually and their contents examined microbiologically. Both *aerobic* and *anaerobic* microbiological techniques are undertaken, decisions as to rejection or approval being based on bacterial plate counts (Sampling and Inspection Procedures for Microbiological Examination of Meat Products in Hermetically sealed Containers, Codex Alimentarius Commission of FAO/WHO 1983).

## OTHER METHODS OF MEAT PRESERVATION

### Antioxidants

An *antioxidant* is defined in the UK Miscellaneous Food Additives Regulations 1995 No. 3187 (as amended in 1997) as 'any substance which prolongs the shelf-life of a food by protecting it against deterioration caused by oxidation, including fat rancidity and colour changes'.

Antioxidants often improve flavour in cooked meat and some prevent colour changes.

### Preservatives

A *preservative* is defined in the above regulations as any substance which prolongs the shelf-life of a food by protecting it against deterioration caused by micro-organisms.

Schedule 2 of the 1995 regulations gives a list of permitted preservatives and antioxidants.

In the assessment of any additive for use in a food, three criteria have to be considered:

1 benefit or need accruing to the food industry, retailers and customers;
2 safety in use;
3 satisfactory standard of purity of the chemical.

Other substances are added to foods for specific purposes, e.g. emulsifiers, stabilisers, acids, non-stick agents, air excluders, phosphates, humectants, sequestrants, firming agents, anti-foam agents, colouring agents, flavours and solvents, in addition to nutritive substances such as vitamins A, $B_1$ (thiamin), C and D, nicotinic acid and calcium. While some of these additives contribute to the shelf-life, they are not normally regarded as true preservatives.

## Irradiation

Electromagnetic radiation is known to inhibit the growth of microorganisms and a considerable amount of work has been expended in an attempt to use it for the sterilisation of foods. Close attention has been paid to the effect on the nutritional value of the treated foods, as well as the possible production of carcinogens and induced radioactivity.

## Infrared radiation

Infrared rays have been mainly used to dry fruits and vegetables and for heat blanching in the same way as high-frequency radiation. Infrared rays have a wavelength of $3 \times 10^{-4}$ cm.

## Ultraviolet radiation

Ultraviolet rays occur at wavelengths of radiation between 100 and 3000 Å and are invisible (the Angstrom, Å, is a unit of length equal to $10^{-10}$ metre or 0.1 nanometre). They have a bactericidal action which is especially valuable for destroying air-borne bacteria, and are utilised in storage vats and other tanks to destroy microorganisms on or above the surface of foods. The penetrating effects of the rays are generally considered to be low and are influenced by factors such as the length of exposure, temperature, pH, relative humidity, light intensity and degree of contamination.

The wavelength for maximum bactericidal activity of ultraviolet rays is about 2500 Å, which can be produced by mercury-vapour lamps. As would be expected, spores and moulds are more resistant than vegetative organisms, yeasts being only slightly more resistant.

Ultraviolet rays are currently used in the *ageing of meat* at relatively high temperatures to control the growth of surface organisms. The bactericidal effect is also due to shorter wavelengths which convert atmospheric oxygen to ozone, an additional bactericide.

## Ionising radiation

Irradiation of food can be achieved by using either gamma-rays produced by a radionuclide, usually cobalt-60, or high-energy machines.

Both gamma-rays and electrons produce ions which induce a sequence of chemical changes in the food, thus causing the particular effect for which the irradiation was applied, e.g. the killing of bacteria. These chemical changes are not unique to irradiation but are also produced by other conventional processing methods such as heating and cooking.

Although the two sources of ionising radiation produce similar reactions in a food, they may not be equally suitable for all food applications because of their different penetrating powers. High-energy electrons are less penetrating than gamma-rays, the extent of penetration being influenced by the energy (maximum permitted level is 10 MeV (mega-electron volt) and density of the product.

Double-sided irradiation allows an increase in the effective thickness of a package, but electrons are not suitable for treating large bulk packages although they can be used for thin packs or for surface irradiation. With gamma-irradiation, pallets of up to 1 m thickness can be used.

The main features of an irradiation plant are the irradiation room, which contains the source of ionising radiation, and an automatic conveyor system which transports the food into and out of the room. Around this room is approximately 2 m of concrete. In the case of a gamma-irradiator, the radionuclide continuously emits radiation and when not in use must be stored in a water pool, whereas machines producing high-energy electrons can be switched off and on. This naturally influences the financial feasibility and a plant needs to be in continuous operation.

**Uses** Some of the uses of ionising radiation are as follows:

1 Decontamination of food ingredients such as spices.
2 Reduction in the numbers of pathogenic microorganisms such as *Salmonella, Campylobacter* and *Listeria* in, for example, meat and meat-type products.
3 Extension of shelf-life of fruits, vegetables, meat and meat products.
4 Insect disinfestation of grain, grain products and tropical fruits.
5 Inhibition of sprouting in potatoes, onions and garlic.

**Effectiveness** The effectiveness of the process depends on the quality of the raw material, the dose applied, temperature during irradiation, type of packing and storage conditions before and after irradiation.

Pathogens such as *Salmonella* and *Campylobacter* are sensitive to fairly low levels of ionising radiation. As the radiation dose increases, more microorganisms are affected, but a higher dose may simultaneously introduce organoleptic changes, and there needs to be a balance between the optimum dose required to achieve a desired objective and that which will minimise any organoleptic changes. With *fresh poultry* carcases, an irradiation dose of 2.5 kGy (kilogray) will virtually eliminate *Salmonella* and extend the shelf-life of the food by a factor of about 2 if the storage temperature post-irradiation is maintained below 5°C. (The gray is the SI unit of absorbed radiation dose, equivalent to transfer of 1 J of energy per kg of product being treated (1 J/kg).). Irradiation of poultry was approved in the USA in 1990.

**Organoleptic changes** Higher doses will give an even greater reduction in the numbers of microorganisms, but at doses of about 5 kGy or above, odour and flavour changes may be produced in the food during storage which will render it unacceptable. These are caused by the formation of volatile sulphur-containing substances – hydrogen sulphide, carbonyls, amines, etc. Hydrogen sulphide odour is lost on subsequent storage, and different odours develop. While beef is especially susceptible to the development of these unpleasant odours and flavours, pork is much less affected.

Irradiation doses up to 10 kGy can be applied to frozen poultry (−18°C) without causing any unacceptable organoleptic changes because in the frozen state the chemical reactions that bring about the desired effects of irradiation are hindered and a higher dose is necessary to achieve the same objective.

When treating *frozen* products, time in the irradiator should be kept to a minimum so that any temperature rise is not significant. Similar considerations regarding dose and irradiation conditions also apply to other products such as frogs' legs and shellfish.

**Other requirements** The benefit to be gained from using irradiation whether, for example, to control food-poisoning microorganisms or to disinfect grain, will only be achieved if the food being treated is of excellent quality and is stored under suitable conditions before and after irradiation. This often involves chilled or even frozen storage, and, depending on the product, humidity control may also be necessary. The need to combine irradiation with suitable storage highlights the point that irradiation is not a technology that can stand alone. It is one technology among many others which in some cases may have advantages over the more conventional food preservation methods.

The UK Food (Control of Irradiation) Regulations 1990 require licensing of premises which can carry out irradiation. The seven permitted descriptions of food are: fruit, vegetables, cereals, bulbs and tubers, spices and condiments, fish and shellfish and poultry.

## High pressure

An interesting development, currently attracting a great deal of worldwide interest, is the use of high pressure. The pressures involved are immense, greater than at the bottom of the deepest ocean, which is over 6.5 tons per square inch. Work in Australia has shown that the cooked tenderness of meat can be improved by such treatment, either before or after rigor mortis, and Japanese workers have demonstrated that the time required for conditioning can be decreased. The microbiological quality of comminuted meat products can be improved, offering potentially increased shelf-life. The water binding of beef patties is increased. However, all of this work is very much in its infancy and is likely to involve further capital investment and many hours of development to bring high-pressure-treated meat and meat products into the market place.

# Chapter 5
# By-products Treatment

The economics of the world's meat industry require that animal by-products are utilised so that the livestock industry generates viable products. Whenever possible, this means creating added-value foods or products, which entails further processing. The cost of the live animal often exceeds the selling price of its carcase and therefore the value of the by-products must pay for the cost of slaughter and provide a profit for the meat plant. Even when some by-products are worthless, they must be disposed of in a hygienic, environmentally-friendly, cost-effective manner.

By-products are divided into *edible* and *inedible*, although the distinction is not absolute. Bovine liver is a valuable edible by-product when passed as fit for human consumption, but when affected with fascioliasis it is inedible, although it can still be utilised by the pharmaceutical and pet food industries.

For animal by-products to be effectively utilised there must be a practical commercial process for converting the animal by-products into a usable commodity, and there must be a large enough volume of economically priced animal by-product material in one location for processing. Highly trained operatives with specialised technical skills are needed. Satisfactory storage of the perishable product prior to processing is critical, as the material used is very susceptible to bacterial contamination and decomposition. Storage post-manufacture will depend on the type of by-product, some requiring refrigeration and some only ambient storage, e.g. dried greaves. Once produced, there must follow an actual or potential market for the commodity.

## EDIBLE BY-PRODUCTS

The yield from meat animals ranges from 20% to 30% of the liveweight for beef, pork and lamb and from 5% to 6% of the liveweight of chickens. Biologically, most non-carcase material is edible, with appropriate cleaning, handling or processing, but variable use is made throughout the world owing to custom, religion, palatability and reputation of the product. The most commonly used organs for human consumption are liver, heart, tongue, kidney, tripe and, in areas free from BSE, sausage casings, sweetbreads and brain. Some cultures will use other parts of the animal – pig and poultry feet, pigs' ears, etc.

Additional non-carcase material is usually separated into categories of decreasing value to provide sausage material and other edible by-products, e.g. fat; pet food; animal feed; and fertiliser.

Edible by-products, in general, owing to their higher glycogen content and lesser fat covering, are more perishable than the carcase and they must be chilled quickly and handled hygienically. They should be kept at a temperature of not more than 3°C. Freezing does not significantly decrease the bacterial numbers in edible by-products but a temperature of −12°C will arrest all microbial growth. Vacuum packaging will also increase the shelf-life, which in some cases can be doubled using this technique. Some of these products can also be cured, smoked, pickled and/or canned.

The *pet food industry* utilises many materials which are not suitable for human consumption and those which, although edible, have a low monetary value, such as sow's liver. The handling and storage should be as for products intended for human consumption but there must be complete separation from edible material as some of the pet food products will not have passed veterinary inspection, e.g. bovine liver with fascioliasis, which could pose a potential risk.

Although chilling, followed by cleaning and trimming and a final freezing of offals for dispatch to pet-food manufacturers was the normal practice, there is now a preference for fresh chilled product generally sent to the manufacturer fresh, chilled in insulated containers for processing to be carried out within a few days of slaughter.

The use of specialised glands for *pharmaceutical* purposes, although still carried out, has decreased owing to the biotechnical manufacture of medicines, which allows for a more consistent product.

By-products of the meat industry and their uses are given in Appendix I.

## BY-PRODUCT PREMISES

Premises should be situated so that raw material can be conveyed to them with minimum handling. They should be spacious, well lit and ventilated, with impervious walls and floors. Floors should be sloped to open channels leading through fat traps to the drains. There should be a good supply of hot and cold water and steam. Although steam is no longer used in the cleaning process, it is required for heating water and in the production of fat. Offals should be treated quickly as storage space is expensive. There should be separate rooms for *green offal*. The room for handling *stomachs* and *intestines* should be adjacent to the slaughterhall but completely separate from it, the only open space being sufficient to allow the hygienic movement of the gastrointestinal tract for further processing. If not processed in a separate room, stomachs should only be treated by means of closed-circuit mechanical equipment which ensures no cross-contamination. Another room will be required for the handling of *edible red offals* such as liver, heart, kidneys, tongues, heads, ox tails and thick skirt. Alternatively, a separate area of the slaughterhall may be acceptable. These meats can be transported via mechanical overhead rails or hung on stainless steel racks for manual movement to trimming and packing rooms. *Feet* and *heads*, not required for edible purposes or for inspection, are either conveyed by shutes into skips on the outside of the slaughterhall or put into wheeled trucks, marked condemned material, and removed to a designated area as soon as possible, and certainly during all breaks and at the end of the day's production.

A room will also be required for the storage of *hides* and *pelts*. The size will depend on whether salting takes place on the premises or if they are removed at the end of each day.

Although, in the United Kingdom, processing of bovine intestines for *sausage casings* is illegal, as they are included in specified risk material (SRM), there is still a demand for further processing of sheep and pig intestines and, of course, also bovine in other parts of the world. This can be an unpleasant task but is greatly facilitated when the room or rooms in which it is carried out, are supplied with good ventilation and drainage.

*Condemned material* should be deposited in clearly labelled bins or trucks and forwarded as soon as possible to the condemned chill or condemned skip to await disposal. It is essential that it should not come in contact with edible product and the chill and containers should be kept locked. Staining of the material will allow it to be easily identified and will prevent improper usage.

The secret in the production of high-grade animal by-products lies in the prompt treatment of the raw material. As animal offals decompose rapidly, it is essential that no raw material is left untreated for any length of time after a day's slaughtering.

## BY-PRODUCT TREATMENT

The by-products that must undergo some forms of processing before final use are fat (edible and inedible), hooves, horns, hides, skins, glands, condemned material and offal.

It has been calculated that of 170 kg of *bovine* by-product going for inedible rendering there is 45 kg carcase bone, 10 kg head, 7 kg manifold, 30 kg intestines, 10 kg feet and 5 kg spleen, thymus, spinal cord and tonsils.

In *pigs* there is a relatively higher percentage of edible fat and a greater amount of edible product, the figure for carcase and edible product is often as high as 80%.

### Fats

With the exception of the hide, the most important abattoir by-product is the fat trimmed from the intestines, kidney area, channel and other internal organs of cattle. Fats

**Table 5.1** Average breakdown of 450 kg steer and a 25 kg lamb.

| | Steer (%) | Lamb (%) |
|---|---|---|
| Carcase and other edible products | 62–64 | 62–64 |
| Edible raw fat | 3–4 | 5–6 |
| Blood | 3–4 | 3.5–4 |
| Inedible raw material | 8–10 | 6–7 |
| Stomach and intestine contents | 8 | 5.5 |
| Hide (pelt and wool in lamb) | 7 | 15 |

are graded 1 edible fat and 2–6 inedible fat. The grades are dependent on free fatty acid (FFA) content and colour. Caul (omentum and its contained fat droplets) and kidney fat are rendered to produce premier jus, which is separated into oleo oil and oleo stearin (suet). Dripping is made from caul, kidney and body fat. Grades 2–6 are used in animal feeds, soaps (mainly 2–4), and the chemical industry (predominately 6). The latter uses them in such diverse products as toothpaste, lubricating oils (where they can be used in two-stroke marine biodegradable fuel), plastic, cotton and liquid washing detergents. More traditionally they have been used in the dressing of leather, and production of commercial glycerine, which itself is used in medicinal preparations, nitroglycerine, gunpowder, cordite and dynamite.

Fat occurs in many regions of the *pig carcase*, the best quality fat being obtained from the peritoneal lining (leaf fat), the next best from the back fat, mesentery and omentum. The surplus fat of pigs is worked up into various qualities of lard. A pig of 90 kg liveweight yields about 6.3 kg of lard.

*Sheep fat* is rendered in the same way as beef fat or lard and, though it is not converted into oleo oil or oleo stearin because of its flavour, it may be used as dripping when blended with other fats. Mutton fat is firmer and contains more stearin than ox or pig fat, and is used as a preservative layer on the top of glass jars of meat paste.

## Edible fat rendering

High-quality fats have low FFA values and are usually stable. Efficient rendering processes ensure that the FFA content remains low by means of initial cold storage of the raw material where it is not immediately used, followed by keeping the processing temperatures as low as possible and the cooking times minimised. There are three main methods of processing edible fat: wet rendering, dry rendering and continuous low-temperature rendering.

The *wet rendering* method involves the use of pressure batch cookers in which the pre-cut raw material is injected with live steam to a temperature of 140°C under pressure, for 3–4 h. After this time the pressure is slowly released and the fat is run into a receiver and further purified by gravity or centrifugation to settle out the water and fines. The proteinaceous solids or greaves are emptied from the cooker, and the fat is removed by pressure and solvent extraction. They are then ground and dried.

The *dry rendering* process uses heat in the form of steam and water over a period of 1½ h at atmospheric pressure to drive off water indirectly from the fat in the cooker. The rest of the process is the same as for the wet rendering method.

The *continuous low-temperature wet rendering* system uses heating, separation and cooling on a continuous basis, and is usually regarded as the ideal process (Fig. 5.1). The process involves mincing of the raw material; melting by live steam injection at 90°C; continuous separation of solids from the liquid fat in a decanter centrifuge; further heating; centrifugation to remove the fines; and cooling in a plate heat exchanger to below solidification point.

An important principle in the rendering of fat is the prevention of the breakdown of fat into fatty acids and glycerides by the action of the enzyme lipase, which is active at temperatures of 40–60°C. Above 60°C lipase is inactivated. The continuous low-temperature system utilises this action and at the same time minimises undesirable chemical activity, burning, oxidation and off-flavours.

## Stomach and intestines

The contents of the rumen/reticulum are generally emptied in the gut room and the intestines are separated from the stomachs. In the UK the bovine intestines are collected, along with the other *specified risk material* (SRM) and rendered and/or incinerated. Specified risk material also includes the bovine head,

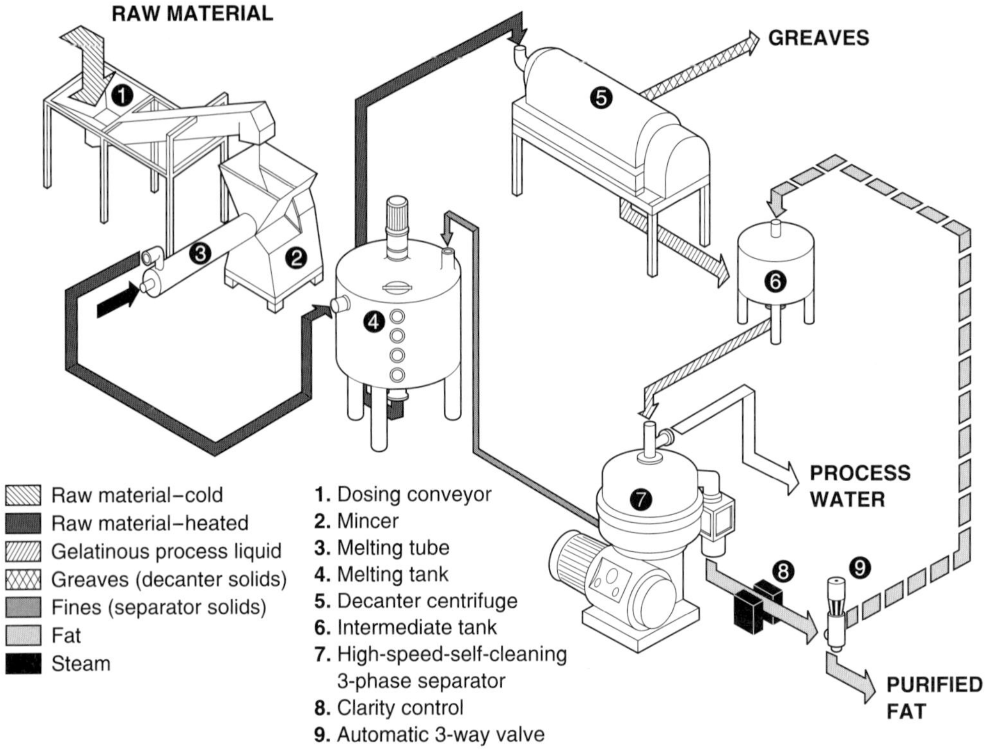


**Fig. 5.1** Continuous low-temperature wet rendering system. (By courtesy of Messrs Alfa Laval Fish & Meat Engineering AS, Copenhagen, Denmark)

including the tonsils but excluding the tongue, spinal cord, thymus, spleen and intestines, and in the sheep the head, excluding the tongue, the spleen, and the spinal cord of sheep over 12 months.

The ruminal contents are transferred via a rotating screw, which removes most of the water, into a skip. Methods of disposal of rumen or paunch contents include the following:

1 Land fill, which is an undesirable and uneconomic approach, and is becoming less common.
2 Use of lagoons and waste-water treatment is usually impractical and costly.
3 Spreading of untreated raw paunch manure directly on to agricultural land is environmentally questionable but still a quite common approach.
4 Use of ensilaged/silaged paunch manure as a feed for livestock has cost implications and the unfavourable perception of feeding waste to animals.
5 Burning, which is not cost effective.
6 Composting of paunch waste into an organic fertiliser. This method of disposal is simple and part of the natural cycle of life, but it requires special equipment and ample space to produce compost commercially.

*Tripe* is produced from the first stomach (rumen, paunch) and second stomach (reticulum) of the ruminant. It can also be derived from the stomach of the pig. The stomachs are first emptied and washed and the fat is trimmed off. The pillars of the rumen (mountain chain) may be removed, trimmed, packaged and frozen for consumption in Japan, and other countries. The remaining material is cleaned in one 'Parmentiere' and then transferred to a second 'Parmentiere' (which has a roughened interior) where the external fat is removed. A 'Parmentiere' is a stainless steel drum which operates rather like a cylindrical washing machine. The stomachs are then scalded in water containing washing soda, scraped and placed in cold water to clean them, and finally cooked for 3–3½ hours at a temperature of 49–60°C. In some countries the omasum is made into tripe, in others it is considered uneconomical because of the difficulty of removing the mucous membrane. *Rennet* is manufactured from the abomasum of the calf.

### *Intestines*

Animal small intestines can be utilised for a variety of purposes such as surgical sutures, collagen sheets (used for burn dressing), strings for musical instruments and sports equipment, sausage casings, human food, pet food, animal feed, tallow or fertiliser. The cleaning and removal of various internal and sometimes external layers, is necessary to convert the intestines into a useful casing. Although there are many factors which influence the quality of the casing, such as the animal's health, species, age, breed, feed and environment, and the portion of the intestinal tract utilised, the most important factor is how the product is handled and processed after the animal is slaughtered. Quality is based on cleanliness, strength, length, caliper, curing and packaging.

### *Casing preparation*

After the intestines have been separated from the attached organs, they are dispatched to an area in the meat plant where further processing can take place. They are highly contaminated and fragile and therefore cleaning must be carried out immediately after slaughter of the animal.

The first operation in handling intestines is 'running', that is separating them from the mesentery. This is by means of a hand-operated knife. The next step is to run the intestine through a 'stripper' comprising large rollers (which resemble a laundry wringer), to squeeze out the residues within the intestines. This step requires the use of a great quantity of potable water to wash the casings and to keep the operation clean. The casing should then be soaked in water for approximately 30 minutes at 38–42°C. In some areas of the world, casings then go through a fermentation cycle, but in other countries (e.g. UK, USA) casings processed by fermentation are no longer acceptable. Intestines which have not been fermented are run through a crushing machine and soaking tank. This breaks the intermucosal membrane and separates it from the rest of the intestine. Next, the intestine goes through a mucosa stripper, which looks and acts essentially like the 'manure' stripper above. Potable water at 42°C is again used to keep the operation sanitary. Any remaining string-like material and mucosa are removed by rolling. After cleaning, the casings are placed in a cold salt solution and held overnight. The next day they are graded, salted with fine salt until they have absorbed 40% salt and packed into barrels.

## Blood

If blood can be collected hygienically, it can be utilised for human consumption. To be cost-effective this can only be achieved in a meat plant with a high throughput. Smaller plants generally have blood spread on land, a practice not appreciated by environmentalists or neighbours.

Approximately 4.5% of the liveweight of an animal is collectable blood, which represents around 10% of the protein available in an animal. Dried blood is high in protein (80–90%) and rich in lysine.

### *Edible blood*

Blood is collected via a hollow knife inserted into the blood vessels where sticking is performed. Normally an anticoagulant such as sodium citrate (0.2% w/v) is supplied to the knife-point through a hollow pipe in the knife handle. It should be collected in a primary tank and held there until the animal from which the blood originated has passed meat inspection. Should the animal not pass meat inspection, only the small holding tank of blood need be condemned.

A typical blood meal plant is shown in Fig. 5.2 in which the actual separation of the two fractions is accomplished in the high-speed centrifuge or separator. After separation, the plasma is frozen or spray-dried at low temperature in order to maintain its solubility and binding properties. The red cells can be used for black sausages or blood puddings or dried into blood meal.

It is important to prevent haemolysis or rupture of the red cell membranes during processing. Haemolysis will occur if the red cells come into contact with solutions of lower

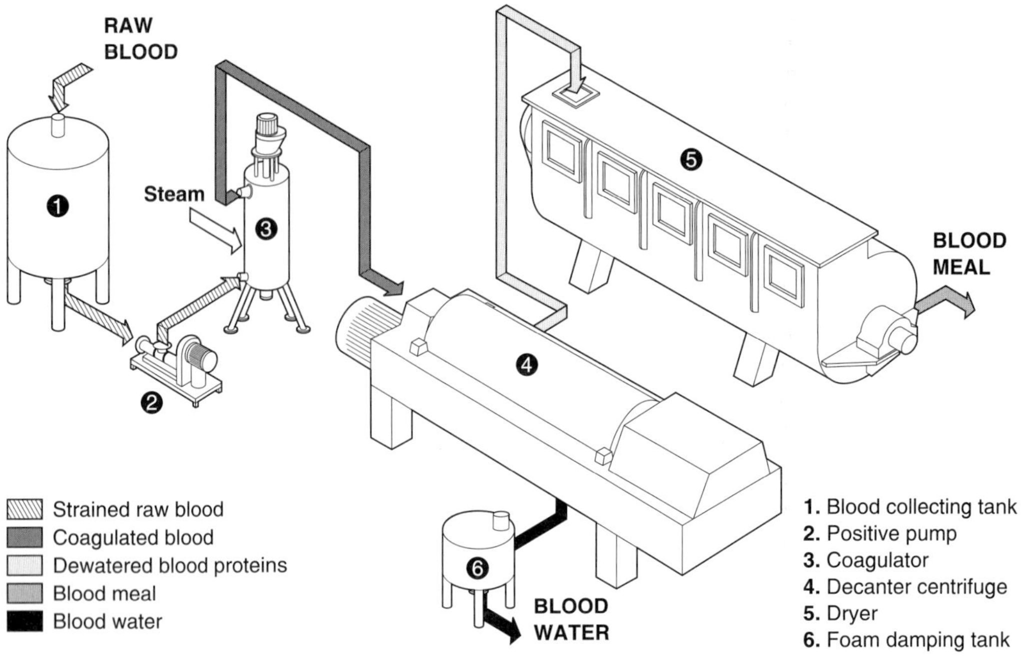


**Fig. 5.2** Blood meat production. (By courtesy of Messrs Alfa Laval Fish & Meat Engineering AS, Copenhagen, Denmark)

osmotic pressure, causing the absorption of water and bursting of the corpuscles, and the presence of fat, which will dissolve cell membranes, bringing about haemolysis. The same problem can be caused by sudden variations of temperature, freezing and damage through rough handling.

### *Inedible blood*

For inedible purposes blood can be collected very easily by placing troughs below the carcases. They should be designed so that they are easily dry-cleaned with rubber squeegees. It is essential that water does not come in contact with the blood for two reasons: (1) water will cause haemolysis of the red blood cells and prevent the adequate separation of plasma and red blood cells, and (2) should blood get into the plant effluent system it will greatly increase the BODs by around ten times and the suspended solids by three times.

Before being allowed to enter the collecting tank, inedible blood should be strained to exclude foreign matter.

*Drying of blood meal* by removing the water is carried out in three main ways:

1. *Direct batch drying* carried out in batch dryers similar to rendering batch coolers. The raw blood is dried to 2–10% moisture by simply boiling off the water.
2. *Batch coagulation followed by batch drying*. The raw blood is initially coagulated by injecting direct steam into an open tank containing the raw blood. The coagulum, which is around 25% total solids (TS) is then separated by draining or hand pressing and dried in a batch dryer.
3. *Continuous coagulation before drying*. This is the most common method of processing blood. Strained blood from a blood holding tank is pumped into an intermediate pre-heating tank equipped with a low-speed agitator and the blood is pre-heated to 60°C by steam. The blood then passes to the coagulator and as a result of steam injection nozzles, positioned at several points in the coagulator, at the exit, the blood is at an optimum temperature of 90°C. A decanter then separates the solids, which are dried, and the liquid.

## Bones

The amount of *bone* available for processing depends on the type of operation being carried out, i.e. whether or not deboning is performed. If the abattoir is concerned solely with slaughter, the small amount of bone produced is usually consigned to an outside inedible rendering plant, where it is mixed with other raw materials, such as fallen animals, condemned meat and offal, and meat and fat trimmings.

Bone maybe classified as 'edible' or 'inedible' depending on its source and its handling. 'Edible' bone must be handled speedily in a hygienic manner. Today there is an increasing amount of 'edible' bone available because of the large amount of boneless meat being produced at source. The end-products of edible bone processing are fat, bone meal and gelatin, with meat-and-bone meal being produced when there is meat in the original raw material. Some, mainly pig bone and chicken necks, are emulsified and used in pet food.

Owing to its high calcium and phosphorus content, bone meal is used as a constituent of poultry feeds and fertiliser. Calcined bone, obtained by roasting in air, is used in the manufacture of high-class pottery and china, in the refining of silver and in copper smelting. Bone charcoal is utilised in bleaching, sugar refining and case-hardening of compounds in the manufacture of steel. Special bone powders are employed for the removal of fluorine from drinking water.

*Gelatin* is produced from 'edible' bones subsequent to the extraction of fat and under carefully controlled pressure. It is used in making brawn, pies, ice cream and capsules for medicines, in photography, as a culture medium for bacteria and in the production of smokeless gunpowder. Some of the gelatin used for these purposes comes from veal and a smaller amount from beef. Nowadays pig skin supplies a large quantity of gelatin.

## Hides and skins

The quality of leather to a large degree depends on the techniques used for hide removal (flaying) and the processing that follows.

*Bovine* hides can be removed manually, which requires great skill to avoid damage, but nowadays in commercial meat plants hides are removed mechanically by hide-pulling machines following initial knife work.

*Pig* hides are scalded and dehaired and this generally makes their skin unsuitable for further processing. Pigs can be skinned with a knife, but considerable skill is required owing to the softness of the fat. Mechanical pulling of the hides is gaining popularity because of energy and labour savings when compared to scalding. However, it results in a 6–8% loss in carcase weight and it is slower (150–300 per hour) than scalding (150–850 per hour).

*Goat* skins are more valuable than sheep skins because they are larger and produce a better-lasting leather. *Sheep skins* require a longer time (up to several hours) to cool after slaughter than other hides owing to the insulating properties of the wool and the presence of grease.

As well as for leather, hides and skins are used in food, cosmetic ingredients and medicinal prosthetics such as skin grafts and sutures. In the case of pig skins, food is the main use, where it is utilised as a major source of gelatin, snack foods and sausages, as well as being part of primary pork and cured cuts.

After flaying, hides and skins should be cured quickly to arrest bacterial and enzymatic decomposition or spoilage. In areas with low relative humidity they may be air-dried for preservation, but salt is mainly used as the curing ingredient. Salt-pack curing involves a flesh-side up stack of hides, usually 90–130 cm high, with an equal weight of salt to hide spread evenly over the flesh-side of each hide in the stack. This draws moisture out of the hides. Preservatives are often used with salt-pack curing. Curing takes 20–30 days for cattle.

Hides and skins constitute the most valuable material removed from the animal carcase. *Skins* come from smaller animals e.g. sheep, calves and goats, while larger skins such as those from cattle, horses, elephants are called *hides*. Leather from cattle hides is used to produce shoes, garment leather, upholstery leather and accessory leather. *Pig skin*, the second most common leather-making raw material worldwide, is thinner than cattle hides and is primarily manufactured into garment leather. The largest producer of pig skins is the People's Republic of China. In other countries pig skin is emulsified and used in the manufacture of sausages. Cattle hide can be used to make reconstituted collagen sausage casings. Sheep and goat skin leathers are produced in many areas of the world primarily for garment leathers.

*Hide curing*

Ox hides arrive at the tannery either fresh from the abattoir or more usually salted and dried to prevent putrefaction. After soaking in water to cleanse and soften them, they are placed in pits filled with milk of lime for 1–4 weeks to loosen the hair and open up the fibre. The hair on the outside, and flesh and meat on the inside, are then scraped off and, after removal of lime by washing in weak acid, the hides are tanned. Tanning may be done by a vegetable process using the barks of trees, or by a chemical process known as 'chrome tanning'. The tannery process, from raw hide to finished leather, takes about three months. The hide from bullocks and heifers, when tanned, is used as sole leather or for belting. Sole leather is obtained from the butt, the area of the hide lying on either side of the backbone.

## TREATMENT OF CONDEMNED MEAT AND OFFALS

The main purpose of meat hygiene is to ensure that only food fit for human consumption is allowed to pass inspection. A properly trained officer will be able to separate the following categories:

1. Meat and offal that are sound and wholesome and can be placed on the market without any restriction.
2. Meat affected with some condition which requires further treatment before it can be released.
3. Meat and offal that does not pass meat inspection owing to public health concern or aesthetics.

The meat inspection laws of the EU, United States, Canada, Australia, New Zealand and Switzerland, as well as the Codex Alimentarius (FAO/WHO), recognise the economic and public health justification for the second classification, their legislation allowing for release of the meat subject to further treatment, which may be boiling, adequate refrigeration or other means.

### High- and low-risk animal waste

Material can be divided into high- and low-risk animal waste. Examples of *high-risk animal waste* are:

1. Animals that have died, or been killed on the farm but were not slaughtered for human consumption.
2. Animals killed in the context of disease control.
3. By-products, including blood, originating from animals which have been condemned on meat inspection.
4. Carcases that have not passed meat inspection, including those with unacceptable levels of residues.
5. Contaminated meat.
6. Parts of the carcase, except hides, skins, hooves, feathers, wool, horn, hair, blood and similar products, of animals slaughtered in the normal way which are not presented for post-mortem inspection.
7. Fish which show signs of disease.

*Low-risk animal wastes* are animal products other than high-risk animal waste, including hides, skins, hooves, feathers, wool, horns, hair, blood and similar products when used in the manufacture of feedingstuffs.

Animal waste must be collected and transported in suitable containers or vehicles which prevent leakage. The containers or vehicles must be adequately covered and all must be maintained in a clean condition. The container should be labelled *'Not for human consumption'*.

The *high-risk material* should be *processed in a high-risk processing plant*, which has been approved by the governmental authorities or disposed of by *burning* or *burial* where transport to the nearest high-risk material processing plant might expose a risk to the environment or the quantity and distance to be covered does not justify collecting the waste. Burial must be deep enough to prevent carnivorous animals from digging it up and must be in suitable ground to prevent contamination of water tables or any other environmental problems. Before burial the waste must be sprinkled with an approved disinfectant.

*Low-risk material* must be processed in a high-risk or low-risk processing plant, in a petfood plant or in a plant preparing pharmaceutical or technical products, or disposed of by burning or burial.

## HYGIENE REQUIREMENTS FOR ANIMAL-WASTE PROCESSING PLANTS

The premises of the processing plant must be adequately separated from the public highway and other premises such as meat plants. Premises for the processing of high-risk material must not be on the same site as meat plants, unless in a completely separate part of a building. Only authorised personnel should be allowed access.

The plant should have a clean and an unclean section, which must be clearly separated. The unclean section must have a covered area to receive the animal waste and must be constructed so that it is easy to clean and disinfect. Floors must be laid to facilitate the draining of liquids. The plant must have adequate lavatories, changing rooms and washbasins for staff. In the unclean section, where required, there must be adequate facilities for de-skinning or de-hairing of animals and a storage room for hides.

The plant should be of sufficient size, and have enough hot water and steam to process hygienically the waste received. The unclean section must, if appropriate, contain equipment to reduce the size of animal waste and equipment for loading the crushed animal waste into the processing unit. A closed processing installation is required in which to process the waste, and where heat treatment is required this installation must be equipped with measuring equipment to check temperature and, if necessary, pressure at critical points, recording devices to record continuously the results of measurements and an adequate safety system to prevent insufficient heating.

To ensure that there is no cross-contamination of finished processed material by incoming raw material there must be clear separation between the area of the plant where the incoming raw material is unloaded and processed and the areas set aside for further processing of the heated material and the storage of the finished processed product.

There must be adequate facilities for cleaning and disinfecting the containers in which animal waste is received and the vehicles in which it is transported. The wheels of the vehicles carrying high-risk material must be disinfected before departure or before leaving the unclean section of the processing plant.

There must be a waste-water disposal system which hygienically removes waste-water and a laboratory to carry out the required testing or of the services of an outside agency.

### Hygiene requirements relating to the operation of animal-waste processing plants

Animal waste must be processed as soon as possible after arrival. It must be stored properly until processed.

Containers, equipment and vehicles used for the transport of animal waste must be cleaned, washed and disinfected after use.

Personnel working in the unclean section must not enter the clean section without changing their clothes and footwear. Equipment and utensils must not be taken from the unclean to the clean area.

Waste-water originating in the unclean section must be treated to ensure no pathogens remain.

There must be a systematic method to prevent the ingress of birds, rodents, insects or other vermin.

Animal waste must be processed under the following conditions.

1 High-risk material must be heated to a core temperature of at least 133°C for 20 min at a pressure of 3 bar. The particle size of the raw material prior to processing must be reduced to at least 50 mm by means of a prebreaker or grinder.
2 Recording thermographs must be provided at the critical points of the heating process to monitor the heat treatment.
3 Pressure-monitoring devices should be installed to record pressure at different stages in the process.
4 The particle size should be monitored regularly and corrected when wear or damage to the breaking equipment is noted that could allow particles larger than 50 mm to enter the process.
5 For continuous systems a residence time-test should be completed under normal operating conditions. Markers, e.g. manganese dioxide ($MnO_2$), should be introduced into the continuous systems at time zero. Samples of

product leaving the process are taken to monitor the recovery of the insoluble marker until the majority of the marker is expected to have passed throughout the system.

The installation and equipment must be kept in a good state of repair and measuring equipment must be calibrated at regular intervals.

The finished products must be handled and stored at the processing plant in such a way as to prevent recontamination and the hides must be salted using sodium chloride.

### Quality control

In the case of high-risk materials, samples of the finished products, taken directly after heat treatment, must be free from heat-resistant pathogenic bacterial spores (*Clostridium perfringens* must be absent in 1 g of the product).

Samples of the final products from both low-risk and high-risk material taken during or upon withdrawal from storage at the processing plant must comply with the following standards:

*Salmonella*: absence in 25 g: $n = 5$, $c = 0$, m = 0, $M = 0$

*Enterobacteriaceae*: $n = 5$, $c = 2$, $m = 10$, $M = 3 \times 10^2$ in 1 g

where $n$ = number of units comprising the sample; $m$ = threshold value for the number of bacteria – the result is considered satisfactory if the number of bacteria in all sample units does not exceed $m$; $M$ = maximum value for the number of bacteria – the result is considered unsatisfactory if the number of bacteria in one or more sample units is $M$ or more; and $c$ = number of sample units the bacterial count of which may be between $m$ and $M$, the sample still being considered acceptable if the bacterial count of the other sample units is $m$ or less.

## INEDIBLE RENDERING PROCESSES

While some meat plants have rendering departments for the treatment of condemned and other inedible material, it is better, from a public health standpoint as well as the efficiency of processing that the premises should be located away from food outlets and be large enough to handle material from a large area.

The best and most economical method of processing unfit meat and offal is by heat treatment in a jacketed cylinder, which gives complete sterilisation and maximum return from the rendered material. A number of different methods are available for handling inedible material, all of which are concerned with the separation of the three main constituents, fat, water and fat-free substance, and the production of sterilised technical fat and meat-and-bone meal.

There are four categories of rendering systems, three of which are:

1. Conventional batch dry rendering with mechanical and/or solvent defatting.
2. Continuous dry rendering with screw press defatting (Fig. 5.3).
3. Semi-continuous wet rendering with centrifugal defatting.

The batch systems are more labour intensive but less expensive to install than continuous systems.

In these three systems the raw material is cooked to sterilise the components (water, fat and meal) for separation, the fat being finally purified. There are major differences in the type and order of the various operations.

In the *continuous dry rendering process* (which resembles batch dry rendering except that the operation is continuous), the system operates at atmospheric pressure. After cooking, the material is pre-strained and discharged to a screw press for defatting. The length of the cooking process depends on the method of filling and the cooker size.

4. Continuous wet pressing and centrifugal defatting.

Various models of this process have been developed but the main principle consists of mincing of the raw material, melting to liberate the fat, wet pressing and drying/sterilising. Water, fat and fine solids are separated by centrifugation. A disadvantage of this process is that, similarly to continuous to dry rendering with screw press defatting, it does not fulfil existing sterilising regulations in some countries, necessitating a further sterilisation of the meal.

The Commission of the European Union has set out minimum conditions concerning

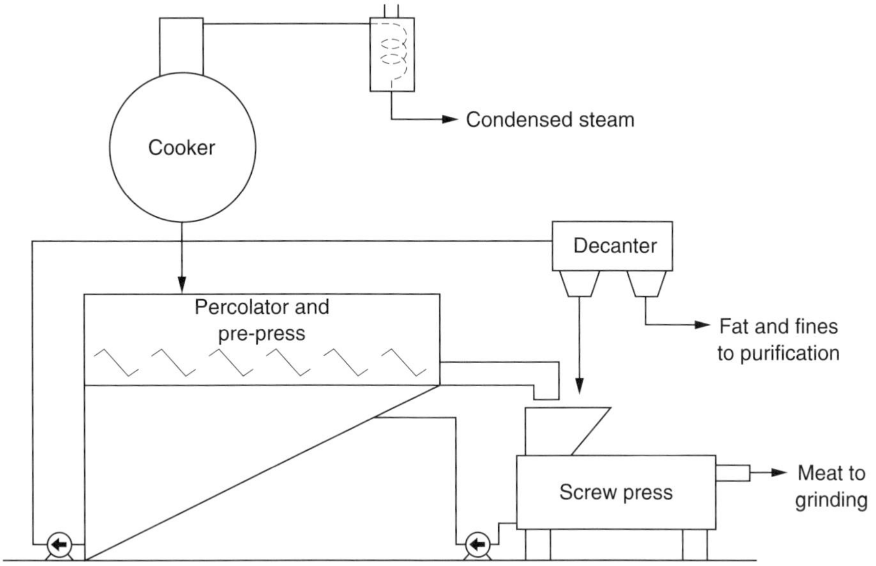


**Fig. 5.3** Continuous dry rendering process. (By courtesy of Messrs Alfa Laval Fish & Meat Engineering AS, Copenhagen, Denmark)

processing waste of ruminant origin by six different methods. These do not apply to the production and processing of:

1 Pet food containing only low-risk material
2 Gelatin
3 Hides and skins
4 Glands and organs for pharmaceutical use
5 Blood and blood products
6 Milk
7 Rendered fats
8 Casings

The production of feather meal requires feathers to be hydrolysed and cooked under pressure.

## TREATMENT OF EFFLUENT

The processing of carcases and the resultant by-products give rise to large amounts of highly polluting waste-waters, semi-solids and solids, which must be separated and treated before being discharged into the environment.

The objective of effluent treatment is to produce a product that can be safely discharged into a waterway or sewer in compliance with the recommended limits for discharge.

*Effluents* can be divided into four categories:

1 Non-toxic and not directly pollutant but liable to disturb the physical nature of the receiving water.
2 Non-toxic and pollutant due to organic matter content of high oxygen demand.
3 Toxic – containing highly poisonous materials.
4 Toxic and pollutant due to organic matter of high oxygen demand and toxic in addition.

The first priorities are to separate effluent from storm water, to lessen the quantity of material requiring treatment, to separate solids from fluid and to lessen the amount of treatment required.

This can be achieved by the use of grills over drains, fat traps and other preliminary treatments, along with continuous dry cleaning or 'clean as you go' during the operation of the plant and at breaks in production.

### Pollution parameters (see also p. 160)

*Biochemical oxygen demand* (BOD) is a measure of the readily biodegradable material in an effluent. It is obtained by measuring the oxygen consumed by aerobic organisms, when a known volume of the effluent is added to a known volume of oxygen-saturated water and incubated at 20°C for 5 days. It is generally used to determine the concentration of pollutant remaining after treatment and prior to discharge.

*Chemical oxygen demand* (COD) is a measure of the oxygen required for the oxidation of all organic matter in a known volume of effluent, using a standard technique. The COD is often used as a cheaper and more accurate means of determining the oxygen requirements of an effluent before treatment.

BOD values vary greatly in the various food processing operations (Table 5.2).

It is the biodegradable material which will have a more direct effect on flora and fauna and therefore BOD is a more appropriate measurement than COD for discharge consents.

*Chloride* (Cl) is a measure of salinity.

*Dry matter* (DM) or *total solids* (TS) is the final weight of a known amount of effluent that has been dried to a constant weight at 105°C over 24 h. It is measured in g/litre or mg/litre.

*Grease, fat and oil* are a group of substances having common properties of immiscibility with water and a lower specific gravity, which cause them to float. Concentrations are measured by the amount of solvent required for the effluent to become soluble. Some water authorities in the United Kingdom will accept a level of 100 mg/litre. The substances tend to coat treatment systems, clogging pipes, pumping systems and screens. They reduce oxygen transfer and can seriously reduce the efficiency of aerobic treatment systems.

*pH* is a measure of the acidity or alkalinity of an aqueous solution. Pure water has a pH value of 7.0.

*Nitrogen* (N) occurs in three forms in effluents: organic nitrogen, ammonium salts and dissolved ammonia gas, and as nitrates which are found in aerobically-treated effluents. *Ammonia* in solution is toxic to aquatic life; the maximum discharge to sewers is 40 mg/litre. High nitrate concentrations in natural waters encourage algae and other plant growth, thus blocking water courses. The maximum level in potable water is 0.5 mg/litre.

**Table 5.2** Average BOD values for some food processing operations.

| Source | BOD mg/litre |
|---|---|
| Poultry meat plant | 1000–1200 |
| Pig meat plant | 1500–2000 |
| Cattle/sheep meat plant | 1400–3200 |
| Fish processing | 1000–3000 |
| Dairy (washings) | 600–1300 |

*Pathogenic bacteria:* Potable water should not contain any coliform organisms.

*Suspended solids* (SS) refers to matter which is insoluble and is suspended in the water. It consists of both organic and inorganic components. The organic material will eventually be degraded and add to the BOD.

*Temperature* should not be more than a few degrees above the temperature of the receiving water in order not to disturb the natural biocycle.

*Turbidity and colour:* Effluent should be clear and colourless

*Volatile solids* (VS) are used as a measure of biogas production.

## Treatment

Standards are set for the discharge of effluent, and these will depend on the volume and strength of the effluent and the sensitivity of the water course or underground stratum to which it is being discharged.

Air pollution with regard to odours is measured subjectively and is related to the effect the odour has on the public, i.e. the degree of 'nuisance'.

### Preliminary treatment – screening

Preliminary treatment is based on the removal of solids and this is best done by letting all water pass through one or more screens. These screens should be non-clogging and self-cleaning, adaptable to different water flows, easy to clean automatically or manually (when required) and noiseless. After the removal of coarse solids, the effluent stream still contains finely suspended solids, fats and grease. For small quantities of low-grade material, a simple fat trap is all that is required. This is in the form of a minimum-turbulence, flow-through tank. Settlable solids can remain long enough to settle out on the bottom of the tank, while grease and fine solids rise to the surface. Continuous sludge removal and skimming of the surface to remove scum are essential.

*Dissolved air flotation* is a successful method of removing suspended solids, fats and grease, and is particularly useful when disposal is to a sewer. It causes a physical separation of suspended matter, fats and grease by the production of micro-bubbles of air that attach themselves to the suspended material, lifting it to the surface to form scum, which is removed, while the supernatant liquor is discharged continuously either to a sewer or for further biological treatment. The addition of chemicals that aid flocculation makes the process easier to control automatically and assists in the production of a more consistent effluent. A large range of flocculants is available, e.g. ferric chloride/sulphate, ferrous sulphate, aluminium sulphate (alum), sodium carbonate (soda ash), calcium carbonate (lime), polyelectrolytes and others. The pH of the effluent has to be maintained and varies depending on the flocculant used. The addition of caustic soda or hydrochloric acid controls this.

*Balancing tanks* may be required when strict control of hourly and daily flow rates is required or when production is cyclical throughout a 24-hour period.

## Secondary treatment

Secondary treatment is carried out using *biological treatment systems*, which involve maintaining under controlled conditions a mixed culture of microorganisms which utilise the continuous supply of organic matter present in the effluent to synthesise new cells.

*Anaerobic digestion* is carried out in totally enclosed systems to prevent the entry of air. It will result in a fast reduction of organic material with the production of biogas. With a BOD higher than 2000 mg/litre it becomes advantageous. The system operates as a two-stage fermentation process in which the stages occur simultaneously within the digester.

During the first stage, bacteria break down complex organic substances into simpler compounds, the most important being volatile fatty acids (VFA). In the second stage, methanogenic organisms utilise the VFA to yield methane and carbon dioxide. Maintaining the pH at around 7.0–7.2 is very important. Overproduction of VFA will lower the pH and stop the process, which can be difficult to re-start. This is very much a 'living' process and the addition of a balanced effluent is essential. Too much protein can destroy the process and therefore blood must not be introduced. There is a high capital cost, the operatives require extensive training and the surplus treated effluent requires further aerobic treatment before it can be discharged into water courses.

### *Activated sludge process*

*Aerobic digestion* is less sensitive to shock loading; the retention time is shorter and therefore the tanks are smaller and cheaper. Air can be forced in through compressed-air systems or surface aerators. The factors which affect aeration of the reactor are concentration of dissolved oxygen, the hydraulic retention time and substrate-loading rate, pH, temperature and toxic substances.

The dissolved organic matter, colloidal residues and fine solids are oxidised to carbon dioxide and water. Proteins are broken down into nitrates and sulphates by a mixed culture of microorganisms in the reactor. The major product of the process is new cells (biomass). The biomass, together with material which has resisted biodegradation, is separated out from the treated effluent in settling tanks (clarifiers). The supernatant liquor from the clarifier is discharged over a weir for disposal or further treatment, if required. A proportion of sludge which settles out at the base of the clarifier is returned to the reactor vessel to maintain the critical concentration of biomass. The remainder is drawn off to be concentrated and may require further treatment before disposal. Where sludges are to be applied to land which is fallow or is to be seed-bed for arable crops, the application is unlikely to become a problem unless the land is close to urban development, when odours may cause a nuisance. Low-trajectory agricultural slurry spreaders can be used. When sludges are to be applied to grassland, there is a greater risk of grazing stock ingesting any pathogens present. In the UK a minimum holding period of 4–6 weeks is required for animal slurries. However, in some EC Member States a period of 6 months is mandatory. Alternatively, sludge can be injected into the soil; application rates will vary with soil type, field capacity and type of crop. Rates in excess of 120 $m^3$/ha are most likely to lead to run-off by leaching or via land drains.

# Chapter 6
# Plant Sanitation

## Reasons for cleaning and disinfecting plant

It should not be assumed that all the reasons for cleaning and disinfecting meat plants are fully understood and appreciated by those responsible for plant hygiene. The technology of plant cleaning and disinfection is complex and changing, with many details to be constantly observed and acted upon. It is, more than ever, essential that the importance of plant hygiene is recognised and that the scientific principles and professional management techniques are understood and employed by all concerned.

Food plants are cleaned for many reasons:

- To meet national and EU legislation.
- To reduce the risk of litigation.
- To engender and maintain a general quality ethos.
- To meet customers' quality expectations.
- To satisfy the increasing number of customer Hygiene Audits.
- To allow maximum plant productivity.
- To project a hygienic visual image.
- To ensure the safety of operatives and maintenance staff.
- To help secure the shelf-life of the products.
- To avoid food poisoning or foreign body contamination.
- To avoid pest infestation.
- To protect marketplace reputation.

Although the most subjective of all, the *visual image* that a factory projects to a visitor can strongly influence getting or losing a customer contract or an EU licence and has a direct bearing on employee morale and the development of a Total Quality ethos. For these reasons, visual cleanliness and the absence of deposits in the plant are goals as important as the control of actual microbiological risks.

Cleaning incurs costs and is often seen as a necessary but unproductive evil, but it is rare to find these costs being fully analysed and controlled in a meat plant. Often only the obvious elements such as chemicals are stressed rather than the complete context of the hygiene budget. Full hygiene budgeting should properly include a factor relating to the possible catastrophic effects of hygiene failure and the protection of investment made in plant and brand image. Only with a full understanding of the business risk can the direct costs of hygiene be seen in their genuine context.

Typical costs for hygiene in a meat plant break down as follows:

| | |
|---|---|
| Labour and supervision | 65% |
| Water supply, treatment, purchase | 2% |
| Water heating | 8% |
| Cleaning equipment | 8% |
| Chemicals | 7% |
| Corrosion | 2% |
| Monitoring | 5% |
| Effluent | 3% |
| Downtime | +? |

Often, cost pressures on the large labour element are brought to bear upon cleaning teams, whether contract cleaners or in-house cleaners. These may encourage the cleaners to combine or leave out individual steps in the cleaning sequence. This action may appear to save money in terms of the cleaning costs alone. However, it may easily lead to increased indirect costs in terms of the shelf-life and safety of the food product and the hygienic image of the factory. All of these factors could affect the viability and profitability of the meat plant.

Chemicals and water (purchase, heating, treatment and disposal) costs may also be significant, but it is important to understand the overall cleaning programme and the related effects of changing these variables.

Over the last 10 years, under pressure more from commercial quality factors than from legislation, the average standards of design of food plants and their maintenance and cleaning have risen markedly. It is still definitely the case, however, that the standards reached and maintained, and the professionalism with which hygiene is managed, vary greatly between different sectors of the food industry, between different plants in the same sector, and between countries.

EU legislation has had (and will continue to have) an important effect on the design of new meat plants or the refurbishment of older plants. EU directives also have something to say about the requirement for routine cleaning and disinfection of food plants. But enforcement of the EU norms varies greatly internationally and some of the directives are vague and inadequate as practical guides to hygiene. It is true that poorly designed, outdated and badly run plants should and can be closed down owing to failure to meet the legislative requirements. Any food plant 'worth its salt', however, will see legislation as a bare minimum set of standards and will, through a total quality ethos and good manufacturing practice, aim for a consistent level of hygiene well above this minimum.

### 'Scotoma' or 'factory-blindness'

It is well known that any person working routinely in an environment such as a meat plant can gradually become mentally 'blind' to hygiene standards and potential problems in their plant. This 'scotoma' effect can be surprisingly powerful and can mean that visitors (be they EU inspectors or customers) to the plant will often see serious hygiene inadequacies missed by the plant personnel themselves. The scotoma can only be overcome by vigilance, training and systematic monitoring and inspection procedures, perhaps with the help of outside assistance.

## THE CHEMISTRY OF CLEANING

Cleaning is essentially a physiochemical process involving a wide range of reactions which depend greatly on a number of variables, which we will now consider.

### The soil

In a meat plant the most common soils or deposits originate from the animals themselves and from any other ancillary additives or components used in the manufacturing process. These product-derived soils include the following:

#### *Fats, oils and greases*

These are often triglycerides of fatty acids and can vary from waxy solids to liquids. They are insoluble in water and can vary in their structure and properties depending on their origin, differing between different parts of the same animal species and between different species. Poultry evisceration fats are very waxy and difficult to remove, for example, compared to beef tallow. Fats, oils and greases can change when exposed to air for some time (particularly those containing unsaturated fatty acids) and may oxidise or polymerise to become harder and more closely bonded to the surface. Exposure to very high temperatures, such as in ovens, will cause fats to carbonise. Fatty or greasy deposits can be recognised by their greasy feel and water repellence and, when aged and oxidised, they take on a cheesy, opaque nature which can be scraped fairly easily with a fingernail. Polymerised oils can become almost plastic in feel and hardness. (This effect is utilised when linseed oil is applied to cricket bats.)

#### *Proteins*

These are complex, large molecules that are normally too large to dissolve easily in water. They have a specific shape that may change when exposed to high temperatures, a process known as denaturation, usually making them harder and more insoluble. (The best known example is the white of an egg.) This property of proteins is important in the processing of foods and in the temperature of water used to wash off protein deposits. In meat plants, the bile proteins and other gut-based soils may give rise to a green or yellow tenacious deposit on evisceration equipment. In pig-dehairing equipment, heavy, hard protein deposits are common. Blood proteins in abattoirs can create particular problems on porous surfaces, often giving rise to green/brown, very resistant staining. Aged protein deposits can be quite hard, normally not scraping off easily with a fingernail.

### *Carbohydrates and starches*

These, too, are large molecules, which may be insoluble, especially after exposure to heat. Their source is usually plant-derived materials such as may be used in producing sauces, coatings, etc. Carbohydrate deposits can vary from soft and powdery to quite hard.

Other soils may originate, not from the food production process itself, but from water, surface corrosion, vehicles and other outside materials. Such deposits include:

- *Limescale* from water drips and leaks or in hot water tanks, cooking kettles, etc.
- *Corrosion deposits* of steel, zinc, aluminium, brass, etc.
- *Rubber marks* from fork lift trucks, etc.
- *Adhesives* from labels, etc.
- *Inks and dyes* from stamps.
- *Algae* in moist areas with high condensation.
- *Fungi* in cold moist areas, especially near chills and freezers and in silicon sealants throughout the plant.

These deposits may or may not present hygiene risks in themselves but are at least unsightly and at worst can act as absorbent substrates for other soils or microorganisms. Chemically they are very different from each other and may therefore need very different cleaning approaches. This is especially true because multiple types of soil are found frequently in the same plant, often combined in the same deposits. Physically this usually makes them harder, more adherent and more difficult to remove. It is important, therefore, to identify the soils present in each plant area by their origins and by their appearance. Only then is it possible to design the correct cleaning regime.

## The substrate: materials of construction

Many different materials may be found in meat plants and while none is perfect, they do vary very considerably in their ease of cleaning and their resistance to corrosion either by the factory environment itself or by contact with cleaning chemicals. Smooth, non-porous, abrasion-resistant, inert surfaces are ideal.

*Stainless steel*, of a high grade, is the best choice for many surfaces, but, especially in its cheaper forms, is liable to pitting corrosion in the presence of chlorine and stress corrosion/cracking at elevated temperatures.

*Mild steel* will rust rapidly in moist and salty environments and should normally be avoided in meat plants.

*Zinc* (as a sacrificial coating on steel) and *aluminium* are both commonly found but are problematical because of their susceptibility to attack by strong alkalis, acids and some process fluids. At worst they can be heavily corroded, embrittled or encrusted, none of which is helpful in maintaining hygienic surfaces. As a rule they should be avoided where the nature of the production or cleaning process poses a corrosion risk

*Terrazzo* and *concrete* may both become porous and cracked if mistreated and are liable to damage by acids.

*Paints* and other similar coatings can vary enormously in their resistance to attack by chemicals and hot or pressurised water and, once flaking, present a risk of foreign body contamination to the food. Chemical-resistant resins are available but it is important to match the coating to the production and cleaning environment expected.

*Plastics* and *rubbers* also vary greatly. At their worst they can swell on contact with some detergents (which may affect smooth running of machinery) or become embrittled by heat, light or chlorine. Some are surprisingly absorbent of soils, especially colourings, mineral oils, smoke, etc., and may even play the generous host to moulds and fungi.

The main point to look for in choosing surface materials is compatibility with the production environment (physical and chemical) and with the cleaning regime. Compatibility with each other is also very important, particularly when two different metals (such as mild steel and stainless) are in contact in a moist environment. *Galvanic corrosion* invariably takes place, causing the 'lower' metal to corrode rapidly. This will also occur in poorly executed welds.

## Energies of cleaning

A principle of prime importance is that every cleaning process, of whatever kind, always involves a combination of four factors:

1. *Thermal energy*, in the form of hot water or steam. As a rough guide, an increase in temperature by 10°C in a detergent solution *doubles* the rate of the chemical reactions involved in cleaning.
2. *Mechanical energy*, in the form of brushes, water jets, turbulent flow in pipes or even the microagitation produced by the bursting of foam bubbles. In circulation (CIP) cleaning of pipe systems, a flow rate of about 2 m/s is needed to ensure turbulence and avoid laminar flow.
3. *Chemical energy*, which depends on the nature and concentration of the detergent used.
4. *Time*, which varies from hours in the case of soak cleaning to seconds in the case of tray or crate washing.

It is essential to understand the interrelation between these factors. Failure to do so will often lead to very poor cleaning results. While it is impossible, because of the complexity of the cleaning reactions, to be absolutely mathematical about it, there must be a balance between the four factors. If one or more factor is limited by the cleaning conditions (e.g. mild chemicals must be used to avoid corrosion of a surface and/or contact time is very limited), then one or more of the other factors must be raised to compensate (e.g. high-pressure water jets at high temperature).

## Chemical and physical reactions of cleaning

Detergency involves many different reactions, physical and chemical, which depend on the nature of the soils to be removed and the nature of the detergent employed to remove them.

### *Physical reactions*

The primary physical reactions are the following:

*Wetting*. Wetting is defined as the displacement of one fluid from a solid surface by another. The displaced fluid may be air or some liquid or semiliquid such as grease. The fluid displacing it is, for the purpose of our discussions, water or a detergent solution.

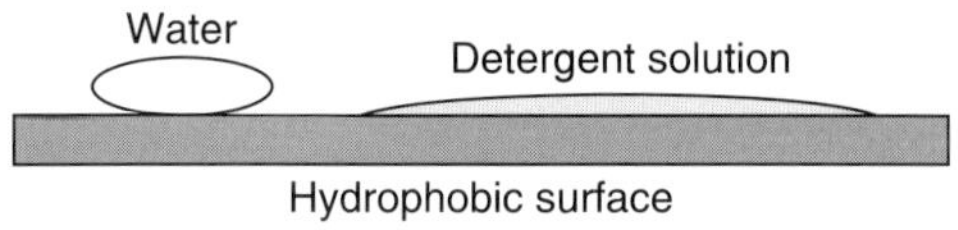


Wetting of hydrophobic surfaces.

Water alone is not sufficiently wet to displace many types of soils or even to displace air from water-repellent or 'hydrophobic' surfaces (for example, water droplets on a Teflon frying pan). In these cases the water curls up under its own surface tension into droplets. Lack of wetting will prevent cleaning taking place.

To achieve wetting of such surfaces, chemical agents which have particular surface properties are employed: 'surfactants' or 'wetting agents'. These are organic molecules which are different at each end. One end is essentially hydrocarbon in nature and closely resembles grease, oil or fat (i.e. 'hydrophobic'). The other end is either ionised to give a positive or negative charge or consists of oxygen-containing groups. In either case this end strongly attracts water (i.e. it is 'hydrophilic'). The result is a dual-nature molecule which concentrates itself at the interface between the water and the surface and allows wetting to take place as shown above.

The nature of the surfactant – whether it foams or defoams, how it wets different surfaces and emulsifies different fats, or how biodegradable it is – depends upon its exact design. There are many hundreds commercially available, which may be used in detergents and disinfectants, either alone or in combination.

*Penetration*. Wetting is the first essential step in the removal of the soil. As wetting agents allow the detergent to displace air from surfaces, detergents are able to penetrate deep into porous dry deposits much faster than water alone. In doing so, the other active components of the detergent are enabled to react with soil components deep in the deposit at a much earlier stage.

*Emulsification*. Emulsions are suspensions of small droplets of one fluid in another. Milk, for example, is an emulsion of milk fats in water, stabilised by other molecules present in the milk. Fats, oils and greases will not naturally disperse in water. First the oil needs to be released from the surface it is resting on. Wetting is the first stage in this as the detergent undermines the oil–surface attraction and starts

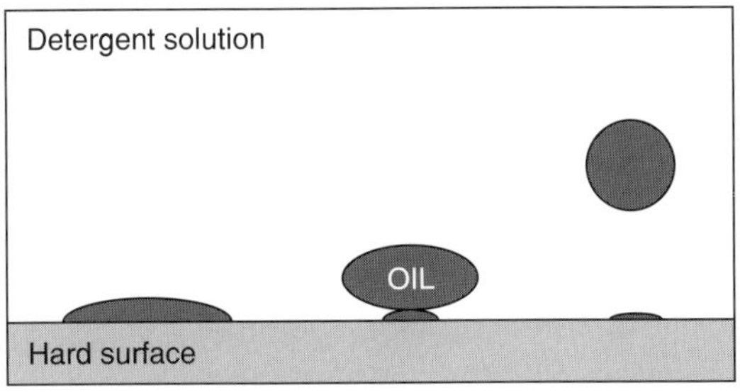


Wetting, roll-up and formation of emulsion.

to displace the oil, which starts to roll up into droplets. This is accelerated if the temperature is high enough to soften or fully liquefy the oil or grease and/or if mechanical energy is applied to the soil. The oil droplets break away from the surface and float freely. Unless prevented from doing so, these droplets would coalesce as they contacted each other at random and would eventually become large enough to redeposit elsewhere. To prevent the coalescence, surfactants, either those involved in the wetting or other specialist emulsifiers, coat the surface of the oil droplets and stabilise the emulsion.

*Dispersion*. This is similar to emulsification except that it involves the breaking up and suspension of solid particles rather than fluid droplets. Dispersion is often carried out in a detergent by components other than surfactants, usually inorganic materials such as carbonates, silicates or phosphates or, in more advanced formulations, by special water-soluble charged polymers. The mechanism of maintaining a stable dispersion, thus allowing the soil particles to be rinsed freely away without re-deposition, involves coating the particles with electric charges which mutually repel. Dispersion is particularly important in circulating cleaning systems (CIP) where sludge can build up, unless dispersed, in slower-moving parts of the system.

*Solubilisation*. This process is simply the taking up of soil components into a true solution (rather than an emulsion or a dispersion). While some soil components are naturally water-soluble under the right conditions, others need the assistance of solvents in the detergent solution. These solvents must be taint-free and of low toxicity and are usually based on alcohols, glycols or glycol ethers. They assist most where greasy soils are too hard to emulsify easily. Here the solvents penetrate the grease and soften or liquefy it.

### *Chemical reactions*

The most important chemical reactions include the following:

*Hydrolysis* of proteins and carbohydrates. These large molecules are made up of smaller subunits (peptides and amino acids in the case of proteins). Hydrolysis involves splitting the molecules at the joints of the subunits, thereby releasing smaller, water-soluble molecules. Hydrolysis takes place most rapidly at extreme pH and is the main reason why alkalis and acids are used in detergents. While alkaline hydrolysis is usually more effective, bile proteins in evisceration areas respond very well to acid hydrolysis. In some cases the acid and alkaline hydrolyses may snip the larger molecule in different locations, neither of which alone is enough to produce small enough molecules. In such circumstances (e.g. old blood stains), alternation of alkaline and acid detergents may help dramatically.

*Saponification of fats, oils and greases* is a particular form of hydrolysis in which an alkali reacts with triglyceride fat molecules, cutting the molecule in three places to give glycerol and soap, both water-soluble. In practice, the formation of the soap can be either helpful, because it acts as a wetting and emulsification agent in its own right, or harmful, because it produces unwanted foam in machine or circulation cleaning. In hard water the foam is less of a problem, but formation of scum (i.e. calcium soaps) may make the clean less efficient.

*Chelation* of insoluble metal ions such as calcium, magnesium and iron. These ions may be present in scale already formed on a surface where they provide anchorage for soil deposits and may become incorporated in the matrix of the deposit itself. Alternatively, they may be a problem in hard water which undergoes heating or evaporation. Chelating agents (sometimes known as chelants or sequestrants) bind the metal ions in water-soluble cages, removing scale or preventing it. In mixed scale/soil deposits the chelates can have a very pronounced effect on the break-up of the deposit. These typical chelating agents (e.g. EDTA (ethylenediamine tetraacetic acid), NTA (nitrilotriacetic acid), gluconate, etc.) are restricted in their economy by the fact that they must be present in ratio to the metal ions needing to be chelated. In very hard water or in large volumes of water this may be prohibitively expensive. In recent years, these conventional chelants have been supplemented by what are known as substoichiometric chelants, usually water-soluble-charged polymers. These act in two ways: (1) They inhibit the growth of scale microcrystals by blocking the corners of the crystals (where growth occurs), forcing the crystals to become spherical. Any scale which does form is thus made soft and powdery and non-adherent to surfaces. (2) They act as dispersants, stringing microcrystals like pearls on a necklace and preventing them from sticking together and precipitating. Whatever the mode of action, these polymeric chelating agents do not need to be present in fixed ratio to the metal ions, but instead function at only several parts per million, even in very hard water. Their main action takes place at low alkalinity, e.g. during the rinse stage. They normally do not actively remove previously formed hard scales.

*Oxidation* of coloured materials, starches etc. Some soil components respond well to chlorine, in the form of alkaline sodium hypochlorite. Coloured deposits may be bleached and some protein or fat deposits may be readily broken down.

*Corrosion inhibition.* Certain chemical components may inhibit the corrosion which normally takes place when aluminium (and to a lesser degree, zinc) come into contact with detergents at very high or low pH. Silicates, for example, in the presence of caustic soda, can render the latter practically non-corrosive on aluminium although this is usually associated with a less effective clean with the risk of scale formation.

*Enzymolysis.* Protease, lipase or amylase enzymes may find use in specialist detergents where they can be quite effective at mild pH conditions. They split the large organic molecules similarly to hydrolysis but sometimes more thoroughly. They are generally difficult to formulate in a stable product.

## DETERGENTS: DESIGN AND CHOICE

It can be seen, from the physical and chemical tasks needed for detergents to remove deposits, that the design of a detergent may be quite complex. In general, the more complex and varied the soil, the more different components need to be employed in the detergent. Other critical variables are the water hardness, the temperature and method of application, the safety considerations for operators and plant surfaces and the possible effects on the effluent system. To meet these varying requirements, the detergent manufacturers will have a range of different formulations. The main components, which may or may not be jointly present, include:

- Alkalis: caustic soda, caustic potash, carbonate, silicate, phosphate.
- Acids: phosphoric, nitric, citric, glycolic, sulphamic, hydrochloric.
- Chelating agents: EDTA, NTA, gluconate, glucoheptonate, citrate, polymeric.
- Solvents: isopropanol, propylene glycol, butyl diglycol, ethers.
- Surfactants: anionic, cationic, nonionic, amphoteric (hundreds of different types exist).
- Inhibitors: organic, inorganic.
- Enzymes: protease, lipase, amylase.
- Oxidising agents: hypochlorite, isocyanurates.
- Stabilisers.
- Viscosity modifiers.

Any one detergent formulation may contain between 2 and 15 components, blended carefully to the application and all its variables.

In order to cover all the needs of the food and beverage industry, a detergent product range may comprise several hundred different formulations, but for any one plant the choice is usually narrowed down to 2–10 products. The skill of the user, in conjunction with the supplier, is in choosing which of the many products to use. In meat plants, the biggest single volume of detergent used is normally an alkaline foam cleaner of some sort, with non-foaming cratewash detergent, manual neutral detergents and acidic foam descalers also finding use. Depending on the degree of further processing, other specialist products may be needed. As a rule, when choosing products for particular applications, the mildest, safest, least corrosive options should be tried first, with the 'heavier guns' being brought in as needed.

Detergent formulations may vary very substantially in their effectiveness; failure to perform is usually not a question of a 'poor' product (though active ingredient levels can be inadequate in some cases) but rather of the choice of the wrong product, applied and controlled in an inappropriate fashion.

While a 'detergent' is designed to remove soils, another term – 'sanitiser' – is often used for some products of a similar type. In Europe, the term 'sanitiser' is taken to mean a combined detergent–disinfectant, while 'disinfectant' means a product designed to kill microbes, but without deliberately employing a soil-removal effect.

## PRINCIPLES OF DISINFECTION

Soil deposits in a food plant would be bad enough if the problem was simply their rather unsightly appearance. But the fact that they harbour, nourish and protect spoilage or pathogenic microorganisms that are invisible to the naked eye makes the job somewhat harder. The soil must, of course, be removed as completely as possible by effective cleaning using the detergents discussed above. Typically the reduction in the total viable bacteria count achieved by cleaning is of the order of 3–4 logs per $cm^2$. If the initial loading was $\sim 10^6/cm^2$, which is frequently the case, there will remain counts of $10^2$–$10^3/cm^2$ after cleaning. It is often necessary to reduce the bacterial numbers further, by the process of *disinfection*, to levels of less than a few hundred. Complete *sterilisation* (elimination of all microorganisms) is neither practical or necessary in the disinfection of food plant surfaces.

### Biocidal active components

The class of chemicals known as *disinfectants* share some components with detergents but others are very different. Their function is to kill bacteria and other microorganisms that are left on the surface after cleaning. They can kill the microbes by several different methods, depending on which components are used in the disinfectant. Some affect the integrity of the cell wall, while others interfere with critical metabolic reactions inside the cell.

Some disinfectants are *oxidising* and will tend to react with most organic material, whether meat residues or bacteria. These oxidising disinfectants include *chlorine*, *iodophors* and *peracetic acid*. These agents are usually rapid-acting and broad-spectrum in terms of the organisms they can kill, but they typically lack a residual effect. They may not be stable in hot water and may be corrosive on a range of metals and other surfaces, but they are usually low-foaming.

It is sometimes wrongly assumed that a chlorine foam can act *fully* as a cleaner and a disinfectant and that subsequent disinfection is not needed. This is partly a false assumption, based on the perception of chlorine as a disinfectant. Depending on the pH, there is an equilibrium in chlorine solutions between $HOCl$ and $OCl^-$. The active biocide in chlorine products is the hypochlorous acid molecule $HOCl$, which, as it is uncharged, can penetrate the bacterial walls. In chlorine foam cleaners, the pH is usually around 10–11. The chlorine is therefore mostly present as the hypochlorite ion $OCl^-$, which acts principally as a detergent and oxidising agent, helping with the removal of proteins and grease and the bleaching of some coloured substances. This pH effect and lack of free $HOCl$ makes the disinfectant properties of alkaline chlorine solutions much weaker (up to a hundred times) than a straight hypochlorite disinfectant solution without alkalis, etc. The better cleaning performance of the chlorine foam physically removes much of the bacterial load along with the dirt, but in areas where a very low surface bacterial count is desired, a separate disinfection stage is needed. This should normally not be a hypochlorite solution because of the risk of corrosion (even on stainless steel) of the breakdown products of the hypochlorite. The lack of heat and light stability of the chlorine means that no residual bactericidal effect is maintained after a relatively short time.

*Non-oxidising* disinfectants are typically based on *quaternary ammonium compounds* (or *'quats'*, a class of cationic surfactant), amphoterics (another class of surfactant with twin positive and negative charges), alcohols, biguanides or aldehydes. The non-oxidising agents are usually heat-stable and less corrosive and have a residual biocidal or biostatic effect if left on surfaces. The surfactant-based disinfectants are often high-foaming, which may prevent their use in some applications.

## DISINFECTANTS: DESIGN AND CHOICE

The method of kill and the point of attack on the defences of the microorganisms may be different in each case. Unless carefully formulated, disinfectants could have weaknesses at lower temperatures or against some more difficult to kill bacteria such as pseudomonads. This could be critical, for example, when disinfecting a chill.

Well-formulated disinfectants may employ several different biocidal components, often with surfactants and chelants to help in the killing action. This also helps eliminate the possibility of resistance developing among the population of microorganisms. (Such resistance to antibiotics is well known and increasing in the medical and veterinary fields, but to date is rarely seen in food plant disinfection.)

Disinfectants can be affected by residues of detergents left on surfaces, perhaps owing to inadequate rinsing. Anionic surfactants in the detergent may neutralise the cationic surfactant of quats, rendering them ineffective.

Disinfectants should be chosen in conjunction with the supplier, taking into full account the surface materials to be disinfected, the soil residues likely to be present after cleaning, the safety to operators and product, the specific organisms, if any, to be controlled, the ambient and solution temperature and the time scale (rapid or residual) required. Cleaning and disinfection may in some cases be adequately combined into one operation using a sanitiser, which has the action of both a detergent and a disinfectant. Usually this is a quat-based neutral or mildly alkaline product for manual use. In general, however, the one-stage product approach does not give as consistent or as effective a final result as the two stages separately.

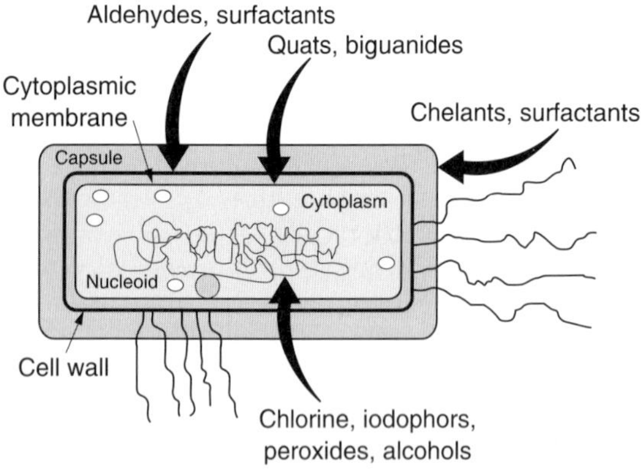


Action of biocides on bacteria.

Under no circumstances should phenolic, pine or other highly-perfumed disinfectants be used in a food plant, even in the offices. The risk of taint, even from very small airborne concentrations, is high, especially in fatty foods. The risk is compounded by the presence of chlorine, even at low levels in factory water. Chlorocresols and chlorophenols may be formed which can taint meat at levels as low as parts per billion (ppb).

## HYGIENE EQUIPMENT AND APPLICATION METHODS

Detergents and disinfectants can often be applied in a number of different ways, dictated by the nature of the cleaning task.

### Manual cleaning

The agents may be applied manually, using cloth, mop, squeegee, brush, green pad, etc. This is usually reserved for small areas on machinery that is non-waterproof or which needs dismantling. It is labour intensive and usually requires safe, neutral chemicals. Detergents or sanitisers (combination detergent–disinfectants) may be used in this way, but not normally disinfectants, as the repeated immersion of the brush, pad or cloth in the solution after contact with the surface would tend to reduce or nullify the disinfectant. Manual cleaning varies significantly with the skill, commitment and time available to the operator. While once common, it is not normally used today for cleaning large plant areas.

### Foam cleaning

This is the established method for the cleaning of large or intricate plant and equipment and is standard procedure in the vast majority of meat, poultry and other food and beverage plants worldwide. A foam blanket, created using a wide range of available equipment (see later), is projected from a nozzle, and allowed to act on the soil for 15–30 minutes, after which it is rinsed off with the released deposits. Large areas such as floors, walls, stands, conveyors, and tables and intricate machinery such as fillers, defeatherers, blackscrapers, etc. are normally suitable for foaming.

The foam itself is merely the carrier for the detergent, to enable it physically to function. The quality of the foam may differ greatly, the best being creamy in consistency rather than either too dry or too wet. The foam should be applied as a thin, uniform layer. Coverage rates are quite rapid and overall economy is good as manual scrubbing is unnecessary and a little detergent concentrate generates a lot of foam (up to 500-fold).

Only specially designed chemicals are suitable for foam cleaning. The foam itself is created by a special surfactant system which is present in the product in addition to the actual cleaning components. Normal detergents which at first may appear quite foamy will give a very rapidly collapsing foam and should not be used for this purpose. Many speciality foam detergents and foam sanitisers are available, from caustic through neutral to acid, plus chlorine or quat, etc., if needed. Recently developed advanced foams give a much improved cling to smooth vertical surfaces and can remain in contact with complete coverage for 20–30 minutes or more. Older or less well-designed formulations can often collapse rapidly and slide off before the cleaning action is complete.

*Foam application equipment*

This can be classified as mobile, centralised or satellite, although there is some overlap.

*Mobile foamers* may be based on pressure vessels (like beer kegs), air-driven pumps, or venturi injector attachments to pressure washers. Advantages include low capital cost and versatility in using different chemicals in different areas. Disadvantages include potential lack of chemical solution strength control, maintenance problems due to abuse, waste of unused chemical solution and preparation and put-away time.

*Centralised foam systems* are based on an automatic chemical dilution, tank and pump station which pumps the solution, as a liquid under pressure, to numerous outlets on a pipework system throughout the factory. Compressed air is injected into the outlet 'foam boxes' to create the foam of the desired flow rate and air content. Advantages include consistent chemical strength throughout the plant with single-point control, no handling of concentrated chemical and the avoidance of drums of chemical in the factory production areas. The elimination of preparation and put-away time is also of benefit, saving about 30 minutes per operator per day. Chemical usage is typically 20–25% lower than with mobiles owing to the lack of waste. Disadvantages include capital cost and the versatility of the chemicals, but the latter can be remedied by using hybrid centralised/satellite foam boxes at chosen locations (Fig. 6.1).

*Satellite foam systems* are normally driven by centralised rinse systems using wall-mounted or trolley-mounted foam boxes equipped with venturi injectors at each outlet. Compressed air is injected at each box in low and medium pressure rinse systems (<40 bar water pressure) to create the foam, but with high-pressure rinse systems (> ~70 bar) atmospheric air alone can be drawn using special venturi foam lances. Advantages of satellite foam systems include low capital costs (in addition to those of the rinse system) and complete versatility of chemical choice and concentration at each outlet. Disadvantages include chemical drums in the production area and lack of central control-of-use rates. As mentioned previously, hybrid central/satellite systems are available which combine all the advantages of the two systems (see Fig. 6.1).

## Gels

Gel cleaning uses special chemicals and spray equipment to give a thick, viscous layer of detergent that clings strongly even on vertical surfaces. This is normally confined to small areas where very long contact time of several hours is needed for burnt-on or otherwise very stubborn deposits. Gel chemicals may sometimes be foamed with certain types of foam equipment, but the high viscosity of the gel is effectively increased within the foam even further. This leads to a slowing down of the cleaning reactions (which depend greatly on

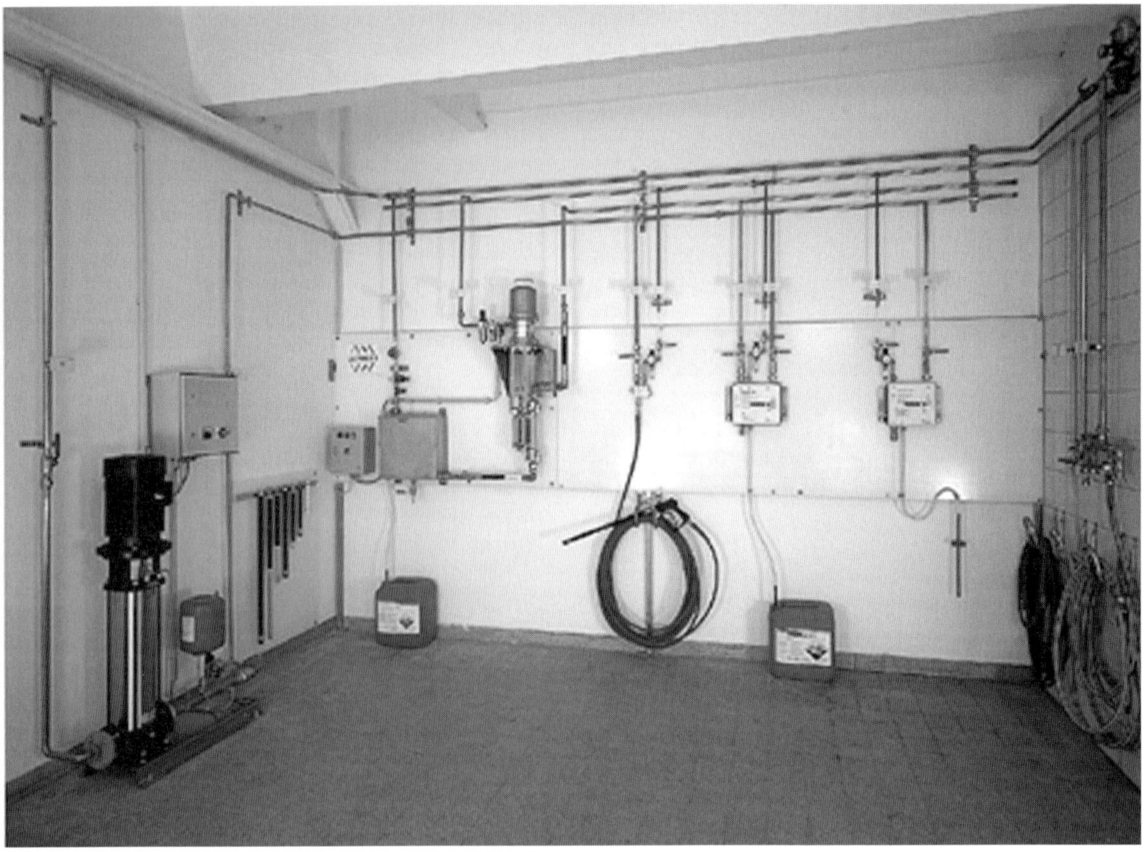

**Fig 6.1** Demonstration room showing installations of central and satellite foam and rinse stations.

diffusion of detergent components into the soil and of soil components out of the deposit). For this reason, gels are not economical for routine general cleaning of large factory areas, where time constraints usually dictate contact times of 15–30 minutes. Ensuring complete rinsing of gels can sometimes be difficult.

### Spray

Spray cleaning uses a lance on a pressure washer (with chemical induction by venturi) or a backpack sprayer. This method is often wasteful of chemical, which runs off rapidly, is slower than foaming, and produces more aerosol. Cleaning performance is inferior to that of foaming. The foaming nature of the chemical is usually not critical in this application as air is not injected into the liquid.

### Fogging

Aerial fogging uses compressed air or other equipment to generate a fine mist of disinfectant solution, which hangs in the air long enough to disinfect airborne organisms and which settles on walls and surfaces to give a bactericidal/bacteriostatic effect. Fogging systems can be small portable devices or built-in automatic central systems. Fogging is only worthwhile if the rest of the hygiene programme is properly carried out. The important parameters for effective fogging are the matching of the volume of liquid being fogged to the volume of the room, the temperature, relative humidity and rate of air change. Ideally saturation of the air with very fine droplets which stay suspended for a long time gives the best results. Failure to saturate or to have fine enough droplet size can mean that only the uppermost surfaces of the plant receive the disinfectant as it rains down and the air itself may remain largely unaffected.

## Machine washing

Industrial machine washing is typically done with an automatic or semiautomatic continuous traywash or buggywash machine with spray nozzles arrayed on booms in separate chambers of the machine or in separate cycles (for detergent, rinse and sometimes disinfectant). An alternative machine design uses submersion tanks or flumes, through which the trays are slowly pulled. A less effective design is the circular carousel (which runs the risk of contamination of clean trays by dirty ones as there is only one entry/exit point). Other machines, especially for buggies, may wash each item individually in a batch process. All machine types represent an expensive capital investment and are critical to the hygiene of direct food contact surfaces. Wash machines generally are large consumers of chemicals and water, especially if not properly maintained and controlled. Filters should be cleaned regularly and blocked nozzles cleared. Prevention of liquid carry-over from one chamber to the next is also important. Traywash machines can also be a contamination risk to the rest of the factory as they can produce large quantities of fine, contaminated aerosols which may drift with natural air flows into critical areas. Chemicals used in these machines must be low foam or even actively defoaming and should be automatically controlled and dosed by conductivity probe, with the probe being cleaned regularly and the concentration checked. Location of the probe is important in obtaining representative readings.

## Cleaning-in-place (CIP) (Fig. 6.2)

CIP, or cleaning-in-place, is used very extensively for the interior cleaning of pipes, vessels, tankers, heat exchangers, fillers, etc. in liquid product plants such as breweries and dairies. The technique is increasing in use in meat and poultry plants where giblets or other materials may be automatically transferred through pipe systems or where sauces, marinades and other liquids are used in added-value products. CIP involves a programmed cycle, including timed pre-rinse, cleaning and rinsing stages, and is nowadays usually automated or semiautomated with a system of valves, pumps and detergent tanks, often controlled by microprocessor. The main points to consider include:

1 The *flow velocity*, which in all parts of the system should be sufficient to cause turbulent flow. This is generally around 1.5–2 m/s. Where pipe diameters vary in the one system, the largest pipe should have this flow rate. Failure to comply with this flow rate means laminar flow at the boundary layer close to the pipe surface, with little or no mechanical energy to help the cleaning.

2 The *spray pressure and pattern* where sprayballs or rotating jets are used for the interiors of large tankers or vessels. Again, if impingement is too gentle or blind spots are protected from the impact of the spray, there will be insufficient energy to have an effective clean. Typical pressures are 1–3 bar for low-pressure systems and 6 bar for high-pressure systems. Flow rates of approximately 2 times the vessel's volume per hour are normally needed to achieve the desired results.

3 The *temperature*, which has a big bearing on the rate of the cleaning reaction. Generally, temperatures of 85°C are used.

4 *Detergent control*, which is typically by a temperature-compensated conductivity probe and pump. Conductivity closely follows free caustic levels in CIP solutions and allows for fully automatic control. Manual dosing, in contrast, runs the risk of chemical strength being too high or too low.

5 *Chemical energy and foam control* depend on the choice of detergent type. The main detergent in CIP is normally an alkali, frequently caustic-based. The additional components, such as surfactants (for preventing foam and aiding

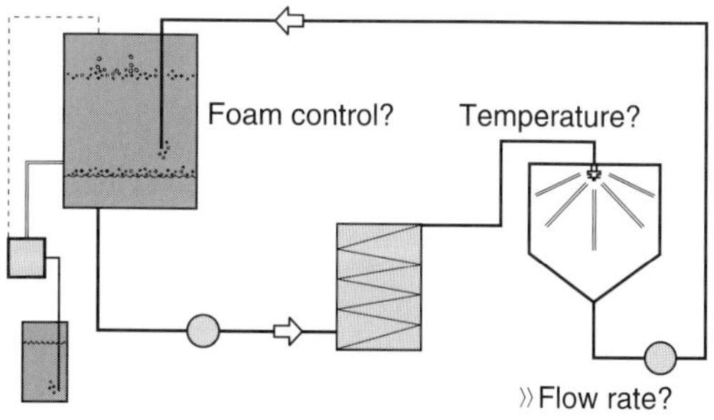


CIP parameters.

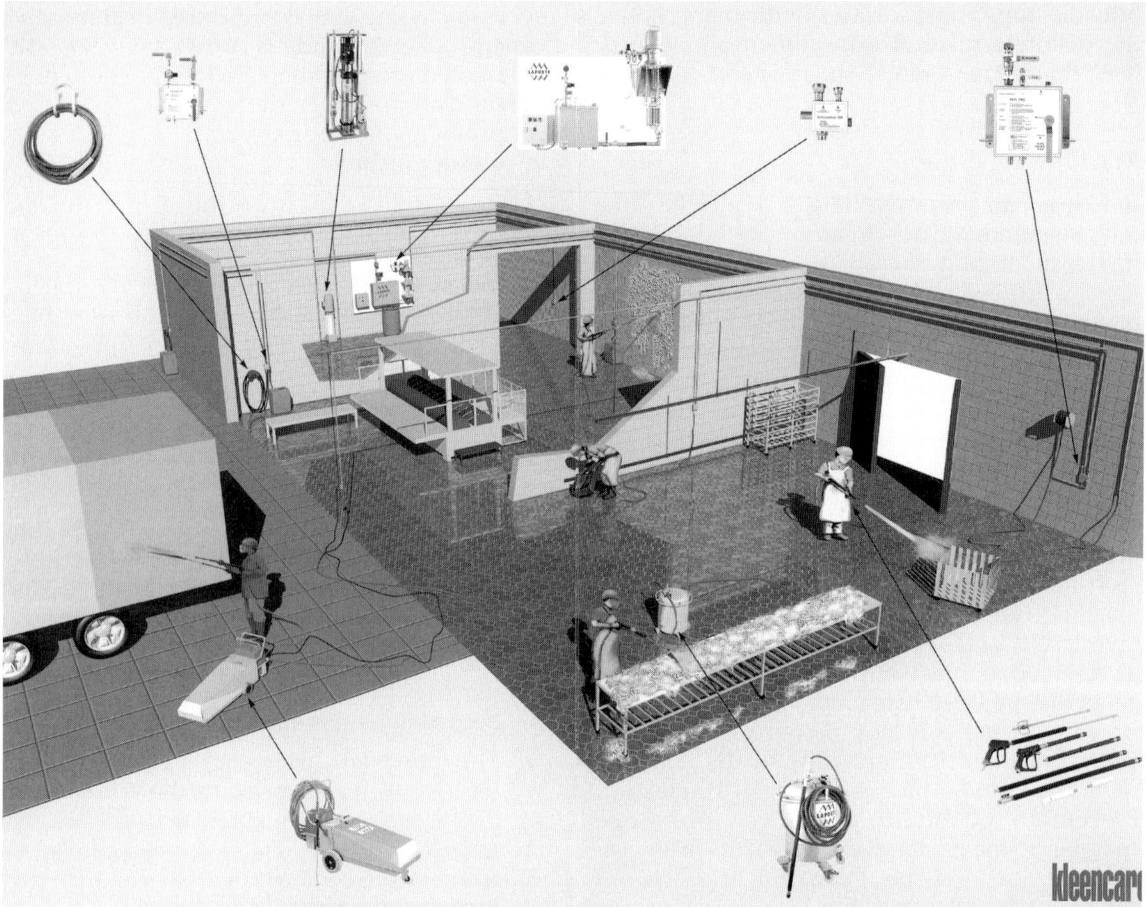


**Fig. 6.2** Various foam and rinse systems in use. (By courtesy of Kleencare Hygiene, Cheadle, Cheshire, UK)

wetting) and chelating agents (for removing scales such as calcium phosphate) may be included in the detergent formulation as supplied (when it is called a built detergent) or they may be supplied separately as a caustic additive. For formulation reasons, additives are technically superior and more economical but require parallel dosing pumps for caustic and additive.

6 *Recycling* of detergent solutions is economical, environmentally-friendly and reduces the loading on effluent plants. Solutions may normally be used many times, depending on the amount of dirt they pick up on each cleaning cycle and on the suspension and chelating power of the detergent. If too heavily loaded, detergent solutions may redeposit old soil or scale in slower-moving parts of the system. Filtration or centrifugation can sometimes be used to extend the life of the solution.

## Rinse systems

Meat and poultry plants need effective rinse systems for washing down the plant before and after the foam application and in some cases for generating the foam itself and applying disinfectant. A number of different systems are possible. The rule governing them all is that the cleaning impact of a water jet on a surface is proportional both to the pressure of the liquid at the point of contact and to the volume of liquid per second in the jet.

Traditional *steam hoses*, which mixed live steam with cold water are now out of favour for a number of reasons, principally cost, safety, humidity and condensation. Although it may be thought that the very high temperature of a steam hose had a disinfecting effect, this is in fact not the case, as expansion at the nozzle causes rapid cooling even at short distances, while conduction of heat away from the point of impact by the surface (usually a metal) means that sufficiently high temperatures are never reached. Live steam can also carry corrosion products from pipelines or carry-over of boiler treatment chemicals, neither of which is desirable hygienically.

Similarly, *low-pressure* (around mains pressure or less than 10 bar) water systems are inadequate for rinsing meat or poultry plants, because the water jet lacks sufficient energy to assist in the cleaning process.

At the other extreme, *high-pressure* rinse systems, based on either mobile pressure washers or built-in pump systems have been widely used. Their use is now in rapid decline for a number of safety, maintenance and hygiene reasons. These systems typically function at 60–120 bar using piston or plunger type pumps. These create a vibration in the system, which can affect the life of the pipework, which is narrow-bore and expensive. The design of the pumps (positive displacement) causes pressure in the system to drop precipitously if the maximum flow rate is exceeded, e.g. if one person too many uses an outlet simultaneously or if one nozzle is missing or worn out. The high velocity of the water from the nozzles causes the jet to break up at a distance of about 1 metre into a fine mist, which has lost virtually all its momentum and impact. Rinsing of surfaces therefore needs to be carried out at close range. This is time-consuming for the operators and in addition causes the soil deposit to be broken up violently, creating contaminating aerosols. High-pressure water is also dangerous and may penetrate the skin or damage eyes.

*Medium-pressure* rinse systems (25–50 bar) are the currently favoured option. Using relatively inexpensive multistage (boiler feed type) pumps and wider bore, medium pressure-rated pipework, these systems are vibration-free and insensitive to sudden fluctuations in water usage at the various outlets. The nozzle used is usually adjustable from a conical flood to a fine concentrated jet and, as the water velocity is lower and the volume per second higher, the jet retains most of its impact even at several metres distance. This means that rinsing can be faster, with a better sluicing-away effect. The extra water consumption per second is more than compensated for by a shorter rinse time. Water consumption in total, compared to a high-pressure system, is more or less equivalent, but labour savings (in the most time-consuming stage of the cleaning sequence) are significant.

### Water temperatures

Although the EU regulations call for 82°C water to be used for knife sterilisation, such high temperatures are impractical for most plant cleaning operations (with the main exception of CIP) for a number of reasons:

- The steam, humidity and condensation obscure vision and encourage microbial growth.
- Proteins are denatured on the surfaces and hard-water scale formation is increased.
- The load on the extraction and cooling systems is increased.
- Thermal shock can damage surfaces owing to differential expansion.
- Pipework lifetime is reduced.
- The lances are too hot to hold and the water jet is dangerous.
- Energy costs are too high.
- Foam quality deteriorates at very high temperatures.

The temperature which gives the best compromise between effectiveness and economy is 60–65°C which is enough to soften the fats encountered in meat plants, without the drawbacks shown above. In fish plants, because of the low denaturation temperature of the proteins, rinse water at ~35°C is used.

## CONTAMINATION AND RECONTAMINATION

Meat plant surfaces will be exposed to microbial contamination by direct contact with the exterior of the animal prior to and after slaughter and to the gut contents during and after evisceration. The dressing process and subsequent production stages are designed so as to reduce further direct contamination of food product with these microorganisms. While viscera are kept physically separate from edible materials, plant surfaces in evisceration areas will have high bacteria counts. Personnel and external material such as pallets, vehicles, etc. also bring microorganisms into the plant, especially on to the floors.

During cleaning these microorganisms, whether spoilage, pathogenic or harmless, may be disturbed in such a way as to be transmitted, perhaps directly on to food product itself or on to previously cleaned surfaces. This accidental *recontamination* is carried by a number of possible *vectors*, which, unless understood and controlled, can nullify the effectiveness of the cleaning procedure.

*Air* can carry dust from hide-pullers, fleeces, feathers, etc., especially in dry weather. This dust is likely to contain faecal bacteria, among others. Air can also carry aerosols created by water jets during rinsing or by washing machines. Such aerosols can be very fine and can drift with natural air movement for considerable distances. *Listeria*, *E. coli* and *Salmonella* are very frequently found on floors and drains, which makes the rinsing of these potentially problematic. Hot water or steam can also create aerosols which condense on cold overhead surfaces, later to drip on to unprotected foodstuffs positioned below. For these reasons, great care must be taken to ensure that all product is removed from areas being cleaned. Differential air pressures must cause air to move from clean to dirty areas and not vice versa. Pressure hoses must not be inserted into drains.

*Water* collecting in hollows on the floor or in blocked drain openings can quickly become highly contaminated. Splashes caused by people or vehicles going through the puddles can directly contaminate surfaces. Water used in washing the plant may be stored in holding tanks feeding the pumps. These may also become contaminated and, with warm water driving off chlorine reserve, the rinse water itself may become a source of recontamination. Hoses supplying product make-up water to bowl choppers and the like can support microbial (especially fungal) growth on their insides.

*Personnel* are the biggest single source of contamination risk in a plant, from dirty protective clothing, inadequate handwashing, hair, jewellery, sneezes, coughs, cuts and sores. All plant personnel must be trained in hygiene and the proper clean protective wear supplied. Hand-washing facilities must be conveniently located close to production stations and entrances. Bactericidal, non-perfumed soaps must be supplied, together with alcoholic hand disinfectant in high-risk areas.

*Surfaces* which are inadequately cleaned may recontaminate entire pieces of equipment. For example, one badly cleaned roller on an otherwise spotless conveyor belt can, in one rotation of the belt, smear it with grease and dirt. Similarly, cutting blades in saws, slicers, dicers, etc. must be very effectively cleaned.

## CLEANING PROCEDURES

The previous sections on soil, substrate, detergents, equipment, methods and recontamination should demonstrate that the cleaning of a meat plant is a complex job. Only with systematic procedures can a consistently hygienic plant be maintained. These procedures form part of the *Cleaning Schedule*, a working reference document which defines standards, methods, frequencies and materials for all cleaning and disinfecting operations in the plant. The schedule should form part of the Quality Manual of the plant and be available for consultation or inspection. Simplified extracts of the schedule, employing pictograms, may be used as wall charts for individual plant areas. Hygiene suppliers often assist in the preparation and upkeep of the hygiene schedules.

To secure a Due Diligence defence in the case of prosecution it would normally be necessary to show that a properly designed cleaning schedule was in place and was being followed.

As mentioned earlier, cost pressures may encourage the cleaners to combine or leave out individual steps in the cleaning sequence. This should be avoided. Anyone responsible for food industry hygiene, and in particular in the methodology of cleaning, should have a clear understanding of what methods are correct for the cleaning of food plants and the dangers of incorrect or inadequate cleaning procedures.

### The cleaning sequence

The correct sequence for general routine surface cleaning of a food plant is:

1 Gross clean/preparation
2 Pre-rinsing
3 Detergent application
4 Post-rinsing
5 Disinfection
6 Terminal rinsing.

Some of these steps may sometimes be skipped or combined (perhaps where the nature and quantity of the soil is light, or during brief intermediate cleaning in production breaks) but for systematic daily cleaning the sequence is very important. We look at each step in more detail.

### *1. Gross clean/preparation*

This is the step that is most often incorrectly carried out or completely ignored. Food residue that is left on the equipment, surfaces and floors has many negative effects on the cleaning performance:

- It protects surfaces and the bacteria on them from the attack of the detergent.
- It reacts with and consumes the detergent so that its function is weakened or chemical wasted.
- It holds bacteria (often at very high levels) which can recontaminate surfaces at a later stage in the cleaning, especially during the rinsing stage.
- It can directly recontaminate surfaces with grease and protein which can act as nutrient for microorganisms and as a barrier to disinfectant. This is particularly true on moving machinery such as conveyors.
- It can end up washed into the drainage system, either causing blockage in traps or high solids/BOD (biological oxygen demand) in the effluent.
- It encourages the cleaning team to miss areas, not to check their work, and also to cut other corners.

*A poor gross clean is the single biggest reason for poor or inconsistent bacterial counts on surfaces and for high bacterial contamination in aerosols caused by rinsing.*

In a properly managed cleaning programme, all pieces of food product, meat, etc., which are larger than a fingernail are removed before application of detergent. Where possible this should be carried out dry by hand-picking, scraping and shovelling. All rubbish/waste collected should be put in bags/bins and removed entirely from the area. It should go without saying that all edible foodstuffs and product packaging should be removed at or before this stage. (It is a constant source of amazement how often this simple fact is ignored.)

### *2. Pre-rinsing*

The purpose of pre-rinsing is to remove deposits which cannot easily be removed by picking/scraping/shovelling, e.g. blood, manure, small meat pieces and particles, etc. The rinse waterjet should not be used as a brush for chasing large amounts of pieces around the floor and towards the drain. This would result in waste of water and time, blockage of drains, loading of effluent water with high BOD/COD, and unnecessarily high humidity.

Pre-rinsing is particularly important in the case of cutting boards, where the thick deposits of grease would make true cleaning of the surface grooves and crevices impossible. Where fresh blood is a problem, the rinse temperature should be below 50°C to avoid coagulation.

After pre-rinsing it is important to remove any water that may be lying in pools on flat surfaces as these would dilute the detergent solution and make it less effective. Any squeegee used to scrape off the excess water must be used only for food contact surfaces and not for floors.

### *3. Detergent application*

The purpose of a detergent is to remove the thin tenacious layers of protein, grease etc. that are still on surfaces which may already look fairly clean. Detergents are not designed for removing large pieces of meat or thick layers of fat. Although they may seem to help in the removal of such large quantities, they will usually fail to remove the last residues actually bonded to the surface if these residues are protected by the thicker layers above them. It is in these thin residues that many bacteria can easily survive and grow and they can also make any disinfectant, which is applied later, ineffective.

Foaming should be methodical and thorough and the operator should check to see that all surfaces have been covered in the foam, both top and bottom. Foam concentration, dryness, thickness of application and contact time are all very important in ensuring the correct results at a controlled, optimised cost.

*4. Post-rinsing*

Post-rinsing is again a very important stage. Care should be taken to minimise the amount of splash and aerosol formed, which may recontaminate previously cleaned surfaces or blast particles of dirt high up on walls and ventilation socks, etc. After post-rinsing, the surfaces should be free of all visible particles, layers of soiling and residues of detergent and should be 'optically clean'. (The soil and detergent residues and any soaps formed by alkaline hydrolysis of fats, will tend to neutralise the disinfectant properties of quats.) It is important to check the efficacy of the rinse, especially where parallel production lines are cleaned in sequence and splash could recontaminate previously cleaned surfaces. The rollers of conveyors are particularly important. After rinsing, any pools of water should be removed from surfaces and vessels, whether disinfection is to follow or not.

*5. Disinfection*

Disinfection should only be carried out on a visually clean, well-rinsed surface, with minimal amounts of surface water. Direct food contact surfaces should be disinfected at least daily, with other surfaces (such as walls, doors, etc.) disinfected on a regular basis. The concentration of the disinfectant is very important.

*6. Terminal rinsing*

Most (but not all!) disinfectants are safe to leave on surfaces without final rinsing. The residual disinfectant often helps maintain a low microbial count for a considerable time after the cleaning sequence is finished. In some sections of the food industry, EU directives and national regulations require rinsing of *food-contact* surfaces with potable water after the disinfectant has acted *unless* the disinfectant is specifically designed to remain unrinsed. If terminal rinsing is being done, it should, if possible, be at such a time as to allow surfaces to dry before production (if necessary) but not so early that remaining microorganisms are able to recover and multiply significantly before production recommences.

This rinsing should be much quicker than post-rinsing after foaming or pre-rinsing before foaming, as no contaminating particles of soil should be present. The microbiological quality of the water is very important. It must be potable or else it can be a source of recontamination itself.

## MONITORING OF HYGIENE

Monitoring of cleaning and disinfection effectiveness is partly a matter of trained *visual assessment* and partly of *microbiology*. A plant that is not visually clean still presents a risk of microbial contamination. The control and avoidance of these risks are best achieved using a HACCP (Hazard analysis by critical control points) approach. Legislation strongly recommends the use of HACCP principles to secure a Due Diligence defence, but a simple logical approach is preferable in practice to an over-ornate, unwieldy bureaucratic system. The critical points in the cleaning and disinfection programme should be identified and measurement and control protocols set up. Some of the CCPs (critical control points) will be readily measurable, e.g. the solution concentration of a detergent or disinfectant, while others involve checking the procedure itself. After each CCP stage in the cleaning procedure, the operator should check for effectiveness and thoroughness. This check should be backed up by the hygiene supervisor, who, if not satisfied, should ask for a repeat of the stage. Quality assurance and/or production personnel should also check the plant regularly, looking in particular for old soil deposits not removed at the last clean, and build-up of fungi, corrosion or scale deposits. The hygiene supervisor and his or her team should also be periodically audited to ensure that the cleaning and disinfection procedures are being followed. Chemical solution strengths should be regularly checked by titration, test kit or conductivity meter. The internal monitoring can be usefully supplemented by audits from external experts, such as hygiene chemical/service suppliers, consultants, etc.

The microbiological assessment should be carried out on representative and random sampling points using skilled personnel. Results should be reported regularly to management and fed back to the cleaning team for remedial action. The advent of rapid methods has meant that results are real-time and allow action to be taken almost immediately. Most systems are based on the measurement of adenosine triphosphate (ATP), a coenzyme which functions in many enzyme-catalysed reactions in animals, plants and micro-organisms, acting as a carrier of energy from oxidative processes to cells requiring it. Food residues are rich in ATP, which bacteria, yeasts, moulds, etc., need to grow and multiply. When ATP is brought into contact with luciferin-luciferase, a reaction takes place with the production of light – bioluminescence. The sensitive light meters in the systems accurately measure the concentrations of ATP and thus of the microorganisms and food residues. The fact that ATP test kits do not (unless a special stage is included) differentiate between somatic (meat-derived) cells and microbial cells is largely irrelevant, as the result is a measure of overall 'cleanliness' and either actual or potential microbial contamination. Techniques such as ATP can be used to optimise the cleaning protocols, evaluate different chemicals, solution concentrations and rinse water temperatures, and so on. Statistical analysis of results over a period of time can identify trends more meaningfully than simply observing daily variations.

Fig 6.3 shows a range of total counts on equipment monitored Mon–Fri.

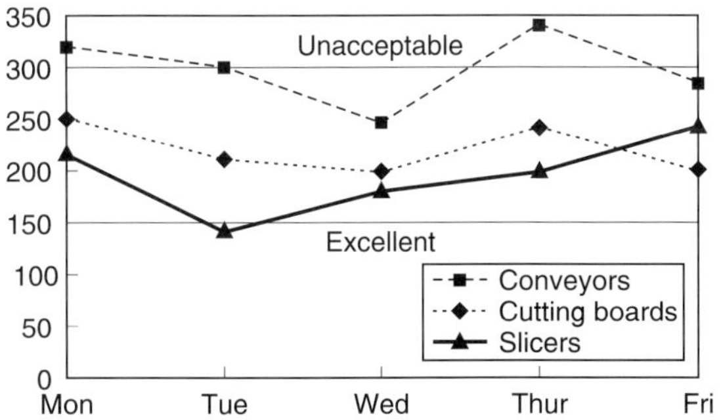


**Fig 6.3** Trend analysis of total counts.

## TRAINING

Training of all operatives and managers involved in plant cleaning is *critically important*. It helps develop and maintain a high self-esteem and status in the cleaning team (traditionally seen, wrongly, as less skilled than production workers) and a problem-solving, self-assessing quality attitude to the job. Training should cover the theoretical background in sufficient depth, particularly the microscopic 'enemy', the risks of recontamination, the importance of procedures and the safe use of chemicals and equipment. Practical, on-the-job training should be continuous, especially when new plant or equipment is introduced or procedures are changed. For protection of Due Diligence, training should be recorded on the personnel records of those trained.

## SAFETY

Industrial detergents and disinfectants are generally, because of the nature of the job they are designed to do, more concentrated and more extreme in pH than domestic products. They should always be applied using the correct protective wear; gloves, goggles (or full-face protector), apron, boots, etc. In areas where high aerosol levels may be created, with a risk of heavy microbial contamination, a suitable face mask should be worn. Chemicals must not be mixed unless under the express instructions of a competent person. All chemical containers must be clearly labelled with product-specific identification and safety information as per EU standards. Safety data sheets on all chemicals must be available which conform to the legislation. All equipment must be properly maintained.

## EFFLUENT AND ODOUR CONTROL

It is beyond the scope of this discussion to deal in depth with these two complex hygiene-related issues. A number of general points, however, may be usefully made.

*Effluent systems* in meat plants may be affected by the misuse of some detergents and disinfectants. If 'slugs' of concentrated or high-volume, high- or low-pH chemicals are let to

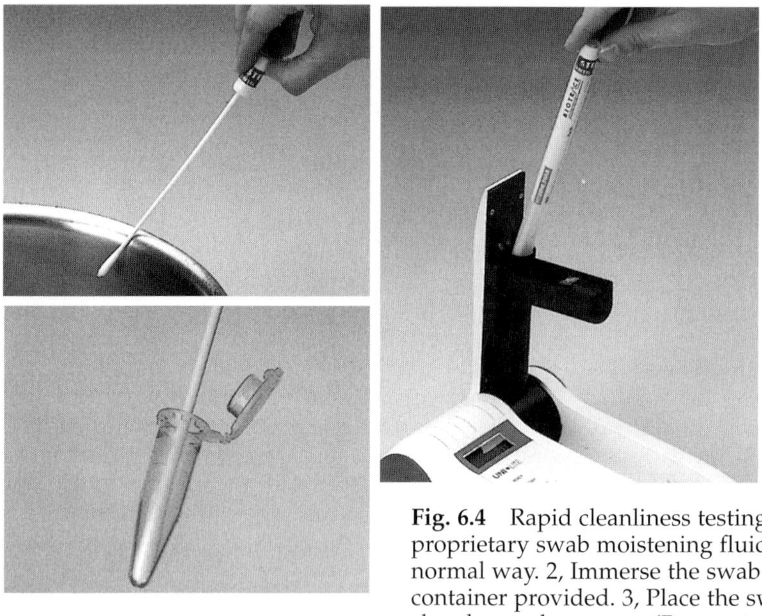

1 2 3

**Fig. 6.4** Rapid cleanliness testing. 1, Wet the swab with the proprietary swab moistening fluid and swab the surface in the normal way. 2, Immerse the swab in the enzyme solution using the container provided. 3, Place the swab into the UniLite sample chamber and measure. (By courtesy of Biotrace Ltd, Bridgend, Glamorgan, UK)

drain, they may (if not neutralised in the balance tank) upset the microbes in biological treatment plants. The same is true for chlorine, quats and some other disinfectants. If a treatment plant (especially the balance tank) is undersized for the effluent it receives at peak periods, it is possible for 'breakthrough' of organics, including some surfactants, to occur. This means that instead of being fully biodegraded in the plant, they survive to give possible foaming problems (especially where aeration occurs) plus high COD/BOD (chemical and biological oxygen demand, respectively), plus increased suspended and dissolved solids. This may result in higher charges from the water authorities or possible penalties. It is important in the factory pre-clean to remove as much organic matter (such as food residues) as possible from production areas before detergents are applied. These larger pieces of organic material are not readily biodegradable and may block or blind the biological treatment plant. No bio-plant likes varying BOD loadings. Steady conditions are preferred if 'shedding' of filamentous growth is to be avoided. In activated sludge plants, the sudden ingress of high-COD material will result in low dissolved oxygen levels, thus potentially turning the plant anaerobic (with resulting malodours) or, by increasing the potential for filamentous growth, causing settlement problems in the final clarifier.

By definition, cleaning chemicals will dissolve, emulsify and disperse organic materials and carry perhaps excessive amounts to the effluent plant. It is also important not to discharge sudden, very large quantities of heavily-loaded water, such as from scald tanks or cooking kettles. The risk is even higher if the water is hot, as fats and oils may be temporarily emulsified by the heat and may pass unhindered through the grease trap prior to the effluent system.

The biodegradability of the detergents and disinfectants themselves is also important, but not because they contribute greatly to the total COD/BOD of the plant effluent. Their contribution, in comparison to that of the food process effluent and residual soil carried away by cleaning, is minor. There are some surfactants, previously common in many detergents and disinfectants, which are now suspected of partly biodegrading to slightly simpler, but more environmentally-damaging, molecules. One group in particular, the alkyl phenol ethoxylates (or APEOs), are believed to have oestrogenic effects in river waters, possibly affecting the reproduction of aquatic organisms.

They are being phased out of detergent and disinfectant formulations. The chemical supplier should be asked to supply chemicals, backed up by specific product data, which conform to the latest environmental regulations.

*Odour control* may be particularly important if the factory is situated close to residential areas. Odour may arise from the effluent plant itself, if aeration is inadequate, loading is excessive (see earlier) and anaerobic bacteria are flourishing. Such problems may be helped by improving aeration and reducing the COD/BOD loading to the plant. Other methods to assist the breakdown of proteins and other organics include the addition of *enzyme* preparations in the effluent stream as it leaves the plant or even in the factory drain system. The enzymes begin the biodegradation process early and assist the main treatment plant in handling its burden. Other odours may arise from exhausts from rendering plants and from waste skips, etc. The most common chemical treatments used here involve 'scrubbing' the exhaust gases with fine showers containing oxidising disinfectants such as chlorine dioxide or peracetic acid or spraying the disinfectant into the skips themselves. These chemicals act to oxidise and breakdown the malodorous molecules (which are usually relatively small volatile molecules containing sulphur). An alternative approach is to use essential-oil-based sprays to destroy the molecules. Attempting to mask the malodour with a perfumed agent is usually not successful.

## CONCLUSION

Plant cleaning and disinfection has a much higher profile than ever before. Cost pressures on one side, versus legislative and quality pressures on the other, contrive to make the hygienist's job more difficult and the cost of failure higher. All persons involved in plant hygiene must appreciate that it is a skilled multidisciplined management task to ensure that the general methods and the fine details are kept under constant attention and that potential problems are highlighted and dealt with early enough to avoid them becoming real and damaging.

# Chapter 7
# From Farm to Slaughter

All modern meat hygiene systems should endeavour to take into consideration the entire process of production and processing which is involved in producing meat or meat products as a food from farm animals. Only by ensuring that the animals on the farm are managed in a responsible manner with respect to drug use, husbandry and welfare can the high standards demanded by the modern consumer be assured. These demands have changed over the last decades in the western developed countries from the immediately post-war call for cheap meat, to the present requirement for a guaranteed wholesome, environmental and animal welfare-friendly, product.

## PRODUCTION OF CLEAN HEALTHY LIVESTOCK (See Figs 7.1, 7.2)

The monitoring of all aspects of husbandry practices on the farm should be the first step in a meat hygiene system. The Richmond Committee on the Microbiological Safety of Food (Part II) concluded that '*farmers can contribute to food safety by producing healthy, clean and unstressed animals for slaughter, and we believe that this simple truth should be borne in mind by livestock producers and stressed by all who provide them with advice*'.

### Levels of faecal contamination of cattle hides

Some idea of the degree of manurial pollution of cattle hides can be gained from the excellent surveys carried out by the British Leather Centre in their Hide Improvement Project. In their 1996 survey (Stosic 1996), which covered the whole of the British Isles, showed the following main findings:

| | |
|---|---|
| Total number of hides inspected | 15268 |
| Average amount of dung per hide | 3.7 kg |
| Percentage of hides affected | 73% |
| Percentage of hides with over 4.5 kg dung | 36% |
| Largest amount of dung/hide recorded | 16 kg |

There were significant variations between the different regions of the British Isles as follows:

| | |
|---|---|
| Scotland | 1.85 kg |
| England & Wales | 2.42 kg |
| N. Ireland | 4.32 kg |
| S. Ireland | 5.57 kg |

The above average weight (3.7 kg) of cattle hide faecal contamination may be compared with that recorded by the author (JFG) in February 1965 of 4 kg, an indication that there has not been much improvement over a period of over 30 years. The worst month for the Irish and Scottish hides was February, while the peak for England and Wales was in April.

In addition to conveying the various food poisoning pathogens (*E. coli* O157 H7, *Salmonella*, *Campylobacter*, *Yersinia*, *Giardia*, *Listeria*, etc.), faecal contamination of hides and fleeces is responsible for damage to hides and eventual leather ('coarsened grain') by excoriating the surface layers of the skin and exposing sensory nerve endings and causing pain, thereby making this a serious *welfare* problem. *Hazards* are also created for operatives engaged in carcase dressing through knife slips. The entire problem is costing the meat industry many millions of pounds anually and deserves immediate attention at farm (mainly), transport and meat plant levels.

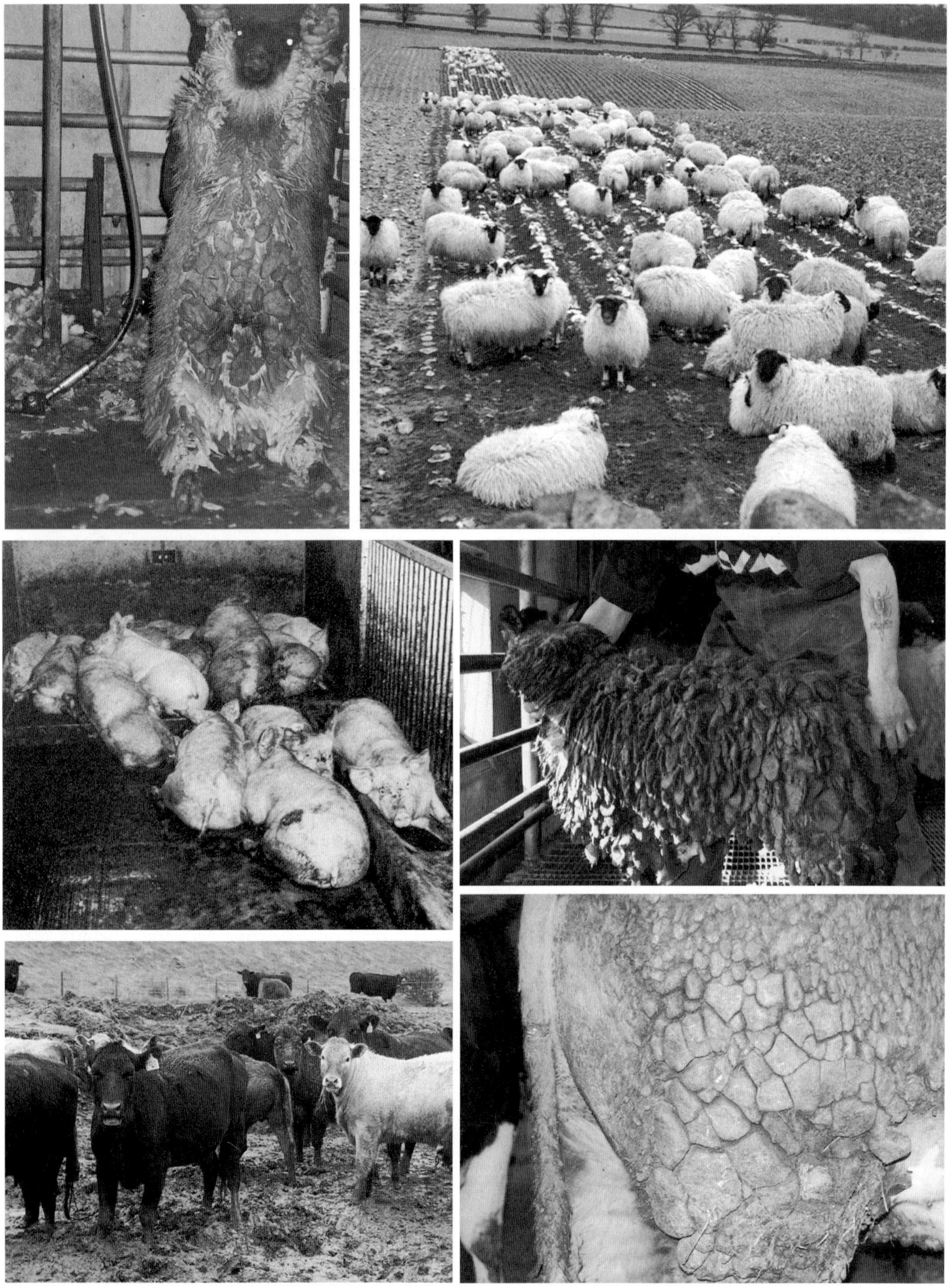

**Fig. 7.1** Unacceptable faecal/soil contamination. (By courtesy of J.A. Ross MRCVS)

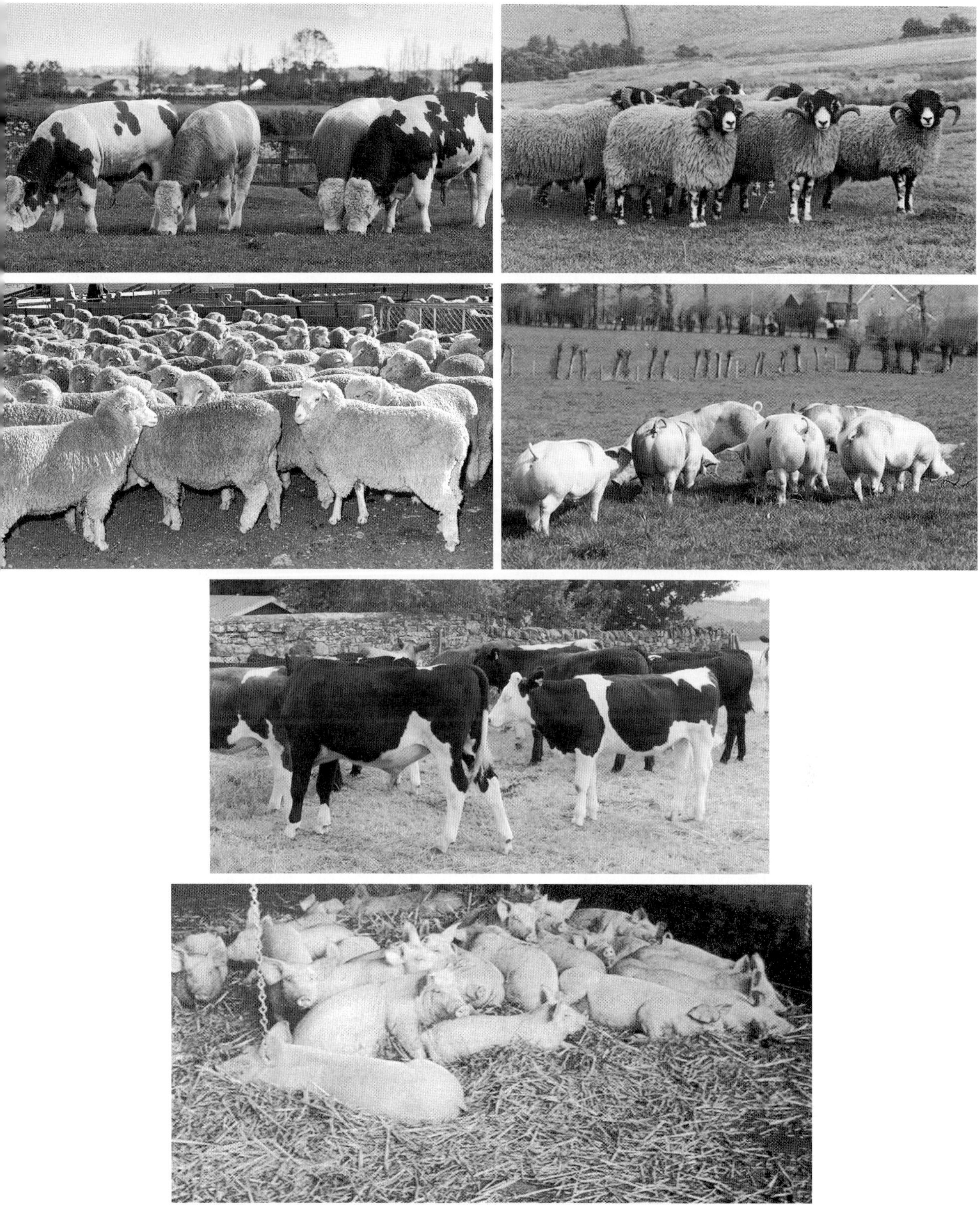

**Fig. 7.2** Excellent standards of animal cleanliness.

*Causes of dirty livestock*

Under typical weather conditions in the British Isles the production of clean cattle and sheep for slaughter is relatively easy where the animals are at grass during the warm summer months. However, in wet weather cattle and sheep all too frequently arrive at the meat plant in a very dirty condition. This is especially the case in those countries in the more northerly latitudes where livestock are housed during the winter months.

A survey carried out in Northern Ireland (Ingram, 1972) showed that the problem of dirty cattle was mainly related to bedded courts with or without open yards. The principal cause was found to be lack of bedding, aggravated by high stocking densities, poor ventilation causing condensation, poor drainage, inadequate floor gradients and infrequent removal of slurry. In some instances deficiencies included incorrect cubicle size, improperly positioned or overflowing water bowls or troughs, blocked slats due to non-removal of slurry, and cattle lying outside the cubicle or bedded area. The problem appeared to be worse on farms where heavier cattle were housed and fed silage. The growth of long hair during the winter months contributed greatly to the accumulation of muck on the cattle.

The following points should be given due attention by farmers producing stock for slaughter:

1 *Housing structure and layout* Defects in design, layout, cubicle size and design, drainage, water bowls, slats, ventilation, etc. should be corrected. Regular maintenance is essential.
2 *Bedding* Adequate bedding is essential. It is best to commence with a deep layer and subsequently to bed with large amounts at regular intervals. A concrete area that is frequently scraped will serve to reduce bedding requirements. Regular and frequent removal of slurry is essential.
3 *Housing density* Either overcrowding or understocking of pens can lead to cattle becoming dirty. If there are insufficient cattle in a slatted pen, the manure will not get tramped through and will accumulate.
4 *Clipping* It is good practice to clip the bellies, briskets and flanks of cattle before housing to prevent the accumulation of matted muck on the hair. The practice of clipping the backs of cattle cosmetically for sale purposes is a waste of time and should be replaced by *brisket, belly and hip clipping for slaughter stock.*
5 *Management* A high level of stockmanship, especially when animals are first housed, is essential. Individuals who do not settle in a particular system should be removed if possible. It is often necessary to encourage or train cattle to lie in cubicles.
6 *Internal parasitism* A veterinary-audited anthelmintic programme should be followed to prevent outbreaks of parasitic gastroenteritis in housed cattle. Attention should be paid especially to the risk of type II ostertagiasis in cattle.
7 *Transport and abattoir lairages* Animals should leave the farm in a clean condition, and be transported under conditions which allow them to arrive at the abattoir clean. In New Zealand, the use of trucks with expanded-metal floors with a 5 cm clearance over solid bases for all of the decks means that the lambs are standing clean and dry during transit.

Internal parasitism can also cause severe problems in *sheep*, with staining and clumping of the wool in the perineal region. Sheep folded on root crops, especially during inclement weather, can become heavily contaminated with soil, making hygienic dressing of the carcase difficult. *Sheep for slaughter should be given a ventral clip at least 16 cm wide from the neck to the anus.* Those folded on root crops should be put on clean grass for at least one week before dispatch for slaughter. Cases of scouring in sheep from whatever cause should not be sent for slaughter until cured. There can also be a potentially serious problem where sheep arrive dirty but dry, from clouds of dust which are produced during the removal of the fleece. To counteract this, it is normal practice in New Zealand to pass sheep through a plunge dip as they enter the lairage. It has been demonstrated, however, that although this practice results in carcases with less visible contamination there is in fact an increase in the total aerobic bacterial and *E. coli* count (Biss and Hathaway, 1996)

The Richmond Committee suggested that 'abattoir managers should pay farmers a premium to take account of the cleanliness of the animals as one of the components of quality'. In New Zealand it is an offence to present dirty stock for slaughter.

In Finland, the problem of excessively dirty cattle being presented for slaughter has been greatly reduced by the application of a series of rules agreed by meat inspection veterinarians, farmers, the meat industry, the leather industry and the state veterinary department. Under this agreement, excessively dirty animals are detained to be slaughtered separately after the clean animals. The scheme has resulted in a decrease in the numbers of excessively dirty cattle by 85% (Ridell and Korkeala, 1993).

The text of the Finnish Agreement (which is combined with detailed advice given to all parties through education, instruction and the press) is as follows:

1 All the parties aim at a situation where the animals offered for transport to slaughterhouses are as clean as possible.

2 If, however, excessively dungy animals are offered for transportation, the owner of the animals is requested to clean them. Animals are transported after cleaning when the next opportunity arises.

3 However, if excessively dungy animals must be received for transportation to a slaughterhouse, the procedure is as follows:

   **3.1** If dung can be removed through cleaning, animals will be cleaned before slaughter.

   **3.2** If dung cannot be removed through cleaning (solid dung layer), the animals must be slaughtered in the sanitary slaughter department. If this is not possible, the animals may be slaughtered in the common slaughterhall after clean animals have been slaughtered. All the slaughter facilities and equipment must be cleaned thoroughly afterwards according to the instructions of the inspection veterinarian.

   **3.3** The extra reasonable costs caused by the treatment and slaughtering of the excessively dungy animals are billed to the seller of the animals.

4 The inspection veterinarian on duty at the slaughterhouse decides which animals have to be slaughtered in the sanitary slaughter department or in the common slaughter room after the slaughter of the clean animals.

5 The slaughterhouse takes care that the animals do not get unreasonably dirty during transportation or in the lairage of the slaughterhouse.

In the UK, the Clean Livestock Policy was introduced during 1977. Cattle and sheep considered by the official veterinarian to be dirty are rejected for slaughter during ante-mortem inspection.

The washing of pigs (Fig. 7.3) where necessary is very beneficial for reducing scalding tank and carcase contamination.

## Healthy livestock

An *ethos of good husbandry and stockmanship* on the farm is essential if healthy animals are to be produced consistently for slaughter. This is particularly so where animals are cared for under intensive systems of agriculture, where attention to nutritional balance and preventive medicine programmes entailing the use of vaccines, anthelmintics, and feed additives are of particular importance.

Careless and unhygienic use of the *hypodermic syringe* (Fig. 7.4) is responsible for much unnecessary pain in animals and for considerable damage to carcases and consequent partial condemnation due to the production of *abscesses*, and in some cases *necrosis*, at the site of injection. If animals are injected outdoors, a dry day should be selected and the injections should be made on clean animals. It is imperative that needles are changed frequently, e.g. every 6 cattle or 25 sheep, and when there is a break in the work. A survey in the USA (Dexter *et al.*, 1993) recorded the incidence of injection-site blemishes in top sirloin butts to be 10.87% ±2.99%. The average weight per blemish was 123.39 g ±5.48 g.

The *site* of the injection has to be selected carefully and must not be an area which is associated with the more expensive cuts. It is imperative, for example, that piglets are not injected with iron into the ham, and that the hindleg is avoided when injecting lambs with antibiotic. Subcutaneous and intramuscular injections should be given either high up on the neck or on the lower rib cage. In sheep, the fold of wool-less skin behind the foreleg is a useful site. Sharp needles, with a metal rather than a plastic mount are less likely to break during the injecting process. A 16-gauge needle is recommended for use in adult cattle and sheep.

Some anthelmintics which are injected subcutaneously in cattle and sheep can cause a very severe reaction and staining at the site of

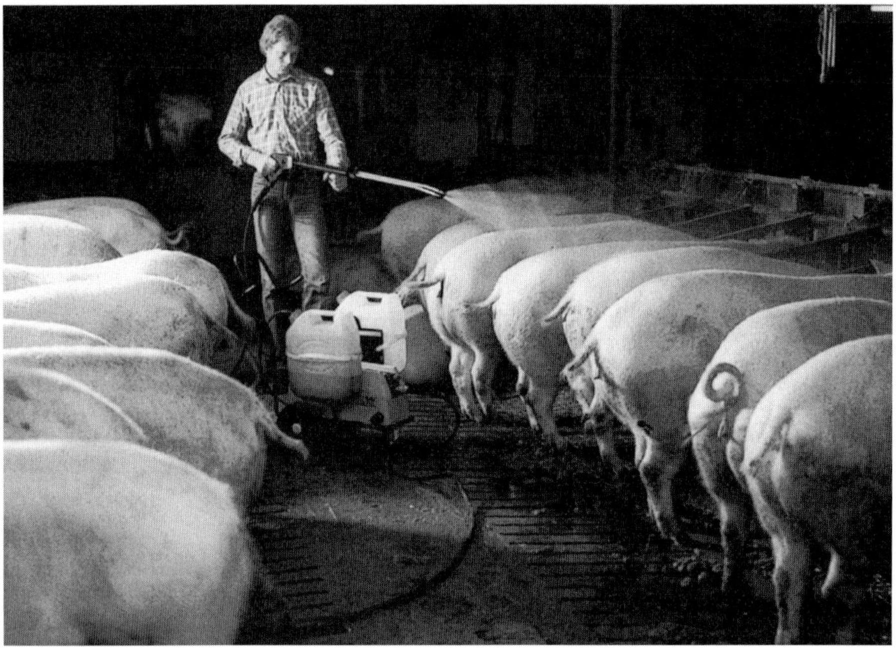

**Fig. 7.3** Pre-slaughter washing of pigs. (By courtesy of KEW Cleaning Systems Ltd, Penrith, Cumbria, UK)

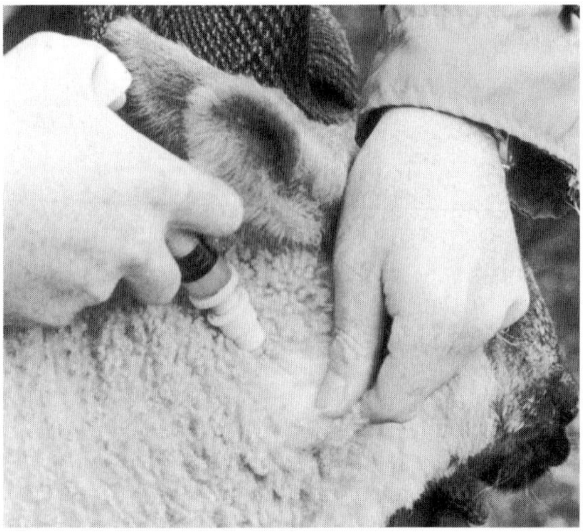

**Fig. 7.4** Sterile injection at proper site in lamb. (By courtesy of Meat & Livestock Commission, UK)

injection. This makes it imperative not only that sterile technique is observed but that the very long withdrawal period, of 60 days in some cases, is adhered to.

With the usual multidose injectors it is impossible for the needle to be disinfected between each injection. However, a sleeve attachment is available which can sanitise the needle, by passing it through a polypropylene cap containing a biocide-impregnated foam, each time the needle is pushed through the animal's skin and withdrawn. The system works well for pigs where injections are made with the syringe at right angles to the surface of the skin, but less well in cattle and sheep where subcutaneous injections require the needle to pass through the skin at an acute angle.

The use of anthelmintics and feed additives requires the producer to be vigilant with regard to *withdrawal periods*. The keeping of good drugs records is both a practical necessity and a legal requirement. The improper use of *drenching guns* may lead to damage to the oral cavity and subsequent abscess formation in the mouth and throat (Fig. 7.5).

Many admirable *livestock assurance schemes* are operating in the United Kingdom, but they represent only a small percentage of the total food animal population and are not always as efficient or complete as they should be.

### Safe disposal of animal waste

An aspect of good management which is worthy of discussion on its own merit is the

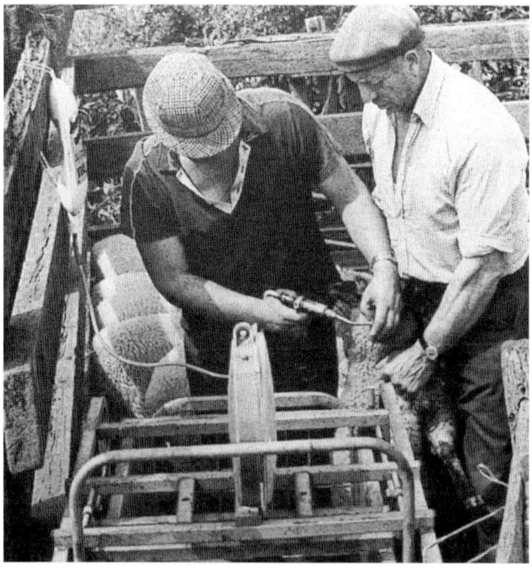

**Fig. 7.5** Efficient restraint of animal is necessary for proper use of drenching guns.

correct and safe disposal of animal waste. Incorrect disposal of farm animal excreta can present a potential hazard to public health, animal health and the environment. In recent years the quantity of slurry in particular produced by intensive systems of agriculture has become, in some cases, the limiting factor to the further expansion of production. This is particularly so with the pig industry in the Netherlands, where it has been suggested that the country is in danger of disappearing beneath a sea of slurry.

Table 7.1 gives figures for the quantities of slurry produced by livestock.

Slurry may be applied to the pasture or arable ground by tanker spreader (Fig. 7.6), rain gun or injection (Fig. 7.7). The production of aerosols by the first two of these methods has been demonstrated as spreading bacteria in a high concentration for at least 5 miles (Jones, 1980). For this reason, as well as for reasons of odour control and contamination of rivers by surface run-off, slurry injection must be the method of choice for application.

The survival of potentially pathogenic microorganisms in farmyard manure or slurry is dependent on several factors including the following:

1 *The microorganism* Some strains or serotypes of a microorganism, e.g. salmonellas, survive longer in the environment than others. Some can assume resistant forms which may survive for several years, e.g. anthrax.
2 *pH* The pH of fresh slurry and farmyard manure varies from 6.2 to 8.0 depending upon the species of origin and the constituents. In the case of slurry, the pH drops to below 6.5 within the first 4 weeks of storage and then

**Table 7.1** Quantities of excreta, as slurry, produced by livestock.

| Type of livestock | Output of livestock (faeces and urine) |
|---|---|
| Dairy cow | 41 kg/day |
| Pigs (fatteners) | 4.5 kg/day* |
| Poultry (1000 laying hens) | 800 kg/week |

*Pigs fed dry. Use of swill or whey may increase this to 14–17 kg/day.

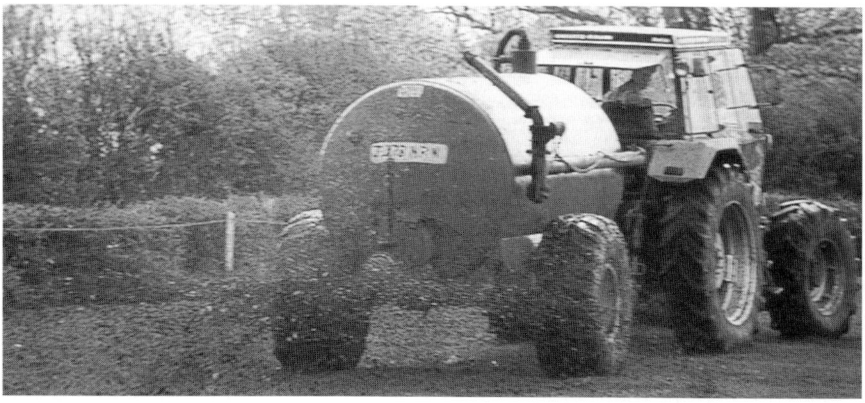

**Fig. 7.6** Application of slurry by tanker spreader. (By courtesy of NW Water, UK)

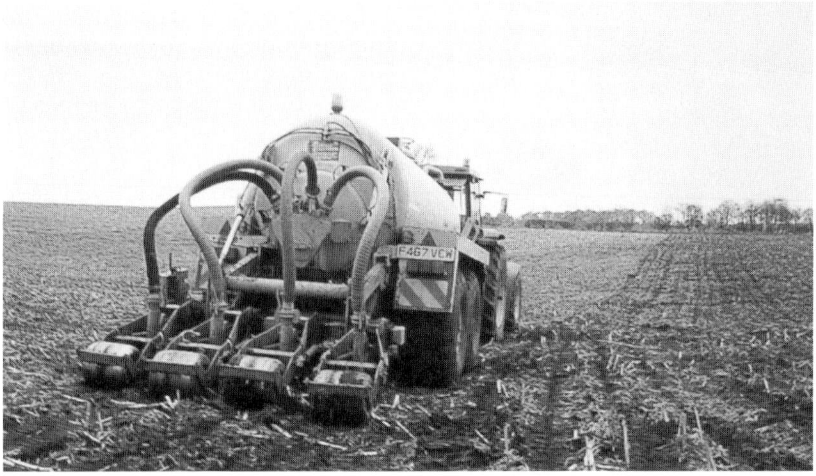


**Fig. 7.7** Slurry application by soil injection. (By courtesy of NW Water, UK)

gradually returns to zero. As a result, the majority of microorganisms, in the case of salmonella over 90%, are destroyed in the first month of storage. The low pH of peat and acid soils creates unfavourable conditions for the survival of many pathogens.
Attempts have been made to sterilise slurry by altering the pH. This has been achieved by the addition of lime, formalin, ammonium persulphate and formic acid, but the expense of the procedure makes these techniques suitable only for situations where there has been an outbreak of a serious disease.

3 *Sunlight* Ultraviolet light can have a bactericidal effect.
4 *Temperature* The rise in temperature which occurs during composting of farmyard manure is generally sufficient to destroy all bacterial and viral pathogens except for bacterial spores. However, since there is no discernible temperature increase within stored slurry, microbiological survival times are generally much longer.

The survival of pathogenic microorganisms in soil is in addition influenced by the initial number of organisms, the available moisture and the presence of competitive bacteria. On pasture, the length of grass is important, organisms surviving longer at the base of the grass than at the top of the leaf. Although salmonellas, for example, have been reported as surviving for many months in soil, it is unusual for them to survive for more than 14 days on grass (Findlay, 1972). *E. coli* have been shown to survive for more than 11 weeks in slurry but for only 7–8 days on the pasture (Rankin and Taylor, 1969).

Comparison of survival times for different organisms is difficult, however, owing to the number of variables to be considered and differences between experimental design and measurement technique.

Experiments have shown that under normal farming conditions infection of adult grazing animals from contaminated slurry on pasture is unlikely. However, if pasture which has been spread with fresh slurry is grazed within a few days by young or stressed susceptible animals, infection may occur.

On the basis of current knowledge the following recommendations can be made:

1 Slurry should be stored for at least 60 days prior to spreading on land.
2 Any disease hazard can be virtually eliminated by spreading slurry or farmyard manure on arable land or grassland used for conservation.
3 Pasture treated with slurry should not be grazed for at least 30 days after spreading.
4 Since young animals are generally more susceptible to disease, they should graze treated pasture only after a prolonged period following application.
5 Utilisation of slurry should be related to the plant nutrient requirements.
6 Slurry, manure and digested sewage sludge should be ploughed in *immediately after*

*application*. Slurry and raw liquid sludge can be injected to a depth of 50–80 mm in grooves 200–300 mm apart.

7 Ground treated with slurry/manure should preferably be ploughed immediately.

### *Sewage sludge*

The solid material in sewage sedimentation tanks is available for agricultural use in raw and dry digested forms. Raw sludge contains potentially harmful bacteria and, on occasions, the eggs of tapeworms such as *Taenia saginata*. In addition, sludge can contain many undesirable heavy metals such as cadmium.

In Great Britain the application of wastes from off-farm sources on agricultural land is controlled by the Control of Pollution (Silage, Slurry and Agricultural Fuel Oil) Regulations 1991, the Collection and Disposal of Waste Regulations 1988, which allow their use, without licensing, providing they fertilise, or otherwise benefit, the land. The use of sludge is governed by the Sludge (Use in Agriculture) Regulations 1989. The aim of these regulations is to prevent the build-up of potentially toxic substances in the soil, the contamination of watercourses, the spread of disease and the creation of noxious odours.

Despite these regulations and associated Codes of Practice, pollution of watercourses is a regular occurrence, as is the stocking of land with farm animals, especially cattle and sheep, after organic wastes have been applied.

## Animal welfare on the farm

Within the United Kingdom, Codes of Recommendations for the Welfare of Livestock have been produced under the provision of the Agriculture (Miscellaneous Provisions) Act 1968 in Great Britain, and the Welfare of Animals (Northern Ireland) Act 1972 for Northern Ireland. There are now codes available for cattle, sheep, pigs, deer, poultry, turkeys and ducks and these are designed to encourage good stockmanship, particularly in young and inexperienced workers.

All the codes are based on the five 'freedoms' or basic animal needs:

1. Freedom from thirst, hunger and malnutrition.
2. Appropriate comfort and shelter.
3. The prevention, or rapid diagnosis and treatment of, injury, disease or infestation.
4. Freedom from fear and distress.
5. Freedom to display most normal patterns of behaviour.

Some intensive systems of agriculture make the attainment of these goals impossible in the short term, but national and European regulations on animal welfare are gradually moving to make them a legal requirement. The banning of all dry sow stall and tethering systems, which restrict the 'freedom to display most normal patterns of behaviour' by January 1999 in the UK was a move in this direction. However, many pig farmers suggest that keeping sows in groups may, in fact, be more stressful on the animals than a stall system by introducing the animals to a competitive environment, the possibility of bullying and fighting, and an introduction, therefore, of '*fear*'. It should be possible, however, to measure up any husbandry system against the principles expressed in the five basic needs. Any animal housing system, for example, should provide the following:

1. Readily accessible fresh water, and nutritionally adequate food as required.
2. Adequate ventilation, to control humidity, irritant gas concentrations and dust, and a suitable environmental temperature. (In controlled-environment houses, e.g. broiler and intensive pig houses, there must be a warning system for electrical failure and a back-up system.)
3. Sufficient light for inspection purposes. Pigs should not be kept in permanent darkness.
4. A dry lying area.
5. A flooring, whether slats or solid, which neither harms the animal or causes undue strain, injury or distress.
6. The correct stocking density. Both overcrowding and understocking can cause problems.
7. Internal surfaces and fittings of buildings and pens with no sharp edges or projections.
8. Internal surfaces of housing and pens which can be cleaned and disinfected effectively.

Intensive methods of husbandry, which involve automatic feeding systems, and slatted houses which require little daily cleaning, greatly reduce contact between people and the animal. This increases the stress on the animal when it has to be handled for marketing, loading and transported. Hauliers report that pigs collected for slaughter from some large birth-to-bacon units are much more difficult to drive and load than those from finisher units where the pigs will have changed premises one or more times. Thought should be given to enriching the pigs' environment by introducing toys, such as rubber balls or chains, or walking through the pens regularly to increase their contact with humans. It has been suggested that leaving a radio on in a pig-finishing house accustoms the animals to human voices and makes them easier to handle.

## TRANSPORTATION OF LIVESTOCK

Having produced healthy livestock in good conditions, and as clean as possible, it is necessary to keep them free from contamination during the subsequent movement to the point of slaughter. It is of equal importance that they be kept free from injury, stress, loss of weight and disease during the journey. For all these reasons it is essential that *livestock be slaughtered as close as possible to the point of production* in order to avoid long journeys. The humanitarian aspects of the transportation of animals are intimately linked with the economic ones and these are of particular consequence in the case of young stock, pregnant stock and casualty animals. Work by Warriss and Bevis (1986) and Warriss *et al.* (1990) in the south of England showed that the average lamb, at two meat plants, spent over 4½ hours in transit and travelled a distance of more than 200 km. Within the UK, Warriss *et al.* (1990) estimated that 94% of slaughtered sheep spend less than 10 hours in transit. A survey conducted in 1985 found that although three-quarters of all pigs were killed within 10 hrs of leaving the farm, over 22% were killed after 8 hours and some not for 32 hours.

### **Loading and unloading** (Fig. 7.8)

Loading and unloading are often the most stressful parts of the transport process, for both animals and handlers. It is imperative that proper thought and planning be given to the procedure before commencing, to avoid the need to use excessive force. For pigs in

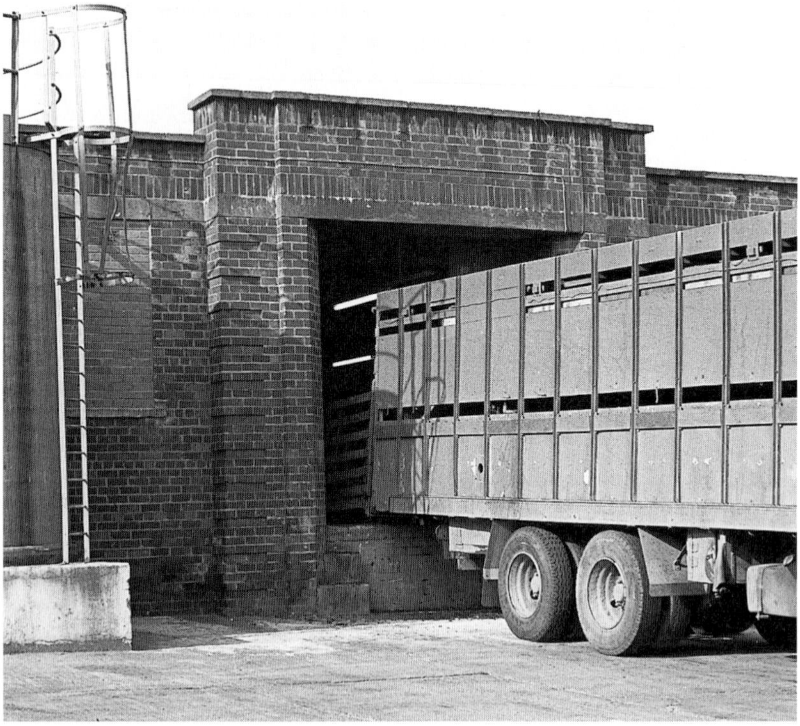

**Fig. 7.8** Excellent floor-level offloading facilities at Dutch pig abattoir.

particular, a proper loading ramp, especially if a lorry is being used, is essential. However, very steep ramps are undesirable because they distress the pigs, may lead to injuries through falling, and by increasing the need for coercion tend to encourage the use of unacceptable force or electric goads.

Work carried out by Warriss *et al.* (1991), indicates that *ramp angles* up to 20° appear to present few problems to pigs whether ascending or descending. Above 20° there is a progressive increase in the time, and thus, by inference, the difficulty with which the ramps are negotiated. Slopes of 30° and above are, from a subjective point of view, obviously difficult for some individuals to ascend and, particularly, to descend. The specification of the Transit of Animals (Road and Rail Order) 1975 (discussed later) that external loading ramp gradients should be no steeper than 30° would seem to be a reasonable maximum, but the specification for internal ramps of 34° may be too steep. When steep ramps are used, the spacing of the cleats may become critical. If it is too wide the ability of the pigs to ascend may be particularly impaired. Philips *et al.* (1988) suggested that a ramp sloped at 20–24° with cleats of 10–40 mm, spaced at a distance of 50–100 mm, was a feasible design.

Lapworth (1990) describes minimum design standards applicable to cattle loading and unloading facilities in Australia. He recommends that ramp floors should be stepped or cleated. Stepped floors should be of concrete with 100 mm rises and 500 mm treads. Cleats on wooden or concrete floors should be 50 mm wide, 50 mm high and 300 mm apart. A maximum slope of 20° is again recommended.

## The journey to slaughter

The personnel responsible for the road transport of livestock have a duty to ensure that the journey is made in a careful manner, avoiding sudden stops and starts, fast cornering and unnecessary delays. Due consideration should be given to all animals conveyed, irrespective of species.

Some transporters have attempted to reduce one of the stressors on *pigs* during transport by providing them with water. The water is provided from an 80-gallon water tank and supplied to the pigs via a pipeline and spring-loaded bite drinkers at 2-foot intervals on each deck. The pipelines are rotated manually by a lockable lever at the rear of the vehicle, allowing nipples to be stowed out of harm's way in a vertical position during travel. Some lorries have also been fitted with cooling sprinklers. Much research is still required to establish categorically basic information, for example, whether different species lie or stand during transport and where and how they prefer to position themselves in the vehicle at different stocking densities. Warriss (1995) suggests a stocking density for pigs during transport of 0.45 $m^2$/100 kg. This provides a slightly greater area than that required for sternal recumbency and will thus ensure enough space for all animals to rest and not become fatigued. Pigs prefer to lie down in transit.

## Transport legislation

Most countries have detailed regulations for the humane transport of animals and in Great Britain a series of orders dating back to the beginning of the century deals with animals being conveyed by road, rail, air or sea. The International Air Transport Association has drawn up a manual which sets standards in this sector and is mandatory and binding on all IATA members – the IATA Live Animals Regulations. The UK Protection of Animals Act, 1911, made it 'an offence of cruelty to convey or carry, or cause or procure, or, being the owner, permit to be conveyed or carried, any animal in such manner or position as to cause that animal any unnecessary suffering'.

Under the Animal Health Act 1981 (Section 37) power is given to make orders relating to the welfare of animals including poultry during transport within, into and out of Great Britain. The main regulations currently in force are:

- Welfare of Animals during Transport Order, 1994 (with amendments)
- Transit of Animals (Road and Rail) Order, 1975 (amended 1988; 1992)
- Welfare of Poultry (Transport) Order, 1988
- The Transport of Animals (General) Order, 1973
- Transit of Animals Order, 1927
- Animals (Sea Transport) Order, 1930
- Horses (Sea Transport) Order, 1952.

*Welfare of Animals during Transport Order, 1994 (with amendments)*

This Order, taken with the other legislation listed, implements Council Directive 91/628/EEC, supplemented by 95/29/EC, on the protection of animals during transport. This legislation applies only to animals transported for distances greater than 50 km and covers those individuals or businesses who transport animals themselves or for a third party, or provide a third party with the means of transport. Non-commercial journeys, journeys with individual animals, and journeys with pet animals when the pet is carried by its owner on a private journey are all exempt from this legislation. General provisions are made for the welfare of animals during transport, loading and unloading, providing protection against exposure to inclement weather and for preventing the transport of an unfit animal. An *unfit animal* is defined as one which is newborn, diseased, injured or fatigued, or has given birth within the preceding 48 hours or is likely to give birth during transport, or for any other reason.

A requirement to unload the animals, and to provide water, food and rest for 24 hours at suitable intervals during the journey is included. For cattle, sheep, goats, pigs and horses the *interval* must not exceed 8 hours, but if the vehicle being used to transport the animals meets certain specified high standards, travelling times may be extended:

- Calves, lambs, kids, foals and piglets may travel for 9 hours before a minimum rest period of 1 hour, followed by a further maximum of 9 hours travel.
- Adult cattle, sheep and goats may travel for 14 hours before a minimum rest period of 1 hour, followed by a further maximum of 14 hours travel.
- Pigs may travel for a maximum of 24 hours, provided that they have continuous access to water during the journey.
- Horses may travel up to 24 hours, provided that they are given liquid and if necessary food every 8 hours.

For journeys undertaken by cattle, sheep, goats and pigs to or from another Member State or third country *where the journey time exceeds 8 hours*, the person in charge of the animal transport must draw up a *journey plan*. This plan must indicate the arrangements for the resting, feeding and watering as outlined above for the various species, and include a strategy for feeding and watering in the event that the planned journey be changed or disrupted. The plan, following approval and stamping, accompanies the consignment. Although these plans are laudable in theory, hearsay evidence suggests that the good intentions contained within this provision are difficult to police and, to date, are widely flaunted.

An interesting development is the imposition of a legal responsibility on the person in charge of any animal transport undertaking which transports animals in the course of a business or trade, to ensure that the animals are entrusted only to persons possessing the knowledge necessary to administer appropriate care to the animals in transport.

*Transit of Animals (Road and Rail) Order, 1975 (amended 1988; 1992)*

This is a comprehensive Order which legislates for the welfare of animals being transported within Great Britain.

*Schedule 1* outlines *general provisions for road and rail vehicles and receptacles*. Road vehicles must be of a durable construction with rigid sides and overhead protection. The interior should be free from any sharp edges or projections which are likely to cause injury or unnecessary suffering to the animal. There must be sufficient distance between each floor and the next floor or the roof to enable each animal to stand in its natural position. *Non-slip surfaces* must be provided and, if necessary, sand or other similar substances must be provided. For calves, i.e. cattle under 6 months of age, and pigs, the floor must be covered with an adequate quantity of bedding. *Internal ramps* (not steeper than 34°) or mechanical lifting gear must be provided to facilitate movement of animals from one floor to another.

If necessary, substantial *partitions* must be used to ensure that the animals are not thrown about during carriage by motion of the vehicle. However, it is the duty of the person in charge of the animals to ensure that the animals are not so overcrowded that injury or unnecessary suffering is caused. Partitions must be 1.27 m high for cattle, other than calves, and horses, and 76 cm for calves, sheep, pigs and goats. The pens must not be more than 2.5 m long for calves, 3.1 m for sheep, pigs and goats, and 3.7 m for horses. If the pen is more than 3.7 m long for cattle, the operator must ensure that the cattle are not injured or caused unnecessary suffering by being thrown about by the motion of the vehicle.

The design and construction of the vehicle must enable the vehicle and its occupants to be inspected. This will require an adequate number of inspection doors and hatches, and adequate light.

Figure 7.9 shows a modern design which caters fully for animal welfare.

Animals must be loaded or unloaded with a ramp, loading bridge or bank, mechanical lifting gear, manual lifting or carrying, except where the distance from the ground to the vehicle is not more than 31 cm. Every ramp which is carried on, or forms part of the vehicle and which is used for loading or unloading animals, must be fitted with treads or other means of providing a foothold to any animals. The gradient of the ramp when in use must not be steeper than 4 in 7 or > 30° when the vehicle is on level ground. The step at the top of the ramp must not exceed 21 cm in height and any gap between the top of the ramp and the vehicle must not exceed 6 cm in width. Barriers, or straps for horses, must be provided to prevent any animal from falling out of the vehicle when the ramp used for unloading is in the lowered position. Protection on each side of the ramp to a height of not less than 1.3 m must be provided and fitted to ensure that any gaps between the side protection, the ramp and the vehicle will not result in injury.

*Schedule 2* deals with the *separation of animals during transport*. The following animals must not be carried in the same undivided vehicle, receptacle or pen as any other animals: a cow with suckling calf or calves; a bull over 10 months of age (except for bulls reared together); a sow and piglets; a boar over 6 months of age; a mare with foal at foot; a stallion. There is a long list of stock which may be carried together in the same undivided vehicle but separately from other animals: horned cattle, polled cattle, calves, bulls reared together, ewes with unweaned lambs, rams over 6 months of age, unbroken horses, etc.

*Schedule 3* concerns *cleansing* and *disinfection*, which must be carried out as soon as practicable after unloading and before any animals or items intended to be used in connection with an animal is loaded into the vehicle. This does not apply where a vehicle is used exclusively, in the course of a single day, for the carriage of animals between the same two points, other than between two markets, provided that the vehicle and its accessories are cleansed and disinfected as soon as practicable after the last journey on which an animal is carried on a particular day.

Powers are given to an inspector to serve notice on owners of vehicles not complying with cleansing and disinfection requirements; if the owners then fail to cleanse and disinfect their vehicles at their own expense, the local authority may carry out the work and recover the cost as a civil debt.

*Welfare of Poultry (Transport) Order, 1988 (amended 1989; 1992)*

*Poultry* includes live birds of the following species: domestic fowls, turkeys, geese, ducks, guinea fowls, pheasants, partridges and quails.

*The Transport of Animals (General) Order, 1973 (amended 1988; 1992)*

This order covers all mammals, except man, and any bird or four-footed beast which is not a mammal, and all fish, reptiles, crustaceans and other cold-blooded creatures of any species except domestic fowls, turkeys, geese, ducks, guinea fowls, pheasants, partridges and quails.

The Order contains a number of general measures that are intended to safeguard the welfare of a wide variety of animals during their carriage by sea, air, road and rail. In relation to carriage by sea or air, the provisions of the Order apply to animals carried on any vessel or aircraft to or from a port or airport in Great Britain whether or not such animals are loaded or unloaded at such port or airport. It is a duty of the owner or charterer of a vessel and of the operator of an aircraft in which animals are being carried by sea or air, and of the carrier or other person in charge of animals being carried by road or rail, to ensure that the animals are:

- fed and watered during the journey and the period of loading and unloading;
- contained in a receptacle which is properly constructed, not overcrowded or liable to

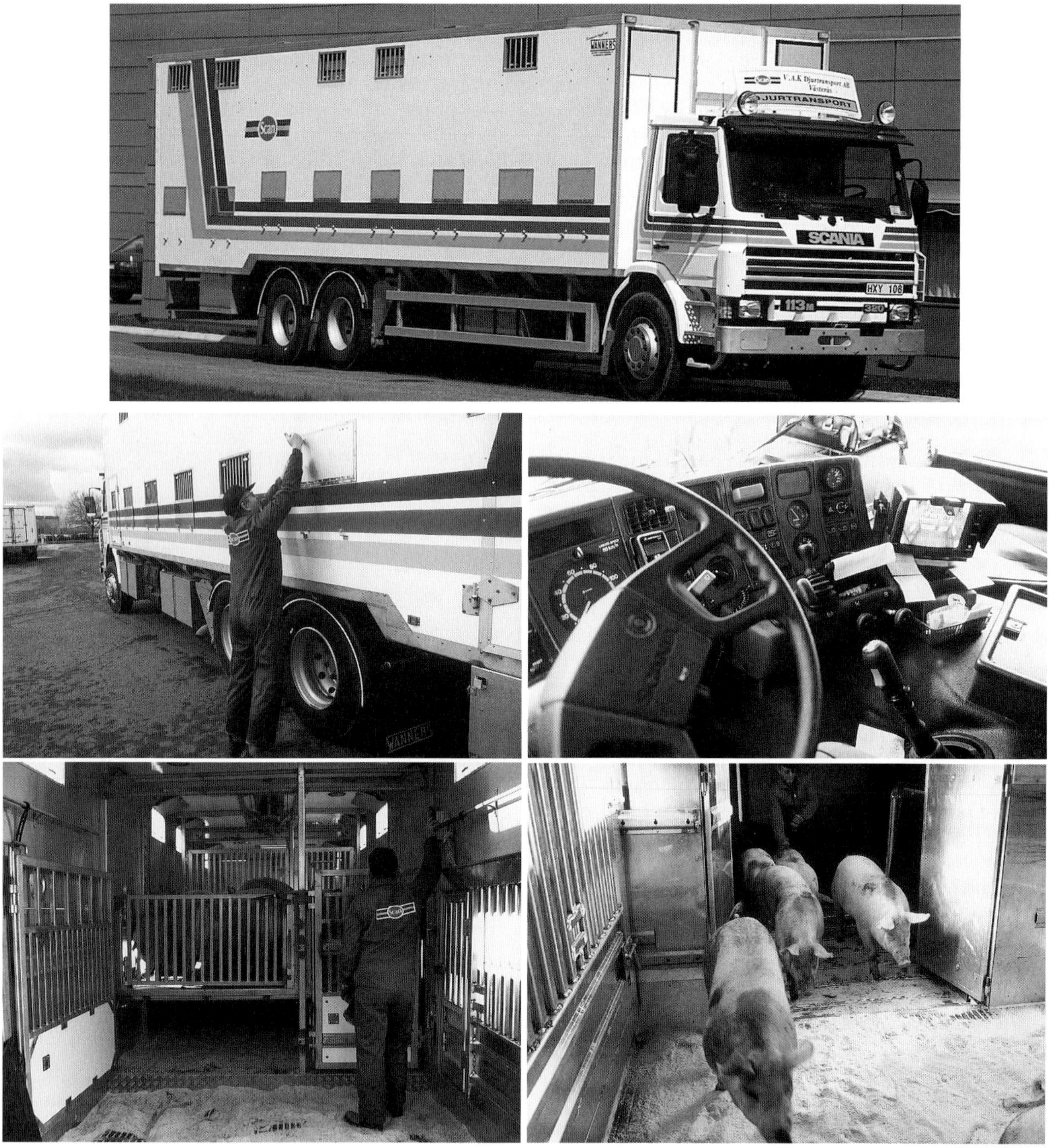

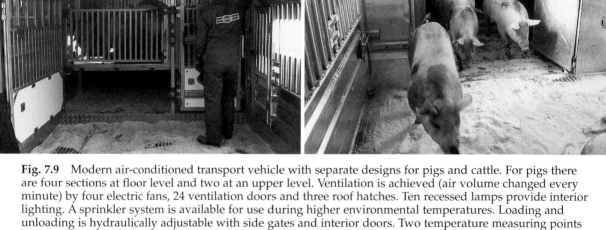


**Fig. 7.9** Modern air-conditioned transport vehicle with separate designs for pigs and cattle. For pigs there are four sections at floor level and two at an upper level. Ventilation is achieved (air volume changed every minute) by four electric fans, 24 ventilation doors and three roof hatches. Ten recessed lamps provide interior lighting. A sprinkler system is available for use during higher environmental temperatures. Loading and unloading is hydraulically adjustable with side gates and interior doors. Two temperature measuring points are located in the vehicle and one in the cab where continuous visual monitoring of the animals during transit is possible. The vehicle is equipped with air suspension on all axles for maximum transport comfort. (By courtesy of Scan Farmek S-532 87, Skara, Sweden)

cause injury or suffering, and must be properly labelled to indicate the species of animal contained therein and the upright position of the receptacle;

- are accommodated in such a way as to avoid any risk of unnecessary suffering, and are not carried in the proximity of any goods the presence of which is likely to prejudice their welfare;
- humanely slaughtered in a manner appropriate to the species if seriously injured, unless the animal can be kept alive and landed from a ship or aircraft without cruelty or receive veterinary treatment without delay.

*Transit of Animals Order, 1927*

This Order covers cattle, sheep, goats, and all other ruminating animals and swine that are carried on vessels, between ports in Great Britain and between ports in Great Britain and Ireland. It contains the structural requirements for penning the animals on deck, for securing receptacles, and welfare conditions to avoid injury or distress to the animals. The requirements for experienced staff, handling of injured animals and cleansing and disinfection are also included.

*Animals (Sea Transport) Order, 1930*

This Order deals with the same areas as the Transit of Animals Order, 1927, described above, but for all other animals.

*Horses (Sea Transport) Order, 1952*

This Order covers specific structural and welfare requirements for horses, including donkeys, mules and jennets, travelling by sea. Food and water must be provided to a horse where a voyage, on average, takes more than 6 hours.

The above regulations, while very comprehensive, require the close cooperation of stock owners, hauliers, attendants and inspectors if satisfactory conditions of animal cleanliness and welfare are to result. A major difficulty concerns their enforcement, which is frequently difficult and not always possible during the hurly-burly of transport, marketing, delivery to meat plants, etc. The legislation is very properly directed towards the prevention of injury, disease and unnecessary suffering, although this is not always achieved. In order to make for better animal cleanliness, it is considered that cleansing and disinfection requirements should be more stringently enforced. There is a need for more thought to be given to the provision of *sumps for liquid manure* and the *sealing of upper floors* in multitiered vehicles, since considerable faecal contamination arises from these sources, leakage occurring through pervious floors. The carriage of sheep on open lorry decks inevitably leads to wet sheep during inclement weather, with consequent problems at slaughter and carcase dressing even if animals are held in lairages for drying out. From an animal welfare standpoint the practice is a questionable one, especially during wet and cold weather when some of the insulating effect of wool is lost.

## Loss of weight during transport

All animals transported to slaughter will suffer some loss of liveweight during the journey. This loss is greater than that which would be lost solely by fasting for a similar period and is due mainly to a loss of water by sweating and respiration, and waste materials in the urine and faeces. The factors affecting this loss are bodily condition, state of repletion, season and journey time. Pigs will lose 2.2–5.4 kg of their liveweight during 24 hours transport; sheep lose 0.9–1.8 kg if kept in a lairage for 24 hours and up to 3.6 kg during transport; a calf of 149.6 kg liveweight loses 4 kg during its first day of travel and 1.8 kg on the second day; a bullock weighing 610 kg will lose 30–40 kg during the first day of travel but only 5–6 kg on subsequent days. Studies indicate that it takes 5 days for cattle to recover this loss.

Studies in New Zealand indicate that in lambs the loss in carcase weight over the first 24 hours in transit is small. However, if the period without food extends beyond 24 hours, the loss of carcase weight becomes significant, amounting to approximately 0.5 kg per animal per day.

Two loads totalling 500 lambs purchased at markets in the UK and transported to southern France, a journey taking 18 and 24 hours, lost 7–8% of liveweight. Much of this was regained in 24 hours, with complete recovery of liveweight and liver glycogen in 96 hours. The behaviour of the lambs indicated that they were alert and physically fit. They were primarily interested in any food that was available upon arrival, and were secondarily interested in drinking, then resting.

Of much greater importance, though difficult to quantify, is the actual loss of flesh during transport. With bacon pigs, the loss in actual carcase weight is about 0.9 kg for every day of their journey, and it is probable that both muscular and fatty tissues are affected, with an abnormal loss of water from the muscular tissues. The effect of overexertion, excitement and strange surroundings on pigs during transit may also cause a loss of 6–7% in the weight of the liver.

The amount of weight loss in pigs is increased with an increase in temperature and decrease in relative humidity. When Large White pigs were sprayed with fine sprays of cold water in an uncovered lorry which travelled 80 km, the weight loss was reduced by 50%. Pigs also lose weight when transported during very cold weather. Relative humidity and temperature also appear to be involved in the development of DFD (dark, firm and dry) meat in cattle, the incidence of which, at least in Britain, seems to be greatest during cold, muggy days of November.

In the United States cattle transported by rail are stated to lose 1.48% of carcase weight on journeys of up to 161 km and 2.1% on journeys of 402–482 km. Tissue shrinkage begins during the early part of a journey, continues at a relatively uniform rate for 90 hours, then tends to diminish. Some shrinkage occurs even if animals receive food and water during transport, but is less if these are provided during long journeys. In the past, cattle from the northern parts of Australia lost so much weight on their long overland trek to the slaughterhouses that they were placed on pastures for up to a year to regain the weight and quality needed to meet export demands.

From work in Australia, Thompson *et al.* (1987) report that in a 35 kg lamb of fat score 3, the losses of hot carcase weight were in the order of 4% and 6% after 24 and 48 hours fasting, respectively, compared to mean losses in 27–32 kg lambs of 2% and 4%.

In relation to *weight loss* suffered during transit, it is possible in many cases to restore some, if not all, of this loss with adequate rest. Cattle transported by rail for 136 km in Zimbabwe and sustaining a total liveweight loss of 12.88% (1.7% tissue loss) regained much of the tissue loss in 24 hours after resting and drinking water, but not eating. Even after rail transport for 4 days in South Africa during mid-summer, cattle recovered rapidly if rested with food and water. In the same country the resting of adult Merino sheep for 24 hours with feed and water after rail transport for more than 3 days had a beneficial effect on carcase yield. Much of the weight loss in pigs during transport is believed to be due to loss of water, so that it is important for these animals to have access to water before and after transport. However, it has been shown in Poland that resting pigs for 24 hours after transport does not help them to recover unless they are fed, and even feeding restores the condition of the muscles and liver but not the loss of carcase weight.

In the case of *farmed deer* it was found that after a journey of 160 km lasting 3 hours, a group of 5 hinds lost 1.09% of their pre-transport weight when weighed within 90 minutes of slaughter. Three similar groups held in a lairage with *ad libitum* food and water for 3, 6 and 18 hours lost 1.93%, 3.19% and 6.22% of their body weight, respectively. Although liveweight loss increased with lairage time, hot carcase weight was unaffected (Grigor *et al.*, 1997).

### Transport mortality

Death during transport, although objective, is, however, a measurement indicating a severe level of distress in transit. A mortality rate above zero must therefore always be considered unacceptable from a welfare perspective. All those involved in the transport of animals must strive to achieve this ideal goal, especially faced with increased consumer awareness of the ethics of food, animal production and transport.

Deaths occur in all classes of livestock during transportation, although in most countries the incidence is less than 0.5%. In a survey of mortality rates in 2.9 million slaughter pigs throughout England, Warriss and Brown (1994) indicated that 0.061% died during transit, while 0.011% died in the lairage. A study of 136 322 pigs in England by Abbott *et al.* (1995) found a death rate during transport of 0.11%. These figures are very similar to those reported in the 1970s by Smith and Allen (1976), suggesting that the position has remained fairly stable over the last 20 years. Figures of mortality rates across Europe, with details of stocking densities, are recorded in Table 7.2. The mortality rate among slaughter sheep transported within the UK was estimated at 0.018% (Knowles *et al.*, 1994).

Extremes of *temperature*, especially heat, can be responsible for many losses in livestock, particularly pigs. More animals die when it is hotter, particularly above 16°C (Allen and Smith, 1974), and when animals are left in a stationary vehicle. It has been noted that in summer, pigs transported in the early morning fare better than those transported in the afternoon. Stress-susceptible strains are much more likely to die and differences in genotype explain much of the variation in mortality recorded in different European countries (Table 7.2). Selection against the halothane gene in Swedish Landrace and Large White breeds was associated with a reduction in mortality in transport and lairage from 0.22% in 1982 to 0.08% in 1987 (Petersson and Gahne, 1988).

The National Livestock Safety Committee of the US Livestock Conservation Inc. has developed a *livestock weather safety index chart* which, in relation to current temperature and *relative humidity*, indicates in hot weather how safe stock in transit may be. They have also devised for low-temperature conditions a *wind chill chart* giving the relationship between actual temperatures and the wind speed, which is particularly important if animals are not sufficiently protected in moving vehicles.

The *post-mortem findings* in *pigs which have died in transit* are usually those of acute cardiac dilation and acute pulmonary hyperaemia. The left ventricle of the heart is no longer conical but more oval, while the papillary muscles and muscular ridges, normally apparent on the endocardium as prominent projections, are much flattened. Pericardial fluid is increased and there is, in severe cases, a diffuse skeletal muscle degeneration. The lungs are heavy and firmer than normal, finger impressions remain on palpation, and a frothy fluid oozes from the cut surface. Acute passive hyperaemia of the liver and spleen may be observed.

**Table 7.2** Pig type, stocking density and mortality during transit in some European countries.

| Country | Pig type* | Stocking density ($m^2$/100 kg) | % Mortality |
|---|---|---|---|
| Denmark | SR | 0.35 | 0.03 |
| UK | SR | 0.37–0.49 | 0.07 |
| Italy | SR | 0.37–0.40 | 0.10 |
| Netherlands | SR | 0.32–0.35 | 0.16 |
| Portugal | Mixed | 0.36–0.38 | 0.16 |
| Belgium | SS | 0.38–0.39 | 0.30 |
| Germany | SS | 0.36–0.49 | 0.50 |

*SR, pig population mainly stress resistant. SS, pig population mainly stress susceptible. Mixed, a range of SR and SS types.

## Conditions induced by transport

*Transit* or *shipping fever* is a catarrhal and often fatal disease which chiefly affects store cattle in poor condition that have become fatigued by a long journey by rail or sea without sufficient food, particularly during the cooler months. It is responsible for severe losses in Canada and the mid-western states of the United States but has also been reported in Europe and Asia. The 'disease' probably consists of a number of related conditions of the respiratory tract in which viruses and bacteria play important roles. Current theories suggest that various biotypes of *Pasteurella haemolytica* are the final cause of the pneumonia but that other pathogens such as viruses and *mycoplasma* may act synergistically to allow the bacteria to become pathogenic.

The *clinical signs* are of an acute, toxaemic bronchopneumonia with a high fever, and a good response to treatment in the early stages. Depression and anorexia are common. Post-mortem lesions are those of consolidated lungs with accumulation of serofibrinous exudate in the interlobular spaces. A catarrhal bronchitis and bronchiolitis and a serofibrinous pleurisy are usually present and may be accompanied by a fibrinous pericarditis. The bronchi may contain fibrin, mucus, blood clots and pus. In chronic cases there are residual lesions of bronchopneumonia with overlying pleural adhesions.

*Transit tetany* occurs under similar circumstances, almost invariably in cows, particularly those in advanced pregnancy and in the warmer months of the year. The disease has also been reported in pregnant ewes and associated with hypocalcaemia and in feedlot lambs. Of 1625 pregnant ewes transported 456 km by road in the United States, 41 died during transport and a further 41 over 4 days following transit. The disease bears a resemblance to milk fever and affected animals usually respond to calcium therapy. There are no specific post-mortem lesions.

*Salmonellosis* in young animals, especially calves and lambs, may be precipitated by transport stress, and compounded by lack of food and water and by chilling. The transportation of young calves from one part of the country to another, exhaustion, dietary changes and chilling on the journey may increase their susceptibility to infection and allow a latent *Salmonella* infection to assume an acute and septicaemic form. Other predisposing factors include intensive rearing and finishing systems, poor cleansing and disinfection of transport vehicles, and poor vehicle design.

It has been found that there is a marked increase in the excretion of salmonellae by pigs and poultry after transport, which is attributed to the rapid passage of faecal matter in response to transport stress and to weakening of the defence mechanisms of the animals. The increase in the numbers of salmonellae isolated with the distance from farm to slaughterhall floor is occasioned by a combination of stress, lack of hygiene and crowding in vehicles, markets and lairages. In Israel in 1970 it was found that of 17 *Salmonella* serotypes isolated from poultry after transport, six were the most prevalent in man at that time. *The transport of animals, therefore, has an important connection with public as well as animal health.*

## LAIRAGE CONSTRUCTION

During the rest period in lairages, animals must be kept under conditions which prevent any further contamination of feet, hides, fleeces or skins. Most lairages have solid non-slip floors, suitably sloped to adequate drains. Slatted floors have also been considered for cattle but, while contamination is reduced in most cases, there are problems in manure removal and disinfection, for example, after outbreaks of anthrax and salmonellosis, or where tuberculosis or brucellosis reactors are routinely slaughtered.

Movable slats, and especially expanded-metal floors, are particularly useful for sheep, where circulation of air below the floor can be useful for drying wet fleeces. Straw-bedded pens also provide a satisfactory environment for sheep, as long as there is good ventilation and drainage, while solid floors with no bedding, combined with regular hosing and good drainage, provide satisfactory conditions for cattle and pigs. Adequate hose points conveniently placed and providing sufficient volume and pressure of water are absolutely essential. So also are hoses with nozzles giving a fishtail spray which can quickly remove soil. The provision of pens with gates which can be used for closing pens and passageways assists the handling of stock and their transfer from one pen to another, thereby facilitating the cleansing operation.

The detail of design of animal walkways and races is important if animals are to move easily through the lairage. The positioning of a drainage gully in the middle of a walkway frequently causes animals to baulk, as do harsh shadows, puddles of water or shafts of light. It is well established that, owing to their natural curiosity, animals move more readily along curved rather than straight passageways, and that sharp corners slow movement considerably. A bend in a raceway of 45° slowed the progress of pigs by about 10%; a bend of 90° or 120° slowed progress by 19%; and a 180° bend slowed their progress by 44% (Warriss *et al.*, 1992a).

Pigs rest more contentedly if they can lie against a solid wall rather than rails, and there is less fighting if they are confined to long narrow pens rather than square ones. Either rails or walls are satisfactory for cattle and sheep. With walls it is possible to wash out a pen without causing stress, by splash and noise, to animals in neighbouring pens. However, animals are much easier to inspect in railed pens, unless an overhead catwalk is provided. Vertical supports should be cylindrical and tubular to reduce the possibility of injury, and the tops capped to allow effective cleansing and disinfection to be carried out. Horizontal rails should also be cylindrical and tubular, as they are easier to clean effectively with a pressure washer than rails of tubular box cross-section.

In Denmark, the development of *automatic systems* to move pigs through the lairage in groups has improved both the welfare of the animals and the efficiency with which the facility operates. The push gates move the pigs in groups of 15 along the passageways at a steady pace from the loading to a holding position. Pigs rest within 20 minutes, contrasted with an hour under normal lairage conditions; and aggression is much reduced (Fig. 7.10)

Facilities should be checked to ensure there are no defects which could cause bruising or even death. Projections and sharp corners are taboo, and if rails are being used for pen partitions it is essential that there is no possibility of animals getting their heads between rails and being strangled; rail gaps must be of the proper width.

In some countries cattle are sprayed with jets of water and walked through foot baths before entering the slaughterhouse area. This practice is of benefit in warmer climates where the hair is short and the skin of cattle is fine, but where hair is long in housed stock and there is a build-up of manure and dirt on the hair, spraying would only serve to make matters worse. A light spraying of pigs is widely considered of value in preventing pigs fighting, and also reduces the build-up of contamination in the scald tank. However, research work has failed to demonstrate that the sprays actually reduce fighting and it has been suggested that the improvement in meat quality in sprayed pigs is due to a cooling effect, rather than a reduction in stress.

The removal of the wool from lambs prior to slaughter would help in the production of clean carcases. However, shearing remains a labour-intensive operation despite efforts to produce shearing robots. The use of chemical defleecing agents, e.g. hydrosulphide, which cause the partial or complete cessation of wool growth, so that it might be removed mechanically, has been an active area of research in Australia. Unfortunately, there is considerable variation in individual animals' response to the chemicals used.

Facilities in the lairage which are required for the carrying out of ante-mortem inspection effectively include:

1 a race, with a crush gate for cattle, where the animal can be identified;
2 an adequate number of well-lit pens, with a system for identification or numbering of pens; for inspection purposes, a light intensity of 220 lux is necessary;
3 an isolation pen, with facilities for examination of individual animals;
4 competent lairage staff to assist with the identification, movement and examination of animals; and

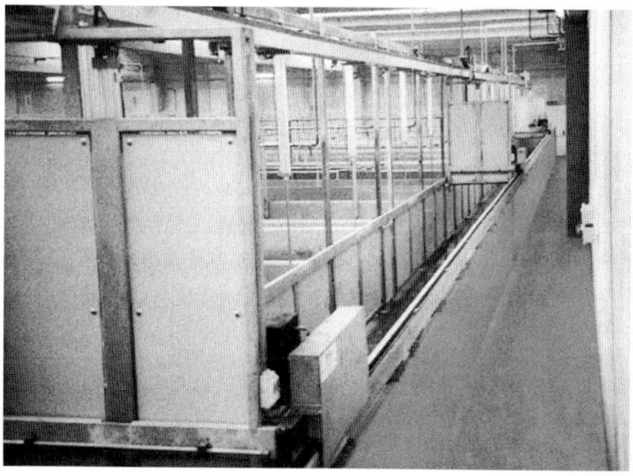

**Fig. 7.10** Automatic lairage system for pigs showing two elevated push gates.

5 an office for the use of the veterinarian is useful for the completion of records.

## ANIMAL HUSBANDRY IN THE LAIRAGE

### Moving animals within the lairage

The avoidance of stress in the animal in the period immediately prior to slaughter is important for economic reasons of meat quality as well as for animal welfare reasons. Animals must therefore be handled with consideration at all times with minimal use of force of any type. Electrical goads have been banned by management from many pig lairages and replaced with gentler driving aids such as solid push boards. The attitude of the lairage attendants can be all-important to the calm and efficient operation of the facility. Persons experienced in animal husbandry know instinctively where to stand when moving stock, and can carry out their task using only encouraging noises and the occasional tap or wave of a stick. Inexperienced operatives frequently excite, confuse and antagonise the animals, making handling at best difficult and at worst dangerous and impossible. The good stockman will automatically recognise the individual characteristics of an animal, and will adapt his or her technique to get the work completed in the least stressful way for both animal and handler.

Good abattoir management committed to high operating standards is essential if animal welfare in the lairage is to be maintained at an acceptable level.

A useful concept which can assist in training lairage staff is that of *'flight zones'*. Each animal can be considered to be surrounded by an imaginary zone or personal space which it will endeavour to maintain. In a semi-wild unhandled animal, such as a range steer, this area will be very large (e.g. > 30 m), while in a dairy cow it will be small. When the handler enters the 'flight zone' the animal will move away to try to re-establish the space between itself and the handler. The direction in which the animal moves depends on where, in relation to the animal, the handler enters the zone; for example, if he enters the zone at a point in front of the animal's shoulder the animal will move backwards, if behind the shoulder it will walk forward.

The movement of sheep through a lairage may be facilitated by the use of a decoy or 'Judas' sheep. This procedure utilises the innate tendency of sheep to follow one another by 'training' one particular sheep, or allowing it to become accustomed to, pass through the lairage leading the others. Use can be made of a mirror, strategically placed, to assist the movement of sheep out of a pen (Franklin and Hutson, 1982). It is particularly important when driving sheep to exercise patience and give them time to move at their own pace. Attempts to rush will result in those at the rear climbing over or riding on those in front, resulting in bruising.

Pigs can be particularly awkward to drive. They move only as a loose group, preferring to move along beside rather than behind their comrades. The maximum number of pigs which should be moved as a group is 15. This is also considered to be the ideal group size per pen at a stocking density of 0.55–0.67 $m^2$/100 kg.

Excessive or strident *noise* can be very stressful to livestock, especially pigs. Measurements indicate that noise levels average 75 dB in lairage pens, rising to 100 dB in the pre-stunning pen. This may arise from human voices, the use of whips, noisy machinery, barking dogs, compressed-air brakes on vehicles, alarm bells, thunder, etc. The manufacturers of meat plant equipment have a duty to ensure that equipment operates as quietly as possible, especially in the stunning area and its immediate surroundings. The provision of rubber baffles on doors and gates is essential.

Cattle are more sensitive to high-frequency sound than are human beings. The auditory sensitivity of cattle is at its greatest at 8000 Hz compared with 1000–3000 Hz in man. Unusual and especially intermittent sounds are upsetting to all classes of livestock. Sheep are visibly frightened by the sight and barking of dogs.

## Social stress

Mixing strange animals together may make them fight to establish a new social order; once this is achieved, fighting ceases. Animals may be mixed several times during the marketing process. Work carried out by Moss and Trimble (1988) in Northern Ireland showed that if cattle were mixed and were active, and their muscle glycogen was depleted, it took at least 2 days, in most cases 3, for this to be replaced.

Aggressive animals and females in oestrus must be isolated, as must horned from polled stock. Although young bulls reared in groups as bull beef may be penned together, breeding bulls and boars should always be penned separately. Larger animals will usually be aggressive to smaller ones. It is important to recognise, however, that both are stressed. This can be seen especially in young bulls which, if mixed in the lairage, can rapidly become exhausted through constant mounting. Mixing of young bulls is therefore contraindicated and they should be slaughtered as soon as possible after arrival in the lairage. It has been noted that if these animals remain in the lairage for only 2–3 hours they may produce dark cutting meat.

## Watering

Animals should receive ample drinking water during their retention in the lairage as this serves to lower the bacterial load in the intestine and facilitates removal of the hide or pelt during dressing of the carcase. Stunning of animals by electrical means is rendered more efficacious if they have received unlimited water during their detention prior to slaughter. The positioning and design of water troughs or drinkers is of particular importance in order that faecal contamination of the water is avoided. Self-filling bowls are generally more satisfactory than large concrete troughs for cattle, and drinkers recessed into the walls of the pens are preferred for pigs. Water nipples are not always readily used by pigs, and some protrude from the pen wall at a height which renders them a welfare hazard.

## Fasting

Among butchers throughout the world the practice of withholding food from animals prior to slaughter has long been observed, it being contended in support of this practice that fasted animals bleed better, that the carcase is easier to dress and that it has a brighter appearance. Scientific evidence for such assertions is lacking and the hungry animal does not settle as well as the animal that has been fed. It is also a known physiological fact that although cattle and sheep are better able to withstand cold than are the other farm animals, resistance to the shock of a severe fall in atmospheric temperature is greater in the fed animal than in one that has been starved.

However, there is a duty to ensure that animals are not presented for slaughter with full stomachs, to prevent carcase contamination due to accidental incision or rupture of the gastrointestinal tract during the dressing procedure. Guise *et al.* (1995) reported that the stomachs from pigs which had been fed 0.64 kg of dry matter and slaughtered 18.5 hours later had on average a wet stomach content of 0.87 kg (0.24–1.33), average dry matter 127.4 g ± 69.1 g.

The withholding of food must be closely considered in relation to the possible loss of body weight, remembering that the fasting period can be considered as beginning at the time the animals leave the farm. If they have been held at a market before consignment, the total period of time may be very long indeed, amounting to several hours, or even days in some countries. It is important to know, therefore, how long animals can be fasted before body weight losses commence and the extent of these losses.

Pigs rested for 24 hours after a journey do not regain normality unless they are fed. Indeed, the fatigue and restlessness engendered by hunger in pigs, in which a definite excitement pyrexia appears to occur in those animals not used to handling, may render the flesh unsuitable for preserved meat products. One authority records a loss of 7% in carcase weight and 30% in liver weight of pigs rested for 72 hours without feeding; feeding of milk and sugar reduced these losses to 3% and 8%, respectively. In sheep detained for 2, 3 or 4 days there is a significant loss in carcase weight and up to a 29% loss in weight of the liver; even 4 days resting and feeding is insufficient to reverse these effects. A series of experiments with lambs, bobby calves and adult cattle conducted in New Zealand, sheds further light on this subject indicating the following:

- Bobby calves were very susceptible to fasting losses, losing about 0.7 kg after one day's removal from their mothers, increasing to 1.8 kg after 3 days removal of food.
- The loss of liveweight in lambs varied from 0.14 kg in the case of North Island lambs to 0.27–0.36 kg for South Island lambs after one day of fasting. (The North Island lambs were very full when taken off pasture.)
- Adult cattle were different: there were no loss for 3 days after removal from pasture, but severe body weight losses after 4 days withdrawal of food.

In general it would appear that the younger the animals the greater the liveweight loss following fasting. Resting periods should therefore be geared accordingly, and stock for slaughter should be drawn from production areas as close to slaughter points as possible.

## Resting of animals prior to slaughter

The actual duration of the resting period necessary to ensure normal physiological changes in the muscle after slaughter depends on many factors. These include the species of animals, age, sex, class and condition, time of year, length of journey, method of transportation, etc. Where different species are handled within the one lairage, it is important to ensure that proper arrangements are made for movement forward for slaughter after an adequate resting period for the particular animals involved. Cows in good condition in temperate countries should not be held for long periods during winter because of the possibility of hypomagnesaemic tetany. Spring lambs require a relatively shorter period of rest than adult sheep, and tend to lose weight with prolonged holding.

However, the quality of the rest encountered in the lairage has been brought into question. Cockram (1991) argues persuasively that the novel environment of the lairage, with people moving around, may not provide optimal conditions for cattle to rest, as measured by lying behaviour. Although conditions may improve overnight, with cattle lying down and resting, he suggests that the evidence is unclear as to whether the meat quality from cattle held overnight in the lairage shows a significant improvement.

It has been determined in Australia that the ultimate pH in steer carcases was lower in animals that had been rested and fed for 4 days than in animals rested for only 2 days after a 320 km (200 mile) journey. In the same country the ultimate pH values in the carcases of rams were higher and the meat colour was darker in animals rested for 120 hours after a journey by road of 1110 km (690 miles). In Bulgaria, blood and muscle values in calves transported by road for up to 450 km were back to normal in 24 hours.

McNally and Warriss (1996) demonstrated that as the time cattle were held in the lairage increased, the amount of bruising increased significantly.

In New Zealand, Purchas (1992), investigated the effect of decreasing the holding time in the lairage from 28 to 4 hours, after 2 hours transport. Overall, the dressing-out percentage based on full liveweights was significantly lower for the 28-hour group, so that for the mean liveweight of 483 kg, the extra 24 hours of holding time led to 4.5 kg less carcase weight, with the rate of loss being slightly greater for the heifers. Perhaps surprisingly, if the lairage is to be considered as a place of rest, the mean ultimate muscle pH was significantly higher for the 28-hour group (0.34 pH units), but this effect was much more apparent for bulls (0.60 pH units) than for steers (0.27 pH units) or heifers (no change), presumably owing to the greater activity that characterises the behaviour of bulls. On the basis of this work it may be suggested that in order to maximise carcase yield and meat quality, holding of cattle in the lairage should be restricted to 4 hours. The number of variables between lairages, however, means that such a recommendation should be treated with caution.

Warriss *et al.* (1992), demonstrated that in pigs blood cortisol and beta-endorphin levels return to normal values after 2–3 hours in the lairage. These blood constituents measure mainly psychological stress and support the observation that the majority of pigs, whether in single or mixed producer lots, cease to fight after the first hour in the lairage and settle down to rest (Moss, 1977). A period of rest of 2–3 hours for pigs has therefore been recommended. It allows sufficient time to recover from previous stresses without significantly increasing the problems of long food deprivation, muscle glycogen depletion and skin blemish seen after longer periods, particularly after holding overnight.

*Excessively long periods of retention* only serve to make the task of lairage cleaning – one of the most difficult tasks in the meat plant – even more difficult, as well as increasing the possibility of cross-infection. *It has been found, for example, that the longer pigs and calves are held prior to slaughter the greater is the build-up of infection, particularly of salmonella organisms, and the greater the risk of cross-infection.* In one experiment with calves awaiting slaughter, it was shown that after a few hours' detention only 0.6% of the animals harboured salmonellae, whereas after 2–5 days 55.6% had salmonella in their intestine. Other authorities have recorded salmonella in 7% of farm pigs, 25% of pigs in the lairage pen, and 50% of pigs at slaughter; 75% of lairage drinking water was also infected. It is recommended, therefore, that young calves be slaughtered as soon as possible after arrival at an abattoir because of the risk of cross-contamination and because it is difficult to induce calves to eat. Small pens with solid bases to the partitions, given regular cleansing and disinfection, will considerably lower the risk of cross-infection with salmonella organisms.

## PRE-SLAUGHTER HANDLING AND MEAT QUALITY

### Stress and the animal

During the process of loading at the farm, the journey to the abattoir or market, the holding at the market, the off-loading, the detention in the abattoir lairage and the subsequent handling up to the point of slaughter, the animal is subjected to a wide variety of stressors, many of which have an adverse effect with subsequent deleterious changes in the carcase. Even death may occur.

Stressors may include physical trauma and fear, and environmental excesses of noise, heat, cold, light, wind chill or humidity. These may make excessive demands on the animal and may result in handling problems which may be reflected in abnormal bodily changes at slaughter.

Fraser (1980) has proposed the following definition of stress: 'An animal is said to be in a state of stress if it is required to make abnormal or extreme adjustments in its physiology or behaviour in order to cope with adverse aspects of its environment and management.' A husbandry system can be said to be stressful if it makes abnormal demands on the animals. An individual factor may be called a *stressor* if it contributes to the stressful nature of a system of husbandry. Amoroso (1967) developed a useful mnemonic for stress: Situations That Release Emergency Signals for Survival.

Seyle (1974) defined stress as a *non-specific response* in an animal attempting to resist or adapt to maintain homeostasis, i.e. the tendency for the internal environment of the body to be maintained constant and in equilibrium. This suggests that, whatever the trigger for the stress, the physiological response is identical. The currently accepted description of stress is that it is the normal and complex summation of a wide variety of responses to any environmental change. Stress is, at most, a short-hand term for the essential characteristic of biological adaptation.

There are two main reactions of an animal to stress: the *alarm or emergency reaction* and the *general adaptive syndrome* (together termed the *fight or flight syndrome*). The alarm reaction is the result of a sudden adverse stimulus and takes place immediately. It is reflected in an increased activity of the sympathetic nervous system which supplies the involuntary muscles, secretory glands and the heart. The result is an out-pouring into the bloodstream of the catecholamines, noradrenaline and adrenaline by the medulla of the adrenal gland, leading to increased heart rate and force of cardiac contraction, constriction of peripheral blood vessels, elevated blood pressure, dilation of bronchi, cessation of digestion and mobilisation of liver glycogen with increases in blood sugar. Glucagon, a peptide produced by the alpha-cells of the Islets of Langerhans in the pancreas, is more powerful than adrenaline in the production of blood glucose by the mobilisation of liver glycogen.

While the alarm reaction is immediate, the general adaptive syndrome is the essential stress reaction and is longer lasting. Adrenocorticotrophic hormone (ACTH) is produced by the anterior pituitary gland and brings about the production of corticosteroids such as cortisone and hydrocortisone (cortisol), which regulate the general metabolism of carbohydrates, proteins and fats on a long-term basis. There is a decrease in carbohydrate metabolism, and an increase in protein metabolism, the amino acids being converted to glycogen in the liver. Fat is metabolised from the fat deposits and is metabolised in the liver, producing ketone bodies. *The overall result is an increase in the level of blood glucose and ketones.* Other changes in the general adaptation syndrome include hypertrophy of the adrenal gland with reduction in its ascorbic acid and cholesterol stores, eosinophilia (reduction in the number of eosinophils), lymphopenia (reduction in the number of lymphocytes), polynucleosis (an increase in polymorphonuclear leukocytes) and an increased susceptibility to disease. Sustained adaptation syndrome leads to reduced growth rate in young animals and loss of weight in adult animals.

This non-specific response of the body, irrespective of the origin of the stress, has been questioned and adapted by Moberg (1983) and others. They suggest that corticosteroids may not be produced as a response to all stressful stimuli, that different species may react differently to the same stressor, and that in some cases other endocrine pathways may be involved. It may be wrong to assume, therefore, that a lack of adrenal response indicates that there is no stress. There appears to be an important role played by the brain, including the limbic system, the pituitary and hypothalamus, especially in the mechanism by which animals cope with stress. *When an animal puts substantial effort and resources into coping with a stressful situation, it can be considered to be suffering distress.*

## Stress and meat quality

The physiological changes described above which occur when an animal is stressed can have a very significant effect on the quality of the meat if the stress occurs in the period prior to slaughter. In order to understand these changes, it is necessary to have some knowledge of the biochemical events which occur in muscle in the period immediately after the animal's death.

After slaughter, the supply of oxygen to the muscle ceases with the cessation of blood circulation. Normal aerobic respiration in the muscle therefore stops, to be replaced by anaerobic reactions. Anaerobic glycolysis, the breakdown of hexose sugars, results in the production and accumulation of lactic acid in muscle, and a characteristic fall in the pH from 7.0–7.2 to around 5.5. This fall normally takes 4–8 hours in pigs, 12–24 hours in sheep and 24–48 hours in cattle.

Anaerobic glycolysis results in the production of much less energy, stored as adenosine triphosphate (ATP), than its aerobic alternative. After death, the levels of ATP therefore fall. Energy is required to keep muscle in its relaxed state. When the levels of ATP fall to a critically low level after death, the relaxed state can no longer be maintained. The muscle's component molecules, actin and myosin, combine irreversibly to form actomyosin, and the muscle contracts slightly in what is known as *rigor mortis* – the carcase 'setting'.

The rate of onset of rigor is therefore dependent on the supply of ATP in the muscle at death. Any external factor which depletes this supply of ATP will hasten the onset of rigor mortis. This fact is demonstrated in exhausted bulls, the carcases of which set rapidly after slaughter owing to low levels of glycogen, and therefore of ATP, in the muscle at the time of death. These animals will, in addition, have a high muscle pH since little lactic acid will have been produced. It is important to recognise that rigor mortis depends only on the availability of ATP, not on the pH of the meat.

Pre-slaughter stress, therefore, affects both the rate of onset of rigor mortis and the rate and the extent of the fall in muscle pH. Alterations in these parameters affect the appearance and eating quality of the meat, the most common manifestations being pale, soft, exudative (PSE) pork, and dark, firm and dry (DFD) beef. These economically significant conditions are described in detail in Chapter 2.

### Pre-slaughter feeding of sugars

In order to ensure adequate pre-slaughter levels of glycogen in the muscle, which will result in sufficient lactic acid being produced to cause the required fall in pH, it is necessary either to minimise stress, fear, excitement, fatigue or excessive exertion on the animal, or to allow for an adequate period of rest prior to slaughter in order for muscle glycogen levels to replenish. Another approach is to feed easily digestible carbohydrates, such as sugar, while the animals are in the lairage. As far back as 1937, experiments in pre-slaughter feeding of molasses to pigs showed a restoration of muscle glycogen and subsequent low tissue pH. Later work emphasised this; the psoas muscle, fillet, had a post-mortem pH of 6.0 when pigs were starved overnight, compared with 5.43 when 1.4 kg sucrose was fed 22 and 6 hours before slaughter. The sucrose-fed pigs also gained more weight during curing, the bacon and ham underwent less shrink while maturing, and a further advantage was a significant increase in liver weight. Better keeping qualities of bacon and ham were also reported.

Sugar solutions have been used to overcome some of the storage, handling and feeding problems of solid sugar. A study at the bacon factory of Cavaghan and Gray in Carlisle showed that carcase yields were increased by 2.8% and liver weights by 27%, and muscle pH was reduced by 0.2–0.3 units, when pigs fed a glucose syrup solution and water and held overnight were compared with those receiving water only. When compared with pigs slaughtered on arrival, the differences were 1.3%, 13% and 0.2–0.3 units, respectively.

In cattle detained for 2 days in the lairage, a 25% loss in liver weight may occur. In one plant in Chicago the effects of stress in cattle are reduced by incorporating molasses in the drinking water. It has also been shown that the feeding of sugar rapidly restores the energy-yielding carbohydrate reserve (glycogen) of the muscles and liver, allowing the development of normal acidity in the former and preventing loss of weight in the latter. The feeding of up to 1.3 kg of sugar for 3 or more days before slaughter of cattle or pigs has increased daily weights. Some workers have found that loss in liveweight can be prevented by feeding sugar.

Under present-day abattoir conditions it is doubtful whether pre-slaughter feeding is always a practical or economic proposition.

## TRAUMATIC INJURY

*Bruising* is defined as traumatic injury without penetration of the skin where blood vessels are damaged to such an extent that there is extravasation into the surrounding tissues. Several studies of cattle bruising have shown that approximately 31% of bruises occur in the loin and hip area, 36% on the shoulder, 13% on the ribs and 20% on other parts of the body. In sheep many of the bruises are due to rough handling, resulting either from animals being lifted by the wool or grabbed by the legs during sorting, weighing and loading on the farm, during unloading or while being handled prior to being stunned.

Fasting has been shown to increase bruising and there is some evidence that chronic stress makes animals more susceptible to it.

### Time of bruising

Although the presence of bruises at slaughter is apparent to the eye, knowledge of the exact time of infliction is necessary if steps are to be taken to prevent bruising. At slaughter a bruise may be dated approximately by the physical criteria listed in Table 7.3.

A more specific method of dating is based on a test which utilises the formation of *bilirubin* from haemoglobin in the area of the bruise. A sample of bruised meat is soaked in Fouchet's reagent (trichloracetic acid and ferric chloride); bruises up to 50 hours old give no reaction; those 60–72 hours old turn the solution light blue; those 4–5 days old give a dark green reaction. The bilirubin test has been used to show, for example, that 90% of poultry bruises are inflicted 0–13 hours before slaughter.

The age of a bruise can also be estimated by measuring the *electrical conductivity* of the tissue, which increases up to a maximum at 40 hours. *Histological methods* have been developed which claim to be able to differentiate between bruises occurring at various times between 48 hours pre-slaughter and stunning (McCausland and Dougherty, 1978)

**Table 7.3** Approximate ageing of bruises by physical appearance.

| | |
|---|---|
| 0–10 hours old | Red and haemorrhagic |
| Approx. 24 hours old | Dark coloured |
| 24–38 hours old | Watery consistency |
| Over 3 days | Rusty orange colour (bilirubin) and soapy to the touch. |

### Rough handling

Observations in over 100 packing stations in the United States have shown that rough handling and the abusive use of clubs, whips and electric goads are responsible for the majority of injuries. If animals become stubborn or fractious, and refuse to enter or emerge from a vehicle, they are all too often beaten and shouted at until they fall, or in the case of pigs are dragged by the ears, sustaining injuries, even fractures and bruises. This senseless form of animal handling is not confined to the United States – it occurs the world over. McNally and Warriss (1996), in a survey carried out in the UK, report that over 35% of cattle bruising was due to stick marks. Giving animals time and space to move is a prerequisite not adopted by all handlers. Some knowledge of animal behaviour, with attention to detail in the design of animal handling/loading/unloading facilities, can remove the stress and danger for both handler and animal.

Three categories of sheep were examined for evidence of bruising: sheep transported direct from farms and those transported from local and distant markets in Scotland (Jarvis *et al.*, 1996). In sheep coming directly from farms, 93% had no bruises compared with 86% from local markets and 74% from distant markets.

Blood biochemistry showed significantly higher levels of serum creatine kinase and plasma osmolality in the sheep from distant markets than in the other two groups, suggesting greater muscle damage and dehydration, respectively. However, there were no substantial differences between the three groups in terms of packed cell volume, total plasma protein and beta-hydroxybutrate.

A survey of 4473 cattle delivered to one slaughter plant from 21 live auction markets in England revealed an overall prevalence of bruising of 8.1% and of stick marking of 2.2%. Differences existed between the prevalences of both bruising in carcase from steers, heifers and bulls. Overall, steers had the greatest amount of carcase damage and young bulls the lowest amount. Variations also occurred in the frequency of bruising (range 2.4–17.9%) and of stick marking (range 0–9.6%) from different markets. There was no evidence that longer journeys (distances ranged from 80 to 464 km) were associated with greater carcase damage. There was a relationship between a high degree of bruising and stick marking at one particular market (McNally and Warriss, 1997).

### Transport and vehicle design

Not enough attention is paid to the design of loading ramps at the farm and unloading ramps at the abattoir. Floor design of vehicles sometimes causes injury and stress owing to absence of non-slip surfaces.

Experimental work with cattle suggests that packing them tightly for mutual support from the sides of the vehicle results in more bruising than allowing them sufficient space to adjust their posture and brace themselves against the movement of the vehicle and to get up after falling. The greater the distance travelled and the greater the number of stops, the higher the incidence of bruising.

It has been suggested that the manner in which the vehicle is driven can have a great influence on both the degree and amount of bruising. The less braking and accelerating and fewer gear changes, the less bruising.

### Presence of horns

An important factor is whether the animal is hornless or horned. The Australian Meat Board has shown that approximately half the bruising in horned cattle is due to the horns and that the incidence of bruising in horned cattle is twice as high as in hornless breeds. The tipping of horns, by the removal of 10–15 cm, has been recommended but was not found to make any significant difference to the incidence of bruising. The only answer is to have all cattle polled, either by dehorning young calves or by breeding naturally-polled stock.

### Temperament

The temperament of cattle obviously has an effect on the incidence of bruising and, as every cattle farmer knows, temperament varies between breeds and individuals. It is considered that the bruising of cattle in a confined space, for example a cattle wagon or lairage pen, is due to the natural 'milling about' of a mob of cattle rather than to malicious aggression. Practical farmers, however, are unanimous in the assertion that a bad-tempered animal can create havoc in a mob of cattle, especially under confined conditions, and personnel in every abattoir have noticed how an old cow may persistently harass its fellows. The same occurs with pigs, where one animal in a group can persistently bully its mates.

Overcrowding undoubtedly increases aggressiveness and may be responsible for a high incidence of bruises in animals awaiting slaughter. Among the food animals, fat pigs are the most likely to be affected during transport as their heat-eliminating powers are very limited and they soon succumb to overexertion.

### Stunning box design

Bruising can be produced in an animal both before and after stunning, but not once the animal has been bled when the blood pressure drops to zero. The design of the stunning box can, therefore, be of importance in the problem of bruising. In Australia it has been shown that over 60% of cattle fall from the stunning box so heavily that they are bruised, the extent of the bruise depending on the severity of the fall and the time between stunning and bleeding.

In Australia, bruising in cattle causes an estimated annual loss of up to $26 million (1976), and horn damage plus stunning box bruising accounts for 48% of this loss. The incidence of stunning box bruising can be reduced by a proper design which ensures that the animal slides out of the box. In some abattoirs the animal is ejected on to a thick rubber mat.

### Mixing of animals

Bruising and bite marks on the surface of the skin of pigs cause depreciation in market value. The incidence of this type of damage, severe enough to result in downgrading, has been recorded as 7.3% (MLC, 1985) with a difference between boars and non-boars of 10% and 5.4%, respectively (Warriss, 1984). Most bruises occur during transport, a minor proportion during loading and unloading. Pigs from different farms loaded on the same lorry behave comparatively quietly once the lorry is in motion but start fighting as soon as the lorry stops. Reducing the stopping periods by 50% reduces the incidence of bite marks by 25%. Pre-mixing of socially unfamiliar groups of pigs in a holding pen for a couple of days prior to transport also considerably reduces injuries from fighting. In the lairage, it is important to avoid mixing pigs from different sources, different social groups, and different ages if at all possible. Spraying pigs with water on arrival has been used to decrease the incidence of pale, soft, exudative (PSE) pork by cooling the pigs, but care must be taken in cold weather not to induce hypothermia by leaving the sprays on for extended periods.

### Breed

Some breeds of cattle, e.g. the Brahmam and Afrikaner, are notoriously excitable. Certain breeds of pigs are so susceptible to the effects of stress, e.g. the Piétrain and Poland China, that steps are being taken to identify the 'stress gene' and remove it from the population by breeding strategy and genetic engineering.

### Incentives and education

The most effective way to educate hauliers and animal handlers about the damage careless handling can do to stock is to allow them to see the results on the carcase. Bruises on cattle, stick marks on pigs and wool pulls on sheep all leave their obvious, permanent and costly marks on the dressed meat. When producers are made aware that they are losing money through the loss of carcase weight due to the trimming of these defects, the pressure to improve handling facilities and stockmanship to prevent bruising is increased.

## ANTE-MORTEM INSPECTION

### The legal requirement

The provision of a veterinary inspection of the live animal prior to slaughter is a basic requirement of most meat inspection systems. The European Directive 91/497/EEC, enacted in Great Britain by the Fresh Meat (Hygiene and Inspection) Regulations 1995, makes the following statements about ante-mortem health inspection:

**1** Animals must undergo ante-mortem inspection on the day of their arrival at the slaughterhouse or before the beginning of daily slaughtering. The inspection must be repeated immediately before slaughter if the animal has been in the lairage overnight. The operator of the slaughterhouse, the owner or his agent must facilitate operations for performing ante-mortem health inspections and in particular any handling which is considered necessary.

Each animal to be slaughtered shall bear an identifying mark enabling the competent authority to determine its origin.

**2** (a) The official veterinarian must make the ante-mortem inspection in accordance with professional rules and under suitable lighting.

(b) The official veterinarian must, in respect of animals delivered to the slaughterhouse, check on compliance with community rules on animal welfare.

**3** The inspection must determine:

(a) whether the animals are suffering from a disease which is communicable to man and to animals or whether they show symptoms or are in a general condition such as to indicate that such a disease may occur;

(b) whether they show symptoms of disease or of a disorder of their general condition which is likely to make their meat unfit for human consumption; attention must also be paid to any signs that the animals have had any substances with pharmacological effects administered to them or have consumed any other substances which may make their meat harmful to human health;

(c) whether they are tired, agitated or injured.

**4** (a) tired or agitated animals must be rested for at least 24 hours unless the official veterinarian decides otherwise.

(b) animals in which one of the diseases referred to in para. 3(a) and (b) has been diagnosed must not be slaughtered for human consumption.

(c) slaughter of animals suspected of suffering from one of the diseases referred to in para. 3(a) and (b) must be deferred. These animals shall undergo detailed examination in order to make a diagnosis.

Where the post-mortem inspection is necessary in order to make a diagnosis, the official veterinarian shall request that the animals in question are slaughtered separately or at the end of normal slaughtering.

Those animals shall undergo detailed post-mortem inspection supplemented, if the veterinarian considers it necessary for confirmation, by an appropriate bacteriological examination and a search for residues of substances with a pharmacological effect which may be presumed to have been administered to treat the pathological state observed.

The Directive also states that the official veterinarian may be assisted by auxiliaries, the meat inspectors, in ante-mortem inspection, the auxiliary's role being to make an initial check on the animals and to help with purely practical tasks.

In the United States the authority for ante-mortem inspection is contained in the Federal Meat Inspection Act, as amended by the Wholesome Meat Act. The regulations state that:

(a) All livestock offered for slaughter in an official establishment shall be examined and inspected on the day of slaughter unless, because of unusual circumstances, prior arrangements acceptable to the Administrator have been made in specific cases by the circuit supervisor for such examination and inspection to be made on a different day before slaughter; and
(b) Such ante-mortem inspection shall be made in pens on the premises of the establishment at which the livestock are offered for slaughter before the livestock shall be allowed to enter into any department of the establishment where they are to be slaughtered or dressed or in which edible products are handled.

## Ante-mortem procedure

Ante-mortem inspection has three main areas of concern: *public health, animal health* and *animal welfare.*

For *public health* purposes the veterinarian must separate normal animals from those which may be suffering from a potentially zoonotic disease or present a hygiene risk to the slaughterhall environment owing to their filthy state. Animals which may contain residues of pharmaceutical product must be detained for testing post-mortem.

It is also very important that the workers within the abattoir are alerted to the presence of any *zoonotic condition*, such as orf or ringworm, or where brucellosis or TB reactor cattle are being slaughtered, so that appropriate protective measures can be taken. In the UK the action to be taken in the event of each condition being identified should be assessed and written down under the 'Control of Substances Hazardous to Health Regulations 1988' which are a series of statutory Regulations made under the framework of the Health and Safety at Work Act 1974.

The *animal health* aspect requires the veterinarian to identify *notifiable disease.* It is recognised within the state veterinary service that it is likely that a serious epizootic, such as foot-and-mouth disease or swine fever, will first be recognised at an abattoir.

The ante-mortem procedure allows the veterinarian to assess the *welfare* implications of the structures and procedures within the lairage. In the ideal situation, this would involve *inspections on the farm of origin*, during transport, as well as in the lairage prior to death.

Following inspection, the veterinarian may make one of the following five decisions.

**1** Animals may progress for normal slaughter.
**2** Animals should not enter the plant or should be condemned ante-mortem. In this group will be dead, moribund, emaciated or excessively dirty animals, and those showing evidence of a septicaemia or other conditions which would result in the meat being unfit for human consumption.
**3** Animals should be slaughtered but may need a special detailed post-mortem examination, or may need to be slaughtered in a special area or at a different time from other animals, owing perhaps to a localised infection or suspicion of a more generalised condition. Animals suspected of being treated with illegal drugs for the purposes of growth promotion, or of having residues of therapeutic substances, may be included in this group. Emergency on-farm slaughtered cases will require particular attention.
**4** Stock should be segregated for slaughter under special conditions, e.g. dirty stock at a slow line speed.
**5** Slaughter may be delayed, e.g. for excessively fatigued, excited animals or those requiring treatment.

## On the farm

From what has been discussed earlier and in Chapter 9, the benefits which can be forthcoming from extending the ante-mortem procedure back to the farm are obvious.

The *integrated approach to meat hygiene* has gained support worldwide, but there are many practical problems to be solved before it can be successfully implemented on a large scale. The most important of these problems, the fast and efficient collection and transfer of accurate information between all stages in the production chain, will be solved by the rapid developments in information technology which will soon allow information to be passed automatically between farm and meat factory by computer and/or fax machine. A direct consequence of this is the requirement for a tamper-proof and easily-read *animal identification system*. European Directive 92/102 requires that all animals, or group of animals, be identified. Although this requirement has more to do with subsidy payments and the avoidance of fraud, it may assist in the development of an improvement on the present metal or plastic tag system for cattle, and ad hoc systems for other farm species. The International Organisation for Standardisation (ISO) has agreed a standard for the electronic identification of animals (January 1996; ISO11784 and ISO11785). This opens the way to a worldwide usage of electronic transponders to record identity and production data about individual animals from birth through to the abattoir.

The most common method of identifying pigs for slaughter in the UK is the slapmark which, if properly applied, is the most satisfactory.

## In the meat plant

Livestock in the lairage should be inspected at rest and while in motion. Both sides of the animal should be observed. In practice this is simple to carry out while the animals are being unloaded, but their excited state during this procedure may mask some conditions such as mild lamenesses, making a second check necessary. In the case of sick or suspect diseased animals, and those in poor condition, the species, class, age, condition, colour or markings, and identification number are recorded. The general behaviour of the animals, whether fatigued or excited, their level of nutrition, cleanliness, obvious signs of disease and any abnormalities should be observed and recorded. In addition to the segregation of diseased and suspect stock, females in oestrus, aggressive animals and horned stock should be isolated. If *unacceptably dirty animals*, i.e. ones which, in the opinion of the veterinarian cannot be dressed at normal line speed without an unacceptable risk of carcase contamination, have been allowed by factory management to enter the lairage, they must be segregated and detained until their condition becomes more acceptable, or they can be dressed at a line speed which decreases the risk of contamination.

Animals showing evidence of localised conditions such as injuries, fractures, abscesses, benign tumours (e.g. papillomata) or conditions which will show up lesions on post-mortem inspection need to be segregated and given a detailed examination. Such animals may pass forward with the normal kill if the condition proves to be a minor one, slaughtered at the end of the day's kill, or slaughtered separately and given a thorough post-mortem examination.

In the case of *sick animals* the temperature should be taken; a rise in temperature may be the first indication of a communicable disease, although in moribund animals the temperature may frequently be subnormal. In sheep, body temperature may be a somewhat misleading guide as, of all the food animals, its temperature is subject to the greatest daily fluctuation; variations between 39°C and 40°C are common and in heavily woolled sheep in summer the temperature can vary between 38.2°C and 40.1°C in healthy animals. Pigs that show a temperature of 41°C or over, and cattle and sheep that show a temperature of 40.5°C or higher should be isolated until the temperature falls for, if they are slaughtered while suffering from this degree of fever, the carcase will be congested and will invariably require condemnation.

*Animals showing signs of systemic disturbance and an elevated temperature should not be slaughtered but retained for treatment, preferably outside the meat plant.*

In the USA, *'suspect'* animals are those suspected of being diseased or affected with certain conditions that might result in condemnation of the carcase on post-mortem inspection. These animals are tagged as 'US Suspect', as are the carcases from such animals, until a final post-mortem inspection is carried out. They include, under USDA regulations, 'downers', cases of leptospirosis, anaplasmosis and tuberculosis reactors, brucella-reactor goats, epithelioma of the eye, anasarca, swine erysipelas, vesicular exanthema, vesicular stomatitis, immature animals, and livestock previously condemned for listeriosis and released for slaughter. A 'suspect' animal must be segregated from other stock, its number recorded and a description made of the animal and the disease affecting it, along with its temperature when this might have a bearing on the ultimate disposition of the carcase.

*Animals that may be condemned under USDA regulations* include dead, recumbent and disabled livestock; those affected with any condition that would entail condemnation of the carcase at post-mortem inspection; any swine having a temperature of 106°F or higher and any cattle, sheep, goats, horses, mules or other equines having a temperature of 105°F or higher (in cases of doubt, such animals may be held for further inspection on the same day); livestock in a comatose or semicomatose condition; livestock showing signs of certain metabolic, toxic or circulatory disturbances; those showing evidence of nutritional imbalances or infectious or parasitic diseases – anaplasmososis, ketosis, leptospirosis, listeriosis, parturient paralysis, pseudorabies, rabies, BSE, scrapie, tetanus, grass tetany, transport tetany, strangles, purpura haemorrhagica, azoturia, infectious equine encephalomyelitis, toxic encephalitis (forage poisoning), dourine, acute influenza, generalised osteoporosis, glanders (farcy), acute inflammatory lameness or extensive fistula, swine fever, anthrax and animals which have been injected with anthrax vaccine within the previous 6 weeks.

In all cases it is absolutely essential that good *records* are kept of the ante-mortem findings. These records must be available to the inspectors at the time of post-mortem inspection so that the findings can be acted upon at that stage. A system which correlates the ante-mortem and post-mortem findings should be kept as simple and transparent as possible. In addition, there must be a simple method, usually *pen cards*, which allows the lairage staff to easily identify which animals have received ante-mortem inspection and what the outcome has been.

## THE CASUALTY ANIMAL

Although the term *'casualty animal'* is in general use by the farming community and the veterinary profession, the word is ill-defined. Legislation within the UK refers to animals as being 'unfit'.

The Ministry of Agriculture, Fisheries and Food, and the Department of Agriculture for Northern Ireland, have both produced notes for 'Guidance on the transport of casualty animals' based upon the Welfare of Animals during Transport Order 1994 and other relevant welfare legislation. This defines casualty animals as 'animals which are suffering from disease or injury where the decision has been made to slaughter them'. The advice given on transporting casualty animals to slaughter is also appropriate for animals which are infirm, fatigued or heavily pregnant, or which have given birth within the preceding 48 hours.

The *reasons for casualty slaughter* of cattle were determined in a comprehensive survey in Switzerland (Wyss *et al.*, 1984). This covered 44 704 cattle, the losses representing 1.83% of all cattle insured. Major reasons, in order of importance, were dystocia (8.84%), tympany (8.44%), respiratory disease (6.49%), joint disease (5.78%), reticular foreign bodies (5.16%), circulatory disease (5.14%), enteritis (4.65%), fractures unrelated to parturition (4.43%), recumbency (4.10%), claw disease (3.46%), abortion (3.39%). Also included were cases of poisoning and spastic paresis. At Belfast Meat Plant the main reasons for casualty or emergency slaughter (1990) were fractures (24%), non-specific injuries (9%), prolapse/ruptured vagina (6.5%), arthritis (6%), CNS lesions (5%), downer cow/hypomagnesaemia (4.6%), digestive disorders (4.6%), spinal injuries (4%). Others were dog worrying, haemorrhages, dislocations, septic injuries, heart abnormalities, cystitis, congenital abnormalities, tendonitis, blindness, radial paralysis, tumours, lameness, laminitis, ovarian cyst, dystocia, respiratory disorders and amputations.

The *conditions governing the admission of diseased or injured animals* into an abattoir in Great Britain, are laid down in the Fresh Meat (Hygiene and Inspection) Regulations 1995, Regulation 17. These conditions are:

1 No person shall send an animal which he knows or suspects to be diseased or injured to a slaughterhouse unless he has given the occupier of the slaughterhouse reasonable notice of his intention to send it.

2 No person shall bring into, or permit to be brought into, a slaughterhouse any animal which he knows or suspects to be diseased or injured unless

(a) he has already ensured that it is accompanied by a *written declaration signed by the owner or person in charge* of it;

(b) that declaration is handed to an inspector or the Official Veterinary Surgeon (OVS) as soon as is practical after the animal's arrival at the slaughterhouse:

3 The occupier of the slaughterhouse shall ensure that, on arrival at the slaughterhouse, the animal

(a) is slaughtered without delay following ante-mortem inspection; or

(b) is taken without delay under the direction of an inspector or the OVS to that part of the lairage provided for the isolation of diseased or injured animals.

The requirement in 2(a) is considered by many veterinarians to be inadequate, especially in the case of diseased animals.

## The on-farm decision

The decision on the farm as to whether or not it is possible to transport an animal to be slaughtered without it suffering unnecessary distress is an important and sometimes difficult one. *The legislation puts the responsibility to ensure that only animals suitable for loading, travelling and subsequent unloading are actually transported for slaughter firmly on the shoulders of the farmer, haulier and veterinary practitioner.*

The animal may not be dragged or pushed by any means, or lifted by a mechanical device, unless this is done in the presence of and under the supervision of a veterinary surgeon who is arranging for it to be transported with all practicable speed to a place for veterinary treatment. This means in practice that in the case of adult bovines, only animals which can walk on to and off the transport, and bear weight on all four legs during the journey, should be transported to an abattoir for slaughter. If the farmer is in any doubt he or she must always take professional advice from a veterinarian. If in turn the veterinary practitioner has any doubts, he or she may consult with the official veterinarian in the meat plant to which the animal is being consigned to seek an opinion or guidance. This approach has the added advantage of helping to reduce conflict of opinion between professional colleagues.

In any case, the welfare of the casualty animal must always be considered as the most important issue when deciding whether a particular animal can be transported live to a slaughter plant. However, the suitability of the animal for food must also be considered. This decision may be based on information such as the species of animal involved, the nature of the animal's affliction, the drugs it has received and when, if recumbent, how long has it been dorsally or laterally recumbent.

When the decision has been made that the animal is a suitable candidate for transport to the abattoir as a casualty, arrangements must be made with the management of the nearest meat plant to ensure that they will accept it, and to ascertain whether the official veterinarian will be present to inspect it on arrival.

## Casualties at the meat plant

As the legislation states, the casualty animal must receive ante-mortem inspection and be slaughtered immediately on arrival at the slaughterhouse or be taken without delay under the direction of an inspector or the OVS to that part of the lairage provided for the isolation of diseased or injured animals. It is a requirement of the Fresh Meat (Hygiene and Inspection) Regulations 1995, Schedule 2, para. 2(d), that the suspected diseased or injured animal be slaughtered, dressed and held in a separate facility from normal stock. Alternatively, it may be slaughtered at the end of the day's kill, or before a break when the slaughterhall and equipment are cleaned and disinfected. This latter option may, however, lead to an unacceptable delay before the animal is dealt with. The small number of UK abattoirs which operate separate casualty slaughter facilities has led to animals having to travel much greater distances to the nearest slaughter-point which will accept them. The provision of a mobile slaughter facility as pioneered in Sweden, which can fit on to a lorry and provide hygienic slaughter and dressing conditions on the farm, would be an ideal answer to this problem.

Both casualties and emergency on-farm slaughtered animals must receive special attention from the meat hygiene team. This point was emphasised as long ago as 1876 when Bollinger pointed out that 80% of the cases of food poisoning in Germany were associated with the consumption of the flesh of animals that had undergone emergency slaughter. Striking confirmation of this was supplied by statistics which showed that the danger from meat of emergency-slaughtered animals, when compared with the meat of those slaughtered commercially, was 80 times greater in cattle, 12 times greater in calves, 100 times greater in sheep, 211 times greater in pigs and 3 times greater in horses. It is essential that the meat hygiene team are alert to the possibility of attempts to market, through the casualty system, animals which may be febrile, bacteraemic or septicaemic or which may contain the residues of drugs which may have been used to treat or mask clinical signs which have now passed. Most carcases from casualty animals must therefore receive bacteriological and residue monitoring.

In a study of 30 cattle in recumbency which had passed a routine ante-mortem inspection under USDA rules, 11 showed histopathological evidence of bacteraemia (Edwards *et al.* 1995), indicating the importance of extreme caution. *Salmonella dublin* was isolated from one of the 30 animals.

## ON-FARM EMERGENCY SLAUGHTER

Where an animal is otherwise healthy but requires on-farm emergency slaughter, owing perhaps to a limb fracture, an uncontrollable haemorrhage, an injury causing severe pain or distress, or a functional or physiological disorder, the animal may be humanely slaughtered on the farm and the carcase transferred to the abattoir. Regulation 18 of the UK Fresh Meat (Hygiene and Inspection) Regulations 1995 states that:

2 No person shall bring into, or permit to be brought into, a slaughterhouse the slaughtered body of an animal, unless

(a) it has been bled;

(b) the animal has undergone an ante-mortem inspection by a veterinary surgeon;

(c) the animal has been slaughtered as a result of an accident or because it was suffering from a serious physiological or functional disorder;

(d) the body of the animal has not been dressed;

(e) the body of the animal is accompanied to the slaughterhouse by a *veterinary certificate;*

(f) the body of the animal is transported to the slaughterhouse in a container or vehicle under hygienic conditions and, if it cannot be delivered to the slaughterhouse within one hour of slaughter, it is transported there in a container or vehicle under hygienic conditions in which the ambient temperature is between 0°C and 4°C.

The veterinary practitioner on the farm therefore plays a pivotal role in the carrying out of the ante-mortem inspection, recording the findings accurately, ensuring that arrangements for the humane slaughter of the animal are made, ensuring its efficient and hygienic bleeding, and hygienic and immediate transfer to the abattoir. As with casualty slaughter, good communications between veterinary colleagues on the farm and in the abattoir are essential.

### On-farm emergency-slaughtered animals at the abattoir

On arrival at the abattoir, the certificate completed on the farm by the veterinary practitioner must be given to an inspector or the OVS. Having checked that the identity of the carcase matches that on the certificate, that the animal has been properly stunned or killed, bled and transported, and that transport has been completed within the hour allowed, skinning and dressing should be carried out immediately.

Post-mortem inspection should seek to confirm the diagnosis suggested by the veterinary practitioner on the certificate which accompanied the animal. The subcutaneous blood vessels, kidney, liver and lungs should be checked for satisfactory bleeding, and the kidney fat, along with the soft tissue organs for greening and autolytic changes.

In most cases, it is often wise to delay the final decision on these carcases for 24–48 hours, to allow rigor mortis to develop, to allow any oedema present to resolve, and to await the results of any bacteriological or residue samples taken. The number of casualty cattle and sheep received at Belfast Meat Plant during 1989–90 whose carcases were ultimately condemned is given in Table 7.4.

**Table 7.4** Casualty animal slaughter, Belfast Meat Plant, 1989–90.

| Class | Number | Condemned | % |
|---|---|---|---|
| Cows | 1156 | 348 | 30.1 |
| Heifers | 264 | 29 | 11.0 |
| Steers | 372 | 42 | 11.3 |
| Bulls | 113 | 9 | 8.0 |
| Calves | 16 | 2 | 12.5 |
| **Total cattle** | 1921 | 430 | 22.4 |
| Sheep | 354 | 74 | 20.9 |
| Lambs | 112 | 26 | 23.2 |
| **Total sheep** | 466 | 100 | 21.5 |

### Animals which arrive dead at the abattoir, without certification

Animals which arrive at the meat plant dead and without certification should on no account be dressed. All should be checked for anthrax as required by the Animal Health Act 1981 and removed from the abattoir for rendering or burial. Observation of the dead animal and the nature and colour of the blood oozing from the natural orifices is of great value in determining the possibility or otherwise of anthrax. The blood is dark and tarry in cases of anthrax; if it is light red and thin in nature it is unlikely to be anthrax. Even so, the onus on the veterinarian is to obtain a blood smear from the peripheral circulation in cattle and sheep, and from the throat in swine and equines.

## ANIMALS WHICH HAVE BEEN SUBJECTED TO SCIENTIFIC EXPERIMENTS

On occasions animals which have been the subjects of scientific experiments may be consigned to the meat plant. This special category of casualty animal must be accompanied by a veterinary certificate which gives full details of the procedures and compounds used under the Animals (Scientific Procedures) Act 1986. While some may present no difficulty with regard to judgement, e.g. cases of rumen and duodenal fistulae used in nutrition experiments, others call for care in making a decision as to the fitness of the meat for human consumption. The latter include those animals used in pharmaceutical and toxicological research.

As far as genetic modification research is concerned, the UK Advisory Committee on Novel Foods and Processes has recommended (June 1991) that, where human genetic material has been used, e.g. in the production of Factor VIII (antihaemophilic factor), the meat from such animals should not be sold for human consumption.

Where there is any doubt as to meat's suitability, the consumer must always be given the benefit of the doubt.

## REFERENCES


Abbott, T. A., Guise, H. J., Hunter, E. J., Penny, R. H. C., Baynes, P. J. and Easby, C. (1995) *Anim. Welfare*, **4**, 29–40.

Allen, W. M. and Smith, L. P. (1974) *Proceedings of the 20th European Meeting of Meat Research Workers, Dublin*, P. **45**.

Amoroso E. C. (1967) *Environmental Control of Poultry Production*, ed. T. C. Carter. Edinburgh: Oliver and Boyd.

Biss, M. E. and Hathaway, S. C. (1996) *Vet. Rec.* **138**, 82–86.

Cockram, M. S. (1991) *Br. Vet. J.*, **147**, 109.

Dexter, D. R., Cowman, G. L., Morgan, J. B., Clayton, R. P., Tatum, J. D., Sofas, J. N., Schmidt, G. R., Glock, R. D. and Smith, G. C. (1994) *J. Anim. Sci.* **4**, 824–827.

Edwards, J. F., Simpson, R. B. and Brown, W. C. (1995) *J. Am. Vet. Med. Assoc.* **207**, 1174–1176.

Findlay, C. R. (1972) *Vet. Rec.* **91**, 233–235.

Franklin, J. R. and Hutson, G. D. (1982) *Appl. Anim. Ethol.* **8**, 457–478.

Fraser, A. F. (1980) *Farm Animal Behaviour*, 2nd edn. London: Baillière-Tindall.

Grigor P. N and Goddard P. J. *et al.* (1997) *Vet. Rec.* **140**, 8–12.

Guise, H. J., Penny, R. H. C., Baynes, P. J., Abbott, T. A., Hunter, E. J. and Johnston, A. M. (1995) *Br. Vet. J.* **151**(6), 659–670.

Ingram, J. M. (1972) *Agric. N. Ireland* **47**(8), 279.

Jarvis A. M. *et al.* (1996) *Br. Vet. J.* **152**, 719.

Jones, P. W. (1979) *Vet. Rec.* **106**, 4–7.

Knowles, T. G., Warriss, P. D., Brown, S. N. and Kestin, S. C. (1993) *Appl. Anim. Behav. Sci.* **38**, 75–84.

Knowles, T. G., Warriss, P. D., Brown, S. N. and Kestin, S. C. (1994) *Vet. Rec.* **134**, 107.

Lapworth, J. W. (1990) *Appl. Anim. Behav. Sci.* **28**, 203–211.

McCausland I. P. and Dougherty, R. (1978) *Aust. Vet. J.* **54**, 525.

McNally, P. W. and Warriss, P. (1996) *Vet. Rec.* **138**, 126–128.
McNally, P. W. and Warriss, P. D (1997) *Vet. Rec.* **147**, 231–232.
MLC (1985) *Technical Notes*, No. 4, 14–16.
Moberg, G. P. (1987) *J. Anim. Sci.* **65**, 1228–1235.
Moss, B. W. (1977) *Appl. Anim. Ethol.* **4**, 4323–4339.
Moss, B. W. and Trimble, D (1988) *Record of Agricultural Research*, Vol. 36 Department of Agriculture for Northern Ireland.
Northern Ireland Department of Agriculture (1984) *Code of practice for the pre-slaughter handling of pigs.*
Petersson, H. and Gahne, B. (1988) *Svinskotsel*, **10**, 18.
Philips, P. A., Thompson, B. K. and Fraser, D. (1988) *Can. J. Anim. Sci.* **68**, 41–48.
Purchas R. W. (1992) *27th Meat Industry Research Conference Hamilton. New Zealand.* Meat Industry Research Institute, NZ.
Rankin, J. D. and Taylor, R. J. (1969) *Vet. Rec.* **85**, 575–581
Ridell, J. and Korkeala, H. (1993) *Meat Sci.* **35**, 223–228.
Seyle, H. (1974) The implications of the stress concept. *Biochem. Exp. Biol.* **11**, 190.
Smith, L. P. and Allen, W. M. (1976) *Agricultural Meteorology* **16**, 115.
Stosic P. J. (1996) *Hide Improvement Project. Dung Contamination of Cattle Hides.* The Leather Technology Centre.
Thompson, J. M., Halloran, W. J., McNeill, D. M. J., Jackson-Hope, N. J. and May, T. J. (1987) *Meat Sci.* **20**, 293–309.
Warriss, P. D. (1984), *Principles of Pig Science.* Nottingham University Press, 425–432.
Warriss, P. D. (1995) *Meat Focus Inter.* Dec., 491–494.
Warriss, P. D. and Bevis, E. A. (1986) *Br. Vet. J.* **142**, 124–130.
Warriss, P. D. and Brown, S. N. (1994) *Vet. Rec.* **134**, 513–515.
Warriss, P. D., Bevis, E. A. and Young, C. S. (1990) *Vet. Rec.* **127**, 5–8.
Warriss, P. D., Bevis, E. A., Edwards, J. E., Brown, S. N. and Knowles, T. G. (1991) *Vet. Rec.* **128**, 419–421.
Warriss, P. D., Brown, S. N., Knowles, T. G. and Edwards, J. E. (1992a) *Vet. Rec.* **130**, 202–204.
Warriss, P. D., Brown, S. N., Edwards, J. E., Anil, M. H. and Fordham, D. P. (1992b) *Vet. Rec.* **131**, 194–196.
Wyss, V., Hartig, J. and Gerber, H. (1984) *Schweizer Archiv fur Tierheilkunde* **126**, 339.

## FURTHER READING

*The Casualty Sheep* (1994): Sheep Veterinary Society.
*The Casualty Pig* (1996): Pig Veterinary Society.
*Salmonella, The Food Poisoner: A review.* A report by a Study Group of the British Association for the Advancement of Science 1975–1977.
MAFF Environment. Codes of Good Agricultural Practice for the Protection of Air and Water, 1991/92.

# Chapter 8
# Humane Slaughter

'A righteous man regardeth the life of his beast.' *Proverbs* 12:10.

The moral and ethical answers to the questions raised when humans kill animals for food can only be answered for each individual according to their own religious, political or economic circumstances. All can agree, however, that if it is to be done, the act of killing must be carried out in such a way as to cause the minimum of stress, or distress, to the animal. There are no 'nice' ways of killing animals. There are only the acceptable and the unacceptable. It is the duty of the veterinarian in the meat plant to have the knowledge and authority to ensure that only acceptable methods are applied.

Thorpe (1965) states that 'there are two opposite pitfalls which beset those who, like ourselves, attempt to decide on the limits of physical injury and restraint which it is not permissible for a civilised people to exceed in their treatment of domestic animals. The first is the error of supposing that domestic animals in their feelings and anxieties are essentially like human beings; the second is the equally serious error of assuming that they are mere insentient automata. To avoid these two pitfalls is relatively easy. To know what path to choose between them is extremely difficult.'

In conventional slaughtering methods in most developed countries, it is normal practice to render the animal insensible by stunning, except in the Jewish and Muslim methods, and then to kill it by bleeding. Stunning has two purposes: to induce an immediate state of insensibility, and to produce sufficient immobility to facilitate the sticking process to initiate bleeding. In this two-stage system of slaughter it is vital that insensibility lasts until anoxia resulting from exsanguination makes the loss in consciousness irreversible. This depends on the length of the interval between stunning and sticking, *which must be as short as possible*, and the efficiency of the sticking itself. It is a matter for great concern that faults occur all too often in both areas owing to lack of training and/or care and supervision and, not least, to the usual high speed of operations in the modern meat plant.

The discovery that satisfactory bleeding can occur where *cardiac arrest* has been induced introduces the possibility of stunning to kill rather than merely rendering the animal insensible. This obviates all risk of cruelty and should be the ideal for the future for all the food animals.

*No legislation is of any value unless it clearly incorporates the ethic that the quest for production must never take precedence over the far more important issues of hygiene, meat safety and the welfare of the animal.*

## PRE-SLAUGHTER HANDLING/RESTRAINT

It is generally regarded as undesirable that an animal awaiting slaughter should view the slaughtering process. Whilst the higher animals undoubtedly share some sensations with human beings, it is questionable whether any trepidation is felt specifically by an animal at the sight and smell of blood. Nevertheless, fear is undoubtedly engendered by strange noises, movements, surroundings and smells, and this fear is accentuated by the separation of the animal from its fellows and the consequent disappearance of the feeling of protection that a gregarious animal enjoys in the presence of its comrades.

The design of the *handling facility in the lairage* which delivers the animals to the point of slaughter should utilise a knowledge of animal behaviour to reduce to a minimum the fear or apprehension felt by the animal. The tendency for one sheep to follow its comrade up a single file race, the preference most animals have to walk up rather than down a slope, and the movement of pigs in optimum-sized groups of about 15 individuals are all examples of good practices. The theory of moving animals within the lairage is dealt with in detail in Chapter 7.

Cattle are usually moved from the pens in the lairage to the *stunning box* via a solid-walled race. Cattle have been shown to move more readily along a race with *curved walls*. A *raised walkway* along one side assists the handlers in their effort to keep the animals moving. The animal should spend the minimum possible time in the actual stunning box where they are finally isolated from their cohorts. They should not be moved into the box until the operative responsible for the stunning procedure is prepared.

Annex B of Council Directive 93/119/EC on the Protection of Animals at the Time of Slaughter and Killing requires that *for mechanical or electrical stunning the animal's head is presented in such a position that the equipment can be applied and operated easily*. There have been a number of types of *head-restraint* for cattle used, but a simple *shelf* which extends to the floor of the stunning box, preventing the animal dropping its head, seems to be the most successful. However, with all head restraints, smaller animals present problems by having sufficient space within the stunning box to position themselves in such a way as to avoid the restraint system. This can be overcome by the provision of a hydraulically-operated *tail pusher* in the back of the box. Personal observations of these mechanisms have shown that, if incorrectly used to force cattle into the head restraint, the animal's spine can be fractured by the pressures applied. The positioning of *lights* above the animal's head to attract its attention is reported as being a useful addition in maintaining the head in a raised position.

Ewbank, Parker and Mason (1992) reported on the use of head-restraints at slaughter and concluded that 'while the introduction of head restraint devices into cattle stunning pens had a positive effect in terms of improving the stunning accuracy, behaviour and cortisol results suggest that enforced usage of this type of head restrainer could be a cause of distress to the cattle involved.' The fixed shelf-restraint was found to improve the accuracy of stunning without increasing the length of time the animal spent in the stunning box and without causing the animal increased stress.

One of the greatest problems in delivering animals to the point of slaughter is presented by the necessity for pigs to be stunned by high-voltage electric current, or in a single-carriage 'Ferris wheel' compact gas stunner, to arrive at the point of stunning continuously at a rate of several hundred/hour, in single file, and to become confined in a 'V'-shaped restrainer. Pigs prefer to move as a group, with their comrades on either side. They resent being forced into single file. The answer, to some extent, has been to utilise a *curved double race* where the pig can see his comrades moving along beside him, but there still comes a point in most cases where the double race must feed into one single restrainer. The single-file chute should be at least 6.1 m long to achieve continuous flow, but no more than 10.7 m long, to keep the pigs moving without excessive goading.

An alternative for high line speeds is to use a *gas stunning system* which allows several pigs to be stunned simultaneously. The pigs may be allowed to move along a passageway with the group size gradually decreasing as pigs progress at different speeds, until the required number is attained. This group, usually of about five or six pigs, is moved into a small pen which descends into the gaseous environment where stunning occurs. Line speeds of 800 pigs/hour can be accommodated by this system.

A relatively recent advance in *restrainer* systems is a double or single moving rail which lifts the animal under its belly and carries it along. The system, which can be used for sheep, pigs or calves, is said to result in reduced struggling.

The effect on pigs of immediate pre-slaughter stress as measured by post-mortem blood biochemistry and meat quality has been studied by Warriss *et al.* (1994). They concluded that these subjective assessments of the stress suffered by pigs correlated well with objective measures, specifically the sound level immediately before stunning, and that as expected higher stress levels were associated with poorer meat quality. They confirmed that the confinement and restraint associated with race-restrainers were stressful to the animals, and that the use of *electric goads* to coerce pigs to move along these systems, particularly at high line speeds, increased the levels of stress.

## THE SLAUGHTERING PROCESS

The European Council Directive 93/119/EEC on the Protection of Animals at the Time of Slaughter or Killing, applies to the movement, lairaging, restraint, stunning, slaughter and killing of animals bred and kept for the production of meat, skin, fur or other products and to Methods of Killing Animals for the Purposes of Disease Control. This Directive has been implemented in Great Britain as The Welfare of Animals (Slaughter or Killing) Regulations 1995.

In the past, all too often, the task of stunning was given to untrained individuals. It cannot be emphasised too strongly that, *in addition to the important matter of animal welfare, proper stunning/killing plays a significant part in preventing injuries to staff engaged in the subsequent shackling and bleeding processes*. Article 7 of the Directive states that 'no person shall engage in the movement, lairaging restraint, stunning, slaughter or killing of animals unless he has the knowledge and skill necessary to perform the tasks humanely and efficiently, in accordance with the requirements of the Directive'. For those operatives employed in the actual slaughtering process, the competent authority must ensure that they possess the necessary skill, ability and professional knowledge. The Official Veterinarian must ensure that this is the case and continuously assess and review the skills and abilities of personnel licensed under the 1995 Regulations.

A licence to slaughter animals is granted to an operative who is over 18 years of age, who is a 'fit and proper' individual for this responsible duty, who has a good general attitude to animal welfare and a good theoretical knowledge of slaughtering procedure, and who can demonstrate competent practical technique. A person may be licensed to slaughter one or more named species of animal using one or more particular methods or techniques.

Slaughter of farm animals is normally a two-stage process of stunning and bleeding, but direct killing can be followed by satisfactory bleeding provided this is effected within 3 minutes.

The permitted methods for *stunning* farm animals, listed in Annex C of the Directive are:

1. Captive bolt pistol
2. Concussion
3. Electronarcosis
4. Exposure to carbon dioxide.

The permitted methods for *killing* are:

1. Free bullet pistol or rifle
2. Electrocution
3. Exposure to carbon dioxide.

Article 2 of the Directive provides an exemption from the need for prior stunning in the case of slaughter required by certain religious rites.

## ASSESSMENT OF UNCONSCIOUSNESS AT SLAUGHTER

The nervous system, composed of a central part, the brain and spinal cord (central nervous system, CNS), and the peripheral nerves, is the important control and communication system of the body. The brain, consisting of two cerebral hemispheres, cerebellum and medulla oblongata, is responsible for coordinating all the activities necessary for the maintenance of life. Situated in the bony cranial cavity, to which it closely conforms, it contains all the vital centres controlling the body's many activities.

The *waking state*, or *state of consciousness*, has been described as 'a dynamic equilibrium between the activation of cerebral neuronal networks maintained by the incessant impact of innumerable ascendant and associative impulses and the cumulative functional depression resulting from the very continuity of this state of excitation' (Bremner, 1954). Consciousness involves an awareness of the environment and the ability to appreciate pain.

Consciousness may disappear as a consequence of sleep, concussion, the administration of an anaesthetic, lack of blood supply to the brain and thereby oxygen (anoxia) and an electroconvulsive shock or death.

In the act of slaughter it is essential that a state of *unconsciousness* or *insensibility* be *instantaneously* produced to ensure total freedom from suffering, this being further ensured by immediate exsanguination. Where *cardiac arrest* has been created there is an almost immediate insensibility which is *permanent*. The discovery that adequate bleeding ensues despite cardiac dysfunction in this method makes this a most important development in the slaughter of animals. It had been always thought that a beating heart was necessary for proper bleeding, but this has been discounted provided sticking is performed soon afterwards.

The *time taken to reach insensibility* due to exsanguination depends upon the technique utilised in sticking, the species, the age of the animal, whether the carcase is suspended or prone and the method of pre-stunning used. Based on electrocephalographic data, sheep have been shown to become insensible in 2–7 seconds, pigs in 12–30 s (average 18 s) and cattle in 20–102 s (average 55 s). The species differences are due to differences in the arteries which supply the blood to the brain via the Circle of Willis. In all cases, in the interests of the animal, it should be assumed that the upper limit applies.

While much of the excellent work on the assessment of the effectiveness of stunning carried out in New Zealand by Blackmore and Newhook, in England by Gregory, Wooton and others and in Denmark and Holland has been based on electroencephalograms (EEG) and electrocorticograms (ECoG), reliance in actual meat plant operations assessment is based on visual observation of behaviour. The animal cannot communicate the degree and type of a painful stimulus in the same way as man. Only by behavioural and biochemical responses can this be done by the animal and reliance has of necessity to be placed on the former.

The *typical signs of effective stunning by electricity* are immediate collapse of the animal with flexion, followed by rigid extension of the limbs, opisthotonus (extreme arching back of the neck and spine), downward rolling of the eyeballs with tonic (continuous) muscular spasm changing into clonic (repeated violent) spasms and eventual muscle flaccidity. The term *electroplectic fit* has been used to describe these signs of an *effective stun*. The tonic spasms last for some 10–25 s, and the clonic phase 15–45 s, in both pigs and sheep.

The *typical signs of an effective stun using percussive methods* in cattle are immediate collapse of the animal followed by tonic spasm lasting about 10–15 s, then slow clonic movements of the hindlegs and eventually vigorous hindleg movements. In pigs the tonic phase lasts 3–5 s. Normal rhythmic breathing must cease, and the eyeball should face outwards with a fixed gaze and not be rotated inwards.

In *carbon dioxide anaesthesia in pigs* the effects are those of a chemical anaesthetic, with the eventual onset of insensibility. A period of increased respiratory rate is followed by slow respiratory movements and final dyspnoea (difficult breathing). Corneal and palpebral reflexes are absent and extreme muscle flaccidity supervenes. The limbs and jaw are consequently relaxed.

The use of palpebral, corneal or pupillary reflexes to ascertain the effectiveness of stunning is inappropriate for most methods of stunning. Palpebral and corneal reflexes are not under cortical control and may therefore be present in an animal or bird which has been rendered insensible. Conversely, the palpebral reflex may be absent in an animal which has been ineffectively electrically stunned. Although complete pupillary dilatation is a reliable sign of total insensibility of an animal nearing the point of death, it is of little practical use since, for example, it has been demonstrated that while sensibility as measured by electrical activity occurs 8 s after the decapitation of a sheep's head, complete pupillary dilatation does not occur until 87 s.

The most reliable objective sign of loss of sensibility is the *absence of respiratory activity*. The return of regular respiratory movement after stunning, but not irregular respiratory gasps, should always be a cause of concern. 'Gagging' respiratory movements are generally a sign of imminent brain death.

## METHODS OF STUNNING

The choice of a particular method of stunning depends on many different factors – class of animal, intended line speed, humane aspects, capital and maintenance costs, efficiency of equipment, ease of operation, safety of personnel, effects on carcase and brain, along with religious and legal requirements.

### **Percussive stunning** (Fig. 8.1)

Many different types of percussive stunning pistol are in use throughout the world, having been introduced at the end of the nineteenth century. They are generally operated by means of a blank cartridge, although some are

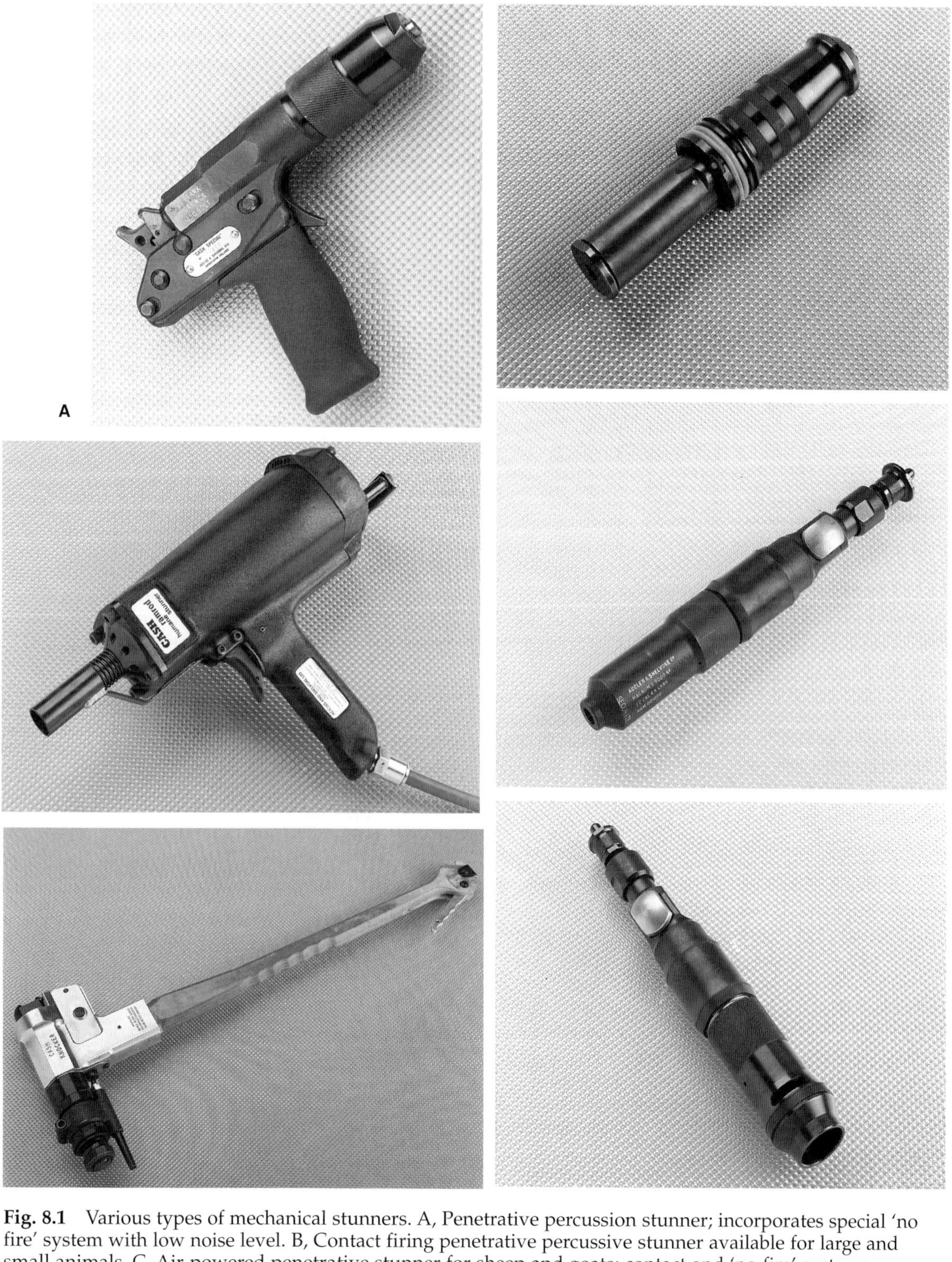


**Fig. 8.1** Various types of mechanical stunners. A, Penetrative percussion stunner; incorporates special 'no fire' system with low noise level. B, Contact firing penetrative percussive stunner available for large and small animals. C, Air-powered penetrative stunner for sheep and goats; contact and 'no-fire' systems incorporated. D, Penetrative percussive stunner .22 calibre; palm- or finger-activated trigger; firing pin pull to cock instrument. E, Contact and failsafe non-penetrative percussive stunner for use in deep stunning pens; suitable for ritual slaughter. F, Non-penetrative percussive stunner incorporating 'no-fire' system; suitable for ritual slaughter. (By kind permission of Messrs Accles and Shelvoke, Witton, Birmingham, UK)

pneumatic in design. With the most common pistol, the *captive bolt pistol*, a bolt is propelled forward on discharge of the blank cartridge and automatically recoils into the barrel. Ideally, the bolt should be recessed into the body of the pistol so that when the muzzle is held firmly against the animal's head, the bolt can gain velocity before penetration of the skull occurs.

It is important when using the captive bolt pistol to ensure that the correct strength of cartridge is used for the different species. With the *Cash* instruments these range in strength from 1 grain for small animals such as milk lambs, up to 3 and 4 grains for large cattle and mature bulls (1 grain = 0.065 grams). In most cases a 0.22 or 0.25 cartridge is used while in horses a 0.64 blank cartridge may be required for certain guns.

Properly used, the captive bolt pistol is very effective in cattle, sheep and calves but less so in bulls and pigs, especially sows and boars, in which the frontal bone structure is very thick.

This *penetrative type of percussive stunner* produces immediate and permanent insensibility by destruction of the cortex and deeper parts of the brain, a rapid rise and then fall in intracranial pressure and the sudden jerk due to the energy the bolt imparts to the head, producing what is known as *acceleration concussion*. These effects result in depolarisation of neurons in the brain, including those of the cerebral cortex.

The important force in producing unconsciousness with the captive bolt pistol is the *actual velocity of the bolt* and the speed at which it strikes the brain, rather than the penetration of the brain *per se*. A velocity of about 55 m/s is recommended for steers, heifers and cows, and between 65 and 70 m/s for young bulls. The strength of the cartridge must be matched with the robustness of the gun to prevent metal fatigue and breaks in washers, buffers, etc.

The captive bolt pistol is a very useful instrument but it cannot be used for slaughter at rates of over 240–250/h owing to difficulties in reloading. In this case an automatically resetting gun can be used.

*Pneumatic stunners*, where the bolt is activated under a pressure of 80–120 p.s.i., require somewhat complicated actions to fire them, and there may be occasions when air pressure is inadequate. With proper pressure, however, a high bolt velocity can be achieved.

*Non-penetrative percussion stunners* using a mushroom head are sometimes used in calves when brains are collected for edible use and these are in regular use in the USA. Properly used, this method is capable of producing immediate insensibility. Much depends on the operative as to whether or not blood splashing results, especially in the case of lambs. If the animals are handled properly and the interval between stunning and bleeding is short, blood splashing in muscle will be minimal. In any case, the period between stunning and sticking should not exceed 30 s with non-penetrative percussive stunning of cattle. This compares with a recommended stun-to-sticking interval of less than 60 s with penetrative percussive stunners in cattle, <15 s for sheep and goats and <10 s for calves.

### **Head sites for percussive stunning** (Fig. 8.2)

With both types of percussive stunners, care must be taken to hold the instrument reasonably firmly against the animal's head at the proper point and direction (Fig. 8.2). In *adult cattle* the correct point is in the middle of the forehead where two lines taken from the medial canthus of each eye to the base of the opposite horn or horn prominence cross. The gun is placed at right angles to the forehead and after firing is lifted away from the falling animal. In *calves* the pistol should be placed slightly lower on the head than for adult cattle, while for *bulls* and *old cows* the muzzle is placed 1.5 cm to the side of the ridge running down the centre of the forehead. Cattle should never be shot in the poll position.

In *hornless sheep and goats* the pistol is placed on the top of the head and aimed towards the gullet, while for *horned sheep and goats* the muzzle is placed behind the ridge which runs between the horns, the direction of aim being the same.

For *bacon weight pigs* the pistol is placed about 2.5 cm above the level of the eyes and fired upwards into the cranial cavity. In older animals captive bolt stunning is less reliable owing to the massive nature of the skulls and the large frontal sinuses of older pigs. The muzzle should be placed about 5 cm above the level of the eyes to the side of the ridge which is in the mid-line of the skull, and at right angles to the frontal surface.

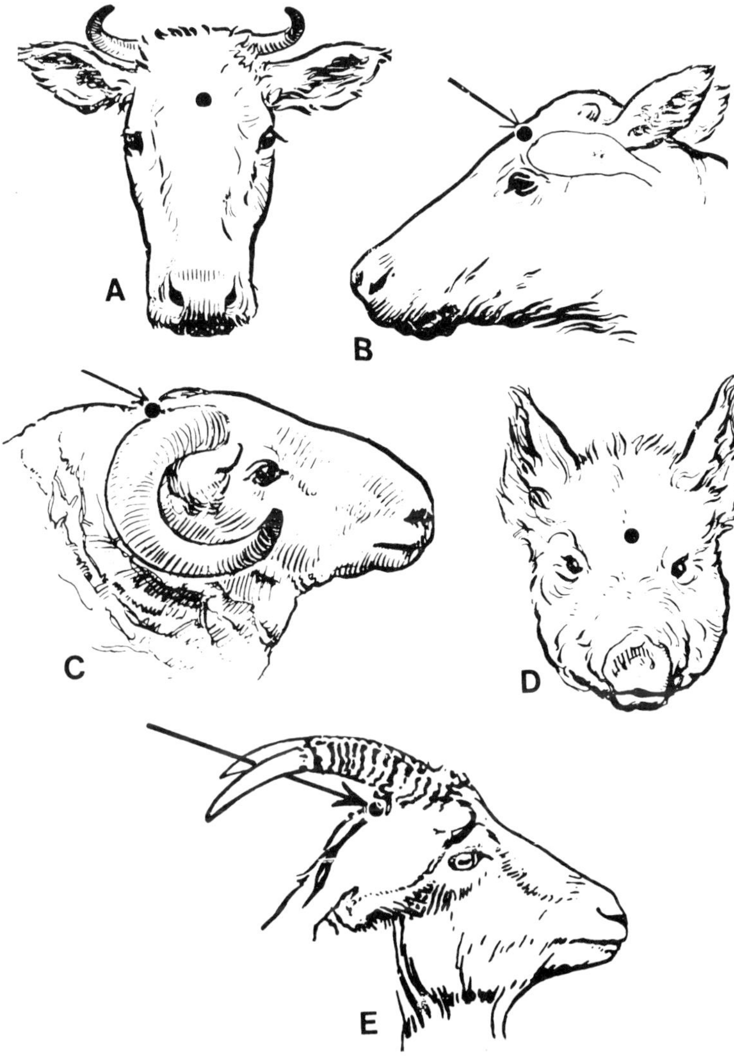


**Fig. 8.2** Points of application for percussive stunning: A, adult cattle; B, calves; C, horned sheep; D, pigs; E, horned goats. (By courtesy of the Universities Federation for Animal Welfare)

In *horses* a special type of captive bolt pistol with a longer and heavier bolt is employed. The muzzle of the pistol is placed at right angles to the frontal surface ~1 cm above the point where imaginary lines from eye to ear cross as the brain is in the upper part of the head.

The *contact-firing types* of *captive bolt pistol* are much more satisfactory than the trigger-operated ones, only a light tap on the animal's head being necessary to fire them. They are quicker and easier to operate and can be loaded and fired 10–12 times a minute. However, if they are dropped on the floor or struck against the stunning box wall, the whole gun can become a dangerous missile.

A defect of percussive stunning and the use of the free bullet is noise.

Most of the really serious defects, however, arise from misuse or from instruments in poor state of repair, as is the case with all forms of stunning. The European Directive on the Protection of Animals at the Time of Slaughtering and Killing, makes it a responsibility of the Official Veterinarian to ensure that the instruments used for stunning, and for restraint, are in a good state of repair.

The importance of *regular maintenance* if the pistols are to function correctly cannot be overemphasised. The velocity of the bolt may be significantly reduced by a build-up of carbon or corrosion on the piston, which drives the bolt forward, or by excessive wear in any of the moving parts. While some manufacturers recommend cleaning every 70 shots, *daily dismantling and thorough cleaning must be carried out*. A common indication that a pistol requires cleaning is the tip of the bolt protruding from the muzzle more than the usual distance between shots. The importance of this is emphasised by the following statement in the European legislation: 'When using a captive bolt instrument, the operator must check to ensure that the bolt retracts to its full extent after each shot. If it does not so retract, the instrument must not be used until it is repaired.' All forms of mechanical stunning devices should be fitted with safety levers to minimise the chances of accidents.

A back-up pistol should always be on hand in cases of emergency.

### *Bolt velocity check*

A device is now available for checking the bolt velocity of all Cash penetrative stunners. The stunner is placed upright in the device and fired, stunning performance of the various cartridges being recorded as FAST, OK or SLOW by means of indicator lights on a separate recorder. Accurate monitoring of stunner performance means more effective stunning, fewer second shots, greater operator efficiency and safety, and a high standard of animal welfare.

### *Neural tissue embolism in cattle*

Embolism with brain tissue in the branches of the pulmonary artery following penetrative stunning may occur but is comparatively rare. Garland *et al.* (1996) in the USA reported the condition in 2.5–5% of cattle stunned by a pneumatic-actuated penetrative captive bolt pistol, the diaphragmatic lobe of the lung being the area most commonly affected. A few cases have occurred in human beings following fatal head injuries (McMillan, 1956).

### *Free bullet pistol* (Fig. 8.3)

The free bullet pistol is frequently used to destroy horses, and sometimes cattle, humanely. Bullets may be of the hollow pointed type, frangible iron plastic missiles or powdered iron bullets fired from a small-bore rifle (.22 calibre) or a small instrument held against the forehead. The benefit of hollow point projectiles is a greater enhancement of the mushrooming effect or expansion on impact; more energy is imparted to the tissues with increased tissue destruction and there is less likelihood of the missile exiting the head.

The points of application are in general the same as those for the captive bolt pistol, in the case of horses this being high up in the forehead immediately below the roots of the forelock where two lines from the medial canthus of each eye to the base of the opposite ear cross. The direction of aim in horses is slightly below the right-angle plane to the forehead.

Great care must be taken to avoid accidents when using free projectiles and each instrument should be fitted with a safety device. In future the use of the free bullet is likely to be increasingly discouraged for reasons of safety.

Because of the destruction of brain tissue by the penetrating bolt or free bullet, the brain cannot be utilised for edible purposes. The commercial drive to recover all edible parts of an animal may well lead to the development of more efficient non-penetrative percussive type stunning instruments. This would also decrease the possibility of aerosol contamination of the slaughterhall environment with brain material, with the potential this may have for the spread of BSE organisms around the slaughter area.

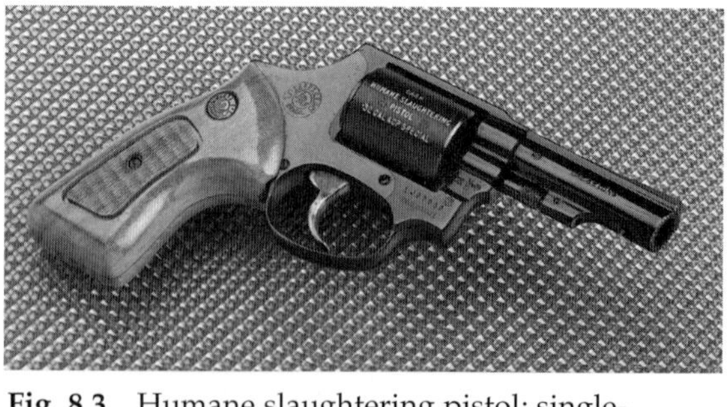

**Fig. 8.3** Humane slaughtering pistol; single-shot/free bullet, .32 calibre. This instrument is not a stunner. (By kind permission of Messrs Accles and Shelvoke, Witton, Birmingham, UK)

*In the case of captive bolt pistols and firearms discharging free bullets, the provisions of the Firearms Act 1968 apply in the United Kingdom, though cartridges for the former are exempt. This requires that all those who possess, carry or discharge a captive bolt pistol (with the exception of slaughterhouse employees working within a licensed slaughterhouse), must have a current firearms certificate. This is not the same as a shotgun certificate, and requires a separate application to a local police station. When the certificate is received, it must be sent to the supplier of the pistol for ratification of sale.*

### Water jet stunning

A novel form of percussive stunning, described by Lambooij (1996), utilises a fine jet of water to penetrate the skull and mechanically destroy the brain by the induction of laceration, crushing and/or shockwaves to such an extent that immediate unconsciousness is induced. The 0.5 mm jet, applied at pressures of 3500–4000 bar at a similar site as for the captive bolt, drills through the skin and skull in 0.2–0.4 s.

Destruction of the brain results in convulsions, which can be controlled using an immobilising current of 400 milliamps applied using 40 volts. Initial work has indicated that it may be possible to produce meat of superior quality, compared to either electrical or $CO_2$ stunning, using this method.

### Carbon dioxide and other gas mixtures

*Carbon dioxide* was first used to induce pre-slaughter anaesthesia in animals in 1904, but not successfully on a commercial scale until 1950. Since then the method has been modified in several different ways and is now used fairly widely throughout the world although not as extensively as it could be, probably because of the high cost of installation and operation. The technique was banned for a period during the 1980s in the Netherlands because it was thought to lead to unconsciousness under very stressful conditions for the animal.

While some authorities suggest that the struggling witnessed in pigs for a period of some 15–20 s when they first come into contact with high concentrations of gas is due to the very irritant properties of carbon dioxide, others are of the opinion that the struggling is equivalent to the induction stages of anaesthesia and that the pig is in fact unconscious during this period. Raj and Gregory (1995) demonstrated that pigs showed no aversion to 30% $CO_2$ in air but a marked aversion to 90% $CO_2$ in air.

Council Directive 93/119/EC on the Protection of Animals at the Time of Slaughter or Killing requires that the concentration of $CO_2$ be at least 70%. It also recommended that the use of other gases, or combinations of gases, for stunning or killing should be investigated. Raj and Gregory (1995) reported that no aversion was shown by pigs to an environment of 90% *argon*, and in 1996 suggested that their ascending order of preference for gaseous environments for stunning pigs would be:

1. 2% oxygen in argon (anoxia) in which the respiratory distress shown by the pigs was minimum but the induction of anaesthesia probably too slow for commercial use;
2. 30% $CO_2$ in argon with 2% residual oxygen, which was intermediate with regard to respiratory distress and rate of induction of anaesthesia;
3. 90% $CO_2$ in air, in which the induction of anaesthesia was rapid and the respiratory distress was severe but short lasting (about 15 s).

Experiments have shown that *nitrous oxide* ($N_2O$) may be an alternative anaesthetic gas for stunning pigs (Monin, 1996). Its density is close to that of $CO_2$ and so it can be used in similar equipment. The indications are that although meat quality may be improved the induction time is unacceptably long.

Currently, however, carbon dioxide is the only gas widely used for stunning animals commercially. It is usually stored in cylinders or bulk tanks as a liquid under pressure. It is also available in solid form for which a converter is necessary. (Solid $CO_2$ is occasionally used for refrigeration purposes.) The gas is non-inflammable and has a higher specific gravity than air, sinking to the bottom of any container, a fact which has to be borne in mind when it is being used for anaesthesia or euthanasia purposes. Properly used it presents no hazard to the operator.

A concentration of 80–95% $CO_2$ in air is the most suitable for pre-slaughter anaesthesia. If the concentration is too low the pigs will not be properly stunned and if it is too high there is a tendency for the pigs to become stiff, show reflex muscular activity and bleed poorly. If the exposure period is too long, superficial congestion of the skin occurs and when pigs are scalded the skin is bluish in colour.

Pigs subjected to carbon dioxide anaesthesia will regain consciousness if they are not subsequently bled, the recovery time varying with the concentration of the gas, but averaging about 90 s. It is important, therefore, that in addition to the correct concentration of gas, the period of exposure should be 45 s and bleeding should take place as soon as possible and certainly within 30 seconds of the pigs leaving the gas chamber. It is possible that some adverse effects observed on occasions are due to incorrect concentrations of gas and air and/or inadequate or too long exposure times. These untoward effects include convulsive struggling and varying degrees of excitement.

The type of *apparatus* employed to administer the gas depends mainly upon the required rate of slaughter. There are three main forms:

1 The *oval tunnel* ('combi') is used for killing rates of up to 600 pigs per hour. As the name suggests the gas tunnel is in the form of an oval through which a slot conveyor carries the pigs, the actual tunnel sloping downwards at an angle of 30° to the anaesthetising chamber. On exit the pigs are shackled, hoisted to an overhead rail and bled. The actual conveyor in the tunnel is divided into ten compartments, one pig being accommodated in each compartment. Pigs up to 113 kg can be handled in this equipment, which is not suitable for other species (Fig. 8.4).

2 The *dip lift* is suitable for any size of pig as well as calves and sheep. It consists of a cage 213 cm long, 68 cm high and 53 cm wide which, when the animal enters it, descends vertically to the $CO_2$ pit where it remains for the pre-set time and then automatically returns to ground level, ejecting the unconscious animal for shackling and bleeding. The greatest advantage of the system is that it allows several pigs to be stunned simultaneously, assisting immediate pre-slaughter handling. This is suitable for small meat plants (Fig. 8.5).

3 The Compact $CO_2$ Immobiliser is a horizontally-revolving apparatus divided into four to eight compartments operating in such a way that, when one section is uppermost for loading, the others are rotating to submerge in the gas chamber. The unit usually has a capacity of up to 300 pigs per hour. In a commonly used design the pigs are exposed to 10% $CO_2$ at the first position, 30% for 10 s at the second, 60% for 10 s at the third and over 90% for 20 s at the fourth and fifth, after which the pigs are discharged from the unit (Figs 8.6, 8.7).

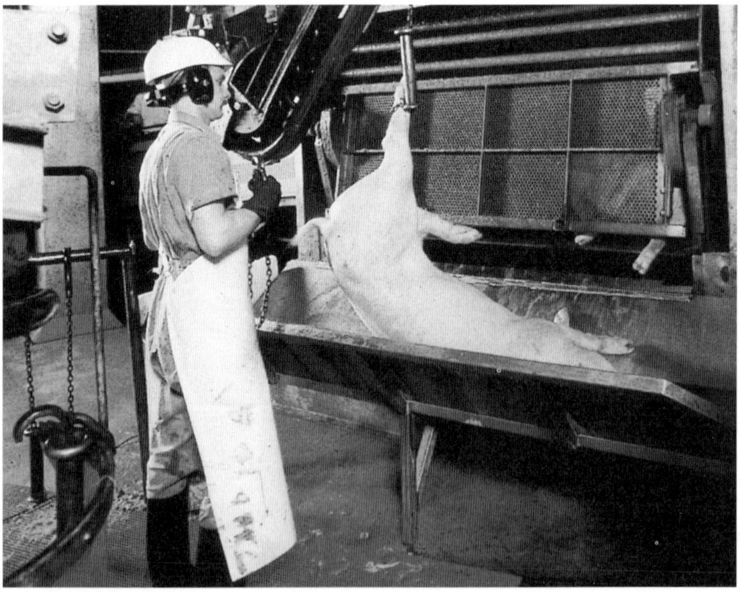

**Fig. 8.4** $CO_2$ anaesthesia. Oval tunnel/Combi system showing convenient shackling position after stunning. (By courtesy of Messrs SFK Meat Processing A/S, Albuen 37, DK 6000, Kolding, Denmark)

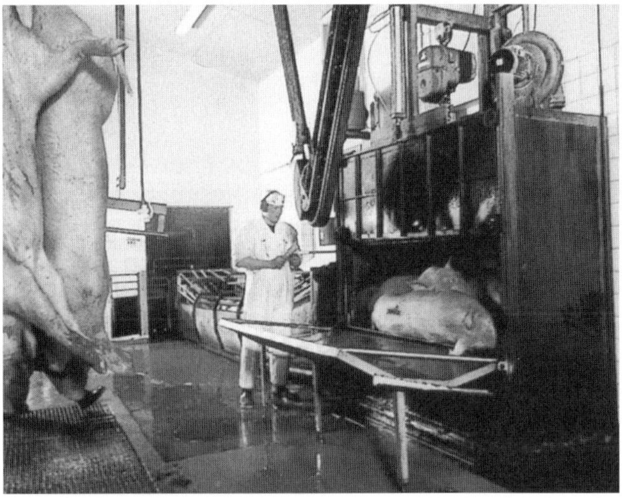

**Fig. 8.5** $CO_2$ anaesthesia. Dip lift system showing discharge of pigs on to receiving stand. (By courtesy of Messrs SFK Meat Processing A/S, Albuen 37, DK 6000, Kolding, Denmark)

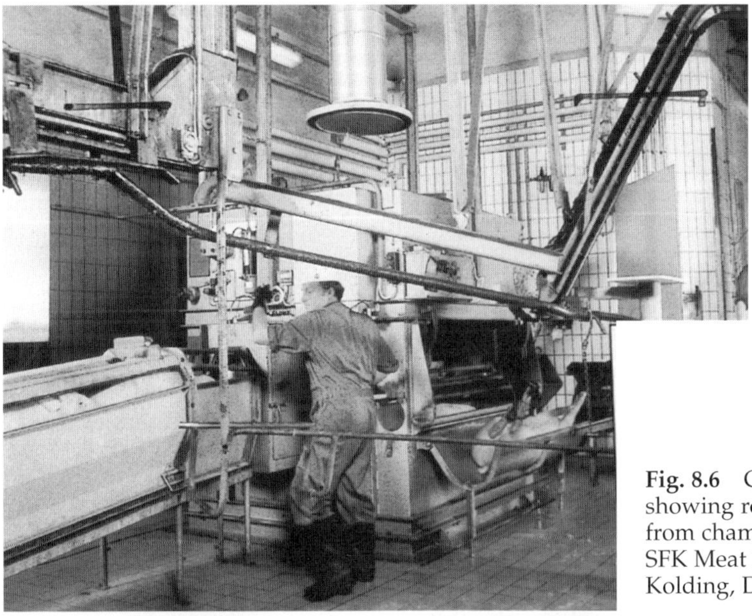

**Fig. 8.6** $CO_2$ anaesthesia. Compact system showing reception of pigs at left and emergence from chamber at right. (By courtesy of Messrs SFK Meat Processing A/S, Albuen 37, DK 6000, Kolding, Denmark)

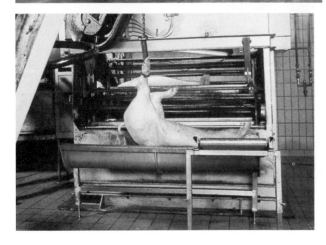

**Fig. 8.7** $CO_2$ anaesthesia. Compact system showing ejection of pigs from chamber and barred pig cradles. (By courtesy of Messrs SFK Meat Processing A/S, Albuen 37, DK 6000, Kolding, Denmark)

With all systems, the chamber must be fitted with *devices for measuring the gas concentration* at the point of maximum exposure and for giving a clearly visible and audible warning if the concentration of the $CO_2$ falls below the required level.

Similar concentrations of carbon dioxide and exposure times are used for sheep, but because of the heavy fleece more gas is required and the operation is, therefore, more expensive. Sufficient information is not yet available to assess the value of the method in calves.

The *advantages* claimed for carbon dioxide anaesthesia include relaxed carcases, allowing easier dehairing and dressing, less noise and reduced labour requirements. It has also been contended that the yield of blood from pigs stunned by this method is 0.75% better because carbon dioxide stimulates respiration and thus favours blood circulation and consequently bleeding. Muscular haemorrhages are said to be avoided, the number of bone fractures is reduced to zero, and the amount of PSE may be reduced.

## Electrical stunning

There are many different types of electrical stunning systems in use, most being manually-operated (Fig. 8.8) while a few are automatic in operation, especially for pigs and poultry.

This method consists of passing an alternating current through the brain and, with some techniques, also the heart of the animal, the instrument most commonly employed being one which resembles a pair of *tongs* (Fig. 8.8). The current causes massive depolarisation of neurons in the brain, resulting in an epileptiform seizure. Since electrical stunning was first introduced in the 1930s, it has received considerable attention from research workers but there is still a lack of knowledge on its efficiency in producing insensibility. It must be agreed that if certain requirements are not complied with, the method, like all others, may be inhumane. If the electrodes are poorly positioned, the electrical current may produce a condition known as *'missed shock'* in which the animal, although paralysed, is fully conscious. Provided it is carried out correctly, however, the electrical method of stunning may be regarded as efficacious and humane since it causes incoordination of the cerebral nerve cells and what may be aptly defined as a confusional state of the brain.

The desiderata necessary for the production of genuine anaesthesia are as follows:

1 The strength of the electric shock should be sufficient to ensure that the animal is killed outright by cardiac arrest or remains insensible until death occurs by exsanguination.
2 Provided sufficient current is applied, a genuine *electroplectic shock* will be induced. The mains voltage may fluctuate considerably and at times fall to a dangerously low level in the stunning apparatus and it is therefore required that every electrical stunning apparatus is fitted with indicators visible to the operator that provide a warning if the current or voltage drops, or the time of application falls short of 7 s for low-voltage systems and below 3 s for high-voltage equipment.

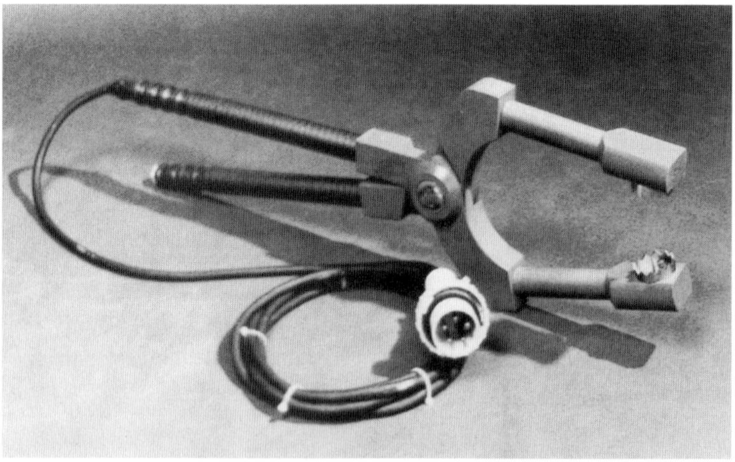

**Fig. 8.8** Electrical stunning tongs.

In order to ensure that the minimum period of application is achieved in every case, the European Council Directive 93/119/EC requires that the stunning apparatus 'must incorporate an *audible or visible device indicating the length of time of its application* to an animal'. The Directive also requires that the tongs should be designed to incorporate a *sensor* or similar *fail-safe device* which would ensure that the equipment did not function if the correct current was not flowing. The fail-safe device operates by setting the maximum impedance that can be sensed by the tongs, given a constant voltage, for a particular species and result in an effective stun. No current will pass through the tongs if the impedance measured across the animal's head is in excess of that set as the maximum.

3 The electrodes should be correctly positioned so that the current will pass through the thalamus and cortex, the chief sensory centres in the forebrain. The electrical resistance of contact with the hair and skin may be lowered by ensuring that the electrodes are kept moist by immersion in brine and the skin of the head is kept clean but dry. The practice of wetting the pig's head should be discouraged since it may result in current tracking over the surface of the pig's skin rather than through the brain. Passage of electrical current is facilitated if the calorific intake of the animal is reduced and its state of hydration increased.

*The animal should be bled immediately after unconsciousness has been produced*, otherwise it may regain consciousness though still remain paralysed. This requirement may be compromised by legislation which delays sticking by making it a necessity for pigs to be bled out of sight of their comrades.

There is little doubt that the failure of operators to observe these criteria has been the cause of much of the criticism of electrical stunning methods, firstly, on the grounds that the method was not always humane and, secondly, because *haemorrhages* were often observed in the muscular tissue of animals stunned by electrical means. Muscular haemorrhages can be obviated or reduced considerably by prior resting, correct stunning and immediate bleeding. In Denmark, great importance is attached to the latter factor, and in pigs the electrical apparatus is kept in position on the head and vasoconstriction is maintained until the moment the throat cut is made.

Electrical stunning is most widely used for pigs, but it is also satisfactory for sheep and calves. Electrical stunning has not proved entirely satisfactory for the anaesthesia of cattle, possibly because of the insulating effect of the fine hairs on the animal's head, although certain continental authorities have found it satisfactory.

A high-voltage *head-to-brisket* system operates in New Zealand for religious slaughter. Electrodes are applied to the animal in a purpose-built stunning pen following capture in a neck yoke. On capture, a chin lift operates from which a nose contact plate is applied. A current of 2.5 A (at 550 V) is applied between the nose and neck yoke for 3 s to stun the animal, with an additional current applied between the neck and a brisket electrode to produce cardiac arrest.

The efficacy of electrical anaesthesia is not dependent on the individual factors of voltage, amperage or time, but on the total quantity of electrical energy supplied, expressed in watt-seconds (watt-seconds = voltage × amperage × time).

It is necessary for an adequate amount of electricity to pass through the brain in a sufficiently short period of time. This depends on the voltage applied and the resistance, or more correctly impedance, present. If too high a current is employed, carcase quality may be compromised by the production of *muscle haemorrhages and broken bones*; if too low a voltage is used, the animal may be paralysed but still conscious of pain. Operator safety also plays a part in determining voltage levels; levels under 150 V are not generally effective, especially allowing for fluctuations in mains voltage.

Since the brains of animals are relatively small, it is important that the electrodes are accurately and firmly placed high up on the sides of the head. The irregular anatomy of the head makes this difficult, especially if the animal is moving. The electrodes are easier to position if the tongs are relatively heavy and if the operator is able to apply them to the animal downwards rather than upwards or horizontally. Placement of tongs is also achieved with less effort in efficient restrainer-conveyor systems. *Head-to-body* equipment should be correctly counterbalanced. The electrodes must be in good repair and not corroded or coated with carbon. It is essential that the equipment be earthed properly for operator safety.

The passage of electric current through the brain results in a rapid rise of blood pressure due to vasoconstriction and increased heart rate, hence the need for immediate bleeding in order to avoid muscle splashing.

For *head-only* electrical stunning systems, a minimum electric current of 400 mA for pigs, and 250 mA for sheep and lambs, has been recommended to produce an effective stun when the tongs are placed in the ideal position. However, most experts set their recommendations considerably higher at 1.3 A for sheep, 0.6 A for lambs, 1 A for pigs and 1.5 A for cattle, having made the assumption that tong placement on the head would frequently be far from ideal.

*Low-voltage electrical stunning*

Low-voltage electrical stunning, i.e. using less than 150 V, is the most common type in operation in Britain and consists of a control panel, on which voltage can be adjusted, meters capable of measuring the current and voltage as it is applied, and a pair of tongs with terminal electrodes for application to the sides of the animal's head. In order to create a better contact, the electrodes are immersed in a saline solution before use or possess in-built water jets.

Since some doubt exists about the overall effectiveness of low-voltage stunning and the length of time for which it should be applied, more use is currently being made of high-voltage systems.

*High-voltage electrical stunning*

Investigations into electrical stunning have shown that high-voltage systems using 300 V or above are more effective than low-voltage systems provided they are used with automatic restrainers and with due regard to operator safety. The application time must be at least 3 s. Fractures (vertebrae and scapula) may occur in pigs stunned on the floor.

High-voltage electrical systems are available in a fully automatic form which incorporates two V-shaped restrainer-conveyors (Fig. 8.6). These are placed in series and move at different speeds so that the pigs are separated sufficiently to present their heads for stunning to a set of specially shaped electrodes suspended on hinged metal plates which hang down inside the second conveyer and contact the animal's head as it passes through. The stunning voltage is of the order 600–1000 V. Ninety per cent of the pigs are killed, the remaining 10% are only stunned. Difficulties may be encountered with this system in maintaining a consistently correct positioning of the electrodes across the brain of the pig. It is particularly important that a back-up stunner is always present to deal with any animal which suffers poor positioning of the electrodes, resulting in only partial stunning.

*Head to back/leg stunning* (Fig. 8.9)

High-voltage electrical stunning in addition to being used for head-only application, may incorporate special tongs through which current is applied simultaneously to the head and back/leg. In this system the brain is anaesthetised and the heart put into arrest, thus cutting off the blood supply to the brain, which suffers death before the anaesthesia ends. Research work carried out at the Meat Research Institute in Bristol, UK, has shown that brain function ceased 23 s after this system of stunning, whereas this time was extended to some 50 s with head-only stunning. The animal

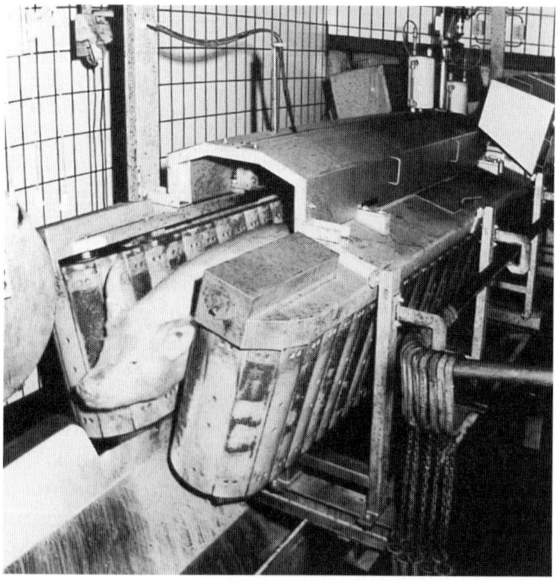

**Fig. 8.9** Automatic head/leg stunning in restrainer/conveyor. (By courtesy of Messrs Nijhuis, Lichtenvoorde, The Netherlands)

is, in fact, killed, thus improving animal welfare and making the stunning-to-sticking interval less important. Provided sticking is performed intrathoracically within 3 minutes, bleeding is satisfactory. A minimum current of 1.3 A applied with a minimum of 250 V is recommended for pigs and 1.0 A at 375 V for lambs.

In order to be fully effective, head-to-back/leg stunning must be combined with automatic restraining systems which prevent adverse reflex muscular movements and the possibility of fractures besides making the task of shackling and bleeding easier for operatives. 'Pelt-burn' in sheep occasionally occurs on the back with this method.

Whatever type of electrical stunning is used, a *back-up stunner*, in the form of a portable captive bolt pistol should be available for use, not only on incorrectly-stunned animals, but also for casualty animals in their transport vehicle or in the lairage. It may be advisable to have an additional set of stunning tongs for use in several electrical sockets positioned throughout the lairage and casualty accommodation. This is particularly useful if sows and boars, which are difficult to stun effectively with a captive bolt, are to be slaughtered.

## EFFECT OF STUNNING ON MEAT QUALITY

Most of the problems associated with penetrative percussive stunning (captive bolt) appear to result from an unduly long interval between stunning and sticking and/or inadequate penetration of the bolt, resulting in *blood splashing in muscles*, particularly of the diaphragm, the abdominal wall, the intercostal muscles and the heart. The all-too-frequent habit of group stunning especially in sheep, is a practice that leads to this result, the animals first 'stunned' being the ones affected. This lesion tends to occur where there is a marked rise in arterial blood pressure, the highest rates taking place in head-only electrical stunning, where the incidence can be markedly reduced by the adoption of a short stun-to-stick interval.

Head-to-back/leg electrical stunning produces a very low incidence of blood splashing but petechiae may on occasions occur in connective tissues and fat. High-voltage head-only stunning in pigs sometimes results in petechial haemorrhages throughout the loin. High-voltage electrical stunning may also result in the *fracture of bones* with associated haemorrhage into surrounding tissue. The fracture is thought to be due to the force of the tonic convulsion induced during and immediately after stunning. Fractures occur in the scapula, pelvis, the neck of the femur and around the fifth or sixth thoracic vertebrae and are much more common in pigs, which have greater muscle mass than sheep.

It has also been demonstrated that the use of tongs with 300 V in a restrainer-conveyor resulted in superior pig meat quality compared with automatic stunning with 680 V, the incidence of PSE being much less in the former method which also showed superior values in relation to pH, temperature, rigor mortis, bacteriological status, etc. It is likely that these differences were due to variations in the amperage and in the number of interruptions in the flow of the current during stunning (Van der Wal, 1983).

Since carbon dioxide-anaesthetised pigs do not exhibit clonic convulsions post-stunning, they are safer to handle for the operators even when blood is being collected for human use. It is generally accepted that carbon dioxide produces the lowest incidence of PSE and blood splash, and that overall the quality of meat produced is superior.

## SLAUGHTER OF POULTRY (see also Ch. 11)

With poultry the speed of operations, which may be typically 6000 birds per hour, complicates the stunning procedure, as it does all other procedures. Indeed *the requirement for speed is a major factor in reducing the standard of all operations in modern slaughter and processing plants for all species of animals.*

Several types of electrical stunning device are utilised for poultry depending on the processing speed. In all cases bleeding is carried out immediately after stunning.

In *hand-stunning devices* one manually operated instrument is fitted with a step-down double-wound transformer to give 50, 70 and 90 V and respective currents of 100, 200 and 250 mA when connected to AC mains of 200–240 V. This device appears to be satisfactory and humane when used on domestic fowls of an average weight of 2 kg with a voltage of 70 V and a shock duration of 1–3 s. For turkeys of 6.8–9.0 kg, 90 V are applied for 10 s. Manually-operated stunning devices are only suitable for low rates of kill up to 1000 birds per hour. Assessment of the effectiveness of stunning with hand-held electrodes can be difficult. This is particularly the case with ducks and geese where the birds may be confined in cones. It is important to emphasise that correctly stunned birds can maintain a nictitating membrane and other eye reflexes.

*Automatic stunning devices* may be of a high- or low-voltage type, and are used on high-speed poultry lines. In the *high-voltage* types, 400–1000 V is carried in a grid over which the shackled birds are conveyed. The current passes through the body to the earthed shackle and needs to be high to overcome the resistance of the scaly comb and legs. Usually only the comb touches the grid but other parts of the body may be involved. Disadvantages of these devices include severe muscle contractions, fractures, imperfect bleeding in killed birds and a possible risk to employees.

*Low-voltage* electric stunners (50–60 V: AC current, 50–60 Hz) markedly reduce the above disadvantages and there is generally satisfactory narcosis with no pain or stress, though much depends on the design and operation of the equipment. As with other forms of electrical stunning, missed shock or electrical paralysis can result.

One form of low-voltage stunning apparatus utilises a cabinet on the conveyor line through which the birds pass while suspended on shackles, electrical contact being made for a period of 5 s. Birds removed from the line and not bled recover in 2–3 min. The stunner uses 50 V and 200 mA for broilers and 70 V for chickens, the birds' heads being drawn through a saline water bath.

The signs of an *electroplectic fit* in poultry are usually taken to be head with raised hackles arched towards back; eyes wide open; legs rigidly extended; body showing constant, repeated muscle tremors; wings, with flight feathers slightly spread, applied close to the body and displaying rapid, short bursts of flapping and tail feathers turned up over the back. Little reliance should be placed on the absent corneal reflex.

Investigations into the stunning of poultry have shown that in many instances birds are not properly stunned before venesection. In 1980 the Farm Animal Welfare Coordinating Executive in England reported that one-third of birds emerged dead from the water bath and another third were unstunned. Schutt-Abraham *et al.* (1983) in Switzerland considered that only about one-third of the chickens passing through the stunner can be looked upon as properly stunned. In addition, automatic neck cutting frequently fails to sever both carotid arteries as is recommended within 15 s of birds emerging from the water bath. It is essential that an operator is always present to check that the birds have been properly stunned and to sever the carotid arteries manually if necessary. Turkeys must not be immersed in a scalding tank or be plucked for 2 min after neck cutting; 90 s for other birds.

In view of these serious findings and because bleeding can be as satisfactory in killed as in stunned birds, it is recommended by Heath (1984) that 'an actual voltage of 200 V can generally be depended on to be accompanied by at least the required mA passing through each broiler'. The recommended current using a water-bath stunner is not less than 120 mA for chickens, 130 mA for ducks and 150 mA for turkeys (Gregory, 1993). This will induce a cardiac arrest in about 99% of the birds. It is further recommended that the birds be immersed in the water bath at least up to the base of their wings.

The use of *gaseous mixtures* for the stunning of poultry in their transport crates prior to shackling has obvious benefits for welfare. Various concentrations of $CO_2$ and argon in air have been trialled experimentally and it has been concluded that stunning with concentrations of $CO_2$ over 30% has no welfare advantages over stunning in argon with 2% residual oxygen, or a mixture of 30% $CO_2$ and 60% argon in air. Birds stunned with argon alone take twice as long to lose sensibility as those stunned using other mixtures, but the birds show none of the behavioural signs, such as gasping and head shaking, associated with the irritant properties of $CO_2$ (Raj and Gregory, 1993, 1994). It is recommended that hanging and neck cutting in broilers should be carried out within 3 min of gas stunning if carcase defects such as red wing tips, wing vein engorgement, wing vein engorgement/haemorrhage, shoulder haemorrhage and red feather tract are to be minimised. However, gas stunning does result in fewer broken bones than electrical stunning, especially the broken wing bones which can enter the breast muscle, the so-called chokers; and breast muscle haemorrhages are eliminated.

It has been discovered that stunning with argon-induced anoxia accelerates the fall in muscle pH during the early post-mortem stage without inducing a PSE-like condition. Used in conjunction with air chilling at 1°C, filleting can be performed at 2 hours post-mortem. The eating quality of this meat was rated in tests as superior to that of control fillets.

### On-farm poultry slaughter

A recent survey carried out by the UK Humane Slaughter Association (HSA) revealed that a significant 25% of poultry producers are not satisfied with the effectiveness of the present method of culling birds on-farm. The majority of producers are killing sick or injured birds on-farm by *neck dislocation* as this is the only method currently available. It is, however, physically difficult especially when performed on large, heavy birds with strong development of neck vertebrae and muscles.

The survey disclosed that 91% of owners supported the need for a new device to slaughter birds. As a result, the HSA along with the UK Ministry of Agriculture and the British Turkey Federation (BTF) will be funding research work at Bristol University to solve this problem. The apparatus will be a portable, practical and cost-effective item which will humanely dispatch birds on the farm and thus considerably improve welfare.

### Effects of stunning on poultry meat quality

As with the larger farm animals, deleterious changes sometimes occur in poultry carcases after slaughter which are attributed to defects in the slaughter methods. These frequently result in downgrading and even condemnation. But conclusions about the effects of stunning are often contradictory and at least some of the changes encountered may in part, if not in whole, be occasioned by the stress of handling and transport.

A broiler is said to be properly bled if it does not show redness on the surface of the skin or engorgement of the visceral blood vessels. Redness of the wing tips and tail is believed to be evidence of *poor bleeding*, as is hyperaemia of the carcase.

Research work has shown that the highest blood loss occurs in broilers stunned at voltages between 50 V and 80 V. Voltages higher than this generally result in lower blood loss but *when cardiac arrest takes place the total loss of blood is much the same compared with non-cardiac arrest, although a longer time is required for bleeding*.

However, Heath (1984) has declared that 'the poultry industry's obsession with the need to withdraw the last drop of blood is unlikely to be founded on scientific, religious, economic or humanitarian grounds'. In view of the fact that many birds are improperly stunned during normal plant operations and because satisfactory bleeding can be achieved in the killed bird, the creation of cardiac arrest would appear to be the method of choice for all purposes and for all animals.

Fractures of limbs and *muscular haemorrhages* may occur, as may ill-defined *variations in colour*. The exact nature and origin of some of these lesions has not yet been determined.

## OTHER METHODS OF SLAUGHTER

Legislation in the major developed countries of the world requires that all animals slaughtered in an abattoir, except those slaughtered by the Jewish and Islamic ritual, shall first be rendered unconscious. In Spain, parts of Italy, Mexico and some South American countries, however, *cattle* were traditionally slaughtered by the *neck-stab* or *evernazione* method, in which a short double-edged knife (*puntilla*) is plunged into the occipito-atlantal space at the nape of the neck, severing the medulla oblongata. This effectively immobilises the animal without inducing insensibility. The technique is banned, and rightly so, by the Council of Europe, since animals slaughtered in this way show a photomotor reflex considered by some experts to be indicative of a state of sensibility (Lumb and Jones, 1973).

In the Arctic, *reindeer* are killed by a curved single-edged knife which after being inserted into the occipito-atlantal space, is directed forwards to destroy the brain.

In India and in the Far East, practically all animals are slaughtered while conscious. In India the majority of sheep and goats are killed by the Halal or Muslim method in which the throat is cut transversely as in the Jewish method of slaughter. The Sikh or Jakta method is also practised, the sheep or goat being decapitated by one stroke of a special sword. The Mohammedan ritual does not forbid stunning of the animal prior to bleeding provided the stunning instrument has never been used on pigs.

There is little doubt that these methods are aesthetically repugnant to some people and, in some instances, are not efficient methods of slaughter. A review of pre-slaughter stunning in the EEC (Von Mickwitz and Leach, 1977) placed enervation (neck-stab, *evernazione*) among the least effective of the six methods of stunning investigated.

The European Directive 93/119/EEC only allows non-mechanical percussive stunning for small batches of *rabbits*. If this is to be done, it must be carried out in such a way that the animal is immediately rendered unconscious and remains so until its death. As with all methods of humane slaughter, the animals must be spared any avoidable excitement, pain or suffering.

## PITHING

After *cattle* are stunned they are sometimes pithed before bleeding by the insertion of a long thin rod or closely coiled wire into the hole made by the penetrating bolt of the pistol. The insertion of this rod destroys the motor centres of the brain so that reflex muscular action does not occur at sticking, thus avoiding injury to operatives and speeding carcase dressing. There is little evidence that this operation interferes to any appreciable degree with the bleeding of the carcase, but the pithing rod or cane should not be any longer than 0.6 m; if it is too long, the spinal cord roots of the greater splanchnic nerve, which is the main vasoconstrictor of the abdominal cavity, are destroyed. The resultant dilatation of the splanchnic blood vessels causes congestion of the liver, kidneys and intestines and, in addition, congestion and enlargement of the spleen, producing the '*slaughter spleen*'.

Pithing was used with the bed system of carcase dressing. *Under modern conditions, it is completely unnecessary provided efficient stunning and shackling are carried out, besides being very unhygienic and time-consuming*. Pithing is also contraindicated in those countries where BSE is known to exist because of the risk of contamination of meat and the infection of operatives. In addition, the complete removal of a damaged spinal cord is rendered impossible. There is some evidence that bacteria can be introduced into the carcase on the pithing cane and subsequently dispersed throughout the carcase before the heart stops beating. It is therefore imperative that if pithing is carried out the cane is sterilised between use on each animal. Again, the consequences of use on potential subclinical cases of BSE should be considered.

## BLEEDING

### Cattle

There are two main methods of bleeding *cattle*:

(1) *bilateral severance of the carotid arteries and jugular veins* by an incision across the throat region caudal to the larynx as in ritual slaughter; and
(2) incision in the jugular furrow at the base of the neck, the knife being directed towards the entrance of the chest to sever the *brachiocephalic trunk* and *anterior vena cava*.

Care must be taken not to pass the knife too far towards the chest for, if the pleura is punctured, blood may be aspirated into the thoracic cavity and adhere to the parietal pleura, particularly along the posterior edges of the ribs. This contamination is known as *back bleeding or oversticking* and, if not washed off immediately, may necessitate stripping of the pleura. In cattle the blood cannot infiltrate between the pleura and contiguous chest wall; this may occasionally occur in pigs but over a small area immediately posterior to the first rib.

Current abattoir practice is to stun cattle and then hoist them, by the shackling of a hind leg, over a bleeding gully. The advantage of a bleeding rail is that it permits centralised collection of blood and also accelerates the throughput of animals, allowing them to be stunned and removed in quick succession through the same stunning pen. Observations in Germany have shown that bleeding was 40% more effective in cattle bled on the rail than in those bled in a horizontal position.

If unilateral sticking at the base of the neck is performed, it is of value to make other small bilateral incisions at the angle of the jaw, severing the jugulars at their division into *internal and external maxillary veins*; this permits easier skinning of heads and also reduces the quantity of blood in the lingual artery. The vertical head-down position of the suspended carcase otherwise causes blood to be retained in the head.

The ordinary bleeding knife severs blood vessels more rapidly if the blade is held at right angles to the direction of the vessels and longitudinal axis of the body.

Whichever method is employed, bleeding should continue for 6 min. The average *yield of blood* obtained in *cattle* slaughter is 13.6 kg. *Cows* yield more blood than bulls or bullocks of the same weight, in some cases up to 22.6 kg in old cows. About 58.3% of the blood is yielded in the first 30 s after sticking, 76.6% after 60 s and 90% after 120 s.

In *calves* the incision was at one time at the side of the neck with the severing of the jugular vein. The purpose of this was to produce slow bleeding after the carcase was hung up prior to dressing, for slow bleeding ensures the desirable white colour of veal. Calves are now bled rapidly at the level of the first rib, and yield 2.7 kg of blood.

## Sheep

In the slaughter of sheep, bleeding is usually carried out by an incision in the jugular furrows close to the head, severing both *carotid arteries* and *jugular veins* and in some cases the trachea, oesophagus and spinal cord at the occipito-atlantal junction. However, *thoracic inlet bleeding* is superior.

Accidental cutting of the oesophagus often results in contamination of the neck, head and blood with ruminal contents. At one time, when cradle dressing was carried out, it was customary to jerk the head back sharply in order to rupture the spinal cord where it enters the skull, the purpose being, as in the pithing of cattle, to obviate reflex muscular action before dressing of the carcase. Like pithing, it is an unnecessary procedure.

The most satisfactory type of knife for the lateral stab method, where the bleeding knife is inserted posterior to the trachea and oesophagus, is one with a blade about 23 cm long and 4 cm wide with a straight back unsharpened except at the tip, and a tapered point on the cutting edge of about 8 cm. The knife is fitted with a circular safety guard between blade and handle. The unsharpened edge is placed in contact with the oesophagus, but it may puncture this organ if the knife is withdrawn at the wrong angle. Even when great care is taken with this technique, both carotid arteries may not be severed.

Approximately 75% of the available blood is lost from ewes within 60 s and in lambs within 50 s. Electrically stunned lambs bleed more rapidly than those stunned with the captive bolt. There was no significant difference in the rates of bleeding between sheep that are not stunned and those stunned with the captive bolt pistol.

*Bilateral severance* is the easiest technique to perform and produces satisfactory bleeding. This is the best method for bleeding sheep in lateral recumbency. When both carotid arteries are severed, the sheep loses consciousness in less than 10 s; if only one carotid artery is severed, insensibility can take more than nine times as long to occur.

In contrast with cattle, which bleed more fully in the head-down position, trials with sheep at the UK Meat Research Institute have shown that sheep bled in the horizontal position lose approximately 10% more blood than those suspended vertically.

Bleeding of the sheep carcase should last for 5 min, the amount of blood obtained from a slaughtered sheep being 1–2.5 kg, lambs having the lower weights.

## Pigs

In pigs the knife is inserted in the midline of the neck at the depression in front of the sternum, and is then pushed forward to sever the *anterior vena cava* brachiocephalic trunk at the entrance of the chest; sometimes the carotid artery is also pierced. Care should be taken not to insert the knife too far as it may penetrate into the shoulder, allowing blood and water from the scalding tank to run back into the shoulder 'pocket' beneath the scapula giving its wall a cooked appearance. Where pigs are bled without being previously stunned, the heart continues for 2–9 min. The carcase should not, therefore, be placed immediately in the scalding tank; too large a sticking wound and contaminated scalding water facilitate the entry of microorganisms into the carcase tissues by way of the jugular vein and may lead to spoilage. In some abattoirs pigs are stunned, then hoisted and bled while suspended. Urination occurring while the pig is bleeding renders the blood unmarketable, but this may be overcome by using the hollow knife. Pigs should be allowed to bleed for 6 min, as during this period the muscles relax and the hair is more readily removed during scalding.

Pork pigs yield 2.2 kg of blood, bacon pigs 3 kg, while boars and sows yield 3.6 kg.

In many abattoirs *prone sticking* of pigs has been adopted. After being rendered unconscious, the animal is discharged on to a conveyor belt and is stuck while lying prone in the tonic phase, the blood draining into a trough running parallel to the conveyor. Immediately after sticking the animals may come under a holding-down belt which continues the full length of the conveyor and restrains the involuntary struggling that occurs during the clonic phase. The advantages of prone sticking of electrically stunned pigs are the more efficient recovery of blood and the elimination of ruptured joints and joint capsules, which are a troublesome condition in pigs bled while suspended and are the cause of the so-called *internal ham bruising*. In addition, a study in Austria found that the incidence of PSE meat was reduced from 62–63% in vertically-bled pigs, to 22–27% in those bled in the horizontal position.

For *sterile collection* of quantities of blood, the necessary equipment (stainless steel hollow knifes, vacuum pump, sterilisation facilities, anticoagulant injection, containers, etc.) must be available. The incision at the base of the neck provides a larger flow of blood evenly and more hygienically than procedures not so geared. Sterile blood collection must be efficient and rapid, otherwise the rate of kill will be considerably reduced (Fig. 8.10).

## EFFICIENCY OF BLEEDING

It was once thought that the efficiency of bleeding had a most important bearing on the subsequent keeping quality of the carcase. Although the validity of this viewpoint is widely questioned, most slaughterplant

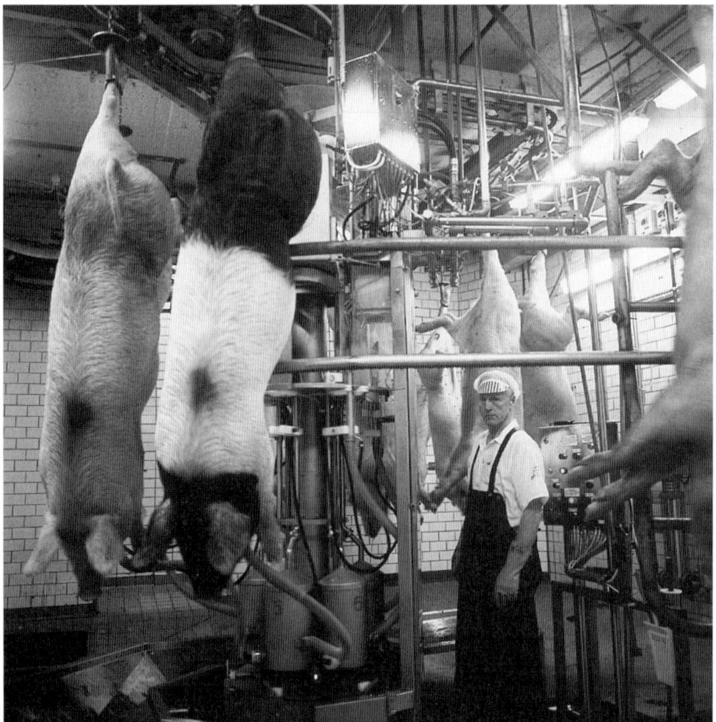

**Fig. 8.10** Hygienic blood collection from pigs showing hollow knives in position and central vacuum system and containers. (By courtesy of Scan Farmek S-532 87, Skara, Sweden)

managers are still convinced of the necessity to extract the last drop of blood from the carcase. Studies have been unable to demonstrate any correlation between the amount of blood lost at the time of slaughter and subsequent pH values, water content, bacterial counts, flavour and tenderness of beef or lamb. The extra blood retained by the poorly-bled animal is retained mainly in the viscera and skin.

Experiments in pigs have shown that if the amount of blood remaining in the carcase after stunning and delayed bleeding is 100 parts, then the amount remaining after stunning and immediate bleeding is 86 parts, that after direct bleeding without previous stunning 70 parts, while after stunning by the electrical method and subsequent bleeding, only 60 parts of blood remain.

The stunning of an animal by any means produces a rise in the blood pressure of the arterial, capillary and venous systems, and in sheep the normal arterial blood pressure of 120–145 mm Hg may rise to 260 mm Hg or over when the animal is stunned prior to bleeding. This is accompanied by a transitory increase in the heart rate. Both of these factors will facilitate immediate bleeding. The importance of *immediate bleeding* is obvious when it is realised that the rate of flow of blood from a cut vessel is five to ten times more rapid than in the intact vessel, and not until 20% of the blood has been lost does the pressure begin to fall. If an undue interval is allowed to elapse between stunning and bleeding, the carcase may be imperfectly bled and may bear blood splashes.

## RELIGIOUS SLAUGHTER

In the United States some 120 million food animals are slaughtered annually, of which 8–10 million are kosher-killed. In Great Britain 1.5 million sheep and 90 000 cattle are slaughtered by religious methods annually.

The Farm Animal Welfare Council (1985) concluded that, even under ideal conditions, a degree of stress, suffering and pain occurred in ritual slaughter. However, it remains a fact that this same accusation could be laid at the door of many of the other accepted slaughter techniques previously described in this chapter. There have been calls, particularly from the animal welfare lobby, that meat produced from animals slaughtered by religious methods should be labelled as such. Although this is accepted and carried out widely for carcases, there are practical and enforcement problems carrying the label through to the retail pack or butcher's shop.

### Jewish slaughter

The Jewish method of slaughter is controlled in Britain by the Jewish Board of Shechita and Jewish slaughtermen have to undergo several years of training before being licensed by the Rabbinical Commission. They are also subject to annual examination of skills by the Commission.

In order for meat to be *kosher*, i.e. right, fulfilling the requirements of Jewish law, animals must be slaughtered and dressed according to ritual methods specified in the Talmud, the body of Jewish law and legend based on the Torah which is the substance of God's revelation to man in the Old Testament (Pentateuch, first five books). The reference to Shechita is said to be found in Deuteronomy 12:21 – 'thou shalt kill of thy herd and of thy flock, which the Lord hath given thee, as I have commanded thee'.

At slaughter the animal must be alive and healthy and have suffered no injury. Prior stunning of the animal is therefore forbidden. Animals that do not conform to these ideals and any defects at slaughter in the form of faults in *shechita* (act of killing for food) or disease lesions discovered in the carcase render the meat *terefa*, i.e. unfit for consumption by Jews. Likewise, animals that lie quietly and cannot be made to rise must not be slaughtered according to Jewish ritual. This early recognition of the inadmissibility of ill or moribund animals for human food is worthy of note.

Shechita is performed by a *shochet*, or cutter, who slaughters the fully conscious animal with a single, deliberate, swift action of a razor-sharp knife, *chalef*, roughly twice the width of the animal's neck and which is devoid of any notch or flaw, and has been examined before the slaughter of each animal. All the soft structures anterior to the cervical spine are severed, including the carotid arteries and jugular veins. It is essential that the neck be fully extended in order to keep the edges of the wound open and thereby prevent any pain.

The *five rules of Jewish ritual slaughter*, in their traditional order, are that the neck incision shall be completed without pause, pressure, stabbing, slanting or tearing. If the knife receives any nick, however small, during the act of shechita, the slaughter is not correctly performed and the use of the meat is not permitted for Jewish food.

The shochet ('cutter') is normally assisted by a sealer (*shomer*) who is responsible for putting the kosher mark on the brisket and on edible offal. In some instances, e.g. large kosher slaughter plants, several shochets may work together in the task of slaughter and tagging meat.

Besides performing the act of slaughter, the shochet offers prayers and carries out a 'post-mortem examination' by making an incision posterior to the xiphoid process and inserting the arm to detect any adhesions in the thoracic cavity ('searching'). Full meat inspection may be performed by a shochet or by the government inspector. Should the carcase be held in the chill room for more than 24 h, it must be washed in order to remove blood, further washing and curing, *mehila*, or broiling being carried out in the home.

Carcases found fit for consumption must have the meat porged by removing the large blood vessels in the forequarter prior to retail sale. Only forequarters are normally used, since the hindquarters, which are said to contain over 50 blood vessels, can only be porged by highly skilled kosher butchers and are therefore rarely eaten. 'Only be sure that thou eat not the blood; for the blood is the life; and thou mayest not eat the life with the flesh' (*Deuteronomy* 12:23).

*Kosher slaughter restraining systems* (Fig. 8.11) (also used for Halal slaughter) were developed to overcome the cruelty associated with the practice of 'shackling and hoisting'. The shackling and hoisting of conscious live animals in the United States has been forbidden since 1958, but kosher slaughter is exempt from this requirement. In acquiring four patents on devices for restraining animals the ASPCA (American Society for the Prevention of Cruelty to Animals) believes it has solved a problem which has plagued humanitarians, religious elements and the slaughter industry for generations. The holding pens meet all Jewish ritualistic requirements and are available to the whole slaughtering industry without royalties or profit to the ASPCA. In 'shackling and hoisting' a chain is slung around one or both hind legs of a conscious animal which then is hoisted and moved, dangling and jerking, along an overhead rail until its life is taken. Occasionally the thrashing animal breaks a leg or its back or suffers internal injuries. More often only indications of pain or fright are observed, but bruises may be detected later at meat inspection. Equally, the Weinberg and similar types of pen, into which it is difficult to persuade animals to enter and which are rotated through 180°, while causing less physical injury than shackling and hoisting, are none the less creators of much discomfort for the animal and have consequently been banned in the European Union.

The ASPCA restrainer pen, first invented by Peter Hoad of Canada Packers, Toronto, Canada, who developed the first 'on-the-line' slaughtering system, has been fully modified by the Cincinnati Butchers' Supply Company and by Temple Grandin (1980). It now takes the form of a metal pen fitted with a belly plate, a rear pusher on a guillotine door and a front neck yoke and chin lift. Hydraulic controls are used to operate the equipment and position the animal for kosher and halal slaughter. The rear pusher and chin lift should be equipped with pressure-limiting devices. While the cut is being made, the hind leg is shackled to withdraw the animal from the pen. There is no doubt that the Cincinnati-Boss (CB) pen is much less stressful on the animal than the Weinberg pen, but it is by no means perfect. One defect is the manner of withdrawal of the animal from the pen, which in some types of CB pen pulls the hind leg in an unnatural manner which must result in hip joint damage. Some stress inevitably occurs due to fixation to the head and raising of the head (see Head restraint). Some means must be found to counter the stress occasioned by the isolation of the animal from its fellows. It has been reported that the presence of blood on the equipment does not appear to upset the cattle and that in fact some animals have been observed to lick the blood.

While most of the normal pens in use can only deal with low slaughter rates, a conveyor-restrainer system has been developed in the USA which can handle rates for kosher slaughter up to 214 cattle per hour. An overhead hold-down rack is placed along the length of a conveyor above the animals until they reach the head holder at the discharge end; the head holder is powered so that it can be

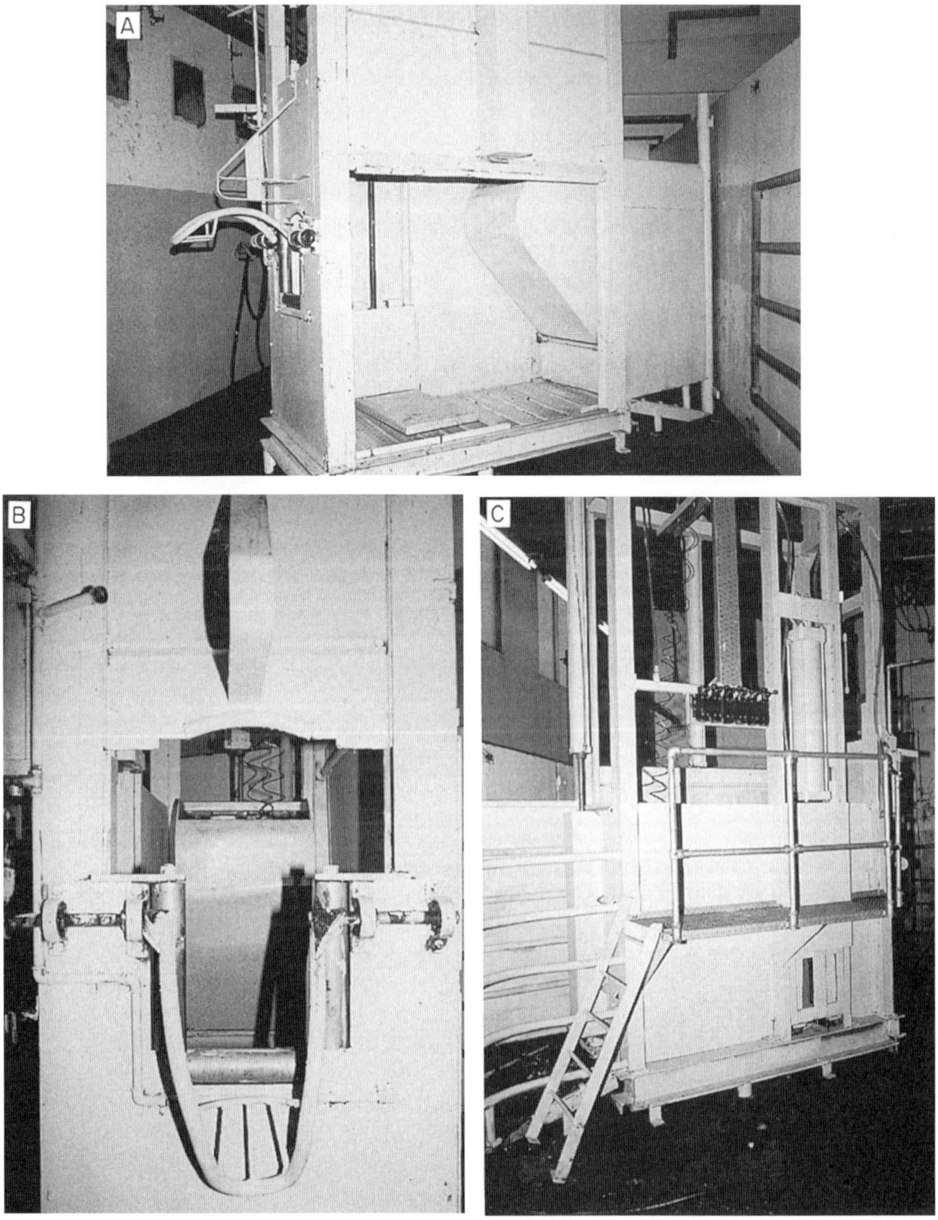


**Fig. 8.11** Cincinnati-Boss restraint pen. A, Interior of pen with elevating belly plate on floor and rear pusher on rear guillotine. B, View from front showing chin lift and neck yoke in raised position. C, Operator's platform and controls for hydraulic cylinders.

raised to position the head and then release it after the cut is made.

Restrainer systems have also been manufactured to deal with *small animals* – calves and sheep. In one of these US items of equipment, which is used for both conventional and religious slaughter, the animal is conveyed straddlewise along a double rail above which is a head cage which positions the head upwards for the neck cut.

It is claimed that the Jewish method of slaughter does not involve any act of cruelty because the knife is particularly sharp, the cut is made dextrously by a trained person, and the severance of the carotid vessels is followed by a very rapid fall in blood pressure within the cephalic arteries. It is therefore suggested that the anoxia from the diminished blood supply to the brain tissues brings about almost immediate unconsciousness. Others contend that it is not anoxia which results in the collapse of the animal but rather cerebral shock due to the sudden fall in pressure of the cerebro-spinal fluid. The persistence of corneal and palpebral reflexes and also the convulsions which occur some time after the neck cut has been made are not associated with consciousness and their significance may therefore be discounted.

Opponents of the Jewish method of slaughter have also contended that additional blood, via the *vertebral artery*, and therefore independent of the carotid supply, may still reach the brain of cattle and prolong the period of consciousness. (The vertebral artery, being enclosed in the spinal canal, is not severed in the Jewish or Muslim method of slaughter.) Anatomical differences in the blood supply to the brain occur in the various species of animals. In the sheep and goat the complete brain is supplied with blood from the common carotid arteries; the vertebral arteries supply only the anterior spinal cord and the posterior medulla oblongata. However, it has been shown experimentally in calves that the vertebral arteries can carry enough blood to maintain consciousness when both common carotid arteries are occluded. Very little blood is required to maintain consciousness, especially in the head-down position and in young animals which have a greater resistance to anoxia. It has been estimated that with religious slaughter sheep may take 14 seconds to lose consciousness and some estimates have suggested that calves can take up to 5 minutes.

A factor of considerable importance, and to which not enough attention has been paid in considering the problem of Jewish slaughter, is that after the carotid arteries of cattle are severed transversely they tend, by virtue of their elasticity, to retract rapidly within their own external connective tissue coat, thus sealing off the cut ends. As the blood pressure in the anterior aorta will then be maintained by the heart action, the blood pressure in the vertebral artery may likewise be maintained at a substantial level and unconsciousness may therefore be delayed. Such sealing can and does occur, in some cases very rapidly, and provides an explanation why some cattle, the throats of which have been cut by the Jewish method, have been known to regain their feet and walk a considerable distance before they have eventually succumbed some minutes later. In the past when such occurrences have been witnessed they have been attributed, perhaps for want of a better explanation, to the fact that all the neck muscles may not have been severed completely, but observations on the Jewish method of slaughter lead one to the conclusion that the cut is invariably made dextrously and the efficiency of the technique is rarely in question. There is, therefore, considerable doubt as to whether unconsciousness always follows rapidly in cattle after the severance of the neck vessels, for by the very nature of the neck cut in Jewish slaughter it is impossible to ensure that self-sealing of the cut ends of the carotid arteries will not occur, although proper neck extension may reduce this likelihood.

The important issue is whether or not the animal is suffering pain during the period of consciousness following cutting of the carotids and jugulars, a matter not readily determined. It is vital that the animal be handled carefully and quietly at this stage. The assertion by supporters of Jewish slaughter that bleeding of the animal is more complete than in other methods of slaughter has been challenged by some authorities who contend that the paler colour of the flesh of Jewish slaughtered animals is due to the violent respiratory efforts which accompany ritual slaughter, these having the effect of increasing the proportion of oxyhaemoglobin in the blood, thus rendering the residual blood in the carcase paler than normal and giving the flesh a well-bled appearance.

Stress created by the CB pen and its chin lift and neck yoke may be more important than the system of bleeding.

### Muslim methods of slaughter

Many of the practices relating to the slaughter of animals and the consumption of meat by members of the Jewish faith also apply to Muslims. The welfare of the animal is a major consideration in both cases and the eating of dead animals, blood and swine is forbidden.

The actual method of slaughter is virtually the same for both religions. The Quran describes the procedure of carotid and jugular section as the 'cutting and draining of blood'. The act of slaughter (*Al-Dhabh*) is allowed in the name of God; therefore pronouncing the name of Allah is the usual practice. This is to remind the slaughterer that he is taking the life of a living creature.

Animals must not be slaughtered in the sight of other beasts and those to be killed are to be fed and watered beforehand. The act of cutting the skin with a sharp knife is regarded as painless, or almost so, and the rapid loss of blood is said to produce instantaneous insensibility. The opinion is held that the brain and the skin of an animal are less sensitive than those of man. Just as defective methods may be used in stunning by mechanical means so also can throat cutting be imperfectly performed with the result that not all four blood vessels are severed. Islamic law demands that the animal is alive at the time of slaughter and that it is slaughtered in a humane manner. The Prophet Mohammed is reported as saying that 'God who is blessed and exalted has declared that everything should be done in a good way; so when you kill, use a good method, and when you cut an animal's throat, you should use a good method; for each of you should sharpen his knife and give the animal as little pain as possible'.

Unlike Shechita, the Muslim method of slaughter is not controlled by a central Board but is overseen by the local Islamic authority (*Muftis*) who decide whether or not particular acts and thoughts conform to the tenets of Islamic Law (*Shariah*). So in some instances prior stunning with electricity or captive-bolt pistol is allowed. (In New Zealand a head-only stun of 0.5–0.9 A for 3 s is performed for sheep, 2.5 A for cattle, the major blood vessels being severed within 10 s of the stun.) It is also understood that non-penetrative percussive stunning has been permitted in some quarters. Provided it can be shown that the heart is still beating after stunning, prior anaesthesia is approved, at least in some instances.

While the actual act of slaughter in Jewish and Halal slaughter can be regarded as painless and humane *if performed efficiently with the wound kept open*, the same cannot be said for many of the methods of restraint currently in use, which would appear to be in conflict not only with modern slaughtering technology but also with the ideals of the Torah and the Quran and, more importantly, with the stricture of the Almighty in Deuteronomy 12:10.

## REFERENCES


Bremner, F. (1954) *Brain Mechanisms and Consciousness*. ed. J. F. Delafresnaye. London: Oxford University Press.

Ewbank, R., Parker M. J. and Mason C. (1992) *Reactions of cattle to head 'restraint at stunning'. A practical dilemma*. Humane Slaughter Association.

Farm Animal Welfare Council (1985) *Report on the welfare of livestock when slaughtered by religious methods*. London: HMSO.

Garland, T. D., Bauer, N. and Bailey, M. (1996) *The Lancet* **348**, 610.

Gregory N. G. (1993) *Outlook on Agriculture* **20**(2) 95–101.

Grandin, T. (1980) Problems with kosher slaughter. *Int. J. Stud. Anim. Prob.* **1**(6), 375.

Heath, G. B. S. (1984) Slaughter of broilers. *Vet. Rec.* **115**, 98.

Lambooij, D. L. O. (1996) *Meat Focus Int.* April, 124–125

Lumb, W. V. and Jones, E. W. (1973) *Veterinary Anaesthesia*. Lea & Febiger, pp. 338–340.

McMillan, J. B (1956) *Am. J. Pathol.* **32**, 405.

Monin, G. (1996) *Meat Focus Int.* April, 123–124.

Munro, R. (1997) *Vet. Rec.* **140**, 536.

Raj, A. B. M. and Gregory, N. G. (1995) *Anim. Welfare* **4**, 273–280.

Raj, A. B. M. and Gregory, N. G. (1996) *Anim. Welfare* **5**, 71–78.

Raj, A. B. M. and Gregory, N. G. (1993) *Vet. Rec.* **133**, 318.

Raj, A. B. M. and Gregory, N. G. (1994) *Vet. Rec.* **135**, 222–223.

Schutt-Abraham *et al.* (1983) In *Proc. Seminar in the CEC Programme of Research on Animal Welfare*, ed. G. Eikelenboom. The Hague: Martinus Nijhoff.

Shewring, J. (1990) Safeguards at slaughter. The new welfare regulations. *The Meat Hygienist*, September.

Thorpe, W. H. (1965) The assessment of pain and stress in animals. Appendix III. Report of Technical Committee to enquire into the welfare of animals kept under intensive livestock husbandry systems. Cmnd 2836. London: HMSO.

Van der Wal, P. G. (1983) In *Stunning Animals for Slaughter*, ed. G. Eikelenboom. The Hague: Martinus Nijhof.

Von Mickwitz, G. and Leach, T. (1977) *Review of Pre-slaughter Stunning in the EEC*. Information on

Agriculture Report No. 30. Commission of the European Communities.
Warriss, P. D., Brown, S. N. and Adams, S. J. M. (1994) *Meat Sci.* **38**, 329–340.

## FURTHER READING

Humane Slaughter Association (1993) Guidance notes 2; *Captive bolt stunning of livestock.*
Humane Slaughter Association (1994) Guidance notes 1; *Electrical stunning of sheep, goats and pigs,* 2nd edn.
Blackmore, D.K. and Delaney, M. W. (1988) *Slaughter of Stock.* Foundation for Continuing Education of the New Zealand Veterinary Association, Publication number 118. Palmerston North, New Zealand: Massey University.

# Chapter 9
# Meat Hygiene Practice

One of the most important roles of the meat hygiene team within the modern abattoir is to ensure that the meat remains free from contamination of all types during the production processes. This involves the inspectors cooperating with factory management, operatives, engineers and quality control staff to ensure that 'Good Manufacturing Practice' is followed at all times, that hygienic techniques are utilised and that effective monitoring of processes and product is carried out.

## SOURCES OF CONTAMINATION (See also Chapter 7)

The classic work of Empey and Scott (1939) in Australia dealt with the sources of contamination of meat. They showed that the main sources of contamination were hides and hair, soil, contents of the stomach and gut, water, airborne pollution, utensils and equipment.

The chief source of bacteriological contamination was found to be the hide and hair of the slaughtered animals, deriving mainly from the microflora of the pasture soil, but with a higher incidence of yeasts. Then, as today, the transfer of microorganisms from the hide to the underlying tissues was found to begin during the first stage of removal of the pelt by means of knives used for skinning. Further transfer occurs via the hands, arms, legs and clothing of operatives.

A similar study carried out in 1996 by Bell and Hathaway in New Zealand demonstrated that there has been little improvement in the general hygienic status of dressed carcases over the intervening years.

### Outer integument – hide, hair, fleece or skin

One of the main sources of carcase contamination in the meat plant is the live animal itself, particularly in winter months when the animals are housed. A survey of 600 cattle hides in Northern Ireland during February 1965 showed that the average weight of manure, soil and other dirt adhering to them was 4 kg, with a range of 0.9–15.8 kg; weights of 36 kg have been recorded in England (Gracey, unpublished data).

Current observations would suggest thats although husbandry practices have changed since the 1960s, the filthy state of many cattle entering the abattoir as a raw material for food has not. It is essential, as discussed in previous chapters, that livestock be presented for slaughter in as clean and dry a condition as possible, this being achieved by hygienic practices on the farm, in transport lorries and in market plant lairage pens.

In Finland, the problem of excessively dirty cattle being presented for slaughter has been greatly reduced by the application of a series of rules agreed by meat inspection veterinarians, farmers, the meat industry, the leather industry and the state veterinary department. Under this agreement, excessively dirty animals are detained to be slaughtered separately after the clean animals, the extra cost incurred being billed to the owners involved. This has resulted in a decrease in the numbers of excessively dirty cattle by 85% (Ridell and Korkeala, 1993).

In the UK, a clean livestock policy was introduced during 1997. It has been very successful in ensuring that only clean cattle and sheep are slaughtered for human consumption. Those considered by the official veterinarian to be in an unacceptable state are sent home.

### Gastrointestinal tract

Accidental puncture of the stomach and intestines is a source of contamination on occasions, as is spillage from the rectum and oesophagus. It has been estimated that the mixed bacterial flora of the gastrointestinal tract may reach $10^{10}$ colony-forming units (cfu) per gram of contents.

### Sticking point

During the act of sticking, bacteria can enter the jugular vein or anterior vena cava and travel in the bloodstream to the muscles, lungs and bone marrow. Many have questioned, however, whether bacterial contamination by this route is of great importance (Troeger, 1994).

### Physical contact with structures

The design of the line must allow for a full range of sizes of stock so that legs do not touch stands or supports and necks or heads do not drag along the floor, walkways or tables. A common weak point occurs at the point on the line where the bovine gastrointestinal tract is dropped on to the gut table, chute or conveyor. Gross cleaning, with squeegee and shovel, etc., must be ongoing throughout the working day to prevent the build-up of blood and debris. Every opportunity must be taken during breaks in production when the slaughterfloor is free of carcases and offal to rinse down the line.

Care must also be taken to ensure that the position and height of offal rails is such as to prevent contact with the floor or structures. Swinging viscera, particularly at corners, may come into contact with supporting structures, while poor positioning of the line frequently leads to operatives dragging viscera across the floor or the line structure for hanging.

### Operatives

All persons working in the slaughterhall are an important, and extremely mobile, source of contamination for the meat. Movement of all personnel about the plant must be strictly controlled, and in the ideal situation movement would occur only from clean to dirtier parts of the plant. In practice this is impossible. To minimise the risk of contamination, upgrade stations must be provided where washing, disinfection and, if necessary, a change of outer clothes can take place. Although the movement about the plant of general operatives making social visits can generally be controlled, practical experience has shown that management, quality assurance staff, but most of all engineers and fitters, can be the greatest problem in this respect.

The commonly held misconception among operatives that protective clothing is to protect them from getting dirty, rather than to protect the product from them, underlines the basic widespread lack of basic knowledge of hygiene matters among workers in the food industry. The EC Hygiene of Foodstuffs Directive 93/43, transposed into law in Great Britain as the General Food Hygiene Regulations, requires that all personnel involved in food manufacture receive an appropriate level of training. This requirement is superseded if a specific training requirement is laid down in a specific food directive, e.g. the Fresh Meat Directive 64/433, Article 10, para. 3 and the Policy Directive 92/116, Article 6, para. 3 both of which state:

> The operator of the establishment, the owner or his agent must establish a staff training programme enabling workers to comply with conditions of hygienic production adapted to the production structure. The official veterinarian responsible for the establishment must be involved in the planning and implementation of that programme.

This duty of the official veterinarian must be taken seriously if satisfactory hygiene standards are to be maintained. It is also an opportunity for the meat hygiene/inspection team to demonstrate their knowledge and training and by doing so improve their status and effectiveness around the factory.

### Equipment and utensils

The equipment used within the slaughterfloor is a potential source of contamination. This includes knives, saws and hockcutters which come into direct contact with the meat and so must be regularly cleaned and sterilised. However, it also involves indirect sources of dirt and debris such as the moving overhead line itself, from which oil or grease may drop on to the meat, the hide-puller from which faeces may flick on to the exposed carcase, and many others.

### The slaughterhall environment

Ventilation in the work-room must be sufficient to prevent the build-up of steam and to prevent condensation forming on the ceiling and overhead structures. A common source of steam emanates from sterilisers which are allowed to operate in excess of 82°C and in which no system is incorporated to discharge the steam. Steam may act as a vector for bacteria and can in addition condense on the carcases, adding to surface moisture and assisting bacterial growth. Condensation dripping on to the carcase from above brings with it dirt, bacteria and moulds.

Water is also a problem if allowed to pool on the floor owing to blocked drains and uneven surfaces. Gullies around the splitting saw frequently become blocked with debris and, if water accumulates, the carcase may be splashed with water from the floor.

Another source of water splash can be poorly positioned *apron washes*. This problem is exaggerated if the water supply does not cut off immediately the operative steps out of the cabinet.

Pressure differences between the workroom and the outside frequently result in draughts which enter if doors are left open. The temptation to leave exterior doors open in temperate climates during the summer is understandable but must be resisted since flies, dust and dirt gain easy access. This is frequently the case when the doors are adjacent to the waste skips, hide stores and green offal rooms.

Poorly maintained structure may result in contamination of the meat from, for example, rust or paint flakes dropping on to the meat or into trays intended for meat. Excessive lubrication of overhead moving chains or cogs is another potential contamination hazard.

### **Vermin** (see also p. 82)

All measures necessary to exclude vermin from the food-producing factory must be taken. Physical exclusion begins with a fence around the entire premises to keep out cats and dogs, and also includes self-closing external doors and fly-screening on windows. Vermin which manage to gain entrance must be systematically destroyed. The official veterinarian must be aware of the procedures in place to carry out this task, including the nature of any poison bait, the bait points and the frequency of the inspections. A regular check should be made of all insectocutor trays and a record kept of the dead fly count. A large fly count indicates that the insectocutor is working, but more importantly, that the exclusion practices are not.

Plant surrounds must be kept clean and tidy so that vermin such as rodents, cats and dogs are not attracted to the site. All external waste bins must be covered, otherwise gulls, starlings and other scavenging birds will be attracted.

### Chemical contamination

Cleaning chemicals may contaminate the meat if they have not been rinsed off the structures correctly. It is not uncommon to find a residue of chemical on sanitised stands and equipment after they have dried. All chemicals used in a meat plant must be stored in a specifically designated store.

The hazard of intrinsic chemical residues in the meat is dealt with in Chapter 13.

## METHODS OF REDUCING CONTAMINATION

### Dealing with the dirty animal

It is almost inevitable that, despite all efforts to prevent it, dirty animals will be presented for slaughter, especially in the winter months in the British Isles. The first option to be considered should always be to reject without slaughtering, but disease restrictions or animal welfare considerations may make this impossible. It is widely agreed that in most cases it is easier to hygienically-dress dirty, dry cattle and sheep than dirty, wet ones. Slaughter should then be delayed until the animals are dry by resting them in strawed yards or, in the case of sheep or lambs, on expanded-metal floors. A technique recommended by one experienced veterinarian is that lambs should be detained until their underside can be rubbed without dirtying the hand. It should be recognised, however, that in warm climates, and where lambs have been fattened on root crops, drying the animals may result in release of dust which adheres to the hot carcase while the fleece is being removed. *In all cases the welfare aspects of the husbandry practices which have resulted in the dirty animals should be borne in mind, and farm inspections by the appropriate agency instituted where necessary.*

In New Zealand, it has been common practice for many years to wash lambs prior to slaughter through plunge dips. A study of this practice by Biss and Hathaway (1996) indicated that, although the carcases of washed lambs showed evidence of less visible contamination than those of unwashed lambs, washing had a detrimental effect on the microbiological load as measured by *E. coli* and aerobic plate counts. Washing heavily cladded cattle is futile from a hygiene perspective, and may be highly detrimental to animal welfare. It is impossible to wash the legs, hooves and ventral aspect of cattle effectively.

A process for *chemically dehairing* cattle between stunning and sticking has been patented in the United States. It involves repeated applications of sodium sulphide and rinses within a closed cabinet and results in the complete removal of dirt, faeces and hair. However, a study of the process by Schnell *et al.* (1995) demonstrated that, although there was less visible contamination on the treated carcases than on conventionally slaughtered controls, total bacterial counts, measured as aerobic plate counts and total coliform counts, showed no decrease in the overall bacterial load.

When the animals are judged ready for slaughter, the inspection team must monitor the operation closely and control the *speed of the line* accordingly. As important as line speed, which gives the operatives sufficient time to carry out the extra washing of hands, arms, aprons and sterilising equipment which will be necessary, is the spacing of the animals. On a moving line, the placing of carcases on every other overhead hanger decreases the possibility of carcases touching each other and also gives the slaughtermen more room to work hygienically. The inspection team must be in a position to control the line, and stop operations if contamination occurs until it can be removed by trimming and the specific problem which caused it is solved.

It goes without saying, however, that the real answer to dirty animals lies primarily with livestock producers on the farm, with hauliers and with meat plant operators. It may well be necessary to provide a bonus payment for suppliers of clean animals or a penalty for the others.

## Protecting the meat from the worker

### *Clothing*

The EC Fresh Meat Directive states in Annex 1, Chapter V, para. 18 that:

> Staff handling exposed or wrapped fresh meat or working in rooms and areas in which such meat is handled, packaged or transported must in particular wear clean and easily cleanable headgear, footwear and light-coloured working clothes and, where necessary, clean neck shields or other protective clothing. Staff engaged in slaughtering animals or working on or handling meat must wear clean working clothes at the commencement of each working day and must renew such clothing during the day as necessary.

Laundry facilities should be provided centrally and the standards monitored by the inspection team. The outdated practice of operatives laundering their own protective clothing at home should be resisted, as the monitoring and enforcement of standards is made impossible.

Headgear must be easily cleanable, and must cover the crown of the head, with the hair restrained within a hairnet and beards within a net or snood. For both hygiene and health and safety reasons, white bump caps are to be recommended for all staff. Easily cleaned footwear means, in effect, that it must be waterproof so that boot washers can be used to remove adherent fat and soils.

### *Hands*

All operatives on the slaughterfloor must have facilities readily available to wash their hands during the working day. The water supply must be premixed to a suitable temperature – too cold and it will not remove the dirt and the operative will not use it; too hot and it will produce steam and the operative will not use it – and must be supplied through a non-hand-operated outlet. This may be controlled by foot, knee or 'magic eye'. Bactericidal soap must be available, with disposable paper towels provided.

Bell and Hathaway (1996), reported that a 44°C water hand rinse removed 90% of the microbial contamination from workers' hands, but rinsed hands, particularly those contacting the fleece, still carried a microbial population exceeding $10^4$ cfu/cm.

### *Gloves*

The wearing of rubber and chain-mail gloves presents a dichotomy between hygiene and health and safety. In the slaughterhall it is likely that with many of the tasks gloves will become grossly contaminated from the hide with faeces and other soils. With rubber gloves of the 'washing-up' type in common usage it is almost impossible to wash the entire length of the glove. There is frequently, therefore, a rim of gross contamination around the top of the glove which is readily transferred to the meat. Attempts to seal the glove to the arm with tape are rarely successful. Chain-mail gloves also become contaminated and can only be effectively cleaned after removal. Although this allows the chain to be cleaned, the fastening tapes frequently remain in a filthy state. The best compromise is probably to cover the chain-mail glove, which is usually worn only on the free hand, with a skin-tight rubber latex type glove.

Cut-resistant polyester yarn gloves are manufactured by several companies for use instead of chain-mail. Some claim that an antibacterial agent has been built into the yarn from which the glove is made which has an activity against Gram-positive and Gram-negative bacteria, including salmonellae. The gloves can be laundered through a washing machine and reused many times.

### *Medical certification*

The EC Fresh Meat Directive states in Annex 1, Chapter V, para. 24 that:

> Persons likely to contaminate meat are prohibited from working on it and handling it. When recruited, any person working on or handling fresh meat shall be required to prove, by a medical certificate that there is no impediment to such employment. The medical supervision of such a person shall be governed by national legislation in force in the Member State concerned.

An example of a staff self-declaration form which may be used to assist a general medical practitioner in the preparation of a Medical Certificate in the United Kingdom is illustrated in Fig. 9.1. The effectiveness of this one-off certificate in preventing persons carrying readily transferable infections is dubious. Some companies require regular faecal samples to attempt to identify salmonella carriers, but since excretion of pathogens is frequently intermittent this is unlikely to be very effective.

The World Health Organisation (Health Surveillance and Management Procedures for Food-Handling Personnel Technical Report Series 785, 1989) concluded that 'the pre-employment and subsequent routine medical examination of food handlers are ineffective and thus unnecessary. Examination may, however, be appropriate in the case of food handlers reporting sick or in the investigation of outbreaks of food-borne disease'. Reference was also made to the policy in the state of Florida in the USA where similar conclusions were reached.

These conclusions were based on a study of the following: physical examination, medical history, throat swabs, blood tests, X-rays and skin tests for TB and other lung infections, and the examination of faeces for pathogens and parasites.

A study of countries where pre-employment and routine periodic medical examinations are mandatory disclosed high costs of medical and laboratory examinations aggravated by the high labour turnover, seasonal employment and the use of part-time staff in the food industry. Many of these countries no longer adopt routine medical examinations.

*The most cost-effective measures were considered to be education and training involving both managers and food handlers.*

It is, however, important that workers who are suffering or who have recently suffered from bouts of gastroenteritis are excluded from duties where they are handling exposed fresh meat. Workers with septic lesions must cover such sores with appropriate waterproof dressings.

## Basic hygienic techniques

### *Hygienic use of knives*

Directive 64/433, Chapter V, para. 18(c) states that:

> Equipment and instruments used for working on meat shall be kept clean and in a good state of repair. They shall be carefully cleaned and disinfected *several* times during the working day, at the end of the day's work and before re-using when they have become soiled.

The most common method of sterilising implements is in a cabinet containing water at 82°C, the knife, saw or whatever piece of equipment is to be sterilised being left *in situ* for at least 2 minutes. It is essential that the level of

**STAFF IN CONFIDENCE**
**HEALTH QUESTIONNAIRE**

Name ..........................................................
Address ......................................................
..................................................................
..................................................................
Job title ......................................................

1. Have you or your family during the past year had contact with:

| | Self | Relative | Date | Place |
|---|---|---|---|---|
| Typhoid Fever | | | | |
| Paratyphoid Fever | | | | |
| Yellow Jaundice | | | | |
| Any severe illness with diarrhoea | | | | |

2. Have you a history of:

| | Yes | No | Comments, e.g. date, treatment, etc. |
|---|---|---|---|
| Septic skin condition e.g. boils, dermatitis, or eczema | | | |
| Discharge from eyes, ears, or nose | | | |
| Bronchitis or a productive cough | | | |
| Poor dental hygiene | | | |

3. Have you been abroad within the last 12 months? **YES / NO**

If YES: Place ......................... Country ......................... Date .........................

Did you have any illness while abroad? **YES / NO**

If YES, please give details

I declare that all the information given above is true and complete, to the best of my knowledge and belief.

*Signature:* ........................................................ *Date:* .........................

**Fig. 9.1** An example of a staff self-declaration form.

the water covers the handle/blade junction and that the knife or implement is visibly clean before being placed in the steriliser. If it is not washed first, the blood and debris will merely harden on to the blade, which should not be considered sanitised. A 44ºC rinse followed by a dip into a steriliser at 82ºC will reduce the contamination on a knife to less than $10^3$ cfu/cm (Bell and Hathaway, 1996). Sterilising equipment without a flow-through of water is not to be recommended as it can quickly become filthy. This is particularly the case for splitting saws where, if a plunge bath is used, the water rapidly takes on the colour and consistency of a thick soup. For this type of equipment a cabinet into which the blade of the implement is placed and sprayed with a foot-operated stream of water is preferred. The water from the cabinet can be positively ducted, reducing steam and splash.

In order that knives in particular spend sufficient time in the water at 82°C it is necessary for each operative to have several knives. This modus operandi is known rather grandly as the *multiple knife technique*. When the operative arrives at the work-station to commence work, he or she places a number of clean knives in the steriliser. Each time a knife becomes contaminated it is washed and placed in the steriliser and another knife is selected. The knives are used serially so that each has spent the maximum possible period in the steriliser.

This technique is suitable for knives and for larger equipment like hock cutters where, however, it may be necessary on some lines for equipment to be doubled up so that each item can spend sufficient time being decontaminated.

### *Hygienic use of the scabbard*

Scabbards of the closed type are in the main unhygienic and a source of contamination to a sterilised knife. The newer open stainless steel scabbard is a considerable improvement.

A scabbard is necessary, for health and safety reasons, for the transportation of knives to the work-station. Once at the work-station, all knives should be unloaded into the steriliser from which they are used for the rest of the working day. The only major exception to this rule on the slaughterline is the operative who removes the head from the bovine. On most slaughter lines he must carry the head from the point of removal to the washing cabinet, where the head is hung, trimmed and washed inside and out with a high pressure spray. It would be unsafe for him or her to do so with the head in one hand and the knife in the other.

### *Hygienic use of the steel*

The steel, which is used to keep the knife sharp, is a source of contamination frequently overlooked in daily operations. A steel which is hanging from the user's belt, dangling either inside or against the outside of a wellington boot, cannot be considered as a suitably hygienic surface against which to rub a knife which has just been removed from a steriliser. The cleanliness of the steel, and its storage when not in use, are therefore very important. On arrival at the work-station, the steel should be removed from the belt or scabbard and sterilised. It is unreasonable to expect the steel to be stored throughout the day in the steriliser, since most operatives believe that this practice destroys the effectiveness of the steel. It should therefore be stored hanging freely from a hook at the work-station where it will remain effectively sterile providing only sterilised knives are used on it. The steel should not be stored in a wash-hand basin, which may contain stagnant water, on ledges, behind pipe-work or in most of the other ingenious places in which it is often found in the workplace.

## Layout and flowlines

The layout of the slaughterfloor and the flowlines for the entry and exit of carcases, operatives, bins and other equipment is particularly important and must be properly designed at the planning stage. There should be a clear demarcation and, if at all possible, physical separation between clean and dirty parts of the abattoir. Operatives must be able to reach their work-station without risking contamination of themselves or the meat by walking through or under carcases on the lines or passing through 'less fit' parts of the abattoir such as green offal rooms, rendering plants or waste storage areas. During breaks, procedures must be in place to ensure that work clothes and equipment remain clean. Insufficient thought in this area frequently leads to workers from different parts of the abattoir using the same facilities during breaks, with the potential for cross-contamination. It is not unknown for food factory operatives to be seen playing football in protective clothing and footwear during their breaks from the line.

It is obvious that waste bins and the hide conveyor should never cross the slaughterline because of the risk of contamination, but poor design, especially in the older factories with twisted lines, sometimes makes this impossible to avoid. It is not only the bin of, for example, bovine feet which is a risk, but also the operative who propels it. He or she will by necessity be passing back and forth from clean work room to the waste skip area. The official veterinarian should be continuously asking the questions of every operative and practice: How did that get there? Where is it going? What is the risk to meat hygiene? Another question, and one frequently omitted, is Where will the tray or buggy be washed before it returns to the work place? The use of chutes removing waste without the need for personnel movements is clearly advantageous.

Another important consideration is the layout of the individual work-station. It is important that the washing and sanitising equipment is sited so that it is simple and convenient to use. To put it bluntly, if the equipment is not positioned so that it is easier for the operative to use it than not, it is inevitable that in the hurly-burly of the workplace and the repetitive nature of the tasks, shortcuts will be taken. Good design is also important.

An apron wash with the steriliser positioned on its outer wall is one such example, where the operative steps into the apron wash, washes the knife as he enters and places it in the steriliser, washes his apron, hands and arms in the apron wash, and collects a clean knife on his way out.

## DRESSING TECHNIQUES – REMOVAL OF HIDE/FLEECE/HAIR

The contamination of the carcase by dirt, debris and hair from the outer integument of the animal must be prevented as far as possible by good dressing technique. In many cases complete prevention is almost impossible, e.g. with deer which have been allowed to wallow, are caked with mud and in addition shed their hair profusely. Details of some recommended techniques are outlined below. These are, however, only suggestions and not all will be appropriate under every circumstance. The skill of the professionally-trained veterinarian is to understand the general principles so that they may be adapted to a particular practical situation or problem encountered.

### *Cattle*

Dry, clean cattle having been stunned, are allowed to slide or tumble from the stunning box. The use of raised slats or metal grid in this area – the dry landing area – is essential in order to keep the animals as clean and dry as possible. The cattle are then hoisted by the leading hindleg on to the line and bled before the removal of the hide commences.

An incision through the skin, the knife moving as it must through the dirty exterior towards and into the clean interior, is always fraught with the hygienic risk of pushing dirt or hair on to the carcase. These initial cuts must, therefore, be carried out with great care and kept as short as possible. Once through the skin, the knife must be washed and sterilised, and/or exchanged for a clean knife. All incisions from this initial one should then be made using a *spear cut technique*, where the blade of the knife is reversed so that its back is against the carcase and the cut is made from the inside of the skin towards the outside, or to put it another way, from clean towards dirty. This results in reduced contamination (Fig. 9.2).

To illustrate the point, consider a common procedure for freeing the hide from the rear quarters during on-line dressing of cattle. An initial short incision is made along the ventral midline between the hindlegs of the suspended animal. The knife used is washed and placed in the steriliser, hands, arms and apron washed, and a clean sterilised knife is collected from the steriliser. The initial incision is extended downwards towards the umbilicus, and upwards along the free hind limb towards the hock, using the spear technique. Skinning then proceeds from these incisions.

During skinning the carcase frequently becomes contaminated from inrolling at the edges of the hide. Small alterations to the positioning of the skinning incisions is often sufficient to alter the way in which the hide hangs and so eradicate the problem. The use of pairs of crocodile clips joined by a plastic cord has been found to be a useful tool in the prevention of inrolling, especially when used at the hide-puller.

A particular problem with hide-pullers, especially those which pull upwards, is dirt flicking from the hide on to the exposed carcase as the hide finally detaches from the carcase and head. These flecks must be removed immediately by trimming (Fig. 9.3).

A particularly important initial cut through the skin is the one which exposes the major vessels in the neck for sticking. As previously described, the knife contaminated while incising the skin must be washed and sterilised, and a clean knife used to sever the blood vessels.

### *Sheep*

Most of the techniques described for cattle are also applicable to sheep. Many of the problems

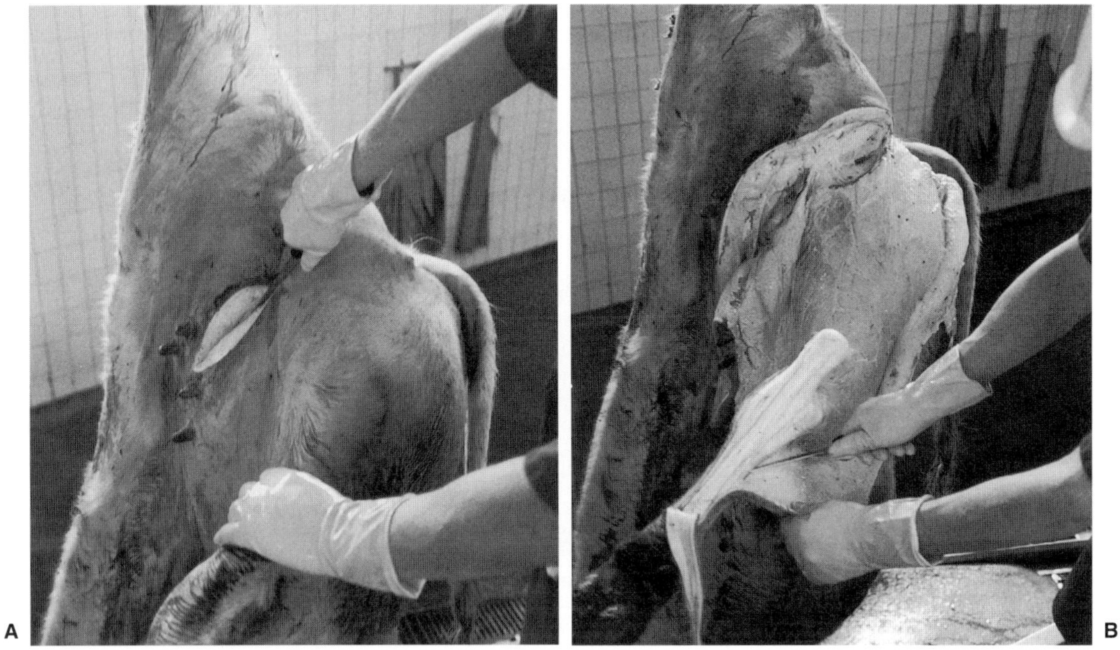

Fig. 9.2 The initial incision, which will be extended using the spear cut technique. Effective outrolling of hide is shown at left in (B). (By courtesy of R. H. S. Moore BA, MVE, MRCVS)

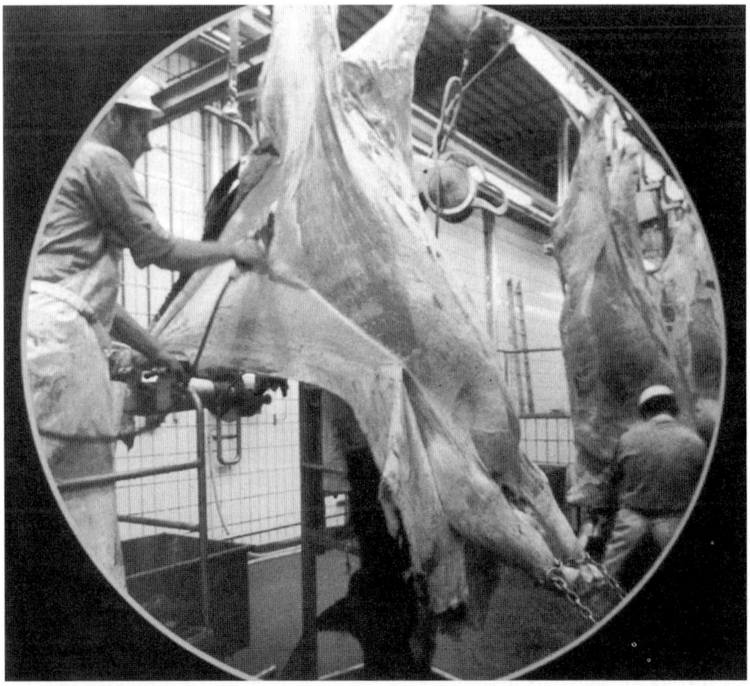

Fig. 9.3 Downward hide puller; more hygienic than upward puller and can also skin head, previously prepared. (By courtesy of Messrs Nijhuis Stachttechniek, Lichtenvoorde, The Netherlands)

occur with the ventral incision and with in-rolling of the fleece. Again the elasticised crocodile clips are useful. Judicious use of glossy paper sheets placed on the sternum and inguinal regions can be very successful. It is imperative that the right sort of paper, which will remain in place but not adhere permanently to the carcase, is used.

A particular problem may be encountered where dry, dirty sheep release dust while the fleece is being mechanically removed. This dust can be virtually impossible to remove from the carcase surface. Pelting machines which allow the pelt to flap about and recoil excessively when it is released from the carcase are most likely to result in the exposed meat surface being showered with loose hairs and other debris from the fleece.

In the *traditional sheep dressing system*, the lamb was suspended initially by the hindlegs. The pelt was freed manually from the hind-quarters and removed to the level of the shoulders by a combination of 'punching out' and pulling downwards from tail to head. The forelegs were then lifted and hung on a rail running parallel to that suspending the hind-feet, and the forequarter was skinned using knife work and a horizontal pull. This technique has been replaced in many sheep slaughterlines by a more hygienic system, known as *inverted dressing*. The lamb is suspended initially by the forelegs, and the pelt is loosened from around the shoulders. Some knife work is utilised to partially free the pelt from the hindquarters, before it is removed by a mechanical pelter pulling from head to tail.

It is common practice, particularly in New Zealand, to wash the carcases after pelting and before evisceration to remove visible contamination such as wool, blood and faeces. It is likely that, although this practice improves the appearance of the carcase, it actually assists in spreading contamination to otherwise clean parts of the carcase and adds water to the warm exposed meat surface to assist bacterial metabolism.

Bell and Hathaway (1996) found that the areas of highest contamination were the forequarter region with inverted dressing and the hindquarter with conventional dressing. In both cases these regions are the sites where cuts are made through the skin. With both systems contamination around these cuts was entirely consistent with direct fleece contact resulting from 'rollback'.

In Italy, mechanical subcutaneous inflation has been used to assist in skinning lightweight lambs. Producers claim that the resultant carcase has a better appearance and that there are fewer cuts in the subcutaneous fat and muscle. The technique has been shown to produce carcases of comparable microbiological standard to those produced by conventional dressing. It is now allowed within the EU under Directive 95/23/EC for lambs with a liveweight of <15 kg.

### *Pigs*

Most pigs in the British Isles are scalded, dehaired, singed and scraped as a preparation for bacon production rather than being skinned. The scalding water may contain many different types of bacteria originating from the pigs' skin and gastrointestinal tract, including *Salmonella* spp. The temperature of the water in the drag-through scalding tank, at 60°C, is generally sufficient to reduce vegetative growth. The skins of scalded pigs have low numbers of both enteric pathogens and spoilage bacteria (Sorquist and Danielsson-Tham, 1986; Troeger, 1994), but the subsequent dehairing process recontaminates the skin. The bacterial content of the muscle and viscera does, however, appear to be affected by the type of scalding equipment.

*Vertical scalding of pigs* on the line with humidified air reduces the opportunity for contamination of the carcase via the stick wound (Fig. 9.4). Humidified air is blown under pressure through nozzles to reach all parts of the carcases. Scalding at a temperature of 61°C continues for about 7 minutes. Water consumption is about 15% of the normal method. There is no cross-contamination, no water in lungs, no infection of thorax through the stick wound and no recirculation of dirty water.

Following singeing, the bacterial load on the carcase surface is of the order of tens of bacteria/$cm^2$, but the scraping and polishing procedures which follow recontaminate the surface to the order of $10^3$ bacteria/$cm^2$. The majority of these are spoilage bacteria, predominantly acinetobacteria, moraxellae and pseudomonads, with enteric organism such as *E. coli* and *Campylobacter* at single figures per $cm^2$.

An apparatus, described by Gill (1996), has been developed and trialled commercially on a

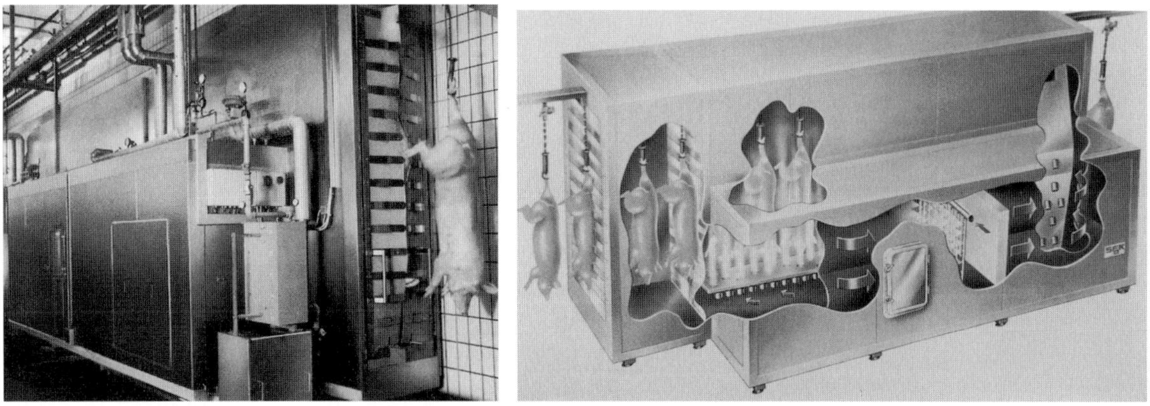

A B

**Fig. 9.4** Vertical scalding of pigs with humidified air. A, Overall view of chamber with exit at right. B, Section of chamber.

pig line operating at 800 pigs/hour, and is capable of reducing the contamination on the surface of uneviscerated pigs by a factor of $10^2$. The machine washes the pigs with sheets of water heated to 85ºC for a treatment time of 15 seconds. Water is recirculated from a tank beneath the line through screens to header tanks which feed the nozzles.

One common problem, or perceived problem, is the failure of the automatic equipment to remove all of the pig's *toe nails* all of the time. Although they look dirty, personal investigation would suggest that toe nails carry no greater a bacterial load than the rest of the carcase.

### Preventing contamination from the gastrointestinal tract

After the outer integument, the gastrointestinal tract is the next most important potential source of contamination. However, if the rectum and oesophagus can be sealed, and the tract removed intact, the contamination can be effectively controlled.

#### *Cattle*

The technique used for sealing the rectum is known as *bunging*. The system depends to some extent on flaying technique and on the type of hidepuller being utilised. If an upwards hidepuller is in use, the skin is pulled away from the perineal region with the rest of the hide leaving the perineal region hygienically exposed. The technique which is recommended involves the operative placing a plastic bag over his left hand with a strong elastic band around his wrist. The exposed end of the rectum is grasped with this hand and a circular incision made around the rectum, freeing it from adherent tissues within the pelvis. The plastic bag is then unfurled over the rectum from the hand grasping it and secured in place with the elastic band. The protected rectum can now be allowed to pass or be pushed down into the abdominal cavity. If a downward hide-puller is utilised, the rectum must be freed prior to removal of the hide. This is a more difficult task to complete hygienically since the circular cut around the rectum to free it has to be made through the contaminated hide.

Recently designed equipment has transformed the task of bung removal, reducing faecal contamination significantly, improving carcase dressing technique and minimising operative fatigue and risk of knife damage (to operative and carcase meat).

A machine developed in Australia known as the Beef Bung Bagging Machine (Fig. 9.5) automatically grasps the rectum, leaving the operative to clear the rectum from its attachments with a circular incision. A plastic bag and rubber ring are applied to make a secure seal on the rectum and all operations are carried out without hand contact with the carcase.

A less sophisticated hydraulically operated elastrator can also be used for sealing a plastic bag with a rubber ring (Fig. 9.6).

The oesophagus (weasand) in cattle is usually sealed by an elastrator ring applied at

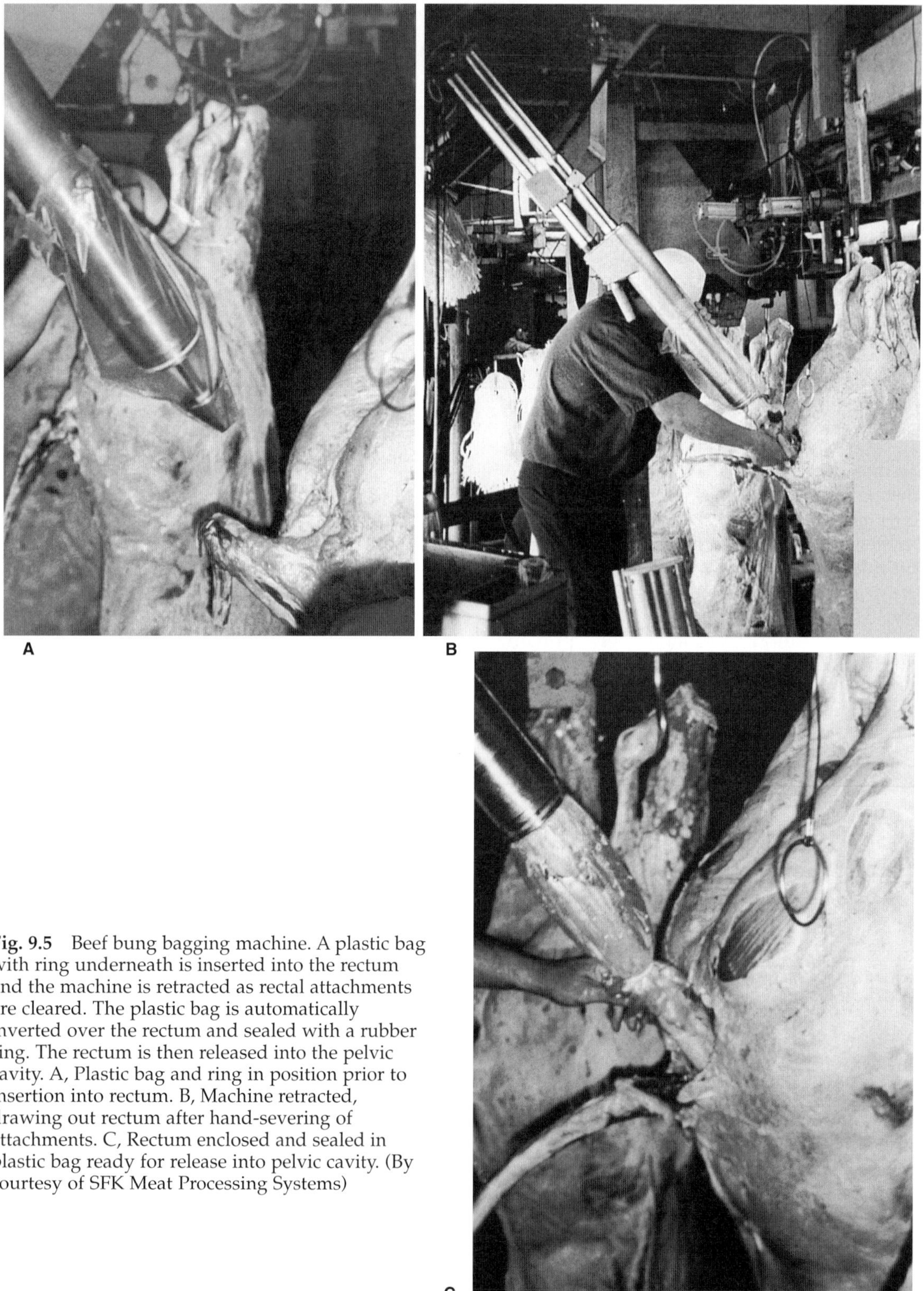

**Fig. 9.5** Beef bung bagging machine. A plastic bag with ring underneath is inserted into the rectum and the machine is retracted as rectal attachments are cleared. The plastic bag is automatically inverted over the rectum and sealed with a rubber ring. The rectum is then released into the pelvic cavity. A, Plastic bag and ring in position prior to insertion into rectum. B, Machine retracted, drawing out rectum after hand-severing of attachments. C, Rectum enclosed and sealed in plastic bag ready for release into pelvic cavity. (By courtesy of SFK Meat Processing Systems)

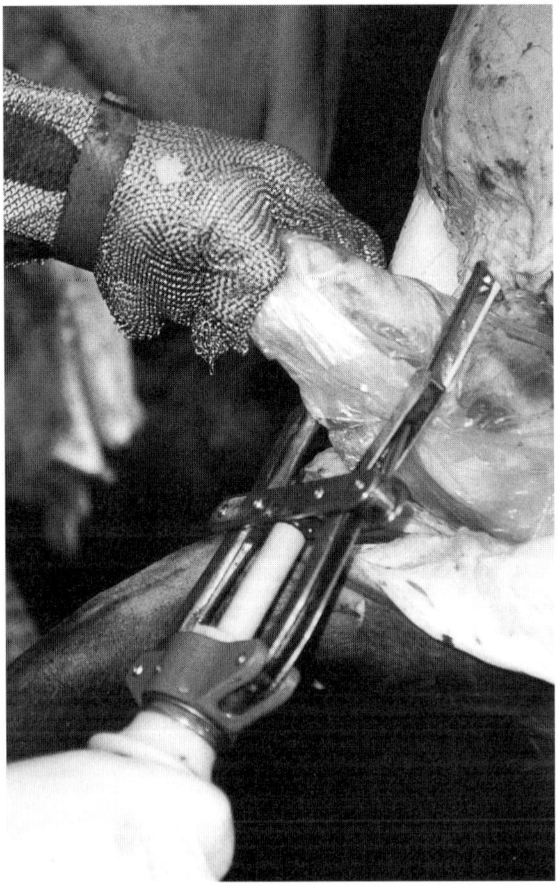

**Fig. 9.6** Elastrators with expanded rubber ring ready for placing over plastic bag or rectum. (By courtesy of R. H. S. Moore MRCVS)

the oesophageal–ruminal junction in a procedure known as *rodding*. The procedure involves the separation out of the oesophagus and, using a stainless steel instrument, forcing a rubber ring up the length of the oesophagus, through the thoracic cavity, to deposit it using a trigger device at the oesophageal–ruminal junction (Fig. 9.7). Rodding is best carried out immediately bleeding is completed to prevent the escape of ruminal fluid, which would contaminate the tissues of the head and neck.

### *Sheep*

In sheep, after the pelt is removed, the rectum is freed from the attachments within the pelvis and a length of 30 cm, or more, is exteriorised. Although several alternative practices exist, it is acceptable to 'milk' the solid faeces back up the rectum, cut off the posterior few centimetres and allow the cut end to drop into the abdominal cavity.

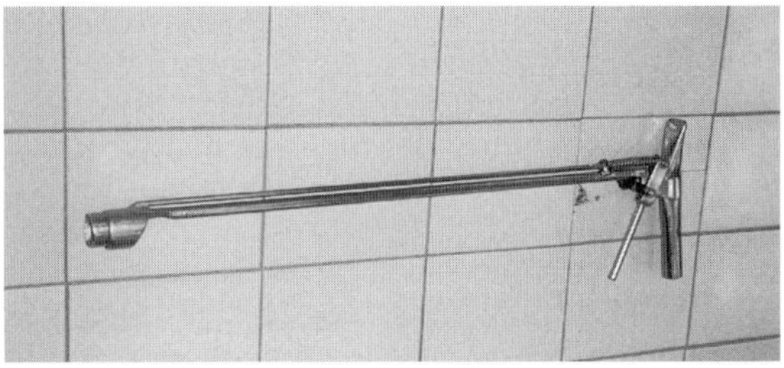

**Fig. 9.7** Stainless steel rodder.

The oesophagus in sheep may be sealed using a smaller version of the bovine rodding equipment, but more frequently clips are used.

### *Pigs*

In pigs, the abdominal cavity is opened and the pubic synthesis of the pelvis is split prior to the freeing of the rectum. The anal sphincter is removed intact and, since the pelvis is split, the rectum can be detached and removed from the abdominal cavity with the entire gastrointestinal tract in one movement. Commonly, the only attempt made to seal the rectum to prevent faecal spillage is a simple knot tied in the posterior rectum. The most common reason for contamination of the carcase is accidental incision of the wall of the rectum while the operative is cutting round to free it. The procedure leaves little margin for error since the operative does not want to cut into the hams, one of the most expensive cuts.

In Denmark this problem has been alleviated by the introduction of automatic bunging. A device with a tubular blade is positioned by a central pin which is placed up the rectum. The blade cuts down around the rectum, loosening it.

No attempt is usually made to seal the porcine oesophagus.

## POST-SLAUGHTER DECONTAMINATION

The emergence of *E. coli* O157: H7, especially in Canada, USA and Scotland, as a significant food poisoning pathogen of animal origin has initiated a search for methods by which the consumer can be given even greater assurances as to the safety of the meat to be consumed. The deaths of children and the elderly who had consumed beef-burgers contaminated with low numbers of the organisms has caused understandable hysteria, especially as it followed upon increased public concern about other food poisoning organisms such as *Salmonella* and *Listeria*. To answer these concerns and in an attempt to improve meat safety, the USDA Food Safety Inspection Service (FSIS), suggest that all carcases must receive at least one antimicrobial treatment before chilling. These treatments may include hot water; organic acid sprays; antimicrobials; hydrogen peroxide; trisodium phosphate (TSP) and chlorinated water.

### Water

In the recent past it was common practice to wash the carcases of both cattle and sheep with large volumes of hot or cold water to remove any visible contamination which had found its way on to the carcase during processing. The general movement has been away from this practice towards the use of the minimal amount of water necessary to remove bone dust from the spinal column, with faecal and other contamination being removed by trimming. This approach was supported by a great deal of scientific research and comment, such as that of Ellerbroek *et al.* (1993), who demonstrated that spray washing did not reduce or increase bacterial contamination of the ventral area of sheep carcases, i.e. a portion of the carcase most likely to be contaminated by slaughter personnel, but led to bacterial contamination of the clean dorsal surface of the carcase. The conclusion was therefore drawn that spray washing with water at 12ºC, 6 bar pressure for 20 s did not improve the microbial status of sheep carcases and that the additional water remaining on the carcase enhanced the multiplication of bacteria in the long run. Many investigators have demonstrated that an improvement in bacteriological results occurs if water at a temperature over 60ºC is utilised with washes of >85ºC frequently being recommended. The USDA have recommended that the water should have a temperature of >74ºC for at least 10 s. Hot water also gives carcases a better bloom than cold water sprays.

One regime for washing carcases recommends water containing 15 ppm chlorine at a temperature of 85–90ºC applied through a fanshaped nozzle at a pressure of 100 psi, at a rate of 18 litres/min for cattle and 9 litres/min for sheep.

Gill (1996) concluded that washing, unaccompanied by heating of the carcase surface to temperatures which will kill bacteria, should be considered as an ineffective means of decontaminating carcases.

### **Steam pasteurisation/sterilisation** (Fig. 9.8)

The Food Safety and Inspection Service of the USDA has approved two novel methods of cleansing beef carcases. The first is a *steam*

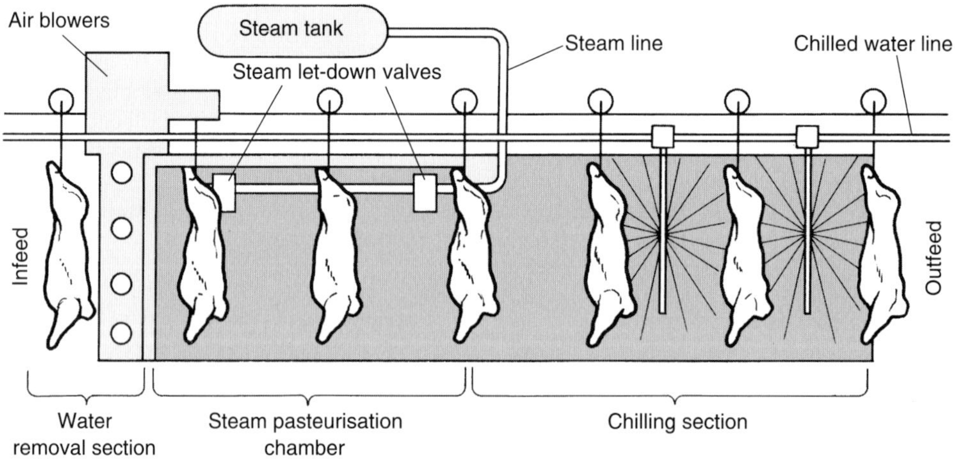


**Fig. 9.8** Steam pasteurisation chamber – water removal, pasteurisation and chill sections.

*vacuum sterilisation process* which uses water at 88°C, vacuum and steam at 45 psi to remove contamination and sterilise the meat surface through means of a nozzle similar to a vacuum carpet cleaner (Dorsa, 1996). The second is a system of *steam sterilisation* in which, after removal of surface water, the split carcases are passed through a sealed chamber where they are exposed to low-pressure steam at over 85°C for 8 s and then cooled with a chilled water spray (Phebus, 1996).

A study by Gill *et al.* (1995) considered that treatment of pig carcases prior to evisceration with water at 85°C for 20 s gave maximum destruction of the surface bacteria present.

### Trimming

Prasai *et al.* (1995) demonstrated that removing visible contamination by trimming and then washing was the most practical and effective method for reducing microbial contamination of the beef carcase. They emphasised that frequent sterilisation of knives and other tools used in the trimming process was essential to reduce or minimise bacterial contamination, and that individual operative technique was the most important factor in the efficiency of trimming.

### Chemical treatments

The following *chemicals* have been used to reduce the bacterial load on meat after slaughter:

| | | |
|---|---|---|
| 1 | Chlorine | |
| 2 | Organic acids: e.g. | acetic acid |
| | | lactic acid |
| | | citric acid |
| | | fumaric acid |
| 3 | Hydrogen peroxide | |
| 4 | Antimicrobials: e.g. | nisin |
| | | bactericin |
| 5 | Phosphates: | trisodium phosphate |

The effectiveness of chemical treatments in reducing the numbers of pathogenic organisms is far from being definitely established. Efficacy may vary with the particular chemical used, the concentration of the chemical, the contact time, the tissue type, the length of time which has elapsed between contamination and treatment, the organism, the temperature of the solution, and the method of delivery.

A study utilising *chlorine* at 20 ppm in a beef carcase wash at 16°C for 10 and 60 s demonstrated that treatments with chlorine at this concentration and temperature were no more effective than water alone for reducing faecal contamination on meat (Cutter and Dorsa, 1995). However, higher concentrations of chlorine up to and above 350 ppm have been utilised and reported to be effective, although such high concentrations of chlorine are neither advisable or acceptable. Chlorine is readily inactivated by organic matter and combines with amino nitrogen to form the less active chloroamines.

Investigations indicate that *acid treatments* are more effective on adipose tissue than lean meat, and that while spray treatments with organic acids do reduce populations of *E. coli* O157:H7 on red meat, neither lactic, citric or acetic acid at concentrations up to 5% reduced the pathogen levels to zero (Cutter and Siragusa, 1994). Brackett *et al.* (1994) confirmed that these acids at concentrations up to 1.5% applied at 20°C and 55°C did not appreciably reduce numbers of *E. coli* O157:H7 on beef. In general it would appear that although organic acids are successful in reducing the numbers of spoilage bacteria present on the meat surface, they are of much less use when required to render meat safer by removing pathogenic bacteria.

*Trisodium phosphate* has been used to reduce the total viable counts on poultry carcases by 50% and the incidence of salmonella-contaminated carcases from 9.5% to 0%. Phosphates are, however, potential environmental pollutants.

The abuse of post-processing treatment to mask sloppy work and inspection processes must be rigorously opposed. The FSIS in the United States recognises this and states categorically that 'antimicrobial treatments will not be permitted to substitute for strict compliance with sanitary slaughter and carcase dressing procedures, e.g. no visible faecal contamination will be permitted on the carcase before the treatment is applied'. Suitably controlled, and as part of an integrated approach to the reduction in the total numbers of pathogenic and spoilage bacteria present on the carcase before it enters the chillers, these treatments may have an important role to play.

Public demand for meat which is naturally produced and residue-free, however, may make the concept of treating meat with antimicrobials, acids or high levels of chlorine, difficult to establish.

### The washing of edible offals

The washing of edible offals such as liver, kidneys, hearts, thin skirt and tails is another important facet of satisfactory abattoir hygiene and it is essential that a continuous flow of clean water be used for this purpose. An excellent device for the washing of tongues is an inclined rotating metal drum with a through-flow of water working on the same principle as a cement mixer though without the central agitating arms.

## ASSESSING OPERATIONAL HYGIENE

Traditionally the meat hygiene inspection team assessed the standard of operational hygiene by utilising a programme of regular checks combined with a random visual and microbiological examination of the end-product. In most meat factories this consisted of regular inspections of the hygiene of structures and equipment, usually utilising check lists. The checks carried out, and the standards of hygiene structure and procedures required were laid down in codes of practice, such as those developed to encourage Good Manufacturing Practices (GMP), directives, decisions, regulations and by-laws enforced by local, national and international bodies.

These *quality control* programmes, however, could at best only identify problems after they had occurred, and put them right. Unless 100% checking took place, which is almost always impossible, quality control systems can only identify problems after they have occurred and, hopefully, before too much substandard product has passed out of the system. All too frequently, a manufacturer only became aware of a problem with the manufacturing process as a result of a complaint of premature spoilage in the marketplace or from reports of illness. Food retailers and their customers increasingly demand a system where there are no errors, and will not accept any risk that food poisoning may occur.

### Hazard Analysis Critical Control Points (HACCP)

To deliver the customer this quality assurance, a more proactive method was sought by which the source of microbiological hazards could be identified and eliminated. What was required was a systematic and targeted approach to food hygiene where the potential problems were identified and the efforts of the inspectors were directed to those areas which could eliminate the deficiency in the process. This approach has become known as *Hazard Analysis Critical Control Points* (HACCP). All federally-inspected meat slaughter plants in the USA must have a plant-specific HACCP plan, and in the EU the principles have found their way into the more recent meat directives. International acceptance of the approach was underlined during the Uruguay Round of the General Agreement on Tariffs and Trade (GATT), when the inclusion of the Codex Alimentarius Commission's recommendations on the application of HACCP were specifically identified as the baseline for consumer protection under the Agreement on the Application of Sanitary and Phytosanitary Measures.

All HACCP systems comprise the following sequential steps:

#### 1. *Hazard analysis*

The first step in applying the HACCP system to a food manufacturing operation is to identify and quantify the microbiological hazards and risks within the operation. The following definitions (ICMSF, 1988) are important:

- *Hazard* means the unacceptable contamination, unacceptable growth and/or unacceptable survival by microorganisms of concern to safety or spoilage and/or the unacceptable production or persistence in foods of products of microbiological metabolism (e.g. toxins, enzymes, biogenic amines).
- *Severity* is the seriousness (magnitude) of the hazard.
- *Risk* is an estimate of the likely occurrence of a hazard.

The analysis requires the specialist knowledge of a multidisciplinary team and should include food microbiologists, engineers, veterinarians, cleaning experts and so on. A step-by-step investigation of the process is carried out , from the specification required for the raw material through the manufacturing process to the distribution chain.

Epidemiological investigation of historical episodes of premature spoilage or food poisoning in which the product was implicated can provide valuable information about potential hazards. All of the data emerging from this analysis should be collated into a flow chart (Fig. 9.9) and all of the hazards identified and evaluated with regard to their severity and likely frequency of occurrence.

2. *Determination of the Critical Control Points (CCPs)*

The classical definition of a *critical control point* (Codex Alimentarius Commission, Codex 1991) is a location, practice, procedure or process at which control can be exercised over one or more factors which, if controlled, could minimise or prevent a hazard. This definition has subsequently been revised and subdivided so that we may now describe:

- CCP1 where the hazard can be prevented or eliminated;
- CCP2 where the hazard can be minimised, reduced or delayed;

or under a different system:

- CCPe where the hazards are eliminated and no further problem exists;
- CCPp where the hazards are prevented but not necessarily eliminated;
- CCPr where the hazard is significantly reduced, minimised or delayed.

The proper identification of CCPs can make the difference between an effective HACCP programme and one that, by the identification of too many points in the system which must be considered as critical, becomes ineffective. The definition of CCPs should, therefore, be amended to mean a point in the process where

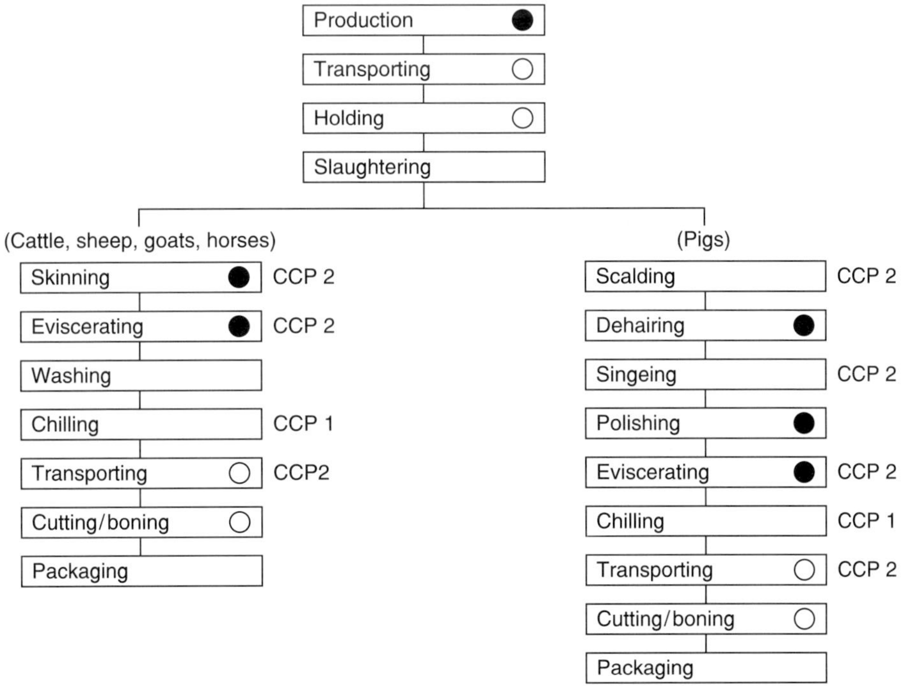


**Fig. 9.9** Flow diagram for fresh meat production and processing. o indicates a site of minor contamination; • indicates a site of major contamination; CCPI effective CCP; CCP 2 not absolute. (International Commission on Microbiological Specifications for Foods (ICMSF) of the International Union of

loss of control has a *reasonable probability* of creating an unacceptable health risk.

*3. Specification of the criteria*

*Criteria* are specific limits of characteristics of a physical (e.g. time or temperature), chemical (e.g. salt or acetic acid) or biological (e.g. sensorial or microbiological) nature. Increasing emphasis has been placed on quantitative, rather than qualitative, criteria which indicate whether or not an operation is under control. Quantitative criteria, such as time, temperature, pH and the concentration of various chemicals, can be measured and indicate definitively that a system is or is not controlled. Qualitative criteria such as colour or smell are more difficult to determine objectively and consequently it is much more difficult to judge divergence from the accepted normal. Microbiological criteria are particularly difficult to quantify in absolute terms under practical conditions. A great deal of standardisation of sampling and laboratory techniques is required before values can be compared. Attempts to quantify in numerical terms the infective dose of a particular pathogen are fraught with difficulties owing to differences in pathogenicity of different strains and varying susceptibility between different groups of consumers.

*4. Implementation of the monitoring system*

*Monitoring* is the systematic checking of the process or procedure, at a particular CCP, in order to detect any deviations from the criteria which have been set. This is best carried out by the operatives themselves or by their supervisors rather than by a special team of quality assurance staff. The integration of the checks into the routine of the manufacturing process and the ownership of the quality assurance by the workers is an important aspect of a successful system. The methods selected for monitoring must give immediate results so that any problems detected can be corrected immediately. Traditional microbiological checks, where the results may not be available for 36 hours or more, are therefore of little value.

A number of new approaches to microbiological monitoring are, however, becoming commercially available. Some of these techniques are suitable for determining total counts of bacteria, while others determine the presence of specific pathogens. Techniques utilising monoclonal antibodies and DNA probes in combination with automatic instruments are being developed which can give results in hours.

A microbial ATP bioluminescence assay has been shown to be an accurate and rapid method for determining the levels of generic bacterial contamination on beef and pork carcases (Siragusa *et al.*, 1995). The technique can distinguish between microbial and non-microbial ATP, but sensitivity is variable at microbial levels below $10^4$ (Siragusa and Cutter 1995). The entire test, including sampling, takes only 5 minutes to complete (see p. 376).

*5. Corrective action*

Procedures must be established so that immediate action can be taken for detection of deviation from the established criteria. This may involve rectifying an out-of-control situation before an operation is allowed to commence, or halting the manufacturing process.

*6. Verification*

*Verification checks* are carried out systematically by the quality assurance staff and the veterinary inspection team. It is important that duplication of effort by the in-house and regulatory inspectors is avoided and that all checks are complementary. Verification may involve some microbiological checks of end-product, structures and equipment. All checks should be carried out at a statistically-significant frequency and in a systematic, targeted manner.

*7. Documentation*

Many HACCP systems in meat plants have died under the weight of paper they generate. If, after implementation has occurred, it is discovered that too many CCPs were identified and that the monitoring process is unnecessarily complicated or cumbersome, there must be sufficient flexibility in the system to allow adjustments to be made. Another risk with cumbersome documentation is that the completion of the form can rapidly become the monitoring personnel's primary objective rather than merely a tool to meet the overall objective of safe food.

A HACCP system is not something which should, or can, be imposed by either the in-house quality assurance staff or the regulatory authority, though both bodies must be intimately involved. For the system to work properly, the entire workforce within the food factory, including all managers, supervisors, operatives, fitters and cleaning staff, must be dedicated to the success of the system and involved in its operation. This requires a considerable investment of time in training for all staff.

## HYGIENE ASSESSMENT SYSTEMS (HAS)

*Risk assessment principles* are also used as a tool for assessing and monitoring hygienic standards. Most of the systems developed depend upon observations being made at each step in a process, with points being awarded according to the degree of compliance with the required standard. Scores are weighted with regard to the risk that partial compliance accords the safety of the final product. A total score at the end of the inspection gives a measure of the hygienic compliance.

In an assessment of the HAS system operated in abattoirs in Great Britain by the State Veterinary Service, a significant correlation was reported between the mean total viable bacterial count for each abattoir and the mean HAS scores. It was concluded that HAS scores were useful in predicting the ability of an abattoir to produce carcases of sound microbiological status, especially the categories concerned with slaughter and dressing, personnel and practices (Hudson *et al.*, 1996).

The score achieved gives a snapshot of the hygienic standard of the process and does provide a useful tool, assisting management in their efforts to improve Good Manufacturing Practice. The assessment has the advantage in that it can be carried out by relatively inexperienced staff.

## REFERENCES


Bell, R. G. and Hathaway, S. C. (1996) *J. Appl. Bacteriol.* **81**, 225–234.

Biss, M. E. and Hathaway, S. C (1996) *Vet. Rec.* **138**, 82–86.

Brackett, R. E., Hao, Y. Y. and Doyle, M. P (1994) *J. Food Protection* **57**(3), 198–203.

Cutter, C. N. and Dorsa, W. J (1995) *J. Food Protection* **58**(12), 1294–1296.

Cutter, C. N. and Siragusa, G. R (1994) *J. Food Protection* **57**(2), 97–103.

Dorsa, W. (1996) *Proceedings of the 49th Reciprocal Meat Conference, Provo, Utah, June 1996*, pp. 114–120.

Ellerbroek, L. I., Wegener, J. F. and Arndt, G. (1993) *J. Food Protection* **56**(5), 432–436.

Empey, W. A. and Scott, W. J (1939) *Council of Scientific and Industrial Research*, Bulletin No. 126.

Gill, C. O. (1996) *Meat Focus Int.* April, 121–122.

Gill, C. O., McGinnis, D. S., Bryant, J. and Chabot, B. (1995) *Food Microbiol.* **12**, 143–149.

Hudson, W. R., Mead, G. C. and Hinton, M. H. (1996) *Vet. Rec.* **139**, 587–589.

Phebus, R. (1996) *Proceedings of the 49th Reciprocal Meat Conference, Provo, Utah, June 1996*, pp. 121–124.

Prasai, R. K., Phebus, R. K., Garcia Zepeda, C. A., Kastner, C. L., Boyle, A. E. and Fung, D. Y. C. (1995) *J. Food Protection* **58**(10), 1114–1117.

Ridell, J. and Korkeala, H. (1993) *Meat Sci.* **35**, 223–228.

Schnell, T. D., Sofas, J. N., Littlefiel, V. G., Morgan, J. B., Gorman, B. M., Clayton, R. P. and Smith, G. C. (1995) *J. Food Protection* **58**(12), 1297–1302.

Siragusa, G. R. and Cutter, C. N. (1995) *J. Food Protection* **58**(7), 764–769.

Siragusa, G. R., Cutter, C.N., Dorsa, W. J. and Koohmaraie, M. (1995) *J. Food Protection* **58**(7), 770–775.

Sorquist, S. and Danielsson-Tham, M. L. (1986) *Fleischwirtschaft* **66**, 1745–1748.

Troeger, K. (1994) *Fleischwirtschaft* **74**(6), 624–626.


## FURTHER READING


(HACCP) principles in food control. Food and Nutrition Paper, 58.

ICMSF (The International Commission on Microbiological Specification Foods) (1988). *Microorganisms in Food, 4. Application of the hazard analysis critical control point (HACCP) system to ensure microbiological safety and quality*. London: Blackwell.

# C0hapter 10
# Red Meat Inspection

It is beyond dispute that the inspection procedures which have served the meat industry since they were first introduced by von Ostertag at the turn of the century are in need of a radical overhaul. The necessity for change has been championed by recognised authorities in meat hygiene worldwide over the last 10 years: Blackmore (1983), Hathaway *et al.* (1987), Berends *et al.* (1993), Johnston (1994) and many others. However, it is essential that any alterations to the existing systems are based on sound scientific principles of food hygiene, and not unduly influenced by political pressures from interested parties either from within the meat industry seeking short-term financial savings, or from the 'inspection industry' seeking to defend their positions and the status quo. Food safety is of paramount importance.

## ANTE-MORTEM INSPECTION

As already discussed in Chapter 7, ante-mortem inspection, as presently carried out in the lairage in many countries, is limited in its effectiveness owing to the often excited nature of the animals, the constraint of the premises, and the fact that there is no requirement for the UK producer, except for casualty slaughter animals, to declare any information with regard to the health status of the animal or group of animals he is presenting for slaughter. The fact is that, as the present system stands, it is in the producer's interest to attempt to conceal all such information in case the inspector should take a particular interest in the animals. This situation means that the Official Veterinarian attempts to make a clinical diagnosis without a history, a situation that could not be tolerated in day-to-day veterinary medical practice.

Many different methods have been tried in an attempt to fill this information vacuum, ranging from the fully integrated production systems operated in Scandinavian countries to small local 'Quality Assured Meat' schemes. The Danish pig system is the pinnacle to which all others should aspire, providing the official veterinarian in the abattoir with detailed information about every production unit, with data on husbandry matters, disease status and drug use. However, it is difficult to see how this system could ever be applied uniformly across all food animal species throughout the European Union or the United States without the introduction of a cumbersome bureaucratic exercise which would be costly and impossible to police, and would result in distortions to trade.

On-farm certification, similar to that introduced by the Poultry Directive 92/116, may be of some finite value. Most of the cattle and sheep production in Europe is still relatively small-scale, and many of the animals slaughtered come to the abattoir via dealers or short-term finishers who can provide only a very limited history. The best hope of progress would seem to lie with 'Producer Groups' or 'Quality Assurance Schemes' where a group of farmers undertake to conform to a set of production standards, but development has been slow owing to the lack of any substantial premium which these animals can attract. This form of producer assurance combined with periodic veterinary inspections to verify the information provided may be the most practical approach.

Without an accurate pre-slaughter history, the preselection of animals for slaughter into disease-risk groups is problematic and at best subjective. Consequently, any suggestion of the introduction of less rigorous on-line post-mortem inspection regimes is difficult to justify. Preselection should, however, remain a long-term aim, and may begin with differentiation by age, young animals in general presenting a lower risk. The requirement of Directive 92/102/EEC for all cattle, sheep and pigs across the European Union to be identified could be coupled with computerisation to form the basis of an animal health system capable of delivering effective pre-slaughter history, for example, concerning the origins of the animals, herd/flock previous post-mortem findings, previous results of residue sampling, health status within government health schemes, membership of 'Quality Assurance Schemes', etc. Such systems already exist in some regions in Europe, one example being the Department of Agriculture for Northern Ireland's 'Animal Health Computer' which holds data relating to all bovine animals within Northern Ireland. This has allowed various assurances to be given to accompany beef exports, e.g. regarding the herd of origin's freedom from bovine spongiform encephalopathy (BSE).

The role of the *auxiliary*, as defined in Article 9 of the Directive 91/497/EEC, in assisting the Official Veterinarian in 'making an initial check on the animals and helping with purely practical tasks' should only go as far as the detention of suspect animals for the veterinarian's attention, and only after the auxiliary has received considerable training in animal production and disease. Effective ante-mortem examination of livestock must be seen as an essential and fundamental monitoring of a Critical Control Point in any HACCP system, ensuring that the meat processor is provided with a healthy, clean, stress-free and, as far as can be determined, residue-free raw material. It must, therefore, remain a basic responsibility of the Official Veterinarian and his appropriately trained team of auxiliaries.

Routine ante-mortem inspection calls for an entirely different procedure in countries such as North and South America, Canada or Australia, where the animals may be range cattle, compared with the United Kingdom and Europe where the animals can usually be approached and handled. In every case an inspection should be carried out daily and the final examination should take place within 24 hours of slaughter.

Close AM and PM liaison is essential.

## POST-MORTEM INSPECTION

### Facilities for post-mortem inspection

In addition to the usual structural and mechanical facilities which provide for good working conditions and enable carcases and their parts to be delivered for inspection in a satisfactory manner, each inspection point should have well-distributed lighting of at least 540 lux in intensity which does not distort colours. There must also be sufficient sanitising units for equipment, hands and aprons, with disinfectant soap and disposable paper towels available. Sterilisers which operate at 82°C and allow for immersion of knives, cleavers and saws to above the blade-handle junction are essential.

These requirements extend to the routine inspection points on the slaughter line and to the 'detained' area where further detailed examination is performed. It is essential that there should be coordination and communication between inspection points and that the inspectors on the inspection line can confidently identify correlated carcases and viscera. For most domestic farm animals, there are normally three main inspection points: head, viscera and carcase. Ideally, the inspection station for the viscera should be slightly before the carcase inspection point so that significant findings can be communicated to the carcase inspector. Synchronisation of conveyorised lines carrying carcases and offal is absolutely fundamental for accurate identification of carcases and their related organs. A fail-safe method must be put in place to ensure that, when a carcase is condemned, the head, viscera and blood can also be retrieved for condemnation. There must also be a mechanism by which, when a carcase is detained, the viscera and other body parts are also sent to the detained room. In many cases, it is almost impossible for the veterinarian to make a proper informed judgement on a carcase without the evidence which the viscera can provide.

A method of communicating the information gained at ante-mortem must be in place and should alert the inspectors at each point of inspection.

*Systems of recording disease data* vary according to the particular operation and the type and rate of slaughter. For low slaughter rates a manual system of recording findings on a washable 'Nobo' board may be satisfactory, but for fast lines computerised systems with automatic recording of the 'kill number' from a transponder on the hook or gambrel, with a touch- or voice-operated information recorder, must be considered. If a *universal microchip* for *the identification of cattle* were to be accepted, this 'number' could be read automatically throughout the animal's life and through to the end of the slaughterline (see Chapter 21).

Every inspection station should have a line stop-button within easy reach. The inspectors must be invested with the authority to stop production immediately in the event of a contamination incident, or if correlation between the inspection points is lost.

## Health and safety

The greatest care must be taken in the handling, slaughter and carcase dressing of animals which may represent a source of zoonotic infection to plant staff. In particular, such animals should be handled separately from normal stock; staff should wash hands and arms frequently; avoid cuts, and contamination of the eyes with body fluids; avoid handling udders and urogenital tracts (hooks to be used instead); avoid incision into these organs and the associated lymph nodes; adopt a high standard of personal cleanliness at all times and seek medical advice if exposure to brucella infection or any other zoonosis has occurred.

Under the UK Control of Substances Hazardous to Health Regulations 1991 (COSHH), the employer is responsible for ensuring that a written assessment of the *hazards* to the potential health and safety of the employee is carried out, that the employee is informed of the risks and given whatever training is necessary, and that suitable protective clothing and equipment are made available and used.

## Carcase identification

It is essential that *live animal identification* be retained on the carcase until it passes over the weighbridge. For the day's kill, or batches within this, a *slaughter programme* will have been compiled giving details of stock, their class, identification, name and address of owner, lot, pen and slaughter sequence numbers, etc., copies of which are made available to appropriate persons including the meat inspection staff. If live animal tags are not actually retained on the carcase because of hygiene concerns, it is important to have a reliable system of substituting 'dead' for 'live' identifications so that accurate details of producer (or wholesaler, retailer), ownership, carcase weight, grade, classification and disease information are maintained.

Practically all the current forms of *meat identification* have drawbacks, from the standpoint of hygiene, legibility or practicality. For example, the commonly used labels with copper-plated clips can cause discoloration of the surrounding meat due to corrosion, necessitating trimming. They may also inadvertently get into packaged meat and for this reason should not be allowed into the cutting rooms, and have been banned by many meat processing companies. Leaving the bovine ear complete with its ear tag on the animal as it travels up the slaughterline has obvious advantages, and equally obvious disadvantages from a hygiene perspective. The use of *transponders* implanted in the ear which can be read at the inspection and grading/weighing points as long as the ear remains with the carcase adds added benefit to this practice. A compromise is to remove the ear during skinning and place it hygienically in a plastic bag which is clipped to the first side of the carcase with a reusable stainless steel hook. Metal and polypropylene stamps with *marking dyes*, which must be approved as being of food grade, e.g. chocolate brown, are in common use for carcase identification, and *roller strips* for indicating grades especially on pigs. *Pigs* are generally identified by a tattoo, or slap mark, applied ante-mortem but legible only after scalding and scraping. Grades on pigs are frequently identified by writing on the exposed dermis with a special pencil.

Probably the most common method of identification in use for *cattle* is gummed numbered *paper labels*, which are stuck on to each of the four quarters as the hide and live animal identification are removed. These labels have not always been stored hygienically, cannot be applied to cold carcases satisfactorily and have to be cut off before the carcase enters the cut-up. Another alternative is a *plastic tag* or *fastener*, applied with instrument which can attach the label to the meat. These tags are not detected by metal detectors, and care must be taken to ensure that they are completely removed so that they do not adulterate the meat.

The search for a tag material which can be left in the meat and made harmless by cooking is now centred on *blood* and *collagen*. Nothing satisfactory has been developed to replace metal or plastic clips which complies with the EC Directive on Materials in Contact with Foodstuffs. A system has been developed in Australia which consists of *gelatin strips* pre-printed with appropriate details and stuck on the carcase fat. This form of identification is said to be edible, waterproof, non-smearing, non-dissolving and abrasion-resistant. If details can be added after the strips are applied, this could be a useful system of carcase identification.

Any good system of carcase meat identification must be clearly legible, easily applied, cheap, non-toxic, non-corrosive and suitable for use with modern data retrieval systems. The UK Meat and Livestock Commission issued a guide on the labelling of carcase meat and prime cuts. It concludes:

1. Do not label, write or stamp unless essential.
2. Fix labels in a consistent position to aid checking and removal.
3. Do not apply labels to parts of the carcase likely to be used for manufacturing, such as flank or brisket.
4. Remove all labels and clips as soon as they are no longer needed.
5. On bone-in cuts apply the label close to the bone and to only one cut in each customer's batch.
6. Label pork carcases high on the front of the hock, away from the ham.
7. Label lamb carcases on the front of the shank.
8. Label beef carcases on the rib cage or chine bone or vertebral column, and veal carcases on the leg.

*Meat detained for re-inspection* must also be identified in a place and by a means acceptable to both the abattoir operator and the Official Veterinarian. The entire process of BSE certification requires that the inspection team be aware of the exact identity and category of every carcase and offal passing through the abattoir. This must involve a system which can ensure that correlation is maintained in order that specified bovine offal is properly removed and that meat and offal from officially BSE-free holdings are separated from those of 'lower' status.

**Current EC post-mortem procedure**

The present on-line inspection procedures as laid down in Directive 91/497/EEC, Annex 1, Chapter VII, and enacted in Great Britain through The Fresh Meat (Hygiene and Inspection) Regulations 1995, Schedule 10 detail the methodology of post-mortem inspection.

This involves the macroscopic visual examination of the slaughtered animal and its organs, the palpation of organs, the incision of certain organs and lymph nodes, the investigation of anomalies in consistency, colour, smell and, where appropriate, taste, and, where necessary, *laboratory examination*, particularly for residues. The inspection is performed throughout the European Union, without regard for the age of the animal, the regional incidence of the conditions being sought or their importance with respect to their public health significance. It should be possible for the inspection procedure to be altered if a region can prove a regional freedom from a disease or condition. This already occurs to a limited degree in that the requirement of Directive 91/497 para. 42 to examine the meat of swine or horses for trichinosis does not apply to all regions.

It is widely agreed that, even when carried out conscientiously, the currently used inspection techniques are ineffective even in detecting the macroscopic lesions they are designed to identify. McCool (1979) reported that <20% of *Cysticercus bovis*, and Heath *et al.* (1985) that only 41% of *Cysticercus ovis*, were detected by on-line inspection. The Dutch research project 'Integrated quality control approach' showed that only 50% of the abnormalities present were detected either by 'regular EEC post-mortem meat inspection or by inspection and palpation only' (Berends *et al.* 1993). Hathaway *et al.* (1987) and Blackmore (1993) suggested that *incision of the lymph nodes*, especially the mesenterics, may result in the cross-contamination of other carcases and organs with *Salmonella* or *Campylobacter* via the inspector's knife. This proposition has been quoted as a reason why incision of lymph nodes as an inspection tool should be abandoned. However, if the inspection points are sufficiently manned, and the inspectors control the speed of the line, there should be no excuse for poor operational hygiene leading to cross-contamination. Lymph node incision should, therefore, remain as a tool in meat inspection where the risk-based assessment mentioned above indicates that it is a worthwhile procedure. Such an assessment carried out on the routine examination of some of the regional lymph nodes of the viscera in lambs in New Zealand (Hathaway and Pullen, 1990) indicated that examination of these nodes added nothing to inspection of the primary organs.

All inspections must be carried out with due regard for hygiene. It is essential that the inspectors set and achieve the highest standards of hygienic dress, appearance and operations if they are to have any hope of enforcing high standards within the plant. Operational hygiene is dealt with separately in Chapter 9.

Before the day's slaughter commences, the inspector must ensure that the premises, equipment and facilities are hygienic and in good working order and that meat operatives are properly clothed and adequate in number. Slaughter should not be allowed to commence until a satisfactory situation obtains. This *pre-slaughter check* may take the form of a visual and microbiological verification of the meat plant's own monitoring system. The preferred system is one where the operatives themselves are responsible for ensuring that the premises are hygienic, the meat inspection team merely verifying their checks.

It is the duty of the inspection staff to arrange for the *stamping of the carcases* when passed, or condemned, and to ensure the proper disposal of the latter. It is particularly important in the United Kingdom that checks to ensure the efficient and hygienic removal of the Specified Risk Material associated with bovine spongiform encephalopathy (BSE) from the carcase and viscera, their marking and disposal.

Many authorities have questioned the use of inspection staff on the line to remove conditions of cosmetic, but no public health, significance. In the case of conditions such as cirrhotic livers due to damage by fluke or ascarid worms, this point of view is generally accepted. However, it has also been suggested that since some of the bacteria involved commonly in abscesses may not be pathogenic to man, identification and trimming of these lesions could be left to plant staff. It is difficult to agree that this would give the consumer the assurance that meat contaminated by purulent material did not end up in the food chain, and, although the causative organism may not be pathogenic to the consumer, the contamination cannot improve the shelf-life or the aesthetic acceptability of the end-product.

The presence of inspectors who are independent from plant management is also important in the maintenance of high standards of dressing and operational hygiene. The wide range of food poisoning organisms which are found in the faeces of apparently healthy animals makes it imperative that, at the very least, visible faecal contamination is eliminated during the dressing process. In practice, high standards are generally maintained by the independent inspectors, who are prepared to slow or stop production during periods when there is increased risk of contamination, for example, when slaughtering dirty cattle or sheep. Inspection staff employed directly by the commercial company may have greater difficulty enforcing such preventive measures in the face of commercial production targets. Since the carcases should be checked individually for contamination, the commercial pressure for less than 100% inspection by the independent inspectors must be resisted.

The prevention of contamination must remain the aim, rather than post-production contamination reduction by means of water, organic acids, other bactericides or irradiation. Washing has been demonstrated (Ellerbroek, 1993), to have no effect in reducing pathogen levels on the surface of the carcase and can, in fact, have a detrimental outcome by spreading the contamination over the surface of the carcase to less contaminated areas and increasing the available water remaining on the carcase. Suitably controlled, organic acids, irradiation, etc., may be useful tools in helping to ensure a safe product, they must not be allowed to mask poor manufacturing practice.

The requirement in the Directive for 'laboratory examination' where appropriate introduces the necessity for *bacteriological examination*. There would be no improvement to the quality or safety of the meat produced by adopting rigid microbiological criteria, owing to variations which would occur in sampling and laboratory techniques, the variation in pathogenicity of different bacteriological strains, the retrospective nature of the results, the effect of storage conditions on the final bacterial count, and the difficulty in interpreting the results. This view was endorsed by Engel *et al.* (1989), who carried out a scrutiny of the effectiveness of the microbiological criteria imposed by the Dutch meat inspection regulations. This bacteriological examination, described by Hobbs (1967), was designed to exclude septicaemic carcases from human consumption, and interprets a positive result as one where there is bacterial growth on media inoculated with muscle tissue or spleen, or where salmonellae are detected in the kidney specimen. They concluded that the strict application of purely bacteriological findings resulted in the condemnation of carcases harbouring a small number of bacteria which have a minimal significance for the health of consumers, whereas animals harbouring organisms potentially pathogenic for man are overlooked. Despite this, the use of microbiological monitoring of carcases to establish trends, especially of potential pathogens, is to be encouraged as a means by which the Official Veterinarian can verify the effectiveness of the dressing techniques and operational hygiene within his abattoir. The limitations listed above, however, must be borne in mind.

*The Official Veterinarian must always bear in mind that he or she alone is responsible ultimately to the consumer for the certification as to the safety of the meat leaving the meat plant. The authority which lies with the Official Veterinarian to stop slaughter and dressing operations on grounds of lack of hygiene, defective dressing techniques or inadequate inspection must be exercised fearlessly when required.*

## Post-mortem inspection of cattle (See also Chapters 16–18)

Inspection of a carcase and its organs, in accordance with regulations currently in place in most countries, should proceed in the following order, though in countries where bovine tuberculosis has been eradicated suitable modifications in the routine technique may justifiably be made.

As has been noted under *T. saginata* in Chapter 18, variations occur in the examination for *Cysticercus bovis* in different countries.

### *Head*

An examination of the outer surfaces and eyes is followed by an inspection of the gums, lips and tongue for foot-and-mouth disease, necrotic and other forms of stomatitis, actinomycosis and actinobacillosis, the tongue being palpated from dorsum to tip for the latter disease. Incisions of the internal and external masseters for *C. bovis* should be made parallel with the lower jaw. After the tongue is dropped, routine incisions of the retropharyngeal, submaxillary and parotid lymph nodes should be made for tuberculous lesions, abscesses and actinobacillosis. The tonsils of cattle and pigs frequently harbour tubercule bacilli and regulations that apply in the United States to federally-inspected establishments and also to abattoirs in the European Community prescribe that the tonsils shall be removed and shall not be used as ingredients of meat products. As part of the BSE controls, tonsils in the UK are classified as Specified Risk Material (SRM), and must be removed and disposed of as such.

### *Lymph nodes*

The detailed examination of lymph nodes, often recommended in different meat inspection codes, is mainly for the detection of tuberculosis and is fully justified where this disease is a problem. But in countries that have had successful eradication campaigns, routine incision of the following lymph nodes can be largely dispensed with:

- *Pigs*: bronchial, mediastinal, gastric, hepatics and mesenterics.
- *Pigs and bovines*: renals, provided kidneys are exposed.

The situation with regard to the *gastric* and *mesenteric lymph nodes* in *cattle* is more problematic, at least in Britain. Examination of TB reactors in 1978 showed that 1.9% of the cattle had lesions in the mesenteric lymph nodes only, *Mycobacterium bovis* being recovered from these lesions. In spite of this finding, however, it is likely that the saving in time and costs of inspection outweigh any slight animal health benefits accruing (Goodhand, 1983). Many countries (among them the USA, New Zealand and Australia) have, because of their virtual freedom from tuberculosis, reduced the number of routine incisions into the lymph nodes without any apparent adverse effect on animal health.

Where an efficient ante-mortem inspection is performed which ensures that, except for casualty stock, all the animals presented for slaughter are apparently normal and where the incidence of tuberculosis is low, detailed examination of all visceral lymph nodes is not justified.

*Lungs*

Visual examination, which should be followed by palpation, should be carried out for evidence of pleurisy, pneumonia, tuberculosis, fascioliasis, hydatid cysts, etc. The bronchial and mediastinal lymph nodes should be incised. The lung substance should be exposed by a long, deep incision from the base to the apex of each lung, and the trachea and main branches of the bronchi opened lengthways, only when they are to be used for human consumption.

*Heart*

The pericardium should be examined for evidence of pericarditis, haemorrhages, etc. The ventricles are then incised and the outer and inner surfaces are observed, particular attention being paid to the presence of petechial haemorrhages on the epicardium or endocardium and to cysticerci, hydatid cysts and occasionally linguatulae in the myocardium. Alternatively, the heart may be everted after cutting through the interventricular septum with four lengthways incisions into the septum and the ventricular wall. This latter procedure lessens the heart's monetary value. A flabby condition of the myocardium is often associated with septic conditions in the cow, while vegetative endocarditis occurs in chronic swine erysipelas and in sheep due to *Streptococcus faecalis* and *Erysipelothrix rhusiopathiae*, the causal organisms of swine erysipelas.

*Liver*

A visual examination with palpation should be made for fatty change, actinobacillosis, abscesses, telangiectasis and parasitic infections such as hydatid cysts, *C. bovis*, fascioliasis or linguatulae. The larval stage of *Oesophagostomum radiatum* may occasionally be found in the ox liver. Observe and, if necessary, palpate the gall bladder. An incision should be made on the gastric surface of the liver, and in bovines an incision at the base of the caudate lobe to examine the bile ducts. Where necessary for a diagnosis, incise as necessary into the bile ducts and liver substance.

In countries where the incidence of fascioliasis is high, e.g. Ireland and the western parts of Great Britain, arrangements should be made for affected livers to be trimmed by factory operatives to avoid the practice of condemning livers only slightly affected with liver fluke.

*Oesophagus, stomach and intestines*

Observe and, if necessary, palpate these organs. The serous surface may show evidence of tuberculosis or actinobacillosis, while the anterior aspect of the reticulum may show evidence of a foreign body. As a result of the virtual eradication of bovine tuberculosis from the United States and much of Europe, it is not now considered necessary to incise the mesenteric lymph nodes in routine examination. Except in reactors to the tuberculin test, the mesentery is now examined by simple palpation.

*Kidney*

Enuculation of the kidney to allow visual inspection and, if necessary, the kidney and renal lymph nodes.

*Spleen*

The surface and substance should be examined for tuberculosis, haematomata and the presence of infarcts with observation, palpation and, if necessary, incision.

*Uterus*

The uterus should be viewed, palpated and, if necessary, incised, care being taken to prevent contamination of the carcase. Evidence of pregnancy or of recent parturition in the well-bled and well-set carcase is not significant. In brucellosis reactors the uterus must not be incised or handled.

*Udders*

The potential for the presence of food poisoning microorganisms in the udder is such, that it is questionable if they should ever be considered as fit for human consumption. If they are, they should be palpated, and each half of the udder opened by a long, deep incision, preferably multiple and about 5 cm apart, and the lymph nodes incised. Abscesses or septic mastitis may be present, and the supramammary lymph nodes, even in a dry cow, should be incised for evidence of abscesses or tuberculosis. In brucellosis reactors the udder is removed intact without incision and without handling.

### *Testis*

If destined for human consumption, the testes should be viewed and palpated.

### *Carcase*

The cut surfaces of bone and muscle, carcase exterior, pleura, peritoneum and diaphragm should be observed, attention being given to condition, efficiency of bleeding, colour, cleanliness, odours and evidence of bruising and other abnormalities. If necessary, palpation and incision of parts may be indicated, e.g. triceps brachii muscle for *C. bovis*. The superficial inguinal, external and internal iliac, prepectoral and renal lymph nodes should be observed and if necessary, palpated and incised. Where a systemic or generalised disease is suspected, in tuberculin reactors and where tuberculous lesions have been detected in the viscera, the main carcase lymph nodes must be examined. The thoracic and abdominal cavities should be inspected for inflammation, abscesses, actinobacillosis, mesothelioma or tuberculosis; the diaphragm should be lifted, for tuberculous lesions may be hidden between the diaphgram and the thoracic wall.

If the above routine examination reveals no evidence of abnormality the carcase may be passed for food.

In 1983 in the United States the number of bovine carcases condemned as a result of post-mortem inspection was 0.37% of the total slaughtered; the affections, in order of frequency, were – apart from 'moribund' and 'dead' – neoplasms (mostly epithelioma of the eye and malignant lymphoma), pneumonia, pyaemia, emaciation and septicaemia/ toxaemia.

## Calves

The routine post-mortem of calves is virtually the same as for adult bovines, with special attention to particular sites. A visual examination of the mouth and tongue should be made for foot-and-mouth disease and calf diphtheria. Attention should also be paid to the abomasum for evidence of peptic ulcers, the small intestine for white scour or dysentery and the liver, portal lymph nodes and posterior mediastinal lymph nodes for congenital tuberculosis. The lungs, kidneys and spinal cord should be examined for melanotic deposits and the umbilicus and joints for septic omphalophlebitis. The consistency of the synovial fluid of the hock can be readily determined by puncturing the protrusion on the inner aspect of the joint with the point of a knife. The appearance and consistency of the renal fat should be carefully noted.

## Sheep and goats

Sheep and goats require a less detailed inspection than cattle, calves and pigs, the routine inspection requiring no incisions. The carcase should be visually examined for satisfactory bleeding and setting, the lungs for parasitic infections, especially hydatid cysts and nematodes, and the liver for fascioliasis. In Australia and New Zealand it is routine procedure to palpate the carcase for evidence of arthritis, caseous lymphadenitis, inoculation abscesses and lesions due to grass seed awns.

## Pigs

Post-mortem examination of pigs follows the same overall routine as for cattle.

Skin lesions are an important diagnostic feature of swine erysipelas, swine fever and urticaria. The skin should also be examined for 'shotty eruption', the tail for necrosis, the feet for abscess formation and the udder for actinomycosis.

The viscera require inspection in the manner detailed for cattle, with particular attention to pneumonia and the secondary complications that develop in virus pneumonia, mainly pleurisy, pericarditis and, to a lesser extent, peritonitis.

The submaxillary lymph nodes should always be examined for tuberculosis. Abscesses in the submaxillary lymph node may be caused by the passage of sharp foreign bodies through the wall of the pharynx or, in some countries, a beta-haemolytic streptococcus which also often causes tongue abscesses. Small yellow, necrotic foci resembling TB but caused by *Corynebacterium equi* are sometimes found in these nodes. The presence of metal spicules in the dorsum of the tongue has been identified as a problem in the UK by the manufacturers of pressed tongue. Some of these fragments have been identified as hypodermic needles, but others are pieces of wire and would appear to have originated from car tyres given to the pigs as 'toys'. The liver need not be incised except when it appears cirrhotic. The kidney surface should be examined for cysts and systemic changes.

Where *Cysticercus cellulosae* is prevalent, the investigation must include examination of the directly-visible muscular surfaces, in particular the thigh muscles, the pillars of the diaphgram, the intercostal muscles, the heart, the tongue and the larynx and, if necessary, the abdominal wall and the psoas muscles freed from fatty tissue. Where trichinosis is known or suspected, appropriate examination and muscle sampling must be carried out.

UK post-mortem inspection in the pig requires that only the submaxillary lymph nodes, and the supramammary lymph nodes in sows, are routinely incised. Within the EU, the mesenteric lymph nodes of pigs are no longer incised because of the frequent contamination of knives with *Salmonella* organisms which may be present in the nodes.

## Equines

Post-mortem inspection of equidae follows the same general pattern for cattle and all other livestock. Although equidae generally possess fewer lesions than other animals, particular attention should be paid to the lungs and liver for evidence of echinococcal cysts and to the muscles and lymph nodes for melanosis. The main carcase lymph nodes should be examined when systemic or generalised disease is suspected, when tuberculosis lesions are detected and when the live animal has shown a reaction to the mallein test. The possibility of glanders requires that the mucous membranes, trachea, larynx, nasal cavities, sinuses and their ramifications are carefully examined, after splitting the head in the median plane and excision of the nasal septum.

## Poultry

Facilities should be available for whole-carcase inspection after defeathering and washing. Cases with obvious disease, fractures, injuries, blood blisters, etc. can be detected and detained at this stage.

Second-stage inspection takes place on the partially eviscerated carcase where it is possible to relate carcase and viscera. The viscera, hock joints and tibias are observed and the latter palpated. The body cavity and internal organs are viewed. In some cases one inspector examines the carcase while another examines the viscera – of value in turkeys but not in broilers. In the United States it is recommended that the spleen of adult birds be crushed. The trimmer is instructed to trim, remove viscera, condemn, etc. as necessary.

It is essential that the inspector in charge arranges for a line speed consistent with the number and competence of his inspectors, type of poultry, presentation methods, incidence of disease, efficiency of evisceration procedures, etc. Line speeds should be reduced in any unfavourable situation and brought back to normal only when conditions are satisfactory. If necessary, operations should cease until the situation is satisfactory. It is recommended that the line start and stop control be within reach of the inspector in charge, who must be totally and transparently independent from the commercial company.

## Traditional versus entirely visual meat inspection procedures

Current meat inspection methods, established at the beginning of the century, are no longer considered adequate to protect the consumer (Anon, 1987, 1990; Berends *et al.*, 1993; Blackmore, 1983; Gracey and Collins, 1992; and others). Manual handling, palpation and incision (which cannot detect all lesions) too often result in cross-contamination. In any case most of the visual lesions encountered, if subjected to microbiological examination, would not yield food-poisoning organisms. Nevertheless, they must be removed for aesthetic reasons.

The present threats to the consumer instead arise not from typical pathological lesions but from microorganisms such as *Salmonella, Yersinia enterocolitica, Campylobacter, Giardia, Listeria* and *E. coli*, etc., which are usually involved with a carrier state in the animal and with serious faecal contamination. Veterinary drugs and chemicals also pose a hazard.

Article 17 of the present EEC Fresh Meat Directive (91/497/EEC) envisaged a change in procedures by stating that 'the Commission shall submit a report . . . on methods of inspection which ensure a level of animal health equivalent to that guaranteed by the methods of ante-mortem and post-mortem inspection described in Chapters VI and VIII of Annex 1'. To this end, an international working group has proposed a revision of the inspection procedures for pigs and recommended that producers should take greater responsibility for livestock quality, that a mandatory feedback system should be instituted, and that meat inspection procedures should be simplified and made purely visual.

Using a quantitative risk assessment approach, Mousing *et al.* (1997) determined the consequences of a change from traditional meat inspection procedures (which included manual handling, palpation and incision) to an entirely visual form of inspection in 183 000 Danish slaughter pigs. Out of 58 lesion codes, 26 (45%) were assessed as merely aesthetic or as the healed stage of an earlier lesion; 9 (15%) were active but local lesions, occurring only in non-edible tissue; 5 lesion codes (9%) were assessed as active, non-septic lesions occurring in edible tissue caused by swine-specific pathogens; 10 (17%) were abscessal or pyaemic lesions occurring in edible tissue. Seven lesion codes (12%) may be associated with consumer health hazards (two frequently and five rarely). One lesion code was associated with an occupational health hazard.

It was estimated that per 1000 pig carcases an additional 2.5 with abscessal or pyaemic lesions in edible tissue containing *Staphylococcus aureus*, $4 \times 10^{-4}$ containing ochratoxin, 0.2 with arthritis due to *Erysipelothrix rhusiopathiae*, 0.2 with caseous lymphadenitis *(M. avium-intercellulare)*, 0.7 faecally contaminated with *Salmonella* species and 3.4 faecally contaminated with *Yersinia enterocolitica* would remain undetected as a result from changing from the traditional to the visual inspection procedure.

These authors concluded that the visual system would result in about 4 additional pigs per 1000 carcases being passed which might cross-contaminate other carcases with *Salmonella/Y. entercolitica*, and that the main direct benefit of the visual system (without manual handling, palpation and incision) would probably be a lower level of cross-contamination with hazardous bacteria, especially from the pharyngeal region and the plucks. In addition, the visual system allows for less labour, with the release of control resources for hygienic surveillance programmes and wider risk assessment strategies.

A significant recommendation was the need to monitor the level of faecal contamination, irrespective of the type of inspection adopted. Such a recommendation is made more vital when the verotoxigenic *E. coli* O157 H7 is included.

## DECISIONS AT POST-MORTEM EXAMINATION (see also Chs 16–20)

The *final judgement* as to the action to be taken with a carcase or parts of a carcase *is based on the total evidence produced by observation, palpation, incision, smell, ante-mortem signs and the results of any laboratory test*. Rarely, but where appropriate, taste may be employed. It is essential, therefore, that the results of ante-mortem and supporting laboratory tests are available to the veterinarian when he is making the final decision.

For some conditions, legislation, such as that based on EC Directive 64/433, Article 5, declares unfit all meat, offal or blood which has originated from animals found on inspection to exhibit signs of the disease. This includes generalised actinobacillosis or actinomycosis, blackleg, generalised tuberculosis, generalised lymphadenitis, glanders, rabies, tetanus, acute salmonellosis, acute brucellosis, swine erysipelas, botulism, septicaemia, pyaemia, toxaemia or viraemia, any carcase showing lesions of bronchopneumonia, pleurisy, peritonitis, metritis, mastitis, arthritis, pericarditis, enteritis, or meningo-encephalomyelitis, generalised sarcocystosis, cysticercosis and trichinosis; animals which have been stillborn or unborn; carcases which show advanced anaemia or emaciation; carcases showing multiple tumours, multiple abscesses or serious multiple injuries; fevered carcases; and any carcase which shows serious anomalies of colour, smell, consistency or taste.

Controversy can, however, surround the specific interpretation of some of these instructions, and decisions require the detailed examination of suspect animals including all parts of the carcase and viscera, even organs and parts whose position is remote from what is considered to be the primary lesion. This will determine whether the lesions are *localised* or *generalised*, and consequently the extent of condemnation necessary.

Similarly, the nature of the specific lesion, along with the entire carcase and viscera, must be considered to decide whether the condition is *acute* or *chronic*.

As a general rule the *acute* and *generalised* condition will require the *total condemnation* of the carcase and the viscera, while the *chronic* and *localised* may require only *local condemnation*, or in some cases *no condemnation* at all. This emphasises the importance of correlation of inspection procedures, and the importance of ensuring that viscera follow the carcase on to the detained rail since there may be significant lesions in both. If we consider some specific lesions, some general guidance can be suggested.

## Abscesses

Abscesses are one of the most common lesions routinely encountered in pigs. A study carried out to map the position of abscesses in 75 130 pigs produced the following findings (Huey, 1996):

1. 2.87% of pigs examined had an abscess at one site.
2. The dominant bacterium isolated from all abscesses was *Actinomyces pyogenes*. It has been argued (Berends *et al.*, 1993) that since this bacterium poses little threat to the consumer's physical health, only local condemnation is ever justified. However, any indication of a bacteraemia or pyaemia can do little for the quality of the meat and nothing to re-assure the public as to the safety of their food. As Norval stated in 1966, 'there can be nothing more disgusting to the butcher or housewife than to slice through an abscess when preparing meat'.
3. 0.26% of pigs slaughtered possessed abscesses at more than one site.
4. Of these, 80% had the tail as one of the sites, indicating the importance of tail-biting in the aetiology.
5. There was a strong statistical interrelationship between abscesses found in combination at tail/lungs, tail/vertebrae, tail/legs, tail/ribs, tail/peritoneum.

As stated above, the following are the two most important questions to be answered.

### *Is the lesion localised or generalised?*

A study of the literature indicates that it is most likely that infection spreads from the tail of a pig to the pelvis via the local lymphatic system, from the tail to the lungs, ribs and legs via the bloodstream, and from the tail to the spinal vertebrae via the cerebrospinal fluid. This would indicate the following in terms of condemnation:

- *Abscesses at a single site:* condemnation of the part is usually sufficient, after careful examination of the rest of the carcase and the viscera.
- *Abscess in the tail and one or more in the spinal vertebrae*: remove the tail and the spinal column only.
- *Abscess in the tail, and one or more in the lungs, ribs, peritoneum, or forelegs:* condemnation of the carcase is justified.
- *Abscess in the tail and hindleg:* local condemnation may be sufficient.
- There is no apparent interrelationship between abscesses in the head or neck and those elsewhere, e.g. the tail or lungs, so only local condemnation is indicated.
- A statistically significant interrelationship was demonstrated between abscesses in fore- and hindlegs. In each case the aetiology must be considered before a judgement can be made. If, for example, the cause is thought to be rough floors, and there is no evidence of haematogenous spread, local condemnation may suffice.

### *Is the lesion acute or chronic?*

If an abscess is in the acute stage of development, in that there is poor or no capsule formation, accompanied by systemic changer it will usually be necessary to totally condemn the carcase and viscera.

### Omphalophlebitis

Omphalophlebitis or navel ill is a relatively common post-mortem finding in countries where very young calves, 4–8 days old, are slaughtered. A study in New Zealand (Biss *et al.* 1994) suggested that there was histopathological evidence that a low-grade bacteraemia was present in approximately 25% of these calves, and that routine condemnation of the carcase was justified in *extended* or *systemic*, but not in *localised* cases. *Localised* was defined where lesions were restricted to the umbilicus, *extended* where lesions were also evident in the umbilical vessels, and *systemic* navel ill where lesions were present in the liver and/or other viscera and the carcase as well as the umbilical tissues. Localised navel ill constituted about 75% of all navel ill cases.

### Arthritis

A small quantity of blood-tinged fluid in a joint is neither unusual nor significant. In all but the most acute cases, the causative agent cannot be cultured from the fluid found in the joint; it can only be isolated from the synovial membrane.

As a basis for judgement:

- If there is purulent material present, the limb should be condemned to the joint above the one affected.
- The limb should be condemned if there is iliac, prescapular or prepectoral lymph node involvement.
- If three or more limbs show lymphatic involvement, the carcase warrants rejection.
- If the popliteal lymph node is enlarged but the iliacs are normal, it may be sufficient to reject only the lower limb.
- If there are systemic changes in the viscera indicating that the arthritis is generalised or acute, the carcase and viscera should be condemned.

### Pneumonia and pleurisy

Carcases must be condemned if there are any signs of systemic change in the viscera, especially the liver, kidney and carcase lymph nodes. If there is no such evidence, condemnation of the carcase cannot be justified, and stripping of the pleura or removal of the rib cage may suffice. In almost all cases where it is necessary to strip the pleura, the diaphragm should be removed.

The possibility of *antibiotic residues* being present must be considered.

### Endocarditis (Plate 1, Fig. 5)

An extensive analysis of the results of bacteriological investigations and judgements of samples obtained from 117 pigs and cattle diagnosed at post-mortem with endocarditis, between 1977 and 1989 in Hungary, was carried out by Szazados (1991). In pigs Erysipelothrix rhusiopathiae, beta-haemolytic streptococci, streptococci belonging to the viridans group, Actinomyces pyogenes and Staphylococcus aureus were isolated in decreasing order of frequency. In cattle, Actinomyces pyogenes was isolated most frequently.

Bacteria were present in the spleen, liver and kidney of over 60% of the samples examined, muscle and lymph nodes were positive in over 30% of samples.

Of the 117 cases, 79 cases (67.5%) were condemned for septicaemia. Without this type of detailed bacteriological examination, however, given these statistics, condemnation of the carcase is justified in all cases of endocarditis.

### Bruising

It is now broadly accepted that:

- Muscle tissue is generally sterile until it is exposed to extraneous contamination.
- Extraneous contaminants grow no faster on bruised than unbruised tissue.
- There is no difference in the microbiological condition of meat from bled and unbled lamb carcases.

The trimming of bruised tissue is therefore purely aesthetic.

### Contamination

Contamination with *faeces* is one of the greatest hazards to public health encountered in meat inspection. This is most commonly due to hurried or poor 'bunging' technique and full stomachs and intestines rupturing on removal. Plant management could greatly reduce this risk by the introduction of mechanical bungers such as the Jarvis or Jupiter systems for cattle and pigs, by tying or bagging the 'bung' in cattle and sheep, or by applying ligatures, clips or elastrator rings, or 'rodding' the oesophagus.

Contamination of the carcase with purulent material, bile or faeces should always be removed by trimming.

Many of the lesions encountered at post-mortem are ill-defined and minute in size, a situation requiring good eyesight and colour differentiation. No one with defective vision which cannot be corrected by means of spectacles or contact lenses should be employed on meat inspection, and those persons requiring these particular aids should receive regular eye examination. Equally important is the inspector's sense of smell, which, if defective, seriously limits his judgement in many instances.

The *decisions made at post-mortem inspection* vary in different parts of the world depending mainly on local disease incidence, local economy and the presence or absence of facilities for the heat treatment of meat conditionally approved for human consumption. The main decisions in most countries, however, are as follows:

1 approved for human consumption;
2 totally condemned;
3 partially condemned.

The category of *conditionally approved for human consumption* is utilised in some countries: carcase meat which is hygienically unsatisfactory or which in some way may be hazardous for human and animal food is treated, e.g. by heating or freezing under official supervision, in such a manner that makes it safe for human consumption.

In certain regions meat classed as *inferior meat*, *viz.* safe hygienically but of a lower standard, may be sold as raw meat without undergoing any treatment. Such meat must be labelled so as to indicate that it is of inferior quality and sold under close supervision by the controlling authority. It includes meat of abnormal colour, odour or taste, with slight oedema or poorly bled and, like the following category, is found in those countries where there is a scarcity of protein.

Lastly, meat may be *approved for human consumption, with distribution restricted to limited areas*. This category also occurs in those countries where meat is at a premium and includes meat from animals in an area under quarantine because of an outbreak of contagious animal disease. In this case there must be no risk to public health and the meat must be restricted in sale to the affected area to avoid the possible spread of disease. The category would also include meat from animals vaccinated in a restricted area.

It has to be said, however, that while every effort must be made to conserve a valuable product such as meat, the provision of several categories of meat for human consumption makes the task of supervision a difficult one and may lead to a situation where malpractice, e.g. in the form of adulteration and substitution, and trade in unfit meat may take place.

## PROPOSALS TO IMPROVE THE CURRENT POST-MORTEM PROCEDURES

As discussed in the introductory paragraphs to this chapter, the current system which operates in most countries, while to a greater or lesser extent protecting animal welfare, and public and animal health, is urgently in need of revision.

The *current post-mortem regime* is generally considered to be too inflexible in prescribing exactly what procedures must be carried out irrespective of the disease status or production standards under which the animals have been produced. The response to this lack of inspection sensitivity should be two-fold: a risk-based assessment to establish whether each inspection procedure needs to be done at all, and, if it does, a targeting of the detailed inspection to the animals assessed through ante-mortem and production records to be at risk. This should improve the detection rate of the lesions and also decrease the number of pointless incisions made, e.g. incision of submaxillary lymph nodes in pigs where there is a negligible regional incidence of tuberculosis. The inspections carried out, and the resulting judgements, must be based on sound scientific research rather than the current system, which is largely rooted in established practice (Johnston, 1994).

Hathaway and McKenzie (1989) in New Zealand concluded that:

> Some countries importing meat and meat products demand absolute replication of their meat inspection law, without recognising the spectrum and prevalence of diseases and defects in the slaughter population in the country of origin or the performance of its meat inspection service. The application of a rigorous risk assessment model for the evaluation of traditional organoleptic inspection procedures for the viscera of *lambs* described in this report should begin to redress this imbalance. Notwithstanding the international inconsistency in ovine meat inspection codes, a number of current procedures have no scientific basis when routinely applied to the viscera of lambs in New Zealand. Thus their continued application is technically unjustified and wasteful. It must be noted that the recommended New Zealand code of organoleptic inspection does not represent any lessening of the guarantees of safety and wholesomeness that accompany lamb meat and offals produced in this country; the risk assessment model ensures that equivalent or better standards to those delivered by traditional programmes are achieved.

It can be suggested that the current inspection system as described could be improved by initiating the following improvements:

1. An *integrated meat hygiene system: the so-called 'byre to buyer', 'gate to plate', 'stable to table' approach is essential with a two-way flow of information between producer and processor, with the involvement of the meat hygiene inspection service and the producer's veterinarian.*
2. *Preselection of stock into risk groups* should be the aim. Use should be made of a computer database carrying details of producer condemnation statistics, residue sampling results, and herd/flock health status within government or local health or quality assurance schemes. Verification of the information should be carried out by periodic veterinary inspections of the producer's premises and records.
3. *Ante-mortem* inspection must remain a basic responsibility of the Official Veterinarian, who may be assisted in making the initial check by suitably trained meat inspectors.
4. The veterinary auxiliary inspector and/or stockman must receive appropriate *training* to allow him/her to assist the Official Veterinarian in the pre-selection of clinically healthy stock at ante-mortem.
5. *Flexibility* must be introduced into the directives to allow risk-based post-mortem inspection. In regions where it has been demonstrated over a reasonable period of time that the incidence of a particular lesion is very low, inspection procedures should be altered to take the risk into consideration.
6. Research must be initiated to confirm the *incidence* and *public health significance of lesions* detected at post-mortem examination. Judgements made on lesions at post-mortem need to be scientifically assessed so that decisions are based on sound principles, rather than established practice.
7. There must always be an *auxiliary*, as defined by Directive 91/497, on the line to carry out a *final hygiene inspection of the carcase* before it is stamped. The presence of the auxiliary is also essential to supervise the speed of the line, and to ensure that trimming is carried out hygienically. Commercial pressure to inspect less than 100% of carcases must be resisted.
8. Post-production decontamination procedures must not be allowed to replace hygienic/good manufacturing practice.
9. The present state of knowledge suggests that the introduction of strict bacteriological criteria for carcases would be of no benefit to hygienic meat production. However, the use of *bacteriological monitoring of carcases* is to be encouraged as a means by which the Official Veterinarian can verify the effectiveness of the dressing techniques and operational hygiene standards as well as the presence/absence of potential food-poisoning pathogens.
10. The Official Veterinarian, and the team of meat inspectors, should be involved in the *identification and evaluation of hazards and critical control points* within the meat plant. They should verify the monitoring of the production process carried out by the abattoir operatives.

The United States, the European Union and other competent authorities worldwide, are considering how best to proceed with the updating of their current inspection protocols. The USA prefaced its proposal by emphasising the importance of the task, stating that there are 5 million cases of food-borne illness, leading to 4000 deaths per year within the United States, attributable to meat and poultry products.

In Europe an *alternative system for the inspection of pigs*, proposed mainly by Denmark, has received much support, and contains the following elements:

1 Only pigs that originate on farms participating in a 'Herd Health Surveillance Programme' may be considered for the alternative inspection regime.
2 The 'Herd Health Surveillance Programme' involves a *monthly inspection* of all the pigs on the production unit by a veterinarian who gives advice on herd health, drug use, animal welfare, nutrition, etc. On the basis of this visit, paid for by a slaughter levy, the veterinarian estimates the number of healthy pigs that will be ready for slaughter over the next month.
3 The farmer then selects the pigs which are fit for the alternative system on a day-to-day basis. On arrival at the abattoir, the pigs receive traditional ante-mortem inspection, which includes an inspection of animal welfare and transportation conditions.
4 If a farm fails to meet the specified minimum requirements for on-farm selection, the pigs undergo traditional meat inspection.

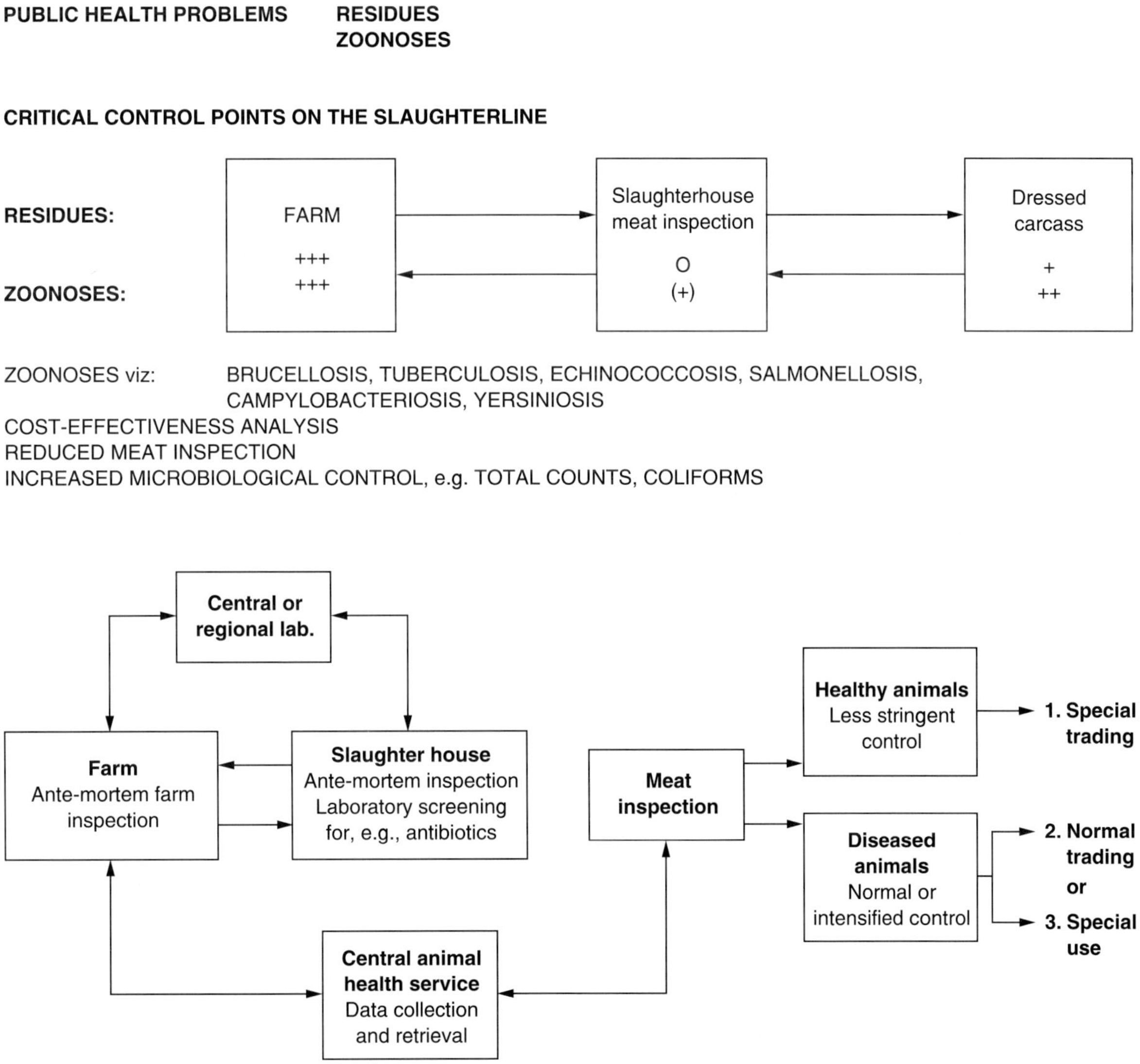


**Fig. 10.1** Integrated meat inspection/hygiene. (After Skovgaard, 1990)

5 Post-mortem of selected pigs, by officially trained auxiliaries under veterinary supervision, will require no incisions, being carried out by visual inspection and palpation.
6 Information gained at ante-mortem and post-mortem will be passed to the producer and the veterinarian carrying out the 'Herd Health Surveillance Programme'.
7 The veterinarian in the abattoir will verify the HACCP control programme set up by the abattoir management to control and monitor contamination of the carcases and offal.
8 Inspection staff, freed from on-line duties, will assist in hygiene control and microbiological verification.

The foundation on which this proposal is built is the regular Herd Health Surveillance by a veterinarian, coupled with a preselection of stock for slaughter by the producer. The participation of a veterinarian on the farm, who is in a position to communicate directly with colleagues within the meat plant, is to be applauded as a suitable *extension of the ante-mortem procedure*. The availability of information on the disease status of the pigs at all stages of their production, together with advice on animal welfare, husbandry, nutrition, and drug use, must be of benefit to both animal and public health.

**Food safety is related to all steps in the food chain** – from livestock producer (whose responsibility is to provide animals which are **healthy, free from undesirable residues and clean**), through manufacturing processes, to retail outlets, hotels and restaurants and the consumer's kitchen. Food-poisoning organisms can be introduced into the food chain at any stage, but the most important is judged to be at primary production where intensive systems of husbandry and with the breeding of stock solely for productivity purposes without regard for disease resistance constitute the main offenders.

Integrated systems of meat inspection (Longitudinal Integrated Safety Assurance – LISA) offer the only means whereby full safety can be guaranteed. At present they appear to be in vogue only in New Zealand and Scandinavian countries (where cooperatives in livestock production/meat inspection/meat processing exist). Without close cooperation between livestock production and slaughter/inspection there can be no improvement in many of today's meat hygiene systems.

Skovgaard (1990) has provided an outline for an integrated meat inspection system (Fig. 10.1).

Throughout the twentieth century, meat inspection procedures have developed as knowledge of disease has increased, and technologies have emerged, which can assist in its detection and control. As we move into the next millennium, this evolution in food inspection must continue to take account of the new risks presented by emerging food-transmitted pathogens and the increased opportunity given for these pathogens to cause illness in consumers by current packaging, storage and eating practices during retailing, and in the home.

## REFERENCES


Anon (1987) National Research Council. *Poultry Inspection. The Basis of Risk Assessment Approach.* Washington DC: US National Academy Press.

Anon (1990) Commission of the European Community. Directorate General for Agriculture. *Draft Report to Scientific Veterinary Committee on Ante-mortem Inspection of Red Meat.* Working Document VI/6346/90 (Dvet/EN/103-0).

Berends, B. R., Snijders, J. M. A. and van Logtestijn, J. G. (1993) *Vet. Rec.* **133**, 411–415.

Biss, M. E., Hathaway, S. C. and Johnstone, A. C. (1994). *Br. Vet. J.* **150**, 377.

Blackmore, D. K. (1983) *Nord. Vet. Med.* **35**, 184–189.

Ellerbroek, L. I., Wegener, J. F. and Arndt, G. (1993) *J. of Food Protection* **56**(5), 432–436.

Engel, H. W. B., Berg, J. van den and Fenigsen-narucka, U. (1997) *Tijdschrift voor de Diergeneeskunde* **112**, 536.

Goodhand, R. H. (1983) *The Meat Hygienist* May/June 1983, No. 38,4.

Hathaway, S. C. & McKenzie A. I. (1989). *Vet. Rec.* **124**, 189–193.

Hathaway, S. C. and Pullen, M. M. (1990) *J. Am. Vet. Med. Assoc.* **196**, 860–864.

Hathaway, S. C., McKenzie, A. I. and Royal, W. A. (1987) *Vet. Rec.* **120**, 78.

Heath D. D., Lawrence, S. B. and Twaalfhoven, H. (1985) *New Zealand Vet. J.* **33**, 152.

Hobbs, B. (1967) *J. S. Afr Vet. Med. Assoc.* **38**(3), 253.

Huey, R. J. (1996) *Vet. Rec.* **138**, 511–514.

ICMSF (1988) *HACCP in Microbiological Safety and Quality*. Oxford: Blackwell Scientific Publications.

Johnston, A. M. (1994) *Br. Vet. J.* **150**, 315.

McCool, C. J. (1979) *Aust. Vet. J.* **55**, 214–216.

Mousing, T. *et al*. (1997) *Vet. Rec*. **140**, 472–477.
Skovgaard, N. (1990) Proceedings of Round Table Conference. The Scientific basis for harmonising trade in red meat. Ante-mortem and post-mortem meat inspection. Need for improvement. WAVFH, Dublin.
Szazados, I. (1991) *Magyar Allatorvosok Lapja* **46**(1), 27–43.

# Chapter 11
# Poultry Production, Slaughter and Inspection

Poultry meat production throughout the world continues to expand both in amount and in sophistication. The *annual* improvements over the last 20 years have seen eggs produced by broiler breeders increase between one and one and a half, increased number of chicks between 0–8 and 1.2, and percentage breast meat by 0.25–0.3%.

In addition the eviscerated yield has gone up by 0.2–0.25% annually, the feed conversion ratio to 2 kg has improved by between 0.04–0.05% and the weight, at 42 days, has increased on average 55–60 g per year. Those trends are expected to continue and broiler selection now involves the criteria of liveweight, liveability, skeletal strength, conformation and feed conversion.

## PRODUCTION OF POULTRY

The *broiler industry* in the UK is concentrated in the hands of fewer than 20 large organisations, most of which have their own parent stock farms and hatcheries. In these companies, broilers may be grown on company farms or on specialist contract units. Other companies do not have breeding farms or hatcheries but purchase day-old broilers, usually on long-term contract, from specialist suppliers. Chickens, turkeys, geese, ducks and end-of-lay hens are processed as well as pheasant, quail, partridge and guinea fowl.

*Broiler chickens* should be placed in houses which have been thoroughly cleaned and disinfected. The surrounding area and the equipment in the house must be clean and disinfected.

Adequate floor space for each bird is essential for its growth, health, quality and general well-being. The amount of space to allow is determined by a combination of the following factors: the weight of the bird at killing age, type of housing, climatic region and time of the year. In the UK the Animal Welfare Code of Practice recommended by the Farm Animal Welfare Council stipulates that at no time should liveweight exceed 34kg/m$^2$ in the interests of welfare and good management. For example, for birds weighing 2 kg there should be no more than 17 per square metre. The stocking density may need to be reduced in summer, especially on units where there are known to have been problems.

*Chicks* should be placed in a house with a temperature of 29–31°C at one day old, reducing by 2°C a week to a final temperature of 18–21°C at 35 days.

A continuous adequate supply of clean water is essential as dehydration must be avoided at all times. Water and feed intake are directly related. There is a trend towards using nipple drinkers, to replace the conventional hanging bell drinkers.

Commercial chicks are generally given a starter ration between 0 and 2 weeks of age containing 23% protein, grower ration between 2 and 4 weeks of 21% protein, and finisher from 4 weeks onwards of 20% protein or less.

As well as the commercial broiler produced intensively in standard poultry sheds, there is a limited demand for speciality products such as 'extensive indoor-barn reared'. This term may only be used where the stocking rate per square metre floor space does not exceed, for chickens 12 birds but not more than 25 kg liveweight; for ducks, guinea fowl and turkeys 25 kg live-weight; for geese 15 kg liveweight. Chickens must not be killed until they are at least 56 days of age, turkeys 70 days and geese 112 days.

The birds are reared in the conventional manner for the first two days, but the temperature of the house is decreased more

**Table 11.1** Slaughterings of poultrymeat.

| | Year | Northern Ireland | UK | EU12 | World |
|---|---|---|---|---|---|
| *Broilers* | | | Number slaughtered (million) | | |
| | 1991 | 43.9 | 522 | N/A | N/A |
| | 1992 | 49.6 | 523 | 3826 | 28 773 |
| | 1993 | 54.1 | 519 | 3803 | 29 688 |
| | 1994 | 57.7 | 553 | 3874 | 31 247 |
| | 1995 | 58.1 | 584 | N/A | N/A |
| *Spent hens* | | | Number slaughtered (million) | | |
| | 1991 | 0.9 | 24 | N/A | N/A |
| | 1992 | 1.4 | 21 | N/A | N/A |
| | 1993 | 0.7 | 20 | N/A | N/A |
| | 1994 | 0.5 | 25 | N/A | N/A |
| | 1995 | 0.9 | 29 | N/A | N/A |
| *Turkeys* | | Number slaughtered (million) | | Dead weight (1000 tonnes) | |
| | 1991 | 0.8 | 33 | 1278 | N/A |
| | 1992 | 0.9 | 33 | 1355 | N/A |
| | 1993 | 1.0 | 35 | 1341 | N/A |
| | 1994 | 1.0 | 35 | 1362 | N/A |
| | 1995 | 1.1 | 38 | 1371 | N/A |

N/A = Not available.
Courtesy of Department of Agriculture for Northern Ireland, Economics & Statistics Division.

quickly so that the environmental temperature is around 21°C at between 14 and 21 days.

The birds are fed a vegetarian diet which is of a lower density than that which is fed to conventional broilers. Some birds are housed in the one building from day-old to processing, while others are reared in conventional sheds and then moved. They have to live in the secondary accommodation for at least 28 days. The lower temperatures promote good feather growth.

*Free-range birds* have the same stocking rate in the house and the age of slaughter is the same as for barn-reared birds except that for chickens the stocking rate may be increased to 13, but not more than 27.5 kg liveweight per $m^2$. The birds, for at least half of their lifetime, must have continuous daytime access to open-air runs comprising an area mainly covered by vegetation of not less than 1 $m^2$ per chicken or guinea fowl, 2 $m^2$ per duck, and 4 $m^2$ per turkey or goose.

Birds are fed a ration of about 24% protein for the first few days but this is soon decreased to 17%. The feed in the fattening stage must contain at least 70% cereals. For chickens the house must be provided with popholes of a combined length equal to or greater than that of the longer side of the house.

Traditional free-range birds must have access to a larger area than free-range and there are extra requirements as detailed in Commission Regulation (EEC) No 1538/91.

The production of these types of poultry obviously adds greatly to the cost and for free-range birds this would be approximately twice that for conventional broilers.

*Poussin* or *Cornish game* are normal conventional broilers which are killed between 21 and 33 days of age.

There are, worldwide, around seven main breeding companies producing different strains of broiler. The companies which produce broiler meat are vertically-integrated. That means they control the production of the eggs which produce the chick, the growing of the birds and the slaughter and further processing of the meat.

## Poultry feeding-stuffs

The raw materials present in the bird's food are carefully sourced and are examined for quality and chemical and microbiological purity. Animal feed is an important source for the transmission of infection to poultry flocks.

The animal feed industry is multifaceted, comprising importers and processors of raw materials, merchants, suppliers of by-products from agricultural operations and food manufacturers, and others such as feed additive and supplement manufacturers, commercial compounders, integrated producers and on-farm mixers.

The feed industry uses numerous products and by-products from other industries. Some, such as cereals, are untreated, whilst others like oil seeds are available as cakes or meals following processing to extract oil. Raw materials may be sourced from all over the world. GATT obligations are serving to further open up the market to Third World country imports. Poultry feed production (some 4 million tonnes per annum in the UK in 1995) accounts for around one-third of the annual production of all compound feeds.

Legislative controls imposed under Part IV of the UK Agriculture Act 1970 require that feeding-stuffs, including raw materials, when sold should be fit for their intended purpose and free from harmful ingredients. Detailed requirements are imposed by the Feeding-Stuffs Regulations 1995 and the Feedings-Stuffs (Sampling and Analysis) Regulations 1982 (as amended).

The Processed Animal Protein Order 1989 requires all processors of animal protein to register with Agriculture Departments and to take samples from their product and have it tested for *Salmonella* in an approved laboratory on each day that material is dispatched from their premises. In the event that *Salmonella* is isolated in the course of testing, movement of contaminated material is prohibited until corrective action has been taken.

*Codes of Practice* for the control of *Salmonella* in animal feed and feed ingredients have also been set up by the UK Government in consultation with industry bodies. The code encourages the application of HACCP principles. In order to ensure that animal feed is of an acceptable quality it is necessary to source the raw materials from registered producers, in the case of processed animal protein, and from those complying with the relevant Codes of Practice in the case of other raw materials.

The raw materials should be stored in suitable buildings which prevent pests gaining access. On-farm storage bins and silos should be similarly treated. Transport of raw materials and finished feeds should be in dedicated vehicles which are thoroughly inspected before use to ensure they are clean and dry. Feed mills must be constructed of appropriate, food-grade, materials and must be regularly cleansed, disinfected and sampled for evidence of contamination. There must be segregation of raw materials from finished feeds to minimise the risk of cross-contamination.

Staff need to know the importance of good hygiene practice and should receive appropriate training.

*Pelleting of feed* improves the overall feed intake and pellets are easier to handle in automated feed delivery system. The process creates temperatures high enough to reduce the numbers of pathogenic bacteria which may be present, although it does not provide a total kill. To achieve this, a separate heat treatment process (i.e. *pasteurisation*) is required. This is an effective way of tackling the problem of *Salmonella* contamination of poultry feed.

## Poultry flock health

All poultry farms should have a *veterinarian*, specialising in poultry, who will advise on the *health and management of the flock*. Visits should be made, at least annually, to ensure a knowledge of practices and facilities on the farm. All events which are outside the normal, for example, increased mortality, poor weights or poor feed conversion, should be thoroughly investigated. The chances of eliminating microbial contamination from poultry meat will be improved if steps are taken to ensure that birds entering the slaughter and processing chain are either free from infection or are identified as contaminated and treated accordingly.

The situation in Sweden where there has been considerable success in tackling the *Salmonella* problem, involves testing all flocks of broilers and turkeys for *Salmonella* one or two weeks prior to slaughter. If *Salmonella* of any stereotype is detected, the flock is not sent for processing but is destroyed and hygienically disposed of. Enlightened processors in the UK are testing broilers before slaughter and this enables *positive* flocks to be handled with special care and attention during processing. This will entail slaughter at the end of the day or week, increased chlorine levels in the water and perhaps lower line speed and/or attention to prevent rupture of the intestines.

Healthier birds are produced on a single-age site ('all-in, all-out' system). The unit is periodically depopulated and thoroughly cleaned and disinfected. Tests are carried out to ensure freedom from, for example *Salmonella*, prior to restocking. Should *Salmonella* be isolated, cleaning and disinfection are repeated until a negative result is obtained.

The need for close liaison with the farm is even more important in the case of poultry than with other species because of their size, large numbers involved in slaughter and dressing, high rates of slaughter and the use of antibiotics, anticoccidial drugs, etc. in their rearing. *Adequate withdrawal periods* are essential for all drugs. This period of time should be adhered to when 'thinning' occurs, i.e. when a number of birds are removed from the house in order to give extra room to allow the remaining birds grow larger.

The *withdrawal of feed prior to loading for transport to slaughter*, in order to reduce crop and intestinal tract contents, can also help to reduce the level of contamination. Published FAO literature recommends a minimum period of 4 hours prior to birds arriving at the poultry plant, but extending the period to 10 hours may result in faeces becoming more fluid, thus increasing the chances of cross-contamination between birds in transit. The UK Advisory Committee on the Microbiological Safety of Food recommends that a period between 6 and 10 hours should be allowed between feeding and kill.

## Catching and crating

This operation should be carried out with care in order to avoid injuries and unnecessary suffering to the birds. Crates must be in good repair and of good design and must not be over- or under-filled, since both situations can lead to injury. The catchers must be well-trained and supervised to avoid injury and downgrading of the birds. Only healthy birds should be crated; diseased or otherwise abnormal birds should be killed on the farm.

One of the most difficult, labour-intensive and unpleasant tasks as far as working conditions and unsociable hours are concerned is that of collecting, crating and loading birds at the point of production. Depending on the quality and commitment of the staff employed, this area can be one where bird welfare is of a high or a low order, the latter often resulting in high levels of downgrading of carcases because of the injuries inflicted.

The majority of *bruises* resulting in downgrading occur during catching and transportation. The incidence of bruising is also directly related to the length of the journey.

In recent years systems have been developed to improve catching (or harvesting) and transportation. For the time being, however, broilers are still caught by hand and carried by one leg. This has to be done with great care to avoid injury. Turkeys must always be carried by two legs.

*Poultry harvesting procedures* can be divided into four basic systems.

*Loose crates* Empty plastic crates are taken from the lorry into the shed, where a team of catchers fill the individual crates. As with all systems, fewer birds are placed in each crate in summer to reduce the risk of heat stress. The birds are passed into the crate through a flapped-opening at the top. For unloading there is a larger aperture in the side or top of the crate through which the birds may be removed. Once a crate has been filled, it is taken to the lorry. Self-stacking crates can be placed on pallets in the shed for handling by a fork-lift vehicle. Loose crates provide a flexible system at low capital cost but a high labour input.

*Fixed crates* The crates are fixed on to the lorry. The birds are carried out of the shed to the lorry and are placed by the handful into one of the lower crates. Numbers in each crate depend on size and weather conditions. When the correct number have been placed in the crate the hinged flap is fastened. For loading the upper crates, a loading platform is attached to the side of the lorry, from which two men can operate. The remainder of the catching team pass the birds to these men. Once again, great care has to be taken to prevent injuries to the birds. The system has the advantage of better protection from inclement weather than provided by loose crates while in transit, but the capital cost is greater although the labour requirements are marginally lower.

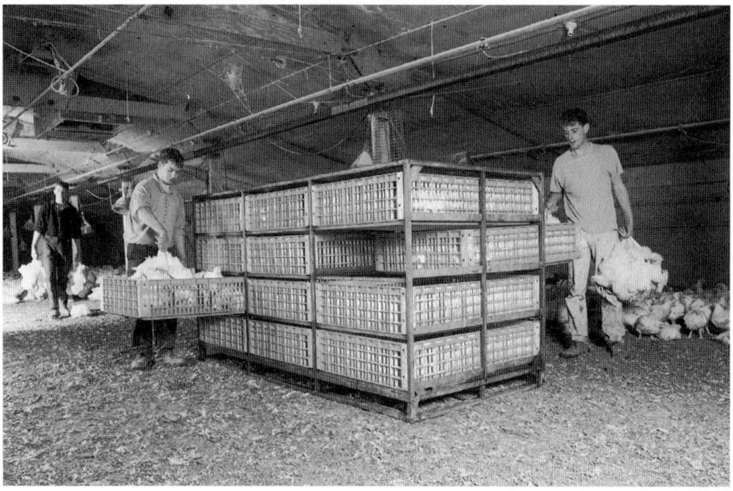

**Fig. 11.1** Modular crates for holding birds.

*Modules* The modular system has been of great benefit in lowering the amount of bruising and other injuries to birds and has obvious improved welfare considerations. Basically, a module is a metal frame containing 4–16 crates or compartments. The empty modules are taken into the house by a fork-lift truck. The birds are caught by hand and put directly into the compartments, thus avoiding the need for multiple handling or carrying the birds for long distances before crating (Fig. 11.1).

Modules tend to be bulky and heavy, weighing about 1 tonne when fully loaded. The floor of the poultry house needs to be firm and 15 m of concrete is needed at the front of the shed for the lorry.

Modules allow for rapid catching and loading and a three-man team can load 6000 birds per hour. They can be loaded from either side and the large open top of each drawer ensures that minimal damage is inflicted on the birds. The modules are stacked two high on the lorry and the outside can have a curtain, which makes them suitable for all climatic conditions.

Dump modules have been used with limited success. In these the birds are off-loaded at the poultry plant by tilting the module and 'dumping' the birds on to a conveyor belt. These were developed with the intention of improving welfare, with expected lessening of fractures and bruising, but present-day thinking is to try to develop methods of stunning the birds in their crates prior to shackling.

Novel *mechanical methods* include herding systems where the birds are herded on to a conveyor, and a fully *automatic harvesting system* which consists of a catching unit, a truck unit and a crate-loading unit. The birds are directed by long rubber fingers, on vertical rotating reels, on to a belt conveyor up to a crating area. The crating system consists of a trailer with a special rotating platform and a loading conveyor which has a hydraulic lifting device so that all drawers of the module can be filled automatically.

## Reception and unloading

The reception area or lairage is the area where birds are held before unloading. It should be under cover and of sufficient size to hold all the transport vehicles awaiting unloading. In warm weather, additional ventilation provided by fans is necessary and evaporative cooling devices are sometimes used to regulate the environment. In addition to good ventilation, control of relative humidity is also essential and this should not be allowed to rise above 70%.

The method of *unloading* will obviously depend upon the type of crate used. Loose crates are unloaded from the vehicle and placed on a conveyor system which carries them to the hanging station. It is important that the crates are not thrown around roughly and that the birds are gently but firmly hung on the rail. The crates continue around on the conveyor, are washed and brought back to the vehicle, which should have been cleaned.

For unloading the birds from fixed crates, the vehicle is driven between two vertically moving platforms. The hangers standing on the platforms open the crates at the side, take out the birds and hang them on the killing line which is behind them. No crate-conveyor system is required but the crates are extremely difficult to clean. In addition, the hangers have to turn through 180° every time a bird is removed and hung on the line.

Some of the modular systems effect unloading through hinged doors in the side in a manner similar to that for fixed crates. Another system raises the modules hydraulically to a high-level unloading platform, so that the drawers are at the required level. The birds are taken from the open drawers and hung on the shackles by a 90° rotation of the unloading operative. The 'Easyload' module is removed from the transport vehicle by a fork-lift truck and fed into an automated system which presents it to a drawer push-out unit. This transfers the plastic drawers to a covered conveyor leading to the hanging station. The open drawer allows unrestricted access for the hanging operatives, greatly reducing bird damage and manpower requirements. The birds are hung directly on the killing line.

Each operator can hang 1500 birds per hour. The hanging area can be enclosed to incorporate dust extraction and light density control, thus aiding health and safety for the operators and welfare of the birds, which allows them to be quiet and lessens stress during transfer on to the killing line.

The empty 'Easyload' drawers are automatically inverted to remove all loose debris and are then immersed in a pre-soak tank before being thoroughly washed and sanitised. The empty drawers continue through the drawer re-inverter to be automatically reloaded into the returning empty module frame. The module frames are also automatically washed.

The layout of this system lends itself to separate clean and dirty areas within the arrival bay.

## Pre-slaughter inspection

On arrival at the plant, every consignment should be checked to determine the condition of the birds and to ensure, for example, that during transit they have not become trapped by the heads, legs or wings.

The lighting in the hanging-on area should be sufficient to enable staff to see the birds and identify problems but not so bright as to disturb the birds. On removal from the crate or module, birds should be checked to see whether they are suffering from a condition which may cause them pain or distress. These birds should be killed immediately either by dislocation of the neck (small birds) or by stunning knife (small and large birds). This must be done by a licensed slaughterman. Runts and diseased birds, which may have been inadvertently crated should also be killed and not shackled.

## Shackling

When correctly handled, most birds remain still after a short period of wing flapping when first placed in the shackles. Broilers will generally have settled within 12 seconds and turkeys 20 seconds. A method of reducing wing flapping is for the shackler to run his hands down the bird's body or to briefly hold on to its legs. A strip of smooth plastic sheeting installed parallel to the conveyor line, along which the breasts of the suspended birds rub also has a quietening effect.

Turkeys must not be suspended for more than 6 minutes and other birds for 3 minutes before being stunned or killed.

## Stunning and slaughter

### *Electrical stunning*

Stunning is usually carried out in an electrically-charged water-bath by dragging the heads of the birds through water in which an electrode is submerged. The shackles of the killing line simultaneously touch an earth electrode, causing an electric current to run through the body of the bird. Effective stunning requires careful observation of the birds and adjustment of the equipment.

The water level is critical and it is essential to avoid water flowing down the inlet chute and causing a pre-stun shock, which may make the birds raise their heads, thus avoiding contact with the water of the actual stunner. Salt may be added to the water to improve the efficiency of stunning.

It is suggested by the UK Humane Slaughter Association that there should be a minimum current of 120 mA to induce cardiac arrest in 90% of birds. However, 105 mA per bird would be acceptable provided both carotid arteries are severed within 15 seconds to ensure death before birds can begin to recover.

Problems with conventional water-bath stunners have been identified through observation in commercial processing plants and experiments in the laboratory. Owing to differences in the electrical resistance of the individual birds, there is little control over the stunning current and hence the effectiveness of stunning. A prototype poultry stunner has been developed which controls the current delivered to individual birds. The machine is capable of operating at typical commercial speeds of 6000 birds per hour. It can provide a constant current to each individual bird provided there is no significant current pathway between adjacent birds. A constant-current stunning system will control the current flow through individual birds at an optimal level which will ensure an effective stun and at the same time minimise the carcase quality problems produced by high currents.

Less commonly used stunning instruments are the dry stunner, usually incorporating an electrically-charged metal grid or plate and hand-operated stunner.

The most reliable indicator that a bird is properly stunned by the low voltage method is the *electroplectic fit*. The characteristics of this condition are: neck arched with the head directly vertically, open eyes, absence of corneal reflex, wings flexed, rigidly extended legs and constant rapid body tremors.

When *cardiac arrest* is induced, these signs are shorter-lasting and less pronounced and are followed by a completely limp carcase, no breathing (absence of abdominal movements in the vent area), loss of nictitating membrane reflex and dilated pupil. The comb reflex can also determine whether sensibility has resumed after stunning or neck cutting.

Although cardiac arrest is preferable from a welfare standpoint, the use of high stunning currents on the quality of the carcase is said by some to be associated with wing haemorrhages, red skin condition, including red wing-tips and pygostyles, poor plucking, broken bones (in particular furculum) and ruptured blood vessels causing blood splashing in the breast muscle.

### *Gas stunning*

Although electrical stunning is the most common method of stunning poultry prior to slaughter under commercial conditions, novel methods of stunning/killing poultry using *gases*, while the birds are still in their transport containers, have been approved under the new EC Directive. Gas stunning/killing will enable shackling to be performed on the freshly killed birds and this would eliminate the live bird handling at the processing plants. The two gas stunning/killing methods that are being approved in the UK are anoxia induced with 90% argon or other inert gases, and a mixture of 25–30% carbon dioxide and 60% argon or other inert gases in air.

The birds would be stunned/killed while they are in their transport containers. This would result in the birds leaving a stunning unit in large numbers, and all the carcases would have to be uncrated and shackled rapidly to allow prompt neck cutting. It is inevitable that the time between the end of gas stunning and neck cutting would be longer than that practised under the conventional electrical stunning system. Although research has shown that the efficiency of bleeding in broiler chickens was not impaired when their necks were cut immediately after gas stunning/killing, delayed neck cutting after gas stunning of broilers could increase the prevalence of carcase downgrading conditions associated with a poor bleed out. This does not happen with turkeys, the difference being attributable to a difference in carcase cooling rate or other factors.

Gas stunning/killing methods accelerate the rate of post-mortem pH fall in poultry and this would allow early filleting in broilers (within one hour after slaughter). Generally with anoxia there are fewer carcase and meat quality defects. Many fewer defects are found in the breast region, including haemorrhages, but there is an increase in defects involving the wings.

### *Neck-cutting*

This should be carried out within 15 seconds of the bird emerging from the stunner. Mechanical neck-cutting is the norm for broilers when the bird's head is guided across a single revolving circular blade or between a pair of revolving blades. Accurate positioning of the head is essential. When cardiac arrest is not produced at stunning, the most humane method of producing rapid brain death is to sever both carotid arteries. In practice this is difficult, but not impossible, to achieve without having an effect on the further processing of the carcase.

Where a mechanical killer is used in the UK it is mandatory to have an operative present to manually kill any bird which has missed the automatic system. Operatives who kill the birds have to be licensed by the local authority.

Birds are killed manually by passing a knife across the side of the neck at the base of the bird's head, which should sever a jugular vein and carotid artery. Again it is better to sever both carotids, but care has to be taken to avoid damage to the carcase.

Whichever method is used, a sharp instrument is essential. Automatic killing of turkeys has not been introduced because of the problem of major variation in bird size within the flock.

## Scalding and defeathering

The minimum time for bleeding between neck-cutting and entering the scald tank in the UK is 1½ minutes for chickens and 2 minutes for turkeys. The birds, on the conveyor, pass through a bleeding tunnel, the blood being collected and pumped into a holding tank.

The birds are scalded either by immersion in hot water or by spray-scalding. Spray-scalding is more hygienic but also more expensive and therefore scald tanks are more commonly installed. The temperature of the water is dependent on the type of final product. For the fresh, chilled market a soft scald of 50–51°C is used as this does not damage the skin, thereby preventing discoloration and drying (barking) on air chilling.

For the frozen market a hard scald at a higher temperature, 56–58°C is used as this facilitates feather removal and the birds need only remain in the tank for 2–2½ minutes instead of 3½ minutes for the soft scald. In the USA there is a statutory requirement for an overflow from the scald tank of about 1 litre/bird for hygiene reasons. Various chemicals can be added to assist feather removal and to try to prevent cross-contamination (but see below).

The scald tank immersion results in large numbers of organisms being released into the water; in addition, faecal material in the tank dissociates to form ammonium urate and uric acid, which form a natural buffer system, thereby maintaining scald tank pH at around 6, the point at which *salmonellas* are most heat-resistant. The overall effect is that *Salmonellas*, *campylobacters* and other organisms, including spores, can survive. Research has shown that the addition of quaternary ammonium, acetic acid, etc. to the scald tank would adjust the pH, the principal controlling factor in the survival of *salmonellas* and *campylobacters*, and therefore improve the hygiene. At present this cannot be used because of the requirements to demonstrate no carcase residues and to use only potable water.

There is no doubt the operation of scalding from a hygiene standpoint is fraught with hazards; the temperature of the scald water, type (immersion, spray with hot water or steam), duration of scalding, static, agitated or countercurrent bath water, type of tank(s), etc. all affect the degree of water-bath contamination. Recent work (Slavik *et al.*, 1995) on the numbers of *Campylobacter* and *Salmonella* on chicken carcases scalded at three different temperatures would appear to confirm that the higher the temperature the greater the contamination (Table 11.2).

Alternative methods of scalding are being devised to improve the situation. Lower bacterial contamination has been achieved with spray scalding and plucking in a single operation (Veerkamp and Hofmans, 1973). Clouser *et al.* (1995) found that a spray scalding system for turkey carcases was superior to traditional scalding.

Improvements in immersion scalding have been made by stirring the water in order to achieve an ideal mixing; division of the scald tank into several smaller ones; and high-

**Table 11.2** Numbers of *Campylobacter* and *Salmonella* (log mpn/carcase) on chicken carcases scalded at three different temperatures.

| Bacterium | Scald temperature (0°C) | Trial 1 | Trial 2 | Trial 3 |
|---|---|---|---|---|
| *Salmonella* | 52 | 3.00 | 3.17 | 3.09 |
| | 56 | 3.16 | 3.17 | 3.34 |
| | 60 | 3.50 | 3.48 | 3.36 |
| *Campylobacter* | 52 | 3.64 | 3.30 | 4.18 |
| | 56 | 3.39 | 2.94 | 3.39 |
| | 60 | 4.08 | 3.59 | 3.98 |

From Slavik *et al.* (1995).

pressure (800 bar) treatment of scald water. All these have shown improvements in scald water quality. Lowering the pH with organic acids may affect product quality and the addition of trisodium phosphate may cause corrosion of equipment. The ideal solution has not yet been found.

## Defeathering

Feathers are removed mechanically, immediately after scalding, by a series of on-line plucking machines. These consist of banks of counter-rotating, stainless steel domes or discs, with attached rubber 'fingers'. Rubber flails mounted on inclined shafts are sometimes used for finishing.

The machines should be close to the scald tank and to each other to lessen the effect of cooling. Generally, birds which have been scalded at higher temperatures require 50% less defeathering capacity. The machines are adjustable to allow for differing bird sizes and this must be carried out to prevent mechanical damage to the carcase.

Continuous water-sprays are usually incorporated within the machines for flushing out feathers. Feathers are commonly taken to a centralised collection point via a fast-flowing water-channel located below the machine. Dry feather systems using a conveyor belt in conjunction with a vacuum or compressed-air arrangement are sometimes used. Any feathers remaining on the bird after plucking, including pin feathers, are removed by hand.

For ducks, *wax stripping* is used. The ducks are dipped in a bath of hot wax and then passed through cool water-sprays so that the wax hardens. The hardened wax, with the feathers attached, is hand-stripped. The plucked carcases are then spray-washed. There is evidence to suggest that the combination of scalding at 60°C followed by immersion in molten wax at 87°C to aid final removal of the feathers has a beneficial effect on the microbiological status of the finished product.

Defeathering machines are major sites of potential cross-contamination in primary processing. Rubber fingers can score the carcase and can also harbour contamination in the 'cobweb' of tiny cracks which form when the rubber becomes brittle. In addition, the spinning action of the plucker heads form aerosols which can spread contamination. Moreover, since the atmosphere inside the machinery is both warm and moist, microbial growth is encouraged.

Following feather removal, the birds are spray-washed and at this point the *whole bird post-mortem examination* takes place. It is here that obviously diseased birds, badly-bled and badly-bruised carcases are removed. The heads of the birds are removed by an automatic head and windpipe puller. By pulling the heads off rather than cutting them off, the oesophagus and trachea are removed with the heads. This loosens the crop and lungs, which assists in their removal by the automatic evisceration machines.

The birds then pass through an automatic foot-cutter. The severed feet remain on the shackles and are removed mechanically on the return line. In the case of large turkeys, retention of the sinews is considered unacceptable. Instead of cutting off the shanks, an automatic sinew-puller is used, and this draws up to nine of the main sinews.

The carcases are re-hung on the evisceration line after removal of the feet. This can now be done automatically, using a transfer system available from several equipment manufacturers. In this case the foot-cutter and transfer device are combined in one unit. This lessens the risk of cross-contamination. The empty, returning, killing-line shackles pass through a *shackle washer* on their way back to the bird arrival area.

## Evisceration (Figs 11.2 and 11.3)

In the EC the evisceration area must be physically separated from the defeathering area.

Chickens are usually suspended from the shackles of the evisceration-line conveyor by engaging the hock joints two-point suspension. Turkeys are commonly hung by a 'three-point' suspension which includes the head as well as the legs. This presents the bird horizontally, making cutting around the vent and evisceration easier.

Evisceration is mainly carried out mechanically, but manual evisceration is still practised. On automatic lines, a cut is made around the vent, a spoon-shaped device is inserted into the opening and the viscera are

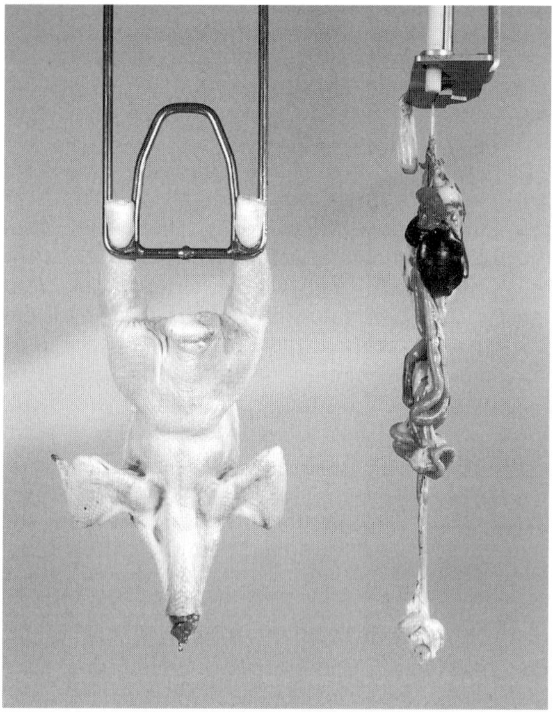

**Fig. 11.2** Separation of carcase meat from offal. (Courtesy of Stork PVM B.V., Boxmeer, Holland)

withdrawn. The viscera may remain attached for inspection, hanging over the back of the carcase connected by their natural tissues or hung separately.

Contamination of the carcase surface with *Enterobacteriaceae* species may ensue if intestines, etc. are damaged. This is not an uncommon occurrence because the machinery used is not able to adjust for the natural variation in the size of birds being processed. A new type of equipment, however, holds the birds horizontally by the head and hocks so that, when the viscera are removed from the body cavity, they emerge sideways. They are placed on a tray beside the bird rather than hung with it and hence do not come into contact with the carcase.

It is at this stage that a further *inspection* takes place which will observe changes in the internal organs. After inspection, the viscera are separated into edible and inedible offal. The edible fraction (sometimes being washed in chlorinated water) is sorted, chilled and packed.

The eviscerated carase is *spray-washed*, internally and externally. This gives a visually-

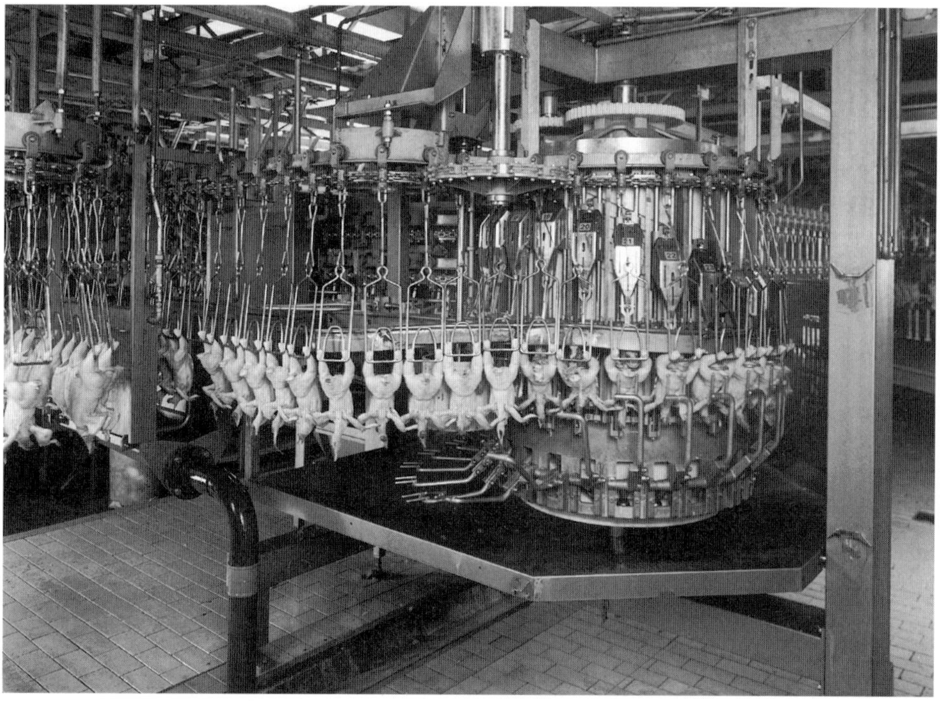

**Fig. 11.3** Evisceration. (Courtesy of Stork PMV B.V., Boxmeer, Holland)

clean bird and also decreases carcase contamination. The carcase should be washed not only after final inspection but between the different stages involved in evisceration, as it has been shown that by doing so the numbers of *coliforms* and *salmonellas* on carcases are reduced because there is insufficient time for attachment to occur. A suitable carcase-washer comprises a small cabinet containing an appropriate arrangement of spray nozzles. The water should contain 40 mg/litre of free chlorine.

The heart, liver and gizzard (the giblets) are often pooled and inserted into the body of the chicken. Giblets are more frequently contaminated with *salmonella* than other sample sites and chickens which contain them are more often contaminated than those without giblets. The carcase and skin of these chickens are more frequently contaminated with *Salmonella enteritidis* PT4 than these sites in chickens not containing giblets, irrespective of whether the giblets themselves were contaminated.

The same study also found that frozen chickens were significantly more regularly contaminated than chilled chickens.

Partial evisceration (or effile) is carried out in Great Britain. In this process, the intestines are removed but the remaining viscera are left inside the carcase. Delayed evisceration is also permissible, where uneviscerated birds are held for up to 15 days under refrigeration at no more than 4°C before evisceration and post-mortem inspection are carried out.

New York-Dressed (NYD) birds are sold uneviscerated and with the head and feet left attached. The EEC marketing of NYD birds from licensed premises is banned from 1 May 1997. However NYD birds may still be produced and marketed by exempt slaughterhouses (i.e. those producing fewer than 10 000 birds per year). NYD birds present a particular hazard owing to the risk of leakage of faeces from the vent and, if evisceration is carried out in a kitchen, the risk of faeces or intestinal contents from ruptured intestines cross-contaminating other foods.

## Chilling

In many plants the high rate of processing (e.g. 7000 birds per hour) is such that there is little loss of heat from the carcase before it reaches the chilling stage, and average carcase temperatures are frequently above 30°C. Prompt and efficient chilling of the bird is essential to delay the growth of psychotrophic spoilage bacteria and prevent any increase in microorganisms of public health significance.

The type of chilling used can have an effect on the type and quantity of microbial contamination of the end-product. Continuous, in-line, *immersion chilling* is still the most widely used method in many countries. Carcases move through a counterflow current of water in a state of constant agitation so that they are constantly moving into cleaner water. This washing effect also removes numerous organisms from both the inner and outer surfaces of the carcases. There may be deleterious effects if there is a significant build-up of blood and carcase material or a rise in water temperature. The addition of hypochlorite or chlorine dioxide to the water might serve to reduce the levels of contamination in the chiller but, because these compounds would quickly be deactivated on contact with skin, there would be little direct effect on carcase bacterial burdens. The main value of chlorinating chiller water is to minimise cross-contamination.

EC regulations state that the carcases must pass through one or more tanks of water or of ice and water, the contents of which are continuously renewed. Only a system whereby the carcases are constantly propelled by mechanical means through a counterflow of water is acceptable.

The temperature of the water in the tank measured at the points of entry and exit of the carcases must not be more than +16°C and +4°C, respectively.

Chilling must be carried out so that the required temperatures of *fresh chilled* poultry meat of not more than 4°C and for *frozen* poultry meat of not more than −12°C are reached in the shortest possible time.

The minimum flow of water throughout the whole chilling process must be:

2.5 litres per carcase weighing 2.5 kg or less;
4 litres per carcase weighing between 2.5–5 kg;
6 litres per carcase weighing 5 kg or more.

Other requirements are the length of time the carcases spend in the tanks (first tank not more than half an hour; others, not longer than necessary); equipment to be thoroughly cleaned and disinfected when necessary and at the end of the day; calibrated control equipment; and the need for microbiological monitoring.

In addition, when chlorine is used it should be monitored to ensure correct levels.

*Static water-chillers* involve the use of static slush ice tanks after immersion chilling and are required for larger birds, especially for turkeys which must also be 'aged' to ensure a tender product prior to freezing. The larger carcases need to be chilled for longer periods. The disadvantages of this equipment are greater than those arising from the use of immersion chillers.

*Spray-chillers* avoid the problems associated with the build-up of contamination in the chill tanks but can give rise to the spread of bacteria through aerosols. They are not suitable for large carcases, e.g. turkeys, and are costly to operate as they use high volumes of water.

*Air-chillers* are generally used where carcases are for sale fresh. Chilling is effected either by batch in a chill room or by continuous air blast. It requires the use of low-scald temperatures to ensure a high-quality appearance. The differences in microbial counts between air and water-cooled carcases are not constant.

Chemical rinsing of carcases with *trisodium phosphate* is used in the USA

## ANTE-MORTEM HEALTH INSPECTION

In the EU the traditional ante-mortem inspection, with its obvious deficiencies of not being able to inspect birds in crates or on the line adequately, has been superseded by on-farm producer declaration or a health attestation signed by a private veterinarian.

Producers with an annual production of up to 20 000 domestic fowl or 15 000 duck or 10 000 turkeys or 10 000 geese complete a declaration which states they do not exceed the above numbers. Birds from their farm receive a pre-slaughter health inspection by the official veterinarian at the plant.

Birds from producers with an annual production in excess of the above can either have a Health Attestation signed by a private veterinarian which states that he has examined the poultry before slaughter, and that in his opinion there are no reasons why they should not be slaughtered for human consumption. The veterinary pre-slaughter health inspection consists of the following:

**(a)** Checking the producer's records, which depending on the type of bird include:
- (1) date of arrival;
- (2) number;
- (3) mortality;
- (4) suppliers of feedingstuffs;
- (5) type, period of use and withdrawal periods of feed additives;
- (6) type of any medicinal product, with dates of administration and withdrawal (this includes vaccines);
- (7) results of any previous official pre-slaughter health inspections of birds from the same specified group;
- (8) number sent for slaughter;
- (9) expected date of slaughter.

**(b)** Any additional examinations needed to establish:
- (1) whether birds are suffering from a disease which can be transmitted to humans or animals;
- (2) whether the birds show disturbance of general behaviour or signs of sickness which may make the meat unfit for human consumption.

**(c)** Regular sampling of water and feed with a view to checking compliance with withdrawal periods.

**(d)** The results of tests for zoonotic agents carried out in accordance with Directive 92/117/EEC.

Alternatively, the veterinarian signs an initial declaration, given to the central competent authority, confirming that the producer's holding is under his supervision. The producer then submits a production report to the manager of the plant at least 72 hours before the birds are due to arrive. The information is then passed on to the Official Veterinary Surgeon (OVS).

If the OVS is not satisfied with the information, he may ask for further information such as details of the hatchery, feedstuffs, growth rates, etc., and if the Production Report is not complete or does not provide the required information or the OVS is not satisfied, he may order an inspection at the farm of origin to enable completion of the report. The inspection is carried out at the owner's expense. The Production Report consists of the following details:

- Holding of origin
- Intended date of arrival at slaughterhouse
- Expected number of birds in consignment
- Mortality data (daily % in final week before slaughter, and weekly mortality before that)
- Results of any on-farm veterinary inspection of flock
- Results of any laboratory tests/diagnosis carried out on birds, litter etc.
- Dates of administration/withdrawal of all medicinal products
- Any other relevant information.

The Production Report should be copied to the veterinary surgeon supervising the holding.

The plant OVS (or a delegated poultry meat inspector (PMI)) is responsible for relaying adverse results of post-mortem inspections and dead-on-arrivals (DOAS) of consignments back to the holding, slaughterhouse management, and veterinarian responsible for the holding as he or she feels necessary.

## POST-MORTEM INSPECTION IN THE PLANT

Plant inspection assistants (PIAs) in the UK are plant employees who have been trained to undertake post-mortem inspection on the whole bird and evisceration inspection points. They can therefore replace PMIs, who now carry out more of a supervisory role, but only with the agreement of the competent authority and after discussion with the OVS. Some purchasers of poultry products insist on the independence of PMIs for inspection.

Poultry inspection assistants are taught the theory and practice of anatomy and physiology, pathology and meat inspection and also poultry welfare and legislation.

Poultry must be inspected immediately after slaughter under suitable lighting (540 lux). The surface of the bird's body, excluding head and feet, except where they are intended for human consumption, the viscera and the body cavities must be subjected to visual inspection and where necessary, palpation and incision.

Attention must also be paid to anomalies of consistency, colour and smell in the carcases, major anomalies resulting from the slaughtering operations and proper functioning of the slaughter equipment.

The OVS must give a detailed inspection of a random sample of the birds rejected in the post-mortem health inspection and examine a random sample of 300 birds, taken from the entire consignment, by inspecting the viscera and body cavities.

He must carry out a special post-mortem if there are other indications that the meat from the poultry could be unfit for human consumption. In the case of partly eviscerated poultry ('effile') whose intestines were removed immediately, the viscera and the body cavities of at least 5% of the poultry from each consignment will be inspected after evisceration. If anomalies are discovered in a number of birds, then all of the consignment must be examined as above.

In the case of New York Dressed poultry, the birds will be examined as above, no longer than 15 days after slaughter, and kept at 4°C or below.

Taking of samples for *residues* must be carried out by spot checks, and in any event of justified suspicion. The OVS also has the authority to ask for laboratory tests to be carried out to aid diagnosis or to detect pharmacological substances. Should the OVS consider that hygienic processing or health inspection is not being adequately carried out, he can lower the line speed or stop production.

The results of the inspections should be recorded and where necessary communicated to the competent veterinary authority (of the holding from which the birds originated), and the owner of the flock of origin who will pass this information to the official veterinarian carrying out the ante-mortem inspection during the subsequent production period.

Many of the diseases listed below will rarely be encountered in the poultry plant.

## DECISION OF THE OFFICIAL VETERINARIAN AT THE POST-MORTEM INSPECTION

Poultry meat is declared totally *unfit for human consumption* where the post-mortem inspection reveals any of the following conditions:

- Generalised infectious diseases and chronic localisations in organs of pathogenic microorganisms transmissible to humans
- Systemic mycosis and local lesions in organs suspected of having been caused by

pathogenic agents transmissible to humans, or their toxins
- Extensive subcutaneous or muscular parasitism and systemic parasitism
- Poisoning
- Cachexia
- Abnormal smell, colour or taste
- Malignant or multiple tumours
- General soiling or contamination
- Major lesions and ecchymoses
- Extensive mechanical lesions, including those due to extensive scalding
- Insufficient bleeding
- Residues of substances exceeding the authorised standards or residues of prohibited substances
- Ascites

Parts of the carcase which show *localised lesions* or contaminations not affecting the health of the rest of meat are *unfit for human consumption*. It is essential that condemned and suspect meat is kept separated from meat for human consumption.

Poultry carcases, in licensed premises, are only allowed to be cut into parts and boned in approved *cutting rooms*. They must be chilled to not more than +4°C before cutting proceeds unless the slaughter room and the cutting room are near each other and located in the same group of buildings and the meat is transferred in one operation by an extension of the mechanical handling system.

Cutting must be carried out immediately and once cutting and packaging are complete the meat is placed in the chilling room. Packaged fresh poultry meat must not be kept in the same room as unpacked poultry meat.

Poultry disease is often multifactorial with, for example, poor ventilation along with a viral disease acting together with bacteria, for example *E. coli*, to produce generalised septicaemia resulting in pericarditis, air sacculitis/perihepatitis and a congested carcase.

Yogaratnam (1995) analysed results of examinations at a poultry processing plant which received 33.65 million birds from 87 commercial broiler growing units in 1992 (Table 11.3). High carcase rejection rates of 3% or more were recorded in birds received from 13.2% of the rearing houses, distributed among

**Table 11.3** Percentages of broiler carcases rejected because they were either dead on arrival or diseased from farms with normal or high rates of rejection of carcases.

| Farm rejection rate | Percentage of carcases | |
|---|---|---|
| | Dead on arrival | Disease conditions |
| Normal | 0.22 | 1.09 |
| High | 0.42 | 5.12 |

48% of the growing units. The higher rates of carcase rejection were found on the units with an average flock size of over 100 000 birds and from rearing houses with a population of more than 30 000 birds. The main cause of rejection were birds dead on arrival (0.24%), disease (1.57%) and miscellaneous conditions (0.28%). The commonest cause of carcase rejection due to disease was colisepticaemia (42.8%). Septicaemia/toxaemia/fevered accounted for 29.63%, emaciation for 19.45% and ascites for 5.91%. Hydropericardium/pericarditis (1.01%), skin lesions (0.62%), joint lesions (0.31%), jaundice (0.16%) and tumours (0.01%) were also seen. The birds from units with high rejection rates had lower average slaughter weights than birds from units with normal rejection rates.

The productivity of intensively-reared poultry falls as a result of disease problems as the size of the flock increases and as the number of rearing houses on one site increases.

## VIRAL POULTRY DISEASES

### IBD

*Infectious bursal disease (IBD, Gumboro disease)* affects young chickens usually up to 6 weeks of age. It is one of the most important diseases because the virus affects lymphoid tissue and acts as an immunosuppressor. Virulent IBD has been responsible for increased mortality and condemnation in recent years. Carcases of birds dying from this infection are dehydrated; there are petechial haemorrhages in the leg and thigh muscles and occasionally on the mucosa of the proventiculus with increased mucus in the intestines.

Colisepticaemia frequently follows immunosuppression.

### Inclusion body hepatitis

Usually seen in meat-producing chickens aged 4–9 weeks, this is characterised by a sudden increase in mortality (2–4%) which can last for 3–4 days. Other birds in the flock often appear bright or they may be depressed for a few days. Overall food conversion and weight gain are usually depressed. The livers are swollen and frequently have haemorrhages.

### Reoviruses

*Reoviruses* have been associated with tenosynovitis or viral arthritis in meat-producing birds over 5 weeks of age. There is bilateral swelling of the digital flexor and the tarsometatarsal extensor tendons. This produces lameness and the birds are reluctant to move. Chronic tenosynovitis may result and this may lead to rupture of the gastrocnemius tendon. Articular lesions may be recognised in long-standing cases. While morbidity is up to 100%, mortality is usually under 1%. Condemnations due to tenosynovitis are usually 1–2%, although, exceptionally, much higher figures have been found.

### Duck virus enteritis

This is caused by a herpesvirus. The disease spreads rapidly and birds affected are disinclined to walk. Post-mortem examination shows the birds to be in good condition. Multiple petechiae are seen throughout the body. Diphtheritic cloacitis and oesophagitis (almost pathognomonic) are seen. There is also an enteritis.

### Turkey rhinotracheitis (TRT)

This commonly affects flocks between 3 and 10 weeks. It has a rapid flock onset together with a high morbidity which frequently approaches 100%. Clinical signs may include depression, change of voice, gasping, moist trachael rales, snicking, coughing, submandibular oedema, swollen infraorbital sinuses, foamy ocular discharge and excess mucus at the external nares.

Uncomplicated cases have rapid recovery but secondary bacterial infection with *E. coli* can cause mortality to exceed 50%. It is more prevalent in areas with a high-density turkey population.

### Swollen head syndrome (SHS)

SHS affects mainly broilers and broiler breeders and is caused by a number of factors. Turkey rhinotracheitis, other virus infections such as infectious bronchitis in conjunction with *E. coli* and other bacteria and poor management have all been incriminated. In broilers the clinical signs consist of severe head swelling giving the face a puffy appearance caused by subcutaneous oedema around the eyes which extends over the head and down into the intermandibular tissues and wattles. Respiratory signs include coughing and sneezing and many affected birds have a severe tracheitis and often die from secondary septicaemia caused by *E. coli*.

Although morbidity is often low, the condition is exacerbated by poor ventilation and high levels of ammonia and dust.

Lesions consist of fine petechiation of the turbinate mucosa which progresses to a severe generalised red to purple discoloration of the mucosa. Removal of the skin over the head reveals yellow, oedematous, subcutaneous tissue.

### Turkey haemorrhagic enteritis (THE) group

There is a variation in virulence among different isolates. Outbreaks may be precipitated by overcrowding, chilling or a low plane of nutrition. Although mortalities of up to 50% have been recorded, they are usually lower. Signs vary from sudden death to depression with wet faeces or, in more chronic cases, dark tarry droppings that make white birds dirty. In these less acute cases there is very little mortality.

On post-mortem examination the intestines are full of blood and mucosal debris, invariably involving the duodenum but extending as far as the caeca in severe cases. The intestinal mucosa of the duodenum has a velvety appearance and may show the occasional necrotic area. Survivors may show a thickening of the duodenal wall and mild catarrhal enteritis and have enlarged mottled spleens. These are often found in the processing plant.

**Judgement** Depends on severity. If localised, partial condemnation; if generalised, total condemnation.

### Chicken anaemia agent (CAA)

A virus which is vertically transmitted and can cause variable mortality in susceptible young chicks. The anaemia–dermatitis syndrome of broilers may be due to combined CAA and reovirus infection and the virus may make chickens more susceptible to other diseases.

### Infectious laryngotracheitis

The more severe forms of this viral disease are of considerable economic importance since they may result in high mortality and greatly reduced production. It is found in domestic fowl and occasionally in the pheasant and partridge.

Signs vary from birds found dead or sudden acute dyspnoea with severe coughing and expectoration of mucus and blood-stained exudate and blood clots, followed by death in 1–3 days. In the acute form, dyspnoea is a feature, but not as severe as in the peracute form. Increasing obstruction of the trachea with exudate causes the bird to breathe with long drawn-out gasps, with a wide-open beak and often a high-pitched squawk and moist rales. In some birds there may be a nasal discharge and conjunctivitis. Cyanosis of the face and wattles can also be seen. Gross lesions vary with the severity but in most cases are restricted to the upper respiratory tract.

### Marek's disease

This is a virus disease of domestic chickens in which lymphoproliferative infiltration and demyelination of peripheral nerves is a common feature. Marek's disease affects chickens from about 6 weeks of age, most frequently between 12 and 24 weeks, but older chickens may also be affected. There are two main forms of clinical disease. In *classical* Marek's disease there is involvement of the peripheral nerves, mainly bronchial and sciatic, leading to progressive spastic paralysis of the wings and legs. Mortality is variable but rarely exceeds 10–15%. These birds should be seen on the farm and should be culled.

Mortality from *acute* Marek's disease is usually much higher than from the classical form and incidences of 10–30% are not uncommon. Outbreaks involving up to 80% of the flock can be encountered. There is diffuse lymphomatous involvement with enlargement of the liver, gonads, spleen, kidneys, lungs, proventriculus and heart. Sometimes lymphomas also arise in the skin in association with feather follicles (known as 'skin leukosis' in the USA) and in skeletal muscles. In younger birds the liver enlargement is usually moderate in extent but in older birds the greatly enlarged liver may appear identical to that in lymphoid leukosis.

### Leukosis/sarcoma group of diseases

This group includes tumours, the main one being lymphoid leukosis. The clinical signs of leukosis are non-specific. The bird may be inappetant, weak and emaciated, diarrhoea may occur, and the wattles may be pale. In lymphoid leukosis, the enlarged liver and bursa may be palpable and occasionally a leukaemia is demonstrable.

On post-mortem examination the most common finding is a grossly enlarged liver – this condition is sometimes called 'big liver disease'. Differentiation from Marek's disease can be achieved by histological examination; several birds should be examined.

Osteopetrosis occurs as thickening of the long bones, especially of the legs and wings while myeloid leukosis affects flat bones (ribs, skull, sternum, etc.). Also included in this group are erythroid and leukosis, haemangiomas, fibro-sarcomas and nephroblastomas, all caused by related retroviruses.

### Lymphoproliferative disease of turkeys

This is a rare disease in the UK. It is mainly seen in growing of turkeys between 7 and 18 weeks of age and occasionally in adults. Affected birds die suddenly. Up to 20% of the flock may be affected.

On post-mortem examination there is marked enlargement of the spleen, which is usually pale pink in colour with a marbled appearance. The liver may be moderately enlarged, with miliary greyish-white foci. Miliary or diffuse tumour infiltration may also occur in the kidney, gonads, intestinal wall, pancreas, lungs, myocardium and thymus.

### Reticuloendotheliosis

Reticuloendotheliosis comprises diseases caused by retroviruses that are distinct from the leukosis/sarcoma group. Neoplastic lesions are seen sporadically in turkeys and more rarely in chickens, ducks, geese, pheasants and quail.

The infection can cause immunosuppression. Post-mortem findings include an enlarged liver and spleen caused by focal or diffuse infiltration by proliferating reticulum cells and sometimes lymphocytes. Similar changes occur in the gonads, heart, kidney and pancreas.

*The judgement of all systemic tumour conditions is total rejection.*

### Newcastle disease

The casual organism of Newcastle disease is a paramyxovirus containing RNA.

Newcastle disease may effect domestic fowls, turkeys, geese, ducks, pheasants and guinea fowl, the period of incubation varying from 2 to 7 days. Birds affected with the *peracute* form are frequently found dead without showing previous symptoms. Occasionally humans may be infected by handling diseased birds, symptoms of malaise and conjunctivitis being evident with fairly rapid recovery.

In less severe outbreaks, affected birds refuse food, are dejected and listless and in some cases show a discharge from the eyes and nostrils. The wings and legs often become paralysed and a characteristic sign is a long, gasping inhalation through the half-open mouth, accompanied by gurgling and a frothy exudate from the beak. Green diarrhoea may be evident, with loss of appetite. In some instances there are nervous signs.

Sometimes the only sign exhibited by adult birds is a fall in egg production and the laying of eggs with abnormal shells, these being either misshapen, soft-shelled, imperfectly shelled or devoid of colour. In the past, mortality was as high as 100%, but vaccination has lowered this considerably. Newcastle disease is no longer subject to compulsory slaughter in the UK, vaccination being widely practised. However, it is a *notifiable* disease and all suspect poultry or carcases must be reported to the regulatory authority.

**Lesions** These vary depending on the virulence of the organism and the organs affected. Respiratory infection may cause tracheitis, often accompanied with haemorrhages, and air sacculitis.

The virulent viscerotropic viruses cause haemorrhagic lesions in the intestinal tract, particularly the proventriculus, at its borders with the gizzard.

### Avian influenza

Outbreaks of this highly virulent disease (previously known as *fowl plague)* have occurred sporadically. The pathogenicity of the various types varies dramatically and mutation can produce extreme virulence from viruses of low pathogenicity. Ducks and waterfowl tend to be refractory, even to the viruses that are highly pathogenic for chickens, although they may be carriers.

Control measures by countries seeking to prevent the introduction of disease include the banning of poultry from affected areas.

## BACTERIAL POULTRY DISEASES

### Necrotic enteritis

Necrotic enteritis is usually a sporadic disease in chickens and turkeys over approximately 4 weeks of age but can also occur in adults.

The small intestine is markedly thickened, owing to extensive velvet-like necrosis of the mucosa, and is deeply fissured and often congested. The condition may follow or be associated with coccidiosis.

**Judgement** Condemnation.

### Ulcerative enteritis or quail disease

This occurs as sporadic outbreaks in intensive systems of management of chickens, bob-white and other quails, pheasants and partridges. There are small, round superficial ulcers with haemorrhagic borders in the mucosa of the small intestine, caeca and upper large intestine which later coalesce and penetrate deeper into the serosa, which may become perforated and cause peritonitis. The liver may have yellowish to grey necrotic lesions and the spleen is usually enlarged and haemorrhagic.

**Judgement** Condemnation.

### Gangrenous dermatitis

*Clostridium septicum* and *Cl. perfringens* type A have been implicated in this disease, but in many outbreaks *Staphylococcus aureus* is also involved. Immunosuppressive organisms, poor management and high stocking rates are predisposing factors. It is primarily a disease of broiler chickens over 4 weeks of age. Affected birds die within a few hours and carcases rapidly decompose with a foul odour. Affected carcases should not reach the poultry plant.

**Judgement** Condemnation.

## Staphylococcal infections

*Staphylococcus aureus*, coagulase-positive, organisms are often found on the skin, nares, beak and on the feet of apparently normal chickens. Injury to the skin may predispose to tissue invasion. Environmental stress and concomitant or earlier infections with other pathogens may result in lowered resistance to the organism.

Conditions in which staphylococci are involved include arthritis and tenosynovitis of the hock joint and bumble foot (subdermal abscess). The synovial membranes of the joints and tendon sheaths become thickened and oedematous and exudate with fibrous deposits is produced within and around the joints and tendon sheaths. There is some necrosis and the exudate may later become caseous. Petechial and larger haemorrhages may be present in the early stages. If the bird survives, the condition becomes chronic with the formation of fibrous tissue.

Gangrenous dermatitis in broiler chickens, most frequently found at the wing tips and the dorsal pelvic region, causes dark moist gangrenous lesions.

Abscesses of the fifth to seventh thoracic vertebrae causing periostitis and osteomyelitis with consequent pressure on the spinal cord leading to paresis or paralysis can also be caused by *S. aureus*.

## Erysipelas

*Erysipelas* is an acute febrile disease, caused by *Erysipelothrix insidiosa*. Although turkeys over 13 weeks of age are most susceptible, it can also occur in ducks, geese, quail and chickens and has caused high mortality in pheasants. The organism is of public health significance because it can cause a skin rash and cellulitis (erysipeloid) and, possibly, endocarditis and encephalitis in humans who sustain a cut while handling diseased carcases.

On post-mortem examination there may be dark crusty skin lesions over any part of the body, especially the head in turkeys. The snood of male turkeys may be swollen and purple in colour. Dark, congested areas are sometimes seen in foot webs of ducks. Lesions are of a generalised bacteraemia and congestion, with small haemorrhages frequently in the skin, muscles, pericardial fat, epicardium, gizzard serosa, mesentery, abdominal fat, liver and under the pleura. An enlarged friable, mottled, congested liver, spleen and kidneys are frequently seen. There is usually a marked catarrhal enteritis. In chronic cases there may be heart lesions and in lame birds a fibro-purulent exudate in the joints.

**Judgement** Condemnation.

## Pasteurellosis

*Pasteurellosis* is a highly contagious disease of domestic fowl, turkeys, ducks and geese caused by organisms of the pasteurella group, mainly *P. multocida*, the cause of fowl or turkey cholera, *Yersinia pseudotuberculosis*, the cause of pseudotuberculosis or yersiniosis, and *Pasteurella (Moraxella) anatipestifer*, the cause of new duck disease, duck septicaemia or infectious serositis.

*Fowl cholera* occurs in several forms: peracute, acute, chronic and localised disease. In the peracute form there may be no premonitory signs and large numbers of birds in a flock are found dead but in good body condition. In the acute form, marked depression, anorexia, mucous discharges from the orifices, cyanosis and fetid diarrhoea are apparent. The *chronic* form can be a consequence of the acute form or infection with an organism of lower virulence. The clinical signs include depression, conjunctivitis, dyspnoea and, later in the infection, lameness, torticollis and swelling of the wattles (*wattle cholera*). Turkeys are more susceptible to cholera than chickens.

**Lesions** In the *peracute* and *acute* forms there is marked congestion of the carcase, multiple petechiation throughout the viscera and multiple pinpoint necrotic foci in the liver. Free yolk may be present in the body cavity. In the *less acute* disease, oedema of the lungs (especially in turkeys) pneumonia and perihepatitis are seen. The presence of lung lesions may help to distinguish, grossly, fowl cholera from erysipelas. *Chronic* lesions include caseous arthritis of the hock and foot joints, swelling with induration of one or both wattles (chickens) and caseous exudate in the middle ear.

### Pseudotuberculosis

*Pseudotuberculosis* is a highly infectious disease of domestic poultry and wild rodents caused by *Yersinia pseudotuberculosis*. It is widespread throughout the world. The disease is especially important in turkeys, in which the mortality rates may be very high. Water fowl are often infected. Overcrowding and debilitating factors predispose to the disease. Infection is probably spread via contaminated food, gaining entry through the intestinal mucosa or possibly through breaks in the skin.

**Lesions** In *acute* cases there is enlargement of the liver and spleen, while in the *chronic* form there are multiple caseous tubercle-like lesions of varying size in the liver, the spleen and sometimes the lungs. Severe enteritis may be observed.

**Judgement** Condemnation.

### Anatipestifer infection

Signs are seen in duckling between 2 and 6 (rarely 8) weeks of age. These appear three days after some stressful circumstance, such as husbandry malpractice or environmental stress, such as a move. The causal organism is *Pasteurella* (*Moraxella*) *anatipestifer,* which is probably transmitted via the egg.

**Lesions** Typical lesions of the *acute* disease are congested lungs, an enlarged pinkish liver and an enlarged spleen which is purple in colour. Externally the vent is stained pale green, the beak is often congested but the bird is usually in good bodily condition. In the *less acute* form, pericarditis and perihepatitis occur with an inspissated caseous deposit in the posterior aspects of the abdominal air sacs. The walls of other air sacs may be thickened. Later the air sacs are more extensively affected and there may be caseous salpingitis. Sinusitis is commonly seen. *P. anatipestifer* may also cause a thickening of the skin, especially around the ventral abdomen.

### Coliform infections

*Escherichia coli* (*E. coli*) is the most commonly isolated organism from condemned carcases. *E. coli* is a normal inhabitant of the digestive tract of poultry and large numbers are often found in the lower part of the small intestine and caeca. The serotypes most frequently causing colisepticaemia (01, 02, 08 and 078) are also likely to be found in the throat and upper trachea. These pathogenic *E. coli* probably invade the bird's body from the respiratory tract to produce the characteristic condition.

The best method of controlling colisepticaemia is to maintain the highest standards of flock management and obtain chicks only from disease-free well-managed breeding flocks and hatcheries. Pathogenic *E. coli* serotypes can be transmitted via the hatchery following faecal contamination of hatching eggs. Chicks should be the progeny of mycoplasma-free stock which have also been vaccinated against IBD, infectious bronchitis and any other disease that is a local threat. The production birds need to be vaccinated against infectious bronchitis and IBD and provided with a coccidiostat in the feed. The birds should be fed a well-balanced diet to avoid the consequences of mineral/vitamin deficiencies and malnutrition. Good litter management and properly ventilated houses are also vital control measures. The litter should be dry, but not dusty, and the air flow should be such that there are no pockets of stagnant air or build-up of ammonia fumes.

**Lesions** The main lesions found in colisepticaemia of broilers, turkeys and ducks are congested muscles, enlarged liver and spleen with pericarditis, perihepatitis and air sacculitis.

### Salmonellosis

There are two specific salmonella organisms which affect only poultry. *Salmonella pullorum* causes *bacillary white diarrhoea*, BWD or pullorum disease, in chicks under 3 weeks of age. The disease is now eradicated from developed countries and because of the age of the bird affected would not be seen in a poultry meat plant.

*Salmonella gallinarum* causes *fowl typhoid*, an acute, subacute or chronic infectious disease of poultry, ducks, turkeys (notably in the USA), pheasants, guinea fowl, pea fowl, grouse and quail. The disease differs from other avian *salmonella* infections in that clinical disease is usually seen in growers or adult birds, although chicks can be affected. In acute outbreaks the first sign will be an increase in mortality, accompanied by a drop in food consumption. Depression, with affected birds standing still with ruffled feathers and their eyes closed, is seen clinically. As with most poultry diseases, the signs of ill health are mainly non-specific. In the chronic phase there is progressive loss of condition and an intense anaemia develops which produces shrunken, pale combs and wattles.

**Lesions** Carcases of birds dying in the *acute* phase have a septicaemic, jaundiced appearance, with the subcutaneous blood vessels injected and prominent and the skeletal muscles congested and dark in colour. A consistent finding is a swollen friable liver that is dark red or almost black and the surface has a distinctive copper bronze sheen. The spleen may be enlarged and there is a catarrhal enteritis.

In *chronic* cases (those most likely to be seen on inspection), greyish areas of necrosis may be seen in the myocardium, pancreas and intestine.

**Judgement** Condemnation.

### *Incidence and control*

In the USA over 150 different salmonellas have been isolated from poultry. Evidence of disease in birds is most common in chicks, poultry or ducklings under 2 weeks of age. The main significance of salmonella infection is as a *zoonosis*. The Zoonoses Directive (92/117/EEC) contains provisions for Community-wide controls for salmonella in domestic fowl and the Poultry Breeding Flocks and Hatcheries Order 1993 reflects monitoring requirements of the Directive. MAFF have a Code of Practice for the Prevention and Control of Salmonella in Breeding Flocks and Hatcheries, supported by Processed Animal Protein Orders.

There was an increased incidence of *Salmonella enteritidis* phage type 4 around 1990 but this has now decreased, probably owing to increased surveillance, and subsequent control measures.

*Salmonella virchow* and *S. thompson* can be invasive in humans and therefore may be as important as *S. enteriditis* and *S. typhimurium*.

Salmonellas gain access to a flock mainly through feed, but infection may also arrive through contaminated stock, wild and feral animals, and personnel. There may also be a carry-over of infection from previous stock. Good biosecurity is essential including an all-in–all-out policy on farms, where all birds are of the same age and are all brought in at the same time and disposed of to allow for proper cleaning and disinfection between crops. Visitors should be discouraged and only essential staff should be allowed access. The perimeter of the farm should be identified, preferably fenced and gated securely, with parking facilities away from the buildings. Good management is dependent on a clean and tidy site. Rodent control is enhanced by the control of vegetation, including in and around ditches, with effective general management. Feed spillages should be avoided and any spills should be cleared up immediately.

Monitoring for salmonella should be carried out to help reduce dissemination and ensure decontamination. Environmental samples are better than faecal and the best sites are nest boxes, slave feed hoppers and fan outlet ducts. Other good sites on breeder farms are egg collection trays, walkways, egg sorting tables and mice. Spillage from egg trays is best in layer houses. Input sampling should include feed, residue from lorry and feed mill audit and chicks; the chick box liners should be put into an autoclave bag with peptone for transport to the laboratory. In the hatchery, trolleys and trays should be sampled as well as fluff samples.

Sampling of cleaned and disinfected houses is essential prior to restocking. Peptone water should be put in cracks on the wall half an hour before swabbing and large fist-sized swabs should be used rather than rectal swabs. The best sites for sampling are floor sweepings, nest box floors, slave hoppers, hydrated walls and fan duct outlets.

### *Culture for salmonella organisms*

Samples should be put into buffered peptone water for 18 hours or overnight for pre-enrichment and then into an enrichment broth such as Rappaport–Vassiliadis (RV), incubated at 42°C and subcultured at 24 and 48 hours on to a selective solid medium such as deoxycholate citrate agar (DCA), brilliant green agar or rambach.

The Poultry Breeding Flocks and Hatchery Scheme Order 1994 requires pooled meconium samples to be taken, 60 samples divided into either 5 groups of 12 samples or 2 groups of 30 samples and taken every 2 weeks for parent stock, a formal sample being taken every 2 months, and every week for grandparent stock, a formal sample being taken every month.

In the hatcheries, surface contamination is the main source of infection. Control can include egg washing, which if carried out must be done meticulously or else it worsens the situation, and fogging of eggs at arrival and in setters. All-in–all-out setters are best. There should be regular fogging and cleaning of floors. At egg transfer from setter to hatcher, manual exchange is better than suction head, although more time-consuming. When using suction head, disinfect the equipment between trays and soak overnight in a disinfectant solution. Continuous formaldehyde evaporation, ensuring correct dilution, during hatching is also helpful.

*Vaccination* against *Salmonella enteriditis* has been used with varying results. Other methods of control have included competitive exclusion (the Nurmi effect), where beneficial bacteria are given to young chicks at day-old to prevent colonisation of the gut with harmful bacteria, and the use of acids in the feed to kill the salmonella organisms.

## Arizonosis

Arizonosis is a disease of turkeys, caused by *Salmonella* var. *arizona*. Clinical signs are virtually confined to poults under 5 weeks of age. Affected birds are listless, tend to huddle, look dejected and have pasty faeces which stick to the vent feathers. There may also be various nervous signs. It is an important disease in North America, but is absent from the British Isles.

## Campylobacteriosis

Campylobacter is the most common cause of diarrhoea in humans in the United Kingdom although not as serious as salmonella food poisoning.

The bacteria (*C. coli*, *C. jejuni*), once swallowed, multiply in the gut and after 3–5 days (usually; range 1–10 days) the patient develops abdominal pains, diarrhoea and sometimes vomiting and fever. Although unpleasant, the illness is rarely fatal and patients usually recover within a few days. The definitive diagnosis is made by growing and identifying the bacteria in the laboratory.

The main sources for *Campylobacter* are raw meat, especially offal, and poultry, where the bacteria may be found in a large proportion of raw broiler chickens sold in shops and supermarkets. Although present in food, they do not usually multiply; therefore, it is rarely the cause of an explosive outbreak of infection. However, the number of bacteria required to cause illness is very small – fewer than 500 can cause infection. About 3000 people are admitted to hospital annually in Britain owing to the disease. Other cases are treated by medical practitioners but the actual figure for those affected in Britain each year may exceed 500 000.

The prevention of infection in humans involves inhibiting transmission through water, milk and food. All animals shed *campylobacters* into lakes, rivers, streams and reservoirs; therefore, all water destined for human consumption needs to be properly treated. In Britain, defective storage tanks have caused outbreaks affecting up to 250 people.

Milk that is not pasteurised or heat-treated may contain the bacteria.

Good kitchen hygiene with the correct handling of raw meat and animal products is essential to prevent infection. Raw poultry and other types of meat should be kept separate from other food and should be properly cooked.

### *Incidence of campylobacteriosis*

In the USA poultry is associated with 50–70% of human cases of campylobacter infection. *Campylobacter jejuni* is the most common isolate found in chickens. Broiler flocks are frequently campylobacter-positive and 100% of birds tested can be positive. Chicken carcases are also often heavily contaminated and numbers of campylobacters per carcase can exceed $10^6$.

In addition, independent investigations have isolated *Campylobacter jejuni* from aseptically-taken muscle samples. In epidemiological studies there has been no effect noticed on the rate of infection in poultry units with concrete floors and surrounds as against those with earthen floors.

Farm studies carried out in Sweden showed that 16% of flocks were colonised with *Campylobacter*. There was a seasonal variation with more positive flocks in late summer and autumn. There were differences in occurrence between farms delivering chickens to different processing companies. This might indicate different levels of farm hygiene and management. Generally only one serotype was found in each flock, which would indicate only one source at a time, instead of infections from several different reservoirs. The most common serotypes in chickens were also the most common serotypes isolated from the surroundings, e.g. ditch water and faeces of wild birds. In general no campylobacters, or new serotypes, were isolated in the following flocks, indicating that the infection was not permanent in the buildings, and that the washing and disinfection of houses between flocks was sufficient to eliminate campylobacters.

Chickens were not colonised with *Campylobacter* before 2 weeks of age. No connection was found between serotypes in broiler flocks and in broiler parents from which the eggs were taken. Broiler parents carried several serotypes in each flock. These epidemiological studies excluded buildings, feed, straw and day-old chicks as the source of *Campylobacter* infection to the broiler flock. It was thought unlikely that water would be a source for the Swedish chicken flocks.

### *Control of campylobacteriosis*

A strict and well-applied hygiene barrier seems to be the most important factor for preventing chicken flocks from *Camplylobacter* colonisation, under the assumption that the chicken house is a closed unit. It was considered that the elimination of disinfectant footbaths and the introduction of changing footwear at a well-defined hygiene barrier, 40 cm high, is essential for keeping *Campylobacter* out of the broiler farms. As *Camplylobacter* may enter from multiple sources outside the rearing units, it is important to prevent all possible ways of transmission into the house. In the UK, the main sources are the environment outside the houses, drinking water, rodents and wild birds. The organism has been found in flies, which could carry it from house to house, and people. Biosecurity of the premises is essential.

Chickens appear to become infected at around 3 weeks of age when the number of salmonella in a flock peak. However, the number of campylobacters continues to increase. When a flock becomes positive, the organism transmits to 90% of the birds in less than one week. After thinning of the flock, more *Campylobacter* are found in the older birds. There can also be a significant increase in the numbers after transport to the plant. The numbers of organisms found in the inside of the bird is relevant to that found on the outside.

In the poultry plant, raising the pH of the scald tank with caustic soda or reducing it with acetic acid has no significant effect. Carcase washes and irradiation have yet to prove successful.

## Tuberculosis

A chronic infectious disease of poultry, pheasants, pea fowl, guinea fowl, ducks and geese, but relatively uncommon in turkeys. Tuberculosis is caused by the acid-fast bacillus *Mycobacterium tuberculosis* var. *avium*.

At one time a common disease of poultry in Britain, tuberculosis is now rare in well-managed modern, poultry units with 'all-in–all-out' stock and disposal of laying stock at the end of the first or second laying year.

The condition is usually chronic and signs may be prolonged over a period of weeks or months before death.

*Post-mortem examination* shows characteristic lesions in the liver, spleen, intestines and at times bone marrow, muscles, ovaries and lungs. The lesions are typically tubercular granulomata. They are irregular, grey-white nodules varying in size from pinpoint to large masses of coalescing tubercular material. When cut through, the nodules are firm and caseous and the centres may be a pale yellow colour, particularly in the bone marrow.

## Chlamydiosis (psittacosis/ornithosis)

*Chlamydiosis* is sometimes referred to as *psittacosis* when it affects humans, mammals and birds of the parrot (psittacine) family and as *ornithosis* for birds other than psittacine. The cause is the intracellular parasite *Chlamydia psittaci*, which belongs to the Group B chlamydias – organisms of uncertain status occupying a position between bacteria and viruses, but probably more related to the former.

The disease is worldwide in distribution, affecting all types of poultry and wild birds. It has a serious public health significance in that man may become affected, usually from close contact with birds of the parrot family. Infection occurs by inhalation of particles of infected dust.

**Lesions** The disease may be either *acute* or *chronic*, which tends to complicate the non-specific post-mortem findings. The lesions range from air sacculitis with thickened inflamed air sacs containing yellowish-white exudate to pneumonia, pericarditis, perihepatitis and enlargement of the liver and spleen.

**Judgement** Affected carcases should be totally condemned. Diagnosis can be established only by laboratory examination, and cases should be reported to the regulatory authorities. Birds suspected at ante-mortem inspection of being affected with ornithosis must not be slaughtered because of the disease risk to operatives.

## FUNGAL DISEASES

### Aspergillosis

Aspergillosis is a fungal disease of the respiratory tract of most species of birds caused, in the main, by *Aspergillus fumigatus*. The disease can be egg-transmitted and mouldy litter, grain and feed, dust and unclean and improperly sanitised hatchery equipment have been associated with outbreaks of aspergillosis.

Young chicks are most susceptible in the first 1–2 days of life, but turkey poults can remain susceptible for several weeks. In *chronic* aspergillosis, which may be found on post-mortem examination of slaughter birds, there may be a large yellowish necrotic area in the lungs, air sacs and any other affected organ. Emaciation and widespread lesions justify total condemnation.

### Candidiasis (moniliasis, thrush)

The main cause is *Candida albicans*. The lesions are usually confined to the upper alimentary tract, especially the crop and mouth. Outbreaks have been reported in chickens, turkeys, pigeons, fowl and gamebirds. Long-term antibiotic therapy can lead to the disease, as can unclean environments, nutritional deficiencies and environmental stressors. It appears grossly as multifocal to confluent mats of white cheesy material, which often adhere to the epithelial lining.

## PARASITIC DISEASES

### Coccidiosis

This is an important disease of poultry affecting domestic fowl, turkeys, game birds and geese caused by protozoan parasites belonging to the genus *Eimeria*. Coccidia are host-specific, e.g. those of the turkey not affecting those of the domestic fowl or other birds. There are seven species in domestic fowl. *E. tenella* (the cause of caecal coccidiosis), *E. necatrix* and *E. brunetti* cause high mortality. Of the others, *E. acervulina* and *E. maxima* have medium pathogenicity and *E. mitis* and *E. praecox* have low pathogenicity, although they may cause unthriftiness.

Broiler chickens and turkeys, up to 8 weeks of age, when the turkeys assume an age immunity, are treated with a coccidiostat in the ration. In most cases there is a withdrawal period for these drugs which must be kept, even for birds which are thinned.

*E. tenella* affects birds around 4 weeks of age. There is sudden death and blood-filled caeca are found on post-mortem examination. *E. necatrix* causes both white and red focal lesions with ballooning of the mid-intestinal walls, and dysentery. *E. brunetti* causes haemorrhagic lesions in the lower intestine. Ecchymotic haemorrhages which are seen routinely in the serosal surface of the intestines of broilers are due almost entirely to coccidioses. Examination and scoring of these lesions can be carried out to help assess the effectiveness of the coccidiostat.

### Histomoniasis (blackhead)

Caused by the protozoan *Histomonas meleagridis*, histomoniasis primarily affects turkeys but may affect chickens and gamebirds. The most important natural route of transmission is within the egg of the caecal worm *Heterakis gallinae*. Parasites are ingested by worms in the caecal lumen. The earthworm may also act as a transport host for *Heterakis*.

The lesions of blackhead are chiefly confined to the liver and caeca. The liver is enlarged and shows numerous yellowish, circular, necrotic areas up to 2 cm in diameter with greyish lines radiating from the centres. These lesions are pathognomonic. Both caeca (the primary site of invasion) may be involved, though more usually only one. The wall is thickened and may show ulcerated areas and the exudate, at first serous or haemorrhagic, becomes caseated and may form a core.

### Hexamitiasis

The flagellated protozoon, *Hexamita meleagridis*, is responsible for this disease, a catarrhal enteritis, an important cause of mortality in turkeys, particularly in some parts of the United States.

In addition to the catarrhal inflammation of the intestine, its wall is thickened, especially in the small intestine. There is marked dehydration of the carcase with dark coloration of the musculature and loss of condition.

Hexamitiasis is unlikely to be encountered on poultry inspection but requires total condemnation.

### Leucocytozoonosis

Some seven species of the protozoon parasite *Leucocytozoon* have been recorded in domestic fowl, turkeys, ducks, geese and guinea fowl.

The disease is rare in the British Isles but serious outbreaks occur in countries where biting fleas of the genus *Simulium* (black flies) and biting midges (*Culicoides*) are found.

The disease may be acute, subacute or chronic in nature. Post-mortem changes vary from severe anaemia and enlargement of the liver to mild enteritis with greenish faeces.

**Judgement** Severely affected carcases warrant total condemnation, but mild cases in good condition may be passed.

### Helminth parasites

Internal parasites, if present in sufficient numbers, may cause emaciation. *Tapeworms* have little significance in today's intensive industry as they require intermediate hosts, such as the earthworm, which are normally not present in indoor systems. *Capillaria*, the smallest of the nematodes, are the most important. *Ascaridia galli*, the largest, will only occasionally be pathogenic in birds on poorly managed litter.

The most important nematode in geese is *Amidostomum anseris*, the gizzard worm, where it causes erosion. Severe disease may occur in goslings, with anorexia, emaciation, anaemia and death.

*Syngamus trachea* causes 'gapes' in gallinaceous birds and the related *Cyathostoma bronchialis* causes a similar condition in geese. The life cycle may be direct or more commonly indirect, involving the earthworm. As a result, soil can remain infected for years and the disease is most commonly seen in birds reared outdoors, such as geese.

### Ectoparasites

External parasites, such as lice, mites and fleas may cause irritation to handlers' hands and arms. Heavy infestations may cause loss of condition, but this reflects poor husbandry. In tropical and subtropical countries, ticks can cause loss of weight due to anaemia and irritation.

## MISCELLANEOUS CONDITIONS

### Dead on arrival

These birds must be condemned and not processed. It is important that the catching team recognise birds which are unfit for slaughter and euthanise them on the farm.

### Bruising and fractures

Causes include improper handling by the catching team, and at the poultry plant careless shackling and defective stunning techniques and wing flapping. Any parts of a carcase with localised bruising are rejected. Severe generalised bruising indicates total condemnation.

Carcase appearance defects include red wing tips, red pygostyles, red feather tracts, engorged wing veins, haemorrhagic wing veins and haemorrhage in shoulders. Haemorrhages may occur in the muscles of the leg and breast and broken bones include the furculum, coracoid and scapula. Unless severe, only local condemnation is required.

Fractures, without bruising, have been caused in the processing after bleeding and are due to defects in processing. It may require resetting of the machinery.

### Breast blisters and hock burn

These are caused when a part of the bird comes into contact with damp litter, which causes a lesion. The *breast blister*, which occurs more often in birds with leg weakness, may become infected and this will require more extensive trimming. The *hock burns* are unsightly and in some processing plants are mechanically removed. The presence of hock burns, in some companies, affects the quality assessment of the bird and therefore the price. Attention to litter management, ensuring adequate ventilation, the avoidance of water spilling from the drinkers and good healthy birds will prevent these conditions.

**Rupture of the gastrocnemius tendon** This occurs when the tendon is unable to support the bird's weight and may be followed by a greening around the area above the hock. Birds being grown to heavier than normal weights, for example, for the Christmas or Easter market, are particularly susceptible. Decreasing energy and protein levels in the earlier stages of growth help prevent this condition. At times infective organisms such as *staphylococci* and/or *viruses* may be responsible.

**Judgement** Condemnation of the affected part; should the bird be emaciated, whole carcases condemnation.

### Ascites

*Ascites* caused by right ventricular failure (RVF) has for many years resulted in significant mortality in broiler chicks raised at high altitude. There has been a dramatic increase in other areas which coincides with a continuing genetic and nutritional improvement in feed efficiency and rate of growth. This rapid growth requires high levels of oxygen which are not available, and combined with restricted space for blood flow through the capillaries of the lungs leads to ascites and death. Right ventricular hypertrophy is a response to the increased workload and this eventually leads to RVF if the volume or pressure load persists.

Most cases of ascites occur as sudden death on the farm, but should any be found on post-mortem examination the carcases should be condemned as the cause, other than pathophysiological, might be *mycotoxins* or polychlorinated biphenyl compounds containing *dioxin*. Liver damage may be the result of congestion of aflatoxin, coal tar products or plant toxins such as cortilaria or rape seed.

In broiler chickens in the USA and the UK, *cholangiohepatitis* (possibly caused by *Clostridium perfringens* or secondary to viral infection in the biliary system) is the most common cause of the liver damage which results in ascites. In both meat-type ducks and breeders, *amyloidosis of the liver* frequently causes ascites. Feed regimes which restrict the early growth of broilers have had a significant effect in decreasing the incidence of ascites.

### Slaughter liver or cholangiohepatitis

This is a condition of enlarged livers. Histologically there is a severe, chronic hepatitis in which bile duct proliferation is a striking feature. It affects all of the liver. This may be accompanied by other changes.

**Judgement** Depends on other lesions and condition of carcase.

### Fatty liver haemorrhagic syndrome (FLHS)

The liver is very enlarged, pale and friable owing to the large amount of fat. There is also increased abdominal fat deposition. It may be due to nutritional imbalances, high temperatures, reduced exercise and strain of bird. It is a disease, predominantly, of older laying birds.

### Vices

Vices in poultry may be considered to be undesirable behaviour, usually precipitated by some aspects of management or environment. Once started by individuals, a vice tends to be copied by other birds and the resulting injuries can often lead to death or downgrading of carcases.

#### *Cannibalism*

Outbreaks sometimes occur without any obvious cause. Predisposing environmental conditions include excessive light in pens and cages, boredom and vent pecking, insufficient feeding and drinking space, high-density stocking, and too much heat during brooding. Blood is found around the vent, through which much of the intestine has been removed by the cannibalising birds.

*Feather pecking or pulling*

This is sometimes precipitated by nutritional deficiencies, but may also be started by the bullying of a weak or sick bird. Overcrowding as broilers and turkeys reach slaughter age may be followed by an outbreak of feather and tail pecking, often leading to serious downgrading of the carcases of affected individuals.

### Contamination

Poultry carcases may be contaminated in various ways, e.g. faecal matter, paints, oils, poisons, biological residues, dirty scalding tank water. All such carcases must be condemned.

### Decomposition

Carcases of poultry that have died from causes other than slaughter must be condemned, as must carcases affected with general *spoilage*.

### Barking

This occurs when the cuticle (the outer layer of the epidermis) is damaged by too high a scald temperature and subsequent plucking. During air chilling there is unequal drying owing to the damage, and brown discoloration of the surface. This is only seen in fresh, non-frozen carcases. Dampening areas which are only slightly affected will remove the abnormal colour.

### Diseases of the female reproductive system

These are relatively common non-infectious disorders in end-of-lay domestic fowl but less so in turkeys, ducks and geese.

*Egg peritonitis* is caused when the ova (yolk) are present in the peritoneum rather than in the oviduct. The yolk is usually viscous and gives the appearance of an 'oily peritonitis'. *Impaction of the oviduct* occurs when a normal egg, or more commonly a mass of inspissated yolk material, obstructs the oviduct to varying degrees.

**Judgement** Condemnation.

### Neoplasms

Tumours other than those mentioned previously may be encountered in all parts of all species of poultry and represent an abnormal and uncontrolled growth of new tissue.

The neoplastic cells are derived from pre-existing body cells and may sometimes closely resemble normal cells, e.g. benign tumours; in other cases they differ greatly in shape, size or morphology, e.g. malignant tumours with the ability to invade tissues aggressively and to form metastases, secondary growths. Benign tumours are slow-growing, generally encapsulated by fibrous tissue and do not form metastases, although they can damage by pressure on surrounding structures, and may on occasions become malignant.

*Haemangioma* is a form of blood tumour occurring as round red-black lesions on the skin of poultry or internally, especially in the muscles, liver and kidneys. The lesions vary from pinhead to a hazelnut in size and large cysts on the skin or in the liver may rupture, causing severe haemorrhage.

If haemangiomas are few and small, a carcase in good condition may be passed: severe haemorrhage and/or emaciation require condemnation.

Many tumours are not evident until post-mortem examination, but conditions such as ascites, often associated with tumour formation, may be seen ante-mortem, e.g. *adenocarcinoma* appears as a firm, whitish or pink cauliflower-like growth. In other cases neoplasia may appear as multiple small nodules on the mesentery, intestines and kidneys.

The liver is frequently affected with single or multiple carcinomata present in the parenchyma or bile duct. The ovary sometimes contains a *fibroma* which appears as firm, whitish or pink nodules, usually small in size.

Malignant *carcinomas* are fairly common in old birds and appear as white nodules frequently in the liver, kidney, intestine or mesentery. *Squamous cell carcinoma* may occur on the skin. Other tumours which may be encountered on poultry inspection include *sarcoma, fibroma* and *lymphoblastoma*.

In cases of benign neoplasms, *judgement* depends on the type and extent of the tumour and the condition of the carcase. Cases with malignant tumours *must* be condemned.

### Oregon disease

A *deep pectoral myopathy* of turkeys and chickens, also called *green muscle disease*, this myopathy is an ischaemic necrosis which develops in the deep pectoral muscle (the fillet).

The condition is only seen at necropsy or at processing, when as many as 40% but usually less, of the spent breeding hens may be affected. It occurs less frequently in males.

The lesion may be unilateral or bilateral and in advanced cases may show a flattening of the normally convex breast muscle ('slab-sided'). The actual lesions are of variable size and are clearly demarcated from the surrounding healthy tissue. Initially there is a swollen, reddish-brown area, often associated with an excess of gelatinous fluid which later becomes green in colour, crumbly and dry. When cooked, the green colour, due to breakdown products of haemoglobin and myglobin, is accentuated.

Advanced lesions can be seen or detected by palpation. More recent ones can be detected by cutting into the muscle or inserting a light into the thoracic cavity after evisceration.

The lesion, although unsightly, is not harmful to the consumer and merits local condemnation only.

### Overscald

Carcases which present a cooked appearance of the flesh owing to an excessively high temperature or being held too long in the scalding tank must be condemned.

### Fevered carcases

Fevered carcases are generally considered to be carcases which have congested musculature but no other signs of septicaemia/toxaemia such as pericarditis, perihepatitis or air sacculitis.

**Judgement** Condemnation.

### Septicaemia

Septicaemic carcases are those which have congested, darkened muscles with some or all of the following: air sacculitis, perihepatitis, pericarditis and enlarged spleen. On bacteriological examination, *E. coli* is found most often but *Salmonella enteriditis* is sometimes isolated. The organisms present tend to be common to the whole flock.

### Insufficient bleeding

In cases where no bleeding has taken place the carcase is very red in colour. There are obvious welfare implications in this condition and it is essential that there is a well-trained, dedicated plant operative as a manual back-up to bleed any bird which may have missed the automatic neck-cutter.

### Emaciation

As in red meat inspection, emaciation is due to some pathological condition. It is important to distinguish emaciation from the poor condition of end-of-lay commercial egg layers, the meat of which is suitable for incorporation into soups, pies, etc., provided it passes meat inspection.

### Viscera absent

Carcases presented for examination with no viscera present should be condemned.

**Relevant EU Legislation** Directives 71/118, 91/495, 92/65, 92/116

**UK Legislation** The Poultry Meat, Farmed Game Bird Meat and Rabbit Meat (Hygiene & Inspection) Regulations 1995.

## REFERENCES

Clouser, C. S. *et al.* (1995) *Poultry Sci.* **74,** 723–731.
Slavik, M. F. *et al.* (1995) *J. Food Protection* **58**, 689–691.
Veerkamp, C. H. and Hofmans, G. J. P. (1973) *Poultry Int.* **12**, 16–18.
Yogaratnam, V. (1995) *Vet. Rec.* **137**, 215–217.

## FURTHER READING

Bremner, A. and Johnston, M. (eds) (1996) *Poultry Meat Hygiene and Inspection.* London: WB Saunders.
Farm Animal Welfare Council (1996) Report on the welfare of boiler chickens.
Farm Animal Welfare Council (1995) Report on the welfare of turkeys.
Jordan, F. T. W. and Pattison, M. (1996) *Poultry Diseases* 4th edn. London: WB Saunders.

# Chapter 12
# Exotic Meat Production

Over recent years there has always been a limited demand for more exotic type meats. Previously these would have included wild-caught rabbits and hares and wild deer. More recently, rabbits, deer and now ostriches are being farmed with the intention of producing consistent hygienic meat and meat products. This demand is sometimes more perceived than actual and the inability to produce a consistent product and constant market has been dominated by supply problems, lack of marketing coordination, cost and unfair competition with other, subsidised, meats.

Cooperatives are being formed which should help to overcome these deficiencies.

## RABBITS

Rabbits are usually reared in small units with a ratio of 1 buck to 10–20 does. The gestation period is 31 days. Stock used are New Zealand White, Californian, 'hybrids' or commercial white. The choice is based on market requirement, performance and personal preference. The does are mated at 16–20 weeks old. The bucks are used when 20–24 weeks old. The rabbits are weaned at 28–42 days old or by weight at 700 g. The average litter size is 8.68 born alive and 6.9 reared to market weight. Re-mating takes place, usually between 10 and 14 days after kindling. It is possible to obtain 6–8 litters per doe per year, giving over 50 rabbits reared per doe per year. Meat rabbits are marketed at 2–3 kg liveweight, which can be reached from 8 weeks onwards. The food conversion ratio is approximately 3:1, but this will increase if they are fed *ad libitum* after 8 weeks of age. They are fed an 18% protein ration and 15% fibre. Rabbits cannot digest starch easily and the diet contains dried grass, small amounts of caustic-treated straw and cereal by-products. Supplementing the diet with hay and straw aids digestion but may slow growth.

A coccidiostat is added to the diet to prevent coccidiosis. The most commonly used one, robenidine, is not effective against *Eimeria steidae*, the cause of hepatic coccidiosis. For treatment of this condition the *sulphonamides* are effective. Ionophores which are used as coccidiostats for poultry are toxic to rabbits. It is essential that there is not a build-up of faeces in cages or beneath them which will allow ingestion of oocysts. Withdrawal periods for coccidiostats as with other medicines must be observed.

Rabbits are more easily housed in poultry-type intensive houses as these give better control over environmental conditions than the natural environment house, in which ventilation and temperature has to be controlled manually, and with the use of micro environments.

Battery cages with wire mesh flooring suitable for rabbits can be used, but it is essential that only those rabbits which do not succumb to traumatic skin diseases such as sore hocks are kept for meat production. Plastic grilles are sometimes used for adult bucks and does. These are less traumatic for the paws and acceptable from a hygiene point of view. Broiler rabbits are housed separately from the does in small groups (4–8 per cage).

### Slaughter

It is estimated that around 500 000 commercial rabbits are slaughtered for meat consumption at three abattoirs in the UK. Commercial slaughter rabbits are usually transported in poultry-type crates, each holding about 12 rabbits. The rabbits are removed one by one from the crates by a single operative, wearing rubber gloves, and each is placed with its head between the arms of the stunner and gently pushed upwards to make contact with the current. *Stunning* is carried out electrically with a minimum stunning current of 140 mA, which can be achieved with an application of 100 V. Following a successful stun, epileptiform activity occurs and the animal will collapse. This is characterised by cessation of breathing, salivation and increased motor activity, tonic (rigid) and clonic (kicking) phase. It is also permissible to stun rabbits by a blow to the head. Following stunning, commercial rabbits are shackled immediately and exsanguination is carried out very quickly, within 10 seconds during the tonic phase, thereby preventing any risk of recovery.

The feet are removed and the carcase passes into the evisceration room where further dressing takes 5–6 minutes.

The *main cause of death* in commercial rabbits is mucoid enteropathy, a non-specific digestive upset. There is impaction of the colon and this condition is precipitated by stress, high-energy feeds and high population densities. *Escherichia coli* is the most common enteric pathogen. It causes diarrhoea in neonatal and weaned rabbits.

## Inspection

In the UK, rabbit plants slaughtering in excess of 10 000 rabbits a year have to be licensed. Inspection is similar to that used in poultry, with ante-mortem and post-mortem being carried out.

## Post-mortem judgements in rabbit meat inspection

### *Death before slaughter*

Rabbits which have died before slaughter should not be presented for processing but detained at ante-mortem inspection. If, inadvertently, they are not detained at the ante-mortem point they may be identified by the muscle, which is darker red than normal along with engorged vessels supplying the viscera, a more pronounced picture than with badly-bled carcases (see below).

**Judgement** Condemn.

### *Badly-bled carcases*

In carcases which are insufficiently bled the blood vessels appear injected, the flesh is dark and the organs including lymph nodes are congested.

**Judgement** Condemn.

### *Injuries including bruising and broken bones*

Injuries are quite common in the form of skin wounds, due to fighting or scratching, and sore hocks. Infection with staphylococci can follow with abscess formation. Bruising and fractures, especially of limbs and thoracic spine, may be sustained ante-mortem, when they are normally associated with haemorrhage.

**Judgement** This should be based on the extent and nature of the lesion and the practicability of carrying out trimming:

**(a)** Extensive injury or bruising, excessive blood or serum in the body tissues or multiple abscesses render the whole carcase unfit.
**(b)** When the bruising is localised, the carcase may be passed following removal by trimming of all affected parts. When trimming, the extension of blood between muscles, bones, etc. should be considered and care must be taken to ensure that all affected tissues are removed.
**(c)** Provided that the carcase is otherwise fit, superficial, discrete, uncomplicated bruises not exceeding 2 cm may be left untrimmed.
**(d)** In the case of fractures, the affected tissues should be trimmed from the carcase. The cut should normally be made at a joint which ensures that all the affected tissue is removed.

### *Enteritis*

Enteritis has many causes including *Bacillus piliformis*. The lesions vary greatly from a mild enteritis involving the whole gut to haemorrhagic enteritis with blood-stained contents. The gut contents may be either abundant and watery or sparse and mucoid, especially in the caecum.

**Judgement** Condemn.

### *Mastitis/metritis*

Mastitis is usually associated with staphylo-cocci or streptococci and metritis with *staphylococci*, *Pasteurella* or *Listeria monocytogenes*.

**Judgement** Judgement depends on the degree and extent of the lesions and condition of the carcase, but usually the carcase is unfit.

### *Tumours*

It is difficult to distinguish between benign and malignant tumours in the meat plant.

**Judgement** Multiple or malignant tumours – reject the carcase and offal. Single benign tumour – reject the tumour and the surrounding tissue.

*Pasteurellosis*

Pasteurellosis is a highly contagious disease of rabbits caused by *Pasteurella multocida*. Rhinitis, bronchopneumonia, middle-ear disease, genital infection and abscesses can occur and may result in septicaemia.

**Judgement** This depends on the degree and extent of the lesions as well as on the condition of the carcase. Animals with mild forms of rhinitis, in good bodily condition may be passed for food, while those with severe forms of pneumonia with fevered carcases and multiple abscesses must be condemned.

*Spirochaetosis*

This is caused by the spirochaete *Treponema cuniculi*. It is a local infection of vesicles, which become moist, scaly crusts on the genitalia.

**Judgement** In the well-nourished rabbit removal of the affected portions is all that is necessary before releasing the carcase for food.

*Tyzzer's disease*

Tyzzer's disease is an acute contagious disease associated with a haemorrhagic enteritis and necrosis of the terminal ileum, large intestine and caecum (typhlitis) caused by *Bacillus piliformis*. Focal necrotic areas may also be found in the liver and heart.

**Judgement** Animals which survive infection are usually in poor condition and normally merit total seizure.

*Myxomatosis*

Characteristic signs are conjunctivitis with a clear discharge which becomes purulent, swelling of the eyelids, base of ears, anus and nose, giving the head a very enlarged appearance. The oedematous ears often droop and condition is rapidly lost. The spleen is enlarged and blackish.

**Judgement** Condemn.

*Coccidiosis*

Coccidiosis is one of the most common diseases of rabbits.

Hepatic coccidiosis is recognised at post-mortem by the presence of numerous small greyish-white nodules or cysts in the liver substance which in older lesions may coalesce to form large cheesy masses. The nodules consist of hypertrophied bile ducts.

Intestinal coccidiosis may show few, if any, lesions at slaughter, especially in early cases. More advanced cases have a thickened and pale intestinal wall.

**Judgement** If condition is good, carcases may be passed for food, but emaciated carcases merit total condemnation.

*Taenia taeniaeformis*

The intermediate larva form of this cat tapeworm occurs as a whitish cyst in the rabbit liver.

**Judgement** Local trimming or condemnation of the affected organ is all that is normally required

*Multiceps serialis*

The cystic stage of *Taenia serialis* of the dog is commonly encountered in the rabbit. Cysts are found in the connective tissue of the lumbar muscles, muscles of the hind legs, and occasionally at the angle of the jaw.

**Judgement** If only one or two cysts are present in the musculature and the rabbit is well nourished, the affected portions may be removed and the carcase passed for food.

*Cysticercus pisiformis*

The cystic stage of *Taenia pisiformis* of the dog is encountered in the peritoneal cavity of the rabbit, especially on the mesentery, the cysts being up to the size of a pea and filled with a clear fluid.

**Judgement** Their presence rarely has any deleterious effect on the carcase. Straw-coloured fluid is present in the above cysts in the early stages, but this usually progresses to pus formation and cheesy inspissated material in older lesions, warranting total seizure.

### Zoonoses

*Salmonellosis*

Salmonellosis occurs occasionally usually due to *Salmonella typhimurium*. There may be virtually no changes to some enlargement of the liver and spleen with general carcase congestion. There is usually no diarrhoea.

**Judgement** Condemn.

*Tuberculosis*

Tuberculosis may affect rabbits due to mainly the avian and bovine types.

**Judgement** Condemn.

*Pseudotuberculosis*

Pseudotuberculosis is characterised by nodules resembling those of tuberculosis in the liver, lungs, spleen and intestines caused by *Pasteurella pseudotuberculosis*.

**Judgement** Condemn.

*Listeriosis*

Infection with *Listeria monocytogenes* may cause serious loss of condition. Some rabbits show torticollis. In addition to the emaciation, there is usually a hepatitis with the presence of numerous fine necrotic foci in the parenchyma.

**Judgement** Condemn.

*Ringworm*

The most common form of ringworm is *Trichophyton mentagrophytes* var. *granulare*, which can also affect man. Typical lesions appear on the head and may spread to other parts of the body.

**Judgement** Provided condition is satisfactory, carcases may be passed for human consumption.

### Guidelines on contamination, missing viscera, trimming

*Contamination*

Rabbit meat, carcases and/or offal affected with general contamination by faecal material, bile, grease, disinfectants, etc. should be considered unfit for human consumption. Where contamination of the carcase is localised, affected parts should be trimmed.

*Missing viscera*

Carcases presented with no viscera should not be passed as fit for human consumption.

*Trimming*

Trimming must be carried out under the supervision of the inspectorate. The selection of lesions or parts which require trimming must not be delegated to the management of the slaughterhouse.

Minor blemishes or bruising may be trimmed at the inspection point.

Trimming of more serious conditions involving infection, for example, septic wounds or moderate contamination by intestinal contents, is usually impractical with high line speeds, and in these cases an adjacent trimming area should be provided.

Trimming of carcases may be delayed until after chilling, provided that:

**(a)** the carcases are segregated and remain identifiable;

**(b)** there is no risk of contamination of other carcases;

**(c)** trimming is done under the constant supervision of an inspector.

Most trimming should be carried out by staff supplied by management. The mode of trimming may be adapted to suit the requirements of management, providing that all affected parts are removed. Care should be taken to ensure there is no unnecessary wastage.

## FARMED DEER

In New Zealand where one in eight farms now produce deer (there are more farmed deer than cattle), velvet antler is harvested and is worth more than the carcase. This is illegal in the UK.

Deer are suited to a variety of management systems, and stratification of the industry is becoming apparent. Many hill farmers sell, in October and November, calves weaned in September, to be finished in lowland units. There is much interest in vertical integration, with many farmers rearing deer, slaughtering them and selling venison on the same premises. Some 60% of farmed venison is sold through farm shops after killing in the field with a rifle.

Value-added products such as roasts with a fat covering, cubed venison for stews, venison burgers, mince, haggis and sausages are being produced.

### *Handling and slaughter*

Deer can be shot with a large rifle at very close range as they stand, unsuspecting, in a field; this has a strong welfare appeal. This should be undertaken, preferably by the regular stockmen, when deer are quiet, as will occur at a selected regular feeding site when they are being hand-fed. Under such circumstances it may be possible to shoot 10 or more deer from a large group before the remainder become unduly disturbed. Alternatively, they can be killed in an ordinary abattoir after transport and this appears to work well with red deer. A third slaughter option is on-farm abattoir.

Successful handling of deer depends upon understanding their behaviour. The dominance hierarchy is very important to deer and handlers must maintain their respect in order to avoid being the object of aggressive behaviour. It is important to be calm, confident and competent. Aggression can take the form of foreleg and hindleg kicks, and male handlers are advised to wear a cricket box or similar protection. Shields may be helpful. Stags in rut should be treated with extreme caution. Regular contact with handlers raises the fear threshold of deer and shortens their flight distance.

Red deer should be deantlered (not while in velvet) about 5 weeks prior to slaughter.

Deer in velvet should not be subjected to abattoir slaughter. Dis-budding of calves destined for slaughter rather than breeding can be carried out.

Deer must be presented for slaughter in a clean condition and therefore access to wallows should be stopped, to reduce mud contamination of the ventral abdomen. By minimising stress, the keeping quality of the carcase is further safeguarded. As in other animals, stress causes glycogen depletion in the muscles. On death, glycogen is converted into lactic acid, creating an acidic environment. Low pH does not favour bacterial growth. An average pH of 5.6, at 24 hours post-mortem, has been recorded for red deer calves and yearlings.

During shedding-out deer must be subjected to minimum stress to ensure no bruising or other injury occurs. They should be kept in familiar groups and should not be in close confinement overnight since fighting can occur when they are left undisturbed, resulting possibly in death.

Suitable facilities are essential for loading when deer are to be transported. Transport trailers should have side-hinged solid gates to prevent the deer from jumping out. Internal partitions should be as high as possible. Some transporters cover eye-level air vents to avoid the deer being frightened by seeing vehicle lights flashing by. Deer should not be left in vehicles overnight. Hinds in late pregnancy, calves under 6 months and stags in rut should not be sent for slaughter. Bedding should be provided.

Deer are unsettled by translocation into an alien environment. On arrival at the slaughterhouse they should not be driven off the vehicle, but allowed to come out quietly by themselves. As they move readily from dark to light, the lairage should be lit, but not to such an extent that the deer are faced with a direct light source. There should be separate facilities for bullied, ill or injured animals which allows them to still see other deer. Those that are in pain or distress must immediately be humanely slaughtered. Sticks and goads should not be used. Partitions in the lairage should be solid and at least 2.5 metres high; long dark passageways should be avoided.

Strange noises, shapes and lights can push deer over the fear threshold. Yorkshire boarding, which throws a broken pattern of light, should be avoided. Deer should be kept in familiar groups in the lairage and allowed time to settle in subdued light. Animals should be brought out individually into the stunning crate for immediate stunning. They should be slaughtered within 3 hours of arriving at the plant. Recent experimental work suggests that where it is advantageous for constant plant throughput, this period may be extended without adversely effecting animal welfare or meat quality.

The *stunning crate* should admit single animals and have solid sides, with a string mesh cover to prevent them jumping out. The top may be draped, but the front shoulder should be left uncovered with a diffused light source to attract the deer forward. A drop-floor restrainer is an alternative to the stunning crate.

Prior to stunning, deer should not be held in the approach passages. One deer at a time must be placed in the stunning crate, and only when the way is clear for it to be stunned, and then bled immediately. Stunning equipment must be properly maintained and reserve equipment readily available. Deer are stunned by frontal head shot with a captive bolt pistol. Pithing is not necessary. The slaughter of a batch must be arranged such that the slaughter of the last deer is not delayed. After hoisting by a hind leg, deer are bled in the same way as cattle. Both forelegs are held to minimise the risk to the slaughterman. Carcases are usually skinned on a modified static sheep crutch. Hide-pullers have been tried and a down-puller for deer is commercially available. As with game venison production, because of their propensity for shedding hair, contamination with hair is a problem. Flood-washing is used to remove hair debris.

*Meat inspection* has followed existing protocols. The possible presence of tuberculosis has to be kept in mind. Blood splashing on the diaphragm and abdominal wall is sometimes seen, but the aetiology is obscure. Bruising provides a good indicator of the adequacy of the handling of the deer and a study of the age and site of lesions can result in the detection of the cause. Focal bruising can be caused by deer placing the forelegs on the backs of other deer or by butting with an antler stump.

Health monitoring can be carried out at the abattoir by the recording and feedback of pathological findings and the taking of liver samples for deficiency estimations.

There is considerable variability in the size of young red deer stags, which may range from 46 kg to 146 kg liveweight and typically kill out at 55%. The carcases must be hung in a chill room so that air can circulate freely between them, drying the surface and cooling the carcase. If chilling is too rapid, cold-shortening of the muscles will occur and produce tough meat. Electrical stimulation of carcases immediately after slaughter hastens rigor mortis and assists in the production of tender meat.

The *field slaughter* of farmed deer is usually practised on farms which operate a farm shop retail outlet. Ante-mortem inspection by a veterinarian must be carried out within a 72-hour period prior to slaughter. After shooting, the deer are bled and transported to an approved dressing facility on the farm. Alternatively, the bled whole carcase can be transported to a licensed abattoir or a farmed game processing facility to arrive and be dressed within 1 hour of slaughter, or if the transporter can be refrigerated to between 0°C and 4°C dressing can take place up to 3 hours after slaughter. In both situations the carcases must be inspected by a meat inspector within 24 hours after slaughter.

## PARK DEER

Wild mammals living within an enclosed territory under conditions of freedom similar to those enjoyed by wild game (i.e. deer parks) are not considered to be farmed game.

Most deer park owners operate a culling system in which the deer are shot as they graze. After shooting, the carcase is immediately bled and eviscerated and transported to the deer larder for completion of dressing. Small numbers of deer handled in this way can be sold direct to the consumer but are subject to public health checks provided in national rules.

Where a deer park culls large numbers of deer or where the carcases are sold to wholesale establishments, the construction and hygiene requirements and the timing of the operation are detailed in the Wild Game Directive 92/45/EEC. In general, after shooting and bleeding the carcase is eviscerated, and the viscera identified with the carcase. It has to be despatched within 12 hours to a processing house. Alternatively, the carcase and viscera can be despatched within 12 hours to a collecting centre where they will be chilled and maintained at a temperature not exceeding 7°C until dispatched to a processing house within a further 12 hours, with certain exemptions for remote areas. All parts must be inspected within 18 hours of entering the processing house. Wild game meat declared fit for human comsumption must bear a health mark.

## WILD DEER

Game venison is seasonal, 50% of the red deer output occurring over a 4-week period.

Venison is low in cholesterol; the fat is not marbled through the muscle fibres although it still has a distinctive flavour.

### Killing

In England and Wales the legal firearm for culling deer is a rifle with a calibre of at least

0.240 inches and a muzzle energy of at least 1700 foot-pounds, firing a soft-nosed or hollow-nosed bullet. Deer are shot either in the neck or chest. A chest shot should ensure rapid unconsciousness due to blood loss. When aiming at the neck, novice stalkers are often advised to err on the high side in order to ensure that the shot does not strike the foreleg. If the vertebral column is hit the animal will immediately collapse.

Sticking should take place as soon as possible.

Deer may be shot two or three miles from the larder and carcases routinely 'gralloched', i.e. have the green offal removed, on the hill. Professional stalkers, as game processors, are aware of public health aspects and grade carcases according to presentation. After gralloching, carcases are dragged to the nearest track and loaded on to transport. Nowadays the Argocat has replaced the traditional deer pony.

On arrival at the larder, the pelvis and sternum are split, the pluck is removed, including the kidneys, and the body cavities are rinsed with clean water and dried with disposable paper towels. The pluck is bagged and tagged and hung with the carcase, which is also tagged for identification. The skin is left on. Red deer like to wallow and so splitting the pelvis, which is done to aid cooling of the haunches, is now discouraged as this can often lead to unacceptable contamination with mud and hair.

The temperature of the venison should be 7°C. Portable air conditioners are now used in many larders.

The carcase should be delivered with its pluck to the game plant within 24 hours of shooting.

After skinning, which is normally performed on a cradle, the carcase is examined by a veterinarian.

Disease is frequently less of a problem than contamination. Contamination with gut contents results from poor shooting and poor gralloching, particularly if the rectum has been imperfectly removed. In the case of poorly-shot animals, large quantities of rumenal contents may be carried in the wake of the bullet under the scapula, leading to forequarter condemnation. Deer shed hair very easily and contamination with hair is another serious problem. Hair debris is best removed with use of copious water. The professional stalker is the key person in the production of clean game venison.

The heart, liver and mediastinal lymph nodes are incised and kidneys and lungs are palpated. Any abscesses are treated as suspect *tuberculosis*, although only 0.1% of carcases have been found to be affected, predominately with the avian strain. Typically lesions range from small, chalky, white foci in the liver or lungs to miliary abscesses, throughout the carcase. TB in deer was made a notifiable disease in Great Britain in May 1989.

Occasionally *tumours, milk spots* and *flukes* are seen in the liver. Fluke infection is rarely serious, not normally producing the same degree of pathology as in cattle and sheep. In the rut, stag livers are often very pale. Cardiac lesions are rare. Pneumonia is also rare, although roe deer are very susceptible to the lungworm *Protostrongylus rufescens. Cysticercus tenuicollis* is another common parasite and *Taenia hydatigena* is occasionally seen.

A major cause of death in wild deer, particularly in February, is the *warble fly, Hypoderma diana*. Young animals may have very heavy warble fly burdens, resulting in extensive meat losses.

*Keds, lice* and *ticks* are common. Ticks may transmit the spirochaete *Borrelia burgdorferi*, which could pose a zoonotic hazard to stalkers and slaughtermen from Lyme disease. *Streptothrix* infections from bone cuts are another hazard, causing 'slaughter finger'.

In a survey carried out by Arun District Council/Forest Commission in 1986/88, 2.13% of 1967 culled deer were totally condemned, in deer larders and 1.77% partially condemned. The main causes were emaciation (10) and tumours (7).

## OSTRICHES

The domestication of ostriches for the purpose of farming for the production of feathers began near Grahamstown, South Africa in 1867. Since that time a greater value has been placed on ostrich skin, which produces a top-quality leather, and a market has been developed, particularly within Europe, for ostrich meat. Although classified as 'Poultry', the ostrich produces a red meat, beef-like in texture, containing lower levels of fat, calories and cholesterol than other red or white meat-producing species, which is particularly attractive to the 'health-conscious consumer'.

*Ostrich production* throughout the world is expanding rapidly. The ostrich (*Struthio camelus*) is the world's largest living bird, belonging to the order Ratitae or running birds. Emus, from Australia and rhea (from S. America) are also ratites. The ostrich is the only living bird with two toes.

The mature ostrich averages 2–3 m in height (to the top of its head). It can weigh up to 150 kg. The ostrich can kick forwards, but not backwards or sideways. The large extended toe has a long nail and can quite easily split a person open from head to foot. No one should underestimate the danger of the captive ostrich, particularly in the breeding season. Ostriches, particularly males, will attack with the minimum of provocation, in fact with no encouragement at all. Placing a hood over the bird's eyes helps to calm it. The ostrich has exceptionally good eyesight and when alarmed stands upright with its long neck extended. Ostriches have a life span of 30 to 70 years.

There are different production systems. Ostriches may be left in colonies, with 8 males and 12 females in 10 acres, or in trios of two females and one male, or in pairs. In Great Britain ostrich farming has to be licensed under the Dangerous Wild Animals Act, implemented by the local authority.

The production of *eggs* by the female is very variable. They seasonally produce from 0–160 eggs, with an average of around 40 per laying hen. The first 3 months is the most critical period in the ostrich's life.

The *mortality* up to 6 months is around 25% and between 6 and 14 months around 5%. Chicks may be fed rations containing 12.5 MJ/kg and 23% protein, although many are fed an 18% protein ration. They must be allowed plenty of exercise and not allowed to grow too quickly in the early stages, in order to prevent leg problems. Older birds are fed a 14.0% protein ration with 9.2 MJ/kg. Different age groups are fed different rations. The feed conversion rate will vary according to the source of the dietary supply, and varies from 2:1 from hatchery to 4 months to 10:1 from 10 to 14 months, when African Black Ostriches will weigh approximately 95 kg liveweight.

In South Africa a high proportion (70%) of the value of the bird is in the skin. Any damage, e.g. kick mark scars, bruising or fresh wounds, results in downgrading by the tannery and therefore the welfare of the ostrich is of prime importance to the abattoir staff. Birds arriving at the abattoir with fresh wounds are generally returned to the farm to heal. Ostriches should always be moved in a calm and unhurried manner. They should not be separated from each other, as this is known to be stressful. Birds may be led by an operative moving ahead of the birds, calling encouragement, occasionally reinforced by the use of the arm and hand to mimic an ostrich. A further operative follows behind the group being moved.

In the UK it is likely that, in the immediate future, slaughter will take place mainly on the farm of origin.

If ostriches are transported to a meat plant, unloading facilities must be suitable for their purpose and have non-slip flooring and the minimum possible incline. Horizontal surfaces should be provided with solid sides or barriers to a height of 2.0 m for unloading ostriches.

*Lairages or holding pens* should be provided without right-angled corners (e.g. octagonal pens constructed of metal tubes which are round in cross-section), be constructed so as to prevent birds slipping or falling, and without gaps in which birds might trap their legs, toes, head or wings and without steps or other obstructions which may cause them to jump and fall or cause other injury.

If larger numbers of birds are handled, they should be moved in small groups (up to 6 birds) through a pre-stun race. The race should be wide enough for one bird and have solid sides up to a height of 2.0 m and be designed so that head, neck or wings cannot become trapped.

## **Restraint** (Fig. 12.1)

Before stunning, animals must be restrained in an appropriate manner in order to ensure avoidable pain, suffering, agitation or injury. Restraint is required to ensure that stunning is carried out accurately and effectively, it does not mean that the bird must be immobilised before stunning. To assist in hoisting and shackling after stunning, birds may be loosely hobbled at this point, although their legs must not be tied in any way that may cause them to fall.

The birds should be brought up the raceway one at a time. When the bird goes through the door, one operative, wearing rubber gloves, holds the beak, or uses a crook to bring the head down into a position easily accessible to the stunning equipment.

## Stunning

The electrodes should be designed and applied to ensure maximum contact area with the head and must be cleaned regularly to maintain optimum current flow. The use of saline sponges in the stunning tongs may increase contact area and current flow. The stunning tongs must span the brain, either laterally (on either side of the head and around the eyes) or vertically (to the top and bottom of the head). If the birds are hooded during stunning, allowance must be made for the possible effect of the hood directing current away from the brain, especially if the hood is wet. An application of 400 mA or greater, with 11 V for 2–6 seconds causes insensibility for 60 seconds. There will be a short phase of initial kicking after which the bird will fall; it will be rigid with its legs flexed beneath it and the neck may arch over the back before falling forward (the tonic phase). This is followed by kicking of varied intensity (the clonic phase). An effectively-stunned bird will not show any signs of rhythmic breathing. A return to rhythmic breathing in a stunned bird indicates that it may be recovering from the stun.

Existing knowledge of mechanical stunning of ostriches suggests that the tonic phase does not occur and stunning produces an extended period of up to 4 minutes of severe convulsions. Mechanical stunning should only be used for emergency slaughter when electrical stunning is not available.

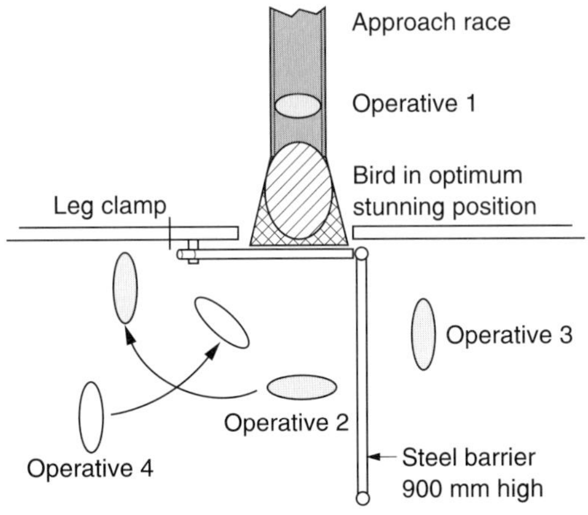


**Fig. 12.1** Stunning area and approach race. (By kind permission of Dr Steve Wotton)

At Grahamstown RSA, four operatives carry out the stunning procedure: one guides the bird into the stunning area, one holds the beak, one applies the electric current, and the fourth rocks the bird backwards with legs flexed into the body during the tonic phase, assisted by the first operative from behind. This enables the application of a leg clamp at the tarso-metatarsal bone, thus restraining the bird sufficiently to permit shackling. At this point the stunning tongs are removed and the fourth operative ring/chain shackles the bird via the big toes and attaches the shackle to a chain hoist.

Extended application of the stunning current, for up to 10 seconds, has been shown to delay the onset of kicking (clonic phase), facilitate restraint of legs and reduce the risk of injury during shackling and hoisting.

*Bleeding must be carried out without delay* after stunning and the cut must sever at least one of the carotid arteries or the vessels from which they arise. The ostrich, like other birds, has an asymmetric arrangement of blood vessels in the neck and bleeding should be achieved by a complete ventral cut of the neck immediately below the head to sever both carotid arteries and the jugular veins, or by thoracic sticking to sever the major blood vessels from which the carotid arteries arise. Although bleeding from a high neck cut is initially profuse, the total bleed-out time is prolonged and birds should be allowed to bleed for approximately 14 minutes in a bleeding area before manual plucking takes place.

## Dressing

The birds are then skinned, which should be done carefully to prevent dander contamination.

A longitudinal incision is made in the neck, the skin is reflected and the oesophagus is exposed and tied. The neck is kept for edible purposes and placed at the inspection point. Electronic identification devices must be removed from the carcase at the time of slaughter to prevent entry into the food chain.

The vent is freed from its attachments, tied and placed in a plastic bag. *Evisceration* is performed by a mid-abdominal incision above the breast plate. Ribs are cut on both sides of the breast plate. Thoracic viscera are exposed by pressing the breast plate down. The bagged vent is pulled into the abdominal cavity and the intestinal tract is removed, together with the liver and spleen. Intestines are placed in a separate tray for inspection and the liver and spleen are placed in the viscera inspection tray adjacent to the head and neck. The lungs may stay on the carcase or they may be eviscerated with the heart. They are then placed in the viscera inspection tray. Kidneys are visually inspected in the carcase and after removal. Different evisceration procedures may be carried out provided they are carried out hygienically and allow for proper inspection.

Ratites are susceptible to similar diseases as other poultry. The digestive tract is the most common site of infection by pathogenic bacteria. Necrotic enteritis caused by *Clostridium* spp. affects ostriches 2 weeks of age and over.

Ostriches should be observed at rest and in movement. This inspection procedure is similar to that for other animal species. A healthy bird is alert, has an erect neck and at times lowers and raises its head. It walks with a springy gait, and appears as if walking with its heels in the air. It is inquisitive, and pecks at its environment. It may be aggressive. The urine is thick, white and clear and the faeces are firm. The feathers are clean and well separated, and the body appears well rounded. The tail is fluffed up and erect.

The main reason for condemnation is *air sacculitis*.

### Changes after slaughter

The pH decline patterns of ostrich muscles are very rapid, with pH 5.85 in some muscles 1.5 hours after post-mortem. Shortly after this the pH rises so that in general the pH is not much below 6.0, which may be considered between normal and moderately DFD meat. It is not known whether this is due to pre-slaughter stress or an inherent ostrich muscle characteristic. The effect will be a shortened shelf life.

Since the subcutaneous fat layer is either absent or very thin when present, and is concentrated in specific areas only (mainly abdominal), cold shortening of muscles may be anticipated if carcases are chilled below 10°C while the muscles are still physiologically reactive. Electrical stimulation of the carcase normally provides a solution for this problem, allowing even hot deboning without inducing shortening.

## COMMERCIAL SQUAB PRODUCTION

Squab, a young pigeon just before it starts flying, is a speciality poultry product which can be raised on either large or small commercial scale. Squabs are very tasty because the meat is very tender, and lend themselves very well to barbecuing and other methods of cooking. About 2 million squabs are marketed each year in the USA.

Almost all squabbing pigeons are confined; 15–18 pairs can be kept in a 3 × 3.5 m pen. Production is labour intensive as it requires constant attention over the flock. Squabs can be marketed as early as 25 days after birth. A good breeding pair can produce 12 squabs for market each year.

## FURTHER READING

Adams, J. (1986) *The Slaughter and Inspection of Wild Deer*. Arun District Council.

Adams, J. and Dannatt (1989) *The Culling and Processing of Wild Deer*. Arun District Council.

Alexander, T. L. (1990) *Slaughter of Farmed Deer*. Veterinary Public Health Association (VPHA) Proceedings November 1990.

Alexander, T. and Buxton, D. (eds) (1994) *Management and Disease of Deer, 2nd Edn*. A Veterinary Society Publication.

Fletcher, T. J. (1990) *Deer Farming in Britain*. VPHA November 1990.

MAFF (1996) *Farmed Deer: Codes of Recommendation for the Welfare of Livestock*.

MAFF (1996) *Guidance Notes on the Slaughter of Ostriches: Welfare*.

Rafferty, G. C. (1990) *Wild Venison*. VPMA November 1990.

*The Commercial Meat Rabbit Producer's Handbook*. The British Commercial Rabbit Association.

Universities Federation for Animal Welfare (1988) *Management and Welfare of Farm Animals*. London: Baillière Tindall.

# Chapter 13
# Chemical Residues in Meat

A large number of drugs used to control or prevent infections or to promote growth are considered essential by some authorities in modern animal production systems. Additional chemicals may be added to food to ensure maximum utilisation and to delay deterioration. However, there is growing consumer resistance to the presence of unwanted *residues* in food.

The principal consumer concerns are drug resistance, toxicity and potential allergy. Drug resistance has been postulated as a problem both from the effect that trace residues may have in stimulating resistance in, or transferring resistance from non-pathogenic bacteria in the meat to, pathogenic bacteria within the consumer's digestive system. Drugs are intended to be toxic to various forms of parasite and as such may have inherent toxic, mutagenic, teratogenic or carcinogenic effects. Penicillin ranks highly among the known allergens and can invoke an allergic reaction in consumers eating food containing sufficient residual drug.

Residues can occur for a variety of reasons. *Clearance rates* for drugs can vary. Conditions that prolong the process can lead to tissue residues at slaughter. For example, even when drugs are used according to recognised doses and routes of administration and when pre-slaughter withholding times are observed, other parameters, e.g. disease conditions, age of animal and husbandry practices, can result in violative tissue residues. Drugs are also sometimes administered to food-producing animals at a dose rate in excess of the recommended level (Hoffsis and Walker, 1984), by unauthorised routes or at more frequent intervals than specified. These therapies can alter the *withholding time* required to ensure that all tissues are clear of residues (Mercer *et al.*, 1977). Veterinary surgeons can administer drugs, approved for use in one country but not in another, to deal with local disease problems. Successful responses to these treatments may lead to further use in areas where information on withholding times is not readily available. When drugs are used in the prevention or treatment of diseases for which they are not approved, appropriate guidelines may not be available. To reduce these problems, the USDA Extension Service has developed a computer databank, the Food Animal Residue Avoidance Databank (FARAD), to compile a single source of veterinary pharmaceuticals, pharmacokinetics and other properties of drugs or chemicals used in livestock (Sundof *et al.*, 1986).

The *pharmacokinetics* (movement of drugs in the body) of specific preparations has a major effect on persistence in the animal tissue and is dependent on several factors. Formulations can give slow or rapid release. Current trends favour the use of slow-release formulations, both to prolong therapeutically-active concentrations of therapeutic drugs in tissues and to minimise the stress involved in repeated handling of animals. The chemical composition of some drugs prevents rapid metabolism and, in some animals in which the metabolic processes are reduced as result of disease, persistence can occur. The route of administration, e.g. by injection, orally or other means, also affects the rate of excretion. An injection into poorly vascularised tissue can result in slower absorption than expected from studies on normal tissues. The recommended withholding time for the residue to fall into the acceptable range should be based on the tissue with the slowest decay rate.

The *therapeutic products* that cause concern fall into a number of categories. The major ones are *antimicrobials*, which are a diffuse group containing several classes of compounds used to treat or prevent bacterial infection. The *pesticides* are also a diffuse group including anthelmintics used for their activities against roundworms, tapeworms, and fluke, ectoparasiticides used to kill external parasites such as mange, sheep scab mites or lice, and antiprotozoals which are most commonly used for the control and treatment of coccidiosis and babesiosis. *Hormones* are used for therapeutic purposes in various fertility treatments or for growth promotion and are administered as injection or implant. One general category includes *tranquillisers* and *β-agonists*.

Animals are exposed to many environmental contaminants including *herbicides, heavy metals* and *fungicides*. Some of these substances find their way into animal tissues via the feed.

In the preservation and processing of food, *additives* are employed to prevent the onset of spoilage, to promote binding properties and to enhance flavour and nutritive value. These additives include antioxidants, emulsifiers, humectants, firming agents, sequestrants, colouring agents, stabilisers, sweeteners, tenderisers, etc. At both production and processing stages, residues or contaminants may enter the food chain from intentional or accidental exposure to these chemicals.

For all chemicals which may produce residues it is essential to establish an acceptable level in the diet. Calculation of this *acceptable daily intake* (ADI) depends on the toxicology of the compound. These toxicological effects are determined by acute and chronic studies involving genotoxicity, carcinogenicity, mutogenicity, teratogenicity, neurotoxicity, and effects on the immune and reproductive systems.

Detection of these unwanted residues presents a new challenge to meat hygienists. Traditional meat inspection examination ante-mortem and post-mortem described earlier, cannot guarantee the detection of residues since many of the drugs used parenterally are rapidly absorbed from the site and, in common with those that are given orally, do not produce changes or lesions which can be routinely observed. Therefore, to reassure consumers, traditional meat inspection procedures need to be complemented by an increasingly wide range of sophisticated laboratory analyses.

A *residue* is defined in EC Directive 96/23/EC as 'a residue of substances having a pharmacological action, of their metabolites and of other substances transmitted to animal products and which are likely to be harmful to human health'. Almost all chemicals administered knowingly or unknowingly to animals result in some trace residue remaining in the carcase. Increasingly, laboratory technology is able to detect these minute traces. It is therefore important to differentiate between safe and unsafe residual concentrations rather than to insist on zero residues.

## Legislative control of residues

The Fresh Meat Directive 64/433/EEC on the Conditions for the Production and Marketing of Fresh Meat requires that animals containing residues of substances with a pharmacological action should be excluded from trade. In the 1970s controls were introduced for animal feedingstuffs (79/373/EEC) and additives (70/524/EEC). Certain substances having a hormonal action (the stilbene group) and substances having a thyrostatic action were banned in 1981 (81/602/EEC). In the same year the approximation of laws of Member States (81/851/EEC) and the analytical, pharmaco-toxicological and clinical standards and protocols required for the testing of veterinary medicines were agreed (81/852/EEC). In 1985 the ban on the use of certain substances having a hormonal action was extended (85/649/EEC) and in 1996 (96/22/EEC) included the β-agonists in the prohibition. However, Directive 96/22/EEC allows for the therapeutic treatment of animals using a variety of these drugs provided that the treatment is administered by a veterinarian or under his direct responsibility. Treatment of animals with hormones to synchronise oestrus under the responsibility of a veterinarian and the treatment of young fish with androgens during the first 3 months of life to cause sex inversion are also permitted.

The *examination of animals and fresh meat for the presence of residues* was first described in Directive 86/469/EEC and has been updated and extended by Directive 96/23/EC, the 'residues directive'. The methods to be used to detect residues of substances having a hormonal or thyrostatic action were agreed. As a result, national plans for the examination of meat for residues have been approved by a series of Council decisions. In support of these sample collection and testing plans, the Commission has set up a series of conditions to be observed by national reference laboratories and lays down reference methods (89/153/EC, 89/610/EC, 90/515/EC). The work of the national reference laboratories will be supervised by community reference laboratories (89/187/EC). To ensure fair competition, meat imported into the community previously had to come from areas with equivalent testing programmes (90/153/EC). However, international trade obligations have made it necessary to consider the importation of meat and meat products from regions and countries such as the United States where the use of growth promoters is part of normal husbandry practice.

These directives have been enacted within Great Britain by the *The Animals and Animal Products (Examination for Residues and Maximum Residue Levels) Regulations 1997.* These Regulations came into force on 11 August 1977 and revoke all previous residue legislation. They implement Directive 96/22/EC concerning the prohibition on the use in food animal production of certain substances having a hormonal or thyrostatic action and of β-agonists, repealing Directives 81/602/EEC, 88/146/EEC and 88/299/EEC. The Regulations also implement Directive 96/23/EC on measures to monitor certain substances and residues thereof in live animals and animal products and repeal Directives 85/358/EEC and 86/469/EEC and Decisions 89/187/EEC and 91/664/EEC and provide for the enforcement and execution of the prohibition in Articles 5 and 14 of Council Regulation No. 2377/90.

The Regulations make the following stipulations:

**(a)** They prohibit the sale, possession or administration to animals of specified unauthorised substances (stilbenes, thyrostatic substances and β-agonists) except in the case of a β-agonist for a therapeutic purpose under the direct responsibility of a veterinary surgeon (regs 3, 4, 5, 6 and 7).

The same provision applies to allyl trenbolone under reg. 25.

**(b)** They prohibit the possession, slaughter or processing the meat of, animals intended for human consumption which contain, or which have been administered with, specified unauthorised substances (reg. 8).

**(c)** They prohibit the sale or supply for slaughter of animals if the appropriate withdrawal period has not expired and prohibit supply for slaughter or, subject to exceptions, the sale of animals or the sale of animal products which contain unauthorised substances or an excess of authorised substances (regs 9 and 10).

**(d)** They prohibit, subject to an exception, the disposal for human or animal consumption of slaughtered animals containing specified unauthorised substances (regs 11 and 12).

**(e)** They empower authorised officers to inspect and examine animals and to take samples and provide for the analysis of official samples (regs 13–22).

**(f)** They provide for offences and penalties and for enforcement (reg. 23).

**(g)** They provide specific defences (regs 24–29).

**(h)** They deny to processors a due diligence defence in specified circumstances (regs 30 and 31).

**(i)** They specify requirements relating to the keeping of records and provide for the suspension or revocation of manufacturers' licences (regs 32 and 33).

**(j)** They apply, with some modifications, provisions of the Food Safety Act 1990 including the defence of due diligence (reg. 34).

**(k)** They amend and revoke other legislation (regs 35, 36 and Schedule 2).

## The safe use of veterinary medicines

The following advice to farmers has been issued by the Veterinary Medicines Directorate of the UK Ministry of Agriculture, Fisheries and Food:

*Source of medicines*

- The supply of veterinary medicines is controlled by law.
- Buy medicines only from your veterinary surgeon, a registered distributor or a pharmacist.
- Medicines from unauthorised sources may not be safe or effective.
- Only purchase or use licensed products. Under the new regulations you are committing an offence if you use an unlicensed product unless it has been prescribed by your veterinary surgeon.

*Administration of medicines*

- Certain medicines may only be administered under the supervision of a veterinary surgeon or according to a veterinary surgeon's prescription.
- Read instructions for the current use and administration of the medicine and ensure that you understand the directions.
- If in doubt, ask your veterinary surgeon for advice on how to administer medicines.
- Check dosage levels.
- Check route and site for administration.
- Unless it has been prescribed by your veterinary surgeon, use a medicine only in the species of animal for which it is approved. Check the label or leaflet.
- Carry out the complete treatment programme.

*Withdrawal times*

- Check and observe the withdrawal period laid down for that particular medicine. Under the new Regulations you have a legal obligation to observe the withdrawal period. Check the label for details.
- Do not sell for slaughter, or slaughter, animals before the end of the withdrawal period. Under the new Regulations you will be committing an offence if you do.

*Record keeping*

- Record keeping should help to ensure that withdrawal periods for animal medicines are observed.
- You have a legal obligation to keep records of the administration of medicines, including in-feed medication.

REMEMBER

*Farmers who already follow sound management practices have nothing to fear from the new controls.*

## Acceptable daily intake (ADI)

The term *acceptable daily intake* was first used by the joint FAO/WHO Expert Committee on Food Additives (JECFA) in 1958. The most recent definition is 'an estimate of the amount of a food additive, expressed on a body weight basis, that can be ingested daily over a lifetime without appreciable health risk' (FAO/WHO, 1987).

Calculation of the ADI depends on the toxicological effects as determined by acute and chronic animal studies involving genotoxicity, carcinogenicity, mutagenicity, teratogenicity, neurotoxicity and effects on the immune and reproductive systems. These result in a defined maximum quantity which may be consumed daily by even the most sensitive group in the population without any untoward effects. For some groups, e.g. hormones, these studies aim to determine the concentration at which there is no observable effect (NOEL). When this concentration has been determined, it is customary to introduce an additional safety factor ranging from ×10 to ×1000 to ensure greater safety. Based on this figure a *maximum residue level* (MRL, see below) can be calculated so that no consumer, even on an extreme diet, is in danger of exceeding the safe daily intake. In residue analyses this is the standard of quality assurance which is sought. Therefore only analytical methods which are accurate at concentrations lower than the MRL are acceptable.

## Maximum residue levels (MRLs)

No chemical is safe under all conditions of use. It is therefore important that all are fully evaluated for safety, as the parent compound and/or as its metabolites, and that the results of these evaluations determine acceptability. Toxicological studies involve both acute toxic effects of the chemicals and more chronic effects including carcinogenesis and mutagenicity. Increasingly, studies of fertility and fetal development and the effect on the immune system have been added to these assessments of safety.

As international markets become increasingly harmonised, standardisation of acceptable residue levels is required. The *maximum residue level* (MRL) is a concept developed to estimate the maximum acceptable human intake over a lifetime. It is adjusted to accept dietary intakes which are at the extremes of expected consumption of tissues containing the highest residue concentrations. It is generally accepted that the MRL of an analyte of any foodstuff is determined by three factors:

1. A minimum dose which produces detectable effects in experimental animals or which, in a therapeutic preparation used in human medicine, produces a recognisable effect.

2 A safety factor in the range 10:1000 and which is lower (1:10) if a preparation is already acceptable in human medicine or higher (1:1000) if there is any evidence to indicate a special risk from experience with chemically similar compounds.
3 A series of factors to balance the proportions of the particular tissues in the average diet.

An MRL can give no more than a conservative indication of levels that are considered unlikely to pose any toxicological hazard to humans. It is *a figure set for acceptable or tolerable intakes believed, on the evidence available, to be safe for man but which may be modified upwards or downwards in the light of any new toxicological findings*. Since any *acceptable daily intake* is set at a conservative figure and increased by a safety factor, then exceeding the MRL occasionally may not be regarded as undesirable. Examples of *maximum residue levels* in meat reproduced from EC Commission Regulation 2377/90 (consolidated), are shown in Table 13.3.

In the case of *banned* substances there is no permitted limit. Detection of any residue confirms that an abuse has occurred and the product must be excluded from the food chain.

## Detection limit

Residues of drugs can be considered in two groups: *banned* substances, e.g. diethylstilboestrol or *permitted* substances, e.g. sulphonamides. In the case of *banned* substances there is no permitted limit. In practical terms the decision criterion becomes the limit of sensitivity of the analytical procedure. With *permitted* substances a risk assessment will be carried out prior to a making authorization being granted and the *acceptable daily intake* will have been identified. For these permitted substances the detection limit of an analytical procedure is regarded as being the lowest concentration of the analyte that can be distinguished with reasonable confidence from a sample blank containing zero concentration of the analyte. Despite the simplicity of this concept, some confusion arises from different interpretations of the 'reasonable confidence' required to distinguish between response of a sample containing some analyte and the response from a sample containing none. It has been recommended that the *detection limit of an analytical system* should be defined as the *concentration corresponding to a measurement level three standard deviations above the mean value obtained by testing a series of blank samples*. Primary tests are supported by confirmatory tests. These are normally based on mass spectrometry, which provides conclusive evidence of the presence of the drug or a unique metabolite based on information related to structure. Both types of test must be capable of detecting residues at concentrations which are not greater than half the maximum residue limit.

## Principles of sample collection for analyses

It is both economically and practically impossible to sample all carcases for all residues. Quality assurance is therefore based on sampling procedures. These are of two types: *structured surveys* initiated to provide quantitative information on the quantities of any drugs which are in the food chain and *targeted testing* designed to detect and penalise producers or processors who use drugs illegally.

### *Structured surveys*

Samples are normally collected on a national basis from randomly selected points in the distribution chain. There are a number of these ongoing schemes. The *UK National Surveillance Scheme* (NSS) fulfils the requirements of EC Directive 96/23/EC. Samples are collected at abattoirs according to throughput and on farms in proportion to stock numbers. To avoid subjective selection of animals for sampling, a programme that generates a list of random numbers is used. The Official Veterinary Officer in the meat plant is provided with a list of the samples that are required from his or her plant, and at a specific time samples are taken from the next slaughtered animal of the species and type specified. The number of samples required from a species or type is chosen to ensure detection of a problem that affects a specific proportion of the population. The relationship between the sample size, the frequency of residue occurrence and the probability of detection can be calculated from the binomial distribution (Table 13.1).

The sample size specified by the EC Directives is normally 300, which gives a 95%

**Table 13.1** Number of samples required to detect at least one violation with predefined probabilities (i.e. 90%, 95% and 99%) in a population having a known violation incidence rate.

| Violation incidence in the population (%) | Minimum number of samples required to detect a violation with a confidence level of: | | |
|---|---|---|---|
| | 90% | 95% | 99% |
| 35 | 6 | 7 | 11 |
| 30 | 7 | 9 | 13 |
| 25 | 9 | 11 | 17 |
| 20 | 11 | 14 | 21 |
| 15 | 15 | 19 | 29 |
| 10 | 22 | 29 | 44 |
| 5 | 45 | 59 | 90 |
| 1 | 230 | 299 | 459 |
| 0.5 | 460 | 598 | 919 |
| 0.1 | 2302 | 2995 | 4603 |

probability that a 1% violation rate would be detected. More intensive sampling, when a problem is suspected, involves sampling 700 animals, giving a 99% probability of detecting a 1% violation rate. The probability of failing to detect a residue in a large population is related to the number of samples taken and can be estimated for a range of abuse rates. Under the NSS, a positive result requires an increase in sampling intensity, but negative findings during a full year may reduce the sample size to 300. Details of these samplings are listed in the Annex to EC Directive 96/23/EC.

A number of other nationwide surveys were established in the UK to provide information on residues entering the food chain. These were targeted to detect residues of antimicrobials, hormones, heavy metals, pesticides, veterinary drugs and environmental contaminants in samples collected on a national basis and were reported annually. The *Retail Animal Products Survey* (RAPS) was introduced in 1989 to extend the range of surveillance and to provide a statistically valid sampling procedure for retail outlets. The scope of this survey was wider than that of the NSS and included manufactured food products which may incorporate tissues not sampled in other surveys. Samples were purchased from retail outlets in towns throughout the UK stratified in proportion to the population density. These purchases were made on a monthly basis and the results were assessed annually. The UK *Imported Meat Monitoring Programme* (IMMP), which also began in 1989, provided information on imported meat and meat products based on samples taken at the point of entry into the UK. The number collected at a specific entry point was in relation to the annual throughput. The tests are similar to those carried out under the NSS. Later, in conformity with EC Legislation, this programme was altered to the *Imported Meats Point of Destination Sampling* (IMPoDS) survey. The *British Meat Survey* (BMS) supplemented the NSS by testing meat samples collected in a similar way to the NSS for those drugs which were not included in the NSS. These individual programmes have been subsumed into a general programme of non-statutory surveillance work which is commissioned and reported by the Veterinary Medicines Directorate in the Medicines Act Veterinary Information Service (MAVIS).

The NSS includes a requirement for identification of all animals, carcases or products so that detailed investigations can take place on the farms of origin. As samples for the RAPS, BMS, and IMMP surveys are collected at small retail outlets, the identification attached to each sample may not permit these follow-up investigations. Together these surveys provide information on the total quantities of residues that are entering the food chain. When problems are identified, testing can be focused on specific areas and more intensive sampling can be undertaken to obtain evidence of the true level and to suggest methods of avoiding residues. This information is essential if the consumer and retailers are to be assured that meat produced under modern systems is free from all contaminants and safe to eat.

## Results of statutory surveillance programmes in Great Britain

In 1997 it was shown that more than 99% of samples tested under the Veterinary Medicines Directorate surveillance programmes were free of residues of veterinary medicines.

Under the random statutory surveillance programme, some 39.652 samples were tested with some 39.454 (99.5%) free of residues. Only 52 (0.13%) were above the Action Level ('positive') and 146 (0.37%) contained residues below the Action Level. There was no evidence of the use of the banned synthetic steroids or clenbuterol.

The Veterinary Medicines Directorate concluded that 'because of the considerable margins of safety which are applied when establishing MRLs for veterinary medicines at both EU and international levels, we are confident that the very low incidence of residues found do not pose a significant health risk to consumers'.

## Meat inspection

In addition to these national schemes, when *suspicious ante-mortem signs* or *post-mortem lesions* are observed during meat inspection, samples are also taken by meat inspection staff for laboratory tests. These signs vary with the drug which is suspected and are described later with each drug group.

In order that regulatory controls can be effective, it is necessary to have secure control and proof of continuity from *sample collection* to the issue of the test result. This is achieved by ensuring that the authorised officers who collect and despatch the samples from the plant record their activities on a form which will accompany the sample until the final report is issued. At all subsequent stages those who handle the samples must also record their activities on a similar form. This paper chain must allow trace-back of all individual samples, confirming the link between the animal sampled and the result reported, should regulatory action be required. Samples may be sent through normal transport or mail only if in a secure container. These are sealed by tamperproof labels or seals which are opened only within the laboratory.

## Sample handling

The pattern of distribution of a residue depends on the drug used, the time since administration and the species of animal. At the time of collection the specific drug involved may not be readily identified and the time from administration may be unclear. In addition, metabolism of a number of commonly used drugs continues in tissues for a period after death. It is, therefore, important to preserve the residue in the samples by carefully managing all stages from collection to analysis. For example, to provide the greatest flexibility in laboratory analyses in NSS testing, a complete set of samples should contain the following: 50 ml of whole blood, 250 g of rectal faeces, 50 g of liver, 50 g of kidney, 50 g of diaphragmatic muscle, 50 ml of bile and 50 ml of urine. Where the samples are being taken from suspect carcases which are detained after slaughter, these should, at least, contain a specimen from the suspect lesion, the kidney and the diaphragm. It is important that these three specimens are packed separately so that diffusion of the drug cannot occur. After collection, samples should be cooled rapidly, placed in an insulated container containing a frozen Freezella pack and despatched to the laboratory. When received in the laboratory, the samples are recorded and then placed in a 20°C freezer for storage prior to sub-sampling or testing.

These procedures reduce deterioration in the samples to a minimum. In other national surveys the selection of sample is predetermined by the product selected for the survey. In meat inspection it is also necessary to include a sample of the suspicious lesion(s) for testing.

# ANTIMICROBIALS

In mammals the most numerous and most frequently used drugs in this group are the *antibiotics*. An *antibiotic* is a chemical substance, produced wholly or partly by a microorganism (usually a fungus or a bacterium), which has the capacity to inhibit the growth of or to kill bacteria. These drugs can be used therapeutically in short courses of treatment to control disease in animals or, at lower concentrations but over a longer time, to promote growth. The latter use occurs most frequently in young calves, pigs and poultry. In the adult ruminant, alterations in the ruminal flora may reduce efficiency of digestion, growth and weight gain. When used therapeutically, antibiotics can reduce the symptoms of disease and may result in unhealthy animals being accepted at ante-mortem inspection.

*Antimicrobials* are a difficult group to detect chemically because they are diverse and show great variation in their chemical structure and molecular weights. They are also used in a wide range of formulations and are administered by many routes. A common characteristic is their antimicrobial activity and this has been used to develop test systems. However, not all antibiotic residues retain activity after metabolism in animal tissues and in a significant number of cases the drug continues to be metabolised by tissue enzymes during cold storage.

It is essential that the inspection team remain constantly vigilant for the *potential abuse of antibiotics* throughout the inspection procedure. At ante-mortem and post-mortem the presence of disease conditions such as pleuropneumonia or arthritis in pigs and sheep or chronic mastitis in cows, may suggest that an antibiotic has been administered recently. *Particular attention must be paid to suspect casualty animals, which should be sampled as a matter of routine.* Recent *injection sites* may appear as an area of discoloration or bruising, but frequently deep intramuscular injections can only be detected as a very slight swelling or lack of symmetry in the muscle. If there is any suspicion, the carcase must be retained until samples prove negative to laboratory investigation.

Commonly used *antimicrobial agents* include the penicillins, the aminoglycosides (dihydrostreptomycin, streptomycin and neomycin), tetracyclines (chlorotetracycline, oxytetracycline, tetracycline), tylosin, cephalosporins and sulphonamides. The use of chloramphenicol, furazolidone and dimetridazole in farm animals is now strictly controlled in some countries. Nystatin and griesofulvin are useful *fungicides* and a range of other agents, avoparcin, virginiamycin, polymixin B, bacitracin and some sulphonamides have been used as *additives* in feed. The latter result in growth promotion and are considered economically worthwhile when incorporated at non-therapeutic concentrations.

Public concern about the use of drugs in intensively reared livestock has led to a re-examination of this practice with the result that, in Denmark, Danske Slagterier has called for pig producers to stop including antibiotic growth promoters in the rations of pigs weighing more than 30 kg. Examples of maximum residue levels for antibiotics are shown in Table 13.2

In addition, *antibiotic residues* are considered undesirable for several other reasons. They produce *unsightly lesions* when administered by injection. The site of the injection is discoloured, and may be haemorrhagic if treatment was administered shortly before slaughter. In many of these cases the antibiotic is still present in an unmetabolised form. Long-standing injection sites, particularly those that incorporate an oily base, may be hard, fibrous nodules within a muscle. The tetracyclines, when given as long-

**Table 13.2** Antibiotic maximum residue levels for bovines.

| Compound | Target tissue | Concentration (μg/g) |
|---|---|---|
| Sulphonamides | Muscle, liver, kidney, fat | 100 |
| Benzylpenicillin | Muscle, liver, kidney, fat | 50 |
| | Milk | 4 |
| Ampicillin | Muscle, liver kidney, fat | 50 |
| | Milk | 4 |
| Apramycin | Muscle, fat | 1000 |
| | Liver | 10 000 |
| | Kidney | 20 000 |
| Cefquinone | Kidney | 200 |
| | Liver | 100 |
| | Muscle | 50 |
| | Fat | 50 |
| Cloxacillin | Muscle, liver, kidney, fat | 300 |
| | Milk | 30 |
| Erythromycin | Liver kidney, muscle, fat | 400 |
| | Milk | 40 |
| Florenicol | Muscle | 200 |
| | Kidney | 300 |
| | Liver | 3000 |
| Spiramycin | Liver, kidney, fat | 300 |
| | Muscle | 200 |
| | Milk | 200 |
| Streptomycin | Kidney | 1000 |
| | Muscle, fat, liver | 500 |
| | Milk | 200 |
| Tetracyclines | Kidney | 600 |
| | Liver | 300 |
| | Muscle | 100 |
| | Milk | 100 |
| Tilmicosin | Liver, kidney | 1000 |
| | Muscle, fat | 50 |
| Trimethoprim | Muscle, kidney, liver, fat, milk | 50 |
| Tylosin | Muscle, liver, kidney, fat | 100 |
| | milk | 50 |

acting preparations, may leave a yellowish stained area with a distinctive odour. Deep-seated injections can be particularly difficult to detect and require the experienced eye of the inspector detecting a slight lack of symmetry in the carcase. Since these lesions must result in trimming by the inspection staff, it is prudent to administer injectable antibiotics always in non-edible or low-value parts of the carcase.

During meat inspection all carcases with *injection sites* should be retained and judgements made according to case history, the time of treatment and laboratory results. Frequently there is no history of previous therapy, so the best evidence on which to base a judgement is the visual appearance of the lesion and the laboratory result.

Antibiotics may also *interfere with further food processing* if this depends on a fermentation reaction. They may cause *allergic reactions* in highly sensitised consumers. A small number of antimicrobials are suspected of having *carcinogenic* properties. There is also considerable concern regarding the *creation of resistant bacteria* in farm animals which may then pass to the consumer. Experimental studies have frequently demonstrated that sub-therapeutic feeding of antimicrobials to livestock and poultry increases the prevalence of R+ enteric organisms some of which may be pathogenic to consumers. An additional factor, seldom considered during these discussions, is the *additional cost of production* which results from the inclusion of unnecessary antibiotics in feed. Sub-therapeutic levels of antimicrobials in feed are most commonly used in poultry, pigs and young cattle, but, as early lamb production becomes more intensive, the potential for extension to sheep systems will also increase. Tissue residues that result from sub-therapeutic use can arise from a variety of sources including failure to observe withdrawal periods, *cross-contamination* between animals on the farm during transport or in the lairage and cross-contamination of feedingstuffs during the milling process.

Where antibiotics are incorporated in feed to control diseases, producers may be unwilling to withhold the drug for a sufficiently long period to ensure that all residues have been eliminated before slaughter. They may also be guilty of administering the drug at levels greatly exceeding the recommended levels and by routes other than those prescribed, thus altering the withdrawal times significantly. Some antimicrobials are excreted by treated animals in an active form and can be recycled by their pen mates. *Cross-contamination of feedingstuffs* during milling has been recognised as a factor in the frequency with which sulphadimidine isolations occur in pig meat.

*Incorporation in feed* poses particular problems for the meat inspection services for several reasons. First, there are no injection sites to be detected by visual observation. Second, the residue levels are likely to be low, probably close to or below the maximum residue level. The consumption of the parent compound and of the principal metabolites by ingestion of contaminated excreta may result in distributions in tissue which differ from those suggested by studies involving parent compound alone. These factors may require reassessments of current maximum residue levels with particular reference to target edible tissues.

Bacitracin zinc, Spiramycin, Tylosin and Virginiamycin were banned in 1998 as feed additives in Great Britain.

### Tests for antimicrobial agents

The most frequently used tests for antimicrobial agents are based on the detection of residual antimicrobial activity. The basic microbiological method is the *four-plate test* (FPT). This test has the advantage of requiring simple apparatus and limited training for analysts, and of having rapid turnaround and broad spectrum detection. It is an agar diffusion test. Meat samples are applied to four plates of agar medium, three of which are inoculated with *Bacillus subtilis* spores at pH 6, 7.2, and 8 or with *Micrococcus luteus* at pH 8 (Bogaerts and Wolf, 1980). Trimethoprim is incorporated into the pH 7.2 medium to enhance the sensitivity of the test for sulphonamide residues. Diffusion of the active antibiotic is detected by the formation of clear zones of inhibition on one or more plates after overnight incubation. The reliability and sensitivity of the tests are monitored by applying 6 mm diameter filter-paper discs containing standard quantities of known antibiotics in each run. The system lacks specificity and its reliability has been questioned. False positive results arise most frequently from the use of deep-frozen tissues, particularly kidneys. To avoid these problems, each tissue can be tested in duplicate, one piece being placed directly on the agar surface and the other being placed on a dialysis membrane placed on the surface. The membrane prevents the diffusion of inhibitory cell components into the medium.

Despite the incorporation of trimethoprim into the pH 7.2 medium to enhance the sensitivity of the test for sulphonamide residues, it remains relatively insensitive for these and it is now customary to examine for sulphonamides by alternative technologies such as *thin-layer chromatography* or *immunoassays*.

Since antibiotics such as dihydro-streptomycin, neomycin, kanamycin and gentamicin are excreted from kidneys at a lower rate than from muscle, correlations in kidney and meat levels can vary.

Other antibiotics, e.g. chloramphenicol and nitrofurans, are metabolised and remain in kidney and liver as inactive metabolites. For these, immunoassays and chemical methods have been developed.

The FPT is simple, inexpensive to perform and well-suited to routine laboratory work. In general the test is best suited to those antibiotics that are used for therapeutic purposes. The test is qualitative and does indicate the quantity of antibiotic that is present. Regular inter-laboratory testing is carried out as a quality control and there is acceptable agreement both between sensitivity and selectivity of the test.

Further evidence of the identity of the specific antibiotic can be obtained using *high-voltage electrophoresis* (HVE) *bioautography*. Two gels, agar and agarose, are prepared, a piece of meat is placed on each, and the antibiotic is allowed to diffuse into the medium. The high voltage is passed through the medium for a period of 2.5 hours. The plates are then overlaid with media containing sensitive species of bacteria similar to those in the FPT and incubation is carried out overnight. The antibiotics inhibit the growth of the bacteria over the areas in which they are concentrated. The distance and direction the antibiotic has travelled from the origin is used to further identify the growth-inhibitory substance into broad categories. Those antibiotics that are suitable for confirmatory testing can then be chemically identified. This intermediate step before proceeding to chemical analysis can significantly reduce costs of residue testing. Further confirmation and identification are obtained using *high-performance liquid chromatography* (HPLC) of extracts from the tissue.

In surveys designed to identify the frequency of use of antibiotics in the population, *kidney* is normally chosen as a target tissue. However, if a carcase is suspected of having antimicrobials present at post-mortem, samples are taken from any detected lesion, the kidney and diaphragm. These are tested by FPT, HVE and, when appropriate, HPLC. If all three samples are negative, then the site that has been detected is trimmed and the carcase may be passed into the food chain. If only the site is positive, or if the site and kidney only are positive, then the site is trimmed, the offal is discarded and the carcase may be passed into the food chain. If the diaphragm is positive, then the carcase is condemned. By this means, meat from carcases containing antimicrobial residues is prevented from entering the food chain.

The major problem presented to the laboratory service by meat inspection sampling is the rapid turnaround time required for judgements to be made on carcases. In view of the urgency with which test results are required, only the FPT and HVE techniques can provide information within the time-frame required. Current work on the development of alternative technologies may result in confirmatory tests, but these will be required to be equally rapid in performance.

## 1996 GB Statutory Survey results

Out of some 17 000 *sheep* kidney samples tested, *antimicrobials* were detected in six (4 penicillin G, 2 streptomycin), the animals involved probably being casualties.

One positive sample out of 2300 *cattle* samples was found, the antimicrobial residues of oxytetracycline occurring at the completely unacceptable concentration of 7620 μg/kg above the MRL of 600 μg/kg.

The situation in *pigs* was found to be more serious, 64 samples out of over 12 300 containing antimicrobials (chlortetracycline 44 being the most common). Out of 1107 tested, 18 (1.6%) pig kidney samples were found to contain a *sulphonamide*, the concentrations ranging from 120 μg/kg to 7170 μg/kg. A person eating a standard meal of 50 g of kidney at the latter high concentration would be exposed to 358 μg of sulphonamides which is well within the ADI for sulphonamide of 0–3000 μg per person and without any harmful effect.

## GROWTH PROMOTERS (HORMONES AND ANTIBACTERIALS)

- **Natural sex steroid hormones** – Oestradiol, progesterone, testosterone.
- **Synthetic steroid androgens** – Nandrolone, norethandrolone, nortestosterone, phenylpropionate, ethinyloestradiol, laurate.
- **Synthetic non-steroidal oestrogens** – Stilbene oestrogens (diethylstilboestrol (DES), hexoestrol), zeranol, trenbolone acetate.
- **Synthetic steroidal progestens** – Melengestrol acetate (MGA).
- **Peptide hormones** – Growth hormone (GH), growth hormone-releasing factor thryotrophin-releasing hormone (TRH).
- **β-Adrenoceptor agonists (beta-agonists)** – clenbuterol, cimateratol.
- **Antibacterials –** Zinc bacitracin, flavomycin, virginiamycin, ionophore antibotics (lasalocid Na, monensin Na, salinomycin), non-ionophore antibiotics (avoparcin, flavophospholipol), arsanilic acid, gut active growth promoters (enzymes and probiotics).

### Glossary

*Anabolic:* Able to build up tissues; the synthesis of complex molecules from simpler ones with the storage of chemical energy, as opposed to *catabolic*, which is the breaking down of complex molecules into simpler ones.

*Steroid* (lit. 'fatty'): *Steroids* are a group of natural hormones naturally produced by the 'steroid glands' (adrenal cortex, testis, ovary, placenta and corpus luteum) and include the glucocorticoids, mineralocorticoids, androgens, oestrogens and gestagens which have synthetic counterparts – *anabolic steroids* (ethyloestrenol, nandrolone, norethandrolone, etc.).

*Stilbene:* Synthetic non-steroidal oestrogen, e.g. diethylstilboestrol (DES), hexoestrol dienoestrol, currently banned in most countries as anabolic agents because of their carcinogenetic effect and the fact that they are not easily metabolised.

*Androgen:* A steroid hormone that promotes male characteristics.

*Gestagen:* A hormone that promotes progesterone activity, i.e. prepares the uterus for conception, prevents expulsion of the implanted ovum, protects the embryo, encourages placental growth and decreases the frequency of uterine contractions.

*Oestrogen:* A hormone that promotes female characteristics induces oestrus receptivity in the female, creates secondary sex characters.

### Use of hormones

*Hormones* have been used for a variety of therapeutic and growth-modifying purposes in animals. They are a particularly important group because of the reports from toxicological experiments claiming to show that there may be associations with neoplasia. The most commonly cited example is *diethylstilboestrol* (DES) therapy previously given to pregnant mothers with threatened miscarriages. A significant proportion of girls born after this therapy subsequently developed cervical adenocarcinomas. While this example demonstrates that a risk exists, the therapeutic concentrations were considerably higher than those that could arise through the consumption of meat from treated animals. Nevertheless, it is an unnecessary risk and best avoided. In 1981 an EC ban (EC Directive 81/602) was implemented in all member states. Although there have been a number of reported cases of violation, the ban has been effective. When the ban was first introduced, the producers had access to other growth-promoting hormone implants (trenbolone, zeranol and natural hormones) which gave better responses at slightly higher costs. The effectiveness of these implants continued the economic benefits that would have been expected from continued use of DES. The subsequent ban on all growth-promoting hormones (EC Directive 85/649) appeared to provoke more resistance from producers.

The safety of five compounds, *zeranol*, *trenbolone*, *oestradiol*, *progesterone* and *testosterone*, was considered by an EC Expert Committee. This committee reported (Lamming, 1984; Lamming *et al.*, 1987) that these five compounds were not harmful to consumers provided that the implants are used according to accepted husbandry practices, i.e. that they are applied in the correct site and the full withholding period is observed. Indeed, the committee concluded that the products were safe even with a zero-withholding period but did not consider the effect that implantation deep into a muscle mass might have in creating residues.

It was postulated that this subsequent ban would result in a return to the use of stilbenes. However, monitoring as required by EC Directive 86/469 has shown no evidence that this reversion has occurred. The illegal use of β-agonists began shortly after the ban on the use of all growth-promoting hormone implants and may have provided a satisfactory, albeit illegal, substitute.

### *Testing*

Tests for growth-promoting hormones are included in the NSS procedures of all EC Member States and, in addition, samples are taken from animals that are suspected of having been implanted when these are presented for slaughter. The range of tests required for all applications is large and the most appropriate is determined by circumstance. In the live animal, which is tested on-farm, blood or faeces are the most convenient samples to collect. Urine may also be collected but this is not normally used under national control schemes. At slaughter, blood, rectal faeces, liver, kidney and muscle can be obtained from all animals; bile is usually available but the quantity may vary. The urinary bladder is frequently empty and is occasionally damaged during evisceration. To provide the greatest flexibility for laboratory procedures, a complete set of samples is preferable. Samples should be cooled rapidly and despatched to the laboratory in an insulated container also containing a freezer pack. When received at the laboratory, the samples are maintained at 2°C prior to sub-sampling for testing.

*Screening tests* for residues of hormonal growth promoter are based on *immunoassays*. Initially, radioimmunoassays developed for the study of physiological variations in natural hormones were employed. More recently, many of these assays have been modified to *enzyme-linked immunoassays*. These tests are rapid, sensitive, selective and cost-effective. Examples of typical limits of quantification (LOQ) for these assays are shown in Table 13.3. The critical component of each assay is the antibody. These antibodies are prepared by linking the hormone to a larger protein molecule, thereby creating an immunogen which, when injected into laboratory animals, elicits an immune response. High-affinity antibodies can be produced which, when diluted, result in very sensitive and selective tests. The synthetic hormones may be confirmed by liquid chromatography – mass spectrometry or gas chromatography. The confirmatory tests are normally less sensitive than the screening tests.

*Antibodies* produced for screening tests can be used in affinity chromatography to concentrate material for the confirmatory test. Incorporation of these immunoaffinity techniques as part of the extraction procedures presents an opportunity to reduce the number of stages during extractions and to introduce an element of concentration of the analyte. These steps will make the confirmatory tests more sensitive. The development of monoclonal antibodies promises to provide antibodies both with uniform quality and in quantities which will be required for greater use.

Before residue tests were required for endogenous hormones, methods for *natural hormones* had already been developed to quantify concentrations within the normal range. The residue programme relies on these tests to quantify accurately the concentration that is present in the tissues. However, it was necessary to examine the extremes of the normal range before the value of testing for natural hormones could be established.

*Selection of carcases for testing* is part of normal ante-mortem inspection procedures. Paragraph 27(b) of Directive 64/433/EC requires that the veterinarian must be on the look out for 'any signs that the animals have had substances with pharmacological effects administered to them'. In this case, specific

**Table 13.3** Typical limits of quantification for recognised growth-promoting hormones.

| Compound | Matrix | Limit of detection μg/l |
|---|---|---|
| Diethylstilboestrol | Urine | 2.0 |
| Hexoestrol | Urine | 2.0 |
| Zeranol | Urine | 2.0 |
| Trenbolone | Bile | 2.0 |
| Oestradiol | Serum | 0.04 (male) |
| Progesterone | Serum | 0.05 (male) |
| Testosterone | Serum | 2.0 (female) |
| Nortestosterone | Urine | 2.0 |

*observation of the behaviour and conformation of each animal* is necessary, since the objective of hormone implants is to improve both efficiency of lean meat gain and the conformation of the carcase. It has been suggested that the behaviour of treated animals differs from that of normal beef cattle, e.g. frequent mounting, aggression and restlessness demonstrated by the animals continuing to mill around long after other animals have settled down to rest. It is therefore possible that animals may be selected at ante-mortem inspection. However, the value of these inspections will depend largely on the experience, dedication and skill of the observer. There has been no scientific study to evaluate the effectiveness of visual selection. Knowledge of local market conditions and production systems can also be valuable in targeting animals for specific detailed post-mortem investigation. This selection would apply to those growth promoters that are administered by implant or orally. The latter would not be detectable by gross post-mortem investigation.

*Post-mortem examinations* need to be extended to include specific examinations for the presence of *implants* and *lesions that may have been caused by implants*. These are normally placed between the concha of an ear or into the muscle at the base of an ear. The presence of an implant may be suspected if a small knot of granules or small plastic tube is palpated in that area. However, in several cases the small nodules have not contained any hormone residue and have been shown by histological examination to be fibrous tissue. Implantation with growth-promoting hormones does not take place under sterile conditions. Frequently *abscesses* form at a site of implantation. Any abscess in a subcutaneous site requires investigation for residues.

Preliminary investigation consists of the detailed dissection of the area to identify objects that resemble pellets. Allowance must be made for deterioration in size and alteration in the shape of individual pellets which occurs as the interval between implantation and slaughter lengthens. On dissection a presumptive diagnosis may be possible on the basis of number, colour and shape of pellet. However, these diagnoses must be substantiated by definitive laboratory tests. In view of the quantity of drug that remains at the site, these laboratory tests require less sophisticated extraction procedures because significant dilution is necessary prior to identification. Since the regulatory measures were introduced, a small number of producers have attempted to introduce the implants at *unusual* sites, e.g. brisket, legs, lateral to the spine, in the tail or directly into the muscles. Although individual cases have been encountered, the tendency for abscessation at implant sites continues and indicates those carcases that require special attention. At present, confirmation of natural hormone implants is possible only if the injection site is found.

When no implant is found, testing is concentrated on the tissue or fluid that is most likely to provide the optimum detection and/or confirmation rate. In the case of the synthetics or xenobiotics, the concentrations in urine, bile and faeces are higher and more stable than those in kidney, liver and muscle. Blood is usually an unreliable matrix for testing.

The natural hormones (progesterone, testosterone, oestradiol) are also present in normal animals, hence tests are aimed at detecting abnormally high concentrations for the sex or physiological status of the animal. There is a wide range of physiological values within normal animals and therefore confirmation is not possible unless an implant site is found.

A study of over 2000 injection sites collected over a period of 15 years in Belgium demonstrated the illegal use of a wide range of injectable compounds with hormonal action (Vanoosthuyze *et al.*, 1994). Over this period the natural hormones oestradiol and testosterone (mainly present as their esters) were used extensively. From 1990, closterol acetate was the most used exogenous hormone. While the use of nandrolone decreased, abuse of progesterone and certain androgens such as stanozolol and fluxymesterone increased.

## β-AGONISTS

The *β-agonists* have the activities of neurotransmitters and of hormones and as such have both physiological and metabolic activities. They act through binding to receptors on target cells. Those which are important in residue analysis have major metabolic effects by repartitioning energy from fat to lean meat production. They are detected in tissues by immunoassay procedures and confirmed by gas chromatography–mass spectrometry.

There are some 20 β-agonists which can be exploited in production of food animals. The most commonly identified by residue analysis include *clenbuterol, mabuterol, cimaterol, ractopamine* and *salbutamol*. The first of these has been licensed for the treatment of respiratory disease and tocolysis in farm animals but is also abused in altering the growth pattern of ruminants. The net effect when added to the feed of cattle is to reduce the fat content of the carcase, producing leaner meats which are favoured by health-conscious consumers. For this effect the dose required is several times greater than therapeutic. At this concentration significant residues accumulate in edible tissues such as liver or kidney (Meyer and Rinke, 1991; Elliott *et al.*, 1993a, b). On a number of occasions these have caused adverse reactions in consumers which have required hospital treatment (Martinez-Navarro, 1990; Pulse *et al.*, 1991).

*Testing*

In member states of the EU, a battery of tests have been developed using a variety of matrices to detect illegally-treated animals. These have been applied using both randomly selected and targeted sampling procedures. The most useful criterion for targeted selection is the recognition of *superior conformation for breed, age and sex*. An adult male animal of dairy parentage yet with beef breed conformation and light fat carcase cover constitutes the most obvious target. The *optimum tissue for detection* for some of these drugs is the *retina* of the eye because the drug residues persist in this location for very long periods after the abuse has occurred. Persistence in this matrix is much longer than in edible tissues and will identify illegal administration (abuse) after any risk to consumers has passed. However, it is necessary to target abuse to avoid illegal use of the drug. Since there are legalised pharmaceutical preparations available, it is necessary to allow producers to justify the presence as a result of therapeutic use under veterinary supervision.

Using a system based on targeted sampling, laboratory analysis of retinal tissue and owner certification, abuse in Northern Ireland has been prevented (Elliott *et al.*, 1995).

**1996 GB Statutory Survey results**

There was no evidence of the illegal use of clenbuterol in either live or slaughtered animals.

## PESTICIDES (See also Chapter 20)

Pest control chemicals must be toxic to some living organisms to fulfil their role. Depending on the pest being controlled, they may be termed insecticides, fungicides, etc. The *insecticides* that are directly applied to food animals and the *anthelmintics* are regarded as the most important subgroups. Pesticides undergo careful evaluation by the Advisory Committee on Pesticides before being approved for use. This evaluation includes consideration of the safety factors for consumers.

### Insecticides

The *chlorinated hydrocarbons* are extremely durable, persistent and bioaccumulating compounds which find their way into the food chain usually through use in controlling environmental or animal pests. The more recently-developed *organophosphate pesticides* are excreted rapidly and do not persist to the same extent in the environment. They are, however, frequently more toxic in small amounts as their biological activity is greater.

Following its introduction, DDT (dichlorodiphenyldichloroethane) was one of the most successful synthetic insecticides and continued in general use for many years. However, the bioaccumulation that occurred in various food chains eventually resulted in the banning of organochlorine pesticides by the 1970s. In use, the toxicity of DDT was quite low, but the ease with which it could be incorporated into many formulations resulted in a high environmental load. There have been cases of human illness and poisoning as a result of ingesting chlorinated hydrocarbons. These occurred when endrin was incorporated in flour and consumed as bread and when hexachlorobenzene was used on seed grain which was diverted and used as human food. Unacceptably high tissue concentrations have also occurred in broilers fed on treated grain. The experience gained through using these compounds demonstrated the usefulness of synthetic organic pesticides but also ensured that agrochemicals are assessed for biodegradation. As a result, strict powers to control the use of pesticides that could adversely affect food for human consumption have been introduced. Before a pesticide is approved for use, it is examined by independent experts of the Advisory Committee on Pesticides and the precautions that must be observed during use are specified.

The *organophosphates* (e.g. coumaphos, malathion, dichlorophos, diazinon) are extremely toxic to mammals but are highly efficient insecticides. They are less persistent in the environment than organochlorines because they can be hydrolysed chemically and enzymically. The organophosphate compounds therefore produce few tissue residues and have been used successfully in cattle to eradicate warble fly with few adverse effects. A number of the members of this group can be taken up by plants and can enter the food chain unless proper pre-harvest precautions are taken.

Concern about the long term safety of the handler using organophosphates, especially as *sheep dips*, has led to the much wider use of the *synthetic pyrethroid-containing products*. Although safer to handle, they are not as effective at eliminating the sheep scab mite and are potentially very harmful to the environment.

Several agrochemicals based on the phenols are used as *preservatives* or *herbicides* (e.g. 2,4-D, MCPA, 2,4,5-T). Although these are not used on food crops or livestock, they pose residue problems when treated products are used for bedding. When absorbed by animals or poultry they cause disagreeable flavours in meat or egg products. Although they are not individually highly toxic, they have derivatives that are regarded with suspicion (2,4,5-trichlorophenol has a highly toxic condensation product, 2,3,7,8-tetrachlorodibenzo-*p*-dioxin). In these cases restrictions are required, not because of the product, but because of the potential for a metabolite or derivative to be toxic.

### Testing

These pesticides are detected by *chemical techniques*. In the laboratory, spectrographic methods of pesticide analysis using colour-producing reactions were the first to reach sensitivities at the ppm level but these methods have been replaced by chromatographic techniques. The latter are required to cope with extracts that can contain complex mixtures of organic compounds. Although the earliest gas chromatographic techniques required milligram amounts, the introduction of argon-activation and electron-capture detectors has increased the sensitivity to the picogram range. The need for even more specific techniques has been met by the development of gas chromatography interfaced with mass spectrometry. These procedures have expanded since the development of complementary microelectronic computing facilities. These detection systems are capable of simultaneous multiresidue detection but are still in a state of development. Further refinements may lead to greater sensitivity and selectivity.

The importance attached to analyses for pesticide residues can be seen from the requirement that *registration applications need to be accompanied by data on tissue concentrations following use*. These requirements have become more compre-hensive so that an extensive background of toxicological test results is now essential. In some countries there is also a requirement that analytical methods capable of detecting and quantifying 0.1 ppm in meat, 0.01 ppm in food crops and 0.001 ppm in milk are made available to the monitoring authorities before registration. These concentrations have been selected as a result of previous toxicological experience with pesticides and are subject to variation if particular problems either are foreseen or occur after registration.

As pesticides accumulate in the environment and are only slowly degraded, it is important to distinguish between the concepts of absolute freedom from residues and concentrations that are below the detection limits of the methodology. When persistent chemicals have been in use for some time, absolute freedom from residues is highly unlikely, but the concentration may be below that which can be detected by existing techniques. As techniques become ever more sensitive, a spiral can develop in which the acceptable concentration is the detection limit of the tests. These detection limits may be below concentrations that could be hazardous in food. It is important, therefore, that full account is taken of the toxicological evidence when establishing acceptable concentrations.

There are other more durable organic environmental contaminants. The development of the plastics industry required stable materials and the *halogenated hyrocarbons* were well suited to this purpose. Two of the most frequently used were the polychlorinated biphenyls (PCBs) and the polychlorinated naphthalenes (PCNs). An outbreak of disease in *cattle* in the USA in 1941 in which the signs were hyperkeratosis, inappetence, depression and liver damage was traced to the PCNs used as lubricants on machinery. The compounds were excreted in the milk from these animals and were toxic to man (Clarke and Clarke, 1967). Attention focused on the PCBs in the mid-1960s when the first of a series of exposure-associated human diseases was recorded. The variability and subjective nature of the problems made correlation with known exposure difficult even when residues were detected in the fatty tissue. The extreme persistence of the PCBs in the environment has continued to highlight their toxic potential and has halted their manufacture and use. Nevertheless, in some areas the fauna of lakes and rivers can be expected to remain positive for some time.

### Anthelmintics

Pesticides used to remove *internal parasites* such as liver fluke and nematodes are important in animal production systems. The MRLs for a number of common anthelmintics for different species and tissues are shown in Table 13.4.

The salicylanide *flukecides*, oxyclosanide, closantel and rafoxanide, are active against *Fasciola hepatica*. They are commonly used to control infections and are extensively bound to plasma proteins in treated animals. As a result they have long terminal plasma half-lives (14.5, 16.6 and 6.4 days, respectively). These are detectable at a limit of 0.1 μg/ml for 90, 112 and 17 days after normal therapeutic dosing. All are distributed poorly in tissues, the tissue-to-plasma ratio being 1:6 kidney, 1:12 liver, 1:30 muscle and 1:100 fat. These ratios reduce the concern to the consumer which might result from persisting residues in meat.

*Nitroxynil* injection is a bright orange-red compound used widely in the treatment of fascioliasis. It is of particular concern in meat hygiene since the brightly-coloured stain and tissue reaction which accompany the subcutaneous administration persists long after the 60-day withdrawal period. If no reliable treatment history is available, the inspector may have to trim a large number of carcases and detain them until receipt of laboratory results.

*Thiabendazole* was the first highly-effective broad-spectrum anthelmintic and has been followed by the benzimidazole and probenzimidazole compounds which have improved efficacy and provide a wider spectrum of activity (parbendazole, cambendazole, mebendazole and oxibendazole). The introduction of the less-soluble benzimidazoles, fenbendazole, oxfendazole and albendazole secured a leading place for this group in the treatment of nematode infections.

These anthelmintics have high therapeutic indices. They are extensively metabolised in mammals after administration, the parent compound is generally short-lived, and the metabolites predominate in plasma, tissues and excreta. Lethal doses have not been established for overdoses of the less-soluble compounds. The main toxic effect is teratogenicity. This was identified in sheep, making the time of administration to pregnant ewes highly critical. When twice the normal dose of parbendazole was given to sheep in the third week of gestation, *congenital defects* of the skeleton were observed. As residues of benzimidazole compounds can occur in meat and meat products, it is necessary to observe withdrawal times for meat and milk after therapy. In tissues, the benzimidazoles may be unbound or bound to protein. The unbound drugs or metabolites are most likely to be associated with the toxic effects. The tightly-bound protein residues, which persist in the tissues for longer periods of time, are thought to be less significant toxicologically (Delatour and Parish, 1986). In general, therapy of human helminthiasis by benzimidazoles indicates that residues in tissues resulting from proper therapeutic doses in animals followed by adequate withholding periods should not cause undue concern.

The *avermectins* are a family of antiparasitic agents produced by fermentation of the actinomycete *Streptomyces avermitilis* and include ivermectin, moxidectin and doramectin. These have a broad range of activities against internal and external parasites

**Table 13.4** Maximum residue levels for common anthelmintics.

| Anthelmintic | Species | Target tissue | Maximum residue level (μg/kg) |
|---|---|---|---|
| Levamisole | Bovine, ovine, porcine, poultry | Muscle, kidney, fat | 10 |
| | | Liver | 100 |
| Ivermectin | Bovine | Liver | 100 |
| | | Fat | 40 |
| | Ovine | Liver | 15 |
| | Porcine | Fat | 20 |
| Abamectin | Bovine | Liver | 20 |
| | | Fat | 10 |
| Doramectin | Bovine | Liver | 15 |
| | | Fat | 25 |
| Eprinomectin | Bovine | Muscle, fat | 30 |
| | | Liver | 600 |
| | | Kidney | 100 |
| | | Milk | 30 |
| Moxidectin | Bovine, ovine | Fat | 500 |
| | | Liver | 100 |
| | | Muscle, kidney | 50 |
| Closantel | Bovine | Muscle, liver | 1000 |
| | | Kidney, fat | 3000 |
| | Ovine | Muscle, liver | 1500 |
| | | Kidney | 5000 |
| | | Fat | 2000 |
| Febantel, Fenbendazole | All food-producing species | Liver | 1000 |
| | | Muscle, kidney, fat | 10 |
| Oxfendazole | Bovine, ovine | Milk | 10 |
| Triclabendzole | Bovine, ovine | Muscle, kidney, liver | 150 |
| | | Fat | 50 |
| Thiabendazole | Bovine, ovine, caprine | Muscle | 100 |
| Netobimin | Bovine, ovine, caprine | Liver | 1000 |
| | | Kidney | 500 |
| | | Muscle, fat | 100 |
| | | Milk | 100 |

of animals. Ivermectin has been used extensively as an oral dose of 0.2 mg/kg without any adverse drug-related effects. Man has been shown to be less sensitive to this drug than laboratory animals. The therapeutic doses are low and safety margins are increased by the fact that levels in muscle are much lower than those in liver. In the edible tissues, liver and fat, the depletion half-lives are 4.8 and 7.6 days, respectively. Within 7 days, 60–80% of the dose is excreted. Therefore if withdrawal periods are observed, concentrations in edible tissue will be negligible.

*Levamisole* has been associated with a number of undesirable side-effects in animals (Hsu, 1980). Toxic effects have also been observed in man at oral doses of 2.5 mg/ml.

In general, these therapeutic drugs are used to strategically control helminth infections in farm animals and are therefore unlikely to be administered close to the time of slaughter. The most significant problem is with those administered by injection, where there may be an irritant reaction. This may require trimming of the sites and laboratory checks for muscle residues.

## HEAVY METALS

Excessive intakes of *heavy metals* in food have caused intoxications in man. These are most often caused by contaminated cereals or by accidental additions during processing. Occasionally, toxic concentrations occur in animal tissues and products. These can be associated with soils naturally high in the element or through environmental contamination from local industry and are cumulative in animal tissues. They may also occur from feeding grain treated with the toxic metal or from excess amounts remaining in the environment following previous use in paints, etc.

These toxic chemicals are detected by *atomic absorption spectrometry*.

### Lead

*Lead* can accumulate in the tissues of animals grazing close to smelting plants or in animals ingesting paints or substances with high lead contents. Interestingly, samples of soil and herbage collected at the Rothamsted Agricultural Experimental Station do not show a correlation with increased environmental loading caused by the addition of lead as an anti-knock petrol additive (Williams, 1974).

Ruminants are more commonly affected than other farm species. During chronic exposure, e.g. from low-level environmental contamination, the metal accumulates in the bones. Acute cases are rare and occur most commonly after ingestion of lead-containing paint. In these the highest concentrations are found in liver and kidney. In 1989 cattle feed was contaminated in the UK following the importation of a maize gluten substitute. A total of 30 animals died. However, the Department of Health considered that, owing to the acute nature of the episode, even in the worst case of maximum intake there was no hazard to human health. This conclusion is supported by experimental evidence. When 100 ppm was fed to cattle for 100 days, the liver contained 2.3 ppm compared with 0.6 ppm in controls, but no lead was detected in the muscle of the experimental animals. Acutely-affected animals should be detected during ante-mortem inspection At post-mortem the muscle of acutely-poisoned bovines is unusually pale.

Special attention has to be taken when dealing with the carcases of game animals, particularly fowl.

### Arsenic

Although restrictions have been placed on the use of *arsenic* because of its toxicity, this element was once widely used in farm practices and is persistent in the environment. It is probably the second most important poisoning hazard for farm animals.

The animals may be exposed to inorganic or organic arsenic compounds when they are given feed, forage or liquids contaminated with arsenical herbicides, rodenticides or insecticides. Arsenic-containing compounds have been used for parasite control, and for the treatment and control of swine dysentery, but these have largely been removed from the market.

Chronic toxicity can occur when arsenical compounds are fed at low levels because the metal accumulates in the liver, kidney and bones. Arsenic is slowly excreted in the faeces, sweat and milk. Although accumulation occurs in exposed animals, the risk to consumers is small because the concentrations in the muscle are not above the maximum safe level for human consumption. Only the liver approaches the hazard level for man (Clarke and Clarke, 1967). Where it is suspected that toxicity may have occurred after chronic ingestion, then a withholding period of 40 days may be needed. Following normal therapeutic dosing, a much shorter withholding period of 5 days is considered sufficient.

Shellfish can accumulate particularly high concentrations if taken from polluted waters. Bottom feeders from these areas also accumulate the metal but free-swimming fin fish are less affected.

### Mercury

*Mercury* preparations containing inorganic salts or organic mercurial compounds have been used widely in agricultural and horticultural dressings and in veterinary medicines. Although mercury is extremely toxic, cases of poisoning are rare. They have been most frequently associated with feeding to animals of seed grain treated with mercury-containing dressings to prevent fungal growth. Above average concentrations may also occur when industrial pollution contaminates grazing areas or when sewage sludge is used intensively as a fertiliser (Vos *et al.*, 1987).

Absorbed inorganic mercury is stored in the liver and kidneys but organic preparations are more widely distributed. The metal is excreted slowly in the urine, but to a smaller extent in faeces, saliva, sweat and milk.

Mercury-containing products have been replaced by less toxic compounds and therefore there is now only a very small risk to consumers from the meat of farm animals.

### Cadmium

*Cadmium* has received much attention because of its reported toxicity to humans. This metal accumulates in body tissues and is said to cause kidney failure. In farm animals the greatest concentrations occur in kidney and liver.

Random samples of horse kidney reveal levels above the maximum residue level, and there have been recent reports of high levels in bovine and porcine kidney. The origin of these residues may be sewage sludge or organocadmium fungicides. It has been postulated that horses live longer than other farm animals and may accumulate the metal over many years, but more recently residues have been detected at very low concentrations in other species, e.g. pigs.

Concentrations as high as 200 μg/g (dry weight) in kidney have been observed in cattle grazing pasture irrigated with aerobically digested sludge, but there were no signs of disease or pathological conditions in these animals (Fitzgerald *et al.*, 1985). Kidney malfunction in man begins when the concentrations are above 200 μg/g wet weight.

Although a one-off consumption of horse kidneys containing cadmium residues at the usual levels encountered does not pose a hazard for man, there is a voluntary agreement with horse abattoirs for all offal from animals destined for human consumption to be discarded.

### Copper

*Copper*-supplemented feeds are prepared for pigs. The metal tends to be accumulated in the liver and kidney. However, there have been no reported cases of toxicity to humans due to this source. Copper-supplemented feed prepared for pigs has accidentally been fed to sheep and led to chronic copper poisoning in this species. (There are indications that particular breeds, e.g. Texel, are more susceptible.) Cases are usually encountered in veterinary practice, when sudden deaths occur. Non-clinical cases are unlikely to be detected ante-mortem but an enlarged yellow liver, jaundice and haemoglobinuria can be observed during a post-mortem inspection.

### Selenium

*Selenium* is an essential element for animals and man. Although it is widely distributed, areas of deficiency and of toxicity occur. In some cases acute selenium poisoning may occur in cattle grazing pasture that contains plants which accumulate this element (e.g. *Astralagus racemosus*, USA; *Neptunia amplexicaulis*, Australia). Toxicity is unlikely to occur in the UK, where many areas are known to be selenium deficient. The most common sign of selenium deficiency is flaccid white muscle.

## OTHER SUBSTANCES

### Fluorine

Cases of *fluorosis* have been reported in cattle grazing pasture contaminated with industrial discharges. This chronic disease is associated with staining of the teeth and excessive wear and degenerative changes in the skeletal system and internal organs. It has not been associated with illness in man.

### NSAIDs especially phenylbutazone ('bute')

The NSAIDs (non-steroidal anti-inflammatory drugs) are a large group of compounds which can be divided into two main groups – *carboxylic acids* (salicylates, aspirin, propionic acid, ibuprofen, ketoprofen, naproxen, carprofen, etc.) and *enolic acids* (phenylbutazone, oxyphenbutazone, dipyrone, isopyrin, etc.).

Phenylbutazone is a powerful NSAID widely used in the horse to provide symptomatic relief from muscle, bone and joint lesions. The drug can also be used in ruminants and dogs. A pyrazolone-derivative, it is probably used in the horse on occasions which militate against animal welfare – the suppression or partial suppression of pain in animals with severe lesions. Unscrupulous individuals have used phenylbutazone to mask lameness in horses prior to examination for soundness. Although designed for slow intravenous use it is frequently given as an intramuscular injection, when it can cause severe local irritation in addition to cardiac and renal dysfunction and ulceration of the alimentary tract.

Its detection and that of its longer-acting metabolite oxyphenbutazone in racing horse urine samples has given rise to the so-called 'eight-day rule', 8 days being the minimum period suggested between the last treatment and the commencement of racing to ensure a negative urine test.

Because of its toxicity to man, phenylbutazone and similar NSAIDs are not normally approved for use in food-producing animals (except for the horse in the USA), even though they do not accumulate in high concentrations in tissues and are almost completely metabolised. Horses undergoing treatment, however, should not be slaughtered for human consumption.

## NATURAL TOXINS

### Mycotoxins

*Mycotoxins* are products of toxigenic moulds (fungi) growing in food and foodstuffs. These agents have caused many problems in livestock, and the potential for residues in meat, poultry or dairy products is a cause for public concern. However, the risk to human health from direct consumption of contaminated grain is much higher than that arising from animal products.

*Aflatoxins* are produced by *Aspergillus flavus* and *Aspergillus parasiticus*. There are four major types of toxin labelled AFB1, AFB2, AFG1, and AFG2. AFG1 is the most commonly produced and the most toxic. Much of the ingested toxin is excreted within 24 hours and excretion is almost complete within 96 hours after ingestion ceases. Liver and kidneys retain detectable quantities for longer periods than other tissues. Dairy products are considered to be the most vulnerable to residue accumulation (Shank, 1981) and transmission of toxic amounts into human food through meat and meat products does not appear likely (Ciegler *et al.*, 1981). The results of feeding trials using contaminated feed have produced equivocal results on the accumulation of residues in beef cattle, dairy cattle, pigs and poultry.

*Ochratoxins* are produced by some *Penicillium* spp. and some *Aspergillus* strains. Ochratoxin A is the most common and the most toxic to mammals, birds and fish. The kidney is the primary target organ, but liver damage has also been recorded at high concentrations. It has been shown to be a teratogen in laboratory animals but has not been proved to be carcinogenic (Busby and Wogan, 1981). The highest risk for consumers is the potential for residues to accumulate in kidney. Lower concentrations occur in liver, fat and muscle.

The presence of these toxins can be detected by a range of commercially-produced *immunoassay* kits, and, if positive animals are identified, they should be retained on a toxin-free diet for 4 weeks prior to slaughter to ensure that the levels in kidney have decreased. In poultry, residues have been detected in liver, kidney and muscle but not in eggs. A 48-hour withholding period is sufficient to clear muscle (Prior and Sisodia, 1978). In ruminants, ochratoxin A is detoxified in the rumen, hence accumulation in their tissues is highly unlikely.

### Shellfish toxin

Shellfish tissues can contain at least three different groups of natural toxins which are grouped according to the clinical signs produced in the consumer: paralytic shellfish toxins, diarrhoetic shellfish toxin and anamnestic shellfish toxin. These result from the accumulation of toxins produced by algae in the environment which are eaten by the shellfish. These toxins occur in most shellfish harvesting areas and the concentration can vary considerably depending on seasonal conditions. There are no overt signs by which toxin-containing shellfish can be detected. Acceptable limits have been set for these toxins based on the effect on experimentally-injected laboratory animals or chemical quantification of already recognised toxins. Biological testing has been retained because it is believed that all toxins may not yet have been identified. Testing for consumer protection depends upon regular sampling for biological, immunological or chemical testing.

## REFERENCES

Anon. (1967) Report of a new chemical hazard. *Scientist* **32**, 612.

Busby, W. F. and Wogan, G. N. (1981) Ochratoxins. In *Mycotoxins and N-Nitroso Compounds: Environmental Risks*, Vol. II, ed. R. C. Shank. Boca Raton, FL: CRC Press.

Bogaerts, R. and Wolf, F. (1980) A standardised method for the detection of residues of antimicrobial substances in fresh meat. *Fleischwitschaft* **60**, 671–675.

Ciegler, A., Burmeister, R. F., Vesonder, R. F. and Heseltine, C. W. (1981) *Mycotoxins and N-Nitroso Compounds: Environmental Risks*, ed. R. C. Shank. Boca Raton, FL: CRC Press.

Clarke, E. G. C. and Clarke, M. L. (1967) *Garner's Veterinary Toxicology*, 3rd edn, pp. 287–291. Baltimore: Williams and Wilkins.

Delatour, P. and Parish, R. (1986) *Benzimidazole Anthelmintics and Related Compounds: Toxicity and Evaluation of Residues in Drug Residues in Animals*, pp. 175–203, ed. A. G. Rico. New York: Academic Press.

Elliott, C. T., McEvoy, J. D. G., McCaughey, W. J., Shortt, H. D. and Crooks, S. R. H. (1993a) Effective laboratory monitoring for the abuse of the beta agonist clenbuterol in cattle. *Analyst* **121**, 447–448.

Elliott, C. T., McCaughey, W. J. and Shortt, H. D. (1993b) Residues of the beta-agonist clenbuterol in tissues of medicated farm animals. *Food Addit. Contam.* **10**, 231–244.

Elliott, C. T., McCaughey, W. J., Crooks, S. R. H., McEvoy, J. D. G. and Kennedy, D. G. (1995) Residues of clenbuterol in cattle receiving therapeutic doses: implications for differentiating between legal and illegal use. *Vet. Q.* **17**, 100–102.

FAO/WHO (1987) Codex Alimentarius Commission, 1987. Alinorm 87/31.

Fitzgerald, P. R., Peterson, J. and Lue-hing, C. (1985) *J. Vet. Res.* **46**, 703–707.

Hoffsis, G. F. and Walker, F. H. (1984) Therapeutic strategies involving antimicrobial treatment of disseminated infections in food animals. *J. Am. Vet. Med. Assoc.* **185**, 1214–1216.

Hsu, W. H. (1980) Toxicity and drug interactions of levamisole. *J. Am. Vet. Assoc.* **176**, 1166–1169.

Lamming, G. E. (1984) Commission of the European Communities (Agriculture) Report Eur 8913.

Lamming, G. E., Ballerini, G., Baulieu, E. R., Brookes, P., Elias, P. S., Ferrando, R., Galli, C. L., Heitzman, R. J., Hoffman, B., Karg, H., Mayer, H. H. D., Michel, G., Paulsen, E., Rico, A., van Leeuwan, F. X. R. and White, D. S. (1987) Scientific report on anabolic agents in animal production. *Vet. Rec.* **121**, 381–392.

Martinez-Navarro, J. F. (1990) Food poisoning related to consumption of the illicit beat agonist clenbuterol in livers. *The Lancet*, **336**, 1311.

Mercer, H. D., Baggot, J. D. and Sams, R. A. (1977) Application of pharmacokinetic methods to the drug residue profile. *J. Toxicol. Environ. Health.* **2**, 787–801.

Meyer, H. H. D. and Rinke, L. M. (1991) The pharmacokinetics and residues of clenbuterol in veal calves. *J. Anim. Sci.* **69**, 4538–4543.

Prior, M. G. and Sisodia, C. S. (1978) Ochratoxicosis in White Leghorn hens. *Poultry Sci.* **57**, 619–683.

Pulse, C., Lamison, D., Keck, G., Bosvironnais, C., Nicolas, J. and Descotes, J. (1991) Collective human poisonings by clenbuterol residues in veal liver. *Vet. and Hum. Toxicol.* **33**, 480–481.

Shank, R. C. (1981) Mycotoxins: assessment of risk. In *Mycotoxins and N-Nitroso Compounds: Environmental Risks*, ed. R. C. Shank. Boca Raton FL: CRC Press.

Sundof, S. F., Craigmill, A. C. and Riviere, J. E. (1986) Food Animal Residue Avoidance Databank (FARAD): a pharmacokinetic based information resource. *J. Vet. Pharmacol. Ther.* **9**, 237–245.

Vanoosthuyze, K., Daeseleire, E., Overbeke, A. van and Peteghem, C. van (1994) *Analyst* **119** (12), 2655–2658.

Veterinary Medicines Directorate, *Annual Reports on Surveillance for Veterinary Residues in 1996*. Veterinary Medicines Directorate. ISBN 0 95312340 5.

Vos, G., Hovens, J. P. C. and Delft, W. V. (1987) Arsenic, cadmium, lead and mercury in meat, livers and kidneys of cattle slaughtered in the Netherlands during 1980–1985. *Food Addit. Contam.* **4**, 73–88.

Williams, C. (1974) The accumulation of automobile emissions on the lead content of soils and herbage at the Rothamsted Experimental Station. *J. Agric. Sci., Camb.* **82**, 189–192.

# Chapter 14
# Food Poisoning and Meat Microbiology

## Part 1 – Food Poisoning

*Food poisoning* is as old as civilisation itself and man acquired, often by bitter experience, a considerable knowledge as to what was suitable or unsuitable to eat. Many of the 'dietary laws' of the Old Testament Books of *Leviticus* and *Deuteronomy* can be regarded primarily as health injunctions, some being related to the prevention of food poisoning, e.g. 'Ye shall not eat of anything that dieth of itself' (*Deuteronomy* 14:21); 'Thou shalt not eat any abominable thing' (*Deuteronomy* 14:3); 'But of all *clean* fowls ye may eat' (*Deuteronomy* 14:20).

Despite this biblical history, there is still a continuing and indeed increasing attention to food poisoning by the public, health care workers and especially the media. This current interest is set against a background of apparently ever-increasing numbers of reports of food-borne illness, for example, between 1985 and 1996 annual notifications of food poisoning in England and Wales more than quadrupled. Such apparently simple facts, however, need to be treated with considerable caution.

The Public Health (Control of Diseases) Act 1984 gives all doctors in clinical practice a statutory duty to notify, to the proper officer of the local authority, cases or suspected cases of food poisoning. However, 'food poisoning' is not defined in this legislation. The definition of *food-borne disease* adopted by the World Health Organisation, and in use since 1992 throughout the United Kingdom, is *'any disease of an infectious or toxic nature caused by or thought to be caused by the consumption of food or water'*. This interpretation gives a very wide spectrum of disease, ranging from, for example, acute gastrointestinal infection caused by verotoxigenic *E. coli* to chronic toxicity such as that caused by lead in water.

### TYPES OF FOOD POISONING

Food poisoning thus includes bacterial and viral infections, chemical contamination of food, plant or animal toxins and food allergies. Almost all agents capable of causing human infection can be transmitted through food.

*Food allergies*, or hypersensitivity to certain foodstuffs, are not uncommon and together with other allergic diseases may be increasing. The *allergens* are generally protein in nature, e.g. milk, eggs, cheese, fish, shellfish, pork, but also mushrooms, tomatoes, etc. In recent years hypersensitivities to nuts such as peanuts have been well documented and food ingredients are carefully scrutinised by susceptible individuals. In some cases the reaction can be so acute and severe as to require a few individuals to carry acute medical supplies. Nuts and cereals are also vehicles for *aflatoxin* produced during the growth of fungi, either before or after harvest. The tendency to sensitivity to certain foodstuffs may be hereditary and a documented case in the literature describes an allergy to hens' eggs which persisted throughout four generations. As many as 30% of all people may be allergic to one or more foodstuffs.

*Chemical contamination* is not common and usually occurs by accidental contamination, or perhaps some unintentional chemical reaction between a foodstuff and its container. The metals encountered include copper, lead, arsenic and antimony. In England and Wales outbreaks caused by chemical contamination have been due to the presence of zinc in acid fruits which have been stored or cooked in galvanised containers. In Germany the storage of prepared foodstuffs in zinc containers is prohibited by law. Water is at particular risk from chemical contamination (usually accidental) such as by aluminium or phenols. Lead may, of course, be leached from lead pipes or even from soldered lead capillary joints. Not only metals are involved; a large outbreak of illness occurred in Spain following chemical adulteration of cooking oil.

Inherently poisonous substances can occur in normally edible plants and animals including certain fungi, berries, fish and shellfish. This is well-recognised in the case of mushrooms, where some types are toxic. Less well-known are foods that are poisonous unless properly prepared, e.g. red kidney beans. Other foods in the right circumstances can acquire toxins from the environment. This is a particular problem with shellfish, which can filter out the algal toxins that cause paralytic and diarrhoetic shellfish poisoning in consumers. In some instances breakdown products can produce illness, as in the case of scrombotoxin poisoning when bacterial action in scromboid fish such as mackerel and tuna converts histidine to histamine. A similar type of illness has been associated with cheese.

## SURVEILLANCE OF FOOD POISONING

There are several different methods of gathering statistics on food-borne disease and it is important to recognise the limitations posed by each of these. The three most important sources of data are:

1 Notifications of food poisoning.
2 Surveillance of laboratory-confirmed infections.
3 Investigation of outbreaks of food poisoning.

Each of these surveillance methods provides valuable, but incomplete, information and none on its own will measure the true extent of all food-borne disease. Specifically, most of the information gathered relates to infectious causes of food poisoning. It is estimated that only between 1% and 10% of all food-borne illness is even counted by the various surveillance systems, and this varies from cause to cause (Fig. 14.1).

In any population, not all of those who become infected become ill. Of those who are unwell, only a proportion will seek medical help and can be counted as 'notifications'. Those who do not require medical assistance are not included in any surveillance system. If the clinician suspects 'food poisoning' then that patient *may* be formally notified, for which the GP will receive a notification fee. The number of notifications may be supplemented, for example, EHOs including cases they become aware of during their investigation. The doctor may submit appropriate samples for laboratory investigation and this forms the basis of

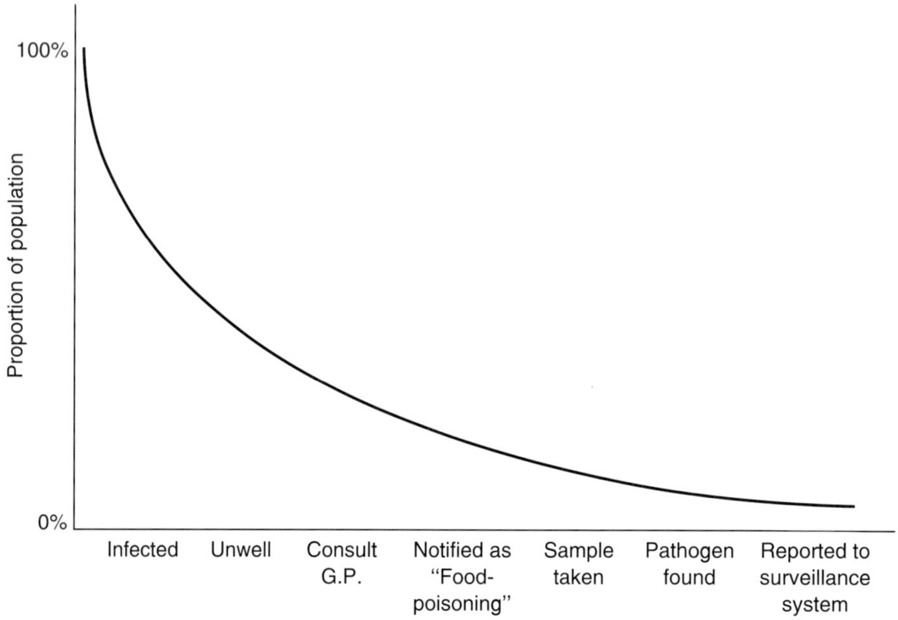


**Fig. 14.1** Surveillance of food-borne illness.

laboratory surveillance. The sample taken may affect the result; for example, vomitus is more appropriate for a viral agent than is a stool sample. Unless the sample is submitted within 24 hours of onset of illness, a viral cause is likely to be missed. If a pathogen is identified then the result should be recorded by the laboratory surveillance. When no pathogen is identified it does not, of course, mean that none were present but rather that the laboratory did not identify anything. This will depend on the organisms under scrutiny. When an outbreak occurs it is likely that there will be greater investigation of the source of infection than might be the case when only a single patient is unwell. Causes of outbreaks may be different from the causes of sporadic infections and it may not be possible to extrapolate.

## NOTIFICATION OF FOOD POISONING

In the UK, notifications of food poisoning have increased very significantly since the 1980s, although the change has been more marked in England and Wales than in Scotland (Fig. 14.2).

It is likely that differences in the way the information has been gathered, or in what is designated as 'food poisoning', at least partly explain the variation between different parts of the UK. Similarly, some of the increase in reports can be attributed to improvements in the way the information has been collected. For example, in Scotland infections with *Campylobacter* spp. were specifically excluded until 1995. Including such infections in the reports for 1996 resulted in notifications rising from 4940 to 10 100, a 100% increase. This was a statistical anomaly, not an increase in illness in the public. There is also no doubt that at least part of any apparent rise is due to ascertainment, which may be self-fuelling. Heightened public and media attention encourages reports which might otherwise not get into the system. It is therefore wrong to claim that there was a four-fold increase in *clinical* disease between the middle 1980s and the middle 1990s.

## LABORATORY REPORTS OF ENTERIC INFECTIONS

Routine reporting from medical laboratories gives a useful picture of the importance of pathogens present in the population. It does, of course, only record the results from *samples* actually submitted to laboratories, and can therefore be distorted by any factors which might influence sampling, e.g. increased media attention. Results can also be influenced by the likely success of identifying a pathogen when

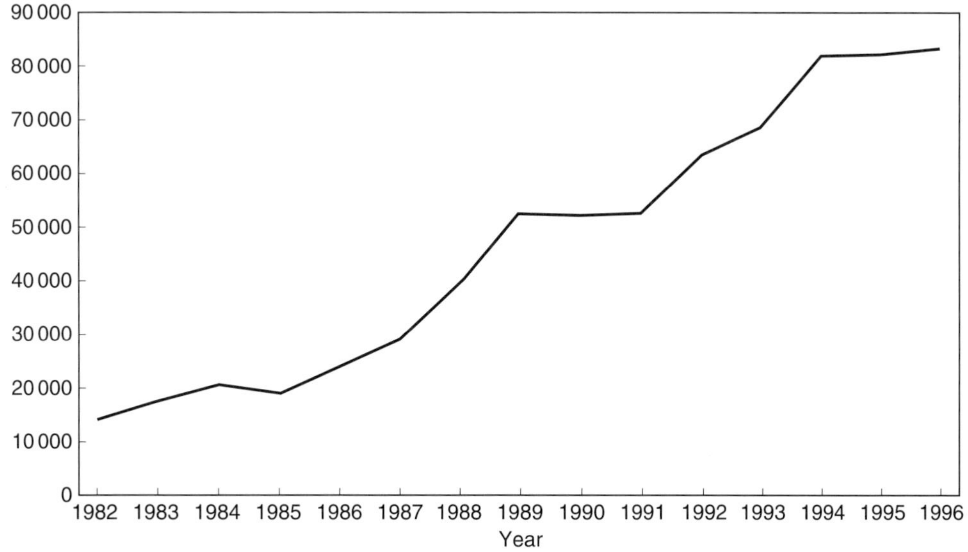


**Fig. 14.2** Food poisoning notifications in England and Wales, 1982–96; includes formal notifications and those cases otherwise ascertained.

present, and this success may change as laboratory methodologies improve. For example, during the 1980s better techniques for the recovery of *Campylobacter* spp. became routinely available and this undoubtedly contributed to the overall increase in numbers reported during the 1980s and 1990s. However, since the early 1990s methods have been standardised and should not be the explanation for the continuing increase for *Campylobacter* spp. (Fig. 14.3).

Similarly, improvements in the methods for isolating verotoxigenic *E. coli* O157 contributed to the rise in reported isolations during the 1980s. The use of further refinements such as immunomagnetic separation may increase the ability to isolate organisms by a factor of 10, especially if the organisms are present in small numbers, as is the case with *E. coli* O157 (Fig. 14.4).

Other extraneous events also play a part when identifying laboratory-confirmed cases. A

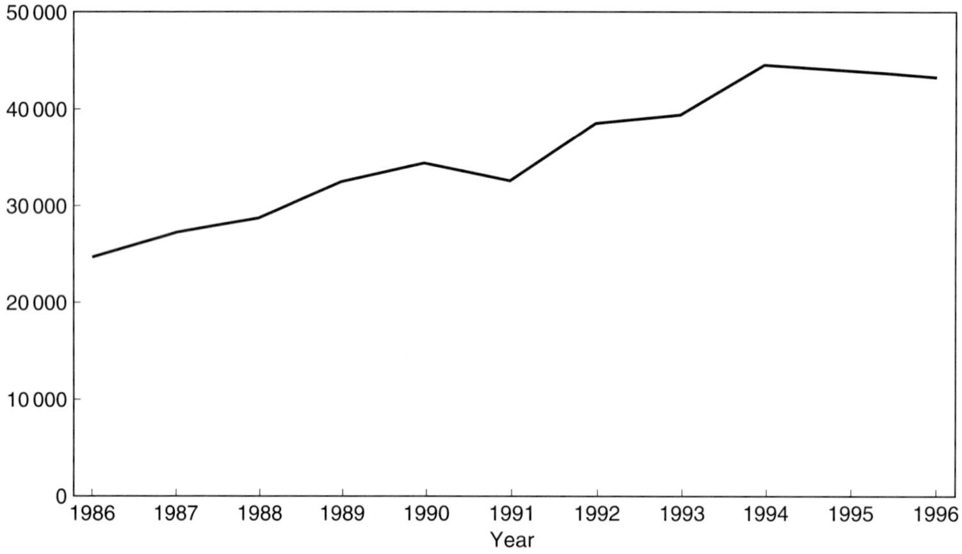


**Fig. 14.3** Laboratory isolates of *Campylobacter* spp. in England and Wales, 1986–96.

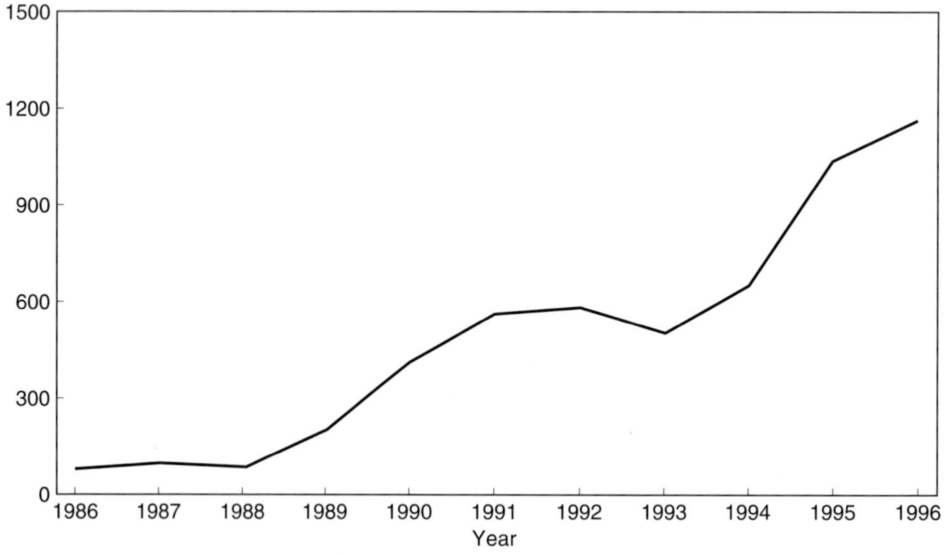


**Fig. 14.4** Laboratory isolates of *E. coli* O157 in England, Wales and Scotland, 1986–96.

change in policy occurred when the Advisory Committee on the Microbiological Safety of Food recommended in 1995 that *all* stool samples be screened for *E. coli* O157. Previously, many laboratories were selective and had perhaps restricted the examination for this organism to stools from children or from patients with bloody diarrhoea.

The variation in laboratory methods and sample submissions may partly explain the geographical differences seen throughout the UK. For example, the average annual rate of *E. coli* O157 infection in England and Wales is approximately 1 per 100 000, yet that for Scotland is more than four times as high. Even within Scotland there is very significant variation between Health Boards, which in 1996 varied between 0 in Shetland and 32.3 per 100 000 in Lanarkshire. This latter rate was influenced by the largest outbreak (496 cases and 20 deaths) recorded in Europe (Fig. 14.5).

Laboratory surveillance is, however, crucial to determining changes taking place within an organism such as *Salmonella* spp. During the 1980s, it became clear that *S. enteritidis* was replacing *S. typhimurium* as the more common serotype and in particular that *S. enteritidis* PT4 was the predominant serotype. In the middle 1990s, *S. typhimurium* has again been increasing in particular definitive type 104. This has become the second most common salmonella in the UK, and is increasingly being reported from other parts of the world (Fig. 14.6).

## OUTBREAK SURVEILLANCE

Investigation into outbreaks can give valuable information on the organisms involved, the food vehicles and the factors contributing to the cause of the outbreak. The main limitation is that the majority of cases of food poisoning occur as single cases or involve a single household only, and it is much more difficult to confirm a source of infection – even if an investigation is carried out.

Outbreaks are investigated in most parts of the world, although there is no common approach in

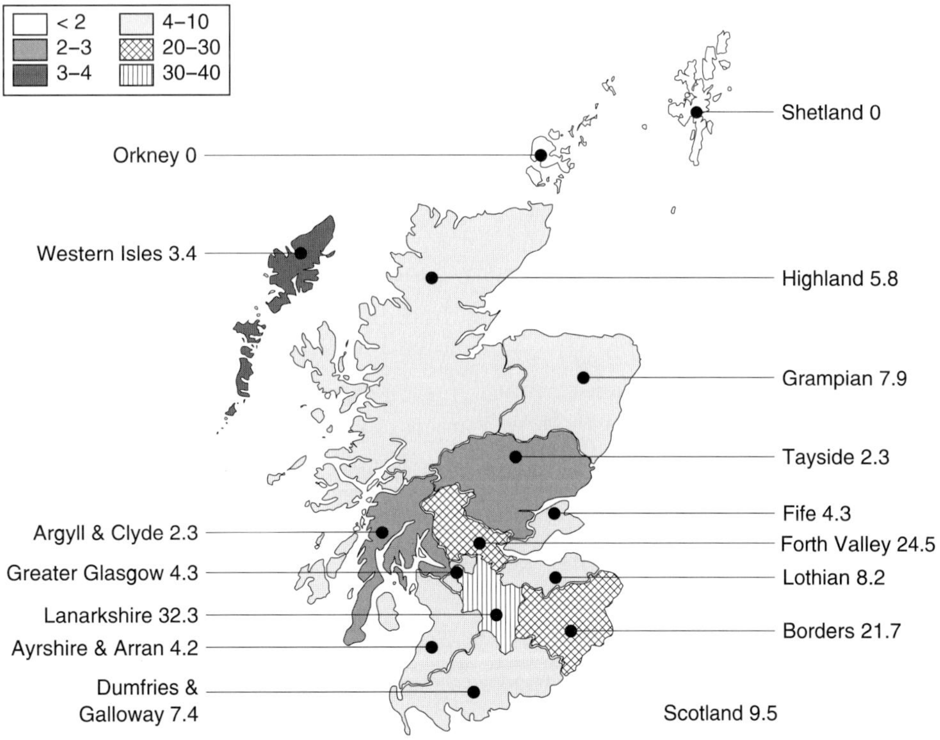


**Fig. 14.5** Rates of *E. coli* O157 in Scotland (per 100 000) by health board of reporting laboratory, 1996.

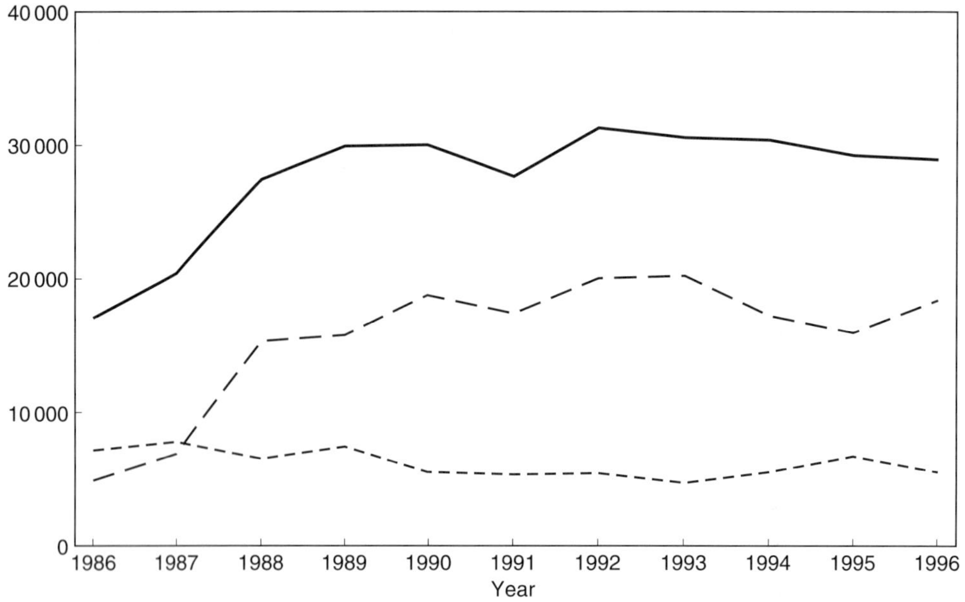


**Fig. 14.6** Laboratory isolates of *Salmonella* spp. In England and Wales, 1986–96: ———, total *Salmonella*; - - - - - -, *S. typhimurium*; — — — — — —, *S. enteritidis*.

the way this is performed. Lack of standardisation makes comparison of reports from different countries very difficult, even though the World Health Organisation in Europe has a coordinating programme. The sixth and latest report was published in 1995 and covered the period 1990–92. It identified a wide and differing range of foods involved in different countries. The relative importance of individual pathogens also varied. While in the UK *Clostridium perfringens* and *Staphylococcus aureus* are now uncommon pathogens, these continue to be important in France. In the UK, poultry and red meat are the most frequently identified foods, while in Germany cakes, puddings and ice cream are the most common and France and Spain report that eggs and egg products are the most important foods involved in outbreaks of food poisoning.

Many of the differences may be due to historical attitudes towards food and how food is handled, prepared and stored. Social practices as well as food preferences contribute towards the different national pictures.

National surveillance of outbreaks of food poisoning in England and Wales is coordinated by the Communicable Disease Surveillance Centre (CDSC) at Colindale, London. During 1992–94, a total of 642 general outbreaks were identified, in 551 of which a bacterial or virus pathogen was identified (Table 14.1).

Many more laboratory reports of gastrointestinal pathogens are received than reports of outbreak investigations and CDSC recorded in the same period 122 388 *Campylobacter* spp. infections, 92 416 *Salmonella* spp. and 1266 *E. coli* O157 (Table 14.2).

## Food vehicles

In England and Wales the food vehicle was identified in 204 (44%) of a series of 458

**Table 14.1** Pathogens from general outbreaks of food-borne infection, England and Wales, 1992–94

| | |
|---|---|
| *Bacillus cereus* | 17 |
| *Campylobacter* spp. | 12 |
| *Clostridium perfringens* | 89 |
| *E. coli* O157 | 9 |
| *Salmonella* spp. | 362 |
| *Shigella sonnei* | 2 |
| Small round structured virus | 42 |
| *Staphylococcus aureus* | 10 |
| Others | 8 |

**Table 14.2** Laboratory-confirmed cases of enteric infections in England and Wales.

| | 1994 | 1995 | 1996 |
|---|---|---|---|
| *S. typhimurium* | 5522 | 6692 | 5573 |
| *S. enteritidis* | 17371 | 16086 | 18296 |
| Other salmonellae | 7518 | 6939 | 5242 |
| *Campylobacter* spp. | 44414 | 43902 | 43240 |
| *Cl. perfringens* | 449 | 342 | 720 |
| *Staph. aureus* | 74 | 59 | 150 |
| *Bacillus* spp. | 87 | 87 | 27 |
| *Listeria* | 112 | 91 | 115 |
| *E. coli* O157 | 411 | 792 | 660 |

**Table 14.3** Food vehicles involved in 458 outbreaks of food-borne disease.

| | |
|---|---|
| Milk/milk products | 9 |
| Meat (unspecified) | 70 |
| Gravy/sauces | 17 |
| Poultry/eggs | 18 |
| Fish/shellfish | 28 |
| Desserts | 32 |
| Salads/vegetables | 25 |
| Water/ice | 3 |
| Other foods | 15 |

**Table 14.4** Reported food vehicles in general outbreaks of food poisoning in England and Wales, 1989–91.

| Food vehicle | *Salmonella* spp. | *Clostridium perfringens* | *Staphylococcus aureus* | *Bacillus cereus* and *Bacillus* spp. |
|---|---|---|---|---|
| Chicken | 23 | 13 | 3 | 2 |
| Turkey | 21 | 5 | – | 2 |
| Other poultry | – | – | 1 | – |
| Beef | 7 | 22 | – | – |
| Pork/ham | 5 | 12 | 3 | – |
| Lamb/mutton | – | 9 | – | – |
| Mixed and other meats, pies and sausages | 24 | 24 | 3 | 2 |
| Gravy/sauces | 1 | 1 | – | – |
| Milk/dairy | 4 | – | – | – |
| Eggs | 50 | – | 1 | 1 |
| Others/not stated | 250 | 59 | 5 | 50 |

outbreaks (Table 14.3). Meat, desserts, salads and fish predominated. In some outbreaks more than one food vehicle was identified.

Some foods are more associated with particular pathogens than others (Table 14.4).

## Risk factors

Between 1992 and 1994, investigations of general outbreaks identified where these occurred and the risk factors involved (Table 14.5).

The common factors contributing to the outbreaks included inappropriate storage, inadequate heating, cross-contamination, and infected food handlers. This indicated that in most outbreaks it was a failure of adequate

**Table 14.5** Location of general outbreaks of food-borne disease in England and Wales, 1992–94

| | |
|---|---|
| Restaurant/cafe/public house/bar | 170 |
| Private house | 101 |
| Hotel/guest house/residential public house | 75 |
| Residential institution | 59 |
| Shop/retailer | 38 |
| Canteen | 35 |
| School | 30 |
| Armed services camp | 20 |
| Hospital | 19 |
| Mobile retailer | 5 |
| Miscellaneous | 90 |

hygiene and food handling practices which resulted in the outbreak.

## GENERAL CONSIDERATIONS

There are many and varied sources of the organisms causing food poisoning. Most originate directly from animals, particularly *Salmonella* spp., *Campylobacter* spp. and *E. coli*. Others not only have animal sources but survive or even increase within the environment. This includes, for example, the *Clostridia* spp., *Listeria* spp. and *Bacillus* spp. Yet others have people as the source or reservoir – particularly *Staphylococcus* and viruses. Other human gastrointestinal infections such as dysentery (*Shigella* spp.) can be passed by contaminated food, although this is not the main route of spread.

Regardless of the origin of the organisms involved, they all have one factor in common. *There has been failure to adequately control the hygiene and temperature control of the whole food chain*. This chain, when it involves animals, can be divided into a number of separate stages:

- Animal feed, e.g. the feed mill
- On farm, e.g. suckled calves
- During processing, e.g. abattoir, cutting plant
- Further processing and distribution, e.g. butchers
- Final preparation, e.g. domestic or commercial kitchen

*Each of these is important in the prevention of food-borne disease and satisfactory practices must be in place. No single part of the food chain bears the total responsibility for the prevention of food poisoning.*

Food-borne disease is not static and constantly changes and evolves. The traditional illnesses such as bovine tuberculosis caused by milk, which have often determined the procedures historically used in meat inspection, have largely been controlled. In the case of TB this has been achieved by reducing the infection in animals, by identifying and removing infected animals, and by treating risk foods, e.g. milk, by pasteurisation.

These traditional zoonotic diseases were usually examples where the food, meat or milk, was itself carrying the pathogen when the animal was slaughtered or milked. The more current problems associated with food poisoning are usually the consequence of the food becoming contaminated either at the time of production or subsequently. This has placed an even greater emphasis on the need for *strict hygiene and temperature control*. That this is not always achieved is emphasised by the continuing and apparently increasing problem of foodborne infections.

Not all food-poisoning organisms cause illness in animals; many bacteria are part of the 'normal' intestinal flora, e.g. *Yersinia* spp, *Clostridium* spp. Even with those which can cause animal illness this may be the exception rather than the norm. Campylobacter infection is a good example of this, the organisms being widespread in animals and birds yet rarely making them ill. But other organisms, such as *Salmonella* spp., do cause considerable animal ill health, although it is not usually the 'sick' animals that enter the food chain, rather recovered or carrier animals which are still shedding the pathogen.

*Most of the organisms causing problems are spread by the faecal route and the main problem is to prevent food becoming contaminated with animal faeces.*

## FOOD-BORNE PATHOGENS

Most cases of food poisoning are caused by bacteria which arise from animal, human or environmental sources. Viral infections are unlikely to be from animals and may be due to direct human contamination or indirectly through the environment, e.g. from shellfish contaminated by discharged human sewage.

Bacterial food poisoning may take one of two forms: infection with living organisms or intoxication with pre-formed toxins such as with *Staph. aureus*. The feature which chiefly distinguishes the two types clinically is the incubation period, that is the interval between eating the food and the development of symptoms. Where *pre-formed toxins* are present, the conditions are somewhat analogous to chemical poisoning and symptoms will develop very rapidly, usually within a few hours. If *living organisms* are ingested, time will elapse before their multiplication in the body has proceeded sufficiently to provoke the usual reactions of diarrhoea and vomiting.

A summary of bacterial causes of food poisoning is given in Box 14.1.

**Box 14.1** Bacterial causes of food-borne infection.

| Agent | Normal incubation period | Normal duration | Main clinical symptoms | Commonly associated foods |
|---|---|---|---|---|
| *B. cereus* emetic toxin | 1–5 hours | < 24 hours | Vomiting | Cereals, rice |
| *B.cereus* enterotoxin | 8–16 hours | < 24 hours | Abdominal pain, diarrhoea | Cereals, rice |
| *Campylobacter* spp. | 3–5 days | 2–7 days | Abdominal pain, diarrhoea (sometimes bloody), headache, fever | Poultry, cooked meats, milk |
| *Cl. botulinum* | 12–36 hours | Extended | Swallowing difficulties, perhaps as respiratory failure | Preserved foods, e.g. canned, bottled |
| *Cl. perfringens* | 10–12 hours | 24 hours | Abdominal pain, diarrhoea | Stews, roasts |
| *E. coli* O157 | 12 hours–10 days | Possibly extended | Abdominal pain, diarrhoea (may be bloody). May lead to renal failure | Beefburgers, meat, dairy products |
| *Listeria monocytogenes* | 3–21+ days | Varies | Fever, headache, spontaneous abortion, meningitis | Soft cheeses, patés, poultry meat |
| *Salmonella* spp. | 12–36 hours | 2–20 days | Abdominal pain, diarrhoea, fever, nausea | Meat, poultry, eggs, dairy products |
| *Staph. aureus* | 2–6 hours | 12–24 hours | Vomiting, abdominal pain, diarrhoea | Cooked meat, human source |
| *Vibrio parahaemolyticus* | 12–24 hours | 1–7 days | Abdominal pain, watery diarrhoea, headache, vomiting fever | Shellfish |
| *Yersinia enterocolitica* | 3–7 days | 1–3 weeks | Acute diarrhoea, abdominal pain, fever and vomiting | Pig meat products |

## *Salmonella* spp.

The salmonellae constitute a large group of over 2200 different serotypes, although only 100–200 different serotypes are identified in any one year in the UK. They are members of the Enterobacteriaceae, are Gram-negative, and can readily grow on a wide range of media including foods. They are temperature sensitive and readily destroyed by cooking.

The different serotypes are identified by means of the somatic (O) and flagellar (H) antigens using the Kauffmann–White serotyping scheme'. Further sub-typing can be carried out by phage typing and, increasingly, molecular methods such as plasmid profiling.

Some salmonellae usually only affect a single animal species including, for example, *S. typhi* in humans, *S. dublin* in cattle and *S. pullorum* in poultry. This is not absolute and cases of human infection with *S. dublin* do occasionally occur, often as a serious systemic invasive infection. Most salmonella species including those associated with food poisoning, can infect many species of animal, although they may not cause illness in all of these. A good example of this is *S. enteritidis*, now the most common salmonella in humans, which is widespread, but usually causes no illness in poultry.

While not as resistant as the spore-forming organisms such as the *Clostridium* spp.,

*Salmonella* spp. can exist for many months in the environment, especially if protected from extremes of temperature and sunlight. This means that recycling through the environment is an important route for animal (and human) infection (Fig. 14.7).

This ability of salmonella to exist within different self-contained compartments makes eradication difficult. Control is a more practical option, although specific salmonellae such as *S. pullorum* have to all intents and purposes been eradicated in commercial poultry. There is considerable ongoing effort being expended by the poultry industry to reduce salmonellae causing human illness, in particular *S. enteritidis*.

### *Infection in humans*

The incubation period in people is variable but is usually between 12 and 36 hours. The typical presenting symptom is diarrhoea but this may be accompanied by nausea and abdominal pain, although vomiting is not usual. There may also be a headache and fever. While the infection is normally self-limiting and does not require antibiotic treatment, occasionally, with more invasive salmonellae such as *S. virchow*, bacteraemia can occur. The infection is rarely fatal in people.

Until the late 1980s, when campylobacter infections increased, salmonella was the most common bacterial pathogen isolated from human cases of intestinal infection. During the 1990s over 30 000 laboratory isolates were reported each year in the UK. Prior to 1986 *S. typhimurium* was the most common serotype reported. However, since then *S. enteritidis*, in particular *S. enteritidis* phage type 4, has predominated and this single serotype in 1996 accounted for over 60% of all human cases of salmonella. This type is largely associated with poultry.

Other serotypes are much less common, with the exception of *S. typhimurium*, which is widespread in different animal species, particularly cattle. During the 1980s, *S. typhimurium* DT 204c was the major animal salmonella, affecting mainly calves. It occasionally caused human infection, usually in people in direct contact with infected livestock. Since the beginning of the 1990s this salmonella type has largely disappeared but has been replaced by *S. typhimurium* DT 104, a major pathogen of cattle of all ages and most other animal species.

Unlike *S. typhimurium* DT 204c, it is also an important human pathogen accounting for about 15% of all human salmonella infections. The difference between *S. typhimurium* 204c and *S. typhimurium* DT 104 is partially explained by the opportunities for the organisms to enter the food chain as a consequence of infection in slaughter cattle, even though they may show no signs of infection.

### *Source of human infections*

People can become infected following a failure of personal hygiene after contact with infected animals (or other infected people). Environ-

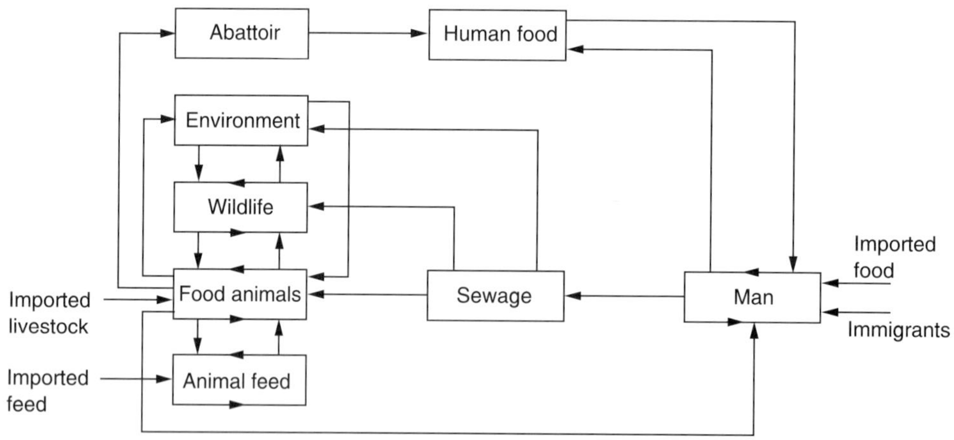


**Fig. 14.7** Salmonella recycling in food animals.

mental contamination, especially *untreated water*, is also important. Most cases are thought to be the result of food-borne infection and highlight the importance of controlling hygiene in the food chain. Meat can become contaminated during the slaughter process either from intestinal contents or from faecal contamination on the hide. As with any faecally-spread organism *it is essential that clean animals are presented for slaughter to help minimise the latter and that the abattoir operates hygienically to prevent both.*

### *Antibiotic resistance*

A particular concern with *S. typhimurium* DT 104 is that it has resistance to many antibiotics and often acquires resistance to others. Most strains are resistant to ampicillin, chloramphenicol, streptomycin, the sulphonamides and tetracycline. Recent resistance additions include resistance to trimethoprim and, of particular concern, to the fluoroquinolones. Resistance to this latter group of antibiotics is a major worry as they are among the drugs of choice for the treatment of invasive salmonella in humans. There is considerable debate as to what factors result in the emergence of antibiotic resistant strains of bacteria, and it is alleged that antibiotic use in animals is part of the problem. Equally the use or misuse of antibiotics, in humans, for example, also lead to the development of antibiotic resistance. The continuing development of antibiotic resistance may lead to sufficient pressure ultimately to restrict the antibiotics available to the veterinary profession for animal treatment.

## ***Campylobacter* spp.**

Campylobacters, although long recognised by veterinarians as a cause of animal disease, were not associated with human enteric infection until 1975. Since then the number of isolates in the UK has steadily increased until they have become the most numerous cause of human bacterial enteric infection. Undoubtedly, improved laboratory methods have contributed to this rise, although, in addition, a true increase has occurred.

The traditional animal strains of *Campylobacter fetus fetus* and *C. fetus venerealis* rarely cause human infection and the most common types in the UK are *C. jejuni* and *C. coli*. Serological subtyping is not as well developed as that for salmonella and most isolates are not further sub-typed. This makes epidemiological investigation very difficult as it is not easy to confirm the origin of human infection.

Unlike many other food-borne organisms *Campylobacter* spp. are fastidious in their growth requirements. They are Gram-negative and microaerophillic, requiring a low oxygen concentration (5%). They are slender, curved and highly mobile and grow best at 42–43°C and not at all below 30°C. They are most unlikely to multiply on food at room temperature. They are not heat resistant and can be killed by cooking. As though to compensate for their inability to grow on food, they have an extremely low infective dose, with as few as 500 cells being sufficient to cause human infection.

### *Infection in humans*

The normal incubation period is 3–5 days, but some evidence exists that this can be considerably extended. A characteristic of infection is acute abdominal pain, which can be so severe as to be mistaken for appendicitis, sometimes precipitating unnecessary surgery. This pain is often accompanied by bloody diarrhoea and fever, but vomiting is rare. Most infections resolve spontaneously within one week while others can be prolonged. Complications during the acute phase are unusual and only exceptionally does death occur. There is, however, increasing evidence that there may be longer-term sequelae to campylobacter infection including both reactive arthritis and even peripheral polyneuropathy (Guillain–Barré syndrome).

In excess of 50 000 infections with *Campylobacter* spp. are now confirmed each year in the UK.

### *Source of human infection*

The lack of a routine discriminatory typing scheme has often hindered investigation of the source of human infections. Unlike salmonellosis, most cases of campylobacter infection are not recognised as part of an outbreak and detailed investigation is not carried out. The exceptions to this are outbreaks associated with milk and water, when hundreds of patients can be involved. In 1995 following contamination of a public water supply with stream water, into which treated sewage was discharged, 711 people reported gastrointestinal illness. *Campylobacter jejuni* of the same molecular type was isolated from a number of those affected. The Advisory Committee on the Microbiological Safety of Food investigated infections with campylobacter and reported in 1993 that poultry was the most common vehicle of infection. However, the types affecting humans can also be isolated from all species of animals (including pets) and a wide range of foods including poultry, milk, water and cooked meats. Person-to-person spread is also important.

The low infective dose for campylobacter means that cross-contamination is a particular risk since a relatively small amount of contamination may be sufficient to establish human infection. This cross-contamination must be prevented throughout the whole food chain.

### *Escherichia coli* O157

Verotoxigenic *E. coli* infections, particularly serogroup O157, were first reported in the UK in 1983. Since then they have become recognised as a major source of human morbidity and mortality.

*E. coli* are ubiquitous inhabitants of the intestinal tracts of animals and man. A variety of serogroups cause infections, usually in a single animal species, for example bowel oedema in pigs. In humans, a number of different disease syndromes are recognised, including:

- Enteropathogenic *E. coli* (EPEC)
- Enteroinvasive *E. coli* (EIEC)
- Enterotoxigenic *E. coli* (ETEC)
- Enterohaemorrhagic *E. coli* (EHEC).

Some of these EHEC have the ability to produce one or more toxins (verotoxins), which can be detected using tissue culture (vero cells), and are often referred to as verotoxin-producing *E. coli* (VTEC). Together with other virulence factors they have the ability to cause human illness but apparently no animal illness. While several serogroups such as O111 and O26 have been involved in the UK, the majority of infections are caused by serogroup O157. In other countries, other serogroups have been reported as more important than O157. As with campylobacter a small infective dose – perhaps as few as 10 cells – is required to cause human illness, but unlike campylobacter they can multiply on food.

#### *Infection in humans*

The low infective dose plays a major part in the spread of these bacteria. Incubation is normally 1–10 days and a considerable spectrum of symptoms can be seen. These range from asymptomatic infection, abdominal pain and diarrhoea, bloody diarrhoea and haemorrhagic colitis to haemolytic uraemia resulting in renal failure. Although the total number of cases, with about 1000 reported each year in the UK, is low, the consequences are serious. In one series of cases in Scotland 59% of cases required hospitalisation, 15% required renal dialysis and 3% died. Serious systemic disease is a particular feature in the old and the young. Following a large milk-borne outbreak in Scotland in 1994, several children required renal transplants. Conversely, many people appear to carry and shed the bacteria yet show no signs of infection.

#### *Source of human infection*

Various studies have identified three main routes of transmission: consumption of contaminated food or water, direct or indirect contact with animals, and person-to-person spread. Beefburgers were recognised as a significant vehicle of infection following a large outbreak across several states in the USA in 1993 in which 732 people were affected and 195 hospitalised with 4 deaths. However, a wide range of foods have been implicated, including apple juice, vegetables, potatoes, bean sprouts and water. Contamination of the food with animal faeces is thought to cause most of the problem.

Early studies in the UK suggested less than 1% of healthy cattle examined at slaughter were excreting *E. coli* O157. When this has been repeated with more sensitive laboratory methods, as many as 40% of cattle have been found to be excreting. Another study demonstrated that 30% of carcases, derived from cattle which were faecally positive in the lairage, were contaminated with *E. coli* O157 in the chill, and 8% of those negative in the lairage were also contaminated. More recent work has shown the presence of VTEC in sheep and goats but not yet in pigs and poultry. Further down the food chain the greatest level of contamination was found in lamb meat products, particularly lamb burgers.

As with all organisms found in animal faeces, control is based on minimising carcase contamination. This begins on the farm by reducing the number of animal carriers, but at present insufficient is known about the natural transmission of *E. coli* O157 to devise a control strategy. *The most important measure is to ensure that only clean animals,* with the minimum of faecal contamination, *are slaughtered.* This was a major recommendation of the Pennington group which reported after a large outbreak in Central Scotland (at Wishaw) in 1996 in which 496 people were affected and 20 elderly people died. Products from a single butcher's premises, including cooked meat, were implicated as the cause of the outbreak.

Slaughter of clean animals must be accompanied by the hygienic operation of the whole slaughterhouse and effective control of the food chain. Ultimately, *thorough cooking* will kill the organisms. The low infective dose means that contamination unlikely to cause problems when *Salmonella* spp. or *Campylobacter* spp. are present may be enough to cause infection if *E. coli* O157 prevails.

### *Yersinia enterocolitica*

*Yersinia enterocolitica* was identified as a human pathogen in the late 1930s. It is a Gram-negative non-spore-forming bacterium which grows over a wide range of temperatures (0–40°C) and optimally at 29°C. The range of growth temperatures allows multiplication at refrigeration temperatures. It is widespread in the intestinal tract of animals and is readily recovered from the environment, including water and soil. It can be divided into biotypes, serotypes and phage types. Different types are associated with different parts of the world. In Europe, serotype O3 is most commonly recorded in humans and is also associated with pigs.

#### *Infection in humans*

The incubation period is about 3–7 days and infection causes acute diarrhoea, abdominal pain, fever and vomiting. It is more common in children, although cases in adults may be followed by longer-term problems including skin rashes and arthritis. Infection is usually self-limiting but, in people with some other underlying pathology, septicaemia with a high mortality may follow. About 500 cases a year are reported in the UK.

#### *Source of human infection*

This organism is often associated with pig meat products, either fresh or cured. The ability to grow at refrigeration temperature means that contaminated food, even if properly chilled, can cause infection. Such foods can also cross-contaminate other foods in the kitchen.

### *Listeria monocytogenes*

Of the several *Listeria* species only *L. monocytogenes* is thought to cause human infection. It is widely distributed in animals, birds, humans and the environment but has only been recognised as a food-borne pathogen since the 1980s. Like *Yersinia* spp., *L. monocytogenes* can grow at a wide range of temperatures (0–42°C) and especially well at 30–37°C. *Listeria* spp. can also grow slowly at refrigeration temperatures. A wide range of serotypes exist, but most human infection is associated with types 4 and 1/2.

#### *Infection in humans*

Most human cases are sporadic and the extended incubation period (several weeks) can make identification of the source very difficult. Unlike the case with most food-borne pathogens, the illness produced is systemic rather than intestinal. Most infected people are symptomless and as many as 5% of the population are faecally excreting at any one time. Illness is most likely to be seen in people with reduced immunity, when the symptoms range from a 'flu-like' illness through fever and septicaemia. There is a particular risk to pregnant women (who have a naturally reduced immune capability) and the unborn child, when the mortality can be as high as 30%.

Although there was a significant rise in reported cases of listeriosis in the late 1980s, this was not maintained in subsequent years. Listeriosis is now relatively uncommon, with about 100 cases reported each year in the UK.

### *Source of human infection*

This is often not identified because of the length of the incubation period. The organisms are ubiquitous and widespread in animals and the environment. Listeriosis can cause animal disease, including abortion in ewes and meningitis in younger sheep. A wide range of foods have been implicated including cheese, paté and poultry meat. Vulnerable groups, especially pregnant women and the immunocompromised, are advised not to eat risk foods such as patés and soft cheeses.

## *Clostridium perfringens*

The mode of action of food poisoning with *Cl. perfringens* is through the consumption of large numbers of bacteria which rapidly form enterotoxin in the small intestine. It is a Gram-positive spore former, requiring anaerobic conditions for growth. In the UK a better understanding of food hygiene, in particular the importance of thorough cooking and rapid cooling, has resulted in a decline in the importance of this pathogen.

Five types (A to E) of *Cl. perfringens* are known to exist but only type A has been implicated in food poisoning. The clostridia form part of the normal intestinal flora of animals and are widespread in the environment.

### *Infection in humans*

The rapid production of enterotoxin in the intestine results in a short incubation period of 10–12 hours. The toxin causes diarrhoea and abdominal pain but not usually vomiting. Illness normally lasts 24 hours and is self-limiting. Subsequent complications and death are rare.

### *Source of human infection*

The clostridial spores survive normal cooking, and the heating process may in fact stimulate them to germinate. As food cools, very rapid multiplication can take place, since optimal growth occurs at 43–47°C. The heating process of cooking also drives off oxygen, creating the anaerobic conditions necessary for growth. These conditions are most likely to be found when large volumes of food are cooked and cooled, particularly large joints of meat or stews and casseroles. Thorough reheating (above 75°C) will kill any vegetative cells present and prevent food poisoning. Most cases occur as outbreaks, which may be large and are often associated with hospital or commercial catering. About 50 outbreaks are reported in the UK each year.

## *Staphylococcus aureus*

Unlike most bacterial food poisoning, illness caused by *Staph. aureus* is due to the consumption of preformed toxin and not the bacteria, which may be absent. The toxin is heat-stable and may survive for 1½ hours at boiling temperature, even though the staphylococci themselves are destroyed. Five major enterotoxins are known to be produced (A to E) of which type A is the most common. The Gram-positive cocci can grow over a wide range of temperatures (10–45°C) with the optimum at 35–40°C.

### *Infection in humans*

The presence of preformed toxin results in a short incubation period of 2–6 hours. The symptoms are primarily nausea and vomiting, with additionally diarrhoea. The illness may also be so acute as to cause fainting or collapse. Most patients recover within 12–48 hours.

### *Source of human infection*

*Staph. aureus* infection usually follows contamination from a human source. The organism can cause wound or skin infections and is present in the nose of up to 40% of healthy people. A failure of basic hygiene, including covering skin lesions, results in contamination of food and subsequent multiplication and toxin production. The foods usually implicated are cooked meats, poultry and dairy produce. This has been an uncommon cause of food poisoning in the UK since the 1950s, with around 10 outbreaks reported each year.

### *Clostridium botulinum*

Botulism is one of the most feared causes of food poisoning because, although it is exceptionally rare, it is a severe disease with a high mortality. *Cl. botulinum* is a Gram-positive spore-forming obligate anaerobe producing one or more of seven toxins (A to G). Toxins A, B and E have been associated with human disease. Types A and B are more commonly linked with meat and vegetables, while type E is associated with fish. The toxin is not thermostable and can be destroyed by cooking at 80°C for 30 minutes.

#### *Infection in humans*

The clostridia produce potent neurotoxins and the symptoms reflect muscular paralysis. Symptoms can appear within 2 hours but may take as long as 5 days. There can be an initial short period of diarrhoea with vomiting and subsequent constipation. Blurring or double vision is often the first systemic sign, accompanied by dry mouth and difficulty in swallowing. The patient is usually mentally alert and there is no loss of sensation. Paralysis can extend to the limbs and eventually result in respiratory failure. The effects of the toxin may persist for several months.

#### *Sources of human infection*

*Cl. botulinum* is ubiquitous and can be found on a wide range of foods. Toxin production only takes place when growth occurs. This can happen during preservation processes, such as smoking or fermentation of fish and meat, which result in a suitable anaerobic environment. Improperly bottled or canned foods can also allow growth to take place.

Botulism is very rare in the UK. The first reported outbreak occurred in 1922 in Loch Maree in Scotland when eight people became ill after eating potted duck paste and all died. The largest outbreak occurred in 1989 when 27 cases (one death) were caused by hazelnut yoghurt. In total only 10 outbreaks have been described in the UK.

### *Vibrio parahaemolyticus*

*V. parahaemolyticus* is a Gram-negative rod usually found in sea water where the temperature is above 10°C. It can multiply rapidly at ambient temperatures but is easily killed by cooking.

#### *Infection in humans*

The incubation period is 12–24 hours, after which profuse diarrhoea and abdominal pain develop. Less commonly, fever and vomiting may be present. The symptoms may persist for 7 days.

#### *Source of human infection*

The organism is found in sea waters, especially if the temperature is greater than 10°C. Fish and shellfish from affected waters may cause illness if inadequately cooked or if subsequently recontaminated. It is rarely acquired in the UK, although one incident involving locally-caught crab was reported on the south coast of England.

### *Bacillus cereus*

*B. cereus* has been recognised as an uncommon cause of food poisoning since the 1970s. It is a Gram-positive, spore-forming, motile bacillus producing two different toxins. A heat-sensitive enterotoxin causes a diarrhoeal illness, while the heat-stable 'emetic' toxin causes vomiting. The spores are heat-resistant and can survive normal cooking temperatures. The bacteria are widespread in the environment, including soil and water, and consequently contaminate many foods, particularly dry foods such as cereals. Any food such as meat, dairy products and vegetables can be vehicles of infection.

#### *Infection in humans*

The two toxins produce different disease syndromes. The more common illness is vomiting caused by the 'emetic' toxin after an incubation period of 1–5 hours. This is particularly associated with rice and pasta. The diarrhoeal illness caused by the enterotoxin has an incubation period of 8–16 hours. Both forms of infection usually last no longer than 24 hours and complications are rare.

*Source of human infection*

Many foods are contaminated with a few spores and these can survive the initial cooking. If food is subsequently kept at ambient temperature, the spores germinate and the vegetative cells multiply rapidly, producing toxin in the food. The 'emetic' toxin is not destroyed by further heating, but the enterotoxin can be inactivated by thorough reheating. This latter toxin can, however, also be produced in the intestine of the patient following consumption of the vegetative cells. The disease is controlled by keeping cooked foods either hot or at refrigeration temperatures. About 30 outbreaks a year are described in the UK.

The protozoa, *Toxoplasma gondii, Giardia lamblia* and *Entomoeba histolytica* are also causes of food poisoning.

## MANAGEMENT OF FOOD POISONING

The investigation and management of outbreaks of food-borne illness in the UK is a shared responsibility between Health Authorities and Local Authorities. These act under specific legislation contained in the Public Health (Control of Disease) Act 1984 and the Food Safety Act 1990. It is this latter act which gives powers to the Local Authority, which has the statutory duty to enforce food safety.

While the responsibility extends to all cases of food poisoning, not surprisingly most effort is expended on the management of outbreaks. However, where the disease is particularly serious, e.g. involving *E. coli* O157 or botulism, the same extent of investigation and management would be carried out.

The objectives of any investigations are three-fold:

1 To prevent any further cases arising from the specific outbreak by identifying and removing the food source.
2 To control further spread, by person to person, from those already infected.
3 To use the information to reduce the likelihood of further outbreaks.

The first of these may be of limited value in a point source outbreak such as a single meal, e.g. at a wedding. However, it is important to identify the source of infection to ensure that the vehicle does not have a wider distribution, e.g. via a widely-distributed product such as cheese, baby infant powder or salami.

Clinical management is important for infections such as campylobacteriosis which can readily be passed from person to person.

The investigations assist the identification of foods or practices which may cause future problems and allow controls to be put in place. For example, eggs have been identified as a vehicle for salmonella: advice is then issued to susceptible groups not to eat lightly-cooked eggs. Similar outbreak investigations highlighted the role of beefburgers as a vehicle for *E. coli* O157 and have led to improved controls such as cooking temperatures and times.

Normally when an outbreak is identified, an 'Outbreak Control Group' (OCG) is created and this group puts into practice an existing Outbreak Control Plan. The membership of the OCG will vary depending on the circumstances but will normally include Public Health, Environmental Health and Medical Microbiologists. Other disciplines can be invited to attend as necessary, e.g. a veterinarian from the State Veterinary Service. It is the role of the OCG to ensure the proper investigation and control of the outbreak, including determination whether there is an outbreak; collection of histories – clinical and food from patients; and collection of samples – stools and faeces.

In some outbreaks the food is immediately identifiable, whereas in others there may only be a statistical association after extensive investigation, e.g. by a case control study. In many outbreaks no food is identified as being responsible.

Often a standard *investigation form* is used to gather the large amount of information required, an example of which is shown in Box 14.2.

The initial information allows a hypothesis to be formed with regard to the source of the outbreak. This can be confirmed microbiologically or epidemiologically by analysis of the data, including food-specific attack rates, odds ratio, etc. Software is available which will not only generate the questionnaires but create the database and carry out the analysis. This is available as a public domain package produced by WHO and CDC Atlanta (Epi Info).

**Box 14.2a**

| Case Ref No | General Outbreak | | Household Outbreak | | Sporadic Case | | Aetiological Agent |
|---|---|---|---|---|---|---|---|
| Name ........................................ | | | G.P. ........................................ | | | | Health Board |
| Address ........................................ | | | Address ........................................ | | | | |
| ............ Tel ........................................ | | | .................... Tel ........................................ | | | | Local Authority |
| Notification by ........................................ | | | Hospital Admission Date ........................................ | | | | |
| Notification date ........................................ | | | Hospital Discharge Date ........................................ | | | | |

DETAILS OF PATIENTS(S) AND HOUSEHOLD

| +ve or -ve | Name | Age | Occupational Details (incl Part time) | Name and Address of Employer/School | Diarrhoea Onset | | Vomiting Onset | | Other Symptoms | Duration of | |
|---|---|---|---|---|---|---|---|---|---|---|---|
| | | | | | Date | Time | Date | Time | | Illness | Incub |
| | | | | | | | | | | | |

Name and details of any other persons similarly affected ____________________

Details of recent travel (including abroad) by <u>any</u> members of household ____________________

**DETAILS OF a) FOOD CONSUMED BY INDEX CASE, AND VENUE, IN 72 HOURS PRIOR TO ONSET OF SYMPTOMS AND b) SOURCE OF PREPARED FOODS PURCHASED FROM COMMERCIAL CATERING OUTLETS DURING 7 DAYS PRIOR TO ONSET**

| DATE | TIME | FOOD AND DRINK | WHERE EATEN | REMARKS |
|---|---|---|---|---|
| | | | | |
| | | | | |

Any type of food not eaten for health, religious or any other reason ____________________

Epidemiological implicated food ____________________ Batch name/Batch No ____________________

Epidemiologically implicated eating outlets of suspected foods ____________________

Details of purchase, storage, preparation, cooking, re-heating etc ____________________

Details of any raw meats, poultry or pet foods prepared in kitchen during 7 days prior to onset ____________________

Place(s) where food apparently contaminated or mishandled ____________________

**Box 14.2b**

**REGULAR AND CASUAL HOUSEHOLD SUPPLIERS OF FOOD**

**(include such details as designation, type, brand name/batch number, fresh, frozen etc)**

| | |
|---|---|
| Milk | |
| Cream | |
| Cheese | |
| Ice cream | |
| Bakery produce | |
| Fish | |
| Shellfish | |
| Meat - raw | |
| Meat - cooked | |
| Meat - tinned | |
| Poultry | |
| Eggs | |
| Fruit | |
| Vegetables | |
| Delicatessen foods | |
| Other | |

**ENVIRONMENTAL FACTORS**

Pets/farm or other animals/vermin ____________________

Water supply - specify: public/private ____________________ Cistern/mains direct ____________________

Source ____________________ Treatment ____________________

Date visited ____________________ Signature ____________________ Designation ____________________

# Part 2 – Meat Microbiology

## BACTERIOLOGICAL EXAMINATION OF CARCASES

In the healthy and physiologically normal animal, those organs which have no direct contact with the exterior may be regarded as virtually sterile, though the actual operation of slaughter and dressing may introduce bacteria to the blood, tissues and organs. These organisms are usually a mixed flora of non-specific organisms of environmental origin but can include *Salmonella, Campylobacter, E. coli* and other food-poisoning organisms. In addition specific pathogens may be present in organs or tissues such as the spleen, muscular tissue or lymph nodes and their presence can only be attributed to a generalised septic or bacteraemic infection in the animal at the time of slaughter. Where such organisms are of intestinal origin, their entry into the systemic circulation may be explained by a breakdown in the natural resistance of the animal with emigration of the organisms from the intestinal tract. Haematogenous invasion may, however, occur from other naturally infected cavities of the body for the same reason. Such systemic invasion is most likely to occur in animals that are ill or exhausted, which should be identified during the pre-slaughter inspection. Subsequent bacteriological examination of the flesh and organs post-mortem would provide definitive material assistance to an inspector charged with assessing the fitness or otherwise of a carcase for human food.

### *Indications for examination*

The examination of food of animal origin for fitness requires the three stages of ante-mortem, gross post-mortem and, where necessary, further laboratory tests.

There is no justification for conducting a bacteriological examination on a carcase or its organs when they exhibit marked pathological changes of a non-infectious nature. Such conditions or evidence of severe systemic disturbance are themselves sufficient to justify condemnation of the carcase. A bacteriological examination can never substitute for a careful organoleptic examination; its value is as a supplementary test to assist judgement when septicaemic or bacteraemic infection is suspected. The only thing to be gained from a bacteriological examination of such overtly unfit material is the identification of the infecting organism – this in itself may be sufficient reason.

A bacteriological examination may be considered obligatory in the case of animals which:

1. have been slaughtered in emergency;
2. have been slaughtered on account of a disease associated with systemic disturbances;
3. show pathological changes on post-mortem inspection that lead to doubt as to the suitability of the meat for human consumption, even though the animal was found healthy on ante-mortem inspection;
4. have been shown by bacteriological tests to have been excreting food-poisoning organisms prior to slaughter, or which emanate from a herd in which the presence of food-poisoning organisms has been officially reported;
5. have not been eviscerated within 1 hour of slaughter or where the parts of the slaughtered animal necessary for post-mortem examination are absent or have been handled in such a way as to make satisfactory judgement impossible;
6. have been slaughtered without the prescribed ante-mortem inspection.

### *Material submitted*

The following samples may be taken for submission to the laboratory for bacteriological examination:

1. Two *complete muscles,* with their fascia, one from a forequarter, and one from a hindquarter, or cubes of muscle, each side measuring not less than 7.5 cm.
2. The *prescapular or axillary lymph node* from the other forequarter of the carcase and the *internal iliac node* from the other hindquarter, including the surrounding fat and connective tissue of the nodes.

3 The *spleen*, which should not be incised except in cases where the organ is considerably enlarged, in which case a piece as large as the hand should be taken.
4 A *kidney*.
5 *In the case of small animals*, the whole *liver* with the gall bladder; in other animals, a portion of liver twice the size of a fist and including the portal vein, or the caudate lobe and including the portal vein, and also the portal lymph nodes and gall bladder.
6 *Parts showing pathological change* and which, in view of their position, are suspected of containing pathogenic bacteria, together with the associated lymph nodes (e.g. in the case of pneumonia a portion of lung and associated lymph nodes).
7 A portion of *small intestine* along with a number of *mesenteric lymph nodes* in those cases where animals have suffered from enteritis and have been reported to be excretors of *Salmonella* organisms, or animals known to emanate from a herd infected with such pathogens.

Laboratory experience has shown that the *liver* frequently contains intestinal bacteria which have gained entry by way of the portal vein. As this invasion may occur after slaughter, the demonstration of organisms in the liver is of no real significance unless the organisms isolated are of a specific pathogenic type. Similarly, the *kidney* should theoretically be of value in bacteriological examinations, but in practice bacterial invasion rarely occurs *post-mortem*.

### *Types of bacteria found*

The bacteria found may belong to a non-specific group that are non-pathogenic or only potentially pathogenic. The most frequently isolated bacteria found on meats and poultry belong to the *Acinetobacter, Aeromonas, Campylobacter, Corynebacterium, Enterococcus, Listeria, Micrococcus, Moraxella, Pseudomonas, Psychrobacter and Vagococcus* genera. Bacteria are present naturally in the intestinal flora and some, such as the non-haemolytic staphylococci, are part of the natural skin flora; their invasion of the bloodstream is of a secondary nature occasioned by some other pathological condition and does not indicate that the animal was affected with a generalised infectious disease.

The bacteria of the specific group regarded as specific pathogens include the haemolytic streptococci, pneumococci, haemolytic staphylococci, *Pasteurella, Salmonella, E. coli, Erysipelothrix insidiosa, Listeria monocytogenes, Campylobacter jejuni, Clostridium perfringens, Yersinia enterocolitica* and *Corynebacterium pyogenes*.

## Laboratory quality assurance techniques of microbiological examination

Provided care is taken in the interpretation of results, microbiological examination of meat is of value in the assessment of wholesomeness; of hygienic methods adopted during slaughter; of dressing and processing techniques and of the efficiency of methods of preservation. It can also indicate the potential shelf-life and help to identify potential health hazards.

One of the difficulties associated with microbiological examination is the lack of a standard technique accepted and applied uniformly between different countries. There are variations in sampling techniques, times of sampling, culture media, parts of carcase to be examined, number of samples, which bacteria to assess, counting methods, etc., all of which require standardisation if comparisons are to be drawn and if the results are to be uniformly interpreted. While it would be useful to have a presence or absence of bacteria approach, the possibility of false positives due to environmental contamination makes this difficult unless special precautions are taken, e.g. use of laminar airflow cabinets.

The bacterial status of the meat is dependent on a number of factors, namely the condition of the animal at slaughter, the spread of contamination during slaughter and the processing and temperature during storage and distribution. Thus, as discussed previously, meat may be contaminated with a range of bacteria which may be significant in spoilage or may be pathogenic. The quality and safety of meat is dictated by the nature and numbers of spoilage and pathogenic species which form the total flora. The microbiology of meat is therefore normally considered under two criteria: *total bacterial counts*, which provide an indication of gross levels of contamination, and *specific counts* of species of spoilage/pathogenic bacteria of significance.

Before microbiological analysis can be carried out it is necessary to obtain samples from the carcase under investigation. This may be achieved by taking either superficial or deep samples, or both if necessary. *Superficial samples* may be taken by removing thin slices, by rinses, swabs or adhesive tape, or by the agar sausage and impression plate techniques. A rapid, but relatively inaccurate, indication of the number and types of microorganisms present on the surface is acquired by pressing microscope slides against the surface which are then either pressed on to a growth medium for culture or fixed and stained on the slide.

Superficial samples provide an indication of the levels of surface contamination present on the carcase. Surface contamination may originate from contact with contaminated surfaces, tools, operatives and airborne contamination. These organisms are all environmental in origin and generally contain the organisms which will form a spoilage flora – *Pseudomonas*, lactic acid bacteria, members of the family Enterobacteriaceae, *Moraxella, Brochothrix, Acinetobacter* and *Alteromonas*.

### *Deep samples*

Deep samples are used to determine the levels of systemic contamination/infection within a carcase. Such contamination is not normally of environmental origin, having resulted from pre-existing disease or infection. Bacteria isolated from deep samples tend to be pathogenic in nature. Deep samples of meat must be taken with care in order to avoid contamination by superficial organisms. Such samples can be obtained using sterile scalpels and forceps or, in the case of frozen meat, a cork borer or an electric drill fitted with a bore-extracting bit. The surface should first be prepared by flaming, followed by an aseptic dissection of about 10 g of meat.

### *Surface slices*

A known weight (usually 10 or 25 g) is removed with sterile scalpels and forceps, then homogenised in a suitable diluent, e.g. Ringer's solution, using a stomacher or other means, to provide a 1:10 dilution before plating on appropriate culture media.

### *Rinses and washes*

Rinses and washes are prepared by washing or rinsing one part by weight of the meat in 10 parts by weight of the sterile diluent. This method is suitable for sausages, beefburgers, whole poultry, etc. Samples of 1:10 dilutions may also be prepared from comminuted forms of the meat since surface washing and rinsing do not give a true picture of the degree of contamination.

The United States Department of Agriculture has mandated a rinse method for sampling poultry carcases for generic *E. coli* as a tool to verify process control. The method requires the poultry carcase, randomly selected after the chill tank at the end of the drip line, to be placed in a 3.5-litre stomacher bag and have 400 ml (in the case of domestic fowl, 600 ml for turkeys) of Butterfield's phosphate diluent poured over it. The bag is then given 30 shakes, taking approximately 1 minute; the bird is removed and 30 ml of diluent is decanted. Counts, established by any validated laboratory method, of over 1000 cfu/ml are considered to be unsatisfactory (cfu = colony-forming unit).

### *Swabs*

Swabs are usually made of sterile non-absorbent cotton wool, 4 cm in length and 1–1.5 cm thick, wound on a sterile thin stick or stainless steel wire and kept in a sterile plugged alloy tube. They are used in conjunction with a sterile template with an opening of defined area, often 100 $cm^2$. The swabs are moistened in dilute (25%) Ringer's solution and applied to the meat surface, using the template; the exposed area is swabbed first in one direction and then at right angles to the original direction. The swabs are then placed in the tubes and, before plating out, 10 ml of 25% Ringer's solution is added to each tube, the swab being rinsed in this solution 10 times. Rinsings (1 ml) are used to prepare plate counts and dilutions can be prepared as required. Colony counts are recorded as the number per square centimetre of surface. The culture medium is usually cooled nutrient agar or other agar medium. The counts are recorded as the number per square centimetre of surface swabbed.

### *Sponges*

As an alternative to swabs, sponges may be used. Such a method is authorised by the

United States Department of Agriculture to verify process control for cattle and pig slaughter by determining the number of generic *E. coli* on carcases sampled in the chillers. Three areas, each of 100 cm$^2$ determined using a sterile 10 cm × 10 cm template, on each carcase are sampled using the sponge, which has been moistened with 10 ml of sterile Butterfield's phosphate diluent. After wiping each of the three sites 10 times horizontally and 10 times vertically, the sponge is placed in a sterile plastic bag with 15 ml of the diluent. Counts, established by any validated technique, of greater than 100 cfu/cm$^2$ for cattle and greater than 10 000 cfu/cm$^2$ for pigs are considered to be unsatisfactory.

*Adhesive tape*

Adhesive tape or labels are used to take superficial samples by pressing a standard area against the surface and then removing it immediately. The tape is pressed against the culture medium and then removed and discarded. The medium is incubated for 24 h at 37°C.

*The agar sausage*

The agar sausage method has proved simple, reliable and valuable. The medium required is poured into a sterile cylindrical plastic casing to fill it. A casing with a diameter of 7.5 cm is suitable for animal carcases but a smaller diameter may be preferred for poultry. The sausage is then placed into a larger casing, the mouth of which is tied firmly, and the whole is sterilised by steaming for 30 min on two successive days, thus ensuring that not only vegetative forms but also bacterial spores are destroyed.

Various *media* may be used in the sausage: nutrient or blood agar for total counts, neutral red lactose agar for *E. coli*, brilliant green phenol red lactose agar for *salmonellae*, and malt agar for *yeasts* and *moulds*. In the assessment of the efficiency of the hygienic procedures in an abattoir it may be considered that the essential tests should be for: (a) total bacterial count, (b) presence of *salmonella* organisms and (c) the presence of faecal *coli*. The method cannot be used for assessing contamination due to anaerobic organisms.

The test is carried out by folding back the outer plastic container and cutting the end of the inner sausage to present a smooth flat surface. The blade is flamed prior to the making of the cut, and between successive cuts is kept immersed in 70% alcohol to avoid contamination during slicing. The cut surface of the sausage is applied to the surface to be tested for 1 second. A slice about 1.5 mm deep is cut from the exposed end and, contact surface uppermost, transferred immediately into a Petri dish. The Petri dish and media are then incubated for 24 h at 37°C. The large surface of the medium renders it easy to count the bacterial colonies.

*Impression plates*

Impression plates are commercial developments of the agar sausage contact method. They consist of sterile, disposable, lidded plastic plates with an inner well filled with agar medium with a convex meniscus which can be pressed against the surface to be sampled.

Perhaps the greatest difficulty associated with any contact method of sampling is that if the organisms are present in high concentration the confluent bacterial growth makes interpretation of the sample impossible. This situation is considerably worsened if any of the organisms present are motile, such as members of the *Proteus* genus. As a result, non-contact methods involving the removal of a small representative sample from the carcase or organ for subsequent analysis form the most frequently employed approach. These samples are analysed as described below.

## Microbiological analysis

The meat sample or the rinse from swabs or sponges form the basis for the microbiological analysis. The solid samples are homogenised in a suitable quantity of diluent to suspend the organisms. A dilution series is then prepared by decimally diluting this original bacterial suspension. This dilution series ensures the growth plates are not subsequently overgrown by a large inoculum of bacteria. All suspensions are then plated out on a suitable growth medium.

A general growth medium such as a total count agar (TCA) will allow the growth of almost all organisms present that are capable of growth under the selected incubation

# PLATE 1

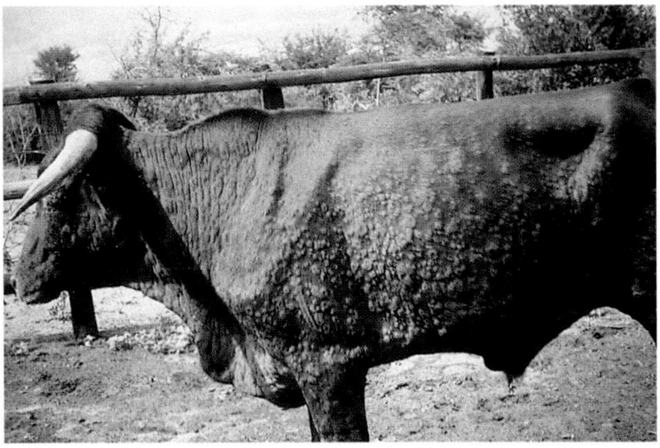

**Fig. 1** Lumpy skin disease. Bovine.

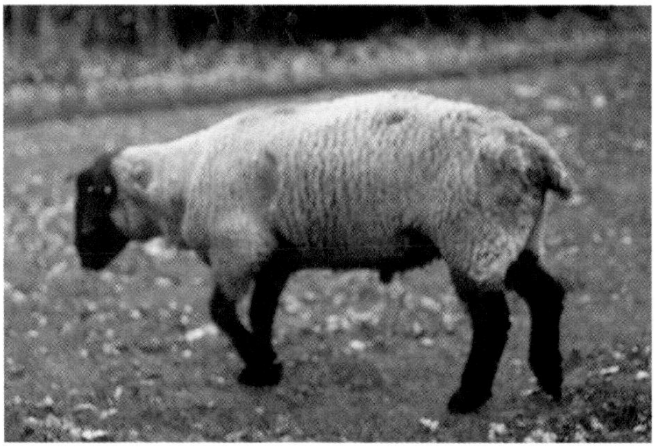

**Fig. 2** Scrapie. Ram.

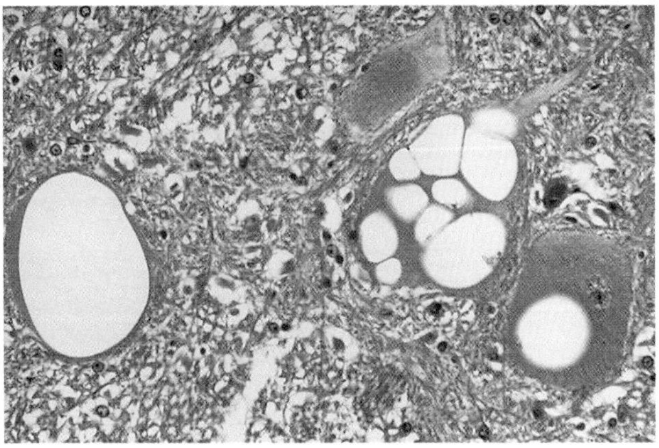

**Fig. 3** Scrapie. Lesions in vestibular nucleus of brain.

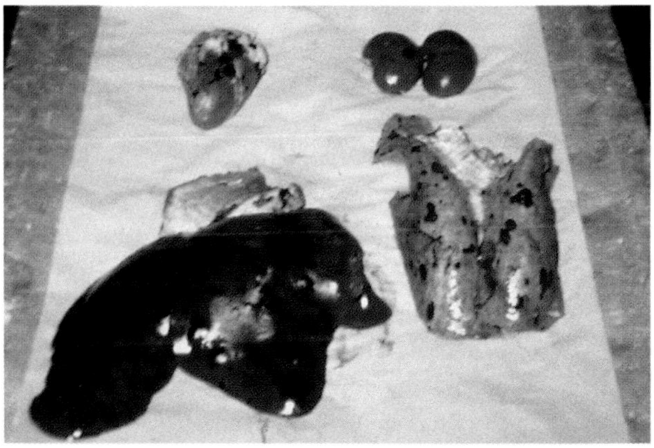

**Fig. 4** Melanosis. Liver, lungs, kidney and heart. Sheep.

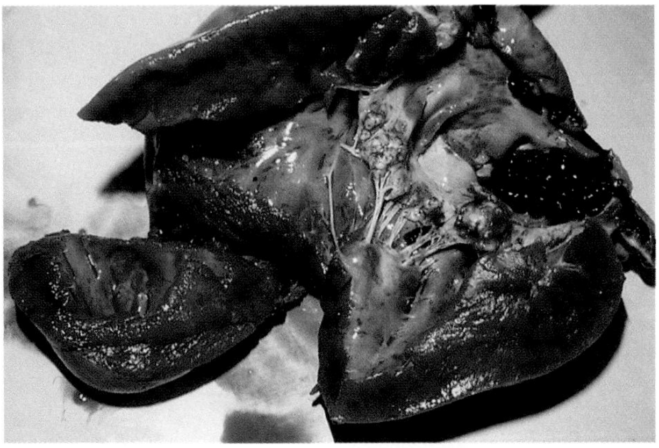

**Fig. 5** Endocarditis. Heart. Bovine.

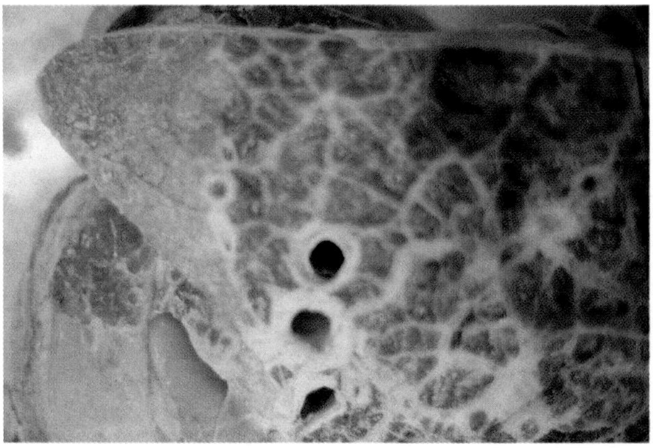

**Fig. 6** Contagious bovine pleuropneumonia. Lung. Bovine.

# PLATE 2

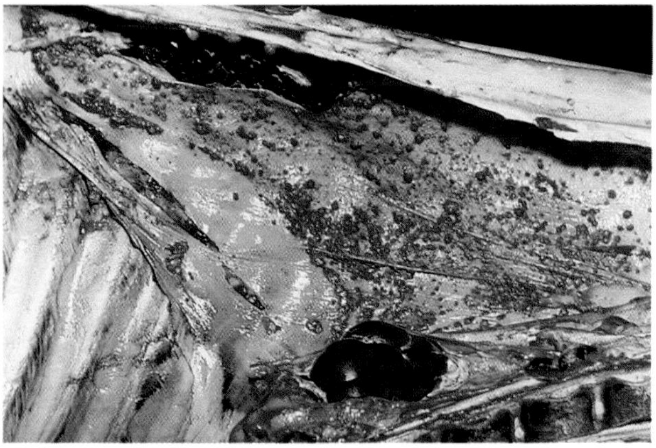

**Fig. 7** Lymphosarcoma. Peritoneum. Bovine.

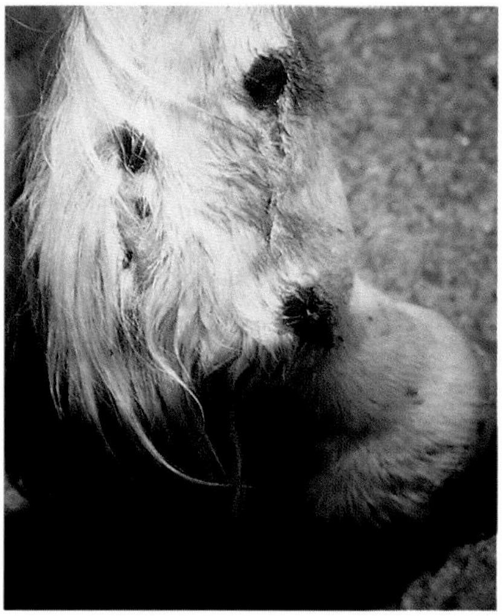

**Fig. 8** Epizootic lymphangitis. Leg. Horse.

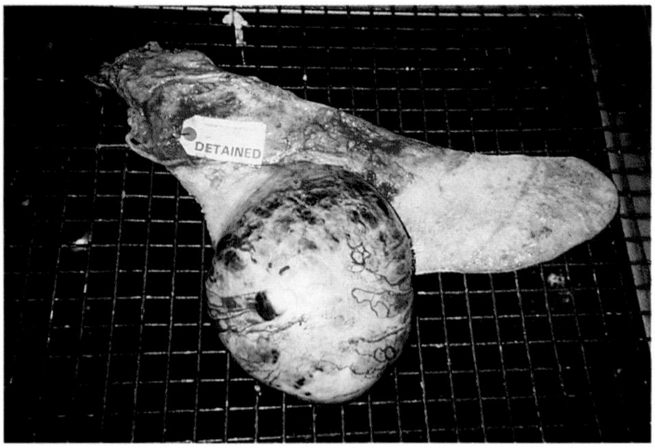


**Fig. 9** Haematoma. Spleen. Bovine.

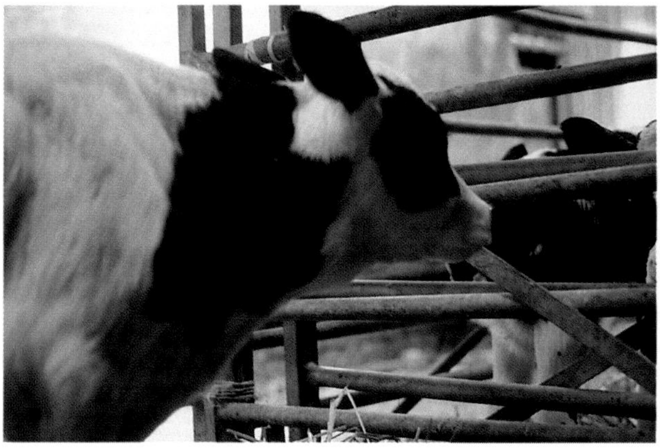

**Fig. 10** Goitre. Thyroid. Calf.

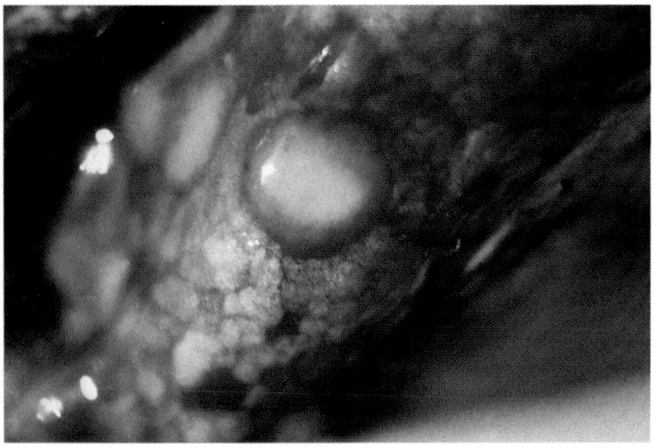

**Fig. 11** Goat pox. Tail. Goat.

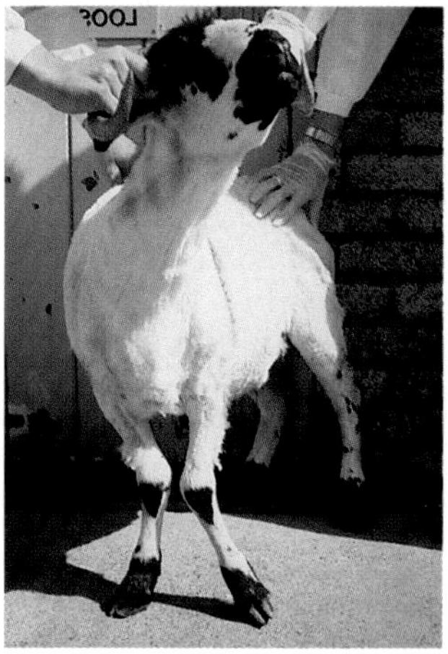

**Fig. 12** Vitamin D deficiency. Sheep.

conditions. TCA is normally incubated aerobically at 20°C and 35°C to assess the levels of mesophilic Gram-positive and Gram-negative organisms present. The plated samples can also be incubated anaerobically to assess anaerobic and facultative anaerobic populations. On completion of incubation the number of organisms per gram of sample or per $cm^2$ may be back-calculated depending on the original sample size and the levels of dilution employed. The colonies on these primary plates can be subcultured to purify bacterial colonies in order to help identify the organisms.

The medium used for growth may be selected specifically to provide information on one particular group/genus of pathogens or spoilage bacteria. Thus, specific agars have been developed for almost every pathogen based on the resistance of those particular pathogens to certain antimicrobial substances. For example, *Listeria monocytogenes* is resistant to naladixic acid, cycloheximide, acriflavine and fosfomycin, and the inclusion of these in the media (Oxoid) restricts the growth of contaminating organisms, allowing a determination of the levels of these target organisms.

Despite being both simple and cheap the *plate count* procedure is not an ideal method for measuring bacterial numbers. The most significant drawback is the time interval before a result is obtained. The incubation period necessary for the development of visible colonies is dependent on a number of factors and may range from 2 to 7 days. In addition, the precision and accuracy of this technique are low, with errors originating from sampling, preparation of dilutions and counting of colonies. In practical terms it is only possible to test a proportion of the product and it must be assumed that this sample is representative of the carcase as a whole. Analytical accuracy also contributes to low levels of reproducibility, and variations in incubation conditions such as time, temperature and humidity may also result in large variations in the results obtained. Thus manually completed plate counts are only accurate $\pm 2\log_{10}$.

In an attempt to improve on the rapidity, accuracy and reliability of the plate count procedure, a number of developments have attempted to automate the plate count procedure, thus removing operator error as a source of inaccuracy. These include media preparators, automatic dilution and spiral plate makers. Automatic video-based colony counters are also available. These are valuable improvements but are, of course, expensive to buy and operate and there is still an unacceptable time delay in obtaining results associated with the analysis incubation time.

In an attempt to reduce the time required to make accurate and meaningful results available, a number of *rapid methodologies* have been developed. These include the use of hydrophobic grid membranes, bioluminescence, electrical methods, radiometry, microcalorimetry, biochemical reactions, immunological and serological reactions, nucleic acid (DNA) probes, DNA amplification (polymerase chain reaction) and flow cytometry. It is outside the scope of this chapter to consider each in detail. However, in general, while these developments must be welcomed, they lack the general applicability and field robustness of the plate count procedure. In addition there are also question marks over the interpretation of the results produced, and they involve considerable capital investment and usually require skilled personnel to operate them. Thus despite the many problems associated with plate count procedure it probably represents the best compromise between cost and performance and is the method which is most widely accepted – in fact it is the standard against which all other techniques are compared.

## Bacteriological standards for meats

Various authorities, for example the EU, WHO and the Codex Alimentarius Commission have attempted to lay down acceptance criteria for different types of meats. Although, as yet, there are no universally accepted criteria for the interpretation of bacteriological findings, the following are frequently used:

- *Microbiological standards*, which are mandatory criteria with legal backing;
- *Microbiological specifications*, which are generally contractual agreements between a manufacturer and a purchaser to check whether the foods are of the required quality;
- *Microbiological guidelines*, which are non-mandatory criteria usually intended as a guide to good manufacturing practice.

The International Commission on Microbiological Specifications for Foods (ICMSF of the International Association of

Microbiological Societies) has stated that any microbiological criterion for a food should contain the following information:

1 A statement of the microorganisms and/or toxins of concern.
2 Laboratory methods for their detection and quantification.
3 The sampling plan.
4 The microbiological limits.
5 The number of samples required to conform to these limits.

The ICMSF recommended that the *total viable count* at 35°C (or at 20°C in the case of chilled meats) should be less than $10^7$/g and that *Salmonella* should be detected in not more than one of five 25 g samples. The ICMSF also recommended that *frozen poultry* when examined by rinsing should give a count at 20°C of less than $10^7$/ml of the rinsing solution and that *Salmonella* should be detected in not more than one of five 25 g samples of the poultry meat.

These microbiological techniques may also be used to assess the nature and degree of bacterial contamination on walls, floors, equipment and fittings and the hands and clothing of personnel. Tests at various operational stages, e.g. at the beginning and end of work and after cleansing procedures, should provide criteria which can be reasonably maintained under everyday conditions. The results should be interpreted carefully and allowance made for factors such as the time of year, time of day, type of stock being handled, cleanliness of animals, staff quality, etc.

While microbial counts form the basis of food microbiological analysis, they are defective indicators for the following reasons:

1 Bacteria in food are not stable like heavy metals; their populations change constantly. Different strains of bacteria vary in toxin and allergen production and in invasiveness:
2 Food usually contains a variety of microorganisms, some or all of which may enhance or inhibit each other:
3 Time of sampling, usually at plant or retail shop, gives no indication of the final microbial count in the consumer's home, long after sale:
4 The number of organisms or amount of toxin or allergen which affect man is not known:
5 Environmental conditions, e.g. temperature, pH and type of sampling, markedly influence bacterial growth:
6 Counting of microbes is a cumbersome and time-consuming procedure.

To remove the reliance on end-product testing, hazard analysis systems were developed. *HACCP* (*Hazard Analysis and Critical Control Point*), is a systems approach to assuring product safety. It is based on identifying and monitoring the most critical points in the production process rather than relying on testing the final product. The Commission of the European Union has produced a Code of Good Hygiene Practices which gives indications on the microbiological checks on the general hygiene of conditions of production in establishments producing fresh meat, giving specifications on the nature of these controls, their frequency as well as the sampling methods and the methods for bacteriological examination.

## DECOMPOSITION AND SPOILAGE

Decomposition is the breaking up of organic matter, chiefly protein, but also fats and carbohydrates, by the action of bacteria, moulds and yeasts, which split the meat up into a number of chemical substances, many of which are gaseous and foul-smelling. All forms of foods in their natural state remain in a fresh and edible state for only a comparatively short time. Foods are rapidly contaminated by bacteria, moulds or yeasts, which are the main causes of spoilage or decomposition. Before terminal decomposition changes occur, however, other factors such as enzyme action and oxidation take place in some foods.

Present in all living cells are *enzymes* which catalyse the complicated chemical reactions taking place in the cells. The process of *autolysis* – self-destruction or self-degradation – is essentially brought about by enzymes and at a rate which varies markedly in the different tissues. In general it is highest in those tissues in which protein is synthesised in large amounts and which have high water contents, e.g. gastrointestinal mucosa, testes, pancreas and adrenals. The *water contents* of some types of meat and offal are given in Table 14.6. Tissues such as the liver, kidneys and endocrine glands

**Table 14.6** Water content of meat and offal.

| | g water/100 g |
|---|---|
| Liver, ox, raw | 73.3 |
| Chicken breast, raw | 73.7 |
| Beef steak, raw | 68.3 |
| Chicken, boiled | 61.0 |
| Beef, corned, canned | 58.5 |
| Bacon, Danish, tank-cured | 46.9 |
| Bacon, English, dry-cured | 36.3 |
| Meat, dehydrated | 7.5 |

have slower autolytic rates and the tissues with the lowest metabolic rates such as skin, muscles, bone, heart and blood vessels have the lowest autolytic rates of all.

All forms of food are subject to natural deterioration, their shelf-life being dependent on their structure, pH, composition, water content, presence or absence of bacteria and/or damage and conditions of storage. It is accepted that meat from fatigued animals spoils faster. The *pH* of the meat from these animals, on the completion of rigor mortis, is in the region of 6.5 rather than the normal value in a rested animal of around 5.6. An adverse (usually low) pH slows the growth of bacteria grown outside their optimal pH range by slowing down the functioning of the enzyme systems and the transport of nutrients into the microbial cells.

Bacteria, moulds and yeasts in turn are affected by factors such as temperature, moisture, availability of oxygen, nutrients and the presence or absence of growth inhibitors. Control of one or more of these factors inhibits microbial growth and lengthens the shelf-life. In addition to microbial spoilage, physical damage which occurs during handling, transportation and processing can be regarded as a form of spoilage, as can the presence of insects, other pests and chemicals. Foods damaged in this way are more susceptible to change by microbial action.

Fresh meats may be initially contaminated from many different sources – soil, dust, faeces, water, equipment – the hands and clothing of personnel subsequently adding to this. And although it was originally thought that the flesh of healthy animals at slaughter was sterile, it is now known that it can harbour organisms, mostly Gram-positive mesophiles. Depending on the types of bacteria present, meat-borne disease or spoilage or both may result, especially if substandard handling methods are adopted.

The various forms of food preservation are designed to prevent decomposition by limiting the activity of enzymes, the process of oxidation and bacterial spoilage.

The main types of bacteria involved in the spoilage of meat belong to genera listed below with their characteristics.

## Gram-positive organisms

1 *Micrococcus*. Some are salt tolerant, some thermoduric and some psychrophilic. Cause spoilage of salted and chilled meats. Optimal growth temperature, 25–30°C.

2 *Staphylococcus*. *Staph. albus* is responsible for spoilage and *Staph. aureus* for food poisoning. Salt tolerant. Optimum temperature 37°C but can grow below this temperature.

3 *Streptococcus*, e.g. *Str. faecalis*, *Str. faecium*, *Str. durans*. Wide temperature range for growth, 10–45°C. Some degree of salt tolerance.

4 *Lactobacillus*. Mainly mesophilic with some thermoduric and psychrophilic strains. $a_w$ limit (water activity) value for growth – 0.91. Can grow at pH of less than 4.5.

5 *Leuconostoc*. Can produce slimes especially in high-sugar foods. Some are salt tolerant and some can elaborate flavours due to diacetyl production.

6 *Bacillus*, e.g. *B. subtilis* (mesophilic), *B. thermophilus* and *B. coagulans* (thermoduric). Very active biochemically with strains that are saccharolytic (able to split carbohydrates), proteolytic and lipolytic. Some forms can cause flat sours in canned meats. Limit of $a_w$ value for growth is 0.95.

7 *Clostridium*. Originate from soil and animal intestine. Proteolytic and putrefactive, e.g. *Cl. sporogenes*, *Cl. histolyticum*. Saccharolytic, e.g. *Cl. perfringens*, *Cl. butyricum*. Limit of $a_w$ value for growth is about 0.95 with no growth at a pH of less than 4.5. An important member is *Cl. botulinum*.

8 *Corynebacterium*. Fine, non-sporing rods. Limit of $a_W$ value for growth, 0.98–0.95. No growth below pH of 4.5. Some strains sensitive to reduced $pCO_2$.

9 *Microbacterium*. Limit of $a_W$ value for growth, 0.98–0.95. No growth below pH 4.5. Psychrotrophic, insensitive to reduced $a_W$ and

able to spoil meat stored at chilling temperature with reduced relative humidity.

Many of the organisms tested above are able to grow under reduced and elevated $pO_2$ (partial pressure of oxygen). The former situation is made use of in vacuum packaging; the latter along with a reduced initial load of spoiling organisms, lowered temperature and $a_W$, and increased $pCO_2$, has enabled chilled meat to achieve a shelf-life of over 6 months within modified-atmosphere packaging.

## Gram-negative organisms

1 *Pseudomonas*. Widely distributed in soil, fresh and sea water and decomposing organic matter. Grow well in protein foods with the production of slime, pigments and odours. Preference is for a high $a_W$. Many are psychrophilic, but temperature range is wide.
2 *Flavobacterium*. Pigmented colonies (orange and yellow) causing discoloration of meat and other foods such as eggs, butter and milk. Some types are psychrophilic.
3 *Acinetobacter*. Able to oxidise ethanol to acetic acid.
4 *Achromobacter*. Similar in action to *Pseudomonas*. Forms slime.
5 *Alcaligenes*. Present in soil, water, dust and manure. An alkaline reaction is produced in some foods, including meat.
6 *Halobacterium*. Obligate halophiles spoiling meats high in salt content.
7 *Moraxella*. Sometimes classified as acinetobacter, e.g. *M. liquefaciens*.
8 *Escherichia*. Abundant in the soil and intestines of man and animals. Commonly found in large numbers in raw foods of animal origin and also in cooked foods that have been contaminated in various ways. *E. coli is* indicative of faecal or sewage pollution. Spoilage of meat by fermentation of carbohydrates to acid and gas causing 'off' odours. The verotoxic strain, *E. coli* O157:H7 is an important food-poisoning bacterium.
9 *Klebsiella*. Non-motile, non-sporing rods. The pathogenic *Salmonella*, *Shigella* and *Proteus* belong to the same group.

The main types of spoilage organisms on chilled fresh meats belong to the above groups, which are responsible for *slime* formation during storage. These particular bacteria are found almost everywhere in nature and it is practically impossible to avoid their contamination of carcases during dressing procedures. The time taken for slime to develop on raw meats is directly related to the initial number of organisms on the carcase surface. It is thus especially important to pay attention to efficient methods of hygiene at slaughter, during carcase dressing, refrigeration, storage and transportation. Chilling procedures do not prevent the activity of spoilage organisms, which can grow at about −7°C; however, temperatures below 2°C will delay the onset of slime formation. Control of the relative humidity in chill rooms, i.e. reducing the $a_W$, can reduce bacterial spoilage, but results in a loss of carcase weight and liability to spoilage by psychrotrophic bacteria (*Micrococcus, Brochothrix, Streptococcus, Lactobacillus*) and some moulds (*Aspergillus, Botrytis, Cladosporium, Fusarium, Thamnidium, Sporotrichum*). A reduced oxygen partial pressure ($pO_2$) in the vicinity of stored meat is of value in curtailing spoilage, as is increased $pCO_2$.

In recent years attempts have been made to counter the adverse action of spoilage bacteria by the use of irradiation, mainly with gamma rays. Using a dose of about 0.1 Mrad immediately before shipping, the storage life of carcases under refrigeration has been prolonged and *salmonellae* eliminated. However, the use of ionising radiation is subject to legislative control in most countries and it is thus used infrequently.

The spoilage process is initially fuelled by the breakdown of carbohydrate. As time passes, however, protein molecules are broken up into simpler substances by acids, alkalis, endogenous enzymes and bacteria, the degree of decomposition varying greatly with the different agencies. Of these agencies the putrefactive bacteria carry the process further, breaking up the protein molecule into proteoses, then peptones, peptides, amino acids, and finally indole, skatol, phenol, together with various gases including hydrogen sulphide, carbon dioxide, methane and ammonia. It is the amino acids, non-toxic in nature, which furnish bacteria with abundant and available nutritive material, and their breakdown products which give the typical appearance and odour of decomposed meat. The recognised everyday signs of decomposition are marked changes of colour to a grey, yellow or green, a softening in the consistency of the tissue, a pronounced repulsive odour and an alkaline reaction caused by the formation of ammonia.

After slaughter of a healthy animal, decomposition eventually develops in the parts exposed to the air, the time taken depending particularly on the temperature and humidity of the environment. The primary surface growth is initiated by aerobic bacteria, among these being *Pseudomonas, Achromobacter* and some coliforms. These organisms extract oxygen from the meat surface and produce conditions suitable for the growth of anaerobic bacteria, e.g. *Clostridium sporogenes,* which can also grow within the deeper tissues where there is no oxygen. After surface putrefaction of meat has commenced, the process spreads gradually by way of the nerve and connective-tissue sheaths and along the surfaces of blood or lymph vessels. The rapidity of the extension of the putrefactive process throughout a carcase is greatly influenced by the condition of the animal before slaughter. In exhausted animals or in those that have suffered from fever (especially from a septic cause) where the meat is alkaline, decomposition sets in very rapidly and quickly reaches the deeper parts.

The condition known in Britain as *'heated beef'*, and in North America as *'sour side'*, is caused by inability of the freshly-killed carcase to dissipate heat rapidly when carcases are hung too close to each other, thus preventing a proper current of air around the sides. This usually affects the prominent areas of the hindquarters and ribs. In mild cases where hot sides of beef have not been in close contact for too long, there is merely a blanching of the surface with no major loss of quality. The condition is also observed in rabbits, hares and game which are packed in hampers or baskets while still warm, and is known in the trade as *green struck.*

In animals that have died and have not been eviscerated, both external and internal decomposition occur simultaneously, owing partly to the high blood content of the meat and partly to the invasion of the abdominal veins by putrefactive bacteria from the intestines. The first bacterium to invade the carcase from the bowels after death is *E. coli,* which in warm weather may reach the joints within 24 hours; these bacteria use up the oxygen in the carcase and pave the way for penetration by anaerobic bacteria, e.g. *Cl. perfringens,* from the bowel. The presence of a greenish hue, first apparent on the kidney fat and peritoneal wall, with the diaphragm soft and flaccid and lying close to the ribs, is a strong indication that evisceration of the animal has been delayed and calls for a severe judgement on the carcase. Lambs coming straight off grass and slaughtered in hot sultry weather have been known to exhibit evidence of incipient decomposition within 1 hour of dressing. Pigs in which evisceration has been delayed, particularly in the summer months, may show a greenness of the abdominal fat in 12 hours, while the kidneys, and also the liver, may exhibit a superficial black coloration; in the kidneys this pigmentation is frequently confined to the anterior poles where blood collects due to hypostasis. This coloration, known as *sulphiding* or *pseudomelanosis,* is due to the formation of iron sulphide by chemical action between hydrogen sulphide from the digestive tract and iron from the blood haemoglobin.

In the case of *shot deer* which cannot be gutted immediately, it is customary among sportsmen to incise the abdominal wall, as a current of air cools the abdominal viscera and delays emigration of putrefactive bacteria from the intestinal tract. Venison, which is particularly rich in connective tissue and therefore exceedingly tough after slaughter, requires conditioning by hanging before it is rendered palatable. It can hang for long periods without decomposition, and it is stated that the muscular tissue of deer possesses antibacterial substances which have an inhibitory action on a great number of putrefactive bacteria as well as on the bacteria responsible for food poisoning; in this way conditioning or ripening can take place in venison unassociated with decomposition.

The smaller animals such as *game* or *hares,* lose heat rapidly after death and at an atmospheric temperature of 16–18.5°C. Small carcases such as rabbits cool to air temperature in about 12 hours, whereas larger carcases such as sheep require about 24 hours. As this rapid heat dissipation inhibits the growth of putrefactive bacteria, it is practicable to consign feathered game and hares to market without removal of the abdominal viscera and packed in crates or baskets.

In British fresh *sausage,* the early stages of decomposition usually take place simultaneously throughout the meat substance, but all the accepted changes associated with decomposition may not be present. Valuable indications of unsoundness in fresh sausage, as distinct from smoked, are stickiness on the surface of the casing; in the early stages, a sour rather than a fetid odour as a result of the activity of lactic acid bacteria and *Brochothrix thermosphactum*; easy separation of the sausage meat from the casing; and a grey colour on section of the sausage. The odour of early decomposition may be detected by a boiling test, especially if a little limewater is added to the water before boiling.

It is important to remember that while the spoilage organisms indicate their presence by off-colours, odours and tastes as well as changes in consistency, most food-poisoning organisms give no indication of their presence in food. Some, such as *Bacillus cereus*, *E. coli*, *Pseudomonas*, *Proteus* and *Citrobacter*, as well as causing spoilage, can also on occasions cause food poisoning. *E. coli* is commonly found in foods of animal origin and is an indication of sewage pollution of water and unhygienic methods of preparation. The factors responsible for the onset of food poisoning (mainly lack of hygiene and careless storage of cooked and uncooked foods at temperatures suitable for bacterial growth) are virtually the same as those that lead to the spoilage of food.

## Decomposition of fat

The problem of *fat rancidity* crops up in the storage of practically every foodstuff. An unpleasant odour or flavour in a fat may be due to absorption of foreign odours, as in the tainting of meat or butter stored in a chamber previously used for fruit, atmospheric oxidation, or the action of microorganisms, which may give rise to extensive hydrolysis of fat. A small amount of free fatty acids, however, has little effect on flavour; it is more likely that the tainted flavour normally accompanying bacterial growth is mainly due to nitrogenous breakdown products of connective tissue.

Rancidity from atmospheric oxidation does not require the presence of microorganisms and is the most common type of deleterious fatty change. The important oxidative lipids in food are the unsaturated fatty acids, particularly oleic, linoleate and linolenate, with the susceptibility and rate of oxidation increasing with their degree of unsaturation. Oxidation continues at low temperature since little energy is required for the biochemical reaction. Exposure to light is another factor which can predispose fatty tissues to oxidation. The natural resistance of some fats, e.g. chicken fat, to the development of rancidity is due to the presence of antioxidants such as vitamin E. Beef and mutton fats are relatively resistant, and cause little trouble except when frozen and stored at −10°C for periods longer than 18 months.

Bacon fat, particularly when exposed to light, is much more susceptible to oxidation. The type of feeding of the bacon pig also affects the rapidity of oxidation, for example, extensive swill feeding produces a soft fat with a high proportion of unsaturated fatty acids which tend to be converted to aldehydes and ketones, imparting the acid flavour associated with rancidity. The rapid onset of rancidity, together with a yellow coloration of the fat, has frequently been observed in carcases of pigs fed on cod liver oil or fish meal. A further deleterious factor in bacon manufacture is that during curing much of the natural resistance of the pig tissues to oxidation is broken down by the specific action of the pickling salts (sodium chloride is known to have a catalytic effect in fat autoxidation), and for this reason bacon fat is more liable to develop rancidity than pork fat. Even at −10°C oxidation of bacon fat is appreciable within a few weeks, though if bacon is smoked subsequently to curing the absorption of phenolic substances confers a certain amount of protection against oxidation during storage. The time factor in the curing of bacon and ham is therefore of particular importance, and bacon which undergoes a long period of manufacture, e.g. Midland cured bacon which takes 3–5 weeks, is more liable to become rancid than Wiltshire bacon which is produced in 2–4 weeks. The still greater length of time taken to manufacture York hams, about 3–6 months, renders it essential that the fat of such hams is of excellent quality, because soft fat, which might be admissible in pork or Wiltshire bacon, will lead to noticeable rancidity before the slowly maturing York ham is ready for the market.

Marked rancidity in pig fat is usually associated with a change in colour of the fat from white to yellow, and the rancid odour may be detected if a piece of fat is rubbed between the hands. Chemical methods of assessing rancidity include the measuring of peroxides produced utilising potassium iodide. The thiobarbituric acid (TBA) test and the Kreis test both rely on the intensity of a colour change to indicate the degree of rancidity which has developed.

As already mentioned, a further factor causing taint in fat is the activity of microorganisms which produce hydrolysis, resulting in the liberation of free fatty acids. Experiments show that the fat of the kidney, brisket and back of the ox develops a taint when the free fatty acids reach 2.5–3.0%. The deep intramuscular fat of meat, as is seen in the marbling of prime beef, is not affected by hydrolysis or atmospheric oxidation and is therefore likely to remain sound for long periods, but the kidney and abdominal fat, being more exposed, is likely to develop rancidity early; it is for this reason that these superficial fats are removed by the retail butcher before the carcase is hung up in the shop. Fats should be regarded with suspicion if they contain over 2% of free fatty acids, although in practice the appearance, odour and flavour are the usual guidelines.

## Bone taint

The rapid dissipation of body heat from a freshly-killed carcase is facilitated when the surrounding air is cool, dry and in rapid circulation. The rate of cooling is slow in heavy carcases owing to their greater thickness and also in those which carry an excessive amount of fat, with the result that a high temperature may persist in the deep-seated musculature of these animals and give rise to deleterious change. This change, known as *bone taint*, is associated with the growth of putrefactive bacteria and occurs most commonly in the region of the *hip joint of the ox and pig*, but occasionally in the *shoulder region of the ox*, especially when ambient temperatures are high. The condition, which was commonly encountered in the days when there was inadequate refrigeration and during the warm summer months, is not a serious problem today.

Bone taint, or deep-seated spoilage of meat, is undoubtedly of bacterial origin. More than one organism may be involved, but the *anaerobic spore-forming bacteria* are the most important and probably emanate from the gut of the animal. It appears likely that the organisms enter the bloodstream before death, rather than during it or at the bleeding stage, and that this entrance is facilitated by pre-slaughter exhaustion, fright, shock or a sudden strain, e.g. the ascent to the top floor of the factory, which predispose the tissues around the head of the femur to bone taint. There is practical evidence that putrefaction can commence in the blood vessels of the bone marrow. The synovial fluid of the hip joint is also a favourable medium for bacterial growth with a pH between 7.0 and 8.0, whereas that of muscle in complete rigor is usually below 6.0. The lymph stream may also be important, for bacteria resembling those in taints have been isolated more frequently from lymph nodes than from bone marrow and muscle. These bacteria may therefore be present in the lymph nodes during life and, under suitable conditions, may spread to the surrounding muscular tissue. The odour of bone taint is apparent in both the musculature around the femur and in the bone marrow; it is very typical, quite unlike that of decomposing meat and resembles the sewage-like smell associated with gut-cleaning. The condition may be associated with a change in the muscle coloration to a grey, or at times a blackish-purple, but frequently the normal red coloration is entirely preserved.

*Bone taint in cattle* can be reduced by avoiding bacterial contamination of the carcase with rapid cooling to 1.5°C. Experimentally, tetracycline injections immediately before slaughter and antibiotic spraying of the carcase can prevent taint. The smaller butcher can aid the dissipation of heat from the freshly-killed carcase of beef by removing the fat from the kidney and the pelvic cavity. Incision of the stifle joint, to promote air access and rapid cooling, will prevent the growth of anaerobic bacteria. To avoid bone taint, the temperature at the centre of the round must not exceed 4.5°C after 48 hours. Bone taint is a local condition requiring condemnation of the affected tissues, but in many cases, when the hip joint or round of beef is affected, generous trimming of the muscle around the femur is all that is necessary.

## Taint in hams

Taint in hams is also known as *souring*, and is attributed by American authorities to contamination by *Clostridium sporogenes*, *Cl.*

*pufrefaciens* and *Cl. putrificum*, which are proteolytic organisms and break down proteins into amino acids and ammonia. The taints in hams and beef are fundamentally similar in origin, being in each case a deep form of decomposition which is unassociated with any surface change. Though the blood, marrow, muscle and bone of normal live pigs are free from ham-souring bacteria, these microorganisms may be present in such tissues soon after slaughter and develop rapidly along connective tissue bands between the muscle bundles. The sticking knife undoubtedly contributes bacteria to the bloodstream, which can be demonstrated experimentally by placing pure cultures of *uncommon* bacteria on the knife blade and isolating them from the tibia and other long bones. The marrow of the femur tends to harbour fewer bacteria than the tibia and, as American authorities note, *'tibia sours'* are much the commoner. Too large a sticking wound also facilitates deep-seated contamination, for the ham-souring bacteria appear to resist the high bactericidal properties of pigs' blood. French experience suggests that heavy eating may be conducive to ham taint as the bacteria then migrate from the intestines – *'la bacteremie habituelle de digestion'*. Other species of bacteria are frequently involved, e.g. faecal streptococci, micrococci and vibrios which are salt-tolerant and *Proteus, E. coli* and *Pseudomonas* which are not salt-tolerant and are associated with 'mis-cured' hams, i.e. hams not properly cured.

A further factor which encourages bacterial growth within the pig carcase is that glycogen is less readily deposited in pig muscle than in other domestic animals, while it is also lost more readily by excitement and fatigue. Pig muscle thus often fails to reach an adequate post-mortem acidity, and the incidence of deleterious bacterial change is therefore high. Adequate and rapid refrigeration of freshly-killed carcases of pork with prompt handling and careful sawing of the shank, together with bacteriological control of the pickling solution have, however, done much to obviate this troublesome condition from commercially prepared bacon and ham, and have reduced all types of taint to a minimum.

## Phosphorescence

Phosphorescence is caused by a number of organisms, e.g. *Pseudomonas phosphorescens*, which are widely distributed in nature, especially in sea water, and may contaminate a chilling room. These organisms are resistant to chilling room temperatures and their invasion of cold stores can be a matter of considerable inconvenience. At the commencement of phosphorescence, which occurs in 7–8 hours when the condition is artifically produced, the surface of the meat, when seen in the dark room, shows luminous areas scattered over its surface and appears as if it were studded with stars. If decomposition develops in the meat, the phosphorescence disappears. Salted or stored meat may show various changes in colour due to bacterial action. Scattered areas, reddish in colour and not unlike beetroot juice, are caused by *Serratia marcescens*, and a similar superficial change, but blue in colour, is seen as a result of surface contamination by *Pseudomonas cyanagenus. Pseudomonas cutirubra* appears to be the primary cause of *'red mould'* on charque, the dried salted beef of South America. Meat affected with phosphorescence or abnormal surface coloration is unsightly and repugnant, but if no putrefactive changes are present it may safely be dealt with by trimming.

## Moulds

In contrast with yeasts and bacteria, moulds are readily seen with the naked eye, appearing typically as fluffy growths on old damp newspapers, walls, rotting fruits, cheese, jam, etc. They can occur in various colours, e.g. white, black, green, blue. Unlike bacteria and yeasts, they are multicellular and typically consist of a mass (mycelium) of branched filaments or hyphae which bear reproductive bodies or spores. Along with yeasts, mildews, rusts, smuts and mushrooms, they belong to the class Mycota or fungi. Like bacteria, they are present everywhere and are responsible for many beneficial and harmful activities.

Saprophytic moulds are largely concerned with the decomposition of organic matter and the decay of foodstuffs. By breaking down complex organic matter they contribute to the rotting of vegetable material and its eventual conversion into soil. Some act as parasites on plants, causing death of the host, while others take part in fermentation processes which are of value in industry, e.g. the ripening of cheese.

The breakdown is due to the secretion of enzymes on to the surface and the mould absorbing the resultant fluid as food. Moulds can produce valuable antibiotics – e.g. penicillin, by several species of the green mould *Penicillium*, one of which is *P. notatum*.

A few moulds are pathogenic: *Aspergillus flavus* causes aflatoxicosis in swine, cattle, sheep and poultry by the production of aflatoxins on groundnuts, soya beans and other cereals during storage; *Claviceps purpurea* causes ergotism in cattle and horses due to the alkaloids ergotamine, ergosine, etc. on rye, rye grasses and other forage plants; and mouldy corn toxicosis is caused by the rubratoxins and other mycotoxins from *Penicillium rubrum*, *Aspergillus flavus* and others.

Moisture, temperature and organic matter are important factors in determining the presence and activity of moulds. The majority are mesophilic and have an optimum growth temperature of 20–30°C, but several types can grow at or just below 0°C, e.g. the so-called *snow moulds* and those responsible for the spoilage of refrigerated foods. Some thermophilic species can grow at 50°C and higher but not below 30°C. Although most favour moist conditions, some, e.g. *Aspergillus*, *Botrytis*, *Cladosporium*, *Fusarium*, *Mucor*, *Penicillium*, *Rhizopus*, *Thamnidium*, *Alternaria* and *Sporotrichum*, are relatively tolerant to water availability (limit of $a_w$ value for growth is 0.88–0.80) and can grow in a pH lower than 4.5.

Moulds first appear and grow most prolifically on the cut surfaces of the lean meat. Although the spores of moulds may have a ubiquitous existence, often in the air attached to dust particles, they cannot germinate without moisture. The growth of moulds can be prevented by low temperatures and attention to humidity; thus, proper ventilation in refrigerating and storage works is necessary so that circulating air may dry the surface of food and containers. The control of moulds in food products with chemicals is neither approved nor successful; the concentration of chemical required to inhibit growth increases rapidly with humidity. The chief *causes* of mould on meat are exposure to dust and variations in temperature causing condensation on the meat surface. Intermittent freezing or temperature fluctuations in a refrigerating chamber are common predisposing causes to mould growth.

## Black spot

This is the most troublesome affection of imported meat and is caused by the mould *Cladosporium herbarum*. *Pullularia* and *Rhizopus* may also be involved. It is liable to attack quarters of chilled beef taken from ships and placed in cold store at a temperature above – 8°C; some varieties grow at – 7.5°C, while all grow well at around 0°C. In beef, black spot is commonly found on the neck, diaphragm and pleura, and in frozen mutton on the legs, inside the neck or in the thoracic or abdominal cavities. The spots are about 6–13 mm in diameter and occur on the surface of the meat. The dark colour is due to the fungal threads in the superficial layers of the meat, and from which the mould derives the moisture necessary for growth.

Black spot cannot be removed by gentle scraping with a knife, and microscopical examination shows that the threads of the fungus, dark green or olive in colour, are interlaced between the fat cells in the connective tissue on the surface of the carcase; they do not penetrate to a greater depth than 3 mm, and the contiguous muscular and connective tissues are perfectly normal. Black spot may at times be accompanied by bacterial spoilage, when decomposition is manifested by a softening, darkening and sliminess of the carcase surface and is associated with the growth of microorganisms of the *Achromobacter* group. Black spot which is not too extensive and which is unaccompanied by decomposition may be removed by trimming. This is invariably practicable in quarters of chilled beef, but in frozen mutton the mould formation may be so extensive on the inner aspect of the carcase, neck and pelvic cavity that total condemnation is required. Mould formation accompanied by bacterial spoilage requires more generous paring and, at times, condemnation of the whole quarter. It has been repeatedly borne out by practical experience that meat affected with mould, and subsequently refrozen after trimming or wiping, will develop mould more rapidly and in greater abundance than meat which, though mouldy, has not been so treated. Meat which has been trimmed or wiped to remove mould therefore requires a quick sale.

## White spot

White spot is caused by *Sporotrichum* and *Chrysosporium* and is the most commonly encountered defect of imported meat. It is seen as small, flat, woolly spots, frequently accompanying black spot of similar size, but it is whitish in colour and entirely superficial in nature. The spores can develop at –8°C, grow more plentifully at –2.5°C, and become profuse when the temperature is above 0°C.

### 'Whiskers'

This fungoid growth belongs to the closely allied genera *Thamnidium and Mucor*. The hyphae grow well at 0°C and may project more than 2.5 cm beyond the surface of the meat, but they collapse in a relatively dry atmosphere. Though the growth of these moulds ceases at temperatures below –7.5°C, they retain their viability and proliferate if the temperature rises above freezing point; thus the presence of 'whiskers' indicates the meat has been exposed during storage to a temperature at or above 0°C.

### Bluish-green moulds

Bluish-green moulds belong to the genus *Penicillium* and are seen frequently on cheese, on unsound fruit, and also on meat. They are superficial in character and grow with difficulty at 0°C, though conspicuous growths will occur at a slightly higher temperature.

The superficial nature of white spot, 'whiskers' and the bluish-green moulds renders their removal easy, either by wiping with a cloth steeped in vinegar or salt water, or by trimming, the latter procedure being often preferable, as mould on meat may be associated with a characteristic musty odour. In imported forequarters of beef affected with mould, particular attention should be paid to the sawn surfaces of the vertebrae, especially the cervical and first four or five dorsal vertebrae; all affected bones should be removed (an affected pleura or peritoneum may be removed by stripping). In spite of the non-pathogenic nature of most moulds, they may impart a mouldy odour and taste if extensive and of long-standing. Moulds, too, may promote rancidity of fat, and in doubtful cases a portion of the meat should be subjected to a boiling test after the meat has been wiped or trimmed.

### The danger of decomposing meat to man

Though decomposition is an index of bacterial growth, it is not an indication that the meat will necessarily be harmful; the question is simply which bacteria and what conditions were concerned in the contamination. *Cl. botulinum* produces serious specific symptoms, but in other illnesses attributed to the eating of decomposed meat there are no specific symptoms and the affection is usually an acute afebrile gastrointestinal inflammation which is frequently of short duration but may on occasions prove fatal.

Another factor which dictates condemnation of decomposed meat is the aesthetic one. The appearance, odour and taste of decomposing meat are repugnant to most of the more civilised nations of the world, and in some individuals its consumption may be accompanied by marked psychological effects. The position may be summarised by the statement that anyone selling a decomposed food is negligent in the legal sense of the word, and, although in most cases eating decomposed meat will do no harm, experience has shown that it can be responsible for human illness. As it is impossible to state beforehand whether the bacteria present are harmful or not, decomposing meat should in all cases be condemned.

## ASSESSMENT OF DECOMPOSITION

The need has long been felt for a laboratory method to establish the extent of spoilage in meat. To be of practical value such a test must be short and simple and must provide unambiguous results which can be interpreted with confidence. During the last 50–60 years, chemical, bacteriological and physical tests have been developed.

**Chemical tests** Various chemical methods have been suggested:

1 Tests based on the detection of free ammonia.
2 The determination of the total amount of volatile bases produced during spoilage.

In neither of these cases does the test give a clear indication of spoilage until the meat itself smells sufficiently to be condemned sensorially.

3 The determination of free amino acid content as an indication of decomposition has been suggested, but it is likewise unsuitable except as a guide to advanced putrefaction.
4 The production of indole, sulphur and other volatile products in decomposing meat has

also been investigated, but although in fish there seems to be a relationship between spoilage and the amount of total volatile reducing substances and total volatile acids present respectively, such a relationship has not been established in meat.

5 Tests for meat spoilage based on either the oxygen requirements of the meat or on its power of reduction have been in existence for some time but have not proved of practical value.

### Bacteriological test

Bacteriological methods have been devised to relate bacterial plate counts to the quality of meat, but these do not show any close relationship between the number of bacteria present and the degree of spoilage as assessed sensorily. It is known, however, that anaerobes cause putrefaction and the desirability of a test for anaerobes in meat comparable with the *E. coli* test in water analysis has been suggested.

Of all the methods suggested to date, none is sufficiently discriminating to replace sensory assessment and there is little doubt that the experienced inspector can arrive at a sound conclusion by estimating the texture, appearance, taste and odour of the food, with the use of a boiling test where necessary. It is, however, contended that in certain cases pH measurements may be of value.

### pH estimation

Meat from freshly-killed cattle has an average pH of 6.4–6.8 and sometimes up to 7.2, i.e. slightly acid or slightly alkaline. The pH then falls rapidly, reaching its lowest level of around 5.6 within 48 hours after slaughter. The pH then remains constant for some time, this period depending on whether the carcase has been properly cooled, the degree of bacterial contamination and the storage conditions. Subsequently the pH rises slowly owing to autolysis and bacterial growth. When a pH of 6.4 is reached, there is suspicion of the presence of incipient decomposition; when muscle reaches a pH of 6.8 or over, the objective signs of decomposition – odour, colour and texture – become apparent. It is an unfavourable indication if the pH does not fall to 6.1 or below within 24 hours.

Estimation of the pH of meat is of value in the judgement of borderline cases, particularly of emergency-slaughtered animals, for it indicates whether or not the meat will possess adequate durability. It is a routine procedure in many continental abattoirs. In animals suffering from febrile disease or exhausted at the time of slaughter, the glycogen content of the muscles is low and the pH of the flesh will remain at a high level. pH can be measured accurately with an electronic meter or, less accurately, by methods employing colour changes using, for example, nitrazine yellow.

In animals slaughtered because of fractures of the lumbar vertebrae, pelvis or hind limbs, it is common to find that the pH of the immobile hind limbs falls to the normal figure of about 5.8, whereas the struggling of the animal causes the forequarters to remain at 6.5 or more.

### Chemiluminescence (see also p. 377)

Chemiluminescence has been studied by the Battelle Columbus Laboratories in Ohio, USA, as a possible 'marker' for assessing the *freshness of food*. As food deteriorates, the unsaturated fats, oils and other lipids emit light. It is suggested the technique could accurately gauge the shelf-life of products which might otherwise be prematurely withdrawn, develop an indicator of the life of oil, thereby improving the flavour of food fried in the oil, and assess the effectiveness of antioxidant additives.

## LEGISLATION AND DURABILITY OF PROCESSED FOODS

The Food Labelling Directive (79/112/EEC) requires most pre-packed foodstuffs to carry a date of minimum durability. This is known as a 'best before' date on the label, which is the date up until which the foodstuff will retain its optimum condition, i.e. it will not be stale. Article 9a of the Directive, which was introduced by amending Directive 89/395/EEC, requires the 'best before' date to be replaced with the 'use by' date on those pre-packed foods 'which, from the microbiological point of view, are highly perishable and are therefore likely after a short period to constitute an immediate danger to human health'. The *'use by' date is the date up to and including which the food may be used safely*, e.g. cooked or processed or consumed, if it has been stored correctly. The 'use by' date is not a voluntary alternative; it must be used instead of the 'best before' date when both of the conditions set out above are met. In addition to the above, pre-packed fresh poultry meat is required to bear a 'use by' date under the terms of Council Regulation (EEC) 1906/90 on marketing standards for poultry meat.

The 'use by' date must be placed on the packaging within the same field of vision as the name of the food. The date mark must be followed by a description of the storage conditions, including a maximum temperature at or below which the food should be stored, and conditions of use which must be observed.

# Part 3 – The Meat Plant Laboratory

Laboratory facilities should be readily available to provide the inspector with the information he requires in doubtful cases involving abnormalities, diseases or residues and in which a macroscopical inspection alone cannot provide the evidence required for passing judgement on a carcase and its viscera.

Of necessity, this laboratory in the slaughter sector must be limited in size and function. Nevertheless it has an important preliminary part to play in disease diagnosis, monitoring of potential pathogens, quality control/plant/staff hygiene standards, assessment of water quality and chemical residues, photography of pathological specimens/livestock disease cases, etc., and the training of staff.

Although at the moment the judgement of carcases assessed as fit for human consumption is usually based on visual inspection in most countries, microbiological assessment may well be essential in future in view of the serious situation regarding incidents of food-borne disease, especially those associated with *E. coli* O157:H7, *Salmonella, Listeria* and *Campylobacter*, etc.

The present high levels of microbial populations on all carcases (cattle, sheep, pigs, poultry) following dressing and occasioned by dirty hides and skins (and sometimes gut contents) may well necessitate on-line carcase pasteurisation followed by microbiological examination of random carcases to ensure absence of potential pathogens and complete fitness for human consumption.

Further detailed work such as histopathological examinations and typing of microorganisms involving serology must be referred to a central laboratory.

The *plant laboratory* should be located at some distance from slaughter/carcase dressing operations in order to minimise the amount of contamination and further steps should be taken in the form of a barrier disinfectant bath near its entrance. Sampling of tissues, equipment, walls, floors, tools, hands and clothing of personnel, etc. is performed on the factory floors thus reducing the traffic to the laboratory.

While the laboratory will be involved mainly with microbiological procedures it will also to a lesser extent be involved with parasitological and clinical chemistry matters.

*Complete sterility of equipment* and *methods is a prerequisite for all laboratory procedures.*

## BASIC LABORATORY EQUIPMENT

- Microscope with ×10 and ×40 objectives and ×90 or ×100 oil immersion objective
- Immersion oil
- Glass slides and cover slips
- Balance
- Bunsen burner
- Camera with close-up facility
- Autoclave
- Incubator
- Refrigerator
- Homogeniser
- Centrifuge with interchangeable heads
- Stomacher Lab Blender
- pH meter
- Thermometer
- Slit sampler, air sampling apparatus
- Colorimeter/photometer/luminometer
- Candle jar (Fig. 14.8)
- Ready poured culture media, e.g. blood agar, MacConkey agar, agar sausages, plate count agar, etc.
- Commercial identification kits
- Ringer's solution
- Anaerobic culture system
- Antibiotic disc dispenser and discs
- Oxoid sensitivity test agar, test organisms (*B. subtilis, Sarcina lutea* and *Staph. aureus*)
- 3% hydrogen peroxide
- 3% potassium hydroxide
- Specimen transport media
- Stains – Gram, Ziehl–Neelsen, polychrome methylene blue, Giemsa, Loeffler's methylene blue, Leishman, etc.
- Test tubes, holding and staining racks
- Durham tubes
- Centrifuge tubes

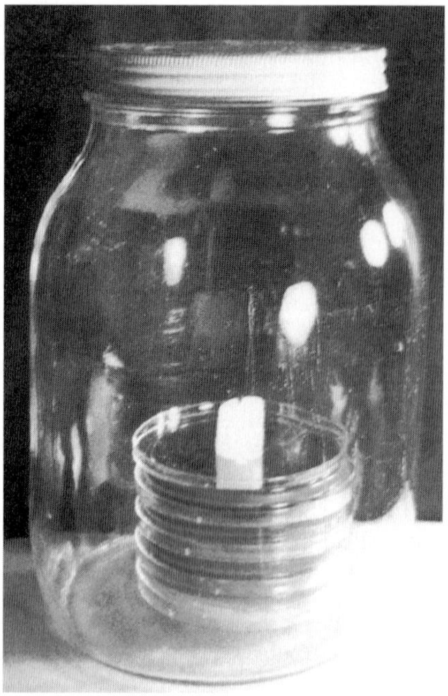

**Fig. 14.8** Candle extinction jar and inoculated plates. (By kind permission of Professors C. Mahon and G. Manuselis)

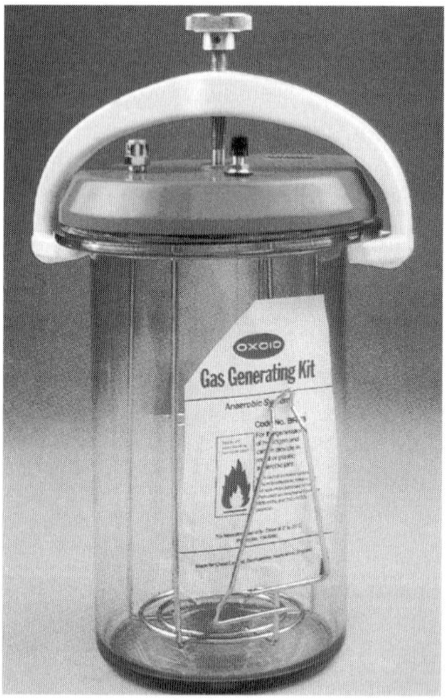


**Fig. 14.9** McIntosh & Fildes anaerobic jar. (By kind permission of Oxoid Marketing)

- Petri dishes (disposable)
- Beakers and flasks
- Measuring cylinders
- Impression plates
- 1 oz, 6 oz, 8 oz bottles
- Universal containers
- Absorbent cotton wool swabs, gauze swabs, alginate swabs
- Metal templates (50 $cm^2$, 100 $cm^2$)
- McIntosh & Fildes jar (Fig. 14.9)
- pH reagent strips, electronic pH meter
- Platinum loops
- Glass wool
- Plastic bags
- Self-adhesive cellophane tape
- Filter pads
- Specimen collection equipment – scalpels, forceps, spatulas, spoons, searing iron, cork borer, skin scraper, metal cylinder

## SAMPLING OF MEAT FOR TESTING

(Reference has been made to the *Manual of Manufacturing Meat Quality* by P. N. Church and J. W. Wood, Leatherhead Food Research Association, Chairman Dr T. Toomey) in the compiling of the following notes.)

A *sample* is a small portion of a larger amount taken for examination (microbiological status, residues/fat/species content, etc.).

The sampling of processed materials (to which most attention appears to have been given) is a complex procedure which requires careful planning, specialised equipment and trained sampling staff and will not be discussed here. The reader is referred to specialised texts on this type of sampling.

Sampling should be as representative as possible, which may mean swabbing several areas of a carcase or re-swabbing with a dry swab.

It should be borne in mind in relation to beef, lamb and pigmeat that the surfaces to be examined are very tacky and do not readily release bacteria. In addition, microorganisms are irregularly distributed over carcases.

The sampling of frozen meats is more complicated than that for fresh meat. Blocks of meats can be cut into 9 cubes from which cores can be removed with an auger or drill.

Chilled and frozen *poultry* carcases can be sampled by rinsing the whole skin, defined areas of skin or the whole carcase.

Full details of the material sampled, site, date, nature of examination required, etc. must accompany the sample.

Care should be taken to ensure that samples arrive at the laboratory in good condition.

## Purpose of microbiological testing

Microbiological testing determines:

1. Types and numbers of microorganisms present.
2. Presence/absence of pathogens.
3. Quality of meat for further processing.
4. Standard of animal hygiene.
5. Standard of slaughter and carcase dressing methods.
6. Standard of personnel and environmental hygiene.
7. Evidence of spoilage due to bacteria/moulds – may be evident on incorrectly stored carcases.

The meat plant veterinarian will be mainly concerned with the possible presence of pathogenic microorganisms, the main ones responsible for food-borne disease in man being:

*Bacillus cereus*
*Campylobacter jejuni*
*Clostridium botulinum*
*Clostridium perfringens*
Enteropathogenic *E. coli* especially O157:H7
*Listeria monocytogenes*
*Salmonella* spp.
*Staphylococcus aureus*
*Toxoplasma gondii*
*Yersinia enterocolitica*

The numbers of these microorganisms present on carcases will be determined largely by the standards listed above, especially that of animal hygiene.

## Colony counts of mesophilic aerobes – agar plate methods

The system of sampling carcases, choice of test method and the interpretation of results requires expertise and experience. Carcases will display vast differences in the number of organisms at different sites, being greater in number at points in contact with faecal material, e.g. the anal region and those areas requiring close contact with the knife and hands of operatives, such as shin and leg.

A representative sample can be achieved by pooling 8–10 smears from these areas, balancing the low and high contamination areas.

**Agar plate counts (APCs)** of *mesophilic* organisms (grow best at 20–50°C) after 30–35°C incubation are useful measures of the bacteriological status of carcases and slaughter hygiene. Taken over a period of time they are a good indication of the overall standard of plant hygiene. Counts of *psychrotrophic* bacteria (grow best at low temperatures: 0–7°C) are a good indication of hygiene practices which affect shelf-life.

**Aerobic plate count (APC)** Also known as the Total Viable Count (TVC), Aerobic Mesophilic Count (AMC) or Standard Plate Count (SPC), this is the most common method of assessing the number of organisms in raw meat.

There are three methods in use: Aerobic Plate Count (Standard Plate Count, Pour Plate Count), Drop Plate method and Surface Plate (Spread Drop Method).

The colonies on plates represent the rapid growth of individual organisms – bacteria, yeasts, moulds – and can easily be counted to give the number of live organisms originally present in the incoculum. Depending on their colour, shape, etc., colonies can often be differentiated to count different types of organisms. This can also be achieved by using selective culture media on which yeasts, moulds, lactic acid bacteria, coliforms and staphylococci can be counted as visible colonies.

The *colony-forming unit* (CFU) is the unit of measurement in this particular test and is usually expressed as 10 cfu ($10^1$ cfu), 100 cfu ($10^2$ cfu), etc., or mean log 10 CFU, all occurring per $cm^2$.

(Refer to *Microorganisms in Foods and Their Significance and Methods of Enumeration*, 2nd edition *1* (1978), *2* (1986)), International Commission on Microbiological Significance for Foods (ICMSF) of the International

Association of Microbiological Societies, University of Toronto, for details of the Aerobic Plate Count methods.)

Although colony counts are the customary methods used, other techniques include Direct Microscopic Count (DMC), electrical methods, Direct Epifluorescent Filter Technique (DEFT) and commercial kits using immunological and DNA-probe hybridisation for rapid detection of pathogens such as *Salmonella* and *Listeria* and some bacterial toxins (staphylococcal and mycotoxins).

## Sampling plans and recommended microbiological limits for raw meat before chilling

The International Commission on the Microbiological Specification of Foods (ICMSF) in *Microorganisms in Foods 2* (1986) classifies the potential hazards in foods into 1–15 *cases* or *degrees* of increasing hazard, raw meat that is to be cooked being regarded as the least hazardous (Case 1). Cooked meats are given higher classification, cooked poultry meat being Case 8. Within each case there are recommended sampling plans for each *lot* of product.

### *Sampling plans*

Each sampling plan has several characteristics, for example:

- $n$ = number of samples to be taken from the lot;
- $c$ = number of samples permitted to fail;
- $m$ = microbial count *below* which the sample is considered to be satisfactory;
- $M$ = microbial count *above* which the sample is considered unsatisfactory.

These characteristics result in three possible classes of microbial contamination (the three-class sampling plan):

(i) samples with counts below $m$;
(ii) samples with counts between $m$ and $M$ and
(iii) samples with counts above $M$.

The three-class sampling plan allows for the known variability of raw meat counts by allowing a certain number to fall between $m$ and $M$ (see Table 14.7).

The sampling plan is the same for all the meats shown in Table 14.7. Only the limits $m$ and $M$ vary. For example, for carcase meat before chilling the target value $m$ is 10/5 and the maximum value is 10/6, while for boneless frozen meat these values are higher at 5 × 10/5 and 10/7, respectively.

A *microbiological standard* is a microbiological criterion that is part of a law or regulation, mandatory and enforceable by the regulatory agency involved.

A *microbiological specification* is a microbiological criterion that is applied a condition of acceptance of a food or ingredient by a food manufacturer.

*Standards of microbial specifications currently used by industry* include levels for:

- Frozen boneless forequarter beef for hamburger production
- Chilled stewing steak for canning with gravy
- Chilled beef for further processing
- Frozen beef head meat for further processing
- Frozen boneless forequarter beef
- Frozen beef suet
- Frozen, rindless, boneless lean pork trimmings for further processing
- Frozen, rindless pork backfat and cutting fat for further processing
- Fresh chicken with giblets
- Frozen mixed hen meat

## EC microbiological standards for meat

These do not exist in the United Kingdom at present except for Directive 88/657/EEC, which deals with the testing of minced meat and meat pieces of less than 100 g and includes a new category 'S' which equals 1000 × $m$, at which the meat must be considered toxic or tainted.

This Directive (not yet accepted) states that five samples per lot will be taken and a three-class sampling plan used.

It lays down standards (legal requirements) in terms of $m$ and $M$ as in Table 14.8.

It is likely that the ICMSF recommendations for the microbiological testing of raw meats will eventually become the standard for the European Commission.

**Table 14.7** Sampling plans and recommended microbiological limits for raw meat[a] (ICMSF, *Microorganisms in Foods*, Vol. 2, 1986).

| Product[b] | Test | Case | Plan class | *n* | *c* | *m* | *M* |
|---|---|---|---|---|---|---|---|
| Carcase meat, before chilling | APC* | 1 | 3 | 5 | 3 | 10/5 | 10/6 |
| Carcase meat, chilled | APC | 1 | 3 | 5 | 3 | 10/6 | 10/7 |
| Edible offal, chilled | APC | 1 | 3 | 5 | 3 | 10/6 | 10/7 |
| Carcase meat, frozen | APC | 1 | 3 | 5 | 3 | 5 × 10/5 | 10/7 |
| Boneless meat, frozen (beef, pork, mutton) | APC | 1 | 3 | 5 | 3 | 5 × 10/5 | 10/7 |
| Comminuted meat, frozen | APC | 1 | 3 | 5 | 3 | 10/6 | 10/7 |
| Edible offal, frozen | APC | 1 | 3 | 5 | 3 | 5 × 10/5 | 10/7 |
| Raw chicken, fresh or frozen | APC | 1 | 3 | 5 | 3 | 5 × 10/7 | 10/7 |

[a] For in-plant quality control use but not at port of entry.
[b] Unfrozen carcases and primal cuts, swab counts per $cm^2$; other meats per g.
* Aerobic plate count.

For example:

$n$ = 5
$m$ = 10/5 cfu per $cm^2$ or gm
$c$ = 3
$M$ = 10/6 cfu per $cm^2$ or gm

**Table 14.8** Provisions of Directive 88/657/EEC.

| Organism | *n* | *c* | *M* | *m* |
|---|---|---|---|---|
| Aerobic mesophile bacteria (total viable count) | 5 | 2 | $5 \times 10^6$ | $5 \times 10^5$ |
| *E. coli* | 5 | 2 | $5 \times 10^2$ | 50 |
| *Cl. perfringens* (sulphite-reducing anaerobes) | 5 | 1 | $10^2$ | 10 |
| *Staphylococci* | 5 | 1 | $5 \times 10^2$ | 50 |
| *Salmonella* | 5 | 0 | Absence in 25 g | |

## SPECIMEN SAMPLING TECHNIQUES
(see also pp. 341–2)

### Swabbing

Moistened cotton or alginate wool swabs used in conjunction with a sterile aluminium template to give a defined surface area (25 $cm^2$) (of carcase, equipment, wall, floor, etc.) for sampling are widely used. Instead of metal templates, disposable paper templates may be used.

The swabs are on the ends of wooden sticks and packed in sterile tubes which are plugged and sterilised.

The cotton wool swab is dipped into a small screw-capped bottle containing 10 ml of diluent (quarter-strength Ringer's solution or MRD) and five small glass beads. (MRD, Maximum Recovery Diluent: a peptone saline solution of 0.1 g peptone and 0.85 g sodium chloride in 100 ml of distilled water.) If sanitising agents have been used for cleaning, 0.05% sodium thiosulphate should be added to the diluent.

Rub the moistened swab over the test surface area, turning the swab while doing so. After use, break off the cotton wool end into the 10 ml diluent. Repeat with another swab and shake the diluent bottle until the swabs are disintegrated.

Examination of swabs should be carried out immediately after sampling by setting up general viable counts using dip slide, pour plate, membrane filtration, spiral plate, etc., methods and incubating at 30ºC for 3 days.

*Interpretation of results*

| General viable count per cm² | Interpretation |
|---|---|
| Not more than 5 | Satisfactory |
| 5–25 | Further investigation required |
| More than 25 | Very unsatisfactory – immediate action necessary |

Swabbing techniques can also be used for poultry but the recovery rate of organisms is usually lower.

Smears should also be made at the same time for staining by Gram's method.

### Preparation of blood smear (Fig. 14.10)

1 Apply a small drop of blood near one end of a clean microscope slide.
2 Place a second slide (with thumb and forefinger) at an angle of 30 degrees on left edge of drop of blood.
3 Spread blood by moving upper slide towards free end of horizontal slide.
4 Dry slide immediately in air and examine.

N.B.: The thickness of the blood film can be modified by varying the size of the drop of blood, the amount of blood drawn and the rate of spread (a fast spread makes a thinner film). A thick film can be made by pooling several drops of blood which are then spread over an area of 1.5 cm.

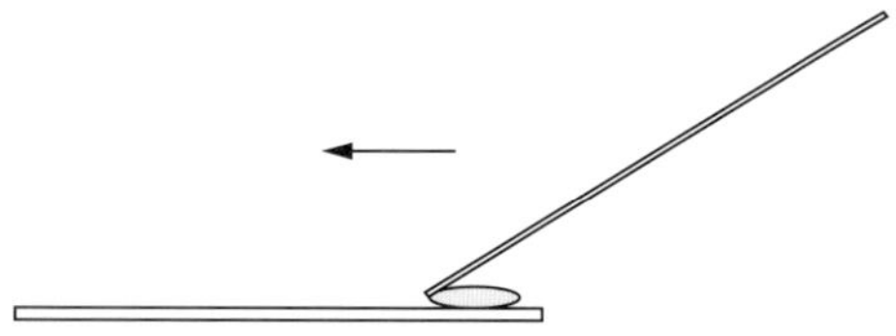

**Fig. 14.10** Preparation of blood smear.

### Diagnosis of intracellular blood parasites
(e.g. *Babesia, Plasmodium, Trypanosoma*)

1 Make thick and thin films.
2 Apply Giemsa stain (5 min) for thick and thin films and Wright stain for thin films. (A thick film is best for *detecting* blood parasites and a thin film for accurate *diagnosis*.)
3 Fix blood smear in methanol for one minute and air dry for 6 hours before staining.
4 Scan first with ×10 objective lens and then with at least ×100 oil immersion.

### Other sampling techniques

**Agar contact or impression,** e.g. Ten Cate agar sausages, can be applied to surfaces and slices cut off for incubation in a Petri dish with the impressed side uppermost. Agar impressions can also be used for poultry in which they are of value in the monitoring of plants for specific organisms.

Cut the end of an agar sausage and squeeze out a small portion from the outer covering. Press the cut end against the test surface and then cut off a thin slice for placing in the Petri dish.

This method is of more value in checking surfaces of equipment, walls, floors, etc., rather than carcases.

**Self-adhesive cellophane tapes or labels** can be applied to surfaces after removal of the backing paper which is then reapplied for transport. The tape, free of backing paper, is applied to an agar plate for incubation. Bacterial counts compare with those achieved by agar contact but are usually less than swab counts. The sterility of the tapes and labels should be checked before use.

**Moistened membrane filters and flamed glass slides** may also be used as contact methods, the latter being pressed on to freshly-cut surfaces after surface sterilisation. The slides can then be used to make an impression plate or pressed on to poured plates of media for incubation. Fixing and staining, e.g. Gram's stain, of the slides should be performed.

**Surface contact or impression plate** The lid is removed from the plate which is then pressed evenly against the test surface (or the skin of poultry). The lid is replaced and the plate incubated according to the requirements of the particular organism.

**Dip slide** The dip slide is removed from its container and the agar surface pressed against the test surface. The slide is then reattached to the container cap and placed in the container which is then incubated at the appropriate temperature.

**Sweep plate technique** This is a useful system for testing surfaces for standard of cleanliness. Air exposure plates with the lids removed are placed face down on the test surface and moved sideways ten times over a distance of 30 cm. The lids are then replaced and the plates incubated.

**Membrane slide cultures** Several commercial kits are available for this method of surface testing. The swab is removed from the receptacle containing 18 ml of buffer solution, excess buffer solution being expressed from it. The swab is then rubbed and rotated over the test area and returned to the container, which is sealed and shaken vigorously. The swab is discarded. The membrane slide sampler in the other container is placed in the test buffer solution and left for 30 s. It is then returned to its original container, which is incubated.

The colonies are counted on the sampler membrane or compared with the kit chart.

Since the sampler absorbs 1 ml of buffer solution, the plate count is multiplied by 18 to give the number of cfu per area sampled.

**Rinses and washes** These have a limited application except for small items like sausages and similar products and poultry. The item is washed in sterile diluent (10 parts by weight) with agitation-comminution of the product will allow more organisms to be recovered.

Various techniques have been used with *poultry* depending on whether skin or whole carcases are being sampled by swabbing. Skin samples of defined areas can be taken from under the wing, near the vent and from the neck. The results from these areas can be combined to obtain an overall body estimation.

The *neck skin flap* is removed aseptically with the carcase in its plastic bag and 20 g is homogenised in 180 ml peptone–saline in a stomacher for 2 min as the primary dilution.

Another method is to press a sharp-edged cylinder against the skin to encircle a known area of skin; 25 ml of diluent is then poured into the cylinder and stirred, with scraping of the skin.

*Whole poultry* are shaken vigorously for 30 s in a plastic bag containing 1000 ml of 0.1% peptone–saline diluent (about half the weight of the carcase). Small glass beads may be used to assist removal of bacteria from the carcase. An amount of fluid is removed from the plastic bag and further decimal dilutions are made in 0.1% peptone–saline. Conversion of the number of bacteria/ml of rinse water to the number per $cm^2$ is made by applying a factor: *the surface of a broiler expressed as* $cm^2$ *equals the weight (G)* × *500.* A high-pressure spray to rinse a defined area of poultry skin can be used to recover surface bacteria.

Rinses may also be used to examine *small items of equipment*, e.g. buckets and other small containers using 500 ml of Ringer's solution (quarter strength).

**Collection of faeces** Faeces can be collected easily from the ground in plastic bags and directly from the animal during defaecation or by the use of a harness to which a plastic bag is attached.

**Collection of material from drains** Gauze swabs or tampons are suitable for suspension in drains for, e.g., *salmonella* examination.

## Potable water samples

A sufficient, clean and wholesome supply of hot and cold water, or water pre-mixed to a suitable temperature, available at an adequate pressure and meeting the requirements of Council Directive 80/778/EEC is required and must be separated from other water used for firefighting, refrigeration and steam boilers. Pipes for the two systems must be separate and clearly distinguishable. The outside and inside of the tap or faucet nozzle must be cleaned and flamed before collection and the water allowed to run for several minutes before filling the container, which should not be opened until the commencement of filling.

If the water supply is chlorinated, a chlorine-neutralising agent, e.g. sterile sodium thiosulphate must be added to the sample before analysis at a rate of 0.1 ml of a 2% solution for each 100 ml of water sample.

Because of the intermittent contamination of some water supplies with certain bacteria in small numbers, it is necessary to have a regular system of testing. Testing should provide an indication of the overall microbiological quality of the water supply as well as evidence of possible faecal contamination.

*Tests*

Plate counts for total and faecal coliforms (37°C and 22°C) in 100 ml are as follows:

| | Maximum concentration* |
|---|---|
| Total coliforms | 0 per 100 ml |
| Faecal coliforms | 0 per 100 ml |
| Sulphite-reducing clostridia | > 1 per 20 ml |
| Faecal streptococci | 0 per 100 ml |
| Colony counts | No significant increase over that normally observed. (Recorded as the number at 20°C or 37°C.) |

Water shall not be regarded as unwholesome solely because the maximum concentration for the total coliforms is exceeded:

1 if, in the preceding 12 months 50 or more samples have been taken in accordance with the regulations (UK Water Supply (Water Quality) Regulations 1989, 1991) in respect of that parameter, and in at least 90% of those samples coliforms were absent; or
2 in any other case, in the last 50 samples so taken, it is established that in at least 48 of those samples coliforms were absent.

## Sampling of air

An overall impression of the density of bacteria and fungi in the meat plant atmosphere may be gained by using air exposure plates in various positions for 15 min. The number of colonies developing on the plates represent the number of individual organisms settling on approximately 0.1 m$^2$ per min.

Special *slit samplers* and *membrane filters* may be used where absolute concentrations of organisms in the air are required.

## COLLECTION OF SPECIMENS OF BLOOD, PUS, MUSCLE, FLUIDS, ETC.

The meat plant will be dealing mainly with the collection of specimens from detained carcases, on occasions from carcases passed as fit for human consumption and also from casualty animals.

It may be necessary, for example, in cases of hypomagnesaemic tetany/milk fever, etc., to obtain blood from an affected live animal in a lairage, but such cases are usually diagnosed on clinical signs. However, the future may demand that blood from live animals be taken for the diagnosis of parasitic diseases such as bovine cysticercosis using the ELISA or other test, a procedure which would obviate much of the present inefficient and mutilating post-mortem examination for this condition.

Various techniques are adopted using sterile syringes for blood, fluids and pus while samples of muscle, lymph nodes, etc., require the use of scalpels and forceps.

The aim of specimen collection is to obtain a sample that is representative of the disease process without contamination.

**Post-mortem cases** If specimens are to be taken at *necropsy* they must be recovered as soon as possible after death especially where rapid decomposition takes place, e.g. in sheep and in most species during warm weather. Opportunistic bacteria will quickly obliterate normal post-mortem changes under suitable environmental conditions making many cases useless for accurate diagnosis. Prior treatment of the animal, e.g. with antibacterials, may also preclude proper bacteriological examination and an accurate diagnosis.

A searing iron must be used on tissues prior to the collection of tissue for bacteriological examination.

Blood, abscesses and fluids from closed body cavities can be aspirated with a sterile syringe which may also be used to obtain urine from the bladder. Swabs may also be used for these specimens in some cases but in general it is advisable to collect larger amounts of body fluids, exudates, blood, etc., since there are usually limited numbers of organisms on swabs.

**Blood** Screw-topped plastic tubes (with separate syringes and needles), evacuated glass tubes ('Vacutainer') and plastic collecting syringes ('Monovette', 'S Monovette') are now normally used for blood collection. The latter two are convenient to use in that they combine container, needle and syringe.

Blood, usually from the jugular vein in the larger farm animals, except the pig in which the anterior vena cava is used, goes directly via the needle (1 inch 19G or 20G) into the container with or without coagulant (sodium citrate), depending on the type of examination required. Blood can be allowed to clot and the serum aspirated for serology testing while the clot can be used for microbiology.

**Faeces** A small metal or wooden spoon is used to place faeces samples in a sterile screw-cap container. Neutral glycerol saline is added to the container if a delay in bacteriological examination is anticipated.

**Serous fluids** are treated in the same way as blood since they are also liable to clot on standing.

**Pus or exudate** Swabs are normally used to collect pus and exudates but syringes or pipettes may also be used.

**Urine** A syringe and needle can be used to collect urine from the casualty carcase and the 'line' carcase before the commencement of evisceration.

In the *live* cow stroking of the skin beneath the vulva with a wisp of hay or straw is often successful. Urination may also be stimulated by flapping together the lips of the vulva. Catheterisation of the cow and mare is sometimes adopted, while holding closed the mouth and nostrils of the ewe will stimulate urination.

These procedures should be carried out with due regard to safety in a crush for the cow and mare.

Urine samples from cattle and horses are sometimes successfully obtained by first providing drinking water and waiting for voluntary micturition. Special harness can be used to collect urine and faeces samples in the large animals.

## TRANSPORT AND STORAGE OF SAMPLES

If the intention is to send the specimens to a regional laboratory it is essential that the samples be maintained in their original state as far as possible in order to limit changes in bacterial numbers. Chilled specimens must be kept at 0–5°C and frozen specimens kept frozen. Specimens taken directly from carcases should be examined as soon as possible.

*Proper identification of the specimens is essential.*

For onward transport, chilled or frozen samples must be sent in special insulated containers. Additional transport *media*, e.g. Stuart's or Amies transport media, which will ensure optimal survival of the bacteria may be required. Special transport media are required for fastidious organisms such as *Chlamydia*, *Mycoplasma* and *Rickettsia* and usually contain antimicrobial agents to inhibit the growth of contaminants. UK postal regulations require that pathological specimens be enclosed in a hermetically sealed container which is placed in a strong wooden, metal or fibreboard case with adequate packing material. The words PATHOLOGICAL SPECIMEN and FRAGILE WITH CARE must be conspicuously marked on the package.

## LABORATORY EXAMINATION OF SPECIMENS

### Types of culture media

**Non-selective media** These are able to support the growth of most bacteria and usually exist in agar plate form. Example: sheep blood agar, nutrient broth, nutrient agar, litmus milk.

**Enrichment media** Where the causative organism is few in numbers or outnumbered by numerous undesirables, it is necessary to enhance the required organism. This is achieved by media such as selenite broth, Gram-negative (GN) broth and xylose lysine desoxycholate agar.

**Selective media** These media contain certain antibacterial or other inhibitory chemical substances which prevent the growth of some bacteria allowing others to grow. For example, MacConkey agar is selective for the Gram-negative coliform organisms, while glucose azide broth is used to isolate faecal streptococci in water supplies and Loeffler's serum agar for corynebacteria.

**Differential media** These types of media produce colonies which are easily recognisable, e.g. haemolytic and non-haemolytic colonies are distinguished on blood agar (a non-selective medium) by the forming of clear zones of haemolysis round the haemolytic colonies. Some media are both selective and differential, e.g. MacConkey's agar which produces red lactose-fermenting coliform colonies and colourless *Salmonella* spp. colonies which are non-lactose-fermenting.

**Elective media** These are used for certain bacteria with special nutritional requirements, e.g. yeasts which need nitrogen are grown on lysine agar.

### Culture methods

Test tubes, flasks, McCartney bottles, etc., contain media in various forms depending on the type of inoculation adopted:

1 *Streak plates* Petri dishes with a thin layer of solid medium, e.g. blood agar. These are used for the separation of mixed colonies of bacteria or the examination of individual colonies. Blood agar containing 5% sheep blood is the most commonly used primary isolation medium since it is able to grow most pathogenic bacteria and is useful for noting colony and haemolysis characteristics.
2 *Pour plates* The inoculum under examination is added to the tube of liquid medium at 45°C, mixed and then poured into a plate.
3 *Shake cultures* are made by dissolving a solid medium in test tubes or bottles, cooling to 45°C, inoculating with the test organisms, mixing and allowing to solidify in the upright position.
4 *Semi-solid cultures* contain sufficient agar to make the culture semi-solid.
5 *Liquid batch cultures* in bottles, flasks, etc., e.g. nutrient broth.
6 *Agar slope* or *slant cultures* are contained in test tubes or small screw-capped bottles in which the medium is allowed to cool in a sloped form for surface inoculation.
7 *Stab cultures* are agar or gelatin media which are allowed to solidify. A long straight wire containing the bacterial inoculum is then plunged into the medium.

**Anaerobic culture media** include Robertson's Cooked Meat Medium; shake culture of nutrient agar, and semi-solid media, e.g. nutrient broth with 0.5% glucose, 0.1% sodium thioglycollate, 0.02–0.25 agar and 0.0002% methylene blue as an indicator of oxidation–reduction potential.

Containers containing media for the growth of anaerobes can be incubated in *McIntosh and Fildes* jar in which the oxygen-free atmosphere is created by the passage of an electric current through a heating coil surrounded by a wire gauze. The *Gaspak* system provides a hydrogen supply in the anaerobic jar by means of a disposable foil envelope which contains sodium borohydride and a mixture of citric acid and sodium bicarbonate. The former generates hydrogen and the second mixture produces carbon dioxide, both when water is added.

### Inoculation of media

Each culture *plate* must be marked on the bottom to indicate the specimen, date, etc.

Most specimens for culture will initially be in the form of swabs. (If tissues collected post-mortem are to be cultured, the surface of the organ must first be seared (but not cooked) and the culture inoculum collected with a swab.) The same swab may be used for the inoculation of several media, the least inhibitory, e.g. blood agar, being used first and the most inhibitory last.

## PRIMARY ISOLATION

*Blood agar* (trypticase soy agar with 5% sheep blood) is probably the most widely used primary isolation medium for all specimens in which pathogenic bacteria are suspected because of its ability to support the growth of most pathogens.

#### *Method 1*

1 Inoculate one-third to one-quarter of the plate with the swab specimen.
2 Make successive light streaks at right angles and overlapping the initial inoculum with the platinum loop for two applications, flaming the loop and allowing it to cool between inocula. (Fig. 14.11)

If several plates are to be inoculated (4 is usual), use the least inhibitory medium, e.g. blood agar, first and the most inhibitory

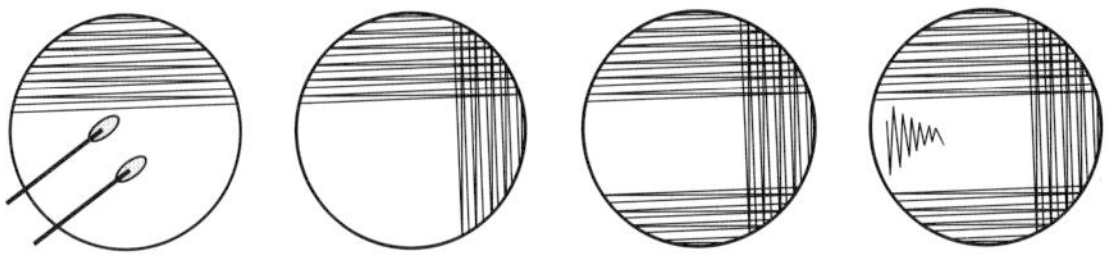

**Fig. 14.11** Streaking method for plate inoculation.

medium, e.g. MacConkey agar, last. (MacConkey is a selective medium for the isolation of Enterobacteriaceae and related Gram-negative bacteria). Subsequent plates can be streaked with the same swab, overlapping a portion of the previous area while flaming the platinum loop and allowing to cool between each plate.

Blood agar, containing 5% sheep blood, is valuable for describing colony morphology as well as determining the presence/absence of haemolysis. Like MacConkey agar, another commonly used primary isolation medium, it can also be used as a differential medium for subcultures.

Primary growth in a broth medium is often difficult to interpret because of contaminants, so liquid media should not be used solely for primary isolation purposes.

For *secondary isolation* (utilising a colony from a solid medium for subculture) the above method may be used.

*Method 2*

1 Make two streaks from the initial inoculum (one extending at right angles across the plate and the second halfway).
2 Succeeding streaks are made parallel and at right angles to the initial inoculum. (Fig. 14.12)

### Incubation of cultures

Inoculated plates are incubated in an inverted position in order to prevent condensation dropping on the medium. Screw-capped containers should be incubated with the cap loosened.

Cultures are incubated at the optimum temperature for the organism under investigation, which for the majority of pathogens is 37ºC. Certain special cultures, e.g. gelatin stabs, however, are usually held at 22ºC.

The usual length of time for incubation is 24 h (overnight) but some fastidious slow-growing types, e.g. *C. pyogenes* may require longer.

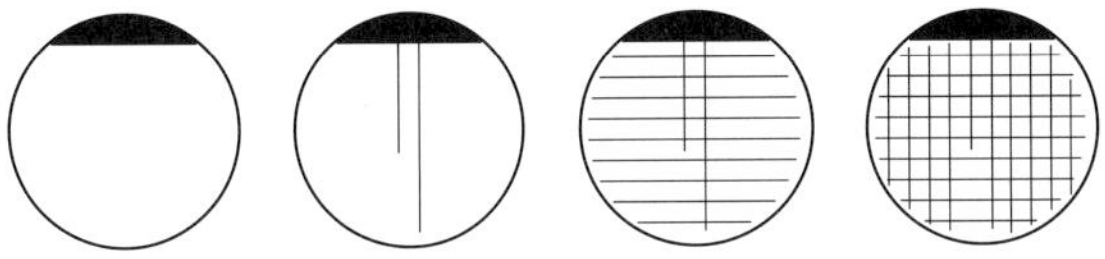

**Fig. 14.12** Plate inoculation. Separation of colonies.

## EVALUATION OF CULTURES

Examination of primary cultures can often provide tentative identification of a bacterium, yeast or mould *but usually requires considerable experience* and *may indicate the need for the assistance of a specialist laboratory.*

Important features to be noted include the number of different types of bacteria isolated, the relative number of each type, the characteristics of the various colonies, and the presence/absence of haemolysis, odour, etc.

The presence of *haemolysis* is often the indication of a possible pathogen, e.g. coagulase-positive isolates of *Staphylococcus* show as double zones of haemolysis. Similarly, *pigmentation of colonies* may also be associated with a possible pathogen.

Colonies which are discrete, raised, convex, opaque or grey with an entire edge are more likely to be organisms of significance, especially if they are in pure culture. On the other hand large, rough, irregular, spreading growths are more often of no importance unless in pure culture. In mixed cultures the most common colony type is not necessarily the most important. *Odours* of cultures are sometimes of value in identification.

The amount of growth of the various organisms in the four streak plates is an important observation.

Knowledge of the characteristics of the more common pathogens and contaminants will assist the bacteriologist who will profit from experience, especially that gained at a specialist laboratory.

An important consideration is to relate the streak plate findings to the *source of the specimen*. If a *carcase*, the body site would be sufficient. But if a *casualty* animal is involved, the body

**Table 14.9** Normal animal body flora.

| Site | Aerobes | Anaerobes |
|---|---|---|
| Ear, skin | Diphtheroids, *Micrococcus*, *Staphs*, faecal contaminants | |
| Mouth nasopharynx | *Actinobacillus*, *Bacillus*, coliforms, *Haemophilus*, *Micrococcus*, *Mycoplasma*, *Pasteurella*, *Proteus*, Staphs, Streps | *Actinomyces*, *Bacteroides*, *Fusobacterium*, spirochaetes |
| Trachea, bronchi, lungs | Transient contaminants | |
| Stomach, S. intestine | alpha-Streps | *Lactobacilli* |
| L. intestine: | *Enterobacter*, *E. coli*, *Klebsiella*, *Proteus*, *Streptococcus* | *Bacteroides*, *Clostridium*, |
| | Diphtheroids, faecal contaminants, *Micrococcus*, *Staphylococcus* | *Fusobacterium*, *Latobacillus* |
| Vulva, prepuce, conjunctiva, udder, uterus | Occasional contaminants | |

site and even a brief description of carcase findings and a tentative diagnosis would be of value. In such cases information regarding antibiotic treatment of the animal is an important element since this may result in poor or no plate growth. If the specimen were taken from a normally sterile site and properly handled, any growth would be considered significant. On the other hand specimens from intestinal sites are usually contaminated with mixed anaerobic types making interpretation difficult.

It is important to be familiar with the *normal flora* of the various organs of the animal body. Some of these are potential pathogens and if identified on the plate(s) and reported may lead to an inaccurate diagnosis (Table 14.9)

**Laboratory records** Accurate *records* of culture characteristics on the various media should be made whether or not a further ouside laboratory is to be involved. Growth, for example, may be present on the first, second, third or fourth quadrant of the streak plate(s).

## PRESUMPTIVE IDENTIFICATION OF ORGANISMS – TESTS (Figs 14.10–14.12)

The characteristics of colony growth, haemolysis, odour, growth on MacConkey, etc., in conjunction with the Gram-staining reaction will materially assist in identification.

*Biochemical tests* can be used to confirm the identity of an organism. Many of these are available in kit form, the powder requiring reconstituting and sterilising before use.

### Potassium peroxide (3%) test

This test may be used as an alternative to the Gram smear.

**Table 14.10** Differentiation of Gram-positive and catalase-positive cocci.

| Organism | Haemolysis | Oxidase | Glucose fermentation | Coagulase |
|---|---|---|---|---|
| *Staph. aureus* | +* | – | + | + |
| *Staph. epidermidis* | ± | – | + | – |
| *Micrococcus* | – | + | – | – |

* Double zones of complete and incomplete haemolysis often observed.

**Table 14.11** Differentiation of small Gram-positive non-sporing rods.

| Organism | Motility | β-Haemolysis | Catalase | $H_2S$ in TSI | Urease | Colonies |
|---|---|---|---|---|---|---|
| *Rhodoc. equi* | - | - | + | - | + | Large, mucoid, pink |
| *C. pseudotuberculosis* | - | V | + | - | + | *Dry, white, grainy |
| *C. pyogenes* | - | + | - | - | - | Very small |
| *C. renale* | - | + | + | - | + | Av. size |
| *E. rhusiopathiae* | - | ± | - | + | - | Very small |
| *L. monocytogenes* | + | + | + | - | - | Very small |

* Brown halo round colony on Tinsdale agar (sheep blood, ox serum, cystine, potassium tellurite).

**Table 14.12** Differentiation of Gram-negative and oxidase-positive bacteria.

| Organism | Motility | Haemolysis | Glucose fermentation | Growth on MacConkey | Urease | Indole |
|---|---|---|---|---|---|---|
| *Actinobacillus* spp. | - | ± | + | ± | + | - |
| *Aeromonas* spp. | + | + | + | + | - | + |
| *Bord. bronchiseptica* | + | - | - | + | ± | - |
| *Brucella abortus*[a] | - | - | - | - | + | - |
| *Moraxella bovis* | - | ± | - | - | - | - |
| *Pasteurella* spp. | - | - | + | - | ± | - |
| *Past. haemolytica* | + | +[b] | + | ± | - | - |
| *Past. multocida* | - | - | + | - | - | + |
| *Pseudomonas* spp. | + | + | - | + | ± | – |

After D. M. McCurnin (1985) *Clinical Textbook for Veterinary Technicians*. W. B. Saunders.
[a] Brucellae exhibit bipolar staining and most require CO for growth.
[b] Haemolysis under colony.

1 Mix a small drop of the reagent with a colony from the blood agar plate with a platinum loop.
2 With the loop, lift the mixture slowly at 5-second intervals to determine whether strands of a viscous gel have formed in 20–30 s.

Formation of a viscous gel is indicative of a Gram-negative bacterium. The Gram-positive organisms mix diffusely in the potassium hydroxide.

### Slide catalase test

This is used to differentiate streptococci from staphylococci and *Erysipelothrix* and *Corynebacterium* from other small Gram-positive rods.

1 Smear a few bacteria from a colony centre on a clean, dry slide.
2 Add a drop of hydrogen peroxide to the smear.

The presence of gas bubbles (splitting of $H_2O_2$) represents a positive test and usually occurs within a few seconds, but may be delayed for up to 2 min with *Pasteurella* and *Actinomyces*.

The test may be difficult to interpret with some weak species – adequate controls are required. False positives may occur with media containing low levels of glucose. Blood agar should not be used.

### Coagulase test

For detection of *Staph. aureus* which produces coagulase that can coagulate plasma, unlike other strains of *Staphylococcus*. The plasma used should not contain citrate, HIV and hepatitis positives.

**Slide coagulase test** detects clumping factor or 'bound' coagulase. Confirm negative results with tube coagulase or DNase test.

1 Emulsify a colony of the test organism with two separate drops of saline on a microscope slide.
2 Mix a loop of plasma with one of the suspensions.
3 Examine second (control) suspension to ensure absence of agglutination.

Agglutination should occur at (1) within 5–10 s to indicate presence of coagulase. Delayed clumping of organisms is not a positive result.

**Tube coagulase test**

1 Mix 0.5 ml of plasma (diluted 1:10 in saline) and 0.1 ml of an 18–24 h nutrient broth culture of the test organism in a test tube (75 mm × 12 mm).
2 Examine after 1, 3 and 6 h and overnight incubation for clot formation.

Clot formation indicates a positive result.

### Oxidase (cytochrome *c* oxidase) test

Detects all Gram-negative bacteria except lactose fermenters which are negative. Useful for identifying *Vibrio, Neisseria, Campylobacter, Aeromonas*. Commercial oxidase reagents are readily available and packaged for use. Alternatively, they can be freshly prepared.

1 Moisten a piece of filter paper with 2–3 drops of oxidase reagent in a Petri dish.
2 Transfer a heavy inoculum of the colony of the test organism to the filter paper using a wooden stick, glass rod or platinum loop (not a nichrome bacteriological loop).
3 Examine for a dark purple colour indicating oxidase production. This should appear within 10 s but may be delayed for up to 2 min with some reagents for *Pasteurella* and *Actinobacillus*.

Alternatively, the oxidase reagent may be dropped directly on to the test colony. A positive reaction is shown by the colony turning pink then black.

### DNAse (deoxyribonuclease) test

Used for confirmation of *Staph. aureus*, which produces heat-stable DNAse, other strains of *Staphylococcus* producing DNAse which is not heat-stable.

1 Prepare DNase medium by mixing a sufficient amount of DNA of known concentration with nutrient agar to give a final concentration of 2 mg/ml. Sterilise by autoclaving at 121°C for 15 min.
2 Prepare plates each containing 15–20 ml of DNAse agar.
3 Place a small spot or streak of the test colony on the plate(s) and incubate for 18–24 h at 37°C.
4 Cover surface of each plate with 2–3 ml of IM (10%) hydrochloric acid and remove excess HCl after 30 s.

*Staph. aureus* organisms will cause medium to become opaque with clear zones round the DNAse-producing colonies.

If dyes such as toluidine blue and methyl green are incorporated into the medium, this is coloured accordingly, the colours changing as the DNA is hydrolysed.

### Hippurate hydrolysis test

This is used to confirm *campylobacters* which can hydrolyse hippurate to form glycine and hippuric acid.

**Reagents** Ninhydrin, a 3.5% solution in equal parts of acetone and butanol. Sodium hippurate, 5% aqueous solution in 0.5 ml volumes stored at −20°C.

1 Grow test organism on blood agar for 18–24 h at 37°C under microaerophilic conditions.
2 Mix a 2 mm loopful of colony with 2 ml of distilled water and add 0.5 ml of sodium hippurate.
3 Incubate at 37°C for 2 h.
4 Add 1 ml of ninhydrin solution and leave for 2 h at room temperature (or 10 min at 37°C).

*Positive reaction* Purple colour indicates the formation of glycine.

### Haemolysis test

Some organisms have the ability to produce haemolysins which can affect red blood cells. *Beta haemolysis* appears as *clear zones* round the bacterial colonies where the RBCs are completely lysed. *Alpha haemolysis* shows as *green* discoloration round the colonies repesenting a partial clearing of blood.

Alpha-haemolysis occurs with *Str. pneumoniae* and certain viridans streptococci; beta-haemolysis with *Str. pyogenes, Listeria monocytogenes, Str. agalactiae.*

### Hydrogen sulphide test

Used to differentiate the Enterobacteriaceae – *Campylobacter, E. coli, Klebsiella, Shigella, Salmonella, Yersinia.*

*Two indicators*: sodium thiosulphate and ferrous sulphate in medium (triple sugar iron (TSI) agar slopes (slants)).

1 Inoculate organism deep into agar slope with a straight wire and streak up the slope.
2 Incubate at 37°C (*Salmonella*) and at 30°C (*Yersinia*) for 18–24 h. Incubate campylobacters in a reduced oxygen and increased $CO_2$ atmosphere for up to 3 days.

*Positive result*: Blackening of medium.

A *rapid test* for *Campylobacters* consists of placing a large inoculum from a 18–24 h blood agar culture incubated at 37°C in a reduced oxygen atmosphere in the upper third of ferric bisulphite pyruvate (FBP) medium (screw-capped tube) which is incubated at 37°C for 2 h.

*Positive result*: Blackening of medium.

### Indole test

Some organisms that possess the enzyme tryptophanase can deaminate the amino acid tryptophan with the production of indole, pyruvic acid and ammonia. These include the *Enterobacteriaceae* and non-glucose-fermenting rods.

*Reagent*: paradimethylaminobenzaldehyde (Kovac's reagent).

1 Inoculate tryptophan broth (1%) which contains trypticase, a peptone rich in tryptophan, and sodium chloride with a pure culture of the test organism and incubate at 37°C for 2 days.
2 Add 5–10 drops of Kovac's reagent, shake and allow to stand for 10 min.

*Indole* is indicated by a *pink* colour at the surface.

### CAMP (Christie, Atkins, Munch-Petersen) test

This test differentiates *L. monocytogenes* from the other *Listeria* species which are CAMP negative. *Staph. aureus* and *Rhodococcus equi* (cause of respiratory infections in animals) are also CAMP positive.

1 Streak the centre of one plate of 5% sheep blood agar with the recommended standard strain of *Staph. aureus* and across the centre of a similar plate with the standard strain of *Rhodococcus equi.*
2 Inoculate each plate with the test organism by streaking at right angles to within 1–2 mm of the standard organisms. Incubate the two plates at 37°C for 18 h.
3 Examine for evidence of *haemolysis* in the form of a clear arrow at the closest points of the two cultures.

*L. monocytogenes* and *R. equi*: haemolysis should be clear but may occur in a reduced or 'block' form which is not to be regarded as a positive reaction.

### Urease test

*Urease* – the first enzyme to be purified and crystallised – catalyses the decomposition of urea to ammonia and carbon dioxide. It is possessed by intestinal organisms and is present in the stomach of man and animals, where it is able act on any excess urea ingested.

A *positive* result in urea broth is indicated by a bright pink colour produced by the presence of ammonia.

## STAINING TECHNIQUES AND MICROSCOPY

Swabs of pus, thin or thick liquids or semisolids, e.g. faeces, are made by rolling the swab backwards and forwards over the slide to deposit a thin, even layer of the sample material.

Thick, granular material, e.g. *Actinomyces bovis*, *Myco. bovis*, or mucoid material should be spread evenly and may require crushing between two slides, rotating the upper slide and finally pulling it off sagittally to spread the material on the under slide. In such cases it is useful to have both thick and thin areas on one slide. Use the better smear or both smears for staining.

Thin fluids, transudates, urine and blood can be dropped on to a slide and spread by using another slide at an angle of 45° drawn from the edge of the material backwards (Fig. 14.11). The thickness of the smear can be varied according to the amount of material drawn by the upper slide.

Smears of *bacteria on culture plates* can be prepared for staining by first placing a drop of water on a clean slide with a platinum loop. Two to four drops may be used. A small portion of a colony on the culture plate is carefully picked off with the loop which has been first flamed and allowed to cool and then transferred to the water drop with the loop, mixed and then spread evenly over its area.

The slide is allowed to dry and fixed gently in the Bunsen flame.

Note that smears of bacteria made from liquid media do not require the addition of water.

## STAINING TECHNIQUES

While the morphology of bacteria can be studied in an unstained condition (unstained wet films, hanging drop for demonstration of flagellae, use of dark-ground illumination, phase-contrast microscopy), special techniques are required for this purpose. Staining of smears is an essential procedure and enables organisms to be more readily seen along with their morphology, spore formation, flagellae, etc., and aids classification when Gram and Ziehl–Neelsen stains are used to differentiate Gram-positive/Gram-negative and acid-fast/nonacid-fast forms.

Staining only colours the protoplasm of the bacteria leaving the *cell wall* or *capsule* unstained and appearing as a clear surround against the stained background. Capsules can be seen in a wet India ink film or with Leifson's flagella stain.

Before a stain is applied, the smear must be fixed by drying in air and heating gently in a Bunsen flame. This action kills the bacteria and allows the stain to penetrate into the cell body.

### Types of stains

*Simple stains* such as carbol fuchsin, methylene blue and methyl violet colour the bacteria, showing shape and size.

*Differential stains* such as Gram's and Ziehl–Neelsen allow the differentiation of bacteria into specific groups and are of great importance in routine microbiology, especially the former.

*Negative or background staining*, e.g. using India ink, colours the background dark and leaves the organisms unstained.

*Silver impregnation* techniques are used to demonstrate spirochaetes.

Some organisms adopt a peculiar beaded form of staining, for example, *Pseudomonas (Actinobacillus) mallei*, *Myco. bovis*, some forms of *Corynebacterium* spp. or bipolar, e.g. *Pasteurella*, *Yersinia* spp.

### Staining of spores

1. Stain with carbol fuchsin for 5 min with gentle heat.
2. Wash.
3. Decolorise with 5% sodium sulphite for 5–10 s.
4. Wash.
5. Counterstain with Loeffler's methylene blue for 8 min.
6. Wash and dry.

Spores stain red or pink and bacilli blue.

In *Gram's method*, spores can be seen as colourless round or oval spaces in vegetative bacteria stained, for example, by Gram's stain.

A *modified Ziehl–Neelsen* method can be applied using carbol fuchsin for 3–5 min with gentle heat, washing in water and then counterstaining with methylene blue for 4–8 min and a final wash and dry. The spores appear bright red and the protoplasm blue, similarly to the acid-fast reaction.

### **Gram's stain** (see Table 14.13)

H. Christian J. Gram (1853–1938), a Danish physician, in 1854 devised the important system of bacterial staining which divides all

**Table 14.13** Some Gram-positive and Gram-negative cocci and bacilli.

| Gram-positive | Gram-negative |
|---|---|
| COCCI | COCCI |
| *Staphylococcus* | *Neisseria* |
| *Streptococcus* | |
| BACILLI | BACILLI |
| *Bacillus* | *Brucella* |
| *Clostridium* | *Pasteurella* |
| *Corynebacterium* | *Escherichia* |
| *Erysipelothrix* | *Vibrio* |
| *Lactobacillus* | *Klebsiella* |
| *L. monocytogenes* | *Campylobacter* |
| *Actinomyces* | *Salmonella* |
| *Nocardia* | *Shigella* |
| *Borrelia* | *Legionella* |
| *B. anthracis* | *Proteus* |
| | *Yersinia* |
| | *Pseudomonas* |
| | *Haemophilus* |

bacteria into Gram-positive and Gram-negative types according to whether or not they resist decolorisation with acetone or alcohol after being stained with a para-rosaniline dye such as crystal violet, methyl violet and dilute iodine.

The Gram-positive organisms (e.g. *Bacillus* spp., *Streptococcus, Staphylococcus, Listeria*) are stained a dark purple/blue/black colour, while the Gram-negative organisms (e.g. *E. coli, Pseudomonas, Salmonella*) appear pink or red when counterstained with basic fuchsin, dilute carbol fuchsin, neutral red or safranine.

The Gram reaction may vary in certain situations, e.g. old cultures, in which some broken Gram-positive bacteria may stain as Gram-negative types while the opposite reaction can occur.

The Gram-positive cell wall, unlike that of Gram-negative organisms, is very thick and composed of a murein layer containing teichoic acid and lipoteichoic acid. This difference in cell wall structure and content also divides the bacterial world into two other groups – Gram-positive bacteria being more susceptible than Gram-negative organisms to the action of antibiotics, acids, detergents, basic dyes, proteolytic enzymes but more resistant to alkalies, proteolytic enzymes, antibody and complement.

As a first step in the identification of bacteria, stains like Gram and Ziehl–Neelsen are also useful in demonstrating the morphology, size and grouping of organisms as well as the presence/absence of spore formation.

*Procedure*

1 Fix smear on slide with gentle heat after drying.
2 Stain with crystal violet for 1 min.
3 Wash slide with water for a few seconds.
4 Flush with iodine solution and allow to stand for 1 min.
5 Wash with water and allow to dry.
6 Wash with 95% ethyl alcohol until stain ceases.
7 Wash with water.
8 Counterstain with carbol fuchsin, etc., for 10 s.
9 Blot dry.

Gram's stain can also be used for some of the smaller bacteria, e.g. *Rickettsia, Coxiella* and *Chlamydia*, but the reactions are generally weak and generally Gram-negative except for *C. burnetii*, which appears Gram-positive.

Care must be taken to ensure that the various reagents are used properly, otherwise false reactions will occur, for example, if the crystal violet is rinsed too vigorously before mixing with the iodine solution or the carbol fuchsin not allowed to act for a sufficient length of time, the Gram-negative organisms will not stain properly. If decolorisation is too strong, the Gram-positive bacteria will be denuded of stain and fail to colour, but if it is insufficient the organisms may be falsely Gram-positive.

## Ziehl–Neelsen stain for acid-fast staining

This staining reaction is a combination of the stains devised by Franz Ziehl (1897–1926), a German bacteriologist, and F. K. A Neelsen (1854–1894), a German pathologist. It is used as a method to distinguish acid-fast (e.g. *Mycobacteria* spp.: *M. bovis, M. tuberculosis*) from non-acid-fast bacteria.

Acid-fastness in microorganisms is attributed to their impermeability due to a high content of fatty acids, lipids and alcohols, which makes them resist decolorisation with strong mineral acids ($H_2SO_4$, HCl) following staining with a strong dye such as hot basic fuchsin.

Acid-fast organisms are stained red with the carbol fuchsin while the non-acid-fast ones are stained blue with the counterstain methylene blue or green with malachite green.

*Procedure*

1 Fix smear with gentle heat after blot drying.
2 Stain with carbol fuchsin for 5 min using gentle heat.
3 Wash with water.
4 Decolorise with acid alcohol until preparation turns pink.
5 Wash with water and dry.
6 Counterstain with methylene blue for up to 2 min.
7 Wash and blot dry.

The Kinyoun and modified Kinyoun stains for acid-fast staining are similar to the above method.

Examples of acid-fast organisms include *M. bovis, M. tuberculosis, M. paratuberculosis, M. kansasii, M. avium, M. leprae, M. marinum.*

### Leishman stain

(0.15 g Leishman powder in 100 ml methyl alcohol)

1 Run or pipette undiluted stain on to slide and allow to act for 2 min. (The methyl alcohol fixes the smear.)
2 Add diluted stain (double the volume with distilled water) and allow to act for up to 10 min.
3 Wash in water to turn film pink.
4 Remove excess water and dry in air.

Along with Giemsa, Castaneda and Michiavello stains this is useful for staining rickettsiae, babesia coxiella and chlamydiae.

### Giemsa stain

(Mixture of several compounds – Azur I, II, eosin in methyl violet)

1 Fix undried smear with pure methyl alcohol for 3 min.
2 Add one part of Giemsa stain to two parts of distilled water and apply to film for 5 min.
3 Wash in water and dry.

### Wright-Giemsa stain (modified)

A rapid stain for films and imprints to colour a large variety of microorganisms. It is a combination of basic thiazine dyes and acid eosin.

1 Prepare smear and fix in alcohol.
2 Dip slide in fixative solution 5 times for 1 s each time.
3 Allow to drain.
4 Dip slide in Solution I five times, for 1 s each time.
5 Allow to drain.
6 Dip slide in Solution II five times, for 1 s each time.
7 Allow to drain.
8 Rinse in water. Dry and examine.

Bacteria stain blue. The nuclei of *protozoa* are coloured red. White cell chromatin stains purple.

### Calcofluor white/Fungifluor Kit

Calcofluor white is a colourless dye that binds to cellulose and chitin. This is a rapid stain for fungi.

The 1% (w/v) stock solution is made by dissolving calcofluor powder in distilled water with gentle heat and then diluting to make a 0.1% solution with 0.08% Evans blue as a counterstain.

1 Place 1–2 drops of Calcofluor white or Fungifluor solution A to fixed smear for 1–2 min.
2 Apply a coverslip or rinse and dry.
3 Examine smear under fluorescent microscope using filters G 365, LP 450 or FT 395.
4 Add Fungifluor solution B if quenching of non-specific staining is required.

*Fungi cells* and *hyphae* show a bright apple-green or bluish-white fluorescence.

### Suspect anthrax blood/transudate smears

1 Allow smear to dry.
2 Stain with polychrome methylene blue for 2–3 min.
3 Wash and blot dry.

Anthrax bacilli show as chains of short, truncated, dark blue rods surrounded by purplish-red 'granular' material which represents disrupted capsules – the so-called 'McFadyean reaction' which is not displayed by other organisms.

## COLONY MORPHOLOGY

When a specimen containing bacteria – from a swab or platinum loop – is inoculated on to a solid culture medium, colonies develop from each individual bacterial cell.

Depending on the species of bacterium, type of solid medium, etc., these colonies vary greatly in size, shape, colour, opacity (translucent, transparent, opaque) and consistency (soft, viscid, granular, buttery) and smell. Colour may be internal or excreted into the surrounded medium. Shape includes round, irregular and rhizoid colonies which may be flat, convex, raised or umbonate in cross-section with entire, dentate, lobate undulate or rhizoid edges. (Fig. 14.13)

Colonies vary in size from being barely visible to several millimetres in diameter. Yeasts and moulds are generally larger than the true bacteria. Bacteria grown on agar slant media exhibit much the same morphology as those in Petri dishes but growth in *liquid media*, e.g. peptone broth, may be confined to the surface as a firm surface pellicle, uniformly distributed through the liquid or appearing as a sediment and sparse or profuse.

Colony morphology should be noted carefully since in some instances it may provide a clue to the identity of the organism under investigation.

## BACTERIOLOGICAL EXAMINATION OF SUSPECT CARCASES

The following procedure is recommended for the examination of cases which would warrant condemnation in the absence of an assurance that they are of an acceptable microbiological standard and is indicated for the following:

1 All emergency and casualty slaughter animals (except obvious injury cases).
2 Imperfect bleeding.
3 Poor setting.
4 pH value higher than 6.5 or more 24 h after slaughter.
5 'Trimmed' carcases, i.e. carcases with organs or parts missing at veterinary examination.
6 Septic conditions.
7 Cases of enteritis.
8 Carcases heavily contaminated during dressing.

**Samples required** Neck muscle, spleen, mesenteric lymph node, carcase lymph node, liver.

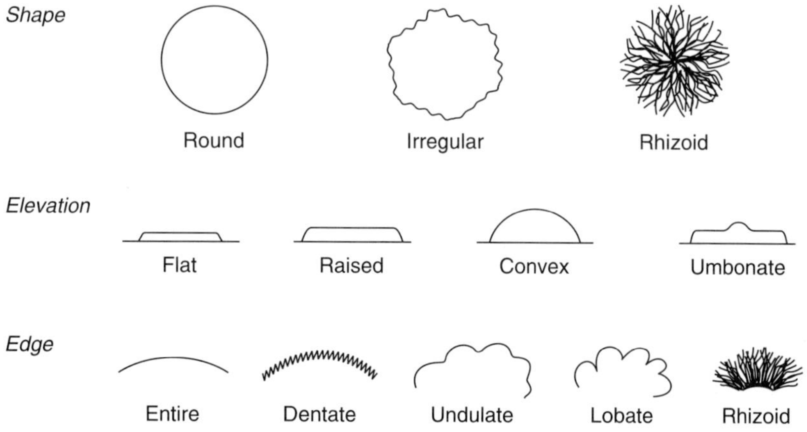


**Fig. 14.13** Colony morphology on solid media.

**Smears** stained by Gram and Ziehl–Neelsen should be made from lesions initially.

**Culture media** Blood Agar, MacConkey Agar, Brilliant Green Agar. Each sample is cultured on these media and incubated at 37ºC for 24 h.

If *Salmonella* spp. are suspected, Selenite Broth at 43ºC for 24 h should also be used for all the samples prior to inoculation on to Brilliant Green Agar.

If *Clostridium* spp. are suspected, anaerobic culture is necessary using the 1% Glucose Agar Stab method, McIntosh and Fildes jar, etc.

*Potential pathogens* which may be isolated include *Staphylococcus* spp., *Streptococcus* spp., *C. pyogenes, Clostridium* spp., enterpathogenic *E. coli, Listeria monocytogenes, Rhodococcus equi, Erysipelothrix insidiosa, Salmonella* spp.

### Interpretation of results

Tentative identification may be based on staining characteristics and colony morphology.

In general, if two out of three samples are positive for one of the bacterial species listed above, this represents a septicaemia or bacteraemia and total condemnation is warranted, action being based on the post-mortem, microbiological and residue findings.

If *Salmonella, Listeria* or *Erysipelothrix* are isolated from samples of neck muscle only, other parts of the carcase should be examined for these bacteria.

(Source: *Laboratory Handbook on Food Hygiene*, Food Hygiene Laboratory. Department of Large Animal Clinical Studies, Faculty of Veterinary Medicine, University College, Dublin, Professors J. D. Collins and J. Hannan.)

## IDENTIFICATION OF BACTERIAL PATHOGENS (see Fig. 14.14)

### Primary isolation media

**Streak for colony isolation** Observe growth rates, colony morphology and haemolytic patterns. Test selected colonies for Gram, catalase and oxidase reactions. Differential and antimicrobial susceptibility tests can be performed from well-isolated colonies.

**MacConkey agar** is a selective, differential medium which selects for *Enterobacteriaceae* (*Citrobacter, Edwardsiella, Escherichia, Klebsiella, Salmonella* and *Shigella*) and other Gram-negative rods and differentiates them into lactose-fermenters and non-lactose-fermenters. It is commonly used as a primary isolation medium as it can provide useful information about bacteria, even group classification and presumptive identification.

Streak for colony isolation: growth is usually Gram-negative. Pink to red colonies with increased redness in medium are lactose-fermenters, e.g. *Escherichia, Klebsiella,*

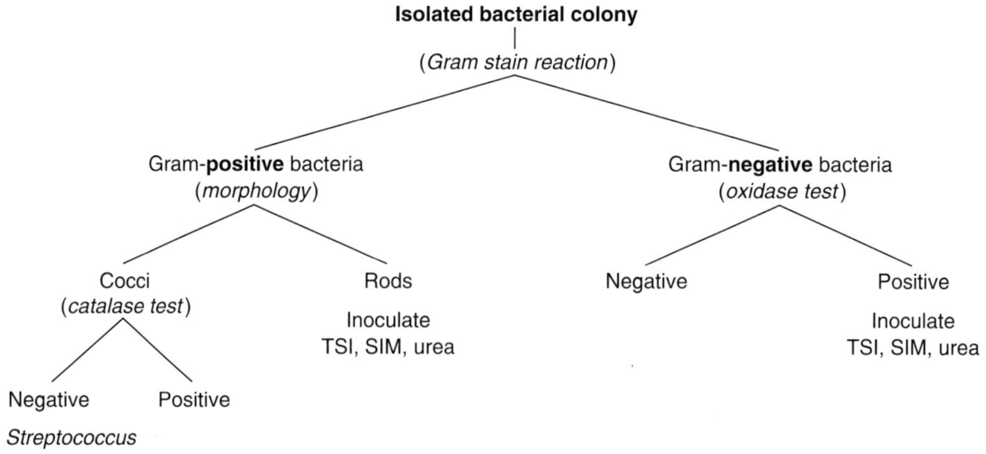


**Fig. 14.14** Flow diagram for bacterial identification. TSI, triple sugar iron agar slant, SIM, test culture to detect sulphide, indole and motility (Esterobacteria reae),

*Enterobacter*. The colourless colonies are non-lactose-fermenters.

**Liquid medium** such as thioglycollate broth is often used as an enrichment broth in the primary isolation procedure. This is an all-purpose medium of value in isolating a wide range of bacteria which were present in small numbers or as anaerobes or facultative anaerobes not recovered on primary plates incubated aerobically. Primary growth in a broth medium is often difficult to interpret: Gram stains of the broth should be compared with growth obtained on primary culture plates.

### Citrate utilisation test

This test indicates the ability of a bacterium to utilise citrate as a source of carbon for metabolism. Most strains of *E. coli* and *Shigella* are unable to utilise citrate, but *Salmonella* is positive to the test.

### Fermentation of sugars (glucose, lactose, mannose, xylose, etc.)

A study of the *production of acid* by various sugars is usually an integral part of bacterial identification. The reaction is shown by a change of colour in the pH indicator present in the culture medium. Lactose is one (the most useful) of a range of carbohydrates which can be used to identify members of the family *Enterobacteriaceae* (Gram-negative bacilli). MacConkey's agar is frequently used to distinguish *lactose-fermenters* (LF), e.g. *Escherichia coli* or *Klebsiellae*, showing as red colonies, and the *non-lactose-fermenting* (NLF) types (*Salmonella*, most *Shigella*, *Proteus* and *Yersinia*), appearing as straw-coloured colonies. *Salmonella* ferments glucose as do all *Enterobacteriaceae*.

Gas formation can be detected when the tests are carried out in liquid media by using small inverted tubes.

1. The basic medium consists of 10 ml of a 10% solution of the required sugar (sterilised at 115°C for 10 min) and 90 ml of peptone water with 1–2 ml of Andrade's indicator solution. This is transferred in 5–10 ml amounts to a series of test tubes or bijoux bottles. (If gas formation is to be checked, Durham tubes are used.) Sterility is checked by incubating overnight at 37°C.
2. Inoculate a pure culture of the organism into the tubes and incubate at 37°C (30°C for *Yersinia*) or up to 7 days.

Acid production is shown by the medium turning *pink*. The Durham tubes will show the presence/absence of gas.

### Methyl red test

This test utilises the metabolism of glucose by the mixed acid fermenters with the production of acids and a low pH. The medium is glucose phosphate broth and the indicator a methyl red solution.

Five drops of indicator are mixed with 5 ml of culture and incubated at optimum growth temperature for 2–7 days.

A *red* colour indicates a positive result.

### Motility test

Motility of bacteria, as demonstrated by their possession of flagella, differentiates motile and non-motile organisms. *Salmonella, Enterobacter*, most *Yersinia* and *Listeria* are flagellate while *Shigella, Klebsiella* and *Yersinia pestis* are non-flagellate.

Motility can be demonstrated fairly easily by examining an unstained drop of fluid culture ('wet preparation') by direct microscopy on glass slide using:

### Urease test

The ability of a bacterium to split urea with the liberation of ammonia and an increased pH is another test applied to enterobacterial strains.

Christensen's urea medium (agar slope or broth) is inoculated with the test organism and incubated at 37°C or 30°C.

The medium changes from yellow to pink or red in positive cases.

### Voges–Proskauer test

This test utilises the ability of certain bacteria to degrade carbon compounds to butylene glycol, acetoin and finally diacetyl, which in the presence of the reagents 40% potassium hydroxide and $\alpha$-naphthol forms a *red* colour.

The medium is glucose phosphate broth as in the methyl red test (q.v.).

## METHODS OF IDENTIFICATION OF BACTERIAL PATHOGENS

Most procedures for the identification of microorganisms in foods follow five main steps, following the use of Gram (and Ziehl–Neelsen) stains. (See also Fig 14.14.)

1. *Pre-enrichment* of the sample in a non-selective broth, e.g. nutrient broth, selenite broth, trypicase soy broth, lactose broth, Gram-negative (GN) broth. (These media contain several nutrients for growth.) Cultures are incubated at 37°C for 24 h.
2. *Selective enrichment* of a portion of the pre-enriched culture using, e.g., glucose azide broth, selenite cystine broth, tetrathionate broth, MacConkey agar, Loeffler's serum agar. (These media contain antibiotics and other inhibitory substances which allow the test organism to grow while restricting competing bacteria.) Cultures are incubated at 37°C or 43°C.
3. Streak selective enrichment cultures on to *selective agar plates*, e.g. MacConkey agar, xylose-lysine-desoxycholate (XLD), bismuth sulphite. Cultures are held at 37°C for 24–48 h and examined for colonies. (Differential media may be used to detect haemolytic and non-haemolytic colonies, e.g. sheep blood agar.)
4. *Biochemical reactions*. Suspect colonies are first tested on differential agars, e.g. triple sugar iron agar slant (TSI) or lysine iron agar butt (LIA). Typical colonies are then tested against a battery of biochemicals for confirmation – fermentation of sugars with, or without, production of gas; indole test, methyl red test, urease test, sodium malonate test, Voges–Proskauer test, etc.
5. *Serology*. The availability of antibodies and antigens of high purity has enabled many different serological tests to be used in the differentiation of bacteria as well as the diagnosis of frank disease in man (AIDS, hepatitis C virus infection and Lyme disease) and animals (TB, brucellosis, etc.).

*Serological tests* include particle agglutination, precipitation assays, double immunodiffusion, counterimmunoelectrophoresis, flocculation, complement fixation, virus neutralisation, indirect fluorescent antibody, immunoassays with labelled reagents (enzyme-linked immunosorbent assay (ELISA)), DNA–DNA hybridisation (gene probe) test, immunoblotting or western blotting, etc. The current high cost of equipment, however, precludes their use in small laboratories.

Many of these tests are commercially available in kit form and take less time than conventional techniques and are capable of being automated. Some, however, are not perfect and reliance has to be placed on traditional methods in some cases. Many, especially the immunoassays with labelled antibodies or antigens, have been improved in quality and will be of value in the future, not only for bacterial and viral diseases, but also for the diagnosis of parasitic disease.

*The field of diagnostics is constantly being improved with the result that many traditional, laborious, non-serological methods fall into disuse with the emergence of tests based on nucleic acid techniques.*

## COMMERCIAL IDENTIFICATION KITS

The development of these systems for the rapid identification of bacteria, assessment of plant hygiene standards, and so on, has been a major advance in food microbiology. For low-volume laboratories they have been a great boon, not only for their rapidity in identifying organisms (often 4–24 h, compared with several days for traditional methods) but also because they are cost-effective and do not require specialist operation.

Prior to 1970, bacteriologists relied totally on the longer methods of growth and isolation of microorganisms on solid agar and broth cultures. Diagnosis of disease was a laborious, complicated and time-consuming task – in reality, a retrospective process. Today the use of many of these systems with their fast identification of pathogens means an early diagnosis and swift action in the judgement of suspect carcases and possible avoidance of outbreaks of food-borne disease. There are now new ways of identifying microorganisms, e.g. by staining them with fluorescein-labelled antibodies (immunofluorescence microscopy), by using immunoelectrophoresis, gas–liquid chromatography, pyrolysis gas–liquid chromatography, electrical impedance monitoring of fluids, microcalorimetry, ELISA (enzyme-linked immunosorbent assay) or biometry luminescence (ATP bioluminescence).

Most commercial kits for bacterial identification consist of a number of test compartments arranged in a compact unit. In one system as many as 300 samples a day (80 samples would be more appropriate for the meat plant laboratory) can be processed simultaneously for salmonella, listeria and staphlyococcal endotoxins. (*E. coli* O157:H7 and other pathogens can also be processed.)

Results for most parameters can be obtained within 60 min (90 min for *Staphylococcus* enterotoxins) after pre-enrichment of samples (which may take 42 h). This system utilises reagents in a closed reagent/sample section which eliminates contamination. The reagent consists of a solid phase and pipetting device and a bar-coded strip containing all the necessary reagents in ready-to-use form. For the larger systems, the unit can be connected to a computer and printer to record results (Fig. 14.15).

### ATP bioluminescence

ATP (adenosine triphosphate) is a nucleotide occurring in all living cells, including bacterial, yeast and mould cells, in which it stores energy in the form of high-energy phosphate bonds.

ATP bioluminescence is based on a reaction that takes place naturally in the American firefly (*Photinus pyralis*). The *Photinus* enzyme, luciferase, uses the energy in ATP to drive the decarboxylation of luciferin with the immediate production of light, which is displayed on the luminometer LCD. The amount of light produced (in Relative Light Units) is directly proportional to the number of microorganisms (plus any residue) in the sample, one molecule of ATP emitting one photon of light. This measurement of ATP is thus a rapid system for detecting microorganisms and is used extensively today in monitoring food plant hygiene and water standards.

The system consists essentially of a sampling swab (for surface sampling) or pen (for water sampling) containing all the necessary reagents and a microprocessor-controlled luminometer.

The ability of ATP monitoring to deal with aerobic, sulphate-reducing and nitrogen-cycle bacteria, *Legionella*, yeasts, fungi and algae compares with standard plate counts for checking only aerobic bacteria and with dual media dipslides for monitoring only aerobic bacteria, yeasts and fungi.

Its portability also adds to its usefulness.

*Steps in ATP monitoring* (Fig. 14.16)

1 Moisten swab with moistening fluid and swab test surface. (For water use sampling pen.)
2 Immerse swab in enzyme solution.

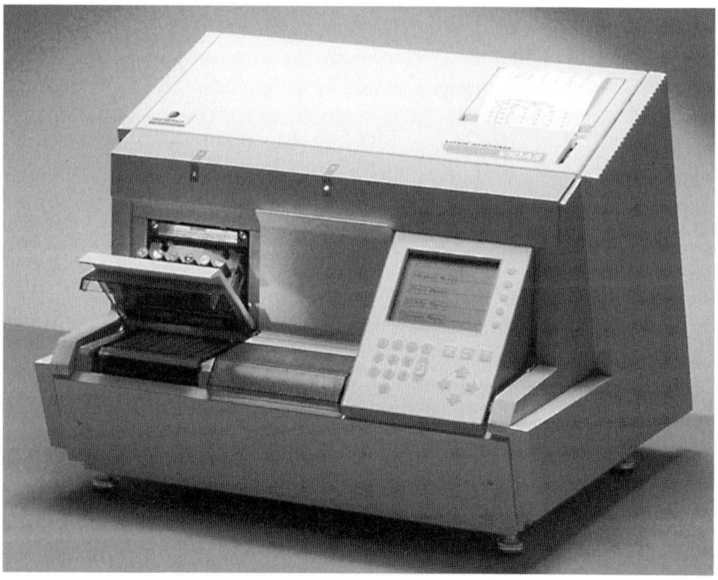

**Fig. 14.15** Automated immunoanalyser (miniVidas) capable of handling 80 samples a day. (By courtesy of bioMerieux Vitek Inc., Missouri, USA)

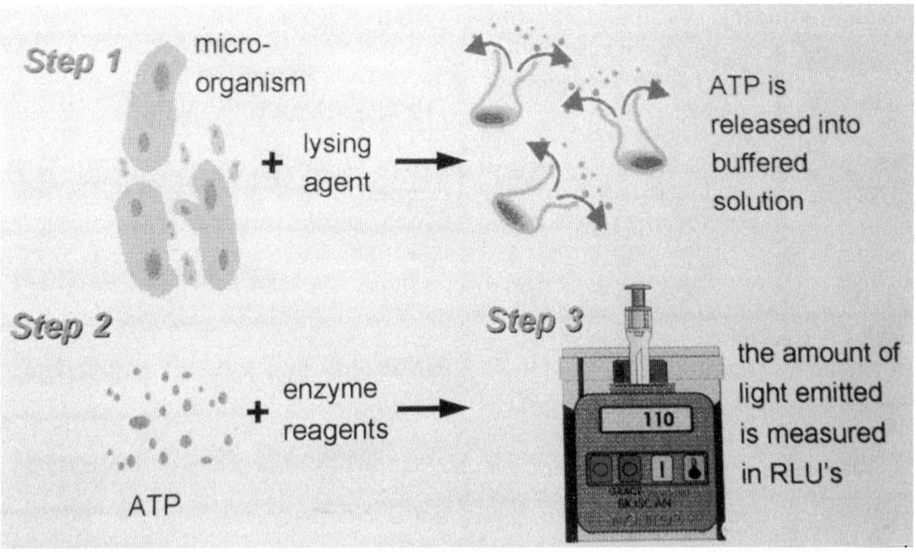


**Fig. 14.16** Summary of ATP monitoring steps. (By courtesy of Biotrace Ltd, Bridgend, Wales, UK)

3 Place swab (pen) in luminometer and read result.

## MONITORING OF PLANT HYGIENE

Aerobic plate counts (30ºC incubation) have been advocated as 'a useful measure of slaughter hygiene and the bacteriological status of carcases' (*Microorganisms in Foods* 6, ICMSF, 1998). The authors further state that 'accumulating such APCs as a trend analysis is a particularly useful measure of hygiene over time'. However, although reasonably accurate gauges of hygiene standards, they are time-consuming, and therefore retrospective, and in any case do not detect food residues. With these methods, results are available when production runs are long completed.

### Assessment of meat plant hygiene using a marker organism

A recent study (Hudson *et al.*, 1998) using a non-pathogenic strain of *E. coli* K12 as a marker organism resistant to nalidixic acid, was carried out to assess the efficiency of slaughter/dressing techniques. Such a marker organism can be detected and counted by direct plating on a highly specific isolation medium and has been employed in poultry processing and in red meat by several workers (Jensen and Hess, 1941; Labadie *et al.*, 1977; Mackey and Derrick, 1979).

Results with beef carcases showed that bagging the excised anus reduced, but did not prevent, the spread of the marker organism from an anal incoculum site. Sheep carcases were found to be contaminated with the marker after the fleece had been inoculated at a single site. The washing of the hands, arms and apron of the operative performing the flaying before and during this operation along with frequent knife sterilisation, however, significantly reduced the contamination ($P < 0.001$). Subsequent washing of carcases had little or no effect on the levels of the marker organism.

It was concluded that the use of the marker *E. coli* may be of value in assessing hygiene control, improving present practices and training abattoir personnel.

What is required is an assessment of plant hygiene standards within minutes rather than days in order that corrective action can be taken quickly. Action may involve an examination of the cleaning methods adopted, the efficiency of equipment and personnel and even the quality of the detergents and disinfectants.

Efficient cleaning/disinfection is the first line of defence against microbial contamination, spoilage of product, infections in staff and poor working conditions and is, therefore, a fundamental part of GMP and HACCP. The condition of the changing rooms, and especially the lockers, will give a good indication of the emphasis placed on hygiene by personnel.

While conscientious inspection using keen eyesight (for all surfaces, especially hidden ones), the sense of smell and the use of a good torch are essential components of examination, they cannot guarantee an efficient cleaning and disinfection level. What may look and smell clean may still harbour bacteria and food residues (which also contain ATP). Efficient cleaning and disinfection involves the removal of *all* ATP (intracellular and extracellular) in soil, debris, faecal material, fat, blood, etc., and product residues in the further processing area.

The results of ATP tests should be correlated with aerobic plate counts, with which they may not tally. The total amount of ATP is first of all determined. When no ATP can be found, the plant is considered clean. If ATP is discovered above a rejection level, the plant is considered not clean; it is an indication of amounts of non-microbial ATP or soil residues although the plate counts may indicate sterility. Therefore, the overall number of microorganisms per se does not necessarily indicate efficient cleaning methods.

### Portable ATP detection system (Fig. 14.17)

Most of these systems consist of a swab, an activator and a luminometer. In some a sampling pen acts as a sampler and activator. A printer can be combined with the luminometer to give an immediate printout. Results, which are delivered in seconds, can be stored for trend analysis. The meat plant can programme the system with its own sampling plans. Plans for every control point can be programmed in, enabling the technician to be led, point by point, through each test point within a process line.

## RESIDUE SAMPLING AND PROCEDURES

This important sector is governed by Council Directive 96/23/EEC which requires random sampling for drug residues by Member States and details the frequency of sampling for the various drugs. In the United Kingdom the relevant legislation is contained in the Animals and Animal Products (Examination for Residues and Maximum Residue Limits) Regulations 1997. The Veterinary Medicines Directorate coordinates a National Sampling and Surveillance Scheme (NSS) in the United Kingdom and specifies the total number of samples required annually.

All these measures are designed to protect the consumer against the consumption of potentially harmful residues of veterinary medicines and apply to cattle, sheep, pigs, horses and poultry (live animals and carcases).

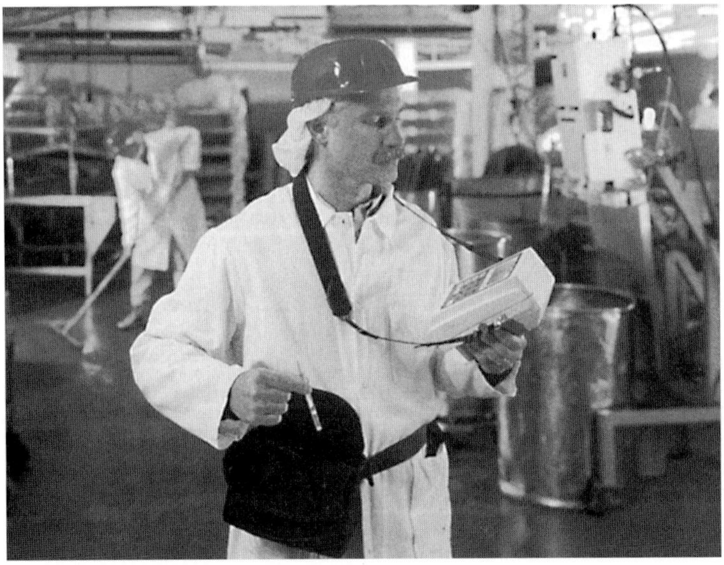

**Fig. 14.17** Plant hygiene monitoring with portable ATP kit. (By courtesy of Idexx Laboratories, Westbrook, Maine, USA)

Annex 1 – Types of Analyses and Samples Required.

Annex 2 – Methods of Collection.

(Full details are given in Chapter 17 of the *Meat Hygiene Service Operations Manual*, to which the reader is referred.)

## MICROSCOPY

### Compound light microscope

This instrument is used for viewing objects as small as bacteria and is the instrument generally used for most microbiological work, the electron microscope being necessary for the study of viruses and large molecules. The light microscope has a resolving power of about ×1500, whereas the electron microscope permits a much greater magnification, ×300 000 or more.

The light microscope consists of a *stand* supported by a horseshoe foot or box containing a built-in *light source* (low-voltage tungsten bulb). The stand carries a *body or draw tube* fitted at its upper end with binocular *eyepieces* and at its lower end with a nosepiece with several *objective lenses* capable of being rotated, depending on the degree of power of magnification required. The body tube possesses coarse and fine adjustment enabling the objective lenses to be brought into focus quickly and accurately – an action which must be done carefully. A monocular tube is often provided near the eyepieces to carry a camera.

The *objective lenses* are normally of low, medium and high power, measured in focal lengths of 25, 50 and 75 mm (low power), 8 and 16 mm (medium power) and 2 and 4 mm (high power). Lenses are often classed as achromats, semi-apochromats or apochromats, the lens for high power being designated *'oil immersion'*. An oil immersion lens is not affected by spherical aberration due to a coverslip, the oil occluding a space between the two.

An arm of the stand is fitted with a mechanical *specimen stage* with knobs for quickly moving the stage in various directions. The coarse and fine focus controls for the body tube are placed near the stage knobs for convenience of operation.

Below the specimen stage is the *condenser*, which may be combined with a *mirror* or *prism* and *iris diaphragm*, enabling light to be directed accurately from the built-in light source.

### Use of the compound microscope

(Variations occur with different models)

The microscope should be clean before use, especially the objective lenses, eyepieces, mirror and condenser.

1. Line up the light source with the microscope.
2. Adjust the condenser to produce a sharp image.
3. Adjust the draw tube to the correct length using coarse adjustment.
4. Place the specimen slide in position.
5. While viewing the object with a ×10 objective lens in position, focus on the slide using coarse and fine adjustments.
6. When focused with the ×10 or ×40 objectives, select a field for the oil immersion lens.
7. Raise the objective, rotate the immersion oil (OI) lens into position, place one drop of immersion oil on specimen and *very gently* lower the OI lens on to the specimen *without touching the coverslip*.
8. While viewing the object, use coarse adjustment and then fine adjustment to produce a clear image.
9. Raise the objective from the specimen and clean off the immersion oil.
10. Place the protective cover on the microscope.

### Dark ground (dark field) microscopy

Ordinary light microscopes are unable to detect certain microorganisms because they are weakly refractile, e.g. leptospires and spirochaetes. These can be viewed with dark ground microscopy by focusing a hollow cone of light from below on to the top of the microscope slide to make the light diverge again and miss the front lens of the objective. The bacteria shine brightly against a dark background because they have been struck by light on the side. The effect can be produced by having water or oil between the condenser and the slide to prevent total internal reflection of light within the condenser as for 'wet preparations'.

The effect is the same as observing fine dust particles when viewing a narrow shaft of sunlight from the side.

### 'Wet preparation' ('Hanging drop')

A drop of a fluid culture is suspended from a coverslip over a hollow-ground slide. It is then examined using a high-power objective with a restricted amount of light by moving the condenser down slightly from its normal position and partially closing the iris diaphragm. Bacteria and other objects that diffract light appear dark against a bright background. Size, shape and motility of organisms can be detected but the motility must be differentiated from *Brownian movement*, which is a continuous agitation affecting all small objects, whereas true motility involves a specific direction using flagella.

### India ink film

This is a negative stain used to demonstrate the capsules of bacteria and yeasts. The fine ink particles are excluded from the capsules which appear clear against a dark background.

1. Pace a drop of India ink on a clean slide.
2. Mix in a little bacterial suspension.
3. Cover with a cover slip and press with blotting paper to make a thin film.
4. Examine with a high-power or oil immersion lens.

## MAIN CHARACTERISTICS OF MAJOR PATHOGENS

### 1. FOOD-BORNE BACTERIAL PATHOGENS (see also Part 1)

#### *Bacillus cereus*

- First diagnosed in Norway in 1947. Considered by FDA to be an emerging pathogen. Two types of illness – diarrhoeal and emetic (resembles *S. aureus* in terms of incubation period and symptoms). Widely distributed in nature – common in soil and vegetables. Can be found on surface of meats, including poultry.
- Gram-positive, motile, β-haemolytic, sporing, aerobic, large rods (3–5 µm × 1.0–1.2 µm). Related to *B. anthracis* and *B. megaterium*. Spores are oval or cylindrical, located centrally or terminally and do not distend the cell.
- Grows well on blood agar and most enriched media – frosted glass colonies.
- Ferments salicin but not mannitol.
- Voges–Proskauer positive. Egg-yolk lecithinase positive.
- Resistant to penicillin and similar antibiotics.

#### *Clostridium botulinum*

The misleading term 'botulism' derives from the latin *botulus*, a sausage, in which food the disease was first described. The extremely potent neurotoxin (of seven different types, A to G), is ingested with the food in which it is formed. Botulism can also occur as a rare wound infection with *Cl. botulinum* infecting a tissue and also as infant botulism in which toxin is formed by the organism in the intestine.

- Gram-positive, obligately anaerobic, motile, sporing large rods (5 µm × 1 µm).
- Spores are oval and subterminal. Motility is achieved by peritrichous flagella.
- Widespread in nature – soil, vegetables, fruits, hay, silage, manure.
- *Demonstration of toxin* in foods, faeces and serum is the test usually adopted for the diagnosis of botulism. The suspect food is homogenised in buffer-gelatin solution and supernatant fluid is centrifuged to produce a test extract. Test extract (0.5 ml) (neutralised with antitoxins A, B and E (main types encountered) and extract (treated with buffer) used as a control) is inoculated intraperitoneally into 2 mice (per sample) which are observed over 3 days. Survival of all mice indicates absence of botulinum toxin. Death of one or more mice along with prior incoordination and dyspnoea indicates suspect botulinum toxin.

*In vitro* neutralisation: Mixtures are held for half an hour at 37°C and then injected (dose 0.5 ml) into separate pairs of mice.

*In vivo* neutralisation: IP dose of 1.0 unit of one of the antitoxin types is given to separate pairs of mice and control mice are given buffer solution. All mice are then challenged 10–30 min later with 0.5 ml of test extract. *Botulinum* toxin is demonstrated by neutralisation of a particular toxin with survival of protected mice.

#### *Clostridium perfringens*

- Normal inhabitant of man and animals and extremely widespread in nature. First isolated in 1890. Now responsible for some

10% of all outbreaks of food-borne disease in man in addition to gas gangrene as well as serious outbreaks of enterotoxaemia in farm animals (Types A, B, C, D, E) and focal symmetrical encephalomalacia in foals (Type D).

- Gram-positive, non-motile, haemolytic, anaerobic (not strict), sporing, capsulated, truncated rods (4–6 μm × 0.8–1.5 μm) usually occurring singly or in pairs. In young cultures the bacteria appear like cocci and in old cultures very long (up to 15–20 μm).
- The spores (rare in laboratory media) are large, oval, central or subterminal and distend the cells.
- Optimum temperature for growth: 45°C with a pH range of 5.5–8.0.
- Ferments a wide range of sugars – glucose, galactose, fructose, lactose, maltose, mannose, sucrose and inositol but not mannitol, sorbitol, trehalose or xylose. Hydrolyses gelatin and reduces nitrate.
- **Recommended media** Egg yolk agar (EYA) detects lecithinase, lipase and proteolytic enzymes. The lecithinase reaction appears as a wide zone of opacity round the colonies. The lipase reaction produces colonies with a multicoloured sheen like mother-of-pearl. On blood agar colonies are normally circular (1–3 mm in diameter), grey or greyish-yellow with glossy appearance, but older colonies may appear umbonate.

Haemolysis is double-zoned.

*Selective media* containing various antibiotics (to which *Cl. perfringens* is resistant), sulphite and iron are used to isolate the organism. These include TSN (tryptose–sulphite–neomycin), TSC (tryptose–sulphite–cycloserine) and SPS (sulphite–polymyxin–sulphadiazine). Colonies turn black with sulphite and iron.

- *Cl. perfringens* in contaminated food samples tends to die off quickly, so these should be examined as quickly as possible.

### *Listeria monocytogenes*

- Listeriosis in sheep and cattle was recognised in Germany in 1925, the first record in humans being in 1926. Since then the incidence appears to have increased although still relatively uncommon. It is, however, a serious disease in animals and humans (especially in neonates, pregnant women and the elderly and immunocompromised, making it an important zoonosis).
- There are six species of *Listeria* (only three of which are virulent) giving rise to 17 serovars.
- The organism has been isolated from a wide range of animals (domesticated and wild), birds, fish, crustaceans, flies, ticks and animal products.
- Gram-positive, motile, aerobic, haemolytic, non-sporing, slightly curved, tiny rods (1–2.0 μm × 0.5 μm) with rounded ends, often occurring in pairs at an acute angle.
- Catalase positive (cf. *Streptococcus*) and β-haemolytic (cf. *Corynebacteria*).
- *Colonies* on sheep's blood agar are very small, smooth, raised, translucent and show a narrow zone of β-haemolysis. The colonies have a close resemblance to those of group B streptococci. Older colonies often have cells that stain Gram-negative.
- Optimum *growth* occurs at 30–37°C (range 0.5–45°C) with a slightly increased $CO_2$ (10%) atmosphere. *L. monocytogenes* is able to grow at refrigeration temperatures and in a high salt medium (up to 10% salt).
- The *motility* of the organism in wet preparations is characteristic, exhibiting a 'tumbling' movement. This is best seen in special motility media in which an 'umbrella' pattern occurs. Motility occurs best at 25°C in young broth cultures in which up to four flagellae can be seen.
- Glucose, maltose (lactose, sucrose slowly) are *fermented* without gas formation, but not mannitol.
- *Thermal death point* is 72°C in 1 s.
- *Isolation media for listeria:*

1. *Cold enrichment method:* Macerate material and add to tryptose broth. Incubate at 4°C (retards growth of contaminants). Sample at intervals on to McBride Listeria Agar (inhibits Gram-negative bacteria). Add sheep blood to medium to show haemolysis. Incubate plates (with 10% $CO_2$, 5% $O_2$, 85% $N_2$) for 48 h at 35°C.
   Screen colonies for motility, biochemical and catalase reactions.
2. Use *trypticase soy–yeast extract enrichment* and selective broth containing acriflavine hydrochloride, naladixic acid and cycloheximide. Store cultures at 30°C and plate after 24 h and 7 days on modified McBride Listeria Agar (without blood).

Transfer suspect *Listeria* colonies to blood agar for haemolysis activity.

3 *Selective enrichment method* (SEP). The antibiotic polymixin B is included with acriflavine, naladixic acid and cycloheximide for selectivity.
Sample cultures after 24 h at 37ºC.

4 *Serology* includes restriction enzyme analysis (REA), bacteriophage typing, ribotyping, multilocus enzyme electrophoresis (MEE) and pulsed field gel electrophoresis (PFGE).

## *Campylobacter* spp. (Fig. 14.18)

- Campylobacteriosis due to *C. jejuni* now regarded as the most common form of acute bacterial gastroenteritis in man. The disease is also important in farm animals, causing sporadic abortion in cattle, diarrhoea and dysentery in calves and enzootic abortion in sheep (*C. fetus*), diarrhoea and colitis in young pigs (*C. coli*). Normal commensals in intestine of cattle, sheep, pigs and poultry – their exact roles in disease are not always clear. Potential zoonotic roles. Species includes *Helicobacter pylori*, recently identified as the cause of type B gastritis and gastric ulcers in man. Formerly classified with the *vibrios* (carbohydrate fermenters).
- *C. jejuni*. Gram-negative, motile (single flagellum at both poles), microaerophilic (requires low levels of oxygen), slender, spirally curved rods (0.5–5 µm × 0.2–0.5 µm) with tendency to form chains (S-shaped, seagull-winged). Appears as coccobacilli in older cultures.
- Grows best at temperatures between 42–45ºC. Sensitive to freezing (– 20ºC to – 5ºC) and heat (thermal death point D value – 55ºC for 1 min in skim milk).
- Samples for testing should be held at 4ºC.
- Catalase-positive. Oxidase-positive.
- No fermentation of carbohydrates.
- Biochemical reactions and the characteristic 'darting' motility in 'hanging drop'

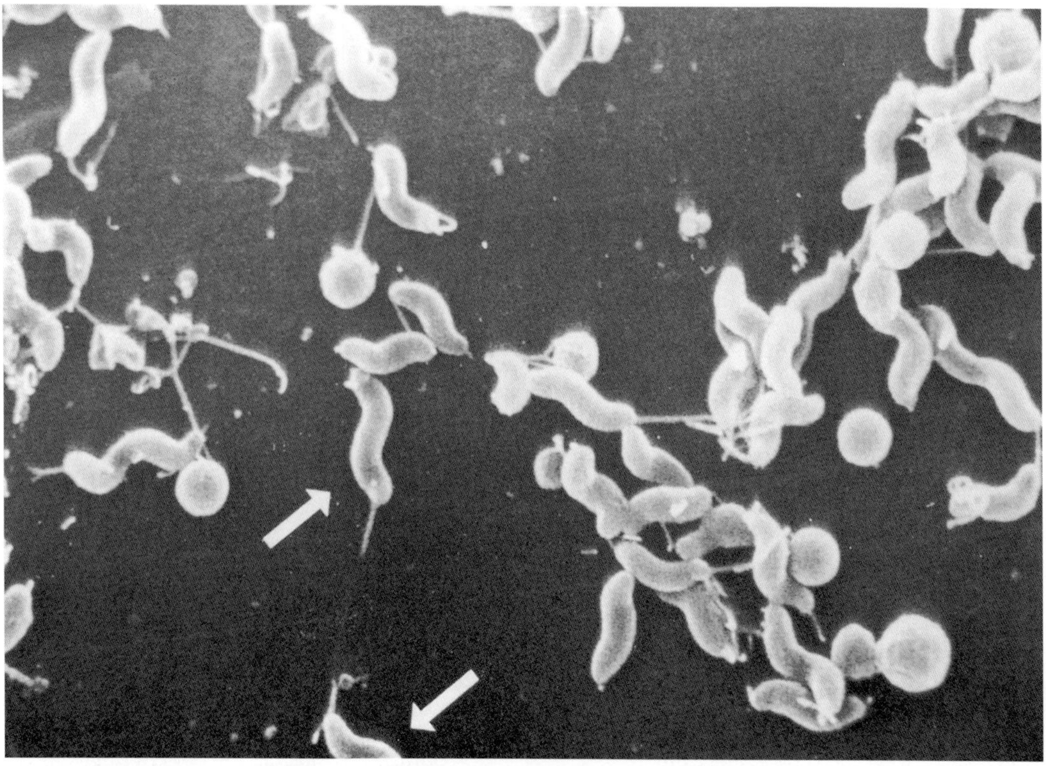

**Fig. 14.18** *Campylobacter jejuni*; electron micrograph showing typical spiral shape and uni/bipolar flagellae. (By courtesy of Professor Diane Newell, Central Veterinary Laboratory, Weybridge, UK)

preparations or phase-contrast microscopy are presumptive evidence of *Campylobacter* spp.

- *Enriched media*: Campy BAP (blood agar plate containing 10% sheep blood and combination of antimicrobials – trimethoprim, vancomycin, polymixin, etc.) or Skirrow medium (Oxoid blood agar base and lysed, defibrinated horse RBCs).
- Ideal atmosphere is 5–10% $O_2$ and 10% $CO_2$.
- *Colony* appearance – moist and spreading, translucent, round, raised or flat.
- Gram stains are faint with safranin – better with carbol fuchsin.
- *Serology:* Latex agglutination tests are now available for rapid identification.

### *Escherichia coli* (Fig. 14.19)

- First described by Theodore Escherich in 1885. An important potential pathogen in man (bacterieria, septicaemia, neonatal sepsis, meningitis and diarrhoeal syndrome) and animals (diarrhoea in newborn animals, especially calves, colibacillosis of newborn, oedema disease, coliform gastroenteritis, cerebrospinal angiopathy, septicaemia, bovine cystitis and pyelonephritis, colibacillosis of poultry).

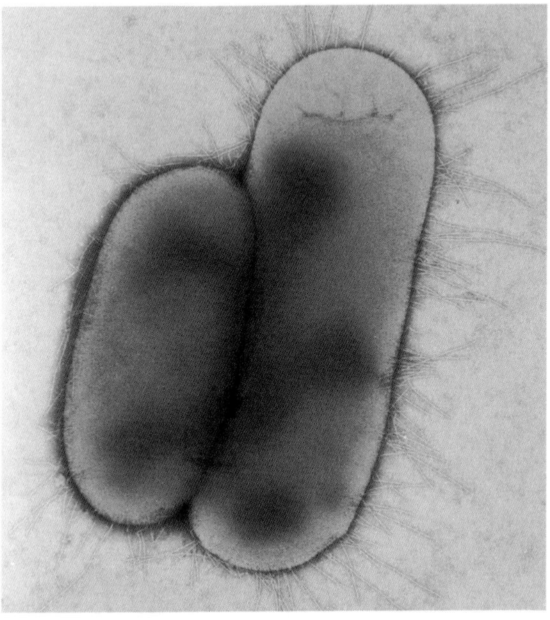

**Fig. 14.19** *Escherichia coli* type 1; electron micrograph. (By courtesy of Central Veterinary Laboratory, Weybridge, UK)

- Gram-negative bacillus, motile and non-motile strains. Possesses O, H and K antigens. Ferments glucose, lactose, trehalose and xylose. Indole and methyl red positive. $H_2S$, DNase, urease and Voges–Proskauer negative. Does not grow in potassium cyanide. Cannot utilise citrate as a source of carbon. On MacConkey agar shows dry, pink, lactose-positive areas of precipitated bile salts.
- There are different types (based on different O:H types, virulence factors, clinical manifestations and epidemiology):

  Enteropathogenic (EPEC)
  Enterotoxigenic (ETEC)
  Enteroinvasive (EIEC)
  Enteroadherent (EAEC)
  Enterohaemorrhagic (EHEC) serotype O157:H7 (verocytotoxigenic – VTEC)

- *Laboratory diagnosis of* E.coli *O157:H7*

1. Faeces culture on highly differential medium, e.g. sorbitol MacConkey agar: heavy colourless growth but no fermentation of sorbitol unlike most *E. coli.*
2. Demonstration of verotoxin in faeces – high levels produced.
3. Demonstration of fourfold or greater increase in neutralising antibody.
4. Demonstration of antigen using antibody-coated magnetic beads. A commercial E. coli *Latex Agglutination Test for serogroup O157.*

A biochemical test is available commercially to screen for O157:H7, this tests for sorbitol fermentation and production of the enzyme β-glucuronidase (*not* produced by O157:H7 but by most other *E. coli*).

### *Salmonella* spp. (Fig. 14.20)

- The natural habitat of the *Salmonella* species is the intestinal tract of man and animals. Most of the 2300 serotypes at present known are non-host-adapted and capable of being carried by many different species. A few are host-adapted, viz. *Salmonella gallinarum* (fowl typhoid) and *Salmonella pullorum* (bacillary white diarrhoea in chicks) occurring only in poultry, *S. cholerae suis* and *S. typhisuis* in pigs and *S. typhi* and *S. paratyphi* in man. Only some 200 of the total number are pathogenic.

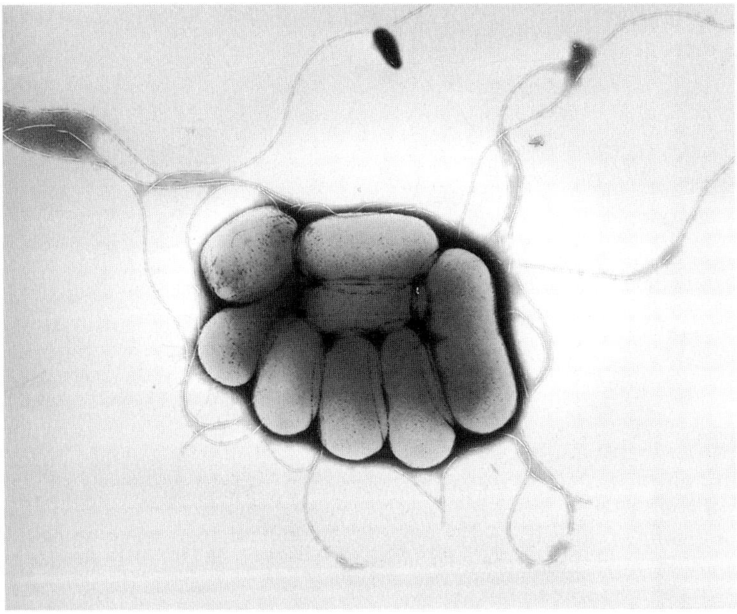

**Fig. 14.20** *Salmonella* spp.; electron micrograph. (By courtesy of Central Veterinary Laboratory, Weybridge, UK)

It has been estimated that the number of reported cases of salmonellosis in Canada is underestimated by a factor of 350:1. At an average cost of about \$700 per case, the annual cost to the Canadian economy for salmonella poisoning is about \$1344 million (or over £6 billion in the UK).

Two types of *Salmonella*, *S. enteritidis* and *S. typhimurium* account for 75% of the food poisoning cases in man, of which *S. enteritidis* accounts for half.

- *Salmonella* are Gram-negative, motile (most by peritrichous or polar flagella), non-sporing, facultative anaerobic, non-haemolytic, straight or curved rods ($2\,\mu m \times 0.5\,\mu m$) indistinguishable under the microscope from *E. coli* and *Shigella*, to which they are closely related genetically.
- Grow best at 37ºC with range of 5–45ºC. pH range: 4–9. Water activity: 0.945–0.999.
- *Colony formation*: Hektoen enteric agar – green/blue green with black centres due to $H_2S$ production.
  Xylose–lysine deoxycholate agar (XLD) – red with black centres due to $H_2S$.
- *Salmonella* and *Enterobacter* are flagellate; *Shigella* and *Klebsiella* are non-flagellate – a useful criterion for differentiation.
- *Classification*: 50 groups based on the O, H and Vi (capsular) antigens.
- Ferment glucose and xylose with gas production (except *S. typhi*) but not sucrose or lactose.
- Dulcitol positive.
- Triple sugar iron agar (TSI) – alkaline red slant and acid yellow butt with or without $H_2S$ (medium black with $H_2S$).
- Lysine iron agar (LIA) – alkaline purple butt with or without $H_2S$.
- KCN broth – no growth.
- Indole negative.
- Lysine decarboxylase positive.
- Methyl red positive.
- Phenylalanine negative.
- Potassium cyanide – no growth.
- Urease negative.
- Voges–Proskauer negative.
- *Serology*: Agglutination assays with antibodies for O, H and Vi antigens, latex and flagellar agglutination assays, grid membrane filtration, DNA–DNA hybridisation (gene) probes.
- Several commercial kits are available for *Salmonella* identification.
- *Presence or absence test*

For detection of the presence of a pathogen, e.g. *Salmonella*, it is the presence of a pathogen, rather than its actual number, that is significant since they are usually expected to be present in small numbers.

- *Routine method for the detection of Salmonella*

This is a simplified version of ISO 3565 1975 Meat and Meat Products – Detection of *Salmonella* (Reference Method) and ISO 6579 1981 'Microbiology – General Guidance on Methods for the Detection of *Salmonella*', except that Rappaport–Vassiliadis Broth is used in place of Muller Tetrathionate Broth and the plating media used are XLD and BSA instead of Brilliant Green (Modified) Agar. It is probable that RV will be incorporated into these ISO methodologies with an incubation temperature of 42ºC. If a high level of background flora is anticipated, it may be desirable to omit the pre-enrichment to avoid overgrowth of *Salmonella*. (Most of the required media are available from several commercial sources.)

1. Pre-enrichment of a 50 g sub-sample in 450 ml buffered peptone water (BPW) (Lab M lab 46) incubated at 37ºC for 18–24 h.
2. Selective enrichment of 1 ml BPW culture in 100 ml Rappaport–Vassiliadis Broth (RV) (Difco 1858–17) at 41ºC and 10 ml in 100 ml Selenite-Cystine Broth (SCB) (Difco 0687–17) at 37ºC, both incubated for 20–24 h.
3. Selective isolation on Xylose Lysine Desoxycholate Agar (XLD) (Oxoid CM 469) and Bismuth Sulphite Agar (BSA) (Difco 0073–01), incubated at 37ºC for up to 47 h.
4. Where appropriate, biochemical confirmation using API 10S or API 20E test systems followed by serological confirmation using polyvalent O and H *Salmonella* antisera.
5. Additional biochemical tests are performed where necessary.
6. Serotyping is carried out if required.

(*Salmonella* antisera: Behring Institute, Difco Laboratories, Wellcome Diagnostics.)

### *Shigella* (Fig. 14.21)

- Obligate parasites of man causing bacillary dysentery or shigellosis mostly in children. Isolated by Kyoshi Shiga in 1896. Closely related to *E. coli*.
- Gram-negative, non-motile (non-flagellate), facultatively anaerobic, non-haemolytic straight rods or coccobacilli.
- *Colony formation:* Large, moist, grey colonies like all Enterobacteriaceae (except *Klebsiella*).

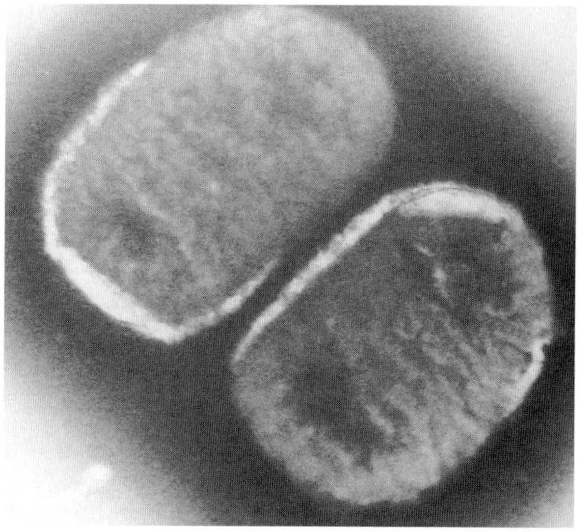

**Fig. 14.21** *Shigella*; electron micrograph showing complete absence of flagellae. (By kind permission of Dr Peter Hawtin)

- Ferment many carbohydrates (except lactose) with acid but no gas.
- Mannitol fermentation: positive by *S. sonnei*, *S. flexneri* and *S. boydii*.
- Lysine decarboxylase negative
- Phenylalanine deaminase negative
- Urease negative
- MacConkey agar: clear, colourless colonies.
- Hektoen enteric (HE) agar: green without black centres (no $H_2S$).
- *Serology*: Grouping (A, B, C, D) based on O antigen by agglutination.

### *Staphylococcus* spp.

- In all there are some 23 species of staphylococci. Besides being responsible for food-borne disease, *Staphylococcus aureus*, a common commensal of man, occurs in the skin, nose, throat, ear and faeces. The relatively mild food-borne disease is caused by the ingestion of a toxin formed in the food.
- *S. aureus* is also one of the most common causes of pyogenic infection in man and animals – skin abscesses, boils, carbuncles, scalded skin syndrome and toxic shock syndrome in man and in recent years has assumed a greater importance because of the emergence of methicillin-resistant strains (MRSA), some of them emanating from hospitals.

- Gram-positive spherical cells appear singly, in pairs or clusters ('bunches of grapes'), non-motile, non-sporing, facultatively anaerobic (most) and β-haemolytic (some species).
- *Colonies* on blood agar are white or golden in colour, round and raised after 24 h incubation.
- *Differentiation of staphylococci, streptococci and micrococci* (Table 14.14).

  Coagulase positive (most strains).

  Maltose: + acid

  Mannitol: + acid

  Mannose: + acid

  Sucrose: + acid

  Xylose: –

- *Detection of enterotoxin in foods*

  Slide agglutination

  Latex agglutination

  Radioimmunoassay

  Enzyme-linked immunosorbent assay (ELISA)

### *Vibrio*

- Thirty species in all, but only some 12 responsible for disease. Found mostly in aquatic environments. Type species is *Vibrio cholerae*, the cause of human cholera, a serious diarrhoeic disease, pandemics of which have been recorded since 1817. *V. cholerae* produces a potent enterotoxin in the small intestine.

Other vibrios, e.g. *V. parahaemolyticus*, are incriminated in human gastroenteritis from contaminated seafoods, especially in Japan and USA. Also causes meningitis, bacteraemia and meningitis. *V. vulnificus* and other vibrios are increasingly being isolated from foods causing enteritis in man.

- *Vibrio* organisms are Gram-negative, motile (polar flagella), facultatively anaerobic, haemolytic (α, β, γ), small, pleomorphic (straight, curved, comma-shaped) rods (0.5 μm × 1.5–3.0 μm).
- *Growth* on thiosulphate citrate bile salts sucrose (TCBS) agar – yellow colonies. This medium differentiates yellow (sucrose-fermenting, e.g. *V. cholerae, V. fluvialis*) from the green (non-lactose-fermenting, e.g. *V. parahaemolyticus, V. mimicus*) vibrios. It is a useful selective medium following enrichment on alkaline peptone water.
- Sheep blood and chocolate agar – fairly large smooth, opaque, iridescent colonies with a greenish tinge α-, β- or γ-haemolysis.
- MacConkey agar – most grow as non-lactose-fermenters.
- Grow best between 30°C and 37°C (range 15–42°C) and pH of 6–10.
- Halophilic, i.e. salt loving, dying quickly in an acid environment. Addition of sodium (at 6.5% NaCl) necessary for optimum growth and accurate identification.

**Table 14.14** Differentiation of staphylococci from streptococci and micrococci.

| | Staphylococci | Streptococci | Micrococci |
|---|---|---|---|
| Motility | – | – | – |
| Strict aerobe | – | – | + |
| Facultive anaerobe | ± | + | – |
| Anaerobic acid/glucose | + | + | – |
| Catalase | + | – | + |
| Growth 5% NaCl | + | ± | + |
| Growth 12% NaCl | ± | – | ± |
| Benzidine test | + | – | + |
| Erythromycin | + | – | – |
| Bacitracin | + | ± | – |
| Furazolidone | – | – | + |

- Oxidase positive (separates *Vibrios* from *Enterobacteriaceae*). The vibriostatic agent 0/129 (150 μg) separates vibrios from *Aeromonas*, the former not growing while the latter do not grow.

### *Yersinia* spp. (Fig. 14.22)

- Of 11 species only 3 are regarded as pathogens – *Y. pseudotuberculosis, Y. pestis* and *Y. enterocolitica. Y. pseudotuberculosis* causes typhoid-like septicaemia/mesenteric adenitis in man. *Y. enterocolitica* – enterocolitis and mesenteric adenitis in man. *Y. pestis* is the cause of bubonic plague ('Black death' of the Middle Ages).

Yersiniosis is the disease in man caused by *Y. entercolitica*. Occurs mostly in children and is of great importance in Europe (Denmark, Germany, Belgium, Norway, Sweden and Canada) but not a major entity in the USA. Contaminated food such as vacuum-packed beef, lamb, pork, shrimps and water have been reported as vehicles of infection.

Reservoirs of infection include many species of animals including pigs, cats and dogs.

- *Y. enterocolitica* and *Y. pestis* used to be classified as *Pasteurellae*.

#### *Y. enterocolitica*

- Gram-negative, facultative anaerobe, non-motile (at 37ºC) but motile when grown under 30ºC (peritrichous flagella), pleomorphic rod sometimes occurring in an ovoid form.
- Psychrotroph, i.e. can grow at temperatures as low as 0ºC and as high as 45ºC (optimum temperature range: 32–34ºC). Optimum pH range: 4.5–9.
- Halophilic at 5% but not 7% NaCl.
- Suitable enrichment media include MacConkey agar, blood agar, cefsulodin–Irgasan–novobiocin (CIN). The organism is more easily isolated at lower temperatures.
- Urease positive.
- Biochemical reaction – acid slant, acid butt on triple sugar iron agar.
- Mannitol – fermented.

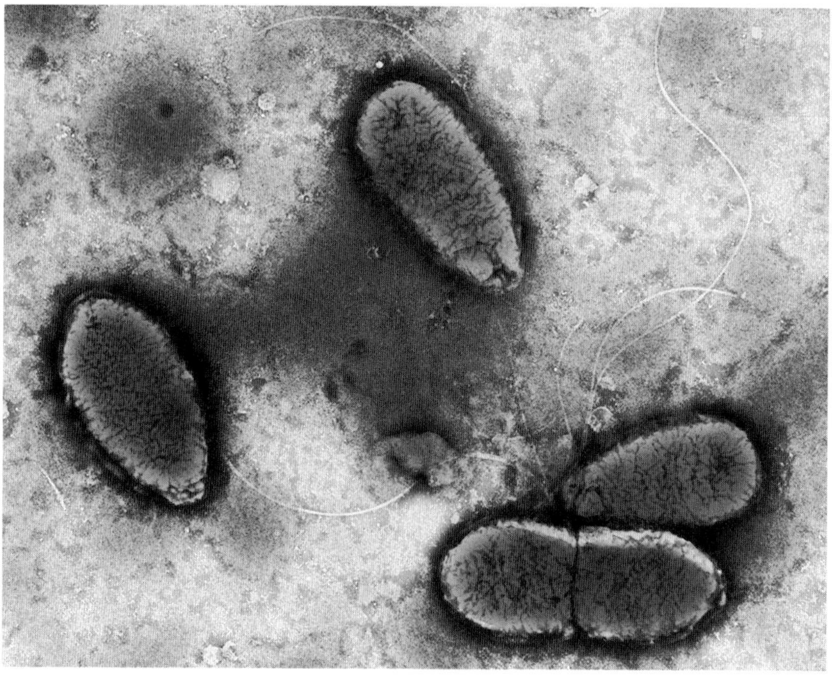

**Fig. 14.22** *Yersinia enterocolitica*; electron micrograph. (By courtesy of Central Veterinary Laboratory, Weybridge, UK)

## 2. Non-food-borne bacterial pathogens (see also Chapter 17)

### *Actinobacillus* (*A. lignieresi*, *A. equuli*, *A. suis*)

- Gram-negative, non-motile, non-sporing, aerobic, haemolytic (variable) small rods or cocci. Urease positive, catalase positive, oxidase variable, indole negative.
- *Growth*

  Blood agar – round, translucent, sticky colonies.

  MacConkey agar – colourless colonies. Growth variable.
- Enhanced $CO_2$ (5–10%) atmosphere required.
- Ferments glucose (with or without gas).

### *Actinomyces* spp.

- Gram-positive, anaerobic, non-sporing, partially acid-fast, straight or slightly curved rods which may form short chains, clusters or long filaments. Staining may show a beaded effect.
- *Growth*

  Blood agar – small, rough, irregularly-shaped, dry, granular colonies slow to develop. Resemble *Nocardia* colonies.
  MacConkey agar – on growth.
- Enhanced $CO_2$ (5–10%) atmosphere required.

### *Bacillus anthracis* (see Ch. 17, Anthrax above)

- Detection of *B. anthracis* is normally confined to use of McFadyean's polychrome blue stain.

### *Bordetella* spp.

- Gram-negative, obligately aerobic, non-motile, non-sporing, haemolytic (variable), small rods or coccobacilli.
- Growth (best at 35–36°C)
  Blood agar – tiny, circular, dewdrop colonies.
  MacConkey agar – as for blood agar.
  Charcoal/horse blood agar – smooth, glistening, whitish-grey colonies.
- Catalase positive.
- Citrate positive.
- Oxidase positive.
- Urease positive.
- *Serology*: Direct fluorescent antibody test. Nucleic acid detection.

### *Brucella* spp.

- Six species – *B. abortus*, *B. canis*, *B. melitensis*, *B. neotomae* and *B. ovis*.
- Gram-negative, non-motile, aerobic, non-sporing, non-haemolytic, non-capsulated coccobacilli (0.5–1.5 μm × 0.5–0.7 μm). Intracellular parasites.
- Gram stain may show bipolar staining.
- *Growth*

  Blood agar – pin-point circular, translucent, opalescent colonies.

  MacConkey agar – no growth.
- Require increased $CO_2$ (5–10%).
- Useful selective media: buffered chocolate-yeast extract agar (BCYE), modified Thayer–Martin.
- Catalase positive.
- Hydrogen sulphide positive.
- Oxidase positive.
- Urease positive.
- Direct smears from exudates may reveal small Gram-negative coccobacilli.
- *Serology*: Based on presence of antibodies in samples. Serum agglutination test (limited in value). Complement fixation test (CFT). Enzyme-linked immunosorbent (ELISA) test. Rose Bengal test (buffered antigen or card test) – an earlier field plate test for infection in serum.

### *Chlamydia* spp.

- Chlamydiae and rickettsiae belong to the grouping between the bacteria and the viruses although they are closer to the bacteria – they possess DNA and muramic acid in cell walls, multiply by binary fission and, unlike viruses, stain by Gram's method. They resemble the smallest bacteria and largest viruses in size. Like viruses, however, they are intracellular parasites and cannot multiply outside host cells.
- Isolation and culture methods resemble those for viruses.
- Gram-negative (better stained by Giemsa, Castaneda or Machiavello), round, minute

bodies with unusual development cycle: elementary bodies (0.3 μm) in diameter are phagocytosed by host cells and develop into larger forms (reticulate bodies, up to 2 μm in diameter) that multiply into more reticulate bodies and eventually large numbers of elementary bodies, all within 40–48 hours. Host cells then rupture to release elementary bodies to infect new host cells.

- Microscopy – as stained organisms, use of fluorescent or electron microscopy.
- *Culture* (fastidious grower): yolk sac, tissue culture or mouse inoculation.
- *Serology*: complement fixation (CF), microimmunofluorescence (micro-IF). Results are often difficult to interpret.

## *Clostridia* spp.

- Causative organisms of serious animal and human diseases – botulism, tetanus, food poisoning, gas gangrene, enterotoxaemia, blackleg, bacillary haemoglobinuria, braxy, etc.
- Gram-positive (most), anaerobic, motile (except *Cl. perfringens*) sporing (spores distend cell wall in most cases), haemolytic, fairly large rods.
- Producers of potent exotoxins, e.g. botulin, tetanospasmin.
- Haemolysis of *Cl. perfringens* is double-zoned.
- Size (4–8 μm × 1 μm) is intermediate between *Corynebacterium* and *Bacillus*.
- Spores: oval and subterminal – *Cl. botulinum, Cl. perfringens, Cl. septicum, Cl. sporogenes, Cl. novyi, Cl. sordellii, Cl. difficile*; large, round and terminal – *Cl. tetani, Cl. tertium.*

  Some *Clostridia* spore freely but others require adverse conditions.
- Indole negative (most pathogenic types).
- Lecithinase negative (except *novyi, perfringens* and *sordelli*).
- Lipase negative (except *novyi* and *sporogenes*).
- DNase variable.
- Glucose positive (except *Cl. tetani*).
- Urease negative (except *sordelli*).
- *Culture*: Grow best at temperatures at or just below 37°C. Most form diffuse, greyish, semitransparent colonies of irregular shape. There is a tendency for colonies of *Cl. tetani* and *C. septicum* to swarm across the plate on solid media.
- *Suitable media*: Anaerobic blood agar (brucella blood agar), anaerobic broth (e.g. thioglycollate, chopped meat), egg yolk agar (EYA), bacteriods bile aesculin agar. Many suitable media for anaerobes are available commercially.
- *Anaerobic culture*: In anaerobic jars with atmosphere of 90% hydrogen and 10% $CO_2$ or 80% nitrogen, 10% hydrogen and 10% $CO_2$ after evacuation of air. Evacuation of air can be achieved with a catalyst, e.g. Anatox (palladium-coated alumina pellets; Don Whitley Scientific, Shipley, Yorkshire, UK).

Anaerobiosis can be achieved by adding reducing agents like glucose or sodium thioglycollate to the medium or using cooked meat medium.

Instead of metal or polycarbonate jars commercially available anaerobic plastic pouches or bags (GasPak Pouch, BioBag, Remel Pouch) can be used. These contain an oxygen-removal system that is activated after one or two plates are inserted and the bag sealed and incubated normally. Growth can be observed through the plastic.

## *Erysipelothrix rhusiopathiae*

- Gram-positive, non-motile, microaerophilic, α-haemolytic or non-haemolytic, pleomorphic thin rods (1–2 μm × 0.2–0.4 μm) often arranged singly, in V-shapes or short chains with a tendency to form long filaments in culture media. V-shapes closely resemble those of corynebacteria.
- Some biochemical reactions resemble those of *Listeria* (Table 14.15).
- Blood agar – dewdrop sized colonies with a smooth surface and haemolytic or non-haemolytic at 24 h. After 48 h there are two types of colonies – smaller, transparent, smooth and convex with entire edges; and larger, flat, rough, opaque colonies with indented edges.
- MacConkey agar – no growth.
- Agar shake – grows best below surface.
- Gelatin stab – 'test tube brush' growth.
- Glucose and lactose – fermented (without gas).
- Sucrose and mannitol – not fermented.
- Indole positive.

**Table 14.15** Characteristics of *E. rhusiopathiae*, *L. monocytogenes* and *Corynebacterium* spp.

| Organism | Motility | Haemolysis | Catalase | Acid from glucose | $H_2S$ production | Nitrate reduction | Urease production |
|---|---|---|---|---|---|---|---|
| *E. rhusiopathiae* | – | none/α | – | + | + | – | – |
| *Corynebacterium* spp. | – | V | + | V | – | V | V |
| *L. monocytogenes* | +(25°C) | β | + | + | – | – | – |

V = variable.

- Oxidase negative.
- Voges–Proskauer – negative.

### *Flavobacterium* spp.

- Gram-negative, non-motile, long, narrow bacilli with bulbous ends that on occasions possess a yellow, green or orange intracellular pigment, sometimes accompanied with a fruity odour.
- On blood agar media – lavender-green discoloration of agar.
- Proteolytic activity – positive.
- DNase positive.
- Indole positive.
- Oxidase positive.
- Penicillin-susceptible (unusual for Gram-negative bacteria).

### *Francisellla tularensis*

- Gram-negative, non-motile, obligately aerobic, capsulated, coccobacilli (0.2 × 0.7 µm) with great tendency to pleomorphism especially in older cultures.
- Intracellular parasites.
- *Culture:* Requires addition of egg yolk or rabbit spleen to liquid media or glucose and cysteine to human blood agar. Infected tissues, e.g. spleen, are used for culture.
- *Diagnosis:* Confirmed by inoculation of mice or guinea-pigs with infected exudates.

### *Klebsiella* spp.

- Gram-negative, non-motile, non-haemolytic, capsulated, medium-sized (1–3 µm × 0.5 µm) rods.
- Most capsulated bacteria are regarded as virulent, the polysaccharide capsule protecting the organisms against phagocytosis.

  Demonstration of capsules is indicative of presumptive identification.
- Blood agar – *K. pneumoniae* grows as large, mucoid whitish, non-haemolytic colonies.
- MacConkey agar – large, mucoid pink colonies.
- Biochemical tests are necessary to distinguish *Klebsiella* from *Enterobacter*.
- *Klebsiella pneumoniae*: indole + ; methyl red +/–; gas from glucose + ; lactose + ; urease + ; Voges–Proskauer +.

### *Legionella*

- Gram-negative, aerobic, thin, pleomorphic rods (1–2 µm × 0.5 µm). On occasion, organisms may reach 20 µm in length.
- Intracellular (macrophage and neutrophil) parasites able to multiply at 20–45°C, with capacity to adhere to pipes, plastics, rubber in water tanks, shower heads, cooling towers of air-conditioning systems. It can survive in the presence of commensal bacteria and algae and within free-living protozoa.
- *Staining characteristics:* Stain weakly with Gram and Giemsa. Gram stain can be enhanced by using safranin counterstain for 10 minutes.
- *Culture*: Fastidious grower. No growth on sheep blood agar. Organism requires the amino acid L-cysteine for growth.
- Chocolate agar (and L-cysteine) and buffered chocolate yeast extract (BCYE) with antibiotics polymixin, anisomysin, vancomycin or cefamandole: greyish-white or bluish-green translucent colonies (2–4 mm) after 3–5 days' incubation. Dissecting microscope: centre of young

colonies is grey and granular and periphery pink and/or blue or green with furrows.

- *Biochemical reactions*

  Acid from glucose – negative.

  Nitrate to nitrite – negative.

  Catalase – positive (weak).

  Peroxidase – positive (weak).

  Urease – negative.
- Commercial media and reagents are available.
- *Definitive diagnosis:* Fluorescent antibody technique. Serological detection of antibodies. Urinary antigen detection.

## *Leptospira*

- *Leptospira* spp. are Gram-negative, obligately aerobic, very tightly coiled spirochaetes in contrast to *Borrelia* and *Treponema*, which are more openly coiled. They are approximately 6–20 μm long and 0.1 μm wide. Unlike *Borrelia* and *Treponema* the leptospires have hooks at one or both ends and possess two periplasmic flagella. The organisms are covered with an external membrane.
- They do not stain readily with the ordinary stains but can be impregnated with silver, e.g. by Levaditi and Fontana. They are readily cultured, although growth is slow, the media requiring the addition of animal serum.
- Dark-ground and electron microscopy in wet preparations show the numerous tight coils and the motility, which is mainly rotary.

## *Moraxella* (e.g. *M. catarrhalis*)

- Gram-negative, non-motile, strictly aerobic short rods often occurring as pairs or in chains.
- Optimum temperature for growth: 32–37°C.
- *Culture*

  Sheep blood and chocolate agar – smooth, opaque, greyish-white colonies.

  Sugars – no fermentation.
- DNase positive.
- Catalase positive.
- Nitrate to nitrite positive.

## *Mycobacterium* spp.

- Some 54 species, only *M. bovis, M. tuberculosis, M. leprae* and *M. ulcerans* being regarded as pathogens and about 12 as potential pathogens.
- Thin, straight or slightly curved, non-motile, non-sporing, non-capsulated, aerobic, acid-fast rods (2–10 μm × 0.2–0.4 μm).
- *M. kansasii* exhibit well-defined cross-banding.
- *Growth*: Slow growth, most pathogenic types requiring up to 6 weeks. Extra (5–10%) $CO_2$ and pH of 6.5–6.8 enhance growth, which is best at 37°C.
- *Staining* (see acid-fast staining): The use of the dye auramine instead of carbol fuchsin or safranin in the Ziehl–Neelsen method, examined microscopically by ultraviolet light, is a better means of detecting the organisms.
- *Microscopy*: Dark-ground microscopy of unstained wet preparations and immunofluorescence may also be used to view mycobacteria and other bacteria. In the latter method, fluorescent dyes, e.g. fluorescein isothiocyanate or lissamine-rhodamine, are coupled with antibodies. When an antibody of this type combines with its appropriate antigen, the antigen–antibody complex fluoresces, the isothiocyanate giving a green and the lissamine-rhodamine an orange fluorescence. Electron microscopy may also be used with ultra-thin sections or material mounted on a thin collodion membrane.
- *Culture*: Lowenstein–Jensen (LJ) medium (eggs, asparagine, potato starch, glycerol, mineral salts and malachite green) is the medium of choice for primary isolation of mycobacteria:

  *M. bovis*: small, round, granular, white colonies with irregular edges.

  *M. tuberculosis*: yellowish, flat, spreading, granular and friable colonies.

  *M. avium:* complex, yellowish, thin, opaque/transparent, smooth colonies.

  *M. kansasii:* Middlebrook 7H10 agar – rough or smooth with dark centres and irregular edges. Grown in dark: pigmented or buff colonies. Grown in light: yellowish colonies.
- Serum albumin agar media, e.g. Middlebrook 7H10 selective (albumin, beef catalase, oleic acid, glycerol, glucose, vitamins, cofactors and mineral salts) and liquid media (in which mycobacteria grow more rapidly) such as BACTEC broth (contains palmitic acid and various antibiotics) are also used for primary isolation.

- Specimens should be collected in wide-mouth jars with screw-cap lids and examined as soon as possible. While tissue specimens do not require decontamination/digestion, fluids such as exudates, CSF, etc., may need the addition of a digestant and/or decontaminating agent such as sodium hydroxide (2–4%), oxalic acid (5%), $H_2SO_4$ (4%). Centrifugation of fluid material may be used to concentrate the mycobacteria into a small volume.
- TCH (thiophene-2-carboxylic acid hydrazide): differentiates *M. bovis* and *M. tuberculosis* (see Table 14.16).
- *Guinea pig inoculation* to detect presence of tubercle bacilli in specimens is now rarely used.
- *Serology*: Undeveloped because of lack of antigen specificity.

## *Mycoplasma*

- Smallest of all free-living organisms, once regarded as viruses. Slow growing, facultative anaerobes, fastidious, pleomorphic organisms that do not possess a cell wall.
- Growth is slow and only on very rich media, which must contain sterols derived from blood and serum, e.g. supplemented PPLO agar.
- *Staining reaction*: Organisms do not stain well with Gram and other stains because of absence of cell wall.
- *Dienes stain* is used by placing a small portion of growth on agar plate on a microscope slide, covering a colony with the stain and examining under low power. Colonies of *Mycoplasma* have a 'fried egg' appearance with a light blue periphery and a dark blue centre.
- *Culture*: Pinpoint, glistening, round, raised colonies with centre of colony embedded beneath the surface (anaerobic blood agar).
- *Serology*: Enzyme immunoassay (EIA) and indirect haemagglutination (IHA) are commercially available.

## *Neisseria*

- Family includes *Neisseria, Moraxella, Acinetobacter* and *Kingella*. *Neisseria gonorrhoeae* is the causal organism of gonorrhoea in man.
- Gram-negative, aerobic, non-motile diplococci shaped like kidney beans. Intracellular parasites. Catalase positive. Oxidase positive.
- *Growth*: Optimum temperature is 35°C in a 3–5% $CO_2$ atmosphere. Small, grey, translucent, raised colonies (*N. gonorrhoea*) on selective agar media.
- *Positive identification of* Neisseria: Rapid carbohydrate degradation and chromogenic substrate tests. Coagglutination and fluorescent antibody (FA) tests using monoclonal antibodies.

## *Nocardia*

- Gram-positive (some weakly acid-fast), aerobic thin bacilli that form branching filaments or hyphae. Gram staining often shows a beaded appearance. Yellowish granules containing numerous organisms in

**Table 14.16** Some distinguishing features of *M. bovis*, *M. tuberculosis*, *M. avium* and *M. kansasii.*

| | *M. bovis* | *M. tuberculosis* | *M. avium* complex | *M. kansasii* |
|---|---|---|---|---|
| Colonies on MacConkey Agar | | See above | | |
| Growth on TCH[a] | – | + | + | + |
| Growth 5% NaCl | – | – | – | – |
| Niacin accumulation | – | + | – | – |
| Nitrate reduction | – | + | – | – |
| Catalase | – | – | ± | – |
| Urease | + | + | + | + |

TCH = thiophene-2-carboxylic acid hydrazide: differentiates *M. bovis* and *M. tuberculosis*.

pus from skin infections (cf. *Actinomyces bovis* when crushed between two microscope slides).

- The *Nocardia* resemble *Actinomyces* and the *fungi* morphologically.
- *Culture*: Most species grow well on normal nonselective media at 25–37°C, colonies appearing whitish, lustreless or velvety in appearance.
  *N. asteroides* ferments only glucose with acid production.
  *N. brasiliensis* ferments glucose, inositol and mannitol with acid production.
- Confirmatory identification of the several species of *Nocardia* is a matter for a reference laboratory.

## *Pasteurella* spp.

- Gram-negative, non-motile, facultatively anaerobic, non-haemolytic, ovoid, pleomorphic coccobacilli. Some strains are capsulated.
  With Gram's stain the organisms may be single, in pairs or as short chains and often show bipolar staining.
- *Culture*: Sheep blood – mucoid colonies with narrow green or brown halo after 48 h incubation.
- *Biochemical reactions*: Most strains are catalase and oxidase positive, ferment glucose and xylose but not lactose and maltose, without gas.

## *Proteus* spp.

- Along with *Citrobacter, Enterobacter, Morganella* and *Providencia*, *Proteus* is an opportunistic member of the Enterobactericaeae, which also includes *E. coli, Edwardsiella, Erwinia, Klebsiella, Pectobacterium, Salmonella, Serratia, Shigella* and *Yersinia*.
- *Salmonella, Shigella* and *Yersinia* are generally considered to be the true pathogens of the family Enterobacteriaceae. *Proteus*, however, can occur in wound infections, bacteriuria and even septicaemia.
- Several of the four species of *Proteus* have a tendency to swarm over many solid nonselective culture media, burying other bacteria, and producing an odour resembling burned chocolate. Colony formation – large, greyish-white, opaque and moist.
- Gram-negative, aerobic, facultatively anaerobic, non-sporing, straight rods or coccobacilli.
- They grow well over a wide range of temperatures.
- The two main types are *P. vulgaris* and *P. mirabilis* differentiated as follows:

| | *Urease* | *Indole* | *H S* | *Sucrose* | *Ornithine* |
|---|---|---|---|---|---|
| *P. vulgaris* | + | + | + | + | – |
| *P. mirabilis* | + | – | + | – | + |

- *Proteus* spp. are often resistant to several antibiotics and are thus able to persist in wounds.

## *Pseudomonas* spp.

*Pseudomonas aeruginosa* has been documented as the cause of mastitis, pericarditis and pneumonia (cattle and pigs), while melioidosis in rodents, and occasionally farm animals, is caused by *P. pseudomallei*. *P. mallei* is the cause of glanders in solipeds. *P. aeruginosa* is involved in man with pneumonia (especially in cystic fibrosis), endocarditis, wound infections, urinary tract infection and bacteraemia.

- Gram-negative, motile with polar flagella (except *Pseudomonas mallei*), aerobic, β-haemolytic (most) bacilli or coccobacilli, many of which produce green or yellowish pigments (pyocyanin and pyoverdin).
- All *pseudomonads* grow well on MacConkey agar. A green metallic sheen is produced on sheep blood agar due to the pigment pyocyanin. A fruity grape-like odour is produced by many strains of *P. aeruginosa*.
- Oxidase and catalase positive. Citrate and cetrimide positive.
- **N.B.** Allied to the *Pseudomonads* is the genus *Acinetobacter*, members of which are ubiquitous in the environment (soil, water, sewage, milk, frozen soups, hospital ventilators and humidifiers, etc.). Some species are opportunistic, being responsible in man for pneumonia, urinary tract infections, septicaemia, endocarditis, cellulitis and meningitis. *Acinetobacter* has recently been advanced by Professors Ebringer and Pirt (King's College, London) as the cause of BSE, genetically susceptible persons producing antibodies against *Acinetobacter*, thus making the disease an autoimmune one. They state that the

organism can cause brain damage similar to that attributed to the prion protein.

### *Rhodococcus equi* (formerly known as *Corynebacterium equi*)

- Gram-positive, non-motile, non-sporing, partially haemolytic, sometimes acid-fast, pleomorphic rods often appearing as V or L formations or branching filaments.
- No fermentation of carbohydrates and reaction to nitrate reduction and urease variable.
- On blood agar colonies resemble those of *Klebsiella* – large, entire, raised, mucoid colonies.

### *Streptococcus* spp.

- Gram-positive, facultatively anaerobic (most) but some anaerobic, non-motile, non-sporing, some capsulated, α-haemolytic, β-haemolytic or non-haemolytic, spherical or oval cocci (1.0 µm diameter) arranged in chains of varying length, depending on the species involved. Catalase negative.
- Chain formation is best seen in fluid cultures or in pathological tissues.
- *Four main groups* are involved as commensals and pathogens in human and animal diseases (abscesses, mastitis, endocarditis, metritis, meningitis, pneumonia, lymphangitis, polyarthritis, septicaemia):

1. Pyogenic streptococci – pus-forming; mostly β-haemolytic.
2. Viridans streptococci – α-haemolytic or non-haemolytic.
3. Enterococci – α-haemolytic, β-haemolytic or non-haemolytic.
4. Lactic acid streptococci – non-haemolytic.

α-Haemolytic: partial lysis of RBCs – green colour round colony.

β–Haemolytic: complete lysis of RBCs – clear zone round colony.

Non-haemolytic: no lysis of RBCs round colony – no change of colour.

#### *Lancefield grouping of streptococci.*

Haemolytic streptococci are divided into Lancefield groups A–H and K–V depending on antigenic structure.

**Group A** (β-haemolytic, *Streptococcus pyogenes*): Can be further divided into a number of Griffiths types (M, T, R) according to antigenic structure. Haemolysis is best seen under anaerobic conditions. Growth is improved by addition of blood or serum at 37°C. Colonies are fine (1 mm after 24 h), dry, greyish-white, opaque or transparent. Granular deposit with clear supernatant in fluid cultures. Susceptible to bacitracin and vancomycin. Hippurate hydrolysis negative. Campo test negative.

**Group B** (β-haemolytic (most); e.g. *Str. agalactiae*): Isolation is made easier by use of selective medium containing aminoglycoside. Haemolysis not as marked as with group A types. Some strains are α-haemolytic and some non-haemolytic. Resistant (usually) to bacitracin. Susceptible to vancomycin. Hippurate hydrolysis positive. Campo test positive (distinguishes *Str. agalactiae* from all other haemolytic streptococci, which are negative).

**Group C** (haemolytic): Mainly animal parasites, e.g. *Str. equisimilis.* Neonatal bacteraemia and septicaemia.

**Group D** e.g. *Str. suis* (meningitis and arthritis in pigs) and *Str. faecalis* (streptococcosis in poultry, neonatal infections, endocarditis in sheep). Resistant to bacitracin. Susceptible to vancomycin. Hippurate hydrolysis negative.

**Group E** (β-haemolytic): Often occurs in chains of 3–16 capsulated cocci. Ferments sugars.

**Viridans group of streptococci** Resemble *Str. pyogenes*. Green pigmentation round colonies on blood agar and heated chocolate agar. Cause of jowl abscesses in pigs. Resistant (usually) to bacitracin. Susceptible to vancomycin. Hippurate hydrolysis negative (usually).

### *Treponema* spp.

- *Treponema* spp. *T. pallidum* is the cause of syphilis in man, while *T. hyodysenteriae* is responsible for swine dysentery and *T. cuniculi* for vent disease (syphilis, spirochaetosis) in rabbits.
- The treponemas are slender, openly coiled organisms measuring 0.1–0.2 µm in thickness and 6–20 µm in length. There are some 4 to 14 regular spirals in each

organism, which bears three periplasmic flagella at each pointed end. Motility is rotational along the longitudinal axis with occasional flexes along their length

- The organisms are microaerophilic but cannot be grown in culture. Staining is difficult, only prolonged contact (24 h) with Gram's stain producing pinkish threads, while other spirochaetes appear deep purple.
- Dark-field microscopy is used to detect the organisms, which appear white against a dark background. India ink can be used in wet films.

### 3. MYCOTA (FUNGI) (mildews, morels, moulds, slime moulds, mushrooms, puffballs, rusts, smuts, stinkhorns, truffles, yeasts, etc.) (see also Chapter 17)

Only moulds and yeasts are of importance in meat hygiene.

*Fungi* are plant-like structures that differ from bacteria in that they possess a nucleus, nuclear membrane and mitochondria, i.e. they are eukaryotic, bacteria being prokaryotic because they lack these structures. Unlike plants they do not possess chlorophyll.

Typical fungi consist of a mycelium which is a mass of thread-like tubular processes (hyphae) that may be septate or non-septate and aerial or vegetative, the aerial forms extending above the colony while the vegetative ones extend downwards to provide nutrients. The cell wall of the hyphae contains chitin or cellulose or both. The mycelium forms the thallus or body of the fungus.

Reproduction is by the formation of spores (conidia) and may be asexual or sexual by the fusion of two sex cells or gametes.

*Moulds* have a hairy or woolly appearance due to the mycelium possessing numerous aerial hyphae.

*Yeasts* are single vegetative cells that form a smooth, yellowish bacterial-like colony without aerial hyphae.

*Identification* of the various species of moulds and yeasts depends on the clinical sites of infection, presence of certain specialised shapes, hyphae structure, absence/presence of dimorphism (tissue and mould phases), use of Wood's lamp, direct examination of specimens (Wood's lamp, KOH, tissue stains and microscopy), culture, biochemical testing (urease test, potassium nitrate and carbohydrate assimilation) and serological testing.

The *germ tube test* is used for the identification of yeasts such as *Candida albicans* that possess germ tubes without constricted bases when grown on media containing serum.

*Wood's lamp* (a source of UV light) is used to diagnose dermatophytosis (ringworm) infections (*Trichophyton verrucosum, T. eqinum, T. mentagrophytes, T. nanum, Microsporon gypseum*, etc.). Infected hair shafts fluoresce under the lamp.

#### Preparation of specimens of dermatophytes

Cleanse the affected area with water or 70% alcohol to reduce contaminating organisms. Remove hairs and scale and place on an agar plate and cover or seal to reduce evaporation. Incubate at room temperature – growth is usually apparent in 3–7 days but may require up to 3 weeks.

A 10–20% preparation of potassium hydroxide is used to detect fungi in skin, hair, etc. Mixed with equal proportions of the specimen on a microscope slide and covered with a coverslip, it dissolves keratin when heated, making the hyphae more readily detected.

**Stains** to detect fungi include India Ink, Giemsa, Masson-Fontana, Calcofluor White, periodic acid-Schiff (PAS), acid-fast.

#### Some characteristics of pathogenic fungi

- *Aspergillus fumigatus*: Septate hyphae; conidia and conidiophores in long chains or easily separated and coloured black, white, yellow, green, pink and tan.
- *Blastomyces dermatidis*: Oval to spherical smooth conidia. Direct microscopy may reveal large, spherical yeast cells with double-contoured walls attached by broad base. Culture (25°C): white to brown fluffy or smooth colonies in ring formation.
- *Candida albicans*: Most common cause of fungal disease in man and animals. Grows well at temperatures as high as 45°C. Produces chlamydoconidia and hyphae. Urease positive (medium turns bright pink). Potassium nitrate assimilation negative.
- *Coccidioides immitis*: Barrel-shaped arthroconidia convert to larger (30–60 μm)

spherules containing endospores. Culture shows moist greyish-white colonies and abundant brown aerial mycelia.

- *Cryptococcus neoformans*: Capsule formation produces typical mucoid colonies. True hyphae not produced on cornmeal agar. Urease positive. Phenol oxidase positive (differentiates from other cryptococci).
- *Histoplasma capsulatum*: Direct Giemsa smear – small yeast cells (5 × 3 μm). Cells often present in macrophages and monocytes. Culture: white to brown mould with colonies showing spiny or tuberculate conidia.
- *Microsporum gypseum*: Culture – abundant conidia produced with powdery, granular, brownish appearance of colonies. Brown or red pigment may form under some strains. Fusiform conidia may contain up to 6 cells.
- *Rhinosporidium seeberi*: Microscopic demonstration of spherules (which may be numerous) in biopsy specimens confirms diagnosis. Spherules vary in size (up to 300 μm) and possess thick periodic acid–Schiff-positive walls and endospores.
- *Sporothrix schenckii*: Direct Gram or Giemsa smear: small, cigar-shaped yeast usually present in small numbers. Cells are small and pleomorphic and often seen in macrophages in tissue exudates or biopsy specimens. *S. schenckii* is dimorphic. Culture: smooth, white mycelial colonies that become darker and mycelial with age. Hyphae bear conidia in the form of a ping-pong paddle in a rosette at the end of the conidiophores.
- *Trichophyton verrucosum*: Most commonly isolated dermatophyte. Culture: rapid grower. Granular and fluffy forms of growth. Macroconidia are thin-walled, smooth, cigar-shaped and appear singly on non-septate hyphae.

## 4. Pathogenic Protozoa

- *Babesia* spp.: Diagnosis depends on demonstration of the causal organism in RBCs using thin blood smears fixed and stained by Giemsa. The organisms appear as tiny purple or blue ring-shaped or pear-shaped trophozoites with a prominent chromatic dot and lighter-staining cytoplasm. Some may be single, double or in the classic tetrad (Maltese Cross) formation.

  Acridine orange stain may be used as an alternative with the smear viewed under UV light.

  The organisms vary in size, *B. bigemina* being large (4–5 μm × 2 μm) and *B. bovis* small (2 μm × 1.5 μm). Early cases in which organisms are few may require thick smears. A red blood cell could contain as many as 12 trophozoites.

- *Besnoitia* spp.: The large (up to 500 μm in diameter), round, thick-walled cysts in the skin, subcutis, lymphatics, blood vessels, mucous membranes, etc., are visible to the naked eye and are fairly characteristic of besnoitiosis. These are filled with crescent-shaped bradyzoites (trophozoites) (5–7 μm in size) which resemble *toxoplasmas* and invade endothelial, macrophages, histiocytic and other cells. Other clinical signs also help to make a presumptive diagnosis.
- *Cryptosporidium* spp.: The round oocysts in faecal samples are small (4–6 μm), transparent, easily broken and resemble a yeast cell. Two forms exist: thick-walled and thin-walled.

  They can be acid-fast stained – oocysts stain bright red whereas yeast cells stain blue or green according to the counterstain used. Use of sugar and zinc sulphate flotation methods aids detection, as does high-power magnification with phase-contrast illumination.
- *Eimeria* spp.: Finding of numerous round, oval or ellipsoidal double-walled oocysts in faecal samples is diagnostic especially if schizonts are present in subepithelial tissues. Colour varies from transparent to brown or green. Numbers can vary greatly, making repeat examinations necessary. Sizes and shapes vary according to species. *Eimeria* oocysts possess four sporozoites (*Isospora* two sporocysts).
- *Giardia* spp.: The trophozoite is pear-shaped and bilaterally symmetrical. It is 9–21 μm × 5–15 μm in size with a rounded anterior and a pointed posterior. The dorsal side is convex and the ventral side concave with a large sucker. There are two oval nuclei and eight flagella arranged in four pairs, which give the organism a 'falling leaf' motility.

  Oval cysts (10 × 14 μm) containing up to four nuclei are formed by which transmission occurs.

  Trophozoites may be detected in smears of loose faeces, but cysts are more readily seen, especially when concentrated by zinc sulphate centrifugal flotation. Staining with iodine, iron haematoxylin or trichrome (Wheatley modification of Gomori stain) enhances detection and differentiation.

- *Hexamita meleagridis*: Diagnosis depends on finding the spindle or pear-shaped, bilaterally symmetrical protozoon parasite (8 µm × 3 µm) in scrapings from the duodenal and jejunal mucosa of turkeys, pheasants, quail, etc. It is a mobile organism (6 anterior and 2 posterior flagella) moving by rapid, darting movements and must be present in numbers to justify a positive diagnosis.
- *Histomonas meleagridis*: Although the liver and caecal lesions of blackhead (infectious enterohepatitis) in turkeys are reasonably diagnostic when occurring together, separately they may be confused with leukosis, tuberculosis, trichomoniasis and mycosis.

  The causal organism can be demonstrated in stained liver sections, which show necrotic holes containing the vegetative form of the parasite which resembles a trichomonad without flagella.

- **Leishmania** spp. Definite diagnosis depends on the demonstration of the organisms as amastigotes in methanol-fixed, stained impression smears of affected tissues in which they occur in reticuloendothelial cells. This particular stage (2–5 µm in diameter) is round or oval. Wright's stain shows a pale blue cytoplasm and large red nucleus and rod-like kinetoplast in the cytoplasm.

  The organisms as promastigate forms are readily cultured on blood agar media.
- *Sarcocystis* spp.: These form cysts varying in size from a few micrometres to several centimeters in the muscles of a wide variety of intermediate hosts – domestic and wild animals and even man.

  Sporozoites are liberated in the small intestine of the intermediate host and give rise to schizonts in vascular endothelial cells. Merozoites from mature schizonts produce a second generation of schizonts that invade striped muscle cells and develop into typical sarcocysts.

  Some sarcocysts are very small but others are large enough (up to several millimetres) to be seen by the naked eye. Those of *S. cruzi* and *S. lindemanni* are 1–2 mm and are similar in shape to *Toxoplasma*. The contained merozoites (12 µm) are banana-shaped in outline.

- *Theileria* spp.: *Theileria* and *Babesia* are piroplasms (*piro* = pear + plasm = matrix) that parasitise RBCs, histiocytes, lymphocytes and monocytes. These schizonts (Koch's blue bodies) occur as round, oval or irregularly-shaped organisms varying in size from 2 to 12 µm or more and during development in the WBC cause it to divide. Giemsa-stained smears of lymphoblasts in lymph node biopsies reveal numerous multinucleated schizonts. Romanowsky stains the organisms blue with red chromatin granules.

- *Toxoplasma* spp.: Infected cats shed oocysts in their faeces. There are three infective forms of the parasite: (1) the crescent-shaped *trophozoite* or *tachyzoite* of *T. gondii* is the actively proliferating form of the parasite and can be found in a wide variety of tissues and measures 4–6 µm × 2–4 µm; (2) the *bradyzoite* or *cystozoite* (10–12 µm) is the resting form found in (3) *oocysts*, which are 50–100 µm in diameter. Confirmation of toxoplasmosis requires demonstration of the organism with Giemsa and/or serological tests (CF, indirect immunofluorescence, haemagglutination) and dye test using methylene blue (now largely superseded).

- *Trichomonas foetus*: This is a pear-shaped flagellated protozoan (three flagella at the anterior end and one posterior flagellum) with an undulating membrane extending the length of the organism (10–15 µm × 5–10 µm).

  Organisms may be found in the placental fluid, the stomach contents of aborted fetuses, uterine and vaginal discharges, and the prepuce and glans penis of bulls. Saline washings can be used to obtain samples. Centrifugation of washings, especially from the prepuce, may be necessary where organisms are sparse. Culture using media containing serum may be used to concentrate numbers.

  The special morphology (pear-shape, presence of axostyle, single nucleus and chromatic granules) and size of organisms along with characteristic jerky motility can be viewed in wet-mount preparations.

  Stained preparations (trichrome, Giemsa, Leishman, Wright) show structures in detail.

- *Trypanosoma* spp.: Diagnosis of trypanosomiasis is confirmed by demonstrating the organisms in wet mounts or stained smears (Giemsa, Leishman, Wright, etc.) of the peripheral blood – fairly easy in the acute stage but not when the condition is chronic. Culture on serum media may be necessary.

A rapid method is to examine a wet mount of the buffy coat area of a PCV tube after centrifugation.

In some cases in man, xenodiagnosis is adopted – i.e. the use of bugs to feed on suspect hosts and the subsequent examination of their stomach contents for trypanosomes.

- *Tyzzeria* spp. Coccidia-like organisms of geese and ducks, domestic and wild. The oocysts (of *T. anseris*) are 10–16 × 9–12 µm, ellipsoidal in shape and, when sporulated, contain 8 banana-shaped sporozoites.

## PATHOGENIC RICKETTSIAE

*Rickettsia* are Gram-negative, short, non-motile bacilli (0.3–2.0 µm × 0.3–0.5 µm) responsible for Rocky Mountain spotted fever, rickettsial pox, boutonneuse fever, endemic typhus and scrub typhus in man, all transmitted by ixodid (hard) ticks. The largest *rickettsias* are about the size of the smallest bacteria.

Diagnosis depends on the isolation of the organism from the peripheral blood and/or the serological (complement fixation) response to infection measured against prototype antigens. Blood films of varying thickness are made, fixed with alcohol for 2 minutes and stained with Giemsa, Wright or new Methylene Blue.

- *Anaplasma* spp. (*A. marginale, A. centrale*) are minute spherical Gram-negative rickettsias occurring at or near the margins of red blood cells in which there may be more than one parasite. Mature forms are 0.3–1.0 µm in diameter. Transfer of the organism from one RBC to another is by puncture of the cell membrane by an initial body that divides into 2, 4, 6 or 8 bodies.

  The organisms stain dark blue or purple with Giemsa.

- *Cowdria ruminantium* is an obligate intracellular pleomorphic rickettsia that inhabits capillary reticuloendothelial cells in cowdriosis (heartwater)

  While clinical signs are presumptive evidence of the disease in acute cases, diagnosis is confirmed at post-mortem by demonstrating the organism in Giemsa-stained smears of cerebral grey matter

- *Coxiella burnetii*, the cause of 'Q' (query) fever, is an obligate intracellular pleomorphic coccobacillus (0.5 µm long) that differs from other rickettsias in several ways (mode of transmission, intracellular development, phase variation).

- *Eperythrozoon* spp. (*E. ovis, E. suis*) appear as minute pleomorphic (rods, rings, cocci) which contain granular material at each end within a single membrane. They occur free in the plasma, around platelets and on the surface of red blood cells.

  When stained with Romanowsky stain the organisms appear red. Giemsa (dark purple or blue), Leishman and new methylene blue stains may also be used.

- *Ehrlichia* spp. (*E. bovis, E. canis, E. equi, E. ovina, E. phagocytophilia*) are tiny pleomorphic coccoid or ellipsoidal parasites with a diameter of 0.2–2.0 µm occurring in leukocytes, especially monocytes. They possess a double membrane wall, contain dense granules and may be present in WBCs singly or in mulberry-like bodies (morulae). Blood smears or smears of cut organ surfaces, e.g. lungs, at post-mortem may be stained with Giemsa for rapid diagnosis.

### Spirochaetales

- *Borrelia* spp. Gram-negative large, slender, microaerophilic, coiled, highly motile organisms varying in thickness from 0.3 to 0.7 µm and in length from 10 to 30 µm. Motility occurs by lashing and rotating

## METHODS OF SPECIMEN COLLECTION AND EXAMINATION (FOR ALL INTESTINAL AND BLOOD PARASITES)

### Faeces

Several specimens taken at intervals of a few days are often required because of sparsity of organisms and/or the frequent intermittent excretion of intestinal parasites.

Methods of *preservation* (10% formalin, formalin–ethyl acetate, polyvinyl alcohol) (PVA) fixative, zinc sulphate, sodium acetate–acetic acid–formalin) are used if immediate examination is not performed. Commercial kits are also available.

Initial gross examination may detect tapeworm proglottids, eggs, oocysts, microfilariae, etc., and presence of blood. Colour of faeces should be noted.

*Microscopic examination*

1 *Direct wet mount, stained and unstained* – to detect motile protozoan trophozoites and cysts, helminth eggs and larvae. Place a drop of physiological saline at one end of a microscope slide and a drop of iodine, e.g. Lugol's, at the other. Add a small amount (2 mg) of faeces to each drop and mix. Cover with coverslip and examine under low- and high-power objectives.

2 *Concentration methods* – wet mount examination. Formalin–ethyl acetate (FEA), zinc sulphate and sugar flotation are commonly used methods of concentration. Zinc sulphate, however, may cause eggs to open and/or collapse and may distort protozoan cysts. High density eggs may be missed due to sedimentation making early examination imperative.

3 *Permanently stained smears* – morphology of trophozoites, cysts, larvae, eggs necessary to identify individual parasites.

- *Stains* – Iron haematoxylin, trichrome. Commercial stains and reagents available.
- Make a thin film of faeces on a microscope slide.
- Fix in Schaudinn or PVA fixative.
- Scan for thick and thin areas under ×10 and ×40 magnifications.
- Trichrome stain: protozoan trophozoites and cysts stain blue-green. RBCs, nuclear chromatin, karyosomes stain dark-red purple; eggs and larvae stain red; background debris and yeasts stain green.
- Iron haematoxylin: organisms stain greyish-black; nuclei stain black; background material stains light blue-grey.

## Blood smears

Giemsa and Wright stains are usually used, especially the former. (Wright stain cannot be used for thick smears.)

- Prepare thin and thick smears – both can be made on the same slide. A thick film (best for parasites) is made by pooling several drops of blood and spreading it on an area of 1.5 cm.
- Fix thin film (but not thick film) in methanol.
- Allow smear to dry for 6 hours before staining.
- Scan first under low power (for microfilariae and larger organisms) and then under ×100 oil immersion for tiny parasites like *Babesia*.

## EXAMINATION OF CARCASE AND ORGANS FOR EVIDENCE OF PATHOGENIC MICROORGANISMS

**Specimen**

(a) Neck muscle
(b) Spleen
(c) Mesenteric lymph node
(d) Carcase lymph node

**Procedure**

- Identify specimen and carcase of origin
- Sear surface with spatula
- Cut into organ with sterilised scalpel
- Insert swab into cut surface and swab on to agar

*Culture on/in*

(i) Selenite broth (to be subcultured on Brilliant Caveen agar (BGA) at 24 hours)
(ii) MacConkey Agar
(iii) Blood Agar (aerobic)
(iv) Glucose Agar (stab)

**Record findings** including Gram stain findings after inoculation

Specimen: _____
BGA: _____
MacC: _____
B/A: _____
Glucose Agar: _____

**Interpretation:** _____

Decision regarding carcase of origin: ——

Source: Collins, J. D. and Hannan, J. *Laboratory Handbook on Food Hygiene*. University College, Dublin Faculty of Veterinary Medicine: Food Hygiene Laboratory.

## THE MICROBIOLOGICAL EXAMINATION OF FRESH MEAT

**Products under examination:** 1. Chicken carcase. 2. Mince meat

1. Mark all plates with its identification.
2. Regarding the chicken carcase, state whether the technique used was (a) neck skin flap; (b) carcase washing.

**Assessment**

1. Organoleptic:
   (a) appearance: _____
   (b) odour: _____
   (c) texture: _____
2. Physical-chemical:
   (a) pH: ____ (b) $A_w$: ____ (c) other: ____
3. Microbiological

| $10^{-1}$ | $10^{-2}$ | $10^{-3}$ | $10^{-4}$ | $10^{-5}$ | $10^{-6}$ | $10^{-7}$ | $10^{-8}$ |
|---|---|---|---|---|---|---|---|

   (a) TVC @ 30°C/3 days
   (b) TVC @ 37°C/2 days
   (c) Total Enterobacteriaceae count @ 37°C/2 days
   (d) *S. aureus* count @ 37°C/2 days
   (e) Presence of *Clostridium perfringens* (presumptive): Take 10 ml of $10^{-1}$ suspension, add to 100 ml of Glucose Agar, heat @ 60°C/10 minutes, to delay vegetative forms, and incubate @ 37°C/2 days.
   (f) Presence of *Salmonella* spp.: Take 10 ml of $10^{-1}$ dilution, add to 10 ml double strength Brilliant Green/Selenite broth, incubate for 24 hours @ 43°C followed by plating onto Brilliant Green agar.
   (g) Microscopic examination
   (h) TVC @ 30°C/3 days _____
   @ 37°C/2 days _____

- Total Enterobacteraceae count: ____
- *S. aureus* count: ____
- *Clostridium perfringens*: present/absent: ____
- *Salmonella* spp.: present/absent ____

**Results and Interpretation:** ____

Source: Collins, J. D. and Hannan, J. *Laboratory Handbook on Food Hygiene*. University College, Dublin Faculty of Veterinary Medicine: Food Hygiene Laboratory.

## THE MICROBIOLOGICAL EXAMINATION OF PROCESSED MEAT

**Microbiological:**

| $10^{-1}$ | $10^{-2}$ | $10^{-3}$ | $10^{-4}$ | $10^{-5}$ |
|---|---|---|---|---|

(a) TVC @ 30°C/3 days

(b) TVC @ 37°C/2 days

(c) Total Enterobacteriaceae count 37°C/2 days

(d) *S.aureus* count @ 37°C/2 days

(e) Presence of *Clostridium perfringens* (presumptive): Take 10 ml of $10^{-1}$ suspension, add to 100 ml of glucose agar, heat @ 60°C/10 minutes, to delay vegetative forms, and incubate @ 37°C/2 days.

(f) Presence of *Salmonella* spp.: Take 10 ml of $10^{-1}$ dilution, add to 10 ml double strength Brilliant Green/Selenite broth, incubate for 24 hours @ 43°C followed by plating on to Brilliant Green agar.

(g) Microscopic examination ______

(h) TVC (10 @ 30°C/3 days _____
(ii) @ 37°C/2 days _____

- Total Enterobacteraceae count: _____
- *S. aureus* count: _____
- *Clostridium perfringens*: present/absent: _____
- *Salmonella* spp.: present/absent: _____

**Results and Interpretation:** _____

Source: Collins, J. D. and Hannan, J. *Laboratory Handbook on Food Hygiene*. University College, Dublin Faculty of Veterinary Medicine: Food Hygiene Laboratory.

## DETECTION OF ANTIBACTERIAL RESIDUES IN FOOD (see also Chapter 13)

MEAT, KIDNEY, LIVER

**Test system:** Incubation of growth of (i) **Bacillus subtilis* and (ii) *Micrococcus luteus* on media with pH of (i) 7.2 or (ii) 8.0

*Note: trimethoprim is added to this medium.

**Procedure:**

1. Take 2 pieces of tissue each approx. 1 $cm^3$
2. Place one piece in a test tube containing 5 ml saline solution and heat in waterbath at 85°C for ten minutes (extract).
3. To each of the pre-inoculated test plates add (i) tissue (direct), (ii) 4 drops of extract into well.
4. Incubate the *B. subtilis* plate at 30°C and the *M. luteus* plate at 37°C for 24 hours.
5. Remove plates and read the results as follows:
   (i) a zone of inhibition 2 mm in radius around any sample is regarded as *positive;*
   (ii) absence of such a zone is regarded as *negative.*

**Test:**

| | *B. subtilis* | *M. luteus* |
|---|---|---|
| Direct: | | |
| Extract: | | |

**Interpretation:** _____

Source: Collins, J. D. and Hannan, J. *Laboratory Handbook on Food Hygiene.* University College, Dublin Faculty of Veterinary Medicine: Food Hygiene Laboratory.

## FAST ANTIMICROBIAL SCREEN TEST (FAST) FOR DETECTION OF ANTIBIOTIC AND SULFONAMIDE RESIDUES IN LIVESTOCK KIDNEY TISSUE. A SELF-INSTRUCTIONAL GUIDE

(This guide is intended for use by FSIS veterinarians and designated food inspectors in a slaughtering plant on tissues from red meat carcases. By courtesy of USDA FSIS Administrative Human Resource Development Division.)

FAST is based on the principle that if animal tissue contains the residue of a previously administered antimicrobial, fluid from the tissues will inhibit the growth of a sensitive organism on a bacterial culture plate. In this test, cotton swabs saturated with tissue fluid from a suspected carcase are placed on a culture plate whose surface has been seeded with spores of a harmless organism (*Bacillus megaterium*). This organism is known to be sensitive to most of the commonly used antimicrobials.

The swabs and plate are incubated to allow growth of the organisms; then the plates are examined for *zones of inhibited growth* around the swabs. The *presence of such zones is presumptive evidence that the carcases tissues contain an antimicrobial residue.*

*Positive* cases are submitted to the central laboratory. *Negative* cases may be released within about 6 hours provided all other inspection criteria are met.

Time required to complete test is 5–10 minutes.

### Equipment

- Clean knife, plastic bags, fine-tipped permanent marker and rubber bands.
- Sterile cotton swabs.
- FAST agar plates.
- *Bacillus megaterium* spore suspension.
- Antibiotic sensitivity N5 discs.
- Thumb forceps.
- Incubator stabilised at 44°C ± 0.5°C.
- Metric measuring device with millimetre graduations.
- 'Retained' tags.

### Storage of reagents

- Agar plates should be kept at room temperature with protection from extremes of heat, cold and moisture.
- N5 discs and spore suspension require to be refrigerated.
- Container for N5 disc dispenser should not be opened until discs are to be used. After use, the dispenser and desiccant pellet should be placed in a sealed plastic bag for refrigeration.

### Sample collection

1. Using a clean knife, collect ~1 lb of kidney from detained carcase and place in plastic bag.
2. Attach 'detained' tag to carcase and record carcase number/pathology details, injection site, if present, plant number, etc.

### Preparation of tissue swabs

1. Open swab pack, remove one swab and jab the sharp end just through the plastic bag containing the kidney tissue, making a ½ inch hole.
2. Macerate the tissue with the sharp end of the swab and completely soak the cotton end in the tissue fluid.
3. Leave swab in place for at least 30 minutes to ensure maximum absorption of fluid.

The cotton swab must not contact anything but the sample fluid and agar plate.

Hands, etc., should be clean and dry but not necessarily sterile.

### Streaking the agar plate with spores

1. Lift plate cover slightly and make an '×' reference mark on outer sidewall (Fig. 14.23A).
2. Place plate bottomside down with reference mark '×' at 12 o'clock.
3. With cap tight, *thoroughly* shake the vial to ensure *even suspension of spores*.
4. Remove cap from spore vial (avoiding touching inside of cap and vial with hands) and holding a sterile cotton swab by the shaft carefully insert it into the spore vial to completely immerse the cotton swab (once only) in the spore suspension.

   Avoid touching the cotton tip with any surface and do not reuse the swab to streak additional plates.
5. Gently touch the side of the vial with the swab to remove excess fluid.
6. Replace screw cap on vial and set aside.
7. Commencing at mark '×' streak spores over the agar surface to opposite side (Fig. 14.23B). Turning the plate ¼ clockwise for three occasions with ½ final turn, streak plate in a similar manner so that whole surface of plate is evenly covered with spores. Discard the used swab.
8. Draw a line with a permanent marker on the bottom of plate from mark '×' to divide plate into two halves (Fig. 14.23C). Identify the plate with last three digits of the tissue sample at 90 degrees at two places on vertical outside of plate.

### Positioning the N5 disc

With thumb forceps, carefully place a N5 disc on spore-covered agar about ½ inch from mark '×' and press gently without breaking agar surface (Fig. 14.23D). Replace the cap on the N5 disc vial and refrigerate.

### Positioning swab on plate

With fingers (*not* forceps) gently place the swab (with saturated end down to prevent fluid flowing down shaft) in the centre of the left-hand side of plate with the shaft end near the N5 disc (Fig. 14.23E). Lightly press the swab shaft with the finger tip to ensure contact with the agar. If two carcases are being tested, place the second swab similarly in the centre of right-hand side of plate.

### Incubation of FAST plate

Incubate plate with cover (and swabs and agar surface uppermost), properly stabilised (44 ± 0.5°C), for a minimum of 6 hours. Record TIME IN and TIME OUT and ensure security during incubation.

Incubation can continue for a maximum of 24 hours without jeopardising results. Prolonged incubation may allow growth of contaminating organisms and/or dissipate antibiotic activity and produce false negative results.

Retest if necessary.

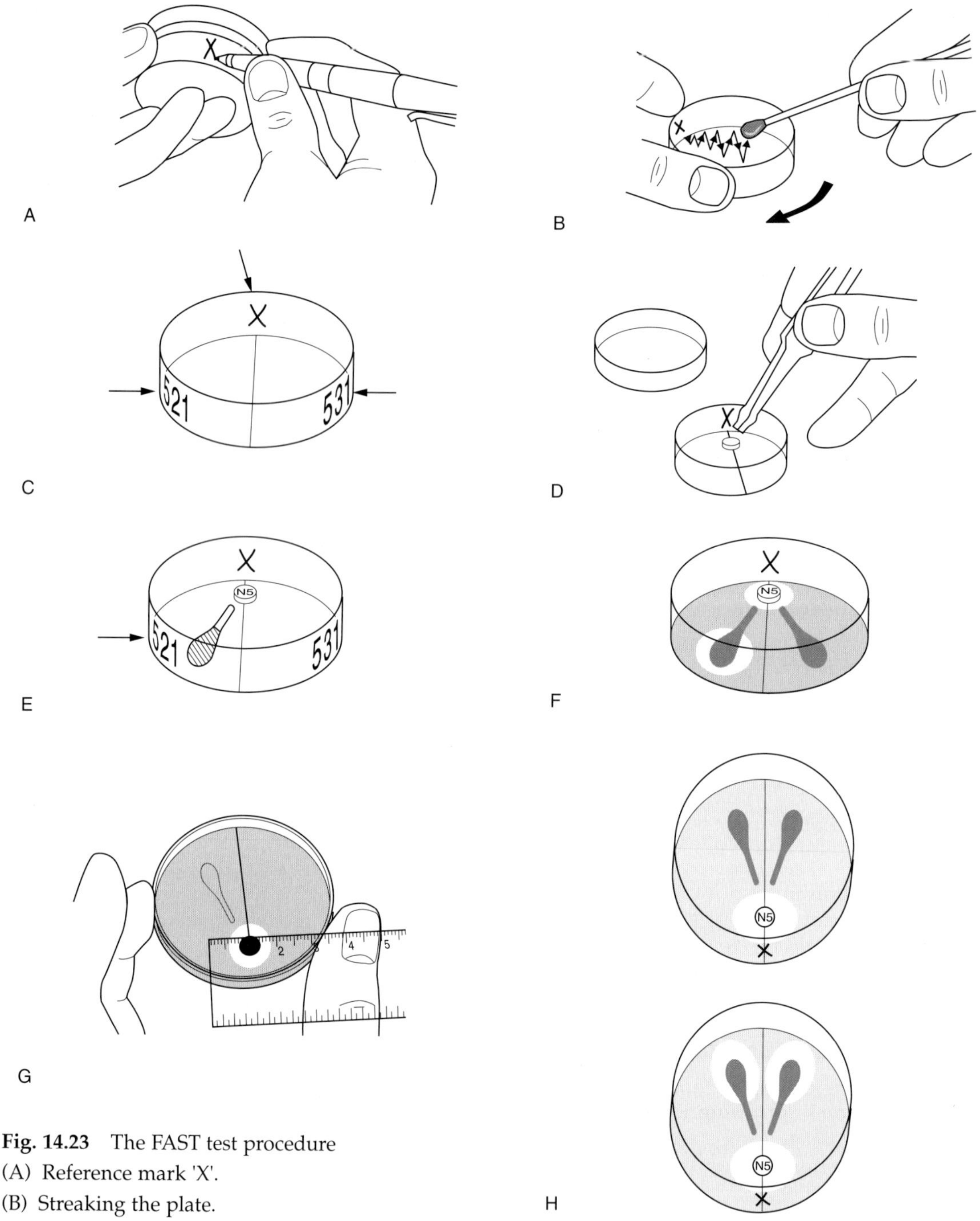


**Fig. 14.23** The FAST test procedure
(A) Reference mark 'X'.
(B) Streaking the plate.
(C) Dividing the plate into two halves and identifying.
(D) Positioning the N5 disc.
(E) Positioning the swab.
(F) Verifying function of the FAST system.
(G) Measuring the zone of N5 disc inhibition.
(H) Interpreting and recording FAST data.

### Verifying function of FAST system (Fig. 14.23F)

- *Growth of test organism* results in an overall yellow or amber colour within 6 hours. This must be verified.
- *A purple zone of inhibition round N5 disc* should be obvious within 6 hours (*clear yellow or amber* after overnight incubation). Determine that this is within the acceptable range of 20–26 mm.
- A zone round of inhibition is an area free of colonies of the test organism (*B. megaterium*) caused by the presence of a growth-promoting substance, e.g. an antibiotic.
- If incubated for 6 hours, the colour will be purple. If incubated for more than 6 hours, the colour will be yellow or amber.
- Turn the plate upside down on flat surface and lightly tap the bottom to dislodge the swab(s) into the cover.
- Observe the plate through the bottom.
- If growth of test organism is evident in at least the areas away from the N5 disc and the swab(s), observe zones of inhibition and measure and record (in mm) the diameter of the N5 zone of inhibition (Fig. 14.23G).
- If the N5 disc zone of inhibition is 20–26 mm, interpret results. If not, rerun test or submit to central laboratory.

### Interpretation of results (Fig. 14.23H)

*Interpretation is based on the presence or absence of zones of inhibition surrounding the tissue swab areas.*

- If no zone of inhibition is present, the test is *negative.* Record.
- If a zone of inhibition is present, the test is *positive.* Measure width of swab zone of inhibition in mm. Record.

### Follow-up action – negative FAST

Release carcases, after appropriate trimming of injection lesion (if present), provided any other reasons for detaining carcase are resolved. Record and notify appropriate authority of action taken.

### Follow-up action – positive FAST

FAST is a screening test and is accurate in determining whether antibiotic or sulphonamide residues are present. Except in the case of bob calves, if the FAST result is positive, tissue samples must be sent to the laboratory for bioassay testing. The purpose of the laboratory testing in larger animals is to confirm that violative levels of antibiotics or sulphonamides are present in the tissues. Carcases other than those of bob calves must be retained pending laboratory results.

**A** If the zone of inhibition is 15 mm or greater and the species code is 21 (bob calf) *condemn* the carcase.

Collect approximately 1 lb each of muscle, kidney and liver from the retained carcase. Place each tissue sample in a separate double bag and freeze. Send to the central laboratory with sufficient coolant to ensure arrival in good condition along with full details.

**B** If zone of inhibition is less than 15 mm for bob calves, test is *negative*: release carcase after appropriate trimming, e.g. removal of injection lesions, etc., provided other reasons for retaining the carcase are resolved. No tissues need be sent to the laboratory.

### Handling culture failures

- Failure of the test *B. megaterium* spores to grow is rare.
- The plate may not have been streaked with spores.
- The plate may be too old or dried out.
- The incubator temperature may have been incorrect.
- Sample tissues may have contained a very high antibiotic level.
- Complete form as 'Failure' under 'Test Results'.
- If the cause of culture failure has been determined, rerun the FAST test.
- If the cause of culture failure has not been determined, submit tissues to the laboratory and proceed as under Follow-up Actions – positive FAST.

### Finishing up FAST test

Maintain an inventory of FAST supplies each time the test is run and follow instructions from Regional Office.

## pH MEASUREMENT (HYDROGEN ION CONCENTRATION)

The pH value is a quantitative measurement of the acidity/alkalinity of fluids, a value of 7 being neutral, with figures less than 7 being acid and those above 7 being alkaline.

Nutrient content, biological structures, oxidation-reduction potential, antimicrobial agents, moisture content and pH constitute the intrinsic parameters of animal tissues.

It is acknowledged that most micro-organisms grow best at pH values of 6.5–7.5. Pathogenic bacteria tend to be more fastidious in relation to pH, while yeasts and moulds are less so.

pH plays an important role in the keeping quality of meats; for example meat from fatigued and stressed animals spoils faster than that from rested animals as a direct result of the final pH on completion of rigor mortis. Detection of PSE and DFD, evaluation of electrostimulation efficiency and suitability of beef for vacuum packaging are among the many reasons for measuring pH.

Effective electrical stimulation of beef carcases should produce a pH of 6.1–6.3. DFD meat (pH above 6.2 at 24 hours post-slaughter) should not be vacuum-packed since conditions favour the growth of *Brochothrix (Microbacterium) thermosphacta*.

### pH indicator papers

These give an approximate measurement of the pH but are suitable for use on the slaughter floor. The colour change in the strips ranges from pH values of 5.2 to 7.2 When used in an incision into meat at a depth of 2 cm for 2 minutes or 10 minutes (pHi), the colour change is compared directly with a given colour chart.

### pH probes and meters

pH probes and meters are the most accurate methods of measuring pH. A wide variety is commercially available. Fibre-optic probes are more accurate than pH meters in the detection of PSE and DFD. The measurement should be performed with spear probes (sharpened metal sheath), which help to prevent the contamination of raw meat from probe breakage.

Before use, the probe (preferably a fibre-optic one) should be calibrated on buffer solutions at the same temperature as the test material unless the pH meter is equipped with a temperature-compensation unit. The probe must also be cleaned in distilled water between readings since blood and fat tend to cause inaccuracies.

The probe measures reflected light in lean meat. Different instruments have different measurements, one commercially available model giving light readings between 0 and 100 (values less than 20 indicate DFD meat and above 50 PSE meat). Readings taken 24 hours after slaughter and greater than 60 are typical of PSE meat, while those below 16 are representative of extreme DFD meat. It is advisable to take several readings at different sites for each of the test samples.

The longissimus dorsi (eye) muscle is normally used for testing purposes. Care must be taken to keep the electrodes from touching other objects. They should be rinsed in distilled water after use.

As an alternative, 10 g samples of meat may be suspended in 20 ml of distilled water and the pH measured after 10 minutes.

### Lovibond Comparator

Meat suspension (5 or 10 ml in distilled water) is added to two tubes of standard size and to one tube is added a standard amount of a suitable indicator. The tubes are placed in the comparator and the colour change is compared against a colour disc rotated until a match is made. Suitable indicators include phenol red (pH 6.8–8.4), methyl red (pH 4.4–6.0), bromthymol blue (pH 6.0–7.6) and bromcresol purple (pH 5.2–6.8).

(The above systems can also be used for the measurement of pH of culture media.)

## DIFFERENTIATION BETWEEN CHILLED AND THAWED FROZEN MEAT

On occasions unscrupulous suppliers have sold thawed frozen meat as chilled meat. Since the former is likely to be of poor quality and liable to spoilage and rancidity, it is important that the two be differentiated.

Two tests are available – *photometric* and *colour* – both of which measure the

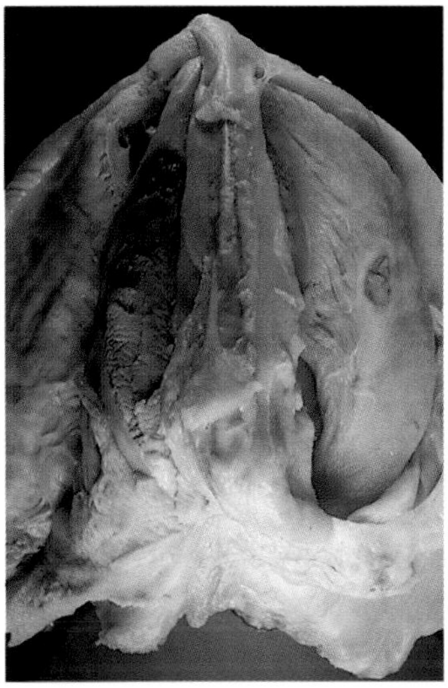

Fig. 13 Deep pectoral myopathy. Fowl.

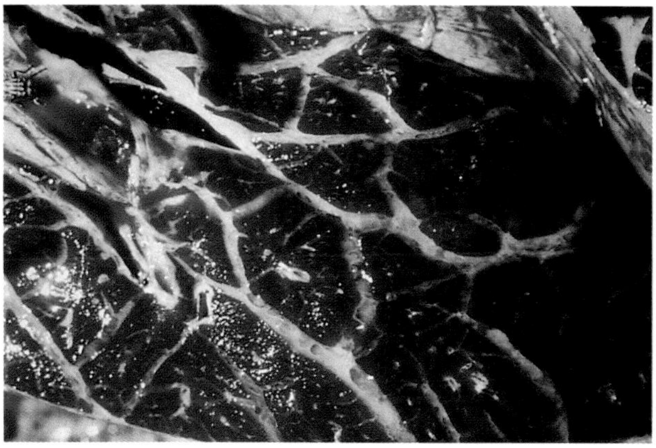

Fig. 14 Haemorrhagic septicaemia. Lungs. Bovine.

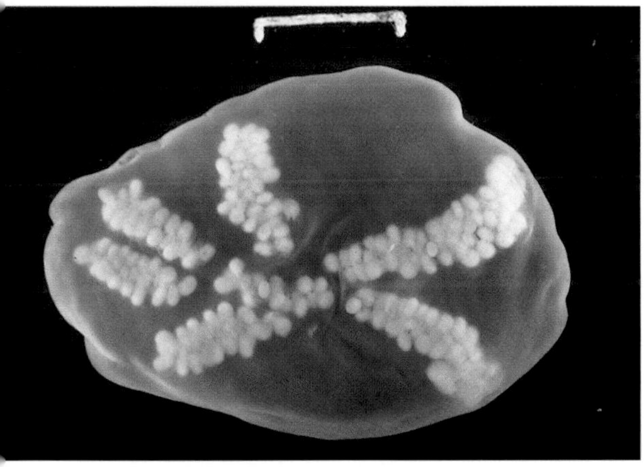

Fig. 15 Coenurus *serialis*. Rabbit.

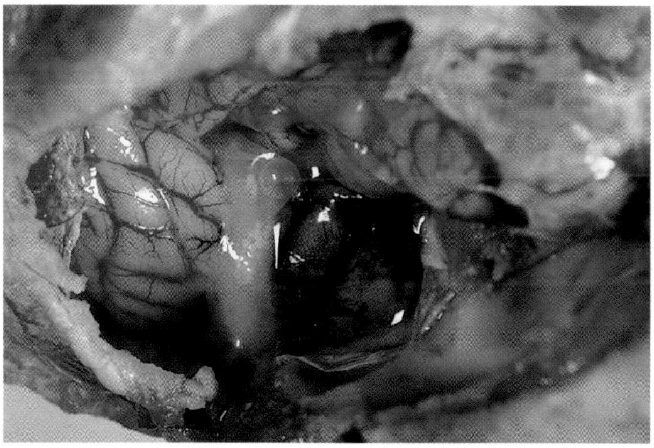

Fig. 16 Coenurus *cerebralis*. Sheep.

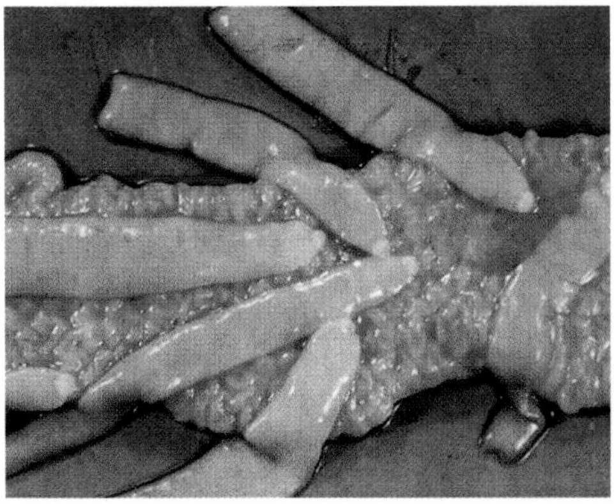

Fig. 17 Anaplocephala magna. Small intestine. Horse (1 year old).

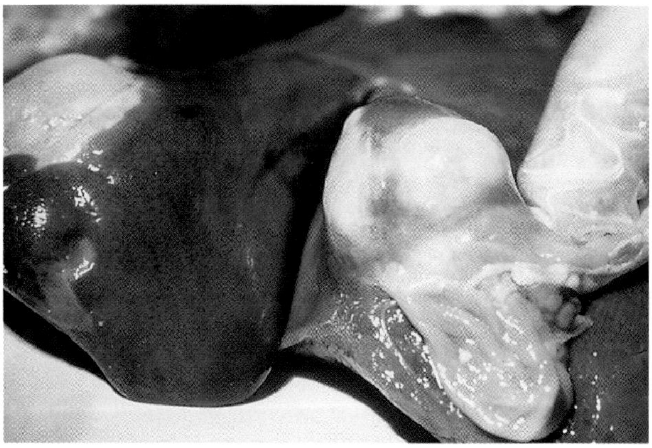

Fig. 18 Hydatid cyst. Liver. Sheep.

# PLATE 4

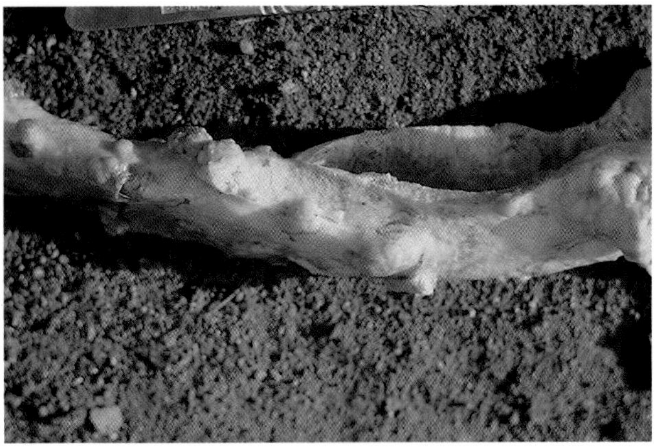

**Fig. 19** *Onchocerca gibsoni*. Oesophagus. Bovine.

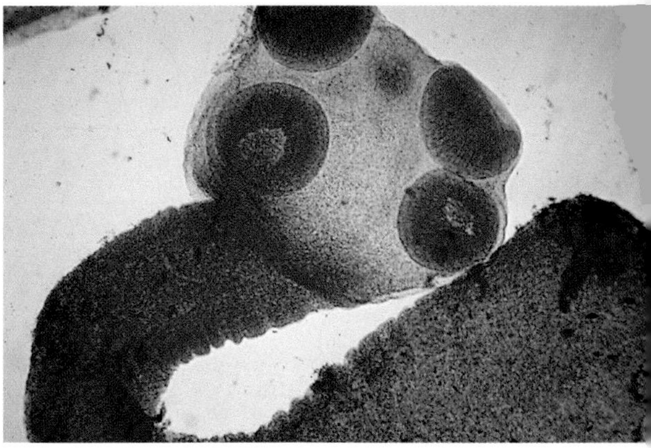

**Fig. 20** *T. saginata*. Scolex and proglottids.

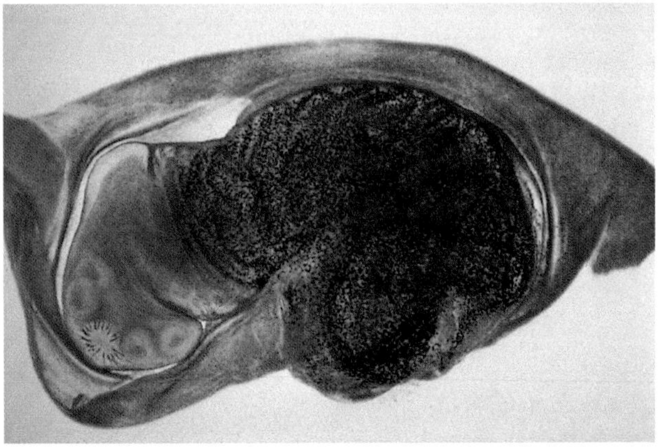

**Fig. 21** *Cysticercus cellulosae*. Diaphragm. Pig.

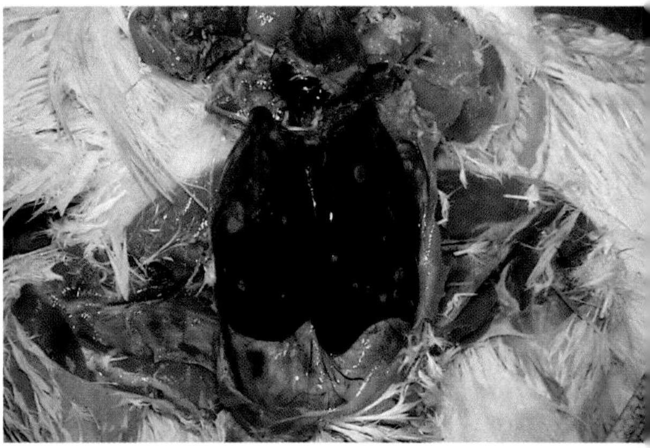

**Fig. 22** Blackhead. Liver. Turkey.

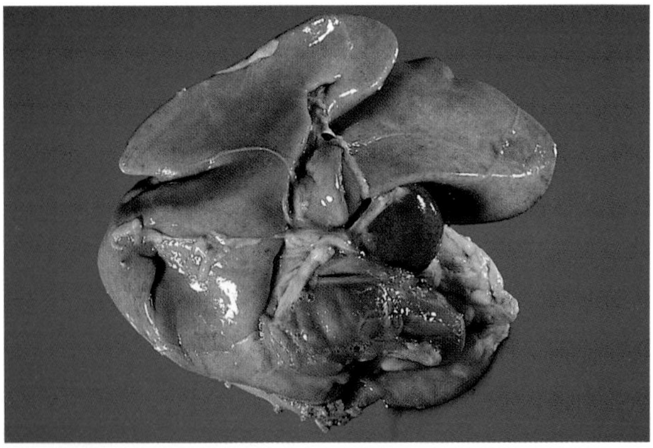

**Fig. 23** Cholangiohepatitis. Broiler.

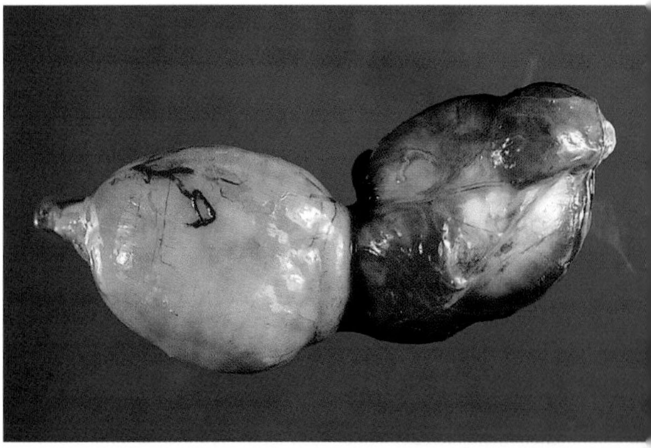

**Fig. 24** Marek's disease. Proventriculus. Broiler.

**Plates 1–4** Grateful thanks for loan of transparencies are accorded to the following: Central Veterinary Laboratory (Fig. 3); D. E. Counter (Figs 5, 10, 12); R. M. Edelsten (Figs 6, 8, 11, 14, 19); M. Fussey (Figs 4, 7, 9); M. Jeffrey (Fig. 13); J. A. Kendrick (Fig. 1); Dr K. A. Linklater (Fig. 2); C. J. Randall (Figs 22, 23, 24); Professor A. J. Trees (Figs 15 to 18, 20, 21).

concentration of a mitochondrial enzyme (β-hydroxy-CoA dehydrogenase, HADH) in meat press juice.

HADH activity is higher in frozen meat because freezing ruptures mitochondria, which release this enzyme in to the meat juice.

## FAT RANCIDITY

Rancidity is a form of spoilage during which an unacceptable taste is produced by the chemical oxidation of unsaturated fats in air and can be accelerated by certain lipolytic bacteria such as *Achromobacter*, *Pseudomonas* and yeasts. Traces of metals such as copper, nickel and iron may cause fat rancidity, as may the action of enzymes such as lipases.

The off-odours are due to aldehydes, ketones and free fatty acids (FFA).

Two tests are available and depend on whether the change is due to hydrolytic rancidity or oxidative rancidity.

### Hydrolytic rancidity – free fatty acids (FFA)

A sample of fat is mixed with neutralised ethanol and titrated directly with standard alkali to obtain a result in terms of percentage oleic acid.

FFA values greater than 3% are considered inedible.

### Oxidative rancidity – Peroxide Value (PV) of fat

This form of fat rancidity is more common than the hydrolytic type. Peroxide and hydroperoxides are produced from unsaturated fatty acids.

The test depends on the release of iodine from potassium iodide in a chloroform–glacial acetic acid solution of the fat. This action is stopped by the addition of water and the released iodine is titrated.

- PV below 5 mEq/kg: the fat is fresh or the hydroxyperoxides have degraded into secondary oxidation products such as ketones. (mEq/kg = milliequivalents per kilogram.) (A chemical equivalent (Eq) is the weight (grams) of a substance that will react with 1 mole of hydrogen ion or 1 mole of electrons.)
- PV between 5 and 10 mEq/kg: commencing rancidity.

## MEAT SPECIES DIFFERENTIATION (see also Chapter 2)

In addition to the normal farm livestock (cattle, sheep, pigs and poultry), the meat of other animals (buffalo, kangaroo, mule, goat, donkey, etc.) is frequently used and is fit for human consumption. On the other hand, substitution can occur, making the product not of the nature and substance demanded by the consumer.

*Serological tests* are utilised to distinguish between the meats derived from the different species of animals and include the precipitin test, ELISA (enzyme-linked immunosorbent assay) and agar diffusion. These serological (immunological) tests are based on the reaction of specific antibodies and antigens.

Commercial kits are available for the serological identification of meat species and the detection of unspecified meats, and even for checking cooked beef, pork and poultry.

In addition to the serological tests, HPLC (high-pressure liquid chromatography), electrophoresis and histology are available but, compared with serology, are less efficient.

## FURTHER READING: Part 1: Food Poisoning

Advisory Committee on the Microbiological Safety of Food (1993) Interim Report on Campylobacter.

Advisory Committee on the Microbiological Safety of Food (1995). Report on Verocytotoxin Producing *E. coli*.

*Management of Outbreaks of Foodborne Illness*. Guidance produced by a Department of Health Working Group 1995. Two Ten Communications, Building ISO, Thorpe Arch Trading Estate, Wetherby, West Yorkshire LS23 7EN, UK. ISBN 011 321662 9.

*The Microbiological Safety of Food*, Part 1, 1990. ISBN 011 321273 9.

*The Microbiological Safety of Food*, Part 2, 1990. ISBN 011 321347 6.

The Pennington Group (1997). Report on the circumstances leading to the 1996 outbreak of infection with *E. coli* O157 in Central Scotland, the implications for food safety and the lessons to be learned.

WHO Surveillance Programme for Control of Foodborne Infections and Intoxications in Europe Sixth Report 1990–92. 1995. ISJN 09480307 ISBN 3 980423174.

## **FURTHER READING:** Part 2: Meat Microbiology

*Clean Catering. A Handbook on Hygiene in Catering Establishments* (1972) London: HMSO.

*EEC Code of Good Hygienic Practices*, Vi/5938/87.

Hobbs, B. C. and Roberts, D. (1987) *Food Poisoning and Food Hygiene*, 5th edn. London: Edward Arnold.

Jay, J. M. (1996) *Modern Food Microbiology*, 5th edn. London: Chapman and Hall.

Parry, R. T., Haysom, L., Thomas, N. L. and Davis, R. (eds) (1982) *A Manual of Recommended Methods for the Microbiological Examination of Poultry and Poultry Products.* London: British Poultry Meat Association.

Public Health Laboratory Service Communicable Disease Surveillance Centre, Weekly Reports.

Roberts, Hooper and Greenwood (eds) (1995), *Practical Food Microbiology*, 2nd ed. PHLS.

Sheridan, J. J., Buchanan, R. L. and Montville, T. J. (1996) HACCP: An integrated approach to assuring the microbiological safety of meat and poultry.

## **FURTHER READING:** Part 3: The Meat Plant Laboratory

Church, P. N. and Wood, J. W. (1990) *Manual of Manufacturing Meat Quality*. Leatherhead: Leatherhead Food Research Association.

Hudson, W. R., Mead, G. C. and Hinton, M. H. (1998). *Vet. Rec.* 142, 545–547.

Jensen, L. B. and Hess, W. R. (1941) *Food Res.* 6, 273.

Labadie et al. (1977) *Zentralblatt fur Bakteriologie, Parasitenkunde, Infecktionskrankheiten und Hygiene* (*Erste Abteilung Originale*) 164, 390.

Mackey, B. M. and Derrick, C. M. (1979) *J. Appl. Bacteriol.* **46**, 355

# Chapter 15
# Occupational Injuries and Infections

## INJURIES

In an industry where livestock are handled, where machinery and knives are used and where floors are often slippery due to water, blood and fat deposits, injuries, sometimes fatal, regularly occur.

By far the most common form of injuries are *cuts* incurred while using sharp knives. Excessive force with a sharp knife, a slip when making an incision (often when cutting through contaminated hides), can result in a severe wound and sometimes death. *Abrasions* are sustained through knocks from equipment, falling gambrels and trolleys often being the cause of contusions and acute injuries. In addition to knives, many injuries are caused by bone splinters, which can be responsible for simple *punctures* or large *lacerations* and are more serious than many knife cuts in that they are more liable to infection.

Newly-employed personnel lacking in efficiency are most often at risk. Most of the recorded fatalities and injuries have been associated with deboning operations in which slips can occur when the knife is drawn towards the operative's body. Fatal stabbings have resulted in penetration of the femoral artery and vein. In addition, modern meat plant operations entail the use of automatic equipment and monotonous tasks which on occasion lead to *repetitive strain injury* (RSI), frequently a tenosynovitis of the hand.

While carelessness and irresponsible behaviour may account for some of these accidents, other reasons include the absence of protective equipment (chain mesh aprons and gloves) and helmets, the use of blunt knives and of steels without guards, holding bare knives while walking, catching falling knives, improper use of steels, use of knives other than one's own, etc. Dangerous machines must be efficiently maintained, fully guarded and properly used by authorised personnel. Rotation of staff should assist in the prevention of RSI. An all-too frequent, and totally unnecessary, cause of cuts is knife slips when skinning filthy cattle on which there are several inches of adherent faecal material.

Inadequate first-aid facilities and lack of proper training frequently add to the problem of injuries and infections. ALL wounds, cuts and abrasions should be *immediately treated* and *tetanus toxoid* should be administered especially in cases of deep penetrating wounds.

## UK LEGISLATION

Health and Safety at Work Act 1974

Factories Act 1961

Prescribed Dangerous Machines Order 1964

The Reporting of Injuries, Diseases and Dangerous Occurrences Regulations 1981

Health and Safety (First Aid) Regulations 1981

The UK *Health and Safety at Work Act 1974* requires all employers to ensure as far as is reasonably practicable, the health, safety and welfare of their employees. The Act provides for a safe workplace, safe machinery and adequate information, instruction, training and supervision. Employees have a duty to take reasonable care of their own safety. Regulations under the Act lay down the accidents which must be reported directly to the Health and Safety Executive (HSE). These relate to deaths, major injury and other dangerous occurrences as defined by the Act. If the injured person goes to hospital, a report is only necessary if he or she is detained for more than 24 hours other than for observation. In all cases completion of the 'Accident Book' is necessary.

The UK *Factories Act* of 1961 lays down specific requirements for *first-aid* arrangements. A first-aid box or cupboard must be provided (more than one if there are more than 150 workers) in every factory. Its contents must conform to certain standards and a responsible trained person must be in charge of it. If the factory employs more than 150 personnel, this person must be either a registered or enrolled nurse or the holder of a certificate in first-aid training issued during the previous 3 years by an approved organisation. Details relating to the siting of first-aid boxes, maintenance of records, situation of ambulance rooms and referral of cases to a doctor or hospital are also included in the Factories Act.

Failure to comply with safety regulations may involve employers in prosecution.

The UK *Health and Safety Executive* (HSE) is responsible for developing standards nationally and for inspection and enforcement in food factories, local authorities being responsible for inspection and enforcement in shops, supermarkets and catering establishments.

Because of the high number (over 1000) of *hand-tool accidents* which occur in the UK meat industry each year, inspectors of the Health and Safety Executive carried out an investigation in 1981 into the nature of knife accidents in meat and fish plants and reported as follows. Out of 254 instances of knife injuries examined 75 (29.5%) involved personnel with more than 5 years' experience of boning-out. In 169 (66.5%) instances there was no protection provided for the non-knife hand and in 228 (89.8%) cases there was no protection for the wrist and forearm. Butchers/boners appeared to be most prone to injury, but slaughterers were involved in about one-third of the total incidents.

It was concluded that injury could have been prevented in 213 (83.9%) of the accidents. In 20% of the cases operatives were wearing plastic or rubber aprons capable of being easily penetrated by a knife.

Usually the non-knife hand is injured, which would tend to indicate that knife-slip is the most frequent immediate cause of injury. Good *knife design*, *proper handle guards* and adequate protection for the non-knife hand, wrist and forearm together with the use of an *apron of chain-mail* are essential items for safeguarding butchers and boners. It is important to keep knives constantly clean and sharp, knife edges being sharpened 'little and often'. Many personnel resist the use of steel-mesh gloves and aprons because of their weight and awkwardness in use. A washable lightweight glove made of high-strength aramid and nylon with a steel core and cut-resistant, but not cut-proof, is now available.

*Safety of personnel in the meat industry* is of the utmost importance – neglect involves injury, pain, possible infection and time off work. Death from knife wounds is not unknown in the meat trade, nor are infection and septic arthritis resulting in finger deformity.

Especially in cutting and boning rooms, *safety gloves* and *aprons* are essential along with a high degree of cleanliness and tidy working conditions, with no extraneous material on floors to cause falls. The collection of blood and fat in slaughter and carcase dressing areas is notorious for causing accidents. *Safety helmets* are essential to prevent injury from moving machinery and falling trolleys and carcases. All machinery must be adequately maintained and in proper working order. Plastic *waterproof footwear with microcellular soles* is of great value in preventing slipping on floors.

Special attention must be given to personnel involved in the handling of BSE-infected animals and those handling heads and spinal cords of all stock.

## ALLERGIES

Some individuals are especially susceptible to animals and their environment. Among the reported allergies are *rhinitis*, which is sometimes combined with *asthma* (now a prescribed industrial disease in Britain) and *skin rashes*. The former two conditions may be related directly to contact with the animals or, for example, to mouldy hay and straw which can set up the condition known as 'farmer's lung'. *'Farmer's lung'* is caused by the inhalation of large numbers of the spores of the bacterium *Micropolysporum faeni*, the antigens of which stimulate antibody production in the alveoli of the lungs. Subsequent exposure to these microorganisms causes a localised inflammatory response, the *Arthus reaction*, producing acute or chronic symptoms of coughing, chills, dyspnoea, fatigue and weight loss. Less commonly, simple chemicals, act in a similar fashion.

In some cases faecal bacteria and Gram-negative bacterial endotoxins in organic dusts cause nose and eye irritation, coughing, chest tightness, headache and nausea. These endotoxins may also play a part in *byssinosis*, which is a bronchoconstriction occurring in workers handling cotton, flax and hemp. These organic dust conditions are not uncommon in intensive livestock farms, especially poultry and pig units.

Severe *dermatitis* of unknown origin affecting the hands of operatives removing pancreases has been observed.

*Occupational skin diseases* are relatively common, forming some 60% of all new spells of certified incapacity for which injury benefit is payable and accounting for twice the number of working days lost compared with all the other occupational diseases together.

Many different causes exist – animal and plant contact, organic and inorganic compounds, trauma, insects, microorganisms, radiation, etc. Factors such as the pattern and intensity of exposure, individual susceptibility, skin pigmentation, presence/absence of skin wounds, cuts and abrasions, skin protection and the presence/absence of efficient first-aid treatment are also of importance.

## ZOONOSES (see also Chapters 17 and 18)

While injuries of various types, including electrocution, are common, workers in the meat industry, especially in the slaughtering sector, are at particular risk in acquiring certain *zoonoses* (*diseases naturally transmitted between animals and man*). A vitiated atmosphere contaminated with microorganisms, poor ventilation and skin injuries contributes to the development of zoonoses.

The zoonoses include anthrax, brucellosis, contagious pustular dermatitis, erysipelas, leptospirosis, listeriosis, louping ill, ornithosis, psittacosis, Q fever (rabies), ringworm, salmonellosis, staphylococcosis, streptococcal meningitis, toxoplasmosis, TB and tularaemia.

### Anthrax

There has been a significant decrease in the number of cases of anthrax in Great Britain in recent years. While in England and Wales in the period 1961–65 there were 56 cases with 4 human deaths, the number of cases per year since 1969 has not exceeded 5 with no deaths in man.

The disease was made notifiable in the UK under the Public Health Act of 1966 in December 1966 and the decline in incidence was most noticeable in persons employed in the hides, wool, hair, bristle, bone flour and meat and bone meal trades. This was mainly due to the introduction of vaccination (cell-free vaccine prepared from a culture filtrate containing the protective antigen) in 1965 for workers at risk and in 1978 to labelling of the unsterilised product. Annual vaccination of grazing stock where disease is prevalent using spore or alum-precipitated antigen vaccine is recommended.

However, workers in the above trades and those handling infected material are still at risk, as indeed are those in the livestock sector. Infection can be introduced with the importation of bone meal, etc., contaminated with *Bacillus anthracis*. Certain environmental events such as floods may cause epizootics.

Cutaneous anthrax appears to occur more often on the hands and arms of meat handlers, while the face and neck are more frequently affected in workers employed in other industries.

The fact that anthrax in animals is not necessarily associated with sudden death is a sufficient reason for great vigilance and for efficient ante-mortem inspection at meat plants.

### Brucellosis

While personnel engaged in the handling of livestock, dressing of carcases and offal and disposal of rejected material and hides are at greatest risk, all abattoir staff are at hazard, especially when infected and reactor animals are being slaughtered, for example, as a result of an eradication scheme. In some instances cases have occurred in meat plant staff unassociated with these duties, making the source of infection difficult to explain – the possibility of personnel having ingested unpasteurised milk has to be borne in mind.

In 1966 a study in Edinburgh revealed antibodies to *Brucella abortus* in 12.5% of abattoir workers and (presumably from the consumption of milk) in 1% of the population in that city.

In the United Kingdom the introduction in 1967 of voluntary schemes for the testing and removal of reactors from individual herds followed by area eradication in 1975 and compulsory eradication in 1979 has ensured a marked decline in the incidence of bovine brucellosis with a parallel reduction of human infection. In 1972 there were 264 cases of human brucellosis in England and Wales, these being reduced in 1986 to 30 isolations of *Brucella* spp. of which 6 were *Br. melitensis*, 11 *Br. suis*, 23 untyped but none proved to be *Br. abortus*. *Br. suis* type 11 is believed to be prevalent in Britain but asymptomatic in pigs and can cause a bacteraemia in man on occasions.

There has been a tendency in the past in disease eradication schemes to rely on the slaughter aspect without paying due regard to the needs of the personnel responsible for handling *infected* and *reactor* animals. Such animals must be handled with great care with strict attention to hygiene at all stages. Workers must attend to personal hygiene, frequently washing hands and arms using a bactericidal soap, and avoid contact with infected organs, discharges and urine. *Uteri* and *udders must not be incised and should not be handled with unprotected hands*. Hooks or other suitable instruments may be used. These organs should be carefully disposed of as rejected offal. Masks and rubber gloves have been advocated but present practical problems.

## Contagious pustular dermatitis (CPD, contagious ecthyma, 'orf')

CPD in sheep and goats is a worldwide disease in distribution caused by a DNA virus of the *parapoxvirus* genus of poxviruses. Lesions on the lips of lambs (mostly up to 1 year old) and udders of ewes are usually apparent, but a more serious form with high mortality may involve the tongue, palate, lungs and digestive tract.

Between 1975 and 1981 in Scotland there were 344 reports of orf in human beings, most cases affecting adults, especially men. In 49 cases those affected were abattoir workers, butchers or meat handlers. Veterinary surgeons may also be affected. It is likely that the actual number of cases greatly exceeds reported ones since many of the lesions, although intractable to treatment, are of minor importance.

The lesions of CPD occur fairly frequently in abattoir workers mainly on the hands, wrists and forearm and sometimes the face. The early vesicle stage is rarely seen, however, and the usual presentation is a chronic, raised, circular dark red *papule* often found on the ulnar border of the hands. This papule is firm to the touch and may reach 3 cm in diameter. Painless at first, the papule becomes dome-shaped with a depressed centre which contains a clear exudate. Pus formation and granulation tissue eventually take place, causing pain.

**Systemic CPD** Although most cases of CPD are local lesions, the virus probably gaining entrance through small wounds or abrasions, there is evidence that a *systemic* form occurs and is becoming more prevalent (Shuttleworth, 1988). The main features of this invasive CPD are a haemorrhagic blister at the site of virus entry, an irregular blotchy rash on various parts of the body with swelling, pruritis of the affected part and axillary lymphadenitis, malaise and a flu-like feeling. Later stages involve aching limbs and joints, fatigue and exhaustion and adenitis of the cervical and inguinal lymph nodes with acute abdominal pain requiring hospital admission. The average duration of clinical signs is 10 months with a range of 2–30 months. The homoeopathic drug *Thuga accidentalis* has been advocated by this author as effective treatment for man, sheep and goats.

Although personnel handling sheep are most often affected, the condition has been reported in engineering staff concerned with the maintenance of equipment, an indication of virus persistence. This ability is further confirmed by the fact that while CPD is most prevalent in sheep and lambs in the spring and early summer, infections have been recorded in abattoir staff in mid-winter. Undoubtedly, indirect as well as direct contact occurs, infection being acquired by both man and animals through intermediate passive transfer from apparently normal animals contaminated by contact, knives, clothing and other forms of equipment. Person-to-person transmission, however, is rare.

Sensible protective precautions should be exercised – strict personal hygiene and prompt attention to cuts and abrasions. Infected animals should be handled carefully in the lairage and, as for all zoonoses, *other staff should be alerted to the presence of CPD*.

The use of a live virulent vaccine applied following scarification of the axilla of sheep would serve to reduce the incidence of CPD in animals and man, but few owners appear to apply it.

### Erysipeloid

A localised cutaneous infection of pig and fish handlers, butchers, cooks and veterinary surgeons, this is caused by *Erysipelothrix rhusiopathiae*, the causal organism of swine erysipelas which may also be associated with arthritis, especially in finger joints.

There is a spreading erythema and oedema at the site which in rare cases may extend to a septicaemia with high fever. The condition responds well to treatment with penicillin or erythromycin.

**Diagnosis** is confirmed by isolation of the causal organism from the local lesion or blood.

### Erysipelas

Erysipeloid must not be confused with *erysipelas*, an acute cellulitis of human beings in the form of a red, painful, oedematous spreading lesion which often has a raised border and is caused by *Group A streptococci*. The lesions occur most often on the face and legs of patients, especially women, who are suffering from a debilitating disease. In some cases the condition is severe with the occurrence of bacteraemia.

### Leptospirosis (haemorrhagic jaundice, Weil's disease, Canicola fever, mud fever, dairy worker fever, swineherd disease)

This is a bacterial disease of varying severity and sporadic occurrence transmitted by contact with the urine of infected animals. The condition is characterised by sudden onset, fever, headache, myalgia, conjunctivitis and sometimes haemolytic anaemia, skin and mucous membrane haemorrhage, icterus, renal failure, meningitis and mental confusion. Fatal cases are not common but may occur where there is jaundice and kidney failure.

In certain parts of the world leptospirosis is an important disease in the livestock industry, e.g. in parts of north and south America, Russia and the near East.

Human infections do occur from time to time, even in the British Isles, and are almost always associated with *rats* in whose urine the leptospires are shed. Hedgehogs, voles, shrews, skunks, opossums, certain reptiles, amphibians and fish also act as reservoirs of infection. Farm and pet animals (cattle, horses, sheep, pigs and dogs) may also act as carriers. The size and movement of the rat population may increase the risk of exposure of human beings to infective material, the disease in man being more prevalent during the late summer and autumn months. Warm humid conditions appear to favour the proliferation of leptospires. Outbreaks of leptospirosis occur where people are exposed to canal, lake and fresh water contaminated with animal urine.

In addition to abattoir workers, livestock handlers, veterinary surgeons, poultry and fish handlers, sewer and canal workers, etc., are liable to infection. Because of improved working conditions, leptospirosis is not now common in miners, sewer workers and fish cleaners, who were at one time frequently infected. The reduction of the rat population and the control of litter with the adoption of hygiene precautions have markedly reduced the incidence of leptospirosis in many areas of the world.

At least 200 different serotypes of leptospires in 23 groups have been recorded in livestock, occurring in two main complexes: *Leptospira interrogans*, including most of the mammalian strains and *L. biflexa*, including the non-pathogenic saprophytic types. Most of the human cases of leptospirosis occurring in England and Wales are of the *icterohaemorrhagiae* serogroup, followed by *hebdomadis* and *canicola* infections.

Serovars commonly identified in causing human infection are *icterohaemorrhagiae, hardjo, canicola, autumnalis, pomona, hebdomadis* and *australis*.

Although infection normally takes place through the skin, especially if cut or abraded, it may also occur via mucous membranes and through inhalation or ingestion.

### Listeriosis (listerellosis, mononucleosis)

This bacterial disease is caused by *Listeria monocytogenes* and manifested in man by meningoencephalitis and/or septicaemia which may be fatal. Sometimes abortion takes place. A cutaneous form of listeriosis is also recognised in adults and appears to be increasing in incidence.

The *reservoir* of *L. monocytogenes* is forage, silage, soil, water and a wide range of animals (domestic and wild) and birds. The organism has been isolated more frequently from the faeces of abattoir workers than from any other class of employees.

The disease occurs mainly in pregnant women, neonates, elderly persons and immunocompromised individuals, including alcoholics.

**Symptoms** in man are usually sudden in onset with fever, nausea, headache, vomiting, mental confusion and sometimes coma, collapse and shock.

**Lesions** of endocarditis are rare but granulomatous lesions may occur in the liver and other organs along with internal and external skin abscesses.

The disease is sporadic in occurrence, human *infection* normally occurring by ingestion of contaminated food (cheeses, vegetables, milk etc.) or contact with infective material (fetuses, fetal membranes, soil etc.). Infection can also be acquired by inhalation and by venereal transmission.

In a few cases the *ingestion* of infected meat by human beings has resulted in listeriosis.

*Primary cutaneous listeriosis* has been recorded by many authors. McLaughlin and Low (1994) cited 17 cases in adults in which the disease appeared as an initial reddish rash which developed into vesicular or pustular lesions 1–2 mm in diameter with either dark or light centres. These cases occurred in a lorry driver, a wholesale butcher and the remainder in veterinary surgeons and farmers. Most cases in the farmers and veterinarians were associated with the manual delivery of aborted bovine fetuses or stillbirths. Various phage types of *L. monocytogenes* were isolated from the cutaneous lesions and the abortion specimens.

**Preventive measures against listeriosis** Pregnant women, immunocompromised individuals, veterinary surgeons and farmers must avoid contact with potentially infective materials such as aborted fetuses and fetal membranes. Only properly cooked meats and pasteurised dairy products should be eaten. Freedom of all foods, especially soft cheeses, from *Listeria* and other food-poisoning organisms should be ensured.

## Louping ill

Louping ill and related tick-borne encephalitides (Central European tick-borne encephalitis, Russian spring–summer encephalitis, Powassan virus encephalitis, etc.) occur mainly in eastern and central Europe, Scandinavia, Asia, Canada and the USA, causing varying severities of encephalitis in man depending on the virus involved, individual susceptibility, and so on.

The frequency of cuts and abrasions undoubtedly predisposes to these infections when acquired occupationally. An incidence of louping ill infection of 8.3% was detected in Scottish abattoir workers in 1966, an incidence which has been markedly reduced in recent years. In addition to infection from biting ticks, louping ill in man may also be acquired through the consumption of infected milk. Adult ticks may procure infection from man.

**Symptoms** usually take the form of fever, headache, flu-like symptoms, conjunctivitis sometimes accompanied with nervous signs. The condition in man is generally mild.

**Preventive measures** should include vaccination of ewes (inactivated vaccine grown in tissue culture).

## Psittacosis and ornithosis (chlamydiosis, parrot fever)

Both diseases are transmissible to man, psittacosis from birds of the psittacine order (parrots, parakeets, etc.) and ornithosis from birds other than psittacines. A sheep strain of *Chlamydia psittaci* can infect pregnant women. The disease is worldwide in distribution and affects a wide variety of birds. Among domestic poultry it is most common in ducks, turkeys, geese and pigeons, which are the main source of human infection.

The first recorded outbreak of ornithosis in the UK occurred in the winter and spring of 1979–80 and was associated with commercially-reared ducks. Some cases involved workers in a duck-processing plant, others occurring in 15 out of 46 veterinary surgeons attending a training course on the supervision of poultry processing premises.

A survey of workers in the British duck industry has indicated a past exposure to infection rate (based on results of complement fixation (CF) tests on blood samples) of 11%. The workers employed on evisceration lines showed the highest titres to the CF test.

Cases of human ornithosis originating from ducks have also occurred in the Czech Republic and Denmark. In the former country it was found that covering the evisceration lines and improving the plant ventilation by the installation of extractor fans solved the problem in the workers.

While the number of human cases arising from psittacine birds has been decreasing since the implementation of the UK *Captive Birds Order of 1976*, the overall number of ornithosis cases has been rising.

Persons may become infected more than once and, while the disease in man is usually mild, occasionally it can be severe. *Human infection* occurs by *inhalation* following exposure to infected aerosols, dust-infected bird droppings and nasal discharges and sheep fetuses and membranes. *Chlamydia psittaci* may also be responsible for cases of conjunctivitis in poultry workers, especially in dust-laden atmospheres.

**Symptoms** in humans include gastrointestinal pain and vomiting, headache, insomnia and pneumonia. Valvular endocarditis may develop. Mild attacks of the disease may be mistaken for influenza. Recovery is usually complete but convalescence may be prolonged. Infection in pregnant women from a sheep source can be very serious.

**Diagnosis** in man is based on serological tests (complement fixation and fluorescent antibody). In birds the organism is demonstrated in stained liver and spleen smears with isolation in tissue culture from fetuses, fetal membranes, etc.

**Preventive measures** should include education of the public on the risk of exposure to infected exotic pet birds and infected ducks, geese, turkeys and pigeons, including feral pigeons; regulation of importation of birds of the parrot family; efficient surveillance of pet shops, aviaries, farms and processing plants; and treatment or destruction of infected stock combined with effective disinfection.

**Treatment** with tetracyclines is usually effective. Antibiotic prophylaxis with chlortetracycline is advocated for control of the disease.

Satisfactory standards of ventilation and the prevention of dusty atmospheres are essential as is the use of dust masks where necessary.

## Lyme disease (Lyme borreliosis, tick-borne meningopolyneuritis)

This is a tick-borne bacterial zoonosis which occurs frequently in eastern and western USA, in Canada (Ontario), Russia, China, Japan and Australia. It also occurs less often in Europe, including England (especially the New and Thetford Forests) and Scotland. The disease is an occupational hazard for farmers, shepherds, deer stalkers, veterinarians and abattoir workers.

The cause is the spirochaete *Borrelia burgdorferi*, which was first identified in 1982. The borreliae are large (10–30 μm long × 0.3–0.7 μm wide), Gram-negative, motile spirochaetes (slender spiral or coiled, very motile bacteria although they possess no flagella). Spirochaetes include *Treponema pallidum*, the cause of human syphilis, and Leptospirae. In addition to Lyme disease, the borreliae are responsible for European and West African relapsing fever (also transmitted by ticks).

The hard tick *Ixodes ricinus*, which has a reservoir in deer (especially white-tailed deer) and a variety of rodents, is responsible for transmitting Lyme disease.

In man the first clinical manifestation is usually erythema chronicum migrans, a redness which extends outwards from the site of the tick bite. Untreated, the infection may extend to a chronic arthritis or to a CNS infection. The latter is manifested by cranial neuritis (commonly involving the facial nerves), transverse myelitis and meningitis. Obvious symptoms are fever, headache, malaise, fatigue, stiff neck, pain in muscles with swelling of joints. Myocarditis may also be a complication. The cases of arthritis are believed to be more common in the USA while the European cases more often assume a neurological form, an unexplained anomaly.

*Diagnosis* is based on clinical signs, association with tick bites and serological tests (IFA, ELISA), although the tests are insensitive during the early stages of the disease especially if antibiotic treatment has been used.

The usual *treatment* is doxycycline for three weeks.

*Control* includes avoidance of tick-infested areas, protection against ticks with proper clothing (arms and legs covered) with use of tick repellents. Adherent ticks should be removed carefully without crushing by gentle traction close to the skin. If the skin is carefully heated beforehand, the mouth parts of the ticks are more easily extracted.

### Q Fever (Query fever, pneumorickettsiosis, abattoir fever, Balkan influenza, Balkan grippe)

In a study of workers in an Edinburgh abattoir (Schonell *et al.*, 1966) it was found that 28.1% showed antibodies to phase 2 antigen of *Coxiella burnetii*, the rickettsial cause of Q fever. An earlier survey in 1953 revealed an incidence of 2.13% in the general population in Britain. In 1966 in Northern Ireland, 28.3% of abattoir workers and 24.4% of veterinarians were positive, although there had been no evidence of previous Q fever infection in animals and man. The disease has been reported worldwide.

Q fever was first officially recognised in the United Kingdom in 1949 and is now routinely tested for in the differential diagnosis of human cases of pneumonia and pyrexia of unknown origin. Between 1975 and 1980 an annual average of 100 cases were reported to the Public Health Laboratory Service in England and Wales. Outbreaks are rare and the source of infection is often difficult to establish.

In recent years in Australia, Q fever has been such a serious disease in abattoir workers that vaccination of susceptible personnel was instituted; 924 non-immune volunteers were inoculated with a *Cox. burnetii* phase 1 vaccine, and while 34 cases occurred in 1349 non-vaccinated workers, there were no cases in the following 18 months. Q fever is a *notifiable disease* in humans in some countries, notably Australia, Israel and Italy.

**Symptoms** The disease in man is an acute febrile condition with sudden onset, pneumonia, coughing, malaise, anorexia, myalgia and weakness lasting 1–2 weeks. Hepatitis, pericarditis and endocarditis may ensue in more severe cases. The mortality rate is low – probably less than 1% in treated and untreated patients. Many cases are asymptomatic. The organisms can survive for long periods in cardiac cases with relapse long after the initial infection. The severity of Q fever increases with age.

**Reservoir of infection** Cattle, sheep, goats, cats and many wild animals and ticks form the reservoir. Cattle and sheep are the main sources of infection, especially at parturition/abortion when numerous organisms are shed in placentae and fetal fluids. Urine, faeces and milk may also be infective. Many infected animals are frequently asymptomatic. The organisms, which can multiply in the genital tract and mammary gland, remain viable in fodder and dust for long periods.

**Mode of infection** Human infection is acquired by inhalation and by direct and indirect contact with infected animals and materials (straw, wool, clothing, fertiliser, etc.). The consumption of raw infected milk may sometimes be responsible. Infection through blood and bone marrow transfusion has been reported.

**Diagnosis** is by complement fixation and ELISA tests. Demonstration of *Coxiella burnetii* in the blood of patients is rarely attempted because of risk to laboratory staff.

**Prevention and control** Along lines enumerated above. Pasteurisation/boiling of milk and hygienic measures, including disinfection, are important. High-risk groups in some countries receive vaccine prepared from inactivated *Cox. burnetii* (Phase 1)-infected yolk sac.

### Ringworm (dermatophytosis, dermatomycosis, trichophytosis, epidermophytosis, micro-sporosis, tinea)

A fungal disease of the skin, this is caused by several species of *Trichophyton* and *Microsporum*, especially *T. mentagrophytes* and *T. verrucosum* (from cattle, horses, rodents and wild animals) and *M. canis* (from dogs).

Spores of ringworm fungi can remain viable for years on carrier animals, tackle and bedding, even longer than the active lesions on animals and man.

**Mode of transmission** Direct and indirect contact with animals and their harness, brushes, combs, clothing, etc. Transmission from person to person is rare. As with many skin diseases, injuries in the form of cuts, abrasions and maceration of the superficial skin layers constitute predisposing factors.

**Clinical signs in man** These resemble those in animals – circular, scaly, pink to red, crusty lesions with slightly raised borders which expand peripherally with loss of hair. The hands, arms and forearms are mostly affected but other body areas may be involved due to scratching.

**Diagnosis** The organisms are identified as characteristic hyaline ectothrix arthrospores in skin scrapings taken from the periphery of the lesion and treated with 10% potassium or sodium hydroxide. Culture should be made for confirmation and species identification. Examination of hairs and scales under Wood's lamp (UV light) shows a yellowish-green fluorescence for *Microsporum* but not for *Trichophyton* species.

**Prevention and control** See also above. Disinfection procedures using formaldehyde are valuable for infected tools and equipment and sodium hydroxide for buildings.

Care should be exercised in handling affected animals. Cattle appear to be more often affected during the winter months in Britain, the condition usually disappearing once spring sunshine arrives. In Russia and some other east European countries a live spore vaccine is used in cattle to protect against *Trichophyton* infection.

Oral griseofulvin is an effective treatment.

## Skin sepsis

Streptococcal and staphylococcal skin infections are fairly common in animal and meat handlers and have become more frequent in recent years.

Outbreaks of skin infection due to *Streptococcus pyogenes* have been recorded among workers in meat processing factories, the first outbreak occurring in Yorkshire, England, in 1978. In this instance there was an attack rate as high as 44% in one department (packing). Altogether there were 103 episodes of infection in 82 workers out of a total staff complement of 347 (Barnham *et al.*, 1980).

Group L β-haemolytic streptococci were also isolated from the clinically infected wounds, impetigo and paronychia of 15 patients involved in the slaughter and dressing of pigs and poultry, *Staph. aureus* being recovered from 8 of these cases (Barnham and Neilson, 1987).

Outbreaks associated with *Staphylococcus aureus* and β-haemolytic streptococci (*Str. pyogenes* being the most common) have been recorded in Scottish abattoirs. In association with these outbreaks a survey of skin sepsis in the different classes of meat handlers revealed that knife injuries constituted the greatest percentage group with slaughterers, inspectors and gut cleaners principally involved. Had this survey been carried out in a processing factory, the main category of worker most at risk would have been boners (Table 15.1).

Meat handlers appear to be particularly susceptible to streptococcal skin sepsis, which takes the form of impetigenous or eczematous lesions, infection round the nail fold and infected lacerations. Second, and even third, episodes of infection may occur. Happily, the extremely serious infected lesions resulting in hand joint arthritis with deformity, common in earlier years, are now of rare occurrence.

## Cutaneous salmonellosis

This condition has been reported in veterinarians following the delivery of dead or emphysematous calves and cannot be excluded as a hazard for meat plant staff. The lesions take the form of pustular dermatitis or folliculitis as small, red, patchy spots on arms and hands apparent within three days of the event. In

**Table 15.1** Survey of skin sepsis in meat handlers, Scotland, 1983–85.

| | Percentage association of each type of skin puncture | | |
|---|---|---|---|
| Occupation | Bone | Knife | Graze |
| Slaughterer | 7 | 75 | 18 |
| Butcher | 31 | 35 | 34 |
| Gut cleaner | 13 | 53 | 34 |
| Loader | 50 | 12 | 38 |
| Packer | 40 | 40 | 20 |
| Inspector | 20 | 60 | 20 |
| Others | 11 | 39 | 50 |

some cases more severe lesions, even ulcerations, have occurred with mild systemic symptoms, headache and fever.

Several types of salmonellae have been isolated – *S. dublin, S. Saint Paul, S. typhimurium* and *S. virchow* (Cameron, 1988; Collyer, 1988; Visser, 1991).

## Clostridial cellulitis

An unusual form of infection occurred in a male worker following a scratch from a bone in a poultry plant in Wales in 1991. The tiny wound become a cellulitis with swelling, pain and an objectionable odour which 'travelled up the arm and eventually enveloped the whole body', making the man a virtual social outcast. Various types of antibiotics were used in addition to UV light, chlorophyll and oxygen without effect. A skin biopsy and microbiological examination revealed the presence of a *Clostridium* bacterium which was secreting toxins, the cause of the foul smell. Recovery took place without apparent reason.

## Streptococcosis (*Str. suis* infection, *Str. zooepidemicus* infection)

*Streptococcus suis* type 2 infection is a disease of pigs, transmissible to man and characterised by meningitis which has been recognised in the United Kingdom, Canada, USA, Brazil and Netherlands. Recent surveys have shown that the disease is widespread in pigs in the United Kingdom, especially in the south and east. It is probably present in all pig-producing countries.

After the first UK outbreak in 1973 there was an increasing number of incidents recorded, to a peak in 1976 after which there was an apparent decline.

Carrier rates for *Str. suis* type 2 in tonsils of pigs from 12 herds in England with a history of *Str. meningitis* varied from 20% to 90%. In two herds thought to be free of the disease, the carrier rates were 20% and 1.5% respectively (Clifton-Hadley *et al.*, 1984).

In Ontario, Canada, *Str. suis* type 2 was detected in 8.1% of 347 pig herds examined in 1985. Microbiological examination of meat operatives' hands and knives showed that eviscerators involved in tongue and lung removal were more at risk of exposure to *Str. suis* infection because of the presence of the organism in palatine tonsils (Breton *et al.*, 1986).

In Australia and New Zealand an examination of 734 pig palatine tonsils showed that 54% were infected with *Str. suis* type 1 and 73% of 959 tonsils with *Str. suis* type 2 organisms. Both forms of bacteria were recovered from the blood and reproductive tracts of 3% of normal pigs (Robertson and Blackmore, 1989).

Streptococcal meningitis in pigs occurs after weaning and when pigs are mixed, the organisms apparently being conveyed by healthy adult carrier animals in the nasopharynx. However, it is possible that human carriers may on occasion be implicated. Stress is probably a precipitating factor.

*Streptococcus zooepidemicus* has been isolated from cases of mastitis in cattle.

### *Human streptococcosis*

Since 1975 there have been several reports of illness in people due to *Str. suis* type 2 (Group R) in England, Wales and Ireland. The persons affected were abattoir workers, meat processing plant operatives, butchers, farmers and veterinary surgeons. In one case there was no history of any occupational involvement. Some of the patients developed meningitis while others suffered arthritis and lymphangitis with bacteraemia. Fever is always present with headache, numbness of the fingers, foot pain, rigors and skin erythema.

*Streptococcus zooepidemicus* infection is responsible for pneumonia and upper respiratory symptoms, cervical adenitis, endocarditis and nephritis.

Humans acquire *Str. suis* infection through handling contaminated meat, while *Str. zooepidemicus* infection occurs in people in contact with sick and carrier animals and by drinking infected milk.

**Prevention and control** See under 'Injuries' earlier.

## Tetanus (lockjaw)

While abattoir workers are probably no more at risk than other occupations, nevertheless in an industry where livestock are handled and where wounds, often deep, penetrating ones, occur, the possibility of tetanus occurring is a very real one.

In England and Wales, reported cases of tetanus usually range from 15 to 24 annually, with deaths varying from 1 to 10 a year, but the actual number is probably four to five times greater. The disease appears to be more common in persons over 45 years of age and in males.

**Prevention and control** See under 'Injuries' earlier.

### Tularaemia (rabbit fever, deerfly fever, O'Hara disease)

Tularaemia occurs worldwide and is especially common in North America where some 2000 human cases, often of rabbit and tick origin, are reported annually in the United States. Japan also has an undue incidence associated with rabbits but the virulence of the causal organism, *Francisella tularensis,* is low. Some strains in North America are more virulent. In general, however, the fatality rate from tularaemia with appropriate treatment is low, normally less than 5%.

In addition to rabbits and hares, muskrats, lemmings, beavers, birds and some domestic animals, especially sheep, are sometimes infected. Ticks and mosquitoes are concerned in the cycle of infection.

The skinning of infected rabbits and hares is a common means of human infection, the organism gaining entrance through small wounds. Insect bites may also be responsible. Ingestion of the organism can cause a pharyngitis. A rarer mode of transmission is via the conjunctival sac.

**Symptoms** in man are variable and include fever, headache, myalgia, pneumonia, pharyngitis, abdominal pain, diarrhoea and vomiting. Where the organism is inoculated through the skin, an indolent ulcer usually develops with an adenitis in the associated lymph nodes.

**Preventive measures** include the avoidance of wounds and cuts especially during the skinning of carcases, control of rodents, dipping of sheep to control vectors and immunisation of persons at high risk. The rodent-proofing of homes in endemic areas is recommended, with the thorough cooking of meat and boiling of water.

## PREVENTION OF OCCUPATIONAL DISEASE IN MEAT PLANT STAFF

1. Education of workers as to the nature of zoonoses and how to minimise the risk of infection by careful handling of potentially infected stock, carcases and offal.
2. Efficient veterinary ante-mortem inspection especially with casualty animals, and the immediate alerting of staff to all disease hazards.
3. High standards of personal and environmental hygiene.
4. Avoidance of cuts, wounds and abrasions with prompt and efficient treatment when they occur.
5. Proper meat plant construction and layout and ventilation with good staff facilities (showers, toilets, handwashing, use of bactericidal soaps, etc.).
6. Good first-aid facilities.
7. Vaccination of staff where appropriate.
8. Where possible, elimination of disease in domestic animals.
9. Close liaison with medical expertise.

## REFERENCES


Barnham, M. and Neilson, D. J. (1987) *Epidemiol. Infect*. **99**, 257–264.

Barnham, M., Kerby, J. and Skillin, J. (1980) *J. Hyg. Camb*. **84**, 71–75.

Breton. J., Mitchell, W. R. and Rosendal, S. (1986) *Can. J. Vet. Res*. **50**, 338–341.

Cameron, I. R. D. (1988) *Vet. Rec*. **123**, 528.

Clifton-Hadley, F. A. *et al.* (1984) *Vet. Rec*. **115**, 562–564.

Collyer, J. H. (1988) *Vet. Rec*. **123**, 476.

McLaughlin, J. and Low J. C. (1994) *Vet. Rec*. **135**, 615–617.

Robertson, I. D. and Blackmore, D. K. (1989) *Vet. Rec*. **124**, 391–394.

Schonell, *et al*. (1966) *BMJ* **2**, 148–150.

Shuttleworth, V. S. (1988) *Brit. Homoeopath. J*. **77**, 12.

Visser, I. J. R. (1991) *Vet. Rec*. **129**, 364.


## FURTHER READING


Andrewes, C. H. and Walton, J. R. (1976) *Viral and Bacterial Zoonoses*. London: Ballière-Tindall.

Bell, J. C., Palmer, S. R. and Payne, J. M. (1988) *The Zoonoses*. London: Edward Arnold.

# Chapter 16
# Pathology

A knowledge of the response of cells, tissues and organs of the living body to injurious agents or deprivations is a prerequisite for efficient meat inspection.

## THE NATURE OF DISEASE

All pathological processes – disturbances in function and structure – are associated with basic cellular changes. When the death of the animal is sudden, e.g. in acute poisoning, aortic rupture, lightning strike, there may be no visible structural changes, while more chronic conditions such as Johne's disease and contagious bovine pleuro-pneumonia (CBPP) lead to well-defined macroscopic changes in cells and tissues, and in whole organs with loss of bodily condition.

The actual *causal agent*, whether it be a bacterium, virus, parasite, etc., produces its specific deleterious effects and these are followed by reactive changes which in many respects resemble physiological changes. These secondary changes may produce resolution of the disease provided resistance, nutritional status and so on are adequate, or the animal may succumb.

### Causes of disease

Disease may be either *acquired* or *genetic* in origin or a *combination* of *both*.

#### *Acquired disease*

Most diseases of animals are acquired, that is they are due to the effects of various environmental factors such as microorganisms, metazoan parasites, etc., which produce infections, or to different forms of malnutrition.

**Infective microorganisms:** These include bacteria, viruses, fungi and protozoa (see also Chapter 17).

Microorganisms are widespread in the environment – in the atmosphere, soil, fresh and sea water, sewage, on the skin, in the mouth and respiratory, genital and intestinal tracts of animals and man where they often exist as normal *commensals*. (The virus of the human common cold in the upper respiratory tract is a typical example.) Commensal microbes on the skin and mucous membranes are capable of excluding more injurious types (*pathogens*). Under certain circumstances, some nutritional in origin and some related to immunodeficiency, but many unknown, commensals are able to multiply, become pathogenic and cause *opportunistic* infections.

*'Infection'* is described as the presence of microorganisms in body tissues where they are normally absent and the term *'infective (infectious) disease'* is applied to the clinical entity. (Microorganisms resembling *L. monocytogenes* have been demonstrated in the brains of 5% of normal sheep in which they have passed several barriers, including the meningeal one (Gracey, 1958).

Only a relatively few of these, however, are capable of causing disease and their ability to produce disease depends on their invasiveness, their multiplication and their potential to be transmitted to other hosts. *Bacteria* produce their harmful effects through poisonous substances termed *toxins*, the exact nature of which largely determines the actual features of the disease. *Viruses* multiply in the living cells of the host and can only thrive in such cells. The type of viral disease depends on which cells are invaded along with the response of the host. Some viruses are involved in the causation of some forms of cancer, where their viral genes become integrated into the genome (genetic inventory) of the host cell.

Whether pathogenic microorganisms are able to invade the animal host depends on many complex factors such as bacterial and viral invasiveness and multiplication as well as specific and non-specific host defence mechanisms (the *immune system*).

The occurrence and treatment of infective disease is further complicated by the phenomenon of *bacterial resistance*. This may be *primary* (innate bacterial resistance) or *acquired* as a result of mutation or genetic change. Resistance to antibiotics by gene transfer is an extremely serious entity, for example, with strains of *Staphylococcus aureus* or *Neisseria meningitidis*. It can also occur between related strains of organisms, e.g. the enteric Gram-negative bacilli, and can be transferred between species, for example, from commensal *E. coli* to *Salmonella* and even from animals to man through the consumption of meat. It is occasioned by the abuse of antibiotic usage in human veterinary medicine such as their prescription for viral conditions on non-completion of courses of treatment, as well as the incorporation of antibiotics in animal feeds for growth-promoting purposes.

**Metazoan parasites** such as liver fluke, warble flies, *Echinococcus granulosus* and other cestodes are important causes of disease (see Chapter 18).

**Chemicals:** Chemical agents are now being increasingly used in agriculture and industry. Substances such as strong acids and alkalis, plant poisons, cyanide organophosphates, pesticides, herbicides, copper sulphate, lead, and various drugs, many of which exert toxic effects on the liver and kidneys (see Chapter 20).

**Mechanical injuries:** These include wounds and contusions, etc.

**Other physical agents** such as excessive heat, cold, electricity and radiation cause local death of cells and an inflammatory reaction.

**Immunological factors:** Hypersensitivity to various microorganisms, parasites, drugs and many other types of allergens (substances capable of producing allergy or specific hypersensitivity) may result in harmful effects, both local and general. Examples are *Purpura haemorrhagica* in horses, urticaria, allergic rhinitis in ruminants, contact allergy and hypersensitivity to helminths, e.g. in parasitic pneumonia and gastroenteritis.

*Anaphylaxis* is an acute antigen–antibody reaction, often resulting in sudden death, which occurs in animals previously sensitised to injections of drugs (lincomycin, erythromycin, sulphonamides, etc.) glandular extracts, blood transfusions or vaccines, and given a second dose of the same allergen after an interval during which the allergen has had time to bind to mast cells.

**Deficiency diseases:** Inadequate intake of high-quality protein, minerals, vitamins and trace elements accounts for much loss in livestock worldwide. Examples are copper deficiency in enzootic ataxia ('swayback'), pica due to salt deficiency, rickets in lambs caused by phosphorus deficiency, hypomagnesaemic tetany in cattle due to inability to mobilise magnesium, nutritional muscular dystrophy (white muscle disease) due to selenium and vitamin E deficiency (see Chapter 19).

## Genetically-determined disease

Genetically-determined disease usually arises from some abnormality of the DNA of the zygote (fertilised ovum). It may also derive from the absence or abnormality of a chromosome. These abnormalities may be inherited from one or both parents (*inherited diseases*) or be occasioned by teratogenic (environmental) factors such as the effects of drugs, chemicals, trace element and vitamin deficiency, viruses, irradiation, toxic plants or hyperthermia. In many cases there is no known cause.

Diseases which arise during fetal life are termed *congenital* and frequently result in fetal death, abortion or stillbirth. But viable and non-viable neonates (newborn animals) may be born only to succumb a few weeks later.

*Congenital abnormalities* include hydrocephalus and neonatal rickets in calves, congenital tremor and various anatomical defects in piglets, mummification, stillbirth and abortion in all species.

*Inherited conditions* may affect all body systems. Examples are freemartins (sterile female twin, usually bovine but sometimes ovine) born with a male; bulldog calves (inherited achondroplasia with hydrocephalus) of the Dexter breed; infertility in all species;

inherited goitre (cattle, sheep and goats); inherited osteoarthritis of cattle; malignant hyperthermia (porcine stress syndrome) in pigs; inherited hydrocephalus in Aberdeen-Angus cattle; Piétrain creeper pigs (muscular weakness).

While genetic defects can produce numerous perceptible anatomical abnormalities (there are some 400 in the dog), it is being more and more recognised that with the current emphasis on productivity in farm livestock with no regard for disease resistance, animals susceptible to general microbial disease are being created. A further concern is the reduction in the diversity of the genetic pool, especially in cattle, with the use of artificial insemination. Embryo transfer is also questionable on the same basis as well as on welfare considerations.

Livestock health, fertility and productivity are inextricably determined by both environmental and genetic factors.

## BODY DEFENCE MECHANISMS

These consist of non-specific and specific immune systems.

**Non-specific immune systems** are comprised of the intact *skin* and the *mucous membranes* of the alimentary, respiratory and urogenital systems. These act as the first barriers to invasion by microorganisms and are assisted by the upward action of the cilia of the columnar epithelium of the respiratory system, intestinal peristalsis and urine flow. Coughing, sneezing and weeping help to clear potential pathogens from the body.

In the skin, blood, tears, internal secretions, intestinal fluid and saliva there is present the enzyme *lysozyme* which, along with sebum produced by the sebaceous glands, has an antibacterial action. *Interferons*, *glycoproteins* released by certain cells to increase phagocytosis, *complement* (a series of enzymatic proteins) and *C-reactive protein* produced in response to inflammation, also play important parts in the body's defensive mechanism.

*Cells* in the form of *leukocytes* (macrophages, neutrophils and eosinophils) phagocytose and kill invading microorganisms while other white blood cells (basophils and mast cells) and natural killer (NK) lymphocyte cells are able to destroy infected tissues by mediating cytotoxic reactions.

These cellular entities can act alone or in association with the specific immune system.

**Specific immune responses** protect only against a particular microorganism or a closely related one. Once infection with a particular organism occurs, protection against a second infection takes place and is normally lifelong (secondary immune response). This response is known as immunological memory. Such a reaction forms the basis for the immunisation against certain infectious diseases with vaccines and sera.

Specific immune responses are activated by substances termed *antigens* which produce specific *antibodies*, a group of proteins called immunoglobulins, to produce *active immunity*. Both humoral (relating to body fluids) and cellular effects are involved in this response. But while the protective effect of antibody can be transferred through the use of serum in a non-immune animal (*passive immunity*), the cellular response can only be transferred by lymphocytes.

*B lymphocytes* (*B cells*), originating from the bone marrow, spleen, fetal liver and fetal yolk sac, are responsible for producing humoral antibodies. (The 'B' in B lymphocyte refers to the bursa of Fabricius in the cloaca of birds where B cell differentiation occurs.) *T lymphocytes* (*T cells*) from the *thymus* generate the cellular immune response. T cells produce a number of substances called *lymphokines* which direct cell functions. Both types of lymphocytes originate from tissues referred to as *primary lymphoid organs*. *Secondary lymphoid organs* (spleen, lymph nodes, tonsils, Peyer's patches in the intestine) are the site of actions occurring during and after the detection of antigen.

Many different types of B and T cells are involved in the specific immune response – Bs (memory, plasma) Ts (cytotoxic, memory, helper, suppressor, dendritic), all with specific functions and acting along with non-lymphocytic forms.

The immune system itself may be involved in disease processes – *autoimmune disease* in which an immune response is generated against 'self' or autoantigens to produce pathological changes; hypersensitivity reactions including anaphylactic shock; immunodeficiency; immunocytic and reactive amyloidosis; allograft rejection.

## INFLAMMATION, HEALING AND REPAIR

### Inflammation (L. *inflammare*, to burn)

Inflammation is the body's most important *defence mechanism* which takes place in tissue cells, blood vessels and blood cells following deleterious injury insufficient to cause actual cellular death.

Its main function is to localise and limit tissue injury and restore the damage to the normal or as near to it as possible. Acute inflammation is essentially a protective response.

Inflammation of a tissue or organ is denoted in most instances by the suffix *-itis*, e.g. enteritis (inflammation of the intestine) and myositis (inflammation of muscle), except in the case of lungs (pneumonia) and pleurae (pleurisy).

*The type of inflammation and it stage of development are important considerations in meat inspection, acute inflammation in general being more serious than the chronic form.*

**Causes** With the exception of the deficiency conditions, these are very similar to the acquired causes of disease, viz. toxins of microorganisms, strong chemicals, mechanical injuries, thermal damage such as frostbite and heat burn, and allergic or immune reactions. In many instances two causes may act in unison; for example, bacterial infection often follows mechanical injury and frostbite.

Should *necrosis* (death of tissue cells) occur in an organ, inflammatory changes in adjacent normal tissues are initiated.

The *main forms* are acute and chronic inflammation.

### Acute inflammation

The cardinal signs of *acute* inflammation were summarised by Celsius (first century AD) as rubor (redness), tumor (swelling), calor (heat) and dolor (pain), to which Virchow in the nineteenth century added *functio laesa* (loss of function).

The acute form is rapid in onset and normally lasts for only days or a few weeks. The chronic form, however, persists for weeks, months, and even years.

Macroscopically, the *redness* and *heat* are due to vasodilatation of the smaller blood vessels due to histamine and serotonin release; *swelling* is occasioned by the escape of protein-rich fluid from the blood vessels into the extracellular tissues and *pain* by the action of plasma polypeptides termed *kinins* (bradykinin and kallidin). *Loss of function* is brought about by reflex inhibition of muscular movement because of pain or by mechanical restrictions due to swelling of the affected part.

Microscopically, there is a temporary contraction of arterioles followed by a dilatation of all arterioles, capillaries and venules (*hyperaemia*). The blood flow initially increases but later gradually slows owing to loss of protein-rich fluid from the venules and capillaries and stops (*stasis*) because of increased vascularity and hydrostatic pressure.

This protein-rich fluid is the *inflammatory exudate* in which tissue factor promotes the formation of fibrin. Leukocytes (polymorphs, monocytes, lymphocytes), through chemotactic action, then begin to stick to the damaged endothelium of the blood vessels and most actually pass through the wall between the endothelial cells by active amoeboid movement (*diapedesis*). Platelets also adhere to the endothelium in clumps or thrombi. Neutrophils dominate the early stages of inflammation (the first few hours) but are superseded by monocytes (macrophages, giant cells and histiocytes) in the later stages. These are active phagocytes and, along with plasma cells, are also the main white blood cells in chronic inflammation.

*Phagocytosis* is the process whereby bacteria, tissue cells and debris and foreign material are ingested by these specialised white cells, usually in the presence of *opsonins* (special plasma proteins).

Should the injury be severe or complicated by bacterial, viral or protozoal infection, systemic changes may result, with the animal being affected with fever/septicaemia/toxaemia and an increased production of leukocytes (*leukocytosis*) by the bone marrow. Certain infectious diseases, however, such as those caused by rickettsiae and certain viruses, are associated with a decrease in the number of circulating leukocytes (*leukopenia*).

#### *Morphology of acute inflammation*

The type of inflammatory reaction depends on a variety of factors – specific cause, tissue involved, presence or absence of microorganisms, metazoan worms, etc., virulence of microorganisms and susceptibility of host. Inflammation may be differentiated according to the type of the exudate produced. The various forms may occur individually or in combination. A change from one form to another may also be observed and all may merge into the chronic condition.

Acute inflammation is normally rapid in onset and of short duration, lasting only a few days or weeks.

**Catarrhal or mucous inflammation** A relatively mild affection of the mucous membranes in which there is excessive production of mucus from mucous glands and goblet cells. The causes are usually benign in character, e.g. bacteria and viruses of low virulence, irritating chemicals and foods, dust and various allergens such as pollen.

*Mucus* is a clear, greyish, slimy, glistening fluid which is normally secreted by the mucosa of the respiratory, alimentary and genital tracts. The increased flow of mucus from the cervical glands during oestrus of the uterus is a natural phenomenon.

In catarrhal inflammation the mucus varies in consistency from being watery to viscid (sticky or glutinous) according to the nature and stage of the infection and the body system involved. Examples are human cold and hay fever, nasal catarrh of calf pneumonia, mucoid colitis, equine and swine influenza. Catarrhal bacterial gastroenteritis in man is often a food poisoning due to *Salmonella*.

**Croupous inflammation** is a form of fibrinous inflammation in which a layer is formed from a fibrinous exudate and becomes loosely attached to the underlying tissue.

**Diphtheritic inflammation (pseudomembranous inflammation)** occurs when the superficial layers of a mucous membrane become necrotic and, together with a fibrinous exudate, form an adherent membrane. It is caused by bacteria which are non-invasive in type but produce potent exotoxins.

Typical examples occur in calf diphtheria, fowl pox, necrotic enteritis and swine fever.

**Fibrinous inflammation** is common on serous and mucous membranes where the exudate is coagulated and fibrin formed. When it occurs on opposed surfaces, e.g. pericardium in traumatic pericarditis, swine erysipelas, the surfaces present an appearance as though two pieces of buttered bread were drawn apart.

This form of inflammation, characteristic of more severe injuries and infections, occurs when the permeability of the small blood vessels is sufficient to allow the passage of fibrinogen molecules from the blood. Fibrin appears as a network of threads or as an amorphous coagulum or clot formed from the fibrinogen of blood by the action of thrombin. Common causal microorganisms are *S. cholerae suis*, *Fusobacterium necrophorum* and the virus of avian laryngotracheitis.

**Haemorrhagic inflammation** is characterized by the presence of excessive numbers of RBCs in the exudate which give it a reddish or brownish colour like clotted or unclotted blood. The exudate itself also contains serum, leukocytes and fibrin. It may be associated with serous inflammation as, for example, in Braxy or in the haemorrhagic enteritis of anthrax and in cases of severe parasitic gastroenteritis.

**Lymphocytic inflammation** Where lymphocytes accumulate in the tissues along with hyperaemia, this term is sometimes applied. The condition may be seen in certain viral diseases of the nervous system, e.g. rabies, Teschen disease and Aujeszky's disease, as well as in listeriosis, leptospirosis and toxoplasmosis. Lymphocytic infiltration is often manifested as an accumulation of lymphocytes round a blood vessel (perivascular lymphocytic infiltration). Blood vessels in the liver are sometimes affected owing to the presence of toxic substances and virulent microorganisms.

**Purulent (suppurative) inflammation** This form of inflammation is characterised by the presence of *pus* or purulent exudate. Pus is a yellowish, greenish or bluish coloured substance which varies in consistency from watery to inspissated (thick) or even solid. Pus is a protein-rich product composed of numerous neutrophils, living and dead, fluid (*liquor puris*) which may become semi-solid or solid, and necrotic cellular debris.

It is caused by certain types of bacteria, especially staphylococci such as *Staph. albus* and *Staph. aureus*, *Strep. pyogenes* and members of the *E. coli* group which are termed pyogenic (pus-producing) bacteria. They produce potent exotoxins which activate neutrophil emigration and the formation of pus by toxic necrosis and the digestion of dead tissue. If the bacterium present is *Pseudomonas aeruginosa*, the pus assumes a greenish-blue colour owing to the production of pyocyanin by the bacterium. Pus can also be produced by *Actinomyces bovis* and *Actinobacillus (Malleomyces) malleus*.

Suppurative changes are among the most serious in pathology since they indicate that local, and sometimes general, defence mechanisms have been overcome. In meat inspection the changes are often associated with septicaemia or pyaemia, which warrant total carcase condemnation.

*Phlegmonous inflammation* refers to the condition in which amounts of pus are scattered throughout a tissue, especially the subcutis, and is similar to *cellulitis*.

An *abscess* is a localised collection of pus in a tissue, organ or confined space. Abscesses may be almost microscopic in size or enormous, containing several litres of pus, and either single or multiple – for example, following metastasis – and can be found in virtually every body system.

In the early stages of abscesss development, toxins released by pyogenic bacteria damage local tissue and cause acute inflammation and oedema. Where the abscess increases in size, coagulative necrosis of dead tissue by cellular (mainly neutrophil) enzymes takes place. The pyogenic bacteria continue to proliferate and produce toxin, resulting in the coagulative necrosis being transformed into pus which tends to increase in amount. Around the edges of the abscess, repair processes commence with the appearance of granulation tissue to form a *pyogenic membrane*, which is eventually transformed into a fibrous capsule in long-standing cases.

Hepatic abscesses in cattle – often unassociated with clinical disease – may eventually heal and leave no scars. Should, however, erosion of the wall of the posterior vena cava occur, great loss of condition with death may take place.

A *pustule* is a small circumscribed collection of pus, usually on the skin.

*Empyema* or *pyothorax* is an accumulation of pus or purulent exudate in a pleural cavity. Sources include infection of the pleura; lung abscess; penetrating injuries of the chest wall or the oesophagus or from the reticulum in the bovine; and via the blood vascular system.

**Serous inflammation** is identified by the production of a thin, clear, watery fluid on the serous membranes of the body cavities (pleural, pericardial, peritoneal) which are well vascularised. This serous exudate often represents the first stages of pneumonia caused by the inhalation of irritants. Later stages may involve the appearance of fibrin, changing the type to *fibrinous inflammation*, or the advent of RBCs (*haemorrhagic inflammation*). A localised form of serous inflammation is seen in the *vesicle* or *blister* and after second degree burns.

Serous inflammation occurs in vesicular stomatitis, vesicular exanthema and aphthous fever.

### *Effects of acute inflammation*

Beneficial effects include the elimination of harmful microorganisms and their toxins by the flow of exudate, action of phagocytosis, dilution of toxins, formation of antibodies and immunity and fibrin production. Along with the accompanying loss of mobility of the part due to the presence of oedema and pain, these are all designed to promote resolution.

Depending on the part involved, however, there may be deleterious results, for example, in acute oedema of the larynx where difficult breathing occurs. Interference with blood flow may result in increased pressure, e.g. in encephalitis/meningitis, and in necrosis. Hypersensitivity reactions, e.g. anaphylaxis, autoimmune diseases such as purpura haemorrhagica, and isoimmune haemolytic anaemia may develop.

### *Outcome of acute inflammation*

There are four possible sequelae of acute inflammation:

**(1) Resolution** with restoration and normal functioning of the part and the overall animal body. Complete disappearance of inflammatory reaction is usual when the injury or infection is minimal and where there has been little tissue destruction. Exudate and fibrin are removed into lymphatics along with cellular debris and neutrophils. Gradually macrophages and monocytes replace neutrophils and actively phagocytose dead tissues and bacterial cells. The vasodilatation and permeability of local blood vessels return to normal. Any fibrin present is lysed by fibrinolytic enzymes and the soluble end-products are removed in the enlarged lymphatics.

**(2) Healing by fibrosis** occurs in cases of significant tissue damage, where fibrin production is excessive or has not been removed by enzyme action and where tissue regeneration in general is failing.

Leukocytes and fibroblasts migrate into the fibrin and vascular endothelial cells form new capillaries (angiogenesis) to create *granulation tissue*. This has a soft, pink, granular appearance on the surface of wounds and is often oedematous. This granulation tissue gradually changes to a scar composed of fibroblasts, collagen and elastic fibres to form rigid *scar* tissue.

*Collagen* is the fibrous protein of the white fibres of connective tissue found in the skin, tendons, ligaments and bone cartilage. *Elastic* tissue is a connective tissue composed of yellow elastic fibres, often formed into sheets.

When a wound heals without complication and with a minimum of connective tissue formation and distortion, e.g. when uninfected, it is said to heal by *first intention* or *primary union*. Where, however, other factors operate, such as suppuration, ulceration and infarction, and where the wound is extensive, the healing process is more complicated and is accompanied by extensive granulation tissue formation – healing is by *second intention* or *secondary union*. Second intention healing is always accompanied by wound contraction and distortion.

**(3) Abscess formation** due to the presence of pyogenic organisms is a serious complication of acute inflammation.

**(4) Chronic inflammation** results from a long-standing (weeks or months) tissue injury and frequently follows the acute form or several acute occurrences. But it can also exist from the outset.

## Chronic inflammation

Chronic inflammation is a sequel to acute forms which are not resolved because of some interference with the healing process, for example in chronic bacterial infections such as tuberculosis where the causal organism is of lower virulence and evokes delayed hypersensitivity; in certain fungal and helminth diseases, and in ulceration, e.g. gastric ulcers associated with some disturbance of gastric secretion.

*Chronic abscesses* with fibrous walls develop granulation tissue on the inside in an attempt to fill the cavity when it is eventually drained. Foreign bodies in the form of dirt, metals, wood, silica, necrotic tissue, etc., can initiate the formation of chronic inflammation.

The persistence of gallstones is accompanied by the chronic inflammatory changes of cholecystitis.

Certain bacteria can persist to produce chronic inflammation from an original acute form.

Chronic inflammation assumes many different forms – chronic abscess, chronic ulcer, chronic sinus (an abnormal channel which permits the passage of pus), fistula (an abnormal tubular passage, usually connecting two internal organs or leading from an internal organ to the exterior) and chronic granulomatous inflammation. This form of inflammation is characterised by greater tissue destruction, by the formation of granulation tissue, and later, fibrous tissue. There is less production of exudate which contains macrophages, lymphocytes and plasma cells but fewer neutrophils.

**Chronic granulomatous inflammation** This is a chronic reaction in which *granulomas* are formed. These are collections of modified macrophages surrounded by connective tissue giant cells, plasma cells, neutrophils, lymphocytes and fibroblasts. In some cases necrosis occurs (*necrotising granulomas*).

Granulomas may arise from the presence of foreign bodies (*foreign body granulomas*) or be associated with bacteria like *Myco. tuberculosis*, parasites, fungi, etc. (*hypersensitivity granulomas*). Examples are the *'grape' lesions* of chronic bovine TB, the granulomata in the lungs and other tissues of coccidiodomycosis, the skin granulomas on the limbs of horses, bovine actinobacillosis, and strawberry footrot of sheep.

**Granulation tissue**, which must not be confused with the term *'granuloma'*, consists mostly of macrophages and fibroblasts and occurs most often in large wounds in which healing has been delayed, the affected area assuming the appearance of numerous red granules making the tissue bulge above the surrounding surface. The red 'granules' are actually small newly formed capillaries (angiogenesis) which later develop into larger capillaries and arterioles. The surface tends to be ulcerated and blood-stained under an overlying brownish scab. Deeper parts of granulation tissues are whitish, tough and firm, while the more superficial layers are more oedematous.

On occasions excessive amounts of granulation tissue – *exuberant granulation* or *proud flesh* – are formed which require surgical excision. The exact cause is unknown.

### Factors influencing wound repair

The complex and orderly processes involved in inflammation (acute and chronic) can be greatly influenced by local and systemic factors.

*Local factors known to reduce healing efficiency* include bacterial infection; inadequate blood supply; excessive movement of the part; increased abdominal pressure; foreign bodies (e.g. sutures, dust, glass, metal, bone); abnormal tissue cells (e.g. necrotic cells); location of inflammatory reaction (e.g. serous cavities and synovial cavities); and ionising radiation.

*Systemic factors which interfere with efficient wound repair* include concurrent bacterial and other diseases, especially diseases of the blood, inadequate nutrition, in particular hypoproteinaemia and deficiency of vitamin C and zinc; certain hormones, especially corticosteroids; and neoplasia.

## IMPORTANT PATHOLOGICAL LESIONS

### Acne (folliculitis, pyoderma)

Acne is a pustular (usually staphylococcal) infection of hair follicles and/or sebaceous glands with a surrounding acute inflammation. Furunculosis refers to abscess formation of a larger size in the dermis. A *furuncle* is sometimes referred to as a *boil* while a *carbuncle* is a deep-seated skin abscess of which *Staph. aureus* is a common cause.

### Bleb (bulla, blister)

A bleb is a large vesicle, usually more than 5 mm in diameter. On the skin it contains clear fluid, while a pulmonary bleb contains air. A *pneumatocele* or *tension cyst* is a fairly large (several centimetres in diameter) air-filled sac in the lungs.

*Erosion* is the superficial loss of an epithelium due to ulceration and or bacterial action.

### Fissure

A fissure is usually a tender crack or cleft in the skin occurring at a point of skin mobility and often overlaid with a scab.

### Papilla

A papilla is a normal small, nipple-shaped projection, e.g. the papillae on the tongue.

### Papule

A papule is a small, circumscribed, raised solid elevation on the skin.

### Ulcer

The localised necrotic destruction of an epithelial surface (skin or mucous membrane) with exposure of underlying tissue, forming an open sore whose surface lies below that of the surrounding tissue. Ulcers may occur in most body tissues and organs and are due to bacterial or viral action, and are sometimes associated with chronic inflammation and stress.

### Vesicle

A vesicle is a small sac (usually less than 5 mm in diameter) on the skin, containing liquid. In pathology it represents a form of acute inflammation caused by injury or microorganisms, usually viruses, e.g. vesicular stomatitis, foot-and-mouth disease, swine vesicular disease.

### Cyst

A cyst is a sac or pouch in the tissues which varies in size but is usually 1–5 cm in diameter. It is lined by a grey, glistening epithelial membrane and may contain clear fluid or solid or semi-solid material of parasitic structures, keratinous debris, sebaceous material, etc. Most are benign structures, but a few are neoplastic. Others tend to become infected.

*Congenital cysts* are frequently encountered in the kidneys of pigs and sheep. They may be single or multiple (polycystic renal disease) and vary in size from being just visible to several centimetres in diameter in cases of single cysts.

*Dermoid cysts* are neoplastic structures of developmental origin which contain material such as sebaceous and sweat glands, hair follicles, bone, teeth, etc., inside a fibrous cell wall lined with stratified epithelium.

*Epidermal inclusion cysts* are small round nodules in the skin which gradually increase in size. They possess a simple cyst wall surrounded by a fibrous capsule.

*Embryonic cysts* develop from portions of embryonic tissue or from organs which normally disappear before birth.

*Exudation cysts* are structures formed by the slow collection of inflammatory exudates in a closed cavity.

*A haematoma* (*haematocyst*) (Plate 2, Fig. 9) is a localised tumour-like collection of extravasated blood (usually clotted) in an organ, tissue or space. Haematomas are normally caused by injury, e.g. a blood blister, bruises which often accompany fractures and more severe injuries.

*Hydatid cysts* are the larval stages of the tapeworms *Echinococcus granulosus* and *E. multilocularis* (Plate 3, Fig. 18).

*Luteal cysts* arise from ovarian follicles which fail to rupture. The cyst wall is lined with a layer of luteal cells.

*Ovarian (follicular) cysts* feature in cystic ovarian disease in which thin-walled follicular cysts develop. These represent ovarian follicles which do not ovulate and are associated with abnormal oestrus behaviour and infertility. They are common in older cows and maps, but less common in sows. They are associated with abnormalities of oestrus – nymphomania, anoestrus and infertility.

*Parasitic cysts* are cysts formed round the larvae of tapeworms, e.g. *Cysticercus bovis*, and trichinae, e.g. T*richinella spiralis, Sarcocystis.*

*Retention cysts* are formed when the outlet of a secreting gland is obstructed owing to, for example, scarring with retention of fluid. They may occur in the kidneys, salivary glands, sebaceous glands, mammary glands and pancreas.

## CELL INJURY AND DEATH

In the healthy animal, cells and tissues possess a *homeostasis* – a state of physiological equilibrium in which cell structure, composition and function are maintained while adapting to conditions optimal for survival. The animal is in harmony within its body and with its external environment.

Homeostasis is essential for life. The blood vascular system maintains the internal environment and works in conjunction with the liver and kidney systems to maintain osmotic levels and remove the waste products of metabolism along with hepatic activity. Hormones, oxygen, enzymes and carbon dioxide are transported by the blood and lymph. The response of the body to disease or injury is a homeostatic activity.

Should any injurious factor upset this balance, local or generalised cell death may ensue. If the injury is minor, the cell has the ability to adapt and recover by atrophy, hypertrophy or hyperplasia. If the damage is irreversible, cell death or necrosis takes place.

### Necrosis

*Necrosis* means the death of cells or tissues while still part of the living body. Autolysis (self-disintegration) of cell contents and membrane takes place through the action of lytic enzymes from lysosomes (derived from the dead cells themselves) to form a mass of debris which is eventually phagocytosed by other cells or macrophages if the animal survives.

*Causes* of necrosis include chemical poisons, plant poisons, toxins, viruses, therapeutic agents, physical damage, heat, burns, ultraviolet rays, ionising radiation, electrical injury, hyperthermia, hypothermia including freezing, ischaemia, pressure, anoxia, hypoxia, nutritional deficiencies.

These injurious agents produce their adverse effects in different ways: anoxia, hypoxia and ischaemia cause *infarction*, the most common cause being artery obstruction due to thrombosis or embolism; bacterial and viral toxins produce lysis of the cell membrane; chemical poisons, physical damage, heat, etc., cause denaturation of cell proteins or inhibition of the cell cytochrome oxidase system; and radiation causes damage by inhibiting cell multiplication, an action utilised in the treatment of cancer.

The term *'cloudy swelling'* (proposed by Virchow in 1860) was used to describe the early degenerative changes in necrosis but is now obsolete because of confusion with other pathological changes. Affected organs – liver, kidney, heart, muscular tissue etc. – are slightly enlarged, paler and softer than normal and, in pronounced cases, have the semblance of having been boiled. On section with a knife, the dull, lustreless tissue bulges on the cut surface.

*Microscopical changes* in necrosis reveal abnormalities in cell nuclei – *karyolysis* (autolysis), *karyorrhexis* (fragmentation) and *pyknosis* (shrinkage with dark staining due to basophilia). The cytoplasm becomes acidophilic due to the loss of nucleoproteins, later less dense with ultimate disappearance. Cell outline fades and finally vanishes along with loss of differential staining.

*Macroscopic* or *gross changes* of necrosis vary greatly in disposition and rapidity of onset in the dead animal. Among the tissues which undergo early autolysis are the intestinal and gall bladder mucosa because of bile action, adrenal gland medulla, the proximal convoluted renal tubules and CNS neurons. Connective tissues, however, are fairly resistant.

Gross changes at post-mortem are markedly affected by the following factors: cause of death; species; body and environmental temperature; length of time the animal has been dead; absence or presence of refrigeration; presence or absence of rigor mortis; type, amount and fluidity of stomach and intestinal contents. Clostridial diseases in ruminants, in particular, bring about early autolytic and putrefactive changes in the carcase. Ruminants develop early autolysis due to fermentation and gas production in the large amount of ingesta, while sheep suffer the most rapid post-mortem changes because of the added insulation from the fleece. Pigs also tend to show early changes, most evident as a greenish discoloration in the flank area, because of the insulating layer of fat. High summer temperatures often make post-mortem examination useless.

Care should be taken to avoid breakdowns and delays during line slaughter as far as possible. Should these occur it becomes necessary to eviscerate as soon as possible or make provision for the escape of stomach and intestinal gases and body heat.

Necrotic tissue is usually pale and firm and may be surrounded by an area of hyperaemia, perhaps best illustrated in the *infarcts* of the kidney or spleen. Necrotic areas which occur superficially, e.g. on the skin or the tails of pigs, may be sloughed off with the formation of an ulcer, while necrosis of deep-seated structures may be followed by encapsulation and eventual absorption of the necrotic tissue with the formation of a scar. The centre of necrotic areas may soften and degenerate, e.g. in bacterial necrosis in the bovine liver associated with *Fusobacterium necrophorum*. Should pyogenic organisms be present, polymorphs accumulate with subsequent liquefaction to form an abscess.

Necrotic or dead tissue is usually paler than normal (unless filled with blood) and is easily torn. On subsequent infection with gas-producing organisms, e.g. clostridia, putrefactive odours become apparent. As a localised entity in a surviving animal, necrosis is disposed of by sloughing, liquefaction with formation of an abscess or cyst, encapsulation with caseation or fibrosis, calcification, gangrene or formation of new tissue.

### *Types of necrosis*

**Caseous necrosis (caseation)** Affected tissues lose their structure and become amorphous; cell outline and contents are lost as is differential staining. The area is converted into a soft whitish, yellowish or greyish, cheesy mass reminiscent of cottage cheese.

The *causes* are locally-acting toxins of bacteria such as *Myco. tuberculosis*, *Corynebacterium pseudotuberculosis (ovis)* and of certain bacteria in granulomas.

**Coagulative necrosis** This takes place in tissues like the heart, spleen and kidney where denaturation of cellular protein and enzymes occurs but autolysis is prevented. Cell outline and nuclei are discernible but pyknotic. The dead area is strongly eosinophilic. The affected part is white, grey or yellow, swollen and firm. It is sometimes depressed below the level of the surrounding tissue.

*Causes* are toxins of bacteria such as *Fusobacterium necrophorum*, *C. pyogenes*, locally-acting poisons like mercuric chloride, infarcts and ischaemia, heat, X-rays, and Zenker's necrosis.

**Fat necrosis** This form of necrosis may be seen in the back fat of pigs and in the mesentery, brisket fat of cattle due to trauma and kidney fat of cattle where it may occur near a liver abscess. It is also encountered in the subpleural, subperitoneal and subcutaneous fat and is attributed to the action of pancreatic enzymes, trypsin and steapsin, which have escaped from the pancreas and liberated fatty acids from triglycerides in the fat cells and with calcium salts form calcium 'soaps'. These appear as whitish, chalky areas in adipose tissue.

Necrosis of brisket fat in cattle, and occasionally sheep, is termed '*putty brisket*', the necrotic tissue being firm, dull white or yellowish in colour and tending to undergo calcification. In New Zealand, fat necrosis is often seen in crutched sheep around the tail.

**Liquefaction (colliquative) necrosis** This is more common in tissues with a high water content, e.g. brain and lungs. It can also occur in abscesses and in tuberculous pneumonia. While most necrotic processes are relatively slow, liquefaction necrosis rapidly forms amounts of water by autolysis. Cavities which look like cysts but are not true cysts are created containing cloudy liquid (pus in the case of abscesses). This liquid is eventually drained away by the lymphatics, the pus in abscesses becoming inspissated.

The causes are similar to those for necrosis in general.

**Zenker's necrosis** is essentially a coagulation of striated muscle proteins causing the affected muscles to be swollen, whitish and shiny resembling hyaline cartilage. The *causes* are believed to be bacterial toxins.

### *Outcome of necrosis*

Much depends on the type, extent and location of the necrosis and the general status of the animal. The prognosis is serious with cerebral and cardiac lesions where infarcts can cause sudden death. Necrotic tissue may be restored to normal but this is unusual.

The usual *sequelae* are liquefaction by autolysis and drainage of fluid by the blood and/or lymph, liquefaction and cavity formation with slow drainage, liquefaction and abscess formation, calcification, encapsulation and fibrosis, desquamation or sloughing especially on epithelia and blood vessel endothelia, gangrene and atrophy.

**Judgement of necrosis** Partial or total condemnation, depending on the overall pathology, disease entity, condition of carcase, etc.

## Gangrene

This refers to the digestion of necrotic tissue by bacterial (usually putrefactive) action. In *primary* gangrene pathogenic bacteria kill tissues by potent exotoxins and then digest the dead tissue. In *secondary* gangrene initial death of tissue is due to some other cause, e.g. ischaemia, followed by digestion by saprophytic bacteria. The terms '*moist gangrene*' and '*dry gangrene*' may be applied to the primary and secondary forms, respectively.

*Primary* or *moist gangrene* includes gas gangrene and is caused by the Gram-positive anaerobic, sporing clostridia (*Cl. perfringens, Cl. oedematiens (novyi), Cl. septicum)* and similar microbes. These organisms are able to flourish in tissues accessible to the air, e.g. limbs, ears, tails, lungs, udder, intestine, and well supplied with blood. The affected part is oedematous, initially very painful but later insensitive, soft, and greenish or blackish in colour with a foul putrefactive odour. It is actually a combination of coagulation and liquefaction necrosis causing a breakdown of tissue protein, carbohydrates and fat. The same changes occur in post-mortem changes and in the putrefaction of meat.

In meat inspection it is most often observed in the udder of the cow as a sequel to septic mastitis, while it also occurs in the bovine lung following septic pneumonia, the faulty administration of drugs or penetration by a foreign body from the reticulum. It may also be seen in the skin, ears and tails of pigs after an attack of swine erysipelas. If gas-forming organisms like *Cl. perfringens* are present the tissue may contain gas bubbles, making it crepitate or crackle owing to the production of $H_2$ and $CO_2$ from the fermentation of sugars (gas gangrene). Gas gangrene can spread through the bloodstream and is always accompanied by severe systemic disturbance.

*Secondary* or *dry gangrene* is found in tissues with a limited blood supply, e.g. due to ischaemia or where the necrosis has developed gradually. Diseased areas show coagulative changes and are denatured, shrivelled, discoloured and leather-like owing to protein coagulation and sulphide production.

All types of gangrene are separated from adjoining living tissues by a line of demarcation seen as a reddish or bluish swollen zone of inflammation.

**Outcome of gangrene** The decomposition of proteins combined with the toxic effects of putrefactive bacteria often result in absorption into the bloodstream with fatal results. Providing resistance is adequate, however, the demarcation zone, and with cellular and humoral defences frequently arrange for an extremity, udder or part of an udder, portion of bone, uterine or intestinal mucosa, etc., to drop off with healing of the separated part.

**Judgement** All forms of gangrene must be regarded as very serious manifestations of disease. Most will have been detected by efficient ante-mortem examination. The judgement will be partial/total condemnation depending on total pm findings, carcase condition, etc., with, however, a definite tendency to favour the latter because of the possibility of toxaemia being present.

### Apoptosis

Whereas necrosis affects fairly large groups of cells, *apoptosis* is a form of cell death which involves single cells or small clusters in the normal process of renewal in certain organs, e.g. the endometrium of the uterus in the oestrous cycle and the thymus where T cells are gradually depleted. Apoptosis, or *programmed cell death*, can also occur in disease conditions – certain virus infections, irradiation, atrophy and tumour formation. The process is activated by an endonuclease which causes chromatin condensation, DNA fragmentation, shrinkage of cell volume and eventual cell disintegration and phagocytosis by macrophages.

### Infarct (L. *in* + *farcire*, to stuff in)

A localised area of necrosis caused by a reduction or loss of blood supply. The part involved is usually supplied by a single *'end-artery'*. (*End-arteries* are blood vessels which have no collateral or adjacent anastomoses which can supply blood should occlusion occur in a distal vessel. They represent single blood supplies and are numerous in the spleen, kidney, brain, lungs and liver, making these organs especially prone to infarction). In the heart the coronary arteries are end-arteries.

The infarct is produced by the thrombotic or embolic occlusion of either the arterial supply of this artery or its venous drainage, mostly the former. Other causes include the twisting of blood vessels to an organ, producing ischaemia; herniation of a portion of intestine; or the entrapment of an organ or portion of organ under a peritoneal adhesion.

The necrotic area is conical with the point of the cone (where the occlusion occurs) directed towards the centre of the organ. Coagulative necrosis normally follows. The *size* of the infarct varies according to the amount of tissue rendered ischaemic, the degree of ischaemia and the susceptibility of tissue cells. Recent infarcts are swollen owing to the absorption of water, but later an acute inflammation occurs at the periphery. This soon subsides and is replaced by a fibrous scar which reduces the level of the infarct below the surrounding tissue and may distort the organ, e.g. infarcts in pig kidney. The infarct is sharply demarcated from the surrounding tissue.

Infarcts may be classified as *haemorrhagic* (*red*) or *anaemic* (*pale*). The former indicate the presence of unhaemolysed RBCs or alternatively represent an early stage of development. *Red* infarcts tend to occur in loose spongy organs such as the lungs and spleen but can also be seen rarely in the liver, brain and ovary. *Pale* infarcts are most often found in solid organs like the kidney although very early stages of these are haemorrhagic.

Coronary thrombosis in man due to atheroma of a major artery results in a pale infarct following coagulative necrosis with eventual fibrosis. Should the embolus causing the obstruction be septic, the infarct becomes an abscess.

**Judgement** Partial/total condemnation.

## INTRACELLULAR ACCUMULATIONS

A large variety of substances may accumulate in tissues on a temporary or permanent basis with innocuous or harmful effects. These infiltrations may assemble in the cell cytoplasm or in the nucleus. In the cytoplasm the substances settle in the *lysosomes* (small intracellular enzymic bodies involved in cell metabolism and phagocytosis). The substances which accumulate may be either *endogenous*, i.e. produced within the animal body, or *exogenous*, i.e emanating from outside the organism – carbon, dusts, carotenoids.

*Endogenous* entities may be produced in excess or may amass because of defective metabolism, e.g. lack of a specific enzyme. In some instances the enzyme deficiency is brought about by an innate error of metabolism giving rise to so-called *storage diseases* (of fats, carbohydrates, proteins, glycogen, etc.). Other endogenous substances include the various pigments – melanin, lipofuscin, haematin, fat, urates, calcium, etc.

## Calcification

Pathological calcification denotes the deposition in tissues of calcium salts together with small amounts of iron, magnesium and other minerals. When it occurs in dead or dying tissues it is termed *dystrophic* calcification but in normal tissues it is called *metastatic* calcification and is associated with hypercalcaemia, hypervitaminosis D, secondary tumour formation and renal failure.

*Dystrophic calcification* is an attempt by the body to repair tissue damage and to enclose and immobilise dead cells and other foreign material. It is encountered in caseous, coagulative and liquefactive necrosis, fat necrosis, infarcts, chronic tuberculous lesions, white muscle disease, metazoan parasitic infestations like trichinosis and *Cysticercus tenuicollis*, certain tumours and granulomas and foci of inspissated pus.

*Metastatic calcification* is related to extensive deposition of calcium salts in normal tissues owing to high blood or tissue levels.

**Judgement** Partial/total condemnation.

## Pathological ossification

On rare occasions bone may be found in extraosseous tissues, e.g. lungs of cattle, lateral cartilages of horses and leg tendons of old turkeys. Damaged muscles affected with inflammation have a tendency to ossify.

## Pigmentation

Pigments may emanate from outside the body (*exogenous* pigments) or from within the body (*endogenous* pigments).

*Exogenous* pigments are normally associated with the grazing of livestock in proximity to certain industries and with urban pollution. The most common is *carbon* or *coal dust* which causes pneumoconiosis in coal miners and various dusts. Carbon appears as black particles in the lung tissue and associated lymph nodes.

*Carotenoid pigments*, derived from carotene A and B (precursors of vitamin A) and *xanthophyll* are of plant origin. These *lipochrome pigments* are normal constituents of many different body tissues – adrenal gland, Kupffer cells of the liver, corpus luteum, testis and the adipose tissue of Jersey and Guernsey cattle as well as the yolk of eggs and butter fat. They are also found in the so-called subcutaneous xanthomas of poultry. These are not true tumours but collections of connective-tissue cells and cholesterol-containing phagocytes.

*Endogenous* pigments in animals include melanin, haematin, haemosiderin, bile pigments, porphyrin, lipofuscin and Cloisonné kidney pigment.

### *Melanin*

All healthy pigmented skin contains a brownish-black protein colouring substance, *melanin*, produced in melanocytes by the oxidation of the amino acid tyrosine. It is especially evident on the surface of the bovine palate, tongue and cheeks and in the hair, horns and eyes of dark-skinned cattle, black and grey horses and black and red pigs. The deposits are black or brown in colour and usually of irregular shape and size, most being about a centimetre in diameter.

Abnormal deposits of melanin (*melanosis*) are encountered chiefly in the bovine and less commonly in sheep and pigs. In the *ox* melanosis is commonly found in the lungs, liver and meninges, where it usually involves the pia mater, more rarely the dura mater, and is termed *'black pith'*. The pigmentation may also be found on the pleura, peritoneum, in cartilages and bone and between muscles. The black coloration of the kidneys of adult cattle, especially the Red Danish breed, may be due to melanin or *lipofuscin*, an endogenous pigment closely allied to melanin. In calves, the liver and the cortex of the kidney are frequently affected but this must be distinguished from the blackish coloration of the kidneys of very young calves due to bile pigments.

In *sheep*, melanosis is commonest in the liver but some black hepatic pigmentation is due to lipofuscin, especially in Australia (Plate 1, Fig. 4).

In the *pig*, the condition is most often seen in the belly fat or in the udder of females, often being revealed as radiating lines or patches distributed along the ducts of the mammary glands.

*Melanomas* are malignant tumours which arise from melanin-forming cells (melanocytes).

**Judgement** Partial or total condemnation depending on the overall evidence. Melanin in itself is not harmful but affected organs should be condemned. Where the condition is generalised, total condemnation is warranted. The presence of a melanoma justifies a very detailed examination; in metastatic cases total rejection is warranted.

## Haematogenous pigments

Haemoglobin (Hb) is a compound protein in red blood cells which consists of the iron-containing porphyrin pigment *haem* combined with the protein globin. Oxygenated haemoglobin (oxyhaemoglobin) is bright red in colour and occurs in arterial blood, while haemoglobin unbound with blood (deoxyhaemoglobin or reduced haemoglobin) is darker in colour and is seen in venous blood which is less saturated with oxygen.

Certain pigments derived from haemoglobin metabolism are encountered in some abnormal conditions.

**Haematin** is a pigment formed by the oxidation of haem from the ferrous to the ferric state. It occurs as a dark brown, black or yellow granular pigment in the parasitised RBCs and reticuloendothelial cells in the spleen, liver, lymph nodes and bone marrow in diseases like babesiosis and malaria in which there is widespread destruction of red blood cells. Several trematodes, e.g. *Fascioloides magna*, and some schistosomes also produce haematins locally in the tissues.

**Haemosiderin**, an iron-containing pigment and store of iron (the other important iron storage pool is *ferritin*), occurs normally in hepatic cells, bone marrow and spleen (in macrophages). It appears in excess as yellowish granules in severe cases of RBC haemolysis as with haematin, in cases of extensive haemorrhage and chronic passive congestion. Haemosiderosis (iron overload) in man is a chronic form of anaemia in which there is excessive deposition of iron in the tissues. Haemosiderin combined with ferritin is occasionally observed in Angora goats in which a brownish or blackish pigmentation in kidneys has the appearance of enamelled jewellery – *Cloisonné kidney*.

## Bile pigments

*Biliverdin* is a green bile pigment formed from porphyrin by the breakdown of RBCs in the liver and bone marrow. It is rapidly reduced, mainly in the spleen, to *bilirubin*, an orange-yellow pigment, and then, bound with albumin, transported to the liver via the reticulo-endothelial system. Most of the bilirubin passes from the liver to the gall bladder and eventually to the small intestine where it is reduced to meso-bilirubinogen and urobilinogen by bacteria. The latter, in association with stercobilin, colours the faeces brown.

### *Icterus*

*Icterus* (*jaundice, hyperbilirubinaemia*) arising from haemolytic, obstructive hepatic or toxic causes, occurs when the balance between bilirubin production and clearance is disturbed. Bile pigments, mainly bilirubin, accumulate in the tissues, which are tinged yellow. The condition is caused by the reabsorption of bile pigment into the circulatory system and displays three main types.

*Obstructive jaundice* may be due to mechanical obstruction to the flow of bile by gallstones, parasites – liver flukes (especially *Dicrocoelium dendriticum*), ascarids or tapeworms like *Thysanosoma actinioides*) in the bile ducts, biliary cirrhosis (especially in the pig but rarely in cattle or sheep), cholangitis (inflammation of the gall bladder) and pressure from tumours, abscesses or granulomas. In pigs the most common parasite in temperate regions to invade the bile ducts from the intestine is *Ascaris suum*.

*Haemolytic jaundice* denotes the excessive destruction of red blood cells by infective organisms, e.g. in babesiosis, eperythrozoonosis, anaplasmosis, equine infectious anaemia and leptospirosis in pigs. The yellow coloration is less marked in this form than in the obstructive and toxic types.

*Toxic jaundice* is brought about by the action of toxic substances on liver cells resulting in fatty change, necrosis and the liberation of plasma bilirubin. *Poisonous plants* incriminated are members of the *Senecio* species (ragwort and groundsel) such as *S. jacobaea* (ragwort, Benweed), *S. vulgaris* (groundsel), *S. burcelli* and *S. cunninghamii* in North America and the latter with *S. quadridenta* and *S. latus* in Australia. These contain pyrrolizidine alkaloids which are potent hepatic toxins also found in certain *Crotalaria*, *Gossypium* (cotton plant) and *Allium* (garlic, onion) species. The mycotoxins associated with some *Lupin* spp. also cause hepatocyte injury and icterus. Some *inorganic poisons*, especially copper and selenium, and *organic compounds* such as phenothiazine can also cause severe jaundice. Excess copper in the diet of calves in Denmark has caused icterus due to toxic hepatitis, cirrhosis and fatty change resulting in carcase condemnations.

A form of hyperbilirubinaemia which is not obstructive, haemolytic or toxic occurs in horses on starvation rations or from anorexia secondary to other diseases, e.g. colic. Most cases are subclinical but some progress to frank disease.

*Rotor's syndrome* and *Gilbert's syndrome* are forms of familial human hyperbilirubinaemia, the former being evident in some natives in the Philipines as well as in Southdown sheep. In these conditions there is an inherent inability for man and animals to oxidise the xanthophylls in the food.

### *Diagnosis and judgement of icterus*

In many cases diagnosis presents a problem. In both the live animal and carcases (especially of cattle and horses), yellow coloration occurs even when serum bile acids/bilirubin levels are normal. Conversely, hyperbilirubinaemia can occur where jaundice is not very evident, perhaps owing to masking by erythema of the mucous membranes. In cases of doubt, therefore, it is necessary to resort to *tests* for *plasma bilirubin*.

There is marked yellowish coloration of the superficial fatty tissues, the fat deposits within the visceral cavities and the serous membranes. Closer inspection may reveal an abnormal colour in connective tissue which varies from lemon to orange-yellow or greenish-yellow. These changes may also be seen in the kidney cortex, calyces and renal pelvis. Yellow pigmentation is often evident in large nerve trunks and in the endothelium of medium-sized arteries such as the internal and external iliacs, brachial and femoral arteries, which are coloured even in slightly icteric carcases. Icteric coloration may also be seen in the lungs, sclera of the eye, tendons and the cartilaginous extremities of long bones.

In doubtful cases, e.g. the presence of slight icterus in a well-nourished carcase, it should be detained for 24 hours and then re-examined since the action of normal muscle enzymes may remove the yellow colour. If the pigmentation is only slightly evident after the 24-hour detention, the carcase may be safely released for food. This is especially so in mild cases of obstructive jaundice, icterus associated with fractures, torsion of the spleen. etc.

Icterus in the pig associated with hepatic cirrhosis may also be accompanied by an abnormal odour and taste; overnight cooling tends to deepen the yellow colour and the skin then appears freckled. Icteric pig carcases should therefore be detained for a similar period and then subjected to a *bile acids* and/or *boiling test*, the latter to detect abnormal odours. In the absence of these changes the carcase may be passed as fit.

In all animals, a marked degree of icterus present after a 24 h detention of the carcase warrants total condemnation. This is the situation in haemolytic, toxic and the more severe cases of obstructive jaundice. Icteric carcases should preferably be examined in daylight since artificial light may distort colours. If, under natural light, carcases show any degree of icterus along with parenchymatous degeneration of organs (the result of bacterial infection) or show an intense yellow or greenish discoloration without evidence of infection, they should be totally condemned.

*Efficient ante-mortem examination combined with reliable veterinary certification should serve to reduce, even eliminate, cases of icterus at post-mortem inspection.*

Jaundice must be distinguished from the yellow colour of fat commonly seen in old bovines and certain dairy breeds like Jerseys and Guernseys in which it is confined to the adipose tissues as the pigment carotene. This yellow coloration is also occasionally met with in pigs and sheep.

*Laboratory tests for icterus*

Icterus index (depth of colour of serum compared with standard solution) and serum bile acids assay are used.

A useful test is to boil 2 g of fat from the suspect carcase in 5 ml of a 5% solution of NaOH for 1 min in a boiling tube. Cool under the tap and carefully add 3–5 ml of ether. Shake and allow to stand. Layers will separate.

**Interpretation** Greenish-yellow colour in the *upper* layer indicates presence of carotenoid pigments; if colour is in the *lower* layer, bile pigments are indicated.

## Porphyrin

Porphyrins are a group of reddish constituents of haem, the red iron-containing pigment of haemoglobin in animals, of green photosynthetic chlorophylls of higher plants, of cytochrome (a red enzyme found in most cells) and of catalase, an enzyme responsible for the breakdown of hydrogen peroxide in mammalian tissues.

The porphyrias are a group of disorders in which there is excessive production of porphyrins or their precursors in the tissues due to enzymic deficiencies in haem biosynthesis. Symptoms include skin fragility and blistering, abdominal pain, paralysis, anaemia, reddish-brown teeth and bones and psychic changes with death in acute attacks.

In man and animals (cattle, sheep, horses, goats and pigs), the presence of photodynamic porphyrins and other substances in the blood (ingested, injected or present as a result of liver damage) causes them to be hypersensitive to sunlight, resulting in dermatitis and oedema – *photosensitisation*.

A rare *congenital* form (pink tooth, congenital porphyria) occurs in cattle, pigs, cats and man in which urine, bones and teeth are discoloured pink or reddish-brown owing to excess porphyrin along with typical skin lesions on exposure to sunlight in cattle but not in pigs and cats. The lesions also occur in the lungs, kidneys, liver and lymph nodes.

The cattle type (*bovine congenital erythropoietic protoporphyria*, BCEP) affects herds in which inbreeding and close line breeding are practised. First recorded in the USA in 1977, BCEP has since occurred in Australia, France and the UK mainly in pure-bred Limousin cattle (Buchanan and Crawshaw, 1995). These authors recorded symptoms of agitation, head shaking and ear twitching in a two-year old Limousin heifer. Scaliness, oozing small scabs and flaking debris affected the pinnae of the ears, which were very sensitive to the touch. A BCEP gene probe has been developed in the USA for use in the eradication of the disease in Limousin stock. The protoporphyria genotype is recorded in the North American Limousin Foundation (NALF) Herd Book. All animals sold at NALF sales and all bulls used for AI must have their genotype recorded.

Various plants contain photosensitising substances, such as hypericin in *Hypericum perforatum* (St John's Wort), fagopyrin in *Fagopyrum esculentum* and *F. sagittatum* (Buckwheat), furocoumarin in *Ammi majus* (Bishop's weed), *Cymopterus* spp. (spring parsley, wild carrot, various clovers, alfalfa and brassicas), and perloline in *Lolium perenne* (perennial ryegrass). Ingestion of these plants in active growth can cause primary photosensitisation.

*Secondary* or *hepatogenous photosensitisation* occurs when liver cells are damaged, for example, in hepatitis or biliary duct obstruction. *Phylloerythrin*, an end-product of chlorophyll metabolism normally excreted in the bile, is then liberated into the blood stream and accumulates in the tissues to cause photosensitisation. *Plants* responsible for hepatoxic damage and secondary photosensitisation include bog asphodel (*Narthecium ossifragum*), Lupin spp. (*Lupinus*), Lantana spp. (*Lantana*), and panic grass spp. (*Panicum*). Various fungi can be responsible, e.g. *Pithomyces chartarum*, which contains sporidesmin, is found in perennial ryegrass (*Lolium perenne*) and is the cause of *facial eczema* in New Zealand sheep (*big head* or *geeldikop* in South Africa). Certain *chemicals* such as phenothiazine, carbon tetrachloride, and corticosteroids may also induce photosensitisation.

The *lesions* of photosensitisation are confined to the white, unpigmented, less hairy and woolly areas of the skin which become reddened and oedematous. Commonly affected parts are the face and ears, but teats, vulva and perineum may also be involved. Skin necrosis and gangrene often ensue. General signs of weakness, fever, anaemia, posterior paralysis and nervous symptoms with death are not uncommon.

**Differential diagnosis** The condition must be distinguished from 'bighead' in sheep caused by *Cl. oedematiens* (*Cl. novyi*).

**Judgement of photosensitisation** When bony structures are affected with pigmentation, consideration should be given to boning-out with release of the unaffected muscular tissue for food. In local affections, the affected part only need be rejected.

### Lipofuscin ('wear and tear pigment', pigment of brown atrophy, lipochrome, haemofuscin)

A yellowish-brown granular pigment which accumulates in the cytoplasm of cells, especially of the heart, liver, adrenal gland and brain and is associated with ageing, apoptosis and chronic wasting diseases. It occurs in Devon cattle, Nubian goats and Hampshire Down sheep, being sometimes described as *ceroid lipofuscinosis*, which is also seen in man. Affected animals show hindlimb ataxia and blindness, post-mortem findings including cerebral and retinal atrophy, neuronal and macrophage granulation and storage of ceroid lipofuscin in nervous tissue especially the brain.

Lipofuscins are derived from the oxidation of tissue lipids and or lipoproteins. Granules of the pigment can be seen in stained sections (Sudan Black and Fontana Silver) as clumps near cell nuclei. They are resistant to fat solvents, acid-fast in reaction and negative to iron stains.

### Xanthosis (xanthomatosis, osteohaematochromatosis, brown atrophy)

Xanthosis affects the heart most often but also involves the diaphragm, masseters, tongue, muscles of the forelimb and organs such as the adrenal gland, liver, kidney, thyroid, parathyroids, ovary and testis. The actual cause of pigment (lipofuscin) deposition is unknown and there is doubt as to its significance.

Xanthosis is encountered especially in old animals but is not confined to them, being seen in otherwise healthy animals. It is being recorded fairly frequently in Ayrshire cattle and their crosses indicating a possible recessive gene.

A survey of 1000 adult cattle slaughtered in North London revealed 10 cases out of 40 Ayrshire cattle (25%) and none in 960 of the other breeds (Hayward and Baker-Smith, 1978).

Duffell and Edwardson (1978) in a survey of 3444 cattle slaughtered in a West Midlands (England) meat plant reported 26 cases among 291 Ayrshires (8.94%). The ages of the Ayrshire cows ranged from 5 to 13 years with a mean of 9.3 years. Three of the latter were generalised cases. Twelve (11 Friesian and 1 Devon) out of 3153 cattle of other breeds had xanthosis. All the animals were healthy and in good condition. Ante-mortem inspection of 9 suspect animals showed an abnormal pigmentation of the skin, the peripheral brown areas of the Ayrshires being darker than normal while the white patches had a yellowish tinge. Suspect Friesian cows displayed a brownish tinge on the black hairs and a yellowish tinge on the white ones. Macroscopic examination of affected carcases confirmed the *heart* to be affected in all cases and the *adrenal cortex* to be involved, except in one Friesian. Of the skeletal muscles, the *masseters* were most severely pigmented but generally less than the heart, the *diaphragm* being the next in order of importance (Bradley and Duffell, 1982).

**Dubin–Johnson syndrome (chronic idiopathic jaundice)** occurs in man, in whom most cases are asymptomatic. It has also been described in Corriedale sheep, the deposited pigment having properties similar to *lipofuscin* and *melanin*. In man there is a high incidence in related families, suggesting an autosomal recessive mode of inheritance, which probably also obtains in Corriedale sheep.

**Yellow fat disease** Yellowish or brownish fat is sometimes seen in pigs fed on fish diets. The staining is due to the deposition of *ceroid*, a waxy substance similar to *lipofuscin*. Ceroid is resistant to fat solvents, is acid-fast and stainable with fat stains.

**Ochronosis (alkaptonuria)** is a rare hereditary disease of cattle, pigs, horses and man in which *homogentisic acid* accumulates in tissues and is excreted in the urine due to a deficiency of its acid oxidase.

Homogentisic acid polymerises to form a brownish-black melanin-like pigment which is deposited mainly in fibrous tissue (tendon sheaths, ligaments, cartilage), kidneys, endocrine gland and lungs. (Homogentisic acid is an intermediate product in the breakdown of the amino acids, phenylalanine and tyrosine.)

**Judgement of xanthosis, Dubin–Johnson syndrome, yellow fat disease, ochronosis** Partial or total condemnation depending on extent of pigmentation and general condition of carcase.

## Fatty change

This denotes an abnormal accumulation of neutral fat or lipid within body cells, especially in the liver, heart and kidney. If moderate, there may be no adverse effect on cell function, as in normal physiological limits, but if excessive, cellular activity may be impaired even to the extent of cell death. Cells can die, however, in the absence of fatty changes. Provided no other adverse changes occur, fatty change by itself is reversible; for example, the acute fatty liver of pregnancy disappears some weeks after parturition. But cell rupture and death can occur.

*Obesity* denotes the deposition of an excessive amount of fat, not only in the organs referred to above but also in the interstitial connective-tissue cells of fat storage depots. It was once acclaimed in livestock grading circles, partly because the animals weighed heavier, as an indication of the superior animal until it was realised that fat was very expensive to produce and that an undue intake in man tended to cause ischaemic heart disease and myocardial infarction as well as cholelithiasis (gall stones), hypertension, etc. Obesity is caused by a prolonged excessive intake of nutrients, especially fats and carbohydrates, reduced energy expenditure due to lack of physical activity, reduced dietary metabolism, endocrine abnormalities, or a combination of these factors.

### *Causes of fatty changes*

Causes are defects in lipid metabolism such as increased free fatty acid synthesis; decreased fatty acid oxidation; diminished triglyceride utilisation and lipoprotein excretion; plant alkaloids (*Senecio*, *Lupinus* spp.); mineral poisonings (copper, phosphorus), carbon tetrachloride; metabolic conditions like pregnancy toxaemia of cows (fat cow syndrome) and of ewes and ketosis; diabetes mellitus; and drugs like phenothiazine, corticosteroids. Many of the extraneous causes resemble those for necrosis (q.v.).

Microscopically, fat appears *in* the cytoplasm of liver epithelial cells as droplets of varying size but mostly tiny. The nucleus may be displaced but is undamaged. In the kidney, the cells of the proximal convoluted tubules are those mainly involved, while the heart shows fat droplets in the cardiac muscle cells. Lipids may also be deposited *outside* cells, e.g. in cases of haemorrhage following fractures with laceration of fatty tissue and release of large amounts of fat into the circulation, resulting in emboli in capillaries with possible infarction.

Macroscopically, the liver is yellowish or yellowish-brown in colour, is larger and heavier than normal and has rounded edges. It is soft in consistency, pits on pressure and is greasy to the touch. On section with a knife, the tissue projects beyond the cut surface and possesses a glistening lustre.

All animals in prime condition tend to show some fatty liver change, which also accompanies advanced pregnancy in all species, especially cows and ewes, and persists for some time after parturition.

Adverse factors such as fractures, severe wounds and rough, prolonged transport frequently result in fatty liver changes. This '*stress liver*' is also associated with the deprivation of food during transport or lengthy detention in lairages.

**Judgement of fatty change** Partial/total condemnation depending on the overall evidence. Partial condemnation is justified where the liver alone is affected, e.g. in cases of 'stress liver', the organ being considered unmarketable. Where generalised changes are evident, total condemnation is warranted.

### Glycogen storage disease

This condition indicates an excessive deposition of glycogen of normal or abnormal structure in tissues, mainly the liver, heart, skeletal muscle, kidneys, brain as well as RBCs and leukocytes.

It affects Corriedale sheep, Shorthorn and Brahman cattle and man (Pompe's disease) as an inherited autosomal recessive disease, the defect being in an enzyme involved in glycogen metabolism. These animals display muscle weakness, especially of the hindlimbs, and haemolytic anaemia. Hyperglycaemia is evident. Only microscopic lesions are evident, taking the form of vacuolation of cells and accumulation of granular glycogen in the cytoplasm.

### Hydropic or vacuolar degeneration

This refers to an increase in fluid *within* cells as distinct from *oedema* where *fluid collects in the intercellular spaces*. It is caused by direct injury to the cell membrane, resulting in increased permeability. Water is present in clear vacuoles in the cell cytoplasm making the cells swell. The cell injury, which is usually a reversible one, attacks epithelial tissues, skin, liver and kidney.

### Hyalin degeneration

*Hyalin* is a dense, white, glassy (hyaline), translucent, homogeneous, albuminoid connective tissue found normally in cartilage. Abnormally it is found in old scars, walls of arterioles (hyaline arteriolosclerosis), corpora lutea and corpus albicans and other connective tissues. In man it occurs in hyaline membrane disease (respiratory distress syndrome) in which excess hyalin is laid down in the bronchiolar epithelium in the lungs, resulting in early infant death due to lack of oxygen.

### Keratinisation

Keratinisation denotes the deposition of *keratin*, a horny, colourless, translucent protein constituent of hair, nails, skin, horny tissues (claws, horns, antlers, hooves, etc.) where it is synthesised by keratinocytes.

Abnormal keratinisation (hyperkeratosis) is manifested in *keratosis* (a horny growth such as a wart or callus caused by friction), bovine hyperkeratosis due to poisoning by chlorinated naphthalenes, parakeratosis in pigs due to zinc deficiency, and inherited parakeratosis (thymic hypoplasia, lethal trait A46, oedema disease) in calves, which responds to oral zinc therapy.

Excessive keratinisation of the ruminal papillae sometimes occurs in cattle fed pelleted feeds. In this condition the ruminal papillae are enlarged, leathery and adhere in clumps.

*Ichthyosis* is a congenital disease of cattle, dogs and man in which horny scales are produced all over the body with desquamation.

*Cutaneous cysts*, which are neoplastic malformations of hair follicles, tend to become keratinised. They are seen in horses, sheep and goats but rare in cattle and pigs.

### Amyloidosis

*Amyloid* is the term applied to several inert fibrillar glycoproteins (immunoglobulin, microglobulin, prealbumin, peptide, procalcitonin, insulin, etc.) which can be deposited in tissues to upset organ function. Almost any tissue may be affected, but kidney, spleen, liver, heart, gastrointestinal tract and brain seem to be most commonly affected. Nodular deposits of amyloidosis can also be found in the lungs, larynx, bladder, skin and tongue as well as the lymph nodes and the suprarenal glands.

Amyloidosis represents a number of disorders or β-fibrilloses and is classified according to the composition of the fibrils (immunoglobulin, microglobulin, prealbumin (transthyretin), peptide, procalcitonin, proinsulin, etc.). Amyloid is composed of non-branching fibrils or rod-like structures arranged in a characteristic intertwined fashion – '*β-pleated sheet conformation*'. In the rod-like aggregates amyloid P-protein (component P) also present except in the CNS. It is synthesised by the liver and circulates in the blood as serum amyloid P (SAP). Amyloid is laid down within or close to blood vessel walls and is stainable dark brown with Lugol's iodine or apple-green with Congo red or Sirius red stains.

Clinically, amyloidosis assumes several forms: *primary*, with no associated general disease; *secondary* when occurring with other disorders, e.g. chronic inflammatory diseases like tuberculosis, osteomyelitis, chronic abscessation, plasma cell tumour, glanders, strangles, peritonitis, chronic parasitic infestations. Renal amyloidosis is the most common form found in animals. A cutaneous type occurs in horses, which have numerous, painless, hard plaques of amyloid on the head, neck, shoulders and nasal passages. The deposit is also sometimes present in horses used for the production of hyperimmune serum.

A *familial* form appears to be most common in man – Mediterranean fever in Shepardic Jews and amyloid polyneuropathy in Scandinavia, Japan and Portugal. In addition to the chronic inflammatory diseases, TB, rheumatoid arthritis, Crohn's disease and Hodgkin's disease, secondary amyloidosis in *man* also features in Alzheimer's disease and several malignant tumours, notably multiple myeloma, renal and thyroid carcinoma and immunoblastic lymphoma.

**Judgement** Partial or total condemnation depending on localised or generalised amyloidosis, carcase condition, etc.

### Mucoid degeneration (mucolipidosis)

This occurs rarely in tissues containing some adipose tissue, e.g. heart, omentum, mesentery and skeletal muscle, the fat appearing translucent and watery.

### Gangliosidosis

Gangliosides are a group of glycolipids found in the CNS. One form, GM1, accumulates in neurons in the brain, spinal cord, ganglia and retina owing to defective lipid metabolism. It has been recorded rarely in Friesian calves, which develop posterior ataxia, stiffness, blindness and eventual prostration. The GM2 form affects pigs and man on occasions. Both are caused by specific enzyme defects and are hereditary in origin.

## DISEASES OF THE BLOOD AND BLOOD-FORMING ORGANS

### Haemorrhage

*Haemorrhage* is the rapid escape of blood from ruptured blood vessels due to injury, section with a knife, fragility and necrosis of the vessel wall, atherosclerosis, rupture due to an aneurysm, action of toxins, chemicals, tumours, parasites and their larvae, ulceration and increase in blood pressure.

Defective blood clotting mechanisms, e.g. deficiencies in blood clotting factors and platelet defects (impaired platelet adhesion or aggregation, platelet deficiency); and liver disease may cause haemorrhage. Various bacterial, viral, rickettsial and protozoal infections are implicated in different forms of haemorrhage. Vascular disorders, especially of the arterial system, are the most common causes of morbidity and mortality in animals and man.

Haemorrhages which are pin-point in size are termed *petechiae*. These are produced by nutritive disturbance of the capillary wall and are encountered in septicaemia and acute infective diseases, especially on serous and mucous membranes, skin, subcutis, fascia, kidneys, muscles and lymph nodes. Almost any organ may be involved – the thymus in calves affected with lead poisoning shows pin-point petechiae. Petechiae are unaffected by the bleeding of the carcase at slaughter. Delayed sticking and some forms of electrical stunning tend to cause petechial haemorrhages and splashing in muscles.

Larger bruise-like haemorrhages are called *ecchymoses*. Extensive haemorrhage occurring over a wide area is an *extravasation*.

A *haematoma (haematocyst)* is a localised tumour-like collection of extravasated blood (usually clotted) in an organ, tissue or space (Plate 2, Fig. 9).

### Anaemia

Anaemia is a condition in which there is a reduction in the concentration of blood haemoglobin with usually, but not always, a decrease in the number of RBCs. It occurs when the rate of RBC production in the marrow fails to balance the rate of destruction or loss of red cells.

Excessive loss of RBCs may be due to extensive haemorrhage and undue destruction of RBCs from haemolysis. *Haemolysis* of red blood cells is mostly due to the destruction of red cells by macrophages in the spleen, liver and bone marrow – *extravascular haemolysis*.

*Intravascular haemolysis* in which haemoglobin escapes from the red cells is occasioned by damage to the cell membrane by antibodies, complement, toxic chemicals or physical trauma. Failure of red cell production results from either bone marrow hyperplasia or hypoplasia.

Anaemia often develops secondary to other conditions – chronic haemorrhage due to bloodsucking parasites like hookworms; viral and bacterial toxaemias (*Cl. perfringens*, *Leptospira*, etc.); haemolytic disease of the newborn; deficiencies of iron, cobalt, copper and certain vitamins (vitamin $B_{12}$, folic acid, pyridoxine, riboflavin); general nutritional deficiency; chronic diseases such as tuberculosis and fascioliasis; action of X-rays and radioisotopes.

*Heritable hypomyoglobinaemia* has been suggested as the possible cause of *anaemic beef carcases*. Three out of nine carcases from year-old Friesian bulls were condemned as 'anaemic'. The animals had been reared intensively and were the progeny of one bull by AI. Except for low vitamin E levels and hyperglycaemia, no other abnormalities were detected in the remaining live animals. (Bowie, 1993).

The mucous membranes and body tissues are pallid and the blood is pale and watery. The carcase may be emaciated, e.g. in terminal bovine TB, or in good condition, e.g. following massive haemorrhage from the liver in acute fascioliasis or rupture of an aortic aneurysm. Hyperplasia of bone marrow shows an increase in the amount of red marrow and a decrease of fatty marrow while the opposite situation obtains in hypoplasia. The main effect of anaemia is a reduced ability of the blood to carry oxygen, leading to tissue hypoxia, cardiac enlargement and failure, fatty liver and heart, with death in severe cases.

**Judgement of anaemia** If associated with severe general disease and emaciation – total condemnation. In less serious cases – conditional approval provided bacteriological and chemical examinations are negative. Heat treatment in areas where facilities exist. Even where carcase condition is good and free from other abnormalities, total condemnation may be indicated because of unmarketability of the carcase.

### Aneurysm

A localised dilatation (usually saccular or fusiform) of the wall of an artery or, less commonly, a vein caused by stretching with weakening or rupture of one or more layers.

A *dissecting aneurysm* is one in which a tear occurs in the intimal layer, through which blood enters to create a cavity within the vessel. It is better described as a *haematoma*.

In the farm animals, aneurysms, although relatively rare, are most common in the horse (aorta, pulmonary artery and cranial mesenteric artery in cases of verminous arteritis) and in turkeys.

Among the *causes* are injuries, vitamin and trace element deficiencies, parasites (*Strongylus* spp.), fungi, necrosis, arteriosclerosis, infectious emboli, lathyrism poisoning, hereditary factors, aflatoxin poisoning in turkeys.

The sequel to an aneurysm is usually spontaneous rupture and sudden death due to increased intravascular pressure. Rupture in horses can follow vigorous exercise or the presence of a thrombus undergoing temporary resolution.

### Arteritis

Inflammation of arteries has many different *causes* – bacterial (*Erysipelothrix rhusiopathiae*, *Salmonella* spp., *Haemophilus* spp.); viral (African horse sickness, equine infectious anaemia, equine viral arteritis, bovine virus diarrhoea, malignant catarrhal fever, blue tongue, Border disease); *Rickettsia* spp.; fungi; protozoa; parasites (*Stongylus* spp., *Schistosome* spp., *Onchocerca* spp.; hypersensitivity, polyarteritis nodosa, serum sickness).

### Endocarditis (Plate 1, Fig. 5)

Myocarditis and pericarditis denote inflammatory changes of the endocardium, myocardium and pericardium of the heart, respectively.

### Phlebitis and lymphangitis

These refer to inflammation of *veins* and *lymphatics*, respectively, while *vasculitis* is a general term for inflammation of blood vessels. *Varicose veins* are veins which are dilated, elongated and tortuous.

### Arteriosclerosis

The term literally means a hardening of the arteries in which degenerative and proliferative changes occur with loss of elasticity and narrowing of lumen. Where the changes are associated with degenerative fatty changes, the term *atherosclerosis* is used, but the two terms are virtually synonymous.

## Ischaemia

Ischaemia represents a partial or complete deficiency of blood in a part. It is usually due to arterial obstruction, venous occlusion being less common. Thrombosis and embolism (q.v.) are the most common causes of ischaemia but *atheroma* (atherosclerosis – thickening of the intima of arteries with fibrous tissue formation) and hyaline arteriosclerosis with the deposition of collagen are also implicated, although more common in man than in animals.

Lack of blood supply often leads to necrosis of the organ or a part of it. In the absence of a collateral circulation, e.g. with end-arteries, an *infarct* (q.v.) is formed. If an alternative circulation is available, compensatory arrangements are possible.

## Hyperaemia (congestion, vasodilatation)

The term refers to an excess of blood in an organ or tissue owing either to more blood being conveyed to it by the arterial system (*active hyperaemia*) or too little blood being drained away from the area by the venules and veins (*passive* or *venous congestion*).

Active hyperaemia is seen in the early stages of acute inflammation, in muscles during exercise and in the alimentary tract following feeding. Passive congestion may be due to venous obstruction and cardiac failure, the inevitable results being chronic pulmonary congestion and generalised oedema.

## Thrombosis (clotting, coagulation)

In the healthy animal, blood is in a fluid state in the blood vascular system. When, however, the lining of a blood vessel is damaged, coagulation changes occur in the blood to repair the damage, ranging from a plug of platelets in minor injuries to a *thrombus, clot* or *coagulum* in more severe injury.

Under the influence of enzymes, some 13 *coagulation factors* (tissue factor, prothrombin, fibrinogen, calcium, proaccelerin, Christmas factor, etc.) are involved in the production of a solid thrombus or clot at the site of injury.

*Tissue factor* is first of all liberated from the damaged tissue, the process ending with the conversion of fibrinogen into insoluble fibrin to form a thrombus or clot and stem the leakage of blood.

Thrombi consist mainly of fibrin and platelets and appear as greyish-red, dull, laminated and roughened when attached to an artery with flowing blood. Where thrombi occur in non-flowing blood, they are dark red in colour and gelatinous in consistency. Thrombi may be large enough to occlude the vessel partially or completely.

Typical thrombi are seen in vegetative (valvular) endocarditis in pigs due to chronic swine erysipelas, in cattle caused by *Str. pyogenes* and in sheep by *Str. faecalis*.

### *Outcome of thrombosis*

Spread of the thrombus along the arterial wall; incorporation into the vessel wall; removal by shrinkage and digestion by plasmin and macrophage enzymes; ischaemia; infarction; formation of an aneurysm; detachment to form an embolus may ensue.

Depending on the location, type of thrombus and degree of vessel occlusion, if complete, death of the animal may ensue. If it is incomplete, reorganisation may occur with recovery. Invasion of the anterior mesenteric artery in the horse by the larvae of *Strongylus vulgaris* may result in arteritis (artery inflammation), formation of an aneurysm or colic with recovery when the larvae depart.

Ante-mortem thrombi must be distinguished from *post-mortem clots (currant jelly clots)* which are dark red in colour, shiny and moulded, but unattached to the vessel intima. The latter are easily removed except when entangled in heart valves.

## Embolism

*Embolism* is the transport in the bloodstream of abnormal material (*embolus*) to a distant part from either the arterial (mainly) or the venous system.

The detached material is most commonly thrombi but it may be fat globules, air or nitrogen bubbles, tissue cells, pieces of tumour, bone marrow, platelet aggregates, fibrin, parasites (*schistosoma* or any other substance gaining entrance to the bloodstream), or even a bullet.

*Septic emboli* are those containing pyogenic bacteria and arise from the fragmentation of vegetations of infective endocarditis or infective thrombi in veins. In newborn animals, detachment of emboli from a septic thrombus in the umbilical vein often leads to multiple abscesses in the liver and other organs. If an infarct becomes infected with a septic embolus, it becomes an abscess.

*Metastasis* is the transfer of disease (usually bacterial or neoplastic) from one organ to another by the blood or lymph, *metastases* being the subsequent growths formed. The organs most often affected with metastases are those with generous blood supply and a fine capillary network, i.e. lungs, liver, kidneys and brain.

*Fat emboli* often occur after fractures of long bones, adipose tissue and fatty liver damage with the passage of fat globules into the circulation. Some of these may lodge in the lungs with fatal results, while some fine fat emboli may pass through the lungs to impact in systemic capillaries, causing multiple petechial haemorrhages in the skin and various tissues.

*Air* or *gas emboli* may originate from extensive wounds, air being sucked into large veins. During routine injections, air may inadvertently be injected into a vein or gain access during surgery. Small amounts are of no consequence. In man, air embolism sometimes occurs in decompression sickness ('bends') or Caisson disease in deep sea divers.

The eventual site of lodgement of emboli depends on their source, size and type as well as the nature of the blood supply of the organ involved. Those from the right side of the heart and systemic veins are arrested in the pulmonary arteries and branches (venous circulation), while emboli from the left side of the heart end up in the systemic arteries (arterial circulation).

Embolism may result in resolution and recovery or in decreased blood flow, heart failure and death. The metastatic, bacterial or neoplastic forms are associated with a poor prognosis.

## Hypostasis (hypostatic or passive congestion)

Hypostasis is the gravitation of blood to the lowermost parts of the body. It may occur during life and includes acute and chronic forms. In the *acute form* animals, especially cattle, sheep and horses, sometimes become recumbent and unable to rise. Oedema is evident, death being due to anoxia, possibly assisted by undue pressure on the heart. The lungs may show evidence of hypostatic congestion with the ventral and anterior aspects of the diaphragmatic lobe affected on the side on which the animal is lying. This lesion can be differentiated from lobar pneumonia by the friable nature of the lung tissue.

If such recumbent animals are given early assistance to rise, recovery is immediate.

*Chronic passive congestion*, on the other hand, mostly due to cardiac failure, is associated with connective-tissue changes. The lungs are indurated owing to interlobular fibrosis (brown induration of the lung) with deposition of haemosiderin providing the colour. The liver is enlarged, hyperaemic and mottled (*nutmeg liver*). The spleen is very enlarged and indurated and the kidneys are congested.

## Oedema or dropsy

In the healthy animal there is osmotic equilibrium between intracellular and extracellular parts. Disturbances of water and sodium homeostasis (sodium retention), hydrostatic pressure or decreased plasma pressure, hypoproteinaemia, heart or kidney failure, lymphatic obstruction, etc., lead to the accumulation of fluid in the intercellular spaces and cavities of the body.

Oedema fluid, with its low protein content, is termed a *transudate* as opposed to an *exudate* of inflammation, which is rich in protein, leukocytes and fibrin.

When this fluid collects in the peritoneal cavity it is called *ascites*; in the pleural cavity, *hydrothorax*; in the pericardial sac, *hydropericardium*; in the brain, *hydrocephalus*; in the subcutaneous and connective-tissue spaces, *anasarca*. The term *effusion* is also used to denote an escape of fluid into a part, e.g. pericardial effusion.

Oedema may be *local*, as in acute inflammation, photosensitisation, cerebral and pulmonary oedema or *generalised* as in severe malnutrition, parasitic gastroenteritis, fascioliasis, '*brisket disease*' of cattle, and *inflammatory* or *non-inflammatory* in origin.

In oedema of the brain there is distension of the perivascular spaces, often with reduction of brain size. In pulmonary oedema, fluid accumulates in the lung alveoli.

In cases of malnutrition and starvation where there is severe protein deficiency, oedema is evident in a generalised form – *nutritional oedema*.

Oedema may also be produced by an *increased permeability* of capillary walls as a result of damage by toxins or to an increased filtrability of the blood. Such changes are evident in allergic conditions like urticaria and purpura haemorrhagica and in bacterial diseases like bowel oedema, malignant oedema, anthrax and mulberry heart disease.

Obstruction to the lymphatic flow from a part, e.g. by tumours or granulomata, may result in oedema.

A peculiar form of oedema (*'bull oedema'*) occurs in young male cattle in Northern Rhodesia and other parts of Africa and is characterised by a well-fleshed carcase with normal musculature but with yellow gelatinous fat in the kidneys and pelvic cavity.

The *'wet carcase syndrome'* of sheep in South Africa described by Brock (1983) is another form of generalised oedema of unknown origin. In this condition non-wool sheep and lambs of good quality are affected by layers of slimy, translucent jelly-like, encapsulated fluid mainly over the buttocks and flanks, and in more severe cases, the brisket area. While not regarded as dangerous food-wise, the condition has warranted extensive total condemnations.

In oedema the affected area is swollen (often several centimetres in depth and mostly well defined), firm, painless and pits on pressure. Section reveals a pale yellowish fluid or gelatinous mass from drips which fluid, which has a tendency to clot.

**Judgement of oedema** Localised, minor forms of oedema and ascites and hydrothorax are of less serious import than anasarca and much easier to judge. Oedema combined with poorness is probably one of the most difficult decisions to make in meat inspection. Detention of the carcase for 12 hours is indicated in all generalised cases while tests are being undertaken.

If the serous cavities have dried out well and the carcase has set properly with reasonable or good condition, the carcase may be passed for food. However, in *anasarca* (oedema) involving the subcutaneous and connective tissues or any form of oedema accompanied by emaciation and non-setting, the carcase should be condemned. (In healthy cattle the bone marrow contains not more than 25% of water, but in anasarca it holds more than 50%.)

Where regional conditions allow for conditional release of carcases, the meat may be passed for cooking or on to the Freibank system. Where no such provision exists, the inspector's decision will be guided by correlating the result of the bone marrow water content test with a visual assessment of the degree and nature of the oedema, carcase condition, whether inflammatory or non-inflammatory in origin, microbiological test, etc.

**Test for estimation of water content of bone marrow** This consists in floating pea-sized pieces of fat from a long bone in alcohol of strengths 32%, 47% and 52%. Marrow containing less than 25% of water will float in each solution of alcohol, in which case the carcase may be released providing there are no other abnormalities; if the water content of the marrow is 50% or more, the marrow sinks in two or three of the solutions and the carcase is judged unfit for food.

An alternative test is to measure the water content of meat samples from the carcase.

## ABNORMALITIES OF DEVELOPMENT

### Anaplasia (Greek, *ana*, back + *plasis*, formation)

Anaplasia is the term applied to the reversion of cells to a more primitive type and is a precursor of neoplasia. The occurrence of many different types of cells (pleomorphism) with abnormal constituents is a feature of anaplasia.

### Aplasia (agenesis)

Aplasia denotes an absence of an organ, e.g. kidney, or part of an organ, owing to failure of development in the embryo. Unilateral renal aplasia, but not bilateral, is consistent with life, providing the single kidney has normal function. The causes are generally genetic in origin but intrauterine infection, drugs like thalidomide and other teratogens are capable of causing physical defects in animals.

### Dysplasia

Dysplasia is a disorderly, but not neoplastic, proliferation of cells and tissues and must be distinguished from *dystrophy*, which is a retrogressive change in cells/tissues which have already reached maturity. It mainly affects epithelial cells but is seen in dyschondroplasia (osteochondrosis) in poultry, where there is an increase in articular cartilage cells.

The causes are similar to those of aplasia and hypoplasia and can include chronic irritation.

### Hyperplasia

Hyperplasia indicates an increase in the overall *number of cells* in an organ or tissue and is closely related to *hypertrophy*, which refers to an increase in cell size and, consequently, organ size. Only cells capable of division are involved. The condition may be physiological, e.g. enlargement of the uterus during pregnancy (in which hypertrophy also occurs), or pathological, e.g. proliferation of connective-tissue cells in wound healing and in hepatic cirrhosis.

### Hypoplasia

Hypoplasia is the failure of an organ to develop to its normal size because of a decrease in cell size or number. It has many of the same causes as aplasia but differs from *atrophy* which is the reduction in size of an already fully developed organ.

### Metaplasia

Metaplasia denotes a change of one kind of adult cells into another type and is occasionally encountered in meat inspection. Examples are the fibrous scar wounds of castrated pigs into bone and the ossification of old ventral hernias in pigs. Ossification in pigs is also seen in the retroperitoneal fatty tissue and in the mesenteric area, especially where the mesentery of the small intestine meets that of the caecum and rectum. In the bovine lung, bony spicules are sometimes found in the alveolar septa while muscle, tendons and cartilage which have been subject to chronic injury are liable to develop bone. The exact reason for metaplasia is unclear but may be an attempt at protection.

### Atrophy

Atrophy is a shrinking and reduction in size of a fully developed organ due to a decrease in the size or number of its cells. Cell death is due to necrosis and autolysis. The *causes* may be physiological, e.g. gradual disappearance of the thymus gland with age, retrogression of uterus following parturition and of mammary gland after lactation, or pathological, e.g. in malnutrition, inadequate blood or nerve supply to a part, ageing, pressure from a tumour. *Pressure atrophy* resulting in a diminished blood supply and inadequate nutrition is commonly encountered in meat inspection, e.g. in hydronephrosis of the kidney as a result of back pressure of urine. In atrophic rhinitis in pigs (q.v.) there is atrophy of the nasal turbinate bones.

In some situations, e.g. ageing, atrophy is accompanied by the intracellular deposition of the granular pigment lipofuscin in tissues, especially the heart, liver and brain – brown atrophy (q.v.).

### Hypertrophy

Hypertrophy represents an enlargement of parenchymal cells which have lost their ability to divide (mainly cardiac and skeletal muscle cells) with a consequent increase in organ size. It is allied to *hyperplasia* (q.v.) which is an increase in cell numbers but the opposite of *atrophy*. Hypertrophy and hyperplasia usually coexist in the same organ.

Both hypertrophy and hyperplasia have similar common *causes* – increased functional demand by the organ (*compensatory hypertrophy*) and hormone stimulation. The former condition is met with in the case of paired organs when one fails to function or is removed, the remaining organ increasing in size to perform the extra work. In human kidney donors, the surviving kidney becomes almost twice its natural size. Increased blood flow in arteries causes a dilatation owing to increases in elastic fibres and smooth-muscle cells in the vessel walls – a situation which obtains in the uterine arteries in pregnancy. Pathological conditions which throw an extra burden on the heart, e.g. increased blood pressure and valvular defects, result in left and right ventricular hypertrophy of the myocardium.

### Judgement of abnormalities of growth

Localised cases of these disturbances normally demand local seizure of the affected organ. Where, however, hypertrophy and hyperlasia are associated with general conditions, regard must be had to the overall disease picture, which may well warrant total condemnation.

## NEOPLASIA

Neoplasia is the process of *tumour* (*neoplasm*) growth. *Oncology* is the study of neoplasms.

A *tumour* (L. *tumere*, to swell) or *neoplasm* is an abnormal growth of new cells which have become insensitive to normal growth-control mechanisms and which (1) usually resemble the cells from which they have derived; (2) proliferate in an unrestrained and disorderly manner; (3) possess no organised structural arrangement; (4) persist after cessation of the causal stimuli; (5) serve no useful purpose, especially in malignancy; (6) result from one or more mutations of the cellular DNA, especially malignant forms. (In some cases tumours need not proliferate progressively and may even regress spontaneously.)

The word '*tumour*' means a swelling, which is an indication of the general gross appearance, although this is not always the case. For example, some malignant carcinomas are relatively small yet capable of causing early death and some mesotheliomas are flattened in appearance. Much depends on the invasive properties (which vary in degree) and location, type of tissue involved, type of tumour, etc.

**Structure** All forms of tumours (benign and malignant) consist of a parenchyma of neoplastic cells and a supporting stroma or matrix of connective tissue, blood vessels and sometimes lymphatics. The parenchyma is responsible for the functioning of the tumour and determines its classification.

### Classes of tumours

*Benign tumours* usually grow slowly by expansion and by compressing or displacing adjacent tissues. They remain localised (although several may appear in an area) and are often spherical in shape with a fibrous capsule. They are thus capable of excision. There is a tendency for benign tumours to resemble the original cells more than malignant tumours.

*Malignant tumours* (cancers) in contrast grow more rapidly by invasion and destruction of the tissues they invade. Although the resemblance to original cells is usual some types differ in cell structure. Pleomorphism (wide variety in cell morphology and staining) is more common with malignant tumours which contain more abnormal products of mitosis (cell division) such as broken chromosomes, huge, dark staining nucleoli and various protein and polypeptide products. They have a great tendency to metastasise, reaching distant sites in the body via the bloodstream, lymphatics and across tissue spaces.

Benign and malignant tumours occurring in endocrine glands may elaborate hormones, e.g. insulin in the pancreas and corticosteroids in the adrenal gland.

### Causes of tumours

Although the exact cause of many neoplasms is unknown, several specific factors, environmental and genetic, are involved:

1 *Physical carcinogens*, e.g. ionising and ultraviolet radiation, chronic irritation, etc., cause DNA damage.
2 *Chemical carcinogens* such as benzene, vinyl chloride, arsenic, chromium, β-naphthylamine, etc., also lead to DNA damage.
3 *Viruses*. Tumour-inducing (oncogenic) viruses which cause tumours in animals include the DNA viruses of the adenovirus, herpesvirus, papovavirus and poxvirus groups and the RNA retroviruses (see Viral and Poultry Diseases).
4 *Hormones*. Disordered hormone metabolism (pituitary, ovary, thyroid, adrenal gland, parathyroid, pancreas) may produce neoplasia (adenomas and carcinomas), especially in man.
5 *Heredity*. Some strains of animals are prone to develop tumours, being inherited in the germ line.
6 *Parasites*, e.g. *Gonglyonema neoplasticum*, can produce gastric carcinoma in the rat and

*Cysticercus fasciolaris* (cystic stage of *Taenia taeniaeformis*) sarcoma in rat livers.

7 *Ageing*. Tumours occur more commonly in older animals. Some, however, like malignant lymphoma, tend to affect young animals more often. Since most food animals are slaughtered at a young age, tumour formation is encountered relatively infrequently in them. The increased incidence with age may be a reflection of the longer period of exposure to carcinogens or to innate changes in metabolism or both.

*Gene mutation (genetic damage) is the basic characteristic in all cases of neoplasia and is associated with the activity of protooncogenes and oncogenes, the former non-transforming genes being converted into transforming cellular oncogenes under special circumstances to initiate the neoplastic events. Fundamental to all tumour formation is the total lack of response to normal growth controls.*

### Effect on host

Cancers are more life-threatening than benign tumours. The latter can occur in animals without any untoward effects, e.g. papillomata. In both types much depends on their location and proximity to vital structures: obstruction of blood vessels, intestine, trachea, oesophagus, bile ducts etc., may result in addition to ulceration of natural surfaces with haemorrhage and secondary infection. Tumours themselves, being well-vascularised, can bleed profusely, even to causing anaemia.

Hormone production can result in excess insulin from the pancreas with hypoglycaemia and overproduction of corticosteroids from the adrenal gland to cause sodium retention and hypertension.

The usual accompaniment of *malignant tumours* with their metastatic effect is severe loss of condition with anaemia, anorexia, weakness and prostration. In some cases, however, e.g. lymphosarcoma (Plate 2, Fig. 7), malignancy does not appear to cause undue loss of weight.

### Nomenclature of neoplasms (Table 16.1)

In general the parenchyma (the essential cellular elements) of the neoplasm determines its behaviour and its name. However, there are serious inconsistencies in the nomenclature of tumours.

*Benign* tumours usually have the suffix *-oma* attached to the cell type from which they originate, e.g. fibroma from fibrous tissue, osteoma from bone, adenoma (Greek, *aden*, gland) from glandular tissue, chondroma from cartilage, leiomyoma from smooth muscle, and so on. *Polyp* is a benign adenoma arising as a projection from a mucous surface. However, the suffix *-oma* can be deceptive since *lymphomas* and *sarcomas* are malignant collections of lymphocytes and melanomas, mesotheliomas and seminomas are also malignant. Some gliomas (tumours of CNS astrocytes and oligodendrocytes), myelomas (plasma cell collections) and teratomas (tumours containing different cell types found in the ovary and testis) are benign and some malignant.

*Malignant* tumours arising from *mesenchymal* tissues (connective tissue, muscle, cartilage, bone, blood and blood vessels, lymphoid tissues, kidneys and gonads) are termed *sarcomas*, e.g. fibrosarcoma, chondrosarcoma, adenosarcoma. Those arising from *epithelial* tissues are called *carcinomas*. The carcinomas can be further differentiated, e.g. squamous cell carcinoma which is a cancer with cells resembling stratified squamous (scaly or plate-like) epithelium.

*Leukaemias* are malignancies in which the normal WBCs are replaced by large numbers of lymphocytes, monocytes or myelocytes.

### Incidence of tumours in food animals

In 1982 a total of 1535 suspected tumours from *cattle* slaughtered in Canada revealed tumours in 1370 cases (89.3%), 165 being inflammatory lesions. Microscopic examination confirmed lymphosarcoma (738), neurofibroma (123), squamous cell carcinoma (101), uterine carcinoma (53), adrenal tumours (38) and hepatic tumours (35). Undiagnosed metastatic carcinomas were recorded in 153 animals.

In Northern Ireland, where regular examination of bovine tumours found on meat inspection is carried out, 61 tumours (0.014%) in 452000 cattle slaughtered in 1995 were found as follows: adenocarcinoma (17), lymphosarcoma (12), carcinoma (7), squamous cell carcinoma (4), biliary adenocarcinoma (3), phaeochromocytoma (adrenal gland) (3), fibrosarcoma (2), osteosarcoma (1), haemangiosarcoma (1), papilloma (1). The 12

**Table 16.1** Origin and character of neoplasms.

| Cell or tissue type | Benign | Malignant |
|---|---|---|
| **1. Connective tissue** | | |
| Adipose | Lipoma | Liposarcoma |
| Bone | Osteoma | Osteosarcoma |
| Cartilage | Chondroma | Chondrosarcoma |
| Fibrous (adult) | Fibroma | Fibrosarcoma |
| Fibrous (embryonic) | Myxoma | Myxosarcoma |
| | – | *Mesothelioma |
| Histiocytes | Histiocytoma | Malignant histiocytoma |
| Mast cells | Mast cell tumour | Malignant mast cell tumour |
| Muscle (smooth) | Leiomyoma | Leiomyosarcoma |
| Muscle (striped) | Rhabdomyoma | Rhabdomyosarcoma |
| **2. Endothelium** | | |
| Blood vessels | Haemangioma | Haemangioendothelioma (Haemangiosarcoma) |
| Lymphatics | Lymphangioma | Lymphangiomasarcoma |
| **3. Epithelium** | | |
| Skin | Papilloma | Carcinoma |
| Skin | Papilloma | Transitional cell carcinoma |
| Glandular | Adenoma | Adenocarcinoma |
| **4. Haemopoietic and lymphoreticular** | – | *Leukaemia, lymphoma |
| **5. Germinal and embryonal** | Benign teratoma | Malignant teratoma<br>Dysgerminoma<br>Seminoma |
| **6. Neuroectodermal** | | |
| Glial cells | – | *Glioma |
| Melanocytes | – | *Malignant melanoma |
| Neurons | Ganglioneuroma | Neuroblastoma<br>Medulloblastoma |
| Meninges | Meningioma | Malignant meningioma |
| Retinal cells | – | *Retinoblastoma |
| Schwann cell | Neurofibroma | Neurofibrosarcoma |
| **7. Placenta** | – | *Choriocarcinoma |

* All benign and malignant neoplasms do not possess counterparts.

cases of lymphosarcoma were all negative for enzootic bovine leukosis virus.

In Edinburgh, Head (1990) recorded a large variety of tumours in *sheep*, mostly old ewes, over a period of 35 years. The pattern was found to be similar to that in several parts of the world. Some tumours were observed by practising veterinary surgeons but others were only detected at carcase inspection.

The anatomical distribution of *891 tumours* was as follows (Table 16.2). Papillomas of the rumen and adenocarcinomas of the small intestine were the most common tumours of the *digestive system*. Generalised and localised lymphosarcomas accounted for almost all the neoplasms of the *lymphohaemopoietic system*, the former disease having a worldwide distribution in sheep with lesions commonly found in lymph nodes, spleen, heart, liver, kidney, intestine, bone marrow, skin and, occasionally, the thymus. In the *respiratory tract*, adenomas represented 96% of the respiratory tumours, while hepatocellular tumours were the most common *liver neoplasms*. (Tumours of cartilage and fibrous tissue are fairly common in sheep but bone tumours are rare. Lymphosarcoma has been transmitted experimentally to sheep and goats using enzootic bovine leukosis (EBL) virus but horizontal spread of the BVL virus from cattle does not occur.)

Bremner (1994) in a survey of *poultry* plant records in England Wales in 1992–93 found that the majority of condemnations in all species were caused by disease, with *leukosis/Marek's, disease* tumours second in importance to *ascites/peritonitis*.

Yogaratnam (1995) in 1992 recorded an overall carcase rejection rate of 3% in *broilers* in a poultry processing plant, with tumours accounting for 0.01% of total disease conditions.

**Table 16.2** Incidence of tumours in sheep (Head, 1990).

| System | Number | Percentage of total |
|---|---|---|
| Alimentary | 325 | (36.5) |
| Lymphohaemopoietic | 118 | (13.2) |
| Respiratory | 107 | (12.0) |
| Liver | 102 | (11.4) |
| Skeletal | 88 | (9.9) |
| Integument | 33 | (3.7) |
| Urinary system | 23 | (2.6) |
| Cardiovascular | 22 | (2.5) |
| Genital | 15 | (1.7) |
| Endocrine | 13 | (1.5) |
| Nervous | 5 | (0.6) |
| Miscellaneous | 40 | (4.5) |
| | 891 | |

## Judgement of neoplasia

Careful examination of the lesions as to shape, size, colour, consistency, location, number, distribution, etc., along with general carcase signs, may give some idea as to identification, whether benign or malignant, to provide a basis for provisional judgement.

However, it is difficult visually to distinguish many tumours, e.g. between fibromas/equine sarcoids, fibropapillomas/fibrosarcomas and between the latter and myxosarcomas and undifferentiated carcinomas. Judgement is usually simpler in poultry, in which poor condition is a common accompaniment.

*An accurate diagnosis can only be made by detailed histopathological examination of samples of suspect lesions, a procedure which should always be resorted to when suspect neoplastic lesions are encountered.*

*Enzootic bovine leukosis* is a *notifiable disease* in the UK and all suspect cases, including those in meat plants, must be notified to the Ministry of Agriculture.

A single or a few localised benign tumours require *condemnation of the affected part or organ*, provided there are no other adverse signs. Numerous benign tumours in different organs and multiple malignant growths warrant *total condemnation*. While poor carcase condition, oedema, etc., may exist to assist in this judgement, it should be remembered that this support is not always present.

### *US FSIS Regulations*

An *individual organ or part* of a carcase affected with a neoplasm shall be *condemned*. If there is evidence of *metastasis* or that the general condition of the animals has been adversely affected by the size, position or nature of the neoplasm, the *entire carcase shall be condemned*.

US regulations allow for total condemnation in cases where certain conditions are detected on *ante-mortem* inspection. Severe *epithelioma of the eye (squamous cell carcinoma) in cattle*, represents one such condition. Squamous cell carcinoma is the main reason for total bovine carcase condemnation in the USA. Where *epithelioma of the eye* occurs at post-mortem inspection, the following decisions are taken:

(a) Carcases of animals affected with epithelioma of the eye or the orbital region shall be condemned *in their entirety* if one of the following three conditions exists:

(1) the affection has involved the osseous structures of the head with extensive infection, suppuration and necrosis;

(2) there is metastasis from the eye or the orbital region to any lymph node, including the parotid lymph node, internal organs, muscles, skeleton or other structures, regardless of the extent of the primary tumour; or

(3) the affection, regardless of extent, is associated with cachexia or evidence of absorption or secondary changes.

(b) Carcases of animals affected with epithelioma of the eye or the orbital region to a lesser extent than as described in paragraph (a) may be passed for human food after removal and condemnation of the head, including the tongue, provided the carcase is otherwise normal.

## CONGENITAL AND HEREDITARY MALFORMATIONS

*Malformations*, which can affect all body systems and all species, are sometimes seen on meat inspection. They are mainly encountered in fetuses but some may be presented as casualty animals. Apparently normal animals and fetuses may show defects.

The system most obviously and frequently involved is the *musculoskeletal*, which occasionally shows various abnormalities of the limbs, head and body. Legs may be absent, twisted, deviated, elongated or affected with osteoarthritis, while the head may display parrot mouth, overshot or absent lower jaw, inherited dwarfism (snorter dwarfs and Dexter bulldog calves), etc. Double muscling as a form of muscular hypertrophy is occasionally met with in calves and lambs. Stress-susceptible Piétrain pigs are often affected with muscular stiffness (Piétrain creeper pigs).

Musculoskeletal deformities are specially common in *poultry* in the form of crooked toes, an extra limb, rotated tibia, spondylolisthesis (kinky back), joint deformities, tibial dyschondroplasia.

**Cardiovascular system** Aneurysms (horses, cattle); aortic stenosis (pigs); persistent R. aortic arch (cattle, horses); ectopic heart (cattle); patent foramen ovale (cattle); patent ductus arteriosus (cattle); ventricular septal defects (cattle, sheep, horses).

**Digestive system** Atresia ani (pigs, calves, sheep); atresia of small intestine and colon (calves, sheep); cleft lip and palate (all species); teeth irregularities (all species); scrotal and umbilical hernias (pigs and cattle); missing diaphragm (calves); double spleen (calves); herniation of liver through diaphragm (calves); rectovaginal constriction (calves).

**Nervous system** Cerebral, cerebellar and brain stem defects – agenesis, aplasia, hypoplasia and atrophy (all species); hydrocephalus (calves); progressive ataxia (calves).

**Reproductive system** Segmental uterine aplasia (white heifer disease); double cervix (cattle); imperforate hymen (cattle); hermaphroditism (all species); freemartinism (cattle); testicular agenesis and hypoplasia (cattle); prolapse of prepuce (cattle); penis defects (cattle); cryptorchidism – failure of testes to descend into scrotum (pigs, horses).

**Skin** Alopecia (cattle); epidermal dysplasia (baldy calves); photosensitisation (Southdown sheep); parakeratosis – adema disease (cattle); hypotrichosis – hairlessness (cattle); ichthyosis – fish scale disease (cattle).

### *Judgement of malformations*

Action will vary from the disposal of dead fetuses to partial condemnation or release of affected older animals depending on the nature and severity of the abnormality.

## GENERALISED SYSTEMIC INFECTIONS

### Mode of spread of infection

Microorganisms present as droplets in the air, in dust particles and in food and water may gain entrance to the animal body by a variety of routes – by the mucous membranes of the respiratory, alimentary and genital tracts or by penetration through the intact skin or via wounds and contusions. Some microbes are able to survive, even multiply, in these mucous membranes while others are repelled.

Whether microbes will spread further depends on their invasiveness, ability to adhere to mucosal epithelial cells, toxigenicity, the resistance of the body's defensive mechanisms and the type of tissue invaded. Microorganisms are specialised in their nutritional demands and are most likely to establish themselves in the animal body if they arrive at a site which best satisfies their biological requirements, although it has to be said that some of the factors that determine microbial colonisation are unknown. Staphylococci are very capable of multiplying in the skin to produce pustules and abscesses but unlikely to establish themselves in the stomach and intestine if swallowed. The reverse is true of, for example, *Clostridium perfringens.* The actual site of infection depends largely on the type of the infective microorganism – bacterium or virus – and their respective capacities for pathogenicity and invasiveness. Viruses, because of their minute size, have a greater capacity for rapid spread within the animal body.

Every infection, of whatever nature, is initially a local one, and its importance in meat inspection is whether it is *acute* or *chronic, localised* or *widespread* and *febrile* or *non-febrile*.

The site of the original infection is of prime importance in determining whether infection will spread or remain localised. While some microorganisms are extremely selective in their *tissue preference* and *predilection sites;* others such as the streptococci, are less demanding and can produce infection in almost any tissue they invade. Pyogenic cocci like *Staphylococcus aureus* and *Streptococcus pyogenes* produce local acute inflammation at the point of entry, while others such as the spirochaetes spread widely through the animal body before the primary lesion at the site of entry is apparent. An *incubation period* is thus created, which is the time that elapses from the entry of the pathogen until clinical signs appear. Salmonellae, for example, after ingestion, penetrate the small intestinal mucosa to reach and multiply in the mesenteric lymph nodes before invading the bloodstream via the thoracic duct. They then arrive at and multiply in the monocytes of the liver, spleen and bone marrow and after a second septicaemia produce frank disease with fever.

On occasion, potential pathogens can exist side by side in a part of the body and yet, when they assume full pathogenicity, take different paths to affect other tissues. This is exemplified in man by the strange actions of *Streptococcus pneumoniae* and *Neisseria meningitidis*, which exist as potential pathogens in the nasopharynx. On becoming pathogenic under suitable conditions, the former invades the respiratory system while the latter causes meningitis.

The reasons for the selective invasion of tissues by microorganisms and the existence of predilection sites by them and by metazoan parasites are largely unknown.

### Bacteraemia/viraemia (literally, 'bacteria/viruses in the blood')

Some types of bacteria, e.g. *Listeria monocytogenes*, *E. coli*, and various protozoa can be demonstrated in tissue smears from healthy animals and are also capable of being cultured from the blood. Lesions produced by bacteria in distant body tissues reach these parts via the bloodstream. So bacteria can be present in the blood but persist as a state of *bacteraemia* for only short periods. Their failure to multiply is due to the presence of antibody, complement and phagocytes in the blood which effectively deal with them.

*Viraemia* means the presence of a virus/viruses in the blood. Both bacteraemia and viraemia (which by themselves cause no systemic disturbance and are of no consequence in meat inspection) may progress to generalised infections, i.e. septicaemia/toxaemia with severe clinical symptoms, when body defences are inadequate.

### Septicaemia

*Septicaemia* is the very serious condition in which highly pathogenic microorganisms, e.g. *B. anthracis*, pasteurellae, *E. coli* (invasive strains), iridovirus of African swine fever, pestivirus of classic swine fever, phlebovirus of Rift Valley fever, are rapidly multiplying in the blood with toxin production and overwhelming the defence mechanisms of the host. The microorganisms are widely distributed and cause extensive tissue damage.

Primary morbid changes may be observed in the original tissue of entry, e.g. metritis, arthritis, enteritis, gangrene of the udder, skin or tail of pigs.

The infective microorganisms of animal septicaemias are numerous – Gram-positive cocci (*Staph. aureus* and *Strep. pyogenes*, the main pyogenic cocci), pasteurellae, salmonellae, leptospirae, erysipelothrix, *Actinomyces pyogenes, C. pseudotuberculosis*, etc., in addition to many viruses and protozoa. It will be noted that many of the septicaemias are zoonoses, e.g. anthrax, salmonellosis, tularaemia.

In addition to microorganisms, septicaemia can also be caused by radiation injury and by immune system defects occasioned by heredity, infections, plant toxins, etc.

*Morbid changes* in septicaemia in the form of extensive endothelial damage and multiple small haemorrhages with high fever are brought about by the action of toxins, except in the case of viruses where the changes are due to the products of damaged tissue cells. Damage to the intima of blood vessels also results in initial clotting and platelet thrombosis but clots and thrombi disappear in the later stages of septicaemia.

### *Clinical signs and lesions*

These are essentially those of multiple small haemorrhages and high fever.

1 *High fever* is always present in the living animal with a temperature up to 41°C or 42°C. As a result the carcase is very congested and bleeds badly, and rigor mortis is reduced or absent. Septicaemic carcases often show signs of icterus as a lemon-white discoloration, especially on the fat and serous membranes.

2 *Petechial haemorrhages* and *ecchymoses* are generally present on the myocardium, kidney cortex, liver and serous membranes, particularly those of the heart, lungs, omentum and mesentery. They are also present as petechiae under the skin, in the conjunctiva and buccal and vulvar mucosae, being due to endothelial damage or representing minute metastatic bacterial foci. Embolic foci of infection may be evident in virtually any organ.

3 *Lymphadenitis* (enlargement and oedema) of the lymph nodes, which may exhibit discrete haemorrhages. In anthrax septicaemia in the pig there may be marked peritoneal effusion and haemorrhagic infiltration around the mesenteric lymph nodes.

4 The liver, heart and kidneys show evidence of *fatty change*. In the early stages of septicaemia the liver is enlarged, its edges are rounded and its capsule is tense, but after two or three days the organ becomes smaller and the cut surface presents dark red portions alternating with those of a yellow colour. Alternatively, the liver may be uniformly clay-coloured.

   The heart muscle is unevenly affected with fatty change, some parts being normal and others greyish-white in colour.

   The kidneys are enlarged, pale and soft in consistency and its capsule is easily stripped off.

   The spleen is usually enlarged and soft in texture with rounded borders, especially in the septicaemias of bovine anthrax (in which it is very enlarged), acute swine erysipelas and *Salmonella enteritidis* infection in calves. In chronic bovine salmonellosis a valuable diagnostic lesion is a marked thickening of the gall bladder wall.

5 Blood-stained serous exudates may be seen in the thoracic and abdominal cavities and the rapid disintegration of red blood cells may frequently give rise to blood-staining of the intima of the large blood vessels.

6 The meat retains a permanent alkalinity and is soft, dark in colour and at times possesses a sweetish, repugnant odour associated with the presence of acetone. This odour can be accentuated by the use of the boiling test. These changes may not be observed in animals which have undergone early slaughter.

### *Diagnosis*

Diagnosis of septicaemia is based on the clinical/post-mortem findings along with the isolation of the causative agent.

### *Judgement of septicaemia*

Septicaemic carcases are unfit for the food of man for two main reasons: the condition may be associated with the entry of food-poisoning microorganisms into the systemic circulation, making consumption dangerous; the congestion of the carcase as a result of hyperthermia, imperfect bleeding and alkalinity impairs its keeping quality and along with its aesthetic quality renders such carcases unmarketable.

In doubtful cases it is wise to detain the carcase for 24 hours and to estimate the degree of congestion and setting at the end of that period. The same procedure can be adopted for the less serious cases of mild fever. Fixation or looseness of the forearm and shoulder in cattle is a useful guide for the degree of setting.

An estimation of the pH value of the meat is also of value, while imperfect bleeding may be demonstrated by the haemoglobin pseudoperoxidase or the haemoglobin extraction tests. Accurate judgement of borderline cases, however, can only be made by bacteriological examination for the presence of salmonellae, listeriae or other harmful organisms.

The benefit of the doubt in all suspect cases (whether septicaemic, fevered or otherwise) must be given to the consumer.

*As with many other serious conditions, effective and responsible ante-mortem inspection should ensure that cases of septicaemia/pyaemia/toxaemia do not reach post-mortem inspection.*

### **Pyaemia** (literally, 'pus in the blood')

In a localised septic focus, thrombus formation may occur owing to endothelial damage to the wall of a vein. Invasion and multiplication of the thrombus by pyogenic bacteria (see Septicaemia) can then take place. Should digestive enzymes cause portions of the septic thrombus to break off, these will be carried in the blood to create metastatic *pyaemic abscesses* in distant tissues by being impacted in arterioles or capillaries. If the impaction occurs in an artery, larger areas of necrosis and pus formation result – *septic infarcts*.

Pyaemic abscesses in the *lungs* usually, but not always, result from septic thrombi in the systemic veins while those in areas supplied by the arterial circulation stem from septic thrombosis in the pulmonary veins.

Like septicaemia, pyaemia can occur with organisms of normally low virulence in immunocompromised animals.

Pyaemia may result in cattle if sharp foreign bodies like pieces of wire, nails, etc., penetrate the myocardium (traumatic pericarditis) and introduce infection into a heart cavity. Infection of the newborn animal, especially calves by way of the umbilicus, may lead to multiple abscess formation. Pyaemia and ulcerative endocarditis are often associated with a haemorrhagic or purulent osteomyelitis in calves in which the bone marrow becomes yellow or chocolate-coloured and later fluid and purulent.

Pyaemia may usually be recognised in the *live animal* by high fever, constitutional disturbance and the presence of an area of local suppuration. Joints like the fetlock, hock and stifle are swollen, hot and painful. In young animals the primary septic focus may be the umbilical vein, while in older animals the uterus, udder and feet may be the source. In the cow pyaemia may take place after parturition, usually arising from thrombosis of the uterine veins secondary to a septic metritis. In pigs tail/ear infections and shoulder wounds resulting from fighting are common causes of pyaemia.

*Post-mortem findings* reveal local suppuration and distant haemorrhagic infarcts, e.g in the liver, lungs, mediastinum, pleural cavity, spleen, kidneys and joints. The area of infarction rapidly becomes purulent. General signs associated with fever may or may not be present.

#### *Judgement of pyaemia*

In most countries authority is available for carcases to be split in cases where abscesses are present or suspected.

*Acute* cases of pyaemia warrant total condemnation.

Care must be taken to distinguish between the acute condition and a longstanding *chronic affection* where abscesses are encapsulated with no evidence of general systemic changes – it is not unknown for some cases of pyaemia to recover. In such instances and with negative bacteriological/residue results, a more favourable judgement may be given.

### **Abscesses in livestock** (see also pp. 499, 500)

In many countries abscess formation and pyaemia have become major problems at post-mortem inspection, accounting for considerable losses of carcase meat in all species of food animals. Where records are available, these conditions are the main causes of condemnation, at least in pig carcases.

Abscesses occur with great frequency in the carcases of meat animals and may be associated with a general condition or exist as isolated lesions. Virtually any body organ can be affected. Especially where they are large in size, great care must be taken to avoid contamination of the carcase.

*Cervical* or *'jowl' abscess* of pigs (streptococcal lymphadenitis) is a common cause of partial rejection in many parts of the world, notably in the United States where annual losses are said to exceed $8 million. These abscesses, caused by Group E streptococci and less commonly *Corynebacterium pyogenes*, *E. coli* and *Pasteurella multocida*, are found in the lymph nodes of the head and neck, especially the mandibular nodes. They are usually small but can measure up to 8 cm in diameter and can completely destroy the lymph tissue, with a greenish exudate which may eventually rupture through the skin. On occasions the abscesses are encountered in the tissues surrounding the lymph nodes. Such lymph node abscesses may be responsible for about 7% of all head condemnations in the USA.

*Injection abscesses* in sheep showed an incidence of 1.36% of all sheep slaughtered in England and Wales in 1984.

In 1988 in the USA pyaemia and abscesses were the most common cause of total (13.7%) and of partial (20.8%) condemnations of pig carcases. The highest incidence was found in hams, followed by bellies, backs and shoulders. Of all pigs slaughtered (79 million) in the USA in 1988, septic lesions were detected in 2%.

Of 354 342 pigs slaughtered in Norway in 1980 *total* and *partial* carcase condemnations were related to pyaemia, followed by pneumonia, polyarthritis and claw and tail lesions. These four affections, which occurred most frequently in the younger pigs, were found to be closely connected with other conditions such as pericarditis, pleurisy and peritonitis (Flesja and Ulvesaeter, 1980).

In an analysis of condemnation data for cattle, pigs and sheep from 1969 to 1975, Evans and Pratt (1978) found the commonest causes of *whole carcase* condemnation in *pigs* were pyaemia and septicaemic conditions/fever, and of *partial* condemnation in the same species were abscess, arthritis and bruising.

In the USA an investigation into an epizootic of abscesses in a commercial goat herd over a 16-year period revealed 518 external and internal abscesses of which 238 were primary and 280 secondary in the same or other anatomic areas. Jaw abscesses (141) were the most common, followed by sternal abscesses (72) with an associated osteomyelitis in a few cases. Cervical lymph nodes and facial areas were frequently involved. Lung abscesses were present in 20 goats. The bacterium most frequently isolated was *Actinomyces pyogenes*, with *Corynebacterium pseudotuberculosis* and *Staphylococci* less prominent (Gezon, 1991).

In cattle, pyaemia and abscess formation are not major reasons for condemnation, being supplanted by bruising and emaciation. However, *hepatic abscesses* are not uncommon in cattle, in which they have various causes – rumenitis and bacteraemia from the consumption of a carbohydrate diet; systemic bacteraemia with infection reaching the liver via the hepatic artery; cholecystitis (inflammation of the gall bladder); foreign body reticulitis in cattle and from the digestive tract in pigs with puncture of the liver capsule; omphalophlebitis in calves with infection reaching the liver by the umbilical vein. The occlusion of veins from pressure of liver abscesses can lead to circulatory disturbances and sudden death may occasionally occur as a result of the release of large amounts of pus from a ruptured abscess into the bloodstream.

Liver abscesses are more common under intensive systems of feeding, e.g. barley beef and feedlot systems. The highly concentrated grain diet has a low pH, which disposes to inflammatory changes in the rumen and the passage of the causal organism into the portal blood system. Such diets are often responsible for the blackening and clumping of the rumenal villi and this and an avitaminosis A may be predisposing factors. The incidence of the hepatic abscesses is reduced when a broad-spectrum antibiotics or more roughage are introduced into the feed.

In about 85% of cases *Sphaerophorus necrophorus* has been isolated, the early lesion being a coagulative necrosis with eventual replacement by purulent material.

Necrosis of the kidneys and the myocardium, manifested by an abnormal paleness of the organs, may accompany liver abscesses in animals kept under intensive conditions.

In addition to the high carbohydrate and low pH diet for cattle, there is no doubt that modern intensive systems of husbandry in pigs can lead to fighting and septic infections from wounds. Careless, unhygienic subcutaneous injection methods also contribute to this huge loss, as does the reckless use of guns for the oral administration of anthelmintics, mineral bullets, etc., pharyngeal abscesses being a common sequel.

*Judgement of abscesses*

Total condemnation is indicated in cases of multiple septic foci; gross accumulation of pus; active pyaemic foci; chronic widespread septic foci; toxaemia; anaemia and emaciation with chronic lesions; widespread septic or gangrenous wounds.

Gross accumulation of pus is often associated with scrotal abscesses. *Scirrhous cord* or *funiculitis* – a necrotic, purulent, granulomatous affection of the spermatic cord following open castration (of pigs, cattle, horses) is invariably associated with systemic changes with toxaemia in the pig, in which it is usually acute but chronic in horses and cattle. The condition is most often caused by *Staph. aureus* and merits total seizure.

Where abscesses are single, encapsulated, few in number and there is no evidence of systemic change, the carcase may be passed following removal of the lesions, providing carcase condition is adequate. Where portions of lung remain adherent to the parietal pleura and contain a small, chronic focus of pus, removal of affected pleura is all that is necessary.

Borderline cases inevitably occur, for example, where there is primary tail necrosis in the pig along with haemorrhagic infarcts in the lungs. These infarcts appear as red, circular areas with a typical conical-shaped form on incision of the lung tissue, which may contain a small abscess. Such cases should be subjected to bacteriological and residue examinations before a final judgement is made.

### Toxaemia and toxic shock

*Toxaemia* (literally, 'toxins in the blood') is the inevitable accompaniment of septicaemia where bacteria are actively multiplying in the blood. But it may also occur with some bacteria, e.g. *Cl. tetani, Cl. perfringens, Cl. botulinum* that have little tendency to spread from their original site but produce exotoxins which diffuse into the blood and lymphatic systems to produce severe vascular endothelial and tissue damage.

*Exotoxins* are produced mainly by Gram-positive bacteria. They are very potent; diffuse out from the living organisms; heat-labile; produce a specific effect on certain target tissues. They can be neutralised by antitoxin.

*Endotoxins* are produced mainly by Gram-negative organisms. They are less potent; are released after death of the bacteria; are heat-stable; and produce a variety of non-specific effects. Antitoxin neutralisation is difficult but capable of stimulating B cells to produce antibodies.

*Toxic* or *septic shock* is a condition in which large amounts of endotoxin, especially from bacteria such as *E. coli, Proteus* spp. and *Klebsiella* spp. gain access to the bloodstream to cause vascular damage and tissue oedema, hypotension due to vasodilatation and reduced blood volume. The mucous membranes are pale, skin is cold, breathing is rapid, heart rate is increased and there is *hypothermia* (low body temperature).

Post-mortem changes in toxic shock include congestion of the lungs, liver and intestine with haemorrhage into the gut lumen. Pulmonary and intestinal oedema may be present along with hydropericardium, hydrothorax and hydroperitoneum.

Causes of non-septic shock include severe trauma, internal bleeding, lightning stroke, severe dehydration, extensive burns, uterine prolapse, extensive surgery, anaphylaxis, congestive heart failure and frostbite.

All cases of septic and non-septic shock are associated with hypothermia, which is also seen in moribund states.

*Judgement of toxaemia and toxic shock*

Judgement is as for septicaemia. Where the situation is reversible, however, as in electrocution or lightning stroke, and the signs less severe, delayed slaughter may be resorted to with re-inspection and, if necessary, laboratory examination. Such cases may justify conditional approval after negative bacteriological and chemical tests.

The possibility of anthrax in the live animal must be borne in mind and, if suspected, a blood smear must be made. Not all cases of anthrax in the live animal result in sudden death. Such animals must be segregated and treated with antibiotics and serum and only slaughtered when a further blood smear is negative.

## IMPORTANT PATHOLOGICAL CONDITIONS

### Hyperthermia (high body temperature)

*Elevation of body temperature* unassociated with acute infection and pyrexia, can occur in animals, the main conditions being *malignant hyperthermia* in pigs (*porcine stress syndrome*, PSS), high environmental temperature and humidity causing heat stroke, dehydration, excitement, excessive muscular exercise, close confinement with inadequate ventilation and various poisons (strychnine, levamisole) and mycotoxins (*Claviceps purpurea*, etc.). The condition is more common in young, fat animals with hairy coats.

Elevated temperatures may occur in animals in overcrowded railway trucks and lorries especially when the environmental temperature is high.

*Lesions* include congestion of the whole respiratory tract including the lungs. The kidneys, heart, muscles and meninges also show hyperaemia while the skin is cyanosed.

#### *Judgement*

Animals affected with hyperthermia must be given adequate rest before slaughter.

If they are slaughtered in a hyperthermic state, total condemnation is called for because of imperfect bleeding – or conditional approval after heat treatment.

### Fever or pyrexia

Acute inflammation, especially of a general type, is associated with systemic effects known as the *acute phase response*, one important aspect of which is the phenomenon of fever – an abnormally high body temperature. It is a response to bacterial, viral, protozoal, parasitic, fungal or chemical pyrogens (agents causing fever) and is mediated by *cytokines* (soluble messenger proteins controlling macrophages and lymphocytes). It is exhibited initially by peripheral vasoconstriction to prevent heat loss and later by vasodilatation, increased metabolic activity in the liver and elevated temperature.

The blood shows a marked leukocytosis – increase in the number of white blood cells, mainly neutrophils – and a lymphocytosis. An increase in the number of circulating neutrophils is an indication of bacterial infection, while an eosinophilia denotes parasitic or allergic reaction.

The animal shows anorexia, thirst, sweating, muscle tremors, increased heart and respiration rates (respiration is usually shallow), reduced urine and bile excretion, constipation (or diarrhoea) and depression. Saliva may be reduced in amount or increased in quantity, e.g. in foot-and-mouth disease and vesicular stomatitis.

#### *Lesions in fever*

The carcase of a pyrexic animal is uniformly congested, giving the carcase a pinkish or reddish hue. Closer examination clearly reveals the fine subcutaneous blood vessels, not normally apparent in the normal carcase. The liver, kidneys and heart display fatty degeneration which varies in degree according to the severity and duration of the fever. There may be marked wasting of muscular and fatty tissues.

Blood vessel congestion in pyrexia is a manifestation of active hyperaemia (vasodilatation) and is accompanied by an increased alkalinity of the muscular tissues and a consequent loss of durability of the carcase. Rigor mortis is absent in fevered carcases.

#### *Judgement of fever*

Total condemnation. In some countries where heat treatment facilities are available, conditional approval is given after negative bacteriological and chemical tests.

### Imperfect bleeding

This condition may be associated with febrile diseases in which there are severe systemic changes in the parenchymatous organs or with physical causes such as poor sticking methods, lightning stroke, electrocution, suffocation, moribund states, conditions promoting stress, females in oestrus, severe indigestion or afebrile affections of the heart and lungs.

In both instances the left ventricle usually contains blood, the subcutaneous blood vessels are injected, the flesh is dark-coloured and the organs are congested and oedematous. The high blood content of the viscera is most apparent in the lungs, while the lymph nodes, especially the prescapular, are suffused with blood but not enlarged.

A useful feature in imperfect bleeding is the easily discernible veins. Incision of the masseter muscle also reveals blood exuding from the cut surface.

### *Judgement*

Where pyrexia and systemic changes are evident, and in advanced cases of afebrile hyperaemia, total condemnation is warranted since badly bled-carcases rapidly undergo decomposition. Less severe afebrile cases may justify a more favourable judgement, e.g. where a sticking procedure has not been fully efficient.

Casualty animals and carcases from animals slaughtered on the farm and subsequent consignment with certification to a meat plant must receive *careful veterinary examination* since such cases may represent febrile conditions, including those of food-poisoning origin.

## Stress

*Stress* brought about by factors unassociated with disease is often encountered on ante-mortem inspection and can be responsible for poor carcase bleeding if immediate slaughter is performed.

The stressors involved are many and varied and include fear, severe pain, excitement, rough handling, overcrowding, mixing of different social groups, high and low environmental temperatures, marked physical effort, strange noises and surroundings, females in oestrus and inadequate transport standards.

Slaughter in these cases must be delayed, adequate rest must be provided and ante-mortem inspection must be repeated to ensure physiological normality. In some cases, however, e.g. young bulls, immediate slaughter may be indicated in order to avoid a potential stressful situation, provided the animals are unstressed on entry.

## Fetuses and immaturity

At one time it was not an uncommon practice for unscrupulous butchers to include the flesh of *unborn* or *stillborn calves* in minced meat or in sausages.

While it is doubtful whether such meat, *provided it is disease-free*, would be prejudicial to human health, nevertheless it would be generally regarded as aesthetically repugnant besides having a low food value with a high water content. The fact that abortion is often associated with many bacterial, viral and protozoal diseases – brucellosis, leptospirosis, salmonellosis, toxoplasmosis, infectious bovine rhinotracheitis, mycosis, etc., gives further support for the non-utilisation of fetuses as food.

Most countries today stipulate that *dead, unborn* and *stillborn animals* be condemned, the US Meat Inspection Regulation further specifying that 'the hide or skin thereof must not be removed from the carcase within a room in which edible products are handled'.

An *undressed fetal or stillborn calf* possesses the following features:

1. The skin presents a sodden appearance, the claws are soft and the soles of the hooves are convex ('golden slipper').
2. Remains of the umbilical cord can be seen attached to the open umbilical ring.
3. Stomach and intestines are free of coagulated milk and the lungs are collapsed (atalectasis) and sink in water. Although the throat may have been cut to simulate bleeding, the edges of the wound are not infiltrated with blood.

The *dressed carcase* will have the hooves detached and the intestines and lungs removed, but the points of origin of the umbilical arteries from the internal iliac arteries will be apparent and the ductus arteriosus and urachus will be wide open. The entire carcase has a sodden appearance and the muscles are loose and flabby.

Occasionally, a newborn calf which has lived for a few days after birth will show some pulmonary alveoli inflated with air and some collapsed due to blocking of bronchioles with amniotic fluid and phlegm aspirated at birth. Such findings indicate that the lungs have not fully functioned after birth.

### *Immaturity*

The only food animal likely to be slaughtered and presented for sale at a very young age is the calf (*'bobby calf'*), although in the past carcases of lambs, kids and piglets were occasionally encountered.

In many countries, including Great Britain, it has been customary to seize very young and 'immature' carcases, in addition to unborn and stillborn animals. The reasons for the rejection of *'immature'* carcases are given as follows:

1 Consumption of the flesh of newborn animals and very young animals, though not prejudicial to health, is thought to be repugnant to the majority of consumers. Meat is usually regarded as unwholesome until the muscle and fat has reached a stage of development which brings it within the definition of meat in the generally accepted meaning of the word.
2 Grounds for seizure may also be based on the fact that immature veal contains little or no fat, has a high proportion of water (usually over 76%) and a high bone ratio. Its value as food is therefore low.

Arbitrary age limits, without real scientific foundation, have been applied to define 'immaturity' in calves in many countries – 14 days (Canada), 15 days (Sweden), 28 days (Austria and Italy) – and minimum offal weights in France.

The US Meat and Poultry Inspection Regulations 1989 stipulate that the carcases of young calves, pigs, kids, lambs and foals are to be condemned if: '(a) the meat has the appearance of being water-soaked, is loose, flabby, tears easily and can be perforated with the fingers; or (b) its color is grayish-red; or (c) good muscular development as a whole is lacking, especially noticeable on the upper shank of the leg where small amounts of serous infiltrates or small edematous patches are sometimes present between the muscles; or (d) the tissue which later develops as the fat capsule of the kidney is edematous, dirty yellow or grayish-red, tough and intermixed with islands of fat'.

Council Directive 91/497/EEC describes 'immature' animals as those 'slaughtered too young and the meat of which is oedematous' and stipulates condemnation.

The GB Fresh Meat (Hygiene and Inspection) Regulations 1995 declare as unfit for human consumption any 'stillborn or unborn carcase and any *immature* carcase which is oedematous or in poor physical condition, together with any offal or blood removed or collected therefrom'.

The Codex Alimentarius Commission (Alinorm 93/16A) recommends that 'fetuses and underdeveloped neonatal animals' be totally condemned or approved as fit for human consumption, with distribution restricted to limited areas.

A recent study was undertaken in New Zealand (Biss *et al.*, 1993) to assess the scientific validity of minimum slaughter ages as arbitrary measures of the *'immaturity'* of meat and offals. The data was derived from 65 Jersey bobby calves in 1-, 2-, 14- and 21-day groups. (Most calves slaughtered in New Zealand for bobby veal in New Zealand are Jerseys.)

The findings of these workers were as follows.

- None of the characteristics commonly ascribed to live calf 'immaturity' were present in the carcases of calves of 5 or more days of age and were inconsistent in the day-old group.
- None of the features commonly regarded as indicative of high water content were present in any of the groups.
- There was a linear relationship between carcase weight and the weights of livers, kidneys and hearts.
- The use of a minimum liver weight as an indirect measure of 'immaturity' had no scientific foundation up to 21 days of age.
- Muscle chemistry: water-holding capacity did not increase significantly with age and this quality along with pH was comparable with that of adult steers.
- Apart from some colour parameters, the quality of the veal remained constant in the age groups despite small changes in muscle chemistry.

This work showed conclusively that the age of slaughtered calves as an arbitrary measure of so-called 'immaturity' had no scientific validity and contradicted previous observations, many of which were probably based on visual assessments only.

### *Judgement of unborn and stillborn animals*

Total condemnation.

### *Judgement of 'immature' animals*

Category I (Meat showing minor deviations from normal but fit for human consumption, provided bacteriological and chemical tests are negative).

*Estimation of age of very young calves*

An examination of the umbilicus, feet and eruption of the incisor teeth will provide a rough idea of the age of very young animals.

The umbilical cord becomes dry and black in 4–5 days and becomes detached from the umbilicus in 8–16 days to leave a sensitive surface which is soon covered by a scab. In 2–3 weeks the umbilicus forms a cicatrix or scar which disappears at about 4 weeks.

The soles of the feet are conical in shape.

*Deciduous* or *temporary teeth* in the bovine (also sheep and goats) have the following dental formula:

$$2\left(Di\ \frac{0}{3}\ Dc\ \frac{0}{1}\ Dp\ \frac{3}{3}\right) = 20$$

(D = deciduous, i = incisors, c = canine, and p = premolars.)

There are usually eight incisor teeth present, although the corner (canine) incisors can erupt at 2–6 days of age. The gum is at first highly reddened and almost covers the incisors but in 7–10 days it retracts and assumes a more rounded form; a calf in which the gum tissue still shows traces of blue coloration is not more than 5 days old. The central incisors and lateral central incisors are free and shovel-shaped at 14 days and the corner incisors at 20 days. By one month all the incisor teeth have emerged from the gums, which are then pale pink in colour.

## Poor condition/emaciation

The difference between *leanness* and *emaciation* is one of degree but both may possess the same basic causes. Thinness may be an expression of physiological normality, but the more serious emaciation is usually associated with other signs of disease.

Both conditions may involve *aphagia* (decreased food intake) in the form of inappetence (reduced appetite), *anorexia* (complete absence of appetite), *pica* (depraved appetite) or complete starvation.

*Decreased food intake (aphagia)* has a variety of different causes; many, however, are unknown. They include all the febrile diseases, stomatitis, pharyngitis, metabolic toxaemia, gastrointestinal parasitism and cobalt deficiency in ruminants, nutritional deficiencies (thiamin in pigs, protein, energy, copper, phosphorus, salt, iron, zinc, manganese, iodine, etc.) thirst, severe pain, stress, and inadequate level of feeding.

Poor condition in sheep arriving for slaughter is currently being seen in parts of Britain and is believed to be due to poor autumn and winter grazings.

*Pica* or *depraved appetite (allotriophagia)* involves the eating, licking or drinking of foreign materials. The materials consumed on occasions are hair, wool, wood, faeces, litter (by all species including poultry), soil, bark, bones, cloth, poisons such as lead and foreign bodies (especially by cattle), cannibalism (fetuses, tails and ears of pigs, etc.). The drinking of urine occasionally observed in dairy cattle is a form of pica but can also be seen in cows deprived of adequate drinking facilities.

*Malnutrition (inanition)* is the state in which the diet contains all the essential nutrients but in reduced amounts – a stage on the way to complete starvation. It is more common than starvation and is associated with some loss of body weight, ketosis, reduced metabolic respiratory and heart rates, hypothermia and sexual activity. Malnutrition commonly occurs during inclement weather in horses, cattle and sheep, in particular where supplementary feeding is absent.

*Starvation* involves complete cessation of food intake (proteins, carbohydrates, fats, vitamins, minerals and trace elements) and quickly leads to a great loss of weight with exhaustion of glycogen stores; breakdown of muscle protein to amino acids and increase in urinary urea; increased fat catabolism with release of fatty acids and formation of ketones; and hypoglycaemia and decrease in insulin production. Starvation does not commonly occur today in developed countries, only being observed in cruelty cases.

In pica, malnutrition and starvation there is an increased susceptibility to infection with higher morbidity and mortality rates.

*Emaciation* is a wasted condition of the animal body that may be pathological, occurring during the course of a disease such as tuberculosis and Johne's disease in cattle, parasitic gastroenteritis, chronic fascioliasis and caseous lymphadenitis in sheep. In old ewes the teeth may be lost and the animal unable to eat. Erysipelas, swine fever, paratyphoid in pigs can produce great loss of condition in pigs. It may also be the result of prolonged starvation.

The *live animal*, especially equines and ruminants, shows a great loss of skin turgor and an increase in skin extensibility owing to the huge loss of subcutaneous fat. The skin *tenting test* (picking up of a fold of skin and noting the time for the fold to disappear) in an emaciated animal usually takes some 45 seconds or more. The eyes are sunken in their orbits because of the reduction of orbital fat, giving the eyes a gaunt, sunken appearance. All the bony prominences – spinous processes of vertebrae, hip bones, ischial tubers, stifle, elbow, shoulder joint, etc. – are conspicuous while the ribs stand out clearly. Weakness is very evident, the heart rate is reduced, the pulse is full and blood pressure is raised. Body weight loss may be as great as 50–60%. Recumbency eventually ensues with death due to circulatory failure.

The blood chemistry changes follow those of starvation. There is abnormal regression of body condition with diminution in size of the organs, especially the muscles, liver and spleen. The outstanding feature, however, is the *loss of body fat* and an alteration in its consistency. The locations that normally carry adipose tissue – mesentery, omentum, perirenal fat, mediastinum, subcutaneous fat, inter- and intramuscular fat, are shrunken and the remaining fat has an abnormal appearance, being oedematous and jelly-like in consistency and of a sickly yellowish colour. The loss of intermuscular fat gives a loose, flabby appearance to the muscles which may be pale in colour if accompanied by anaemia. There is also an increase in muscle connective tissue associated with atrophy of the actual muscles.

Chemical analysis of the meat reveals an increase in water content compared with the normal and a decrease of protein, fat and inorganic salts. In extremely emaciated animals, the water content is about 80% and protein about 19%, giving a ratio of water to protein of over 4 to 1. In lean but healthy animals, the percentage of water is rarely above 76.5% and the protein content about 22%, making the water–protein ratio less than 4 to 1. The ratio between water and protein may be of value in distinguishing between carcases that are very thin and those that are emaciated.

The lymph nodes, especially in young emaciated animals, are enlarged and oedematous. The marrow of long bones is red, watery and poor in fat content, the fat in some cases being replaced by wet, slimy material (*serous atrophy of fat*).

An emaciated carcase does not set in the normal manner and has a moist appearance on its surface and in the body cavities. Changes in the consistency of the fat are best seen around the base of the heart, in the mediastinum, the kidney region or between the spinous processes of the vertebrae.

### *Judgement of poorness/emaciation*

Judgement is based on the degree of loss of condition, efficiency of setting, presence of concurrent disease, and results of laboratory examinations.

Both conditions, especially where unassociated with concurrent disease, are among the most difficult to assess on meat inspection. This is particularly the case in regions where conditional approval for manufacturing purposes and/or heat treatment is not authorised. Regard has to be given to the extent of emaciation, presence/absence of oedema and concurrent disease.

Tuberculosis with emaciation warrants total condemnation.

In borderline cases it is advisable to detain the carcase for 12 hours. If after this time there is considerable drying of the body cavities with absence of serous infiltration of muscles combined with negative laboratory tests, the carcase may receive a more favourable judgement.

Emaciation and oedema frequently coexist and are suggestive of pathological emaciation.

In the absence of disease, confirmed by bacteriological and residue tests, conditional approval may be given with heat treatment.

The Codex Alimentarius Commission Alinorm 93/16A *Recommended Final Judgement* for 'General chronic conditions such as anaemia, cachexia, *emaciation*, loathsome appearance, degeneration of organs' is total condemnation.

Depending upon the *extent* of the condition also:

1 approved as fit for human consumption, with distribution restricted to limited areas; or
2 meat showing minor deviations from normal but fit for human consumption; or

3 conditionally-approved for human consumption after heat treatment, if economically justified.

*Total condemnation is always warranted if the condition is caused by chronic infection and laboratory examination has established presence of infection, recent use of antimicrobial substances or drug residues.*

## Advanced pregnancy/recent parturition/ abortion

Animals, especially bovines, in *late pregnancy* should not be consigned for slaughter since it may involve the loss of a valuable fetus besides subjecting the dam to unnecessary stress.

The hindquarters of a bovine slaughtered in late pregnancy and those that have recently given birth are usually more moist than normal, the genital tract is hyperaemic and the liver shows some fatty change.

*Extra-uterine pregnancy* is a rare condition in which the fertilised ovum develops outside the uterus. Implantation may occur in the fallopian tube which becomes distended and eventually bursts, leaving the mummified fetus embedded in the abdominal wall. Provided no other adverse changes are present, such carcases may be released after removal of the fetus.

*Recent parturition* cases in bovines along with those of advanced pregnancy cases are rarely met with today because of the potential value of the calf.

### *Judgement*

Cases of advanced pregnancy and recent parturition, especially in cattle, should not be sent for slaughter until 10–14 days after parturition or abortion.

If encountered in the meat plant, late pregnancy cases should be withheld from slaughter until parturition occurs. *Cases of abortion must be treated with due care and full laboratory examinations performed. The possibility of brucellosis, listeriosis, toxoplasmosis and campylobacteriosis in cases of abortion must be considered and fetuses, placentae and discharges hygienically handled and disposed of.*

Poor condition with evidence of general disease and positive bacteriological and residue results justify total condemnation. Otherwise judgement involves approval as fit for human consumption, partial condemnation or conditional approval subject to heat treatment where feasible.

## Oestrus

Females of all species in heat undergo considerable stress in lairages. They should be isolated and given adequate rest before slaughter. Heifers in oestrus may have carcases in which imperfect bleeding is evident.

It is sometimes contended that sows and gilts in heat tend to produce bacon of poor keeping quality and liable to taint.

## Livestock used for research

Large farm animals which have been used in toxicology evaluation, production and maintenance of infectious agents/neoplasms/ monoclonal antibodies, breeding of harmful mutants, exposure to ionising radiation, surgical procedures, etc., under the UK Animals (Scientific Procedures) Act 1986 and similar legislation in other countries present considerable difficulty when presented for slaughter for the food of man.

While some, e.g. bovines and sheep with rumenal fistulae used for feeding experiments in farm animals, are suitable candidates for meat inspection, others are unacceptable and should not be consigned to meat plants. Guidance is provided in some countries as to the eventual disposal of such research animals.

The United States Meat Inspection Regulations stipulate that no livestock used in any research investigation involving an experimental biological product, drug or chemical shall be eligible for slaughter at an official establishment unless the following requirements are met:

1 The operator of the establishment, the sponsor of the investigation or the investigator or the Veterinary Services Unit of Food Safety and Inspection Service has submitted data or a summary evaluation of the data which demonstrates that the use of such biological product, drug or chemical will not result in the products of such livestock being adulterated and a Program employee has approved such slaughter.

2 Written approval by the Deputy Administrator FSIS is given to the Area Supervisor prior to the time of slaughter.

3 All investigational drugs, experimental economic poisons, food additives and pesticide chemicals administered to animals must comply with all preparation/distribution standards and with all tolerance limitations under relevant legislation.
4 The Inspector in charge may deny or withdraw the approval for slaughter of any livestock when he deems it necessary to assure that all products prepared at the official establishment are free from adulteration.

## REGIONAL DISTRIBUTION OF LESIONS

(Cross-reference should be made to Chapters 15–18, 20 and 21 and to the Index.)

In general the judgement of a suspect carcase is favourable if the condition is localised, carcase condition is satisfactory and laboratory tests are negative. If, however, the affected area represents part of a general *acute* condition with evidence of systemic disturbance, total condemnation is justified.

## SKIN

Skin is the largest organ in the body, constituting up to 11% of the total body weight and forming the first line of defence against disease and injury. It plays a significant role in homeostasis and its condition is influenced by both internal and external factors and is thus a reflection of the animal's general health. The presence of jaundice provides direct diagnostic evidence of specific disease, while many diseases, especially debilitating conditions, result in skin deterioration with loss of bloom, scaliness, reduction of sebaceous and sweat secretions and of flexibility.

Examination of the skin should determine whether the skin alone is affected with disease or whether the observed lesions are part of a general condition. Many skin diseases *per se* can lead to severe pruritus and great loss of body weight.

The *causes of skin disease* are many and varied and may be primary (local), secondary as a manifestation of systemic disease or a combination of both. They include bacteria, genetic defects, fungi, neoplasms, nutritional deficiencies, physical defects (injuries, contact dermatitis, bites, etc.), parasites, poisons/toxins and viruses.

**Bacteria** *Staphylococcus aureus* and *Streptococcus* spp. (infectious pyoderma), *Dermatophilus congolensis* (lumpy wool), *Dermatophilus pedis* (strawberry foot rot), *Actinomyces pyogenes* (hygromas on knees and hocks) and *Actinobacillus* spp. (hygromas and granulomas), *Mycoplasma kansassii* ('skin tuberculosis').

**Fungi** Ringworm.

**Genetic defects** *Epitheliogenesis imperfecta* (absence/deformity of skin of ears, muzzle, mouth, tongue, palate, oesophagus, lower limbs, claws, atresia ani) in Aberdeen-Angus, Ayrshire, Holstein, Jersey, Shorthorn calves; ichthyosis (fish scale disease and keratinisation) in Holstein, Norwegian Red Poll and Brown Swiss calves; hypotrichosis (partial or complete absence of hair in calves and lambs; epidermal dysplasia (baldy calves – alopecia and scaly, thickened, folded skin); parakeratosis (Adema disease) – exanthema, loss of hair, scaliness round mouth, eyes, jaw, legs; dermatosis vegetans (thickened, oedematous skin of coronets, bellies, inner thighs of piglets; inherited photosensitisation.

**Neoplasms** Cutaneous lymphosarcoma; fibroma; squamous cell carcinoma.

**Nutritional deficiencies** These range from marginal deficiencies of vitamins (especially A and C) and of trace elements (copper, zinc, selenium) to inadequate intake of all nutrients and starvation.

**Parasites** Chorioptic, demodectic, psoroptic and sarcoptic mange mites; lice, keds; blow flies *(Lucilia sericata, Phorma terra-novae)*; warble flies (*H. bovis, H. lineatum, H. diana)*; ticks *(Ixodes ricinus, Dermacentor* spp., *Haemaphysalis* spp., *Boophilus* spp., *Rhipicephalus* spp., *Hyalomma* spp., *Amblyomma* spp., *Ornithodorus* spp.); screw worms (*Callitroga* spp., *Chrysomyia* spp.) (see Chapter 18).

**Physical causes** Injuries, cuts, abrasions, lack of bedding, dirty, dungy conditions, chronic diarrhoea causing scald, eczematous dermatitis in cow with pendulous udders, transit erythema, photosensitisation, urticaria (may also be toxic and viral), *hypotrichosis cystica* ('shotty eruption').

**Poisons/toxins** Excess selenium, molybdenum, arsenic, iodine, ergot, silage additives causing pyrexia–pruritus–haemorrhagic (PPH) syndrome, snake bites. (Certain biting flies are capable of injecting toxins.)

**Viruses** Bovine viral papillomatosis, cow pox, swine pox, sheep pox, pseudo-cow pox, bovine herpesvirus, foot-and-mouth disease, swine vesicular disease, mucosal disease, malignant catarrh.

**Primary skin lesions** (directly associated with skin diseases) include abscesses, bites, wounds, cuts, abrasions, bullae, cysts, haematomas, macules (flattened nodules of colour change, usually less than 1 cm in size), nodules, papules, plaques (circumscribed, elevated, firm, flat-topped areas generally over 1 cm in diameter), pustules, tumours, wheals (localised areas of oedema) and vesicles.

**Secondary skin lesions** (associated with systemic disease): Alopecia, crust (scab), erosion, excoriation, fissure, keratosis (overgrowth of horny epithelium), loss or excess of pigment, ulcer (circumscribed erosion of superficial layers of dermis with depression of eroded area below surrounding tissue), scale, scar.

**Hypothrichosis cystica** ('shotty eruption') in pigs consists of numerous hard, circular papules in which curled-up bristles are found. It is not an infection but a disturbance of growth of the hair follicle, the hair being retained in the hair follicle which is dilated by a dark sebaceous gland liquid and desquamated epithelial cells.

**Equine sarcoid** is the most common cutaneous tumour in horses. Caused by a papillomavirus/retrovirus, it appears as nodules or warts of varying size on any part of the body but most often on the lower limbs, lips, eyelids, base of ears, prepuce and perineum.

**Transit erythema** usually affects pigs on long journeys and those transported in winter after removal from a heated sty. Red patches appear on the skin of the belly and hams in contact with the floor and are attributed to the irritant effects of disinfectant and urine. At meat inspection affected areas may be trimmed off, but severe extravasations of blood into the subcutaneous fat may require extensive removal of all discoloured adipose tissue. Very severe cases may show lymphadenitis and fever sufficient to justify total condemnation.

### *Diagnosis of skin diseases*

A skin scraping is necessary to diagnose the various forms of mange. It is treated with 10% NaOH or KOH and examined under a low power (×40) microscope in a drop of mineral oil. The larger parasites (lice, keds, ticks, etc.) can be examined by direct microscopy.

For bacterial culture, swabs are taken to make smears and culture on blood agar.

The diagnosis of ringworm is achieved by special culture (dermatophyte test medium) of hair and scale scrapings for one week or more, the dermatophyte colonies appearing white to off-white in the medium, which is changed in colour from yellow to red. Wood's lamp may be used to detect the green fluorescence of hairs infected with ringworm spores.

A skin biopsy fixed in 10% buffered formalin is necessary for the differential diagnosis of suspect tumours (Jackson, 1993).

### *Judgement of skin lesions*

Judgement is based on all the evidence obtained at ante-mortem and post-mortem inspection along with a detailed history. It is important to distinguish between local skin diseases and lesions representing systemic disease and to note whether pain or pruritus is present. Providing carcase condition is satisfactory, cases of skin disease *per se* may justify approval or at most local condemnation, but cases of systemic disease showing septicaemia, fever, jaundice, etc. warrant total condemnation.

## Diseases of the subcutis

*Oedema* may occur as an inflammatory oedema – anthrax in horses and pigs, oedema caused by *Clostridia* spp., and bites and stings. A non-inflammatory condition – *anasarca* – in which oedema fluid is widespread throughout the subcutaneous tissues occurs as a sequel to hypoproteinaemia due to intestinal parasitism, starvation, congestive heart failure, etc. *Myxoedema* is a subcutaneous oedema mainly of the neck along with thickening of the skin occurring as a sequel to congenital hypothyroidism in pigs. *Angioedema* is a subcutaneous oedema, mainly of cattle and horses, due to the ingestion of plant allergens.

*Lymphangitis* is an inflammation of the lymphatic vessels. It occurs in *horses* in strangles, glanders, epizootic lymphangitis, sporadic lymphangitis and ulcerative lymphangitis caused by *C. pseudotuberculosis*, in cattle in skin farcy (*Nocardia farcinica*), 'skin TB' (*Myco. kansassii*) and granulomatous lymphangitis due to *Pasteurella granulomatis*.

*Haemorrhage* in the subcutaneous tissues may be present as an extravasation or a haematoma due to trauma or as petechiae, ecchymoses, etc. due to injuries or general conditions such as purpura haemorrhagica in horses, bracken and dicoumarol poisoning in cattle, inherited haemophilia and haemangiosarcoma.

*Abscesses* caused by *C. pseudotuberculosis, C. equi* and *C. pyogenes, Staph. aureus* and *Streptococcus* spp. are encountered in all species, arising from local skin penetration or as metastases from general conditions.

*Cysts* (dermoid, sebaceous, apocrine) may be found in the skin and subcutis.

## ALIMENTARY SYSTEM

### Head/buccal cavity/pharynx/larynx/oesophagus

Bacterial/protozoal/protozoal, fungal, genetic, neoplastic, nutritional, parasitic, physical, poisonous and viral/chlamydial causes of disease are evident as they are in virtually all body regions.

(*This classification of causes will be followed for all body systems.*)

**Bacterial, etc.** Lesions of actinobacillosis, actinomycosis, oral necrobacillosis (*F. necrophorus*), infectious pyoderma (*Staph. aureus*/streptococci), big head in rams (*Cl. oedematiens/novyi*), infectious kerato-conjunctivitis (*Moraxella bovis*), haemorrhagic septicaemia (*Pasteurella* spp.), tuberculosis, atrophic rhinitis (*Past. multocida*). Anthrax. Strangles.

**Genetic** Teeth – malocclusion, defective enamel formation, brownish staining in porphyrinuria, supernumerary (cattle); cleft palate, Dexter bulldog calves, parrot mouth in horses, over- and underdevelopment of mandible, absence of mandible, snorter dwarfs (calves).

**Fungal** Ringworm lesions. Bovine rhinosporidiosis. Mucormycosis.

**Neoplastic** Cutaneous lymphosarcoma, squamous cell carcinoma (epithelioma of eye), papilloma, fibroma, odontoma, osteoma, osteosarcoma, histiocytoma, mast cell tumours, angiomatosis (cattle), congenital neurofibromatosis (cattle).

**Nutritional** Periodontal disease in sheep (broken mouth, premature wear of teeth). Oesophagogastric erosion and ulcers in pigs has been found to be due to the use of very fine commercial diet (ground through a 3 mm or 6 mm screen) (Elbers *et al.*, 1995). (Xanthosis is occasionally seen in the bovine tongue.)

**Parasitic** *C. bovis* cysts (masseter muscles, tongue, heart, oesophagus, diaphragm), eye worms (*Thelazia* spp.), cutaneous habronemiasis (*Habronema* spp., *Draschia* spp.), larvae causing granuloma in skin, conjunctiva), bites of face flies (*Musca autumnalis*), head flies (*Hydrotaea irritans*) and horn flies (*Haematobia irritans*) in cattle, horse flies (*Tabanidae* spp., *Hybomitra* spp.), stable flies (*Stomoxys calcitrans*. Warble fly larvae (*Hypoderma bovis, H. lineatum, H. diana*), *Sarcosporidia* (oesophagus).

Nematodes of the genus *Gongylonema* are sometimes found in the oesophageal mucosa of sheep and cattle as small, spiral, filiform worms lying parallel to the long axis of the oesophagus. In pigs *Gongylonema pulchrum*, 13–38 mm in length, is found in the mucosa of the tongue, pharynx and oesophagus in the southern USA, where all pig tongues used in meat products or shipped from the establishment as 'pig tongues' must be scalded and have the mucosa removed.

**Physical** Cuts, wounds, abrasions due to foreign bodies (pieces of wire, nails, etc.), drenching or balling guns, probang, stomach tube, etc., spines and awns of plants causing traumatic pharyngitis and oesophagitis (lymphoid hyperplasia, erosions and diphtheresis).

Choking with partial or complete obstruction and pharyngeal/oesophageal injury and abscessation, may occur in cattle fed on potatoes, turnips or sugar beet.

**Poisons/toxins** Acute inflammation and ulcers produced by irritant chemicals such as acids, alkalis, mercury, etc., and alkaloids of plants. Fluorosis causes erosion of teeth enamel with yellowish, brownish or blackish mottling of teeth. Sweating sickness (tick toxicosis) causing moist dermatitis at the base of ears from epitheliotropic toxin produced from the salivary gland of the tick *Hyalomma truncatum*.

**Viral/chlamydial** Lesions of foot-and-mouth disease (ulcers), swine vesicular disease (vesicles), contagious pustular dermatitis ('orf'), vesicular stomatitis, papular stomatitis, bovine viral diarrhoea, bovine papillomatosis, mycotic stomatitis, mucosal disease, rinderpest, bovine malignant catarrh, infectious bovine rhinotracheitis, bluetongue, sheep pox, ulcerative dermatosis (sheep), vesicular exanthema (pigs), encephalitis, Aujeszky's disease, rabies, botulism.

## Rumen/reticulum/omasum/abomasum and intestines

**Bacterial diseases** are numerous and usually cause enteritis or inflammation of the intestinal mucosa with diarrhoea and sometimes dysentery – signs that are accompaniments of many systemic diseases – actinobacillosis, anthrax, campylobacteriosis, salmonellosis, Johne's disease, colibacillosis, swine dysentery, entertoxaemia, giardiasis.

Protozoa: *Eimeria* spp.

Non-diarrhoeic disease: gut oedema.

*Fungal* causes include *Candida albicans*, *Absidia* spp., *Aspergillus fumigatus*, *Histoplasma*, *Phycomycetes*, *Penicillium rubrum*, *Mucor* spp. Mycotic infections must be suspected in cases of haemorrhagic inflammation and thickening of the wall of the forestomachs and intestine.

**Neoplasms** Lymphosarcoma.

**Nutritional deficiencies** Copper, cobalt, iron, molybdenum, inadequate intake of nutrients, unsuitable diets.

**Parasites** Parasitic gastroenteritis helminths, coccidia, cryptosporidia, *Strongylus* spp., *Trichonema* spp., *Ascaris* spp., *Trichuris* spp., cryptococci, *Isospora* spp., *Hyostrongylus* spp., *Oesophagostomum* spp., *Strongyloides* spp., *Toxocara vitulorum*, *Chabertia ovina*.

**Physical** Ingestion of sand, soil, foreign material.

**Poisons/toxins** Arsenic, copper, nitrates, molybdenum, fluorine, sodium chloride, poisonous plants, drugs.

**Viruses/ricketettsiae** Mucosal disease, bovine malignant catarrh, rinderpest, winter dysentery, TGE, rotavirus, coronavirus, rickettsiae (ehrlichiosis), bluetongue, classic swine fever, African swine fever.

*Physical abnormalities* encountered in the stomachs and intestine comprise diaphragmatic hernia, L & R displacement of the abomasum, impaction of abomasum, intussusception, obstruction, enteroliths, torsion, volvulus (intestine and mesentery) and rupture.

Cattle, in particular, are notorious for ingesting *foreign bodies* – pieces of wire, nails, umbrella ribs, cloth, rope, pieces of rubber, plastic, coins (which presumably have been present in feed) and even scissors, are constantly being recovered (Fig. 16.1). The smaller pointed bodies are found mainly in the ventral sac of the rumen, sometimes in the reticulum, and occasionally in a tract through the diaphragm to the heart (traumatic

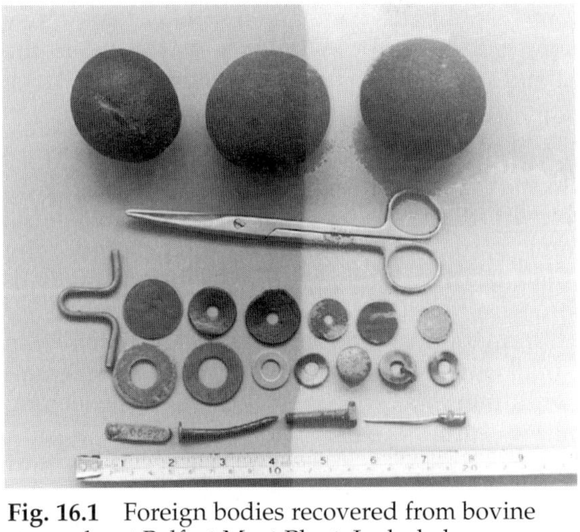

**Fig. 16.1** Foreign bodies recovered from bovine stomachs at Belfast Meat Plant. Included are enteroliths, dressing scissors, nails, a needle, washers, a metal car tag, and Egyptian and Nigerian coins.

reticulopericarditis). Incidences of 70% of dairy cows in Denmark, 52% of cattle over 18 months of age in Czechoslovakia and 49% of cattle in Germany have been recorded. Poulson (1976) estimated that the overall annual loss of cattle and condemnations of meat in Denmark due to traumatic reticulopericarditis was in excess of DKr21 million. Both the rumen and reticulum may be inflamed owing to trauma, frequently resulting in peritonitis and adhesion of these organs to the posterior aspect of the diaphragm with often a large pyogenic tract between the stomach, liver and diaphragm.

**Inflammatory changes** of varying degrees may affect all regions of the alimentary tract – enteritis, gastritis, rumenitis, reticulitis, abomasitis etc. Gastritis and *ulcers* involving mainly the non-glandular mucosa of the stomach are very common in the pig. Round or oval, sharply defined ulcers are often found in the abomasum and rumen of cattle.

**Multiple haemorrhages** in the stomach and intestine of cattle, sheep and pigs are usually associated with the act of stunning and often co-exist with muscle splashing. They also occur in swine fever.

**Abomasal ulcer disease** regularly occurs in calves and adult cattle. A survey of 304 commercially-reared veal calves at slaughter revealed ulceration in 264 (86.8%). Loose-housed calves with access to straw and fed milk substitute *ad libitum* were most often affected but growth rates were apparently not adversely affected. Most of the ulcers were located in the distal pylorus. The consumption of large amounts of milk substitute and straw was incriminated (Welchman and Baust, 1987).

**Acute enteritis in salmonellosis** in cattle shows bloody diarrhoea with high fever, septicaemia and marked constitutional disturbance. The fluid faeces are foul-smelling, intermixed with blood, fibrin and mucous. Post-mortem examination reveals intense congestion of the small intestine, occasionally the abomasum, with petechiae on the mucosae which may show diphtheresis. The mesenteric lymph nodes are enlarged, oedematous and haemorrhagic and there may be enlargement of the spleen and effusion of blood beneath the visceral and parietal pleurae. In more chronic cases necrotic foci may be seen in the liver and kidneys (*miliary organ necrosis*) and are pathognomic of infection with *S. enteritidis* or *S. typhimurium*. Less acute cases of salmonellosis may show only a mild enteritis with few, if any, general signs, making such cases easily overlooked.

**Regional ileitis** (porcine intestinal adenomatosis) of pigs is due to *Helicobacter sputorum* var. *mucosalis* in which there is thickening of the mucous and muscular coats of the ileum. The same organism is responsible for *haemorrhagic bowel syndrome* in pigs and often associated with the feeding of whey. This is characterised by extensive haemorrhage into the lumen and may include the entire large intestine. Haemorrhage into the intestine in pigs may also be caused by shock, stress of various forms, anticoagulants, chemicals and mycotoxins.

**Terminal ileitis** in lambs associated with *Eimeria crandalis* and *E. ovinoidalis* and *Campylobacter coli* exhibits a gross thickening of the terminal ileum with corrugation of the mucosa and vascular proliferation on the serosal surface. The terminal mesenteric lymph node is enlarged (Green *et al.*, 1992).

**Hairballs** (trichobezoars) and round masses of hair and vegetable fibre produced by animals licking themselves are common in the small colon of all animals, especially horses. *Enteroliths* (*faecaliths*) are smooth, rounded, lamellated intestinal calculi composed mainly of ammonium magnesium phosphate and mainly found in the large intestine of horses. Both hairballs and faecaliths may be responsible for intestinal obstruction.

*Rectal prolapse* and *stricture* and *atresia of the colon, large intestine and anus* are *congenital deformities* occurring mainly in pigs and calves.

## Liver

Affections of the liver in the food animals are usually secondary to systemic disease or spread from an adjoining organ. Primary diseases of the liver are relatively uncommon except as a result of certain poisonings and fatty degeneration as a result of fat cow syndrome.

The liver's vital role in intermediary metabolism, synthesis of albumin and fibrinogen, production of enzymes, detoxification of waste products, production and excretion of bile and storage of glycogen, proteins, vitamins and minerals as well as its portal venous circulation (from the gastrointestinal tract and spleen) and arterial blood flow make it an important organ for careful examination in meat inspection. It is the first organ to undergo fatty degeneration in infectious disease and the last to regain normality should the animal survive, making it a valuable guide in determining toxic changes, e.g. fatty degeneration.

Hepatic disorders stem from compromised cellular dysfunction, fatty changes, necrosis, atrophy, intrahepatic or extrahepatic cholestasis (partial or complete reduction of bile flow), fibrosis, cirrhosis, reduced blood flow, congenital lesions, neoplasms and reduced reticuloendothelial function.

### *Causes of liver disease*

**Bacterial diseases** Actinobacillosis, bacterial necrosis *(F. necrophorum)*, BWD, campylobacteriosis, clostridiosis (Black disease – *Cl. novyi*), colibacillosis, hepatic abscesses (*F. necrophorum, C. pyogenes*), bacillary haemoglobinuria (*Cl. haemolyticum, Cl. novyi*), listeriosis, nocardiosis, *Haemophilus* infection, *Pasteurella* infection, salmonellosis, tuberculosis, Tyzzer's disease (*B. piliformis*), yersiniosis.

**Inherited** Hepatic insufficiency in Southdown and Corriedale sheep; congenital bile duct cysts; multiple small serous cysts are sometimes found on the diaphragmatic surface in calves, lambs and foals; inherited photosensitisation; congenital porphyria; Dubin–Johnson syndrome (chronic idiopathic jaundice).

**Fungal** *Periconia* spp., *Pithomyces chartarum, Phomopsis* spp., *Fusarium* spp. As for diseases of the stomach and intestines. Histoplasmosis.

**Neoplastic** Hepatic tumours are the most common of the visceral tumours in the food animals. Except for lymphosarcomas, primary tumours are more common than secondary ones. Lymphosarcomas, arising as metastatic lesions from other areas, are probably the most common tumours in cattle. Adenomas, carcinomas, adenosarcomas and haemangiomas also occur in bovines and melanomas are sometimes encountered in cattle, sheep and pigs, although more commonly in the skin. Adenomas (hepatomas) appear as small brownish or yellowish swellings or larger lobate or pedunculated masses.

**Nutritional** Deficiencies of cobalt, selenium, vitamin E, methionine and cystine have been cited as causes of nutritional hepatitis. Hepatic lipidosis secondary to ketosis.

**Parasitic** Fascioliasis, ascariasis, hydatid cysts, *C. tenuicollis, C. bovis* (rare), *C. cellulosae, Linguatula* larvae, *Schistosoma* spp., *Stephanurus dentatus, Toxocara canis, Toxocara cati, Eimeria stiedae, Histomonas meleagridis.*

*Hydatid cysts* are fairly common in the liver of sheep and cattle and less commonly in the pig and horse. They must not be confused with cystic hyperplasia of the larger bile ducts and gall bladder wall which are sessile or polypoid in shape, contain mucin and may be the result of chronic inflammation.

**Physical** Pressure necrosis from tumours. Cholelithiasis (gall stones).

**Toxic/poisonous** Inorganic poisons – arsenicals, copper, phosphorus, selenium, zinc; Organic poisons – carbon tetrachloride, dioxin, hexachlorethane, aflatoxins, blue-green algae (*Microcystis aeruginosa*); plants and shrubs – ragwort, crotalaria, lupins, Alsike clover, ngaio tree, Yellow wood, *Tribulus, Pithomyces chartarum.*

**Viral/chlamydial** Equine viral arteritis, equine infectious anaemia, equine influenza, equine viral rhinopneumonitis, equine herpesvirus, bovine malignant catarrh, Rift Valley fever, Wesselsbron disease (flavivirus spread by mosquitoes and causing abortion and perinatal mortality in sheep with enlarged orange-coloured, friable, patchily congested liver).

**Telangiectasis** (cavernous haemangioma, 'plum pudding liver') is very common in old cows. Affected livers present circumscribed, bluish-black areas, irregular in shape and varying in size from pinpoint to several centimetres scattered throughout the liver parenchyma. The lesions consist of dilated sinusoids filled with blood and lined with epithelium. They are depressed beneath the surrounding liver tissue and, on section, appear as cavities with a network of residual stroma. Livers containing a few lesions may be seen in heifers and bullocks. The condition is not uncommon in the horse and has been observed in sheep and poultry.

The *aetiology* is obscure but a feeding factor combined with *Fusarium necrophorus* has been suggested. Another theory is that the lesions represent a cell-mediated immune reaction. The condition is more likely to be a benign vascular tumour or a *hamartoma* – a local malformation in which cells normal to the affected part are present in abnormal numbers. The condition occurs in man on the skin (*naevus* or birthmark, 'port wine stains') lips, tongue, liver, pancreas and brain. Slightly affected livers may be passed for food after trimming but severely affected ones must be condemned.

The changes associated with *fatty liver* (q.v.) are due to the mobilisation of lipids from extrahepatic sources and from increased synthesis of lipids in the liver itself. There is also a significant increase in the activity of liver enzymes (malic enzyme, dehydrogenases – malic, glucose-6-phosphate and isocitric) which generate NADP (nicotinamide–adenine dinucleotide phosphate). While increases in the enzymes glutamic dehydrogenase and sorbitol dehydrogenase serve as markers for generalised liver damage, these NADP-generating enzymes appear to be specific for fatty liver change and may serve as a test for the condition (Bogin *et al.*, 1988).

**White liver disease** in sheep, in which the liver is enlarged, pale in colour and shows fatty change with ceroid/lipofuscin deposition, is believed to be associated with a cobalt/vitamin $B_{12}$ deficiency. *Ceroid* is an acid-fast lipopigment found in the liver, muscle and nervous system.

**Hyperplasia of the liver** is usually associated with proliferation of the bile ducts and is normally caused by the action of parasites, especially *Fasciola* and toxins (phomopsin, pyrrolizidine alkaloids and aflatoxin). Acute hepatitis, tumour formation, fatty changes, abscesses and cirrhosis also bring about enlargement of the liver. It also occurs in equine serum hepatitis in horses passively and actively immunised against various diseases, e.g anthrax, tetanus, *Cl. perfringens* and in ovine white liver disease, a form of hepatic lipidosis in which the pigment ceroid is deposited. *Atrophy of the liver* as a result of starvation, poor dentition, etc. leads to hypoplasia and a small, dark liver with wrinkled capsule due to reduction in size of hepatocytes.

**Rupture** of the liver occurs as as result of trauma, neoplasms, cysts and acute fascioliasis (q.v.). *Torsion of lobes*, especially the left lateral, is sometimes seen in sows and may result in strangulation, haemorrhage, atrophy or necrosis and death. *Displacement* (acquired or congenital) of the liver may be caudal or anterior through the diaphragm into the thorax.

## Gall bladder

*Cholecystitis* (inflammation of the gall bladder) and *cholangitis* (inflammation of the bile ducts) may be part of a general disease or local infections. The main infection is salmonellosis, which causes fibrinous cholecystitis (thickening of the gall bladder wall) in cattle, especially calves. Local infections are usually due to *E. coli* and streptococci of enteric origin (gall bladder empyema). In cholangiohepatitis the liver is enlarged, normal or abnormal in shape due to hyperplasia, with a smooth or granular capsule which may bear fibrinous villi. The onset of icterus gives the liver a yellowish, pigmented colour. In long-standing cases chronic fibrosis replaces the liver parenchyma and produces huge enlargement of the organ, which becomes grey and gristly. Alternatively, the fibrosis may occur as wedge-shaped infarcts.

*Cholelithiasis* (choleliths, biliary calculi, gallstones) are fairly common in cattle, less so in sheep and pigs. (If this organ were examined more frequently the incidence would undoubtedly rise.) They occur as tiny grains or large single stones and are usually yellow or dark brown in colour depending on their composition (mixtures of cholesterol, salts of bile acids, calcium salts and a protein matrix). Gall stones have been recorded in poultry. Although equidae have no gall bladders, gall stones may be found in the common bile duct.

Adult ascarids, abscesses and, occasionally, tumours may cause biliary obstruction.

Gall bladder *tumours* are rare as primary entities and are usually secondary to adenomas and adenocarcinomas originating elsewhere.

## Pancreas

*Acute pancreatitis* (inflammation of the pancreas) with abscess formation occurs on rare occasions and probably represents an extension of infection from a peritonitis. The pancreas is slightly swollen and oedematous. *Chronic interstitial pancreatitis* is more common in the food animals and is usually due to the introduction of infection by parasites such as *Strongylus equinus, Stephanurus dentatus, Dicrocoelium dendriticum, Opistorchis sinensis* and *Eurytrema pancreaticum* (small, red flukes) making the pancreas increased or decreased in size.

Nodular *hyperplasia* of the pancreas may be mistaken for tumour formation.

*Fat necrosis* (lipomatosis) appears as chalky deposits with hyperaemic zones around the pancreas, in the mesentery and omentum and sometimes in the subperitoneal fat and the ventral mediastinum. The pancreas may be enlarged and oedematous overall or the oedema limited to certain areas. Yellowish or haemorrhagic adhesions may occur with the omentum and the visceral surface of the liver. Calcareous concretions in the pancreas of the ox and pig represent final stages of fat necrosis and may progress to complete destruction of the organ.

*Calculi* in the form of tiny, hard, whitish stones (carbonates and phosphates of calcium and magnesium) are sometimes found in the pancreatic ducts.

*Tumour* formation is uncommon and consists mainly of adenomas and adenocarcinomas.

## Peritoneum and retroperitoneum

*Peritonitis* may be primary or secondary, the latter being more common and associated with an extension of infection from a lacerated, ruptured or ulcerated abdominal organ (stomach, reticulum, rumen, intestine) or urogenital organ (bladder, uterus, vagina) or through skin perforations and surgical procedures. In some cases infection may arise as an extension from an intact diseased organ, e.g. rumenitis in cattle. Difficult calving, non-sterile surgery and injections into the peritoneum are also incriminated.

*Ingesta* in the peritoneal cavity in cattle and horses indicates a ruptured stomach (possibly due to a perforated ulcer) or intestine and the presence of *urine* to a ruptured bladder. The presence of *blood* in the peritoneal cavity (haemoperitoneum) usually arises from a ruptured liver, spleen or kidney because of trauma, acute fascioliasis in sheep and certain toxaemias. Laceration of the uterus and rupture of a uterine artery at parturition can result in haemoperitoneum as can veterinary extirpation of a corpus luteum and the ingestion of anticoagulant rodenticides and sweet clover hay.

*Ascites* or *hydroperitoneum* is the accumulation of excess fluid in the peritoneal cavity. This is usually a transudate and is clear or straw-coloured and due to obstruction of efferent lymphatics or increased production of peritoneal fluid, biliary cirrhosis, congestive heart failure or generalised oedema, etc. But the excess fluid may represent an exudate of serous peritonitis following urinary obstruction or bladder rupture.

*Bacteria* involved include *Actinomyces pyogenes, Actinobacillus lignieresi, E. coli, Mycoplasma* spp., *Myco. tuberculosis* and *Clostridia* spp. in ruminants; *Act. pyogenes, E. coli, Haemophilus suis, Str. suis* type 2 in pigs.

Bovine TB is an example of a peritonitis occurring secondary to TB pleurisy and appears as numbers of shiny, grey nodules (*'pearl disease'*) similar to those on the pleurae but less nodular and more diffuse. The congenital form of TB peritonitis in the calf is associated with tuberculosis of the hepatic lymph node and may be either lymphatic or haematogenous in origin. TB peritonitis may spread to the uterus and vice versa.

*Traumatic reticuloperitonitis* (hardware disease) is caused by a penetration of the reticulum by sharp foreign bodies, probably aided by the increased abdominal pressure of pregnancy and parturition. The tissue damage may remain as an acute localised peritonitis, but the foreign body may slowly advance forwards through the diaphragm to set up traumatic pericarditis, creating a septic fibrinous tract in the process.

*Parasitic* diseases of the peritoneum are usually the result of larval migration and include *C. tenuicollis, Fasciola hepatica, Gasterophilus* spp., *Habronema* spp., *Stephanurus dentatus, Strongylus edentatus, S. equinus, S. vulgaris and Setaria* spp. (all of which are found as adult worms in the peritoneal cavity and the larvae as microfilariae in the bloodstream – horses *(S. equina)*, ruminants *(S. digitata, S. cervi, S. labiato-papillosa, S. tundrea)*.

Immature *Fasciola* larvae (0.317–3 mm in size) may occasionally be found under the parietal peritoneum. Hydatid cysts (*Echinococcus granulosus*) may develop on the peritoneum following rupture of a mature cyst from the liver.

*Peritonitis*

May be acute or chronic, purulent or non-purulent, haemorrhagic, granulomatous and local or widespread. Acute cases may result in toxaemia and rapid death, e.g. in the clostridial diseases, while septicaemia is the frequent sequel in pyogenic infection.

In *acute peritonitis* there is a straw-coloured inflammatory exudate with fibrinous deposits in the peritoneal cavity with feeble adhesions. Early organisation of the acute state results in fibrinolysis, collagen deposition and healing with some scar formation.

*Chronic peritonitis* cases, however, show a yellowish cheese-like covering of the abdominal organs and a foul smell. These may develop to fat necrosis in the omentum and mesentery with marked hydroperitoneum. Long-standing cases exhibit connective granulation tissue with firm *adhesions* between structures in close apposition. Chronic localised peritonitis is often seen in sheep in the form of adhesion of the liver to the posterior surface of the diaphragm due to extensive chronic fascioliasis and perforation of gastric ulcers in equidae by the larvae of *Gasterophilus* spp. In the bovine adhesions may be seen between the reticulum and the diaphragm as a result of trauma or a hepatic abscess. Widespread lesions of actinobacillosis and tuberculosis are occasionally observed on the bovine peritoneum.

An increase in the number of cows exhibiting peritoneal adhesions following caesarian section has been observed in recent years. This would appear to reflect an increase in dystokia cases occasioned by the use of large continental breeds, especially Belgian Blue, as sires and the development of the practice of embryo transfer. Peritonitis may also follow the research operations of rumen and duodenal fistulae.

Areas of *fat necrosis* are sometimes present in the omental, mesenteric, retroperitoneal and kidney fat of sheep and cattle in very good condition and, less commonly, in pigs and horses. It appears in the form of small whitish or yellowish dry, solid, gritty nodules or large solid masses enclosed in fibrous tissue, the latter being the case in cattle, especially Jerseys.

*Steatitis ('yellow fat disease', nutritional panniculitis)* is an inflammation of subcutaneous adipose tissue with the deposition of ceroid-lipofuscin pigment. Of nutritional origin (feeding of diets high in unsaturated fatty acids and/or low in vitamin E, e.g. fish meal), steatitis is seen in pigs and horses, but not ruminants, the yellowish colour being due to the deposited pigment.

*Mesenteric emphysema* is occasionally met with in the pig, sheep and poultry. It is characterised by single or multiple clusters of thin, colourless cysts, sometimes blood-filled, resembling a bunch of grapes. The condition is usually seen at the junction of the ileum or jejunum and the mesentery and in severe cases may involve the mesenteric lymph nodes. The clusters are lymphatic vessels dilated by gas from sugar fermentation by coliform organisms. Small *serous cysts* (q.v.) are occasionally found attached to the peritoneum and liver capsule.

*Neoplasms* of the peritoneum and retroperitoneum include the *primary mesothelioma* arising from the serosa and appearing as numerous, firm, sessile or pedunculated nodules varying in size from 1 to 10 cm or greater in diameter in cattle, sheep and pigs. Some forms may be fibrous in nature. Other primary tumours are the benign *lipomas* (which arise in the mesentery, mainly of horses, and may be very large with necrotic centres) and the very rare *myxomas, fibromas, neurofibromas* and *ganglioneuromas* occurring mostly in cattle. *Secondary* tumours include *carcinomas* (often a cause of ascites in cattle) and *melanomas* which occur most often in horses.

*Judgement of peritonitis*

Except for tumour involvement (which itself may be generalised), peritonitis must be regarded as bacterial in origin. If localised in form, rejection of affected parts may suffice, but if extensive and combined with systemic changes, total condemnation is indicated.

## RESPIRATORY SYSTEM

Injurious agents in the form of bacteria, viruses and parasites reach the respiratory system by both airborne and haematogenous routes, while noxious substances (gases, particulates) in the air are inhaled.

### Nasal passages and paranasal sinuses

Various bacteria, viruses, allergens, dust and other irritants are responsible for *rhinitis* (inflammation of the nasal passages) which may be localised or part of a specific disease and serous, catarrhal, haemorrhagic, fibrinous, purulent, ulcerative, necrotic, granulomatous and sometimes gangrenous in type.

Both rhinitis and sinusitis are often present in specific *bacterial* diseases such as atrophic rhinitis (*Pasteurella multocida*) of pigs and, less commonly, goats; *C. pyogenes* infection in sheep; tuberculosis, especially in cattle; strangles in horses (*Str. equi, Str. equisimilis, Str. zooepidemicus*); glanders in horses (*Pseudomonas mallei*) and melioidosis or pseudoglanders (*Pseudomonas pseudomallei*) of sheep, goats and pigs and necrotic rhinitis (*F. necrophorum*) of young pigs. *Melioidosis* primarily affects rodents but can cause abscessation in a wide variety of tissues – upper respiratory tract, lung, lymph nodes, spleen, liver, joints, placenta and CNS in other species. In goats the disease is similar to caseous lymphadenitis (*C. pseudotuberculosis*), and in horses the microabscesses in the nasal mucosa resemble those of glanders.

*Necrotic rhinitis* of pigs appears as a necrotic cellulitis of the nose, mouth and face which spreads to the nasal passages causing erosive ulcerative lesions with nasal discharge.

**Fungal diseases** Granulomatous rhinitis (*Aspergillus fumigatus, Cryptococcus neoformans, Penicillium* spp.) and *Conidiobolus* spp.; rhinosporidiosis (*Rhinosporidium seeberi*) and epizootic lymphangitis (*Histoplasma farciminosum*). Rhinosporidiosisis is a disease of cattle and horses in which large polyps are formed in the nasal passages.

**Parasitic diseases** The larvae of *Oestrus ovis* (sheep nasal fly) after two moults attach themselves to the nasal mucosa and that of the sinuses causing catarrhal inflammation, head shaking and sneezing. Erosion of bone and meningitis (rarely) may occur. *Linguatula serrata* (tongue worm) is found in the nasal passages and paranasal sinuses of the horse, sheep, goat and rabbit causing a mucoid inflammation and sneezing. Larvae may also be found in the mesenteric lymph nodes. Larvae of the nematode *Schistosoma nasalis* develop in the veins of the nasal passages and cause dilatation and thrombosis of the veins with catarrhal rhinitis, fibrosis, granulomas and small abscesses in all the food animals. Larvae of the nematode *Habronema*, after burrowing through the skin, may be found in the anterior nares causing granulomas in horses. Larvae of the nematode *Syngamus nasicola* cause rhinitis in the nasal passage of ruminants in tropical countries and the microfilaria of *Elaeophora schneideri* in the USA. *S. trachea* is found in poultry (qv).

**Congenital defects** of the nasal passages and sinuses may be part of a more extensive deformity of the whole skull but can be limited to the cleft palate or deformities of the nasal and turbinate bones. A familial allergic rhinitis in cattle has been reported.

**Nutritional deficiencies** Nasal amyloidosis in which firm, chronic deposits of amyloid are laid down in the nasal passages and sinuses as part of a generalised condition usually associated with a chronic purulent body process.

**Neoplasms** Most tumours are secondary, the most important being the malignant carcinomas (squamous cell carcinoma, adenocarcinoma, transitional carcinoma), neuroblastoma and the benign adenoma and papilloma.

**Viral diseases** may be localised in the nasal and paranasal regions but the more serious conditions are generally associated with the whole respiratory system – bovine malignant catarrh, rinderpest, mucosal disease, sheep pox, contagious ecthyma (orf), equine virus rhino-pneumonitis, Aujeszky's disease, infectious bovine rhinotracheitis, bluetongue, equine viral arteritis, inclusion body rhinitis, swine influenza, classic swine fever, African swine fever, equine influenza, bovine herpesvirus, porcine respiratory coronavirus, calf pneumonia (parainfluenza 3 virus, reovirus, syncitial virus).

### Larynx/trachea/bronchi/bronchioles

*Laryngitis*, *tracheitis*, *bronchitis* and *bronchiolitis* are involved in much the same disease processes, apart from parasitisms, as rhinitis and sinusitis as participants in upper or lower bacterial and viral respiratory disease. Inflammation of all three organs may assume the same inflammatory changes as those affecting the nasal passages and paranasal sinuses. There may be evidence of *ulcers* or healed ulcers on the laryngeal cartilages and in the trachea. Necrobacillosis can occur as part of the oral form.

A useful diagnostic sign in acute classic swine fever is fine *petechiation* of the laryngeal mucosa which may progress to ulceration in later stages. *Deposits* of a *diphtheritic nature* are encountered in calf diphtheria and in laryngotracheitis in pigs.

**Fungal and neoplastic diseases** are relatively rare (see nasal passages and sinuses). *Congenital malformations* are included with those of the lungs.

Flat or pedunculated lesions of actinobacillosis may be seen in the larynx of the ox. Laryngeal *abscessation* may occur due to trauma or to congenital cavitation of the arytenoid cartilage. Laryngeal *oedema* may be traumatic or inflammatory in origin or associated with pneumonia in cattle, gut oedema in pigs or purpura haemorrhagica in horses.

**Parasitic diseases** (see under Pneumonia)

Exposure of the tracheal mucosa by a longitudinal incision through the tracheal cartilages is general practice in some countries, being of value in the detection of aspirated stomach contents, parasitic infections and the ulcers of glanders. Localised infections of the upper respiratory tract *per se*, however, are not generally of importance in meat inspection.

## Lungs and pleurae

The bacterial and viral diseases listed for the nasal passages and paranasal sinuses have the lungs and pleurae as their main areas of assault. To these can be added contagious bovine pleuropneumonia (CBPP) (Plate 1, Fig. 6) and enzootic virus pneumonia of pigs and calves. As with the upper respiratory tract, inflammatory changes may be serous, catarrhal, haemorrhagic, fibrinous, purulent, ulcerative, necrotic or granulomatous in type. Since alveolar cells of the lungs may be involved, a further form – proliferative – can be added.

### *Pneumonia*

*Pneumonia* (pneumonitis) is an inflammation of the lungs in which exudate in the alveolar spaces produces consolidation of the lung tissue. It may be acute, subacute or chronic and occur as a bronchopneumonia (lobular pneumonia), lobar pneumonia or as an interstitial pneumonia. This classification is arbitrary, often making differentiation difficult.

**Causes** Bacteria, mineral dusts, irritant gases, fungi (*Candida albicans, Mucor*), parasites (see verminous pneumonia), viruses, allergens, plant toxins and the aspiration of fluids following vomiting, passage of stomach tube into trachea, dipping operations; rupture of pharyngeal abscess, paralysis or obstruction of the oesophagus, etc.; penetration by foreign body from outside the chest or from the reticulum. Ingesta may be accidentally inhaled under stressful conditions.

In cattle and sheep, ingesta are often regurgitated from the rumen during slaughter and may be inhaled, especially during Jewish and Halal slaughter and if pressure is applied to the flank to facilitate bleeding. Where rodding is not practised, the main bronchi should be incised if contamination is suspected.

The *trachea* may be severed when the neck vessels are cut, especially during religious slaughter, blood being aspirated into the bronchi and lungs. The condition may be detected by the red colour of certain lung lobules on incision, intermixed with normal tissue to differentiate the condition from bronchopneumonia. If blood is aspirated as a fine spray, the lung is studded with fine haemorrhages (petechial blood aspiration). Lungs containing blood and water aspirated during the scalding process should be condemned. In the latter case the lungs are heavy and bulky and the bronchi contain a frothy liquid and blood, skin debris and hair.

### *Types of pneumonia*

**Bronchopneumonia** Infection first affects the terminal bronchi, then extends into the surrounding pulmonary alveoli creating a patchy appearance with numerous discrete foci of *consolidation* (solidification) of lung tissue. The cranio-ventral areas of the lungs are most often affected. The foci are dark red or grey areas about 1–2 cm in diameter and firmer than the adjacent lung tissue. Progression makes these areas of consolidation larger to produce lobular pneumonia. Further extension resembles lobar pneumonia.

**Lobar pneumonia** Infection first attacks the alveoli, then the associated bronchioles, alveoli and lobules, the consolidation being sharply delineated from the normal lung tissue. A whole lobe or part of a lobe is uniformly affected. At the outset the part is *congested* and firm and the alveolar spaces filled with oedema. Later, the affected lobe becomes dark red and solid with greyish strands of fibrin on its surface. Section shows a firm, dry, granular tissue resembling liver which sinks in water – *red hepatisation*. The surface eventually becomes greyish in colour and granular with fibrin in the alveoli and a fibrinous pleurisy – *grey hepatisation*. Should healing occur, fibrin is liquefied and coughed up with eventual aeration of the alveoli and fibrous adhesions between lung and pleura.

Lobar pneumonia is usually the result of infection with the more virulent types of the same bacteria responsible for bronchopneumonia.

**Interstitial pneumonia** Diffuse and widely distributed thickening of the alveolar interstitial septa following an early exudative phase. Infection is usually blood-borne (bacteria, parasites, chemicals, plant toxins and viruses), but can be caused by inhalation of dusts, injury and shock.

**Microorganisms involved** *Bacteria* are the main causes of bronchopneumonia, perhaps following an initial insult from a virus, dust, etc., and include *Pasteurella* spp. and *Actinomyces pyogenes* in cattle and sheep, *Pasteurella multocida, A. pyogenes, Haemophilus* spp., *Actinobacillus pleuropneumoniae, Salmonella cholerae suis, Toxoplasma gondii* and *Bordetella bronchiseptica*.

*Viruses* are also major activators of pneumonia (see Nasal passages and Sinuses).

Both lobar and bronchopneumonia may be associated with sharply defined necrotic foci which vary in size from a pinhead to a fist, become rapidly purulent and produce a *septic pneumonia*. Septic pneumonia due to *Bacterium purifaciens* is often encountered in sheep, the lungs containing several abscesses filled with a thick, yellowish-green pus. Lobar pneumonia tends to become septic very rapidly, making early slaughter and salvage of affected cases advisable. Gangrene may develop if putrefactive organisms are present – it is a common sequel to septic pneumonia or penetration of the bovine lung.

### *Parasitic infestations of the respiratory tract*

Common *lungworms* responsible for varying degrees of inflammation are listed in Table 16.3.

The most common parasite affecting the lungs of sheep in Britain and Europe is *Muellerius capillaris*, which causes little local reaction.

*M. capillaris* causes small greyish-brown fibrous nodules about 5 mm in diameter raised above the lung parenchyma in which the worms can be found. Some of the nodules may be calcified. *Dictyocaulus filaria* and *D. viviparus* cause irritation and blockage with exudate, coughing and loss of weight. Pig lungworms are responsible for bronchopneumonia and emphysema with coughing and loss of weight in the more chronic cases.

Immature forms of *F. hepatica* are sometimes seen in the lungs of cattle and less often in sheep.

### *Pulmonary abscesses*

These usually arise from a local septic pneumonia or from infected emboli transferred by the blood from other septic organs – mastitis, metritis, septic thrombosis of the posterior vena cava in cattle, omphalophlebitis, etc. Haematogenous spread will usually result in multiple abscesses. Penetration of the lung tissue by foreign bodies which may also be aspirated is a further cause. Posterior penetration of the lung from the reticulum will show evidence of a necrotic fibrous tract in the ventral border of the lung in longstanding cases.

In the pig, small, encapsulated abscesses containing pale green pus are sometimes seen on the pleurae in the region of lung abscesses caused by *Corynebacterium pyogenes*.

Specific diseases in the form of actinobacillosis, aspergillosis, tuberculosis, moniliasis, coccidoidomycosis, melioidosis and caseous lymphadenitis may be involved in pulmonary abscessation.

Granulomatous pneumonia may be caused by *Actinobacillus, Actinomyces, Mycobacterium, Nocardia* spp. as well as fungi and aspirated foreign bodies.

*Pneumomycosis* may be due to *Aspergillus* and *Mucor* (see Poultry diseases).

**Pigmentation.** *Melanosis*, congenital and acquired, is probably most common in sheep but also occurs in cattle and pigs. Deposits vary

**Table 16.3** Parasites causing inflammation in the respiratory system.

| Animal | Parasite | Site |
|---|---|---|
| Sheep and goats. | *Muellerius capillaris* | Lung tissue and alveoli |
| | *Bicaulus* spp. | Small bronchioles |
| | *Cystocaulus nigrescens* | Lung and subpleural tissue |
| | *Cystocaulus ocreatus* | Lung and subpleural tissue |
| | *Dictyocaulus filaria* | Small bronchioles |
| | *Neostrongylus linearis* | Small bronchioles |
| | *Protostrongylus rufescens* | Small bronchioles |
| | *Spirocaulus* spp. | Small bronchioles |
| Cattle, deer, reindeer, buffalo | *Dictyocaulus viviparus* | Bronchi, trachea |
| | *(Metastrongylus elongatus)* | Bronchi, trachea |
| Pigs. | *Metastrongylus elongatus* | Bronchi, bronchioles |
| | *M. pudendotectus, M. salmi* | Bronchi, bronchioles |
| | *M. madagascariensis* | Bronchi, bronchioles |
| Equidae | *Dictyocaulus arnfeldi* | Bronchi |
| Deer | *Elaphostrongylus* spp. | Intermuscular tissues of thorax, CNS |
| | *Parelaphostrongylus* spp. | Venous sinuses and sub-dural spaces of CNS |
| Fowls, turkeys, geese | *Syngamus trachea* | Trachea |
| Geese, ducks | *Cyathostoma bronchialis* | Bronchi, trachea |

in size from tiny flecks to sharply defined, bluish-black foci which are lobular in outline and distributed over the lung surface.

**Pulmonary tumours** Secondary tumours arising by metastasis from other organs are much more common than primary neoplasms in the lungs. They involve the pulmonary epithelium and include adenoma, adenocarcinoma, lipoma, squamous cell carcinoma, papilloma and undifferentiated carcinomas. These tumours often extend to the regional lymph nodes. Pulmonary adenomatosis (jaagsiekte) of sheep is an infectious form of adenoma caused by a retrovirus which acts like a low-grade carcinoma.

### *Pleurisy (pleuritis)*

Inflammation of the pleurae is a common meat inspection lesion and is usually secondary to pneumonia or a pulmonary abscess although infective agents can reach it via the bloodstream, lymphatic system and foreign body penetration (from reticulum or oesophagus). Pleurisy may occur as part of a specific disease, *Haemophilus* infection in pigs and chlamydiosis in cattle being common causes in addition to those noted for nasal passages and sinuses above.

The acute stage has a red, velvety appearance. It tends to assume a chronic form with the production of fibrinous *adhesions* between the parietal pleurae and the lung surface.

*Pleural adhesions* are common in pigs, on occasions reaching 100% of pigs slaughtered from certain producers. In an investigation of the prevalence of pleurisy in slaughter pigs, Hartley *et al.* (1988) found the mean batch incidence of pleural stripping in four abattoirs in the east of England to be $0.15 \pm 0.04$ and the average batch proportion of lungs condemned to be $0.23 \pm 0.05$. There was a significant positive correlation between the number of carcases requiring lung condemnation and the number those requiring pleural stripping.

Acute pleurisy in cattle may be confused with *'back bleeding'*, which occurs when the pleura at the entrance to the chest is punctured during sticking, resulting blood being aspirated into the thoracic cavity where it solidifies on the parietal pleurae, especially along the posterior edges of the ribs.

Small *haemorrhages* beneath the parietal or visceral pleurae may be associated with poor stunning operations. They can also occur in many septicaemias, including classic swine fever and acute swine erysipelas. Tuberculous pleurisy in the form of irregularly-shaped tubercles (*'grape lesions'*, *'pearl disease'*) frequently accompanies other forms of bovine TB.

*Pleural effusions* are collections of various types of fluid in the thoracic cavity. They may be inflammatory or non-inflammatory in type. Inflammatory *exudates* (high in plasma protein) are due to increased capillary permeability and are associated with pneumonia, pleurisy, diaphragmatic abscess and diseases like tuberculosis. As with oedema, inflammatory exudates are rich in plasma proteins and may be haemorrhagic, purulent, serous, serofibrinous or purulent in nature.

*Non-inflammatory transudates* (low in plasma protein) are connected with conditions causing increased intravascular pressure – emaciation, hepatic cirrhosis, nephritis, neoplasms, obstruction of lymphatic flow.

#### *Types of n-i transudates*

- *Chylothorax*: The collection of lymph which is creamy in colour due to obstruction of, or injury to, the thoracic or right lymphatic duct, e.g. by tumours.
- *Haemothorax*: Blood in the pleural cavities follows rupture of blood vessels or haemangiomas from trauma, erosion of a blood vessel wall or haemorrhagic inflammation.
- *Hydrothorax*: Collection of oedema fluid due to malnutrition, nephritis, cirrhosis of the liver, obstruction of flow of lymph, extensive tumour formation on pleurae. Hydrothorax is also seen in specific diseases like African horse sickness, black disease in sheep, mulberry heart disease.
- *Pneumothorax*: The presence of air or gas is usually due to trauma – perforation of the thoracic wall or rupture of a lung. Pulmonary emphysema (enlarged terminal bronchioles and alveoli) may be involved because of rupture of the distended bullae). Pulmonary tuberculosis may be an underlying cause.
- *Pyothorax* or *empyema*: Purulent *exudate* or pus in a pleural cavity.

#### *Pleural tumours*

Both primary and secondary tumours of the pleura are uncommon, mesothelioma, affecting the bovine, horse and goat, being most often encountered (see Mesothelioma of peritoneum).

#### *Judgement of respiratory conditions*

**Total condemnation** Conditions forming part of an acute systemic disease; acute septic, necrotic or gangrenous pneumonia; multiple pulmonary abscesses; diffuse fibrinous or serofibrinous pleurisy; purulent and gangrenous pleurisy; widespread tumour formation.

**Approval as fit for human consumption with seizure of affected organs, subject to results of laboratory examinations (microbiological and chemical) and satisfactory carcase condition:** Localised tumour formation; sinusitis; rhinitis; bronchitis; tracheitis; pleural adhesions; catarrhal pneumonia; pleuropneumonia; atalectasis; emphysema; pigmentation; aspiration of blood, fluid and ingesta.

**Conditional approval for human consumption following heat treatment and satisfactory laboratory results, carcase condition, etc.** Subacute cases of pneumonia and bronchopneumonia.

## CARDIOVASCULAR SYSTEM

### Heart

#### *Pericardium*

Most diseases of the pericardium are secondary to specific diseases caused by microorganisms (CBPP, pasteurellosis, clostridial haemoglobinuria, porcine enzootic pneumonia, black disease, blackleg, sporadic bovine encephalomyelitis, tuberculosis, salmonellosis, ornithosis, staphylococcosis in rabbits, *Mycoplasma* spp., *Haemophilus* spp., etc.) or exist as extensions from adjacent thoracic or anterior abdominal organs, e.g. reticulum in traumatic reticulopericarditis in cattle.

*Pericarditis* (inflammation of the pericardium) may be serous (early stages), fibrinous or septic. Early stages show hyperaemia with a thin, clear exudate.

**Fibrinous pericarditis:** In later stages greyish-white fibrin strands are formed, sometimes flecked with blood, and the exudate is reduced in amount. In chronic fibrinous pericarditis, the fibrinous exudate appears as villous strands when the epicardium and pericardium are separated – 'bread-and-butter' pericarditis.

**Septic or purulent pericarditis:** The presence of pyogenic bacteria is indicated by the appearance of pus which varies in consistency and colour according to the types of organisms involved – thin, whitish pus or thick creamy, yellowish, yellowish-green or greenish pus. Putrefactive bacteria produce a foul smelling pus.

*Septic pericarditis* is the form occurring in *traumatic reticulopericarditis* in cattle. (Traumatic pericarditis can also occur in the horse and sheep.) Early forms show the above septic changes but more chronic cases reveal varying deposits of fibrin which fuse the epicardium and pericardium together. The pericardial sac itself is thickened and there is usually a fistulous cord-like fibrous tract (which may contain some pus) connecting the reticulum and pericardium. *Corynebacterium pyogenes* is the most common organism in a mixed flora which may contain anaerobic gas-forming bacteria. A local chronic peritonitis is frequently associated with the fistulous tract and may give rise to adhesions between the diaphragm, pericardial sac and anterior aspect of the reticulum. Pleural and pneumonic changes are frequent associates. Bacteria may pass from the infected pericardial sac into the bloodstream, producing septicaemia, but more commonly the infective material remains encapsulated with toxins being released to cause cachexia.

*Traumatic reticulpericarditis* occurs most often in cows over 4 years of age, often shortly after parturition (Poulson, 1976). Its frequency is related to the bovine habit of licking and swallowing various foreign bodies (see Fig. 16.1) and the close relationship of the reticulum and the heart. These organs are about 5 cm apart during expiration and 2.5 cm during inspiration. The regular movement of the diaphragm during respiration facilitates the forward movement of sharp objects through the anteroventral border of the reticulum and the diaphragm to penetrate the pericardial sac at the apex of the heart. Occasionally, sharp objects may penetrate the myocardium, lung, pleura, liver or spleen.

**Tuberculosis** of the bovine pericardium is usually an extension from the lungs but can be the result of haematogenous spread. It takes the form of small, greyish tubercles, at first translucent but soon becoming caseous.

In pigs, a *fibrinous pericarditis*, often accompanied by adhesions of the parietal or visceral pleura, may result from swine erysipelas and pasteurellosis. Pericarditis associated with salmonellosis in pigs is a fibrinohaemorrhagic type with epicardial haemorrhages.

**Hydropericardium** An excess of clear, serous, slightly yellowish transudate in the pericardial sac is often due to neoplasia (causing venous and lymphatic obstruction), emaciation, generalised oedema and congestive heart failure. Exudates of bacterial or viral origin are seen in African horse sickness, heartwater, oedema disease and mulberry heart disease of pigs.

**Haemopericardium** is an effusion of blood into the pericardial cavity caused by spontaneous rupture of aneurysms of the aorta, coronary artery or an atrium and leads to sudden death. Inherited defects and nutritional deficiencies, e.g. copper-containing enzyme lysyl oxidase can also lead to haemopericardium.

## Epicardium

The serous layer of the heart is a common site for petechial haemorrhages and ecchymoses (q.v.) in all species occurring in septicaemias and toxaemias, mulberry heart disease of swine and in improper stunning, especially electrical stunning.

## Endocardium

Subendocardial *haemorrhages*, especially in the left ventricle, are found in septicaemias and toxaemias but are less common than the epicardial types. They may be of agonal origin at slaughter and are often apparent on the mitral valve of young calves. Subendocardial *fibrosis* (congenital or acquired) in the form of strong whitish strands may be evident in the atria, the acquired form occurring in chronic wasting diseases. Whitish grains or plaques of calcium and phosphorus may be present under the endocardium in cachectic conditions.

*Endocarditis* (inflammation of the endothelial lining of the heart) is bacterial, parasitic or mycotic in origin, most often affecting the valves (Plate 1, Fig. 5). The most common lesion is *verrucose* or *vegetative endocarditis* of pigs, a valuable diagnostic lesion of chronic swine erysipelas. The mitral valve is the main part involved, varying degrees of rough yellowish or greyish-yellow adhering to the valve, sometimes large enough to occlude the atrio-ventricular orifice. The chordae tendineae may also show vegetations. Streptococci, especially *Str. suis* type 2, are common causes of acute endocarditis in pigs (Lamont *et al.*, 1984).

Ulcerative valvular endocarditis due to streptococci or *C. (Actinomyces) pyogenes* is occasionally met with in the bovine, appearing as rough valvular plaques.

In sheep, verrucose endocarditis, when caused by *Streptococcus faecalis*, is usually seen on the bicuspid valve.

*Valve cysts* and *haematomata* of congenital origin, are frequent lesions in the hearts of young calves. In a survey in England of 1000 sows and 500 6-month-old pigs at slaughter, Jones (1980) found abnormalities of the valves (9.8%) and mural endocardium (1.2%). These consisted mainly of atrial ridges and plaques, thickened valves and non-vegetative endocarditis confined mostly to the left side.

## Myocardium

The main lesions encountered are myocarditis, fatty and hydropic degeneration, haemorrhages (see Endocardium), necrosis/abscessation, atrophy and pigmentation.

*Myocarditis* is an inflammation of the heart wall, *myocardosis* being a degenerative non-inflammatory disease of the myocardium. It is always secondary to pericarditis and endocarditis as part of systemic disease and is bacterial/toxaemic, viral or parasitic in origin.

Bacteria causing myocarditis include *Actinobacillus equuli, Clostridium chauvoei, Haemophilus somnus, Listeria, Salmonella pullorum* (see Poultry Diseases) and *Myco. tuberculosis* (rarely). The pyogenic organisms (*A. equuli, H. somnus, Listeria*) produce abscesses while *Clostridium chauvoei* causes lesions similar to those in muscle. Protozoa responsible include *Neospora, Sarcocystis* and *Toxoplasma* (q.v.).

*Fatty changes* appear as irregular light grey or yellow streaks and foci while *hydropic degeneration* assumes a uniformly greyish appearance and a softening of the cardiac muscle.

*Myocardial necrosis* is seen in the febrile diseases, especially foot-and-mouth disease, necrobacillosis due to *Haemophilus somnus* as well as porcine stress syndrome. Deficiencies of vitamin E, selenium and copper and certain plants, e.g. bracken fern and those containing gossypol (a toxic polyphenolic pigment) and glycosides, can cause cardiac necrosis when ingested. Coronary embolism or thrombosis causing obstruction of one or more arteries leads to infarction and necrosis. Affected areas are greyish-brown in colour but some may be so small as to be invisible.

*Abscesses* may be present in the myocardium of cattle as a result of foreign body penetration or resulting from metastases in cases of pyaemia, septic metritis, listeriosis, toxoplasmosis, Chagas' disease (*T. cruzi*) and some clostridial infections.

**Atrophy** of the heart is seen in cachectic conditions and may be associated with *xanthosis* (q.v.).

**Parasites** All the parasites which have an affinity for muscle may be found in the myocardium, especially the cysticerci of *T. saginata (C. bovis)* in cattle, of *T. solium (C. cellulosae)* in pigs and of *T. ovis (C. ovis)* in sheep. Larvae of *Linguatula* have been found beneath the epicardium in cattle, appearing as hard, elastic nodules with greenish-yellow necrotic centres. *Trichinella spiralis* cysts are occasionally encountered.

Lesions which may be confused with *C. bovis* but are due to the nematode *Cardophilus sagittus* are sometimes found in the hearts of cattle, buffalo and wild ruminants in various parts of Africa. The lesions are granulomatous in nature, usually sited in a coronary groove, and contain one or more coiled worms.

**Congenital conditions** of the heart are relatively few in the food animals. They include ectopia cordis (displaced heart), patent ductus arteriosus (pulmonary artery and aorta connected), atrial septal defect (failure of interventricular septum to develop), patent foramen ovale (failure of the fetal opening between the atria to close) and congenital haematomas (haemocysts). Most are unlikely to be encountered on meat inspection.

**Tumours** Most neoplasms occur as metastases from other organs, the most common being lymphosarcoma, mostly as a component of enzootic bovine leukosis. This takes the form of smooth pale yellowish areas which can be nodular or diffuse in form and from which a whitish milky fluid exudes on section. Mesothelioma, leiomyoma, haemangiosarcoma, myxoma, neurofibroma and rhabdomyoma may also be present.

## Blood vessels

While diseases of blood vessels (vasculitis or angiitis, comprising arteritis and phlebitis (inflammation of arteries and veins, respectively) are of little consequence *per se* in meat inspection, they are important entities in a host of infectious bacterial, viral, rickettsial, chlamydial, protozoal and parasitic diseases (see Nasal Passages and Paranasal Sinuses). Several non-infectious diseases – mulberry heart disease, mercury poisoning, serum sickness, staphylococcal hypersensitivity, purpura haemorrhagica (as a sequel to earlier *Str. equi* respiratory infection) and polyarteritis nodosa – also include vasculitis in their pathology.

*Aneurysms* (abnormal localised dilatations of blood vessels and the heart) are occasionally encountered, especially in thoroughbred horses and fast-growing male turkeys. The shape may be saccular, fusiform or dissecting. A *dissecting aneurysm* (more properly named *arterial dissection*) is a tear of the intima (inner endothelial layer) allowing blood to enter between the inner and outer layers and eventually burst through the thinner outer layer. The aorta, pulmonary and uterine arteries and atria of the heart are most often affected. Aneurysms are liable to *rupture*, often after strenuous exercise and parturition in the mare. The type in turkeys are dissecting aneurysms of the aorta or atria and may be associated with atherosclerosis due to copper deficiency, high dietary protein or aflatoxin poisoning.

*Arteriosclerosis* (hardening of arteries with loss of elasticity) and *atherosclerosis* (arteriosclerosis with fatty changes) are common in man but rare in animals.

In old cows the aortic wall may be thickened with calcareous deposits, while miliary TB of the bovine lungs is sometimes associated with an endarteritis of the aorta, the intima at the level of the aortic arch presenting roughened, ulcerated areas having a ridged appearance.

*Polyarteritis nodosa* is a rare condition in all the food animals in which the entire walls of medium-sized arteries and arterioles (hepatic, gastrointestinal, renal, coronary, skeletal) show focal points of necrotising inflammation usually with occlusive thrombosis. Chronic inflammation ensues to replace the necrotic with fibrous tissue. The weakened wall may develop into an aneurysm.

*Parasitic* or *verminous arteritis* is mainly caused by the parasites of the genera *Ascaris* (pigs), *Onchocerca* (ruminants) and *Strongylus* (horses) in the food animals.

In their migration, the infective larvae of *Ascaris suum* reach the liver via the portal vein after release from the adult worms in the small intestine. By breaking through the fine capillaries they cause haemorrhagic tracts in the liver substance which later heal and are replaced by fibrosis causing scars ('milk spots') which may become confluent. Extensive condemnations are often necessary. (*A. suum* may also cause similar lesions in lambs.) Larvae reaching the lungs via the systemic circulation produce focal haemorrhages in the parenchyma.

*Onchocerca armillata* causes lesions in the aorta (thoracic and abdominal), brachiocephalic trunk, brachial arteries and costocervical arteries of ruminants in Africa and Asia in which there are nodules and tracts in the walls.

*Strongylus vulgaris* fourth-stage larvae create necrotic/fibrinous inflammatory tracts in the walls of the cranial mesenteric and sometimes the renal, coeliac, spermatic arteries and the aorta.

Agents of parasitic thrombophlebitis include members of the family Schistsomatidae especially *Schistosoma bovis* and *S. matthei* and *S. japonicum*. They cause damage to the veins and venules of the liver, lungs, intestine and urogenital tracts by forming granulomatous nodules and fibrosis which may lead to occlusion.

## Blood

### *Anaemia*

*Anaemia* may be defined as a reduction in the concentration of circulating haemoglobin (Hb) below the normal range for the particular animal. It is occasioned by either the decreased production, increased destruction or loss of red blood cells (RBCs).

The immediate effect of anaemia is a reduction of the oxygen-carrying capacity of the blood, tissue hypoxia with pallor of the mucous membranes, slight fever, dyspnoea, weakness, weight loss, sometimes icterus and subcutaneous oedema, fatty changes in organs, compensatory heart dilation, etc., depending on the type of anaemia involved and its cause.

### *Classification and causes of anaemias*

1 *Failure of RBC production – bone marrow hypofunction.*

(a) Decreased RBC production: occurs in nutritional anaemia (protein, carbohydrate, cobalt, vitamin $B_{12}$ and folic acid deficiencies) and haematopoietic neoplasia.

(b) Decreased haemoglobin synthesis: occurs in iron and vitamins E and $B_6$ deficiencies.

(c) Viral infections causing marrow dysfunction – enzootic bovine leukosis, avian leukosis, equine infectious anaemia, retroviruses, etc.

2 *Loss of abnormal RBCs*

(a) Enzyme-deficient RBCs, hereditary anaemia.

(b) Immune-mediated anaemia, e.g. haemolytic disease of the newborn.

(c) Haemolytic anaemia causing vasculitis and coagulation.

3 *Loss of normal RBCs*

(a) Haemolysis of normal red cells – bacterial, chemical, plant and physical agents. *Bacterial haemolysis* – anaplasmosis, babesiosis, bacillary haemoglobinuria, ehrlichiosis, eperythrozoonosis, leishmaniasis, leptospirosis, trypanosomiasis, etc. *Chemical haemolysis* – benzene, toluene, lead, arsenicals, copper, molybdenum. *Plant haemolysis* – kale, rape, turnips, onions, castor beans. *Physical agents* – burns, exposure to cold, ingestion of cold water.

(b) External or internal haemorrhage (wounds, lacerations, uterine prolapse, dehorning, castration, tumours, abscesses, ulceration) and *parasitism. External parasitism* – ticks, mosquitoes, black flies, keds, lice, mites, etc. *Internal parasitism* (gastrointestinal parasitism) – *Haemonchus, Ostertagia, Cooperia,* etc.

**Lesions of anaemia** vary according to the basic cause and include pallor of the mucous membranes, occasional jaundice, pulmonary oedema with tracheal foam, hydroperitoneum, hydropericardium, hydrothorax, anasarca with oedema of the throat, pale musculature, cardiac dilation, fatty changes in the heart, kidney and liver, distended gall bladder (which may be empty), periacinar degeneration and necrosis of the liver, enlarged or atrophied spleen.

### *Leukaemia and leukoses*

*Leukaemia* is a primary malignancy of the blood-forming organs in which the leukocytes are replaced by large numbers of WBCs of a single type, e.g. lymphocytes, monocytes. There are two forms: *acute* which involves immature white cells; and *chronic* which involves mature or maturing cells, the most common type in the food animals.

*Leukosis* is the neoplastic proliferation of leukocyte-forming tissues and is sometimes used synonymously with leukaemia, lymphosarcoma, lymphomatosis and malignant lymphoma (see Enzootic Bovine Leukosis, Lymphoid Leukosis of Poultry).

*Acute leukaemia* is fairly rare in the food animals and is manifested by anaemia, pallor of mucous membranes, oedematous lymph nodes normal in size, enlarged spleen, pale marrow fat with haemorrhagic infarction, atrophy of thymus, condition good or slight loss, mild fever.

*Chronic leukaemia* is typified by *enzootic bovine leukosis* (EBL) which affects all ages of cattle (less than 3% are clinical cases) and exhibits anaemia, leukaemia, enlargement (often symmetrical) of the lymph nodes (which may occur throughout the body, especially behind the eye) and enlargement of the intestinal lymphoid tissue. The lymph node enlargement is not inflammatory in type but a generalised lymphoid hypertrophy.

The whitish, greyish or greyish-red tumours resemble bacon fat and are often interspersed with blood spots or larger haemorrhagic areas. In very enlarged lymph nodes, necrotic tissue is often apparent, being dry and orange-yellow in colour and sharply defined, especially in the marginal areas of the node. Although enlarged, these areas retain their shape and do not coalesce. On incision the surface bulges and a milk-like fluid exudes on pressure. The tumours may affect any body organ and may be found even in the spinal canal. In this invasive action the haemolymph nodes may be affected.

The spleen may be normal in size or greatly enlarged. When enlarged it is firm to the touch and there may be subcapsular haemorrhage which can result in death if the capsule bursts. The kidney lesions are nodules in the cortex which vary in size and project above the surface of the organ. The liver is usually affected with the spleen and is enlarged and friable, possessing rounded edges. There is usually a great tendency for the heart to be involved, the tumour assuming a nodular or diffuse form.

In young cattle of 1–2 years of age the thymus and the regional lymph nodes are grossly enlarged with tumours in the bone marrow.

In the *skin* form of EBL there are round, raised lesions, often with ulcerated surfaces, on the head, face and perineum.

*Sporadic* forms of bovine lymphoma occur unassociated with EBL virus infection.

*Sheep* and *goats* may be infected with lymphoma, especially the former, the disease being due to a retrovirus. Unlike EBL, leukaemia is absent, but pale yellow tumours are found in the liver, heart, spleen (which is enlarged) and kidneys.

In *pigs*, external and internal lymph nodes are enlarged with lymphocytosis, anasarca, eyeball protrusion and loss of condition.

In *horses*, lymphoma occurs in two forms: leukaemia with reduced blood RBC, WBC and platelets, anaemia, subcutaneous oedema and fever; and lymphoid tumour formation affecting virtually all parts of the body.

**Haemoglobinaemia** Excess haemoglobin in the blood plasma is manifested in the live animal by a haemoglobinuria, the presence of free haemoglobin in the urine, which appears dark red or blackish in colour. In the true form of the condition the haemoglobin has emanated from RBCs haemolysed in the blood and is commonly seen in diseases such as babesiosis, bacillary haemoglobinuria (*Cl. haemolyticum*), anaplasmosis and post-parturient haemoglobinuria in dairy cows.

### *Judgement of diseases of the cardio-vascular system*

In general, those conditions forming part of a systemic disease with marked circulatory disturbance merit total condemnation. More localised entities may warrant partial condemnation, conditional approval following heat treatment or approval with restricted distribution. All judgements must be based on the overall evidence and carcase condition supported, where necessary, with laboratory tests (microbiological and chemical).

**Total condemnation (T)** Acute septic and bovine traumatic pericarditis with fever and circulatory disturbance (systemic disease). Acute verrucose endocarditis with associated lung and liver lesions (systemic disease). Widespread lymphosarcoma. Anaemia – part of a systemic disease. Haemoglobinaemia.

**Conditional approval following heat treatment (Kh)** Subacute pericarditis with no complications. Ulcerative and verrucose endocarditis without complications.

**Approval as fit for human consumption (A)** Chronic bovine traumatic pericarditis. Chronic pericarditis without complications. Chronic ulcerative endocarditis without complications. All non-infectious heart conditions. Anaemia due to haemorrhage from trauma (possible partial condemnation). Localised abscesses, arteritis, arteriosclerosis, atherosclerosis, aneurysms and tumours without complications.

**Tumours of the haematopoietic (bloodforming) system** Haemangioma, haemangioendothelioma, haemangiosarcoma, lymphangiosarcoma, telangiectasis, leukaemia, lymphoma.

## LYMPHORETICULAR SYSTEM

This system is composed of the thymus gland and bone marrow (primary lymphoid organs), and the lymph nodes, spleen and lymphoid tissues (secondary lymphoid organs) both of which are involved in important body defence mechanisms.

## Lymph nodes

Besides acting as a filter for various foreign agents, the lymph nodes are involved in the immune response (q.v.), supplying B cells from their outer cortex and T cells from their deeper tissues. Although in the normal state they are small and hardly palpable, when affected by disease they become enlarged, sometimes oedematous and haemorrhagic, and react in specific ways to invading microorganisms and other invaders.

An examination of the lymph nodes is a valuable guide to the nature and gravity of many diseases, including tuberculosis, although the form of examination in the bovine and pig warrants modification in many countries today where TB is no longer a major problem. Multiple incisions often create more contamination, often with *Salmonella*, *Campylobacter*, etc., revealing little of pathological value to assist in judgement of the carcase and its viscera.

A survey of lymph node lesions in 171 000 cattle slaughtered in Ontario, Canada in 1987 showed 0.4% to be affected, the principal diagnoses being abscesses (51% of all lesions), actinobacillary granulomas (36%) with smaller percentages of mycotic and parasitic lymphadenitis and tuberculosis (Herenda and Jukes, 1988).

**Lymphadenitis** Inflammation of the lymph nodes may be either acute or chronic. It is a sequel in various infections and must be distinguished from hyperplasia of the lymph node which is not associated with infection.

**Acute lymphadenitis** occurs in the pyogenic infections, e.g. streptococcal lymphadenitis of pigs (cervical or jowl abscesses), and many acute and peracute bacterial and viral diseases, e.g. anthrax, acute swine fever, pasteurellosis of lambs (*P. multocida*), rinderpest, salmonellosis, strangles, tularaemia. It is manifested by swelling, congestion, mobility and oedema of the node which is painful and softer than normal as shown by the so-called 'strawberry' lymph nodes of acute swine fever and anthrax. When the changes are due to pyogenic bacteria, abscess formation is likely.

*Chronic lymphadenitis* is manifested by development of fibrous connective tissue of the node, which becomes enlarged and indurated. Some oedema and congestion may be present, but not regularly, and the nodes may be adherent to adjacent tissues. Such changes are observed in caseous lymphadenitis, bovine actinobacillosis and tuberculosis, and in the supernumerary lymph node in bovine chronic mastitis and brucellosis. Granulomatous cervical lymphadenitis is encountered in the submaxillary lymph node of pigs caused by *Rhodococcus (Corynebacterium) equi* and is sometimes mistaken for TB. The same organism also occurs in cases of bovine lymphadenitis.

**Hyperplasia** of the lymph node indicates an increase in its size due to the formation and growth of new cells. It may be follicular or diffuse in type but is more a reflection of histopathology, being difficult to distinguish from chronic lymphadenitis and, especially, lymphosarcoma.

Lymph node *atrophy* is seen in old animals, especially those in poor condition. The nodes are very small and show dark brown pigmentation.

**Pigmentary changes** in the lymph nodes, especially of the bronchial group, are seen as a result of inhalation of coal dust (anthracosis) in cattle and sheep grazing in urban areas and near collieries. Xanthosis (q.v.) occurs in bovine lymph nodes and melanosis in those of sheep.

**Parasitic infections** are not uncommon in lymph nodes, occurring during migration and lodging accidentally. Larvae involved include those of *Linguatula serrata* (common in the mesenteric nodes of cattle and sheep); *Muellerius* spp. and *Protostrongylus* spp. (bronchial nodes of sheep and goats causing a granulomatous lymphadenitis); *Oesophagostomum columbianum* (mesenteric nodes of sheep) and *F. hepatica* (mesenteric nodes of cattle and sheep); *Strongylus vulgaris* (abdominal nodes of equidae causing a haemorrhagic lymphadenitis).

## Lymphatic vessels

*Lymphangitis* (inflammation of the lymphatic vessels) is prominent in many of the specific diseases affecting the lymph nodes as well as epizootic lymphangitis of equidae (*Histoplasma farciminosus*) (Plate 2, Fig. 8), ulcerative lymphangitis of horses (*Corynebacterium pseudotuberculosis* (*ovis*)), glanders, cutaneous dermatophilosis of cattle, sheep, goats and horses, Jöhne's disease, bovine intestinal TB, mycotic lymphangitis (bovine farcy) due to *Mycobacterium farcinogenes*, sporadic lymphangitis (Monday-morning disease in horses). The normally indistinct lymphatic vessels appear as swollen, firm cords under the skin which may rupture, ulcerate and exude pus (cf. epizootic lymphangitis).

*Lymphoedema* is an abnormal collection of lymph due either to a congenital lymphatic defect (absence of lymphatics) or to lymphatic obstruction, injury, inflammation or tumours. There is extensive subcutaneous oedema seen especially in the limbs, head and neck with hydroperitoneum and hydrothorax. The condition is sometimes seen in Ayrshire calves.

**Tumours of the lymphoreticular system** See tumours of the haematopoietic system and enzootic bovine leukosis above.

## Spleen

*Enlargement* of the spleen (splenomegaly) with hyperaemia occurs in the acute specific diseases (vide RBC haemolysis under anaemia and EBL above). The most important disease in relation to splenomegaly is bovine septicaemic *anthrax* in which the spleen is very large, soft and liable to rupture, exuding very thick, dark-red or blackish blood which brightens on exposure to the air. (Suspect anthrax cases must always be cleared first of all by negative blood smear examination before decomposition takes place.) An enlargement of the spleen is not so marked in the pig.

Splenomegaly is a constant finding in bovine salmonellosis, in which the spleen is congested and contains tiny foci or nodules of necrosis (*'board spleen'*). Similar changes are seen in sheep, pigs and horses. Chronic enlargement of the spleen may also be seen in liver stasis resulting from swine erysipelas, traumatic pericarditis, leukaemia (*'burst spleen'*), lymphoma and virtually all cases of anaemia.

Tuberculosis of the spleen arising from haematogenous spread produces tubercles and an enlarged spleen and is common in pigs, less so in cattle.

*Abscesses* in the spleen may be associated with melioidosis (*Pseudomonas* (*Malleomyces*) *pseudomallei*) in all the food animals, especially pigs. The encapsulated abscesses vary in size but are usually less than 1 cm in diameter and project above the spleen surface. They contain thick, creamy or yellowish-green pus which later becomes inspissated. Clinically normal animals may have splenic abscesses. Caseous lymphadenitis may also show one or two splenic abscesses, goats and sheep being mainly affected.

In addition to these specific diseases, pyogenic abscesses in the spleen may result from foreign body trauma – sharp metal objects from the reticulum of cattle and stomach of horses being responsible. In horses the perforation of stomach ulcers by the worms *Gasterophilus* spp. and extensions of granulomata due to *Habronema* spp. larvae can establish splenic abscesses.

*Congenital defects* are rare. The spleen may be absent or duplicated in pigs, calves and lambs.

*Haemorrhages* and *haemorrhagic infarcts* are valuable diagnostic lesions in classic swine fever. *Haemorrhages* of traumatic or agonal origin associated with slaughter are sometimes seen beneath the splenic capsule in healthy cattle. Haemorrhage and *rupture* of the spleen may be occasioned by severe injuries, e.g. during transportation.

Splenic congestion and enlargement may occur in cattle from the use of an inordinately long *pithing rod ('slaughter spleen')*. Enlargement of the spleen has also been noted in pigs stunned by certain forms of captive bolt pistols and sometimes by electrical methods. The placing of pigs in scalding tanks while still conscious has been known to produce splenomegaly.

*Torsion* of the spleen leads to enlargement and is brought about by the loose attachment of the organ to the stomach, the whole spleen or its lower portion rotating on its long axis to cause passive congestion and acute swelling. Passive congestion with enlargement of the spleen, which assumes a dark bluish colour, can also occur in some haemolytic anaemias and in defects of the systemic and portal circulation. Chronic congestion may result in complete *necrosis* – not uncommon in healthy pigs which are unaffected clinically.

*Parasites* occasionally found in the spleen – echinococci, encysted liver flukes, *C. tenuicollis* and *Linguatula* larvae.

*Cysts*, other than parasitic, are rare in the spleen. They are either neoplastic in type (haemangioma, haemangiosarcoma) or degenerated haematomas.

*Infarcts* caused by occlusion of end-arteries are not uncommon and may be associated with ulcerative endocarditis in the pig. They are initially haemorrhagic in type, conical in shape and raised above the spleen surface, but later become pale and cause considerable shrinkage and distortion of the organ.

*Amyloidosis* may be present as part of a generalised condition without splenomegaly.

*Tumours* are relatively rare, haemangiomata being the most common primary neoplasm. Lymphosarcoma, EBL, haemangiosarcoma, squamous carcinoma, leukaemia and melanoma are occasionally found.

### Thymus

The regression of the thymus with age, although it never completely disappears, makes the organ relatively unimportant in meat inspection except in young animals.

The thymus, like other organs, may be absent (aplasia) in neonatal deaths, or show inflammation, necrosis, atrophy, hyperplasia, hypoplasia and neoplasia. Inflammatory changes are present in classic swine fever (with atrophy in the chronic form), bovine immunodeficiency virus infection and EBL. Numerous fine petechial haemorrhages are evident in cases of lead poisoning.

*Tumours*, most often seen in cattle and goats, include benign thymoma (consisting of epithelial and lymphoid cells and associated with hyperplasia of the thymus) occurring mainly in year-old cattle, lymphoma (unassociated with EBL), lymphoid thymoma, lymphosarcoma (EBL).

#### *Judgement of lymphoreticular lesions*

**Total condemnation (T)** All situations involved with systemic disease and marked circulatory disturbance.

**A, Kh, I** or **L** All other localised and chronic lesions. (I = meat showing minor deviations from normal but fit for human consumption; L = approved fit for human consumption, with distribution restricted to limited areas.)

## URINARY SYSTEM

### Kidney

The functions of the kidneys in metabolism, fluid balance and excretion make it, along with urine assessment, an important system for close inspection, especially in the haemolytic anaemias, toxaemias and uraemia. Regard has to be given to their shape, size, colour, consistency, and presence of abnormalities.

Renal disease is not uncommon in the food animals, especially in cattle. A survey of the prevalence and type of kidney lesions in cattle was carried out in a Dublin abattoir during 1979–80 (Monaghan and Hannan, 1983). Of 4166 animals examined, 173 (4.2%) had abnormal kidneys, the rejection rate in cows, bullocks, heifers and bulls being 7.7%, 1.7%, 2.2% and 28%, respectively. The most common reason for rejection was focal interstitial nephritis (60.1%), followed by cysts (26.0%), pigmentation (6.4%), pyelonephritis (3.5%), amyloidosis (2.9%), glomerulonephritis (0.6%), renal atrophy (0.6%) and agonal haemorrhage.

*Nephritis* is an inflammation of the kidneys and, depending on the part involved, may be broadly divided into glomerulonephritis (glomeruli), interstitial nephritis (interstitial tissues), acute tubular necrosis (tubules) and pyelonephritis (pelvis and calyces), although overlapping occurs. The term *nephrosis* refers to any kidney disease in which degenerative changes occur in the tubules, although it is sometimes used to denote tubular degenerative and inflammatory changes.

*Glomerulonephritis* usually occurs as a part of bacterial and viral systemic disease, e.g. chronic swine fever, bovine virus diarrhoea, campylobacteriosis, trypanosomiasis etc., but it can develop as a primary disease in the *'thin sow syndrome'* (a combination of malnutrition, internal parasitism, too frequent mating and early weaning, etc.) and following the consumption of certain poisons. In the *acute* form the kidneys are enlarged, pale in colour, oedematous and may show fatty changes and petechial haemorrhages. In *chronic glomerulonephritis* the kidneys are shrunken owing to fibrous tissue formation and the surface has a granular uneven appearance.

A hereditary deficiency of the complement-inhibitory protein factor H has been shown to lead to the development of lethal membranoproliferative glomerulonephritis in weaner pigs of the Norwegian Yorkshire breed but not in the Norwegian Landrace breed. The disease is controlled by identifying carriers using an enzyme immunoassay for porcine factor H and preventing them from breeding.

*Interstitial nephritis* may be acute or chronic, septic or non-septic, and focal or generalised. The *acute* type is seen in leptospirosis in cattle and pigs, malignant catarrhal fever, lumpy skin disease, sheep pox and theileriosis and where irritant substances (similar to those causing toxic hepatitis) have been ingested. Kidney enlargement with fatty changes and necrosis result, the colour being very pale, even whitish in colour. In acute leptospirosis in cattle and pigs, the kidneys are enlarged and diffusely dark in colour but later assume a lobular haemorrhagic coloration which finally becomes greyish owing to fibrosis.

Numerous fine foci (initially fine abscesses), which later become nodules, may be found in the kidneys of calves (*'white spotted kidney'*/ nephritis fibroplastica) owing to *E. coli*, *salmonella* or *Brucella abortus* represent infection in the *chronic* form. In this case the kidneys are atrophied due to fibrosis. They affect some 1% of calves in the UK but disappear during the first year of life, usually before 6 months of age.

*Septic interstitial nephritis* is manifested by the presence of abscesses in the cortex, either as a few large foci or as numerous microabscesses (the number is inversely proportional to their size). It may arise from within the kidney (urogenous) or by haematogenous spread by septic emboli from a pyaemia or pyogenic ulcerative endocarditis, the septic emboli lodging in the renal artery or its branches (glomerular or tubular capillaries) to produce septic *infarcts* and *embolic septic nephritis*. If the renal artery is affected, the entire kidney becomes necrotic, while smaller vessels produce the typical conical-shaped infarct. Hyperaemic and red at first, the infarct soon becomes pale, then necrotic and finally fibrosed. A common cause in horses is *Actinobacillus equuli*.

*Pyelonephritis* is a fairly common disease in cows, generally occurring as a sequel to parturition, but it also affects sows (mainly the acute form). It is rare in calves, horses, sheep and goats. It attacks the kidney pelvis and parenchyma and results from ascending infection. As with other kidney infections, it may be acute, chronic, septic or non-septic.

The condition is probably a mixed bacterial one but a prominent organism appears to be *Eubacterium suis*. In 23 cases of porcine pyelonephritis and cystitis examined in 1993, Carr and Walton (1993) isolated *E. suis* in 21, other organisms present being *E. coli*, *Enterococcus faecalis* and a streptococcus.

Pyelonephritis may be unilateral or bilateral and is manifested by catarrh and dilatation of the renal pelvis which is filled with a slimy, detritus which may contain fibrinous clot or pus and possesses a strong ammoniacal odour. The acute form begins with inflammation and necrosis of the renal crest (projection of the renal medulla into the pelvis containing the openings of the tubules). At this stage the parenchyma is swollen, dark red and firm. Haemorrhages may also be present in the acute stage. If infection extends along the uriniferous tubules, it may give rise to abscesses in the cortex and irregular grey areas on the kidney surface. Occasionally, the infection causes complete obliteration of the kidney parenchyma, making the organ a purulent sac.

As the disease progresses in more typical situations, chronic tubulointerstitial nephritis supervenes with progressive fibrosis. Scarring with contraction of the fibrous tissue and loss of kidney tissue produce marked contraction and distortion of the organ even to virtual obliteration of some lobes. In very severe cases, the kidney assumes a greyish, nodular appearance, becoming very small in size.

*Cysts* of congenital origin are common in the kidneys, especially in pigs and sheep, less often in cattle. They may be single or multiple, single cysts being quite large – up to several centimetres in size – while multiple forms vary from tiny translucent specks to about a centimetre in diameter. Clear fluid is contained within their transparent walls which usually protrude from the surface. Cysts, however, may occur deep in the parenchyma. While most cysts are the result of dysplasia some may be caused by obstructive lesions, e.g. retention cysts in chronic nephritis/pyelonephritis.

*Aplasia* (complete absence of kidney) and *hypoplasia* (incomplete development) of one or both kidneys are also hereditary in origin. A survey in England (Wells *et al.*, 1980) showed an incidence of 47.5% in pigs from one producer, all being the progeny of one Landrace boar.

Renal *dysplasia* (abnormality of development) may also take the form of persistence of fetal lobulation (pig), horseshoe kidney and other abnormal shapes.

*Nephrosis* (acute tubular necrosis) is a term used to denote any kidney condition in which there are degenerative changes. *Hydronephrosis*, caused by mechanical obstruction to the flow of urine along the ureters, is seen in all the food animals, but is especially common in pigs. The obstruction, complete or incomplete, originates in the bladder, urethra or ureter, urinary calculi being a common cause. The pelvis and ureters are dilated, often with such pressure as to obliterate the kidney tissue with the formation of a large cyst filled with urine (pressure atrophy). Unilateral hydronephrosis is most commonly caused by twisting and occlusion of a ureter, which results in extensive destruction of parenchyma. Bilateral hydronephrosis may be due to a chronic cystitis or to obstruction of the urethral lumen by calculi and is a more serious condition.

**Urinary calculi (uroliths)** Kidney stones are mainly concretions of carbonate, oxalate, silica, struvite (a combination of magnesium ammonium phosphate hexahydrate), urate and xanthine resulting from metabolic sources – high content of minerals, etc., in feed, pasture and water, deficiency of vitamin A, presence of mineral-precipitating substances such as mucoproteins and mucopolysaccharides. They are fairly common in feedlot cattle in the USA.

Uroliths are more common in males because of their anatomy, urinary calculi being most liable to form in the sigmoid flexure of the urethra of male cattle and sheep. Early castration prevents full development of the genital organs and may contribute to urolithiasis. Uroliths are not uncommon in horses.

Calculi may form in any part of the urinary system, even in the collecting tubules of the kidney. The most common sites are the sigmoid flexure of the penis of steers and bulls and the vermiform appendix of rams and the bladder of horses, all of which sites may be involved in mucosal ulceration with urinary stasis, urethritis, cystitis and clinical signs.

Uroliths vary in size and shape from small, hard, granular material to large, spherical, ovoid, irregularly-shaped lamellated stones. Their colour may be white, yellow, grey, dark brown or brownish-red.

Renal *amyloidosis* in cattle occurs as an enlarged, pale, firm left kidney, deposits of amyloid being present in the medulla and glomeruli (Monaghan, 1982; Monaghan and Hannan, 1983).

**Pigmentations** Accumulations of various pigments are often seen in the course of major diseases, mainly in cattle, e.g. haemosiderin (brown colour), following haemolytic anaemia and haemoglobinuria: lipofuscin (brown) in xanthosis/haematochromatosis (q.v.); haemoglobin (dark brown to black) in acute haemolytic diseases such as babesiosis (the black coloration may be seen in animals long recovered from babesiosis); cloisonné kidney (black); bile pigments in icterus and methaemoglobin in chronic copper poisoning (greenish-yellow) and porphyrin (brown) (q.v.).

**Parasites:** Parasites are not common in the kidneys of the food animals.

*Stephanurus dentatus*, the kidney worm of pigs, is a serious affection of swine in tropical and subtropical countries. Infection occurs by the ingestion of infective larvae, which can also gain entrance via the skin. After a long migration, the larvae reach the liver by the portal circulation and pierce the capsule to arrive in the perirenal tissues, from which they penetrate the ureters (which become thickened and sometimes occluded) and produce cysts in the ureters, kidney pelvis and sometimes the kidney tissue. Cysts may also occur in the adjacent perirenal tissues, pancreas, liver, spleen and psoas muscles. Eggs are laid in the ureters and kidney pelvis and passed out in the urine.

*Dioctophyma renale*, the giant kidney worm, occurs in the pig, ox and horse worldwide. Intermediate hosts include mud-worms, fish and frogs. After ingestion, the infective larvae penetrate the gut wall to reach the peritoneal cavity and finally the kidney where they encyst in the pelvis, producing a haemorrhagic and septic pyelitis. Kidney parenchyma is gradually destroyed in severe cases, only exudate and the capsule being left. Aberrant forms may also create cysts in the bladder, uterus and udder.

The blood fluke, *Schistosoma mattheei*, is sometimes responsible for causing granulomas in the kidney pelvis, having escaped from the portal and mesenteric veins.

*Setaria* spp. filarioid worms of the family Onchocercidae, are usually found in the peritoneal cavity of ungulates. The larval forms of *Setaria digitata*, however, are occasionally responsible for granulomata in the bladder of cattle and buffalo.

The thorny-headed worm, *Macracanthorhyncus hirudinaceus*, occurs worldwide, except in western Europe. It normally inhabits the small intestine of the pig (where it causes an ulcerative enteritis). Aberrant forms may occasionally be found in the kidney pelvis.

In severe infestations, hydatid and *C. tenuicollis* cysts may be present in the kidneys of sheep and cattle.

**Tumours** Primary neoplasms are rare but metastatic forms are fairly common and tend to involve both kidneys. In metastatic lymphosarcoma the kidneys are enlarged and mottled yellowish-white, the projecting growths being either diffuse or nodular. In avian lymphoid leukosis the kidneys are enlarged with diffuse miliary or nodular tumours, while avian myeloid leukosis is diffuse in form, the kidneys being mottled with a granular surface.

Embryonal nephroma (nephroblastoma) is a congenital primary tumour not infrequently seen in pigs at the anterior end of the bovine kidney in contact with the adrenal gland; it is usually localised and well encapsulated. It is normally unilateral and can attain a huge size, but is usually about the size of an orange. Section reveals large areas of haemorrhagic greyish-white necrosis interspersed with yellowish connective tissue resembling the adrenal cortex. In the USA embryonal nephroma is regarded as the most common tumour of swine. Adenomas occur rarely and mainly affect cattle and horses.

Renal carcinomas occur in cattle and sheep and appear as discrete round or oval grey or yellowish growths, often haemorrhagic and necrotic, which can become larger than the actual kidney.

## Urinary bladder, ureters and urethra

The *bladder* may be involved in specific bacterial and viral disease in the same way as the kidneys and other organs, showing cystitis with congestion and haemorrhages in classic and African swine fever, salmonellosis in pigs, purpura haemorrhagica in equidae. Cystitis, often combined with pyelonephritis (see kidney), ureteritis and urethritis, may also occur as a localised infection following trauma, urolithiasis (see Kidney), neoplasia, the ingestion of irritant substances and infection from the urethra.

Acute cystitis produces a mild catarrh with hyperaemia and submucosal oedema or a more severe haemorrhagic, fibrinous or diphtheritic type. The urine is cloudy and contains mucous.

Chronic cystitis shows as irregular thickening and folding of the mucosa, which may also show polyps, and is often associated with tumour formation.

*Rupture* of the bladder may follow urolithiasis of the urethra, difficult parturition, injury or tumour erosion.

## Urine

*Haematuria* (blood in the urine) is present in cases of trauma, septicaemia, purpura haemorrhagica, acute glomerulonephritis, certain poisonings, tumour formation, ulceration of the bladder and urethra mucosa. The blood may be present as clots (red colour) or as a faint reddish or brownish turbidity.

*Haemoglobinuria* (presence of free haemoglobin in the urine, which is coloured brown or deep red) occurs when red cells are lysed in the course of specific diseases such as the parasitic diseases of the blood (anaplasmosis, babesiosis, theileriasis, etc.), haemolytic anaemias, bacillary haemoglobinuria (*Cl. haemolyticum/novyi*) and post-parturient haemoglobinuria in cows.

*Myoglobinuria* follows severe muscle damage, e.g. in azoturia in horses in which the urine is coloured dark brown.

*Uraemia* (*azotaemia*) denotes an excess of nitrogenous end-products (urea, creatinine, etc.) of protein and amino acid metabolism in the urine. It is associated with chronic renal failure, e.g. in urinary tract obstruction by a calculus or tumour, glomerulonephritis, pyelonephritis, interstitial nephritis, hydronephrosis and rupture of the bladder. Azotaemia occurs during the course of several diseases, e.g. equine haemoglobinuria (azoturia, Monday morning disease), visceral gout in poultry, amyloidosis, pericarditis and congestive heart failure.

Uraemic carcases usually emit a strong urinous odour which may persist for a considerable period depending on the degree of uraemia. Suspect carcases should be detained for 24 hours and then subjected to a boiling test.

**Tumours of the bladder, ureters and urethra** follow the same general pattern as for the kidney except for papillomata which occur fairly often in the bladder and lymphomatosis which is of rare occurrence.

### *Judgement of diseases of the urinary system*

Assessment of carcases follows the same lines as for the cardiovascular system, viz. the total evidence is gleaned, including the results of microbiological and chemical tests, carcase condition, etc. If the case is associated with an acute systemic disease with marked circulatory disturbance, total condemnation is warranted. Chronic and localised conditions may merit more lenient treatment.

**Total condemnation** Nephritis associated with uraemia. Septic and embolic nephritis. Pyelonephritis (bovine) with uraemia. Cystitis with uraemia. Rupture of the bladder with uraemia.

**Approved as fit for human food** Cystitis, chronic cystitis, chronic nephritis, renal calculi, renal cysts, pigmentation, pyelonephritis, localised tumours. All without systemic effects.

## REPRODUCTIVE SYSTEM

The reproductive system, apart from the uterus and udder, is generally not given extensive attention in the course of meat inspection. It is, nevertheless, liable to many defects and diseases, some of which can influence a final judgement, apart from providing useful feedback information.

*Abnormalities of genetic development* include hermaphrodites (in which ovaries and testes are present in varying degrees in the same individual), freemartins (sterile females born co-twins with males), agenesis and hypoplasia of the ovaries, imperforate hymen (with distension of the vagina, cervix and uterus with fluid), double cervix, double vagina, absence of uterine cornu. Most of these abnormalities are noted at birth, mainly in calves and piglets, many of which succumb at an early age.

In a survey of 1380 *porcine genital tracts* in Zimbabwe, Obwolo and Lawson (1992) found *abnormalities* in 27.1% as follows: hydrometra in 314 (22.75%), muscular hypertrophy of the cervix in 97 (7.03%), bilateral hydrosalpinx in 21 (1.52%), muscular hypertrophy of the uterus in 16 (1.16%), cervicitis in 7 (0.51%), mucometra in 7 (0.51%), hypoplasia of the vulva in 6 (0.43%), bilateral follicular ovarian cysts in 6 (0.43%), with smaller numbers of unilateral aplasia of the ovary and fallopian tubes, cervical hyperplasia and stenosis of the vulva.

### Ovary and Fallopian Tubes

One or both ovaries may be absent (agenesis) or underdeveloped (hypoplasia) which occurs in the freemartin in cattle.

*Haemorrhage* of the bovine ovary may arise during ovulation or from enucleation of corpora lutea. *Pyometra* – an accumulation of pus in the uterus may result in *adhesions* between the ovary and the oviduct, in which case the oviduct may show septic inflammation (*pyosalpinx*).

The ovary appears to be resistant to most *infections* but may show granulomatous lesions of bovine TB and be affected in some viral diseases, e.g. herpesvirus.

Various forms of *cysts* are probably the most common lesions found in cows and sows and include serous inclusion cysts, follicular cysts and dermoid cysts. *Inclusion cysts* are small epithelium-lined structures not unlike follicular cysts occurring on the surface or deep in the ovarian tissue. *Follicular cysts* (*cystic follicles*) are the most common forms in cows and sows. They develop from graafian follicles which fail to ovulate or undergo regression and may be difficult to distinguish from normal follicles, except when they reach a large size. They may be single or multiple, unilateral or bilateral, and usually possess a thick wall with some adherent lutein tissue but no ovum. *Lutein cysts* (cystic corpora lutea) have partially or completely luteinised walls and appear as single or multiple smooth, spherical bodies.

### *Ovarian tumours*

- *Primary*: Granulosa-theca cell tumour (cow, mare, ewe), a benign tumour arising in the granulosa cells surrounding the ovum; luteoma, haemangioma, dysgerminoma, teratoma and leiomyoma.
- *Secondary*: Lymphosarcoma (probably the most common metastatic tumour); carcinoma.

*Hydrosalpinx* is a collection of fluid in the fallopian tube caused by an obstruction of the lumen resulting in distension of the tube.

*Pyosalpinx* is a collection of pus in the oviduct following septic metritis.

*Salpingitis*, inflammation of the fallopian tubes, is usually associated with serous, catarrhal or septic inflammation of the uterus.

## Uterus

Like other organs, the uterus may be involved in atrophy, hypoplasia or hyperplasia of the endometrium.

*Metritis*, or inflammation of the uterus, is bacterial in origin and usually occurs as a result of a retained placenta, injury or rupture of the uterine mucosa during parturition; less commonly it may arise from decomposition of the fetus *in utero*.

Serous, catarrhal and septic forms may occur. The very serious *septic metritis* is manifested in cows by high fever, very fast pulse, muscular weakness, severe depression and, in many cases, recumbency and inability to rise. The vulva is very swollen and a discharge, at first serous, then yellowish, red or chocolate in colour with a foul odour, is evident. Tympanitis usually occurs if peritonitis is present, and when the temperature reaches 41.5–42°C death often follows in 3–4 days from septicaemia/toxaemia.

Post-mortem examination shows the uterus to be two or three times larger than normal and containing a large amount (sometimes several gallons) of chocolate or greyish-coloured fluid composed of effused blood and the remains of fetal membranes. The mucous membrane of the affected uterine horn is thickened, dirty brown or dark green in colour, softened and covered with diphtheritic exudates and blood clots found mainly at the base of the maternal cotyledons, which are greyish in colour, pulpy and almost detached from the uterine mucosa. The walls of the uterus are thickened owing to inflammatory oedema, while the peritoneum, especially over the uterus, may be highly congested and covered with pseudomembranous layers of fibrin. Toxic infection of the carcase is manifested by gross enlargement of the iliac, lumbar, sacral and ischial lymph nodes. There is generalised congestion of the carcase with degenerative changes in the parenchymatous organs.

*Chronic endometritis*, on the other hand, is a fairly common localised affection in cows and is characterised by a mucopurulent vaginal discharge but without general disturbance.

*Pyometra* (pus in the uterus) due to *Actinomyces pyogenes* also often occurs without systemic change, though longstanding cases may result in emaciation. Pyometra is sometimes seen in maiden heifers suffering from *white heifer disease* which usually affects white Shorthorn heifers and is a partial aplasia of the uterus with retention of uterine endometrial secretions.

*Uterine abscesses* are fairly common in cattle and may follow metritis or injury (sometimes associated with obstetrical manipulations). They are often found on the dorsal wall of the uterine body and may be small and numerous or single and large.

*Contagious equine metritis* (CEM) is a highly contagious disease of mares caused by the coccobacillus *Taylorella equigenitalis*, which can be present subclinically in the prepuce of stallions, infection being transmitted during coitus. A thick, mucopurulent discharge accompanies the endometritis.

*Prolapse* of the uterus commonly occurs in cattle and sheep and is associated with dystocia, retained placenta and forced traction at parturition. There would appear to be an inherited disposition in some ewes.

*Rupture* of the uterus may involve the whole uterine wall or only the mucosa. It is usually due to obstetrical operations but can follow torsion and is accompanied by haemorrhage, which is fatal if extensive.

*Torsion*, or twist of the uterus, sometimes occurs in cows and is responsible for dystocia. It may be complete or incomplete. If the former occurs in a gravid uterus, the uterus become oedematous and congested and any fetus present becomes mummified. Rupture may also be a sequel.

In *brucellosis* there is a placentitis with a fetid seropurulent exudate between the uterine lining and the chorion and in some cases a leathery appearance of the placenta with necrosis of the cotyledons. To minimise human infection and prevent possible contamination of the meat in *Brucella* reactor and other suspect *Brucella* cases, uteri and udders should not be incised or handled with bare hands. The uterine lesions in *campylobacteriosis* resemble those of brucellosis but are not so marked. The areas between the cotyledons are oedematous and opaque (and sometimes leathery), while the cotyledons are pulpy and yellowish in colour.

*Tuberculosis* may affect the uterus, occurring usually as numerous small granulomatous tubercles in the endometrium in the miliary form or as a caseous type with gross thickening of the mucosa. Large amounts of yellow pus-like curdled milk are discharged.

*Mummification of the fetus* occurs without bacteria being involved, in which case there is no constitutional disturbance or adverse effect on the carcase. It occurs most often in the sow which is a multiparous species. The fetus becomes black or brown in colour and leathery in appearance and with further dehydration finally becomes a hard shrunken mass of skin and bones. This mass may be expelled from the uterus in multiparous animals (producing several offspring at a time) or retained indefinitely in uniparous animals (producing one offspring at a time).

The presence of bacterial infection such as *Campylobacter* or *Clostridium chauvoei* results in *fetal maceration and emphysema*, the fetal tissues appearing as a soft, grey mass with gas formation.

*Abortion* is the premature expulsion of a dead fetus from the uterus and occurs during the course of many infectious diseases – brucellosis, bovine virus diarrhoea, classic swine fever, enzootic abortion of ewes, epizootic bovine abortion, campylobacteriosis, equine herpesvirus, equine viral arteritis, mycotic abortion, listeriosis, leptospirosis, Q fever, salmonellosis, toxoplasmosis, yersiniosis, etc. Mycotic abortion may be caused by *Aspergillus, Mucor, Absidia, Rhizopus* fungi.

*Stillbirth* is the delivery of a dead, fully-formed neonate.

*Hydrops amnii (hydramnios fetalis)* indicates an excess of fluid in the amniotic sac and is often associated with fetal deformity in cows and ewes.

*Hydrops allantois (hydrallantois)* is an excess of fluid in the allantoic sac and is usually connected with uterine placental disease in cows.

## Vagina and vulva

Both these organs show inflammation in several infectious diseases: vulvovaginitis due to *Mycoplasma agalactiae* var. *bovis*, infectious pustular vulvovaginitis (IPV) caused by bovine herpesvirus-1, infectious bovine cervicovaginitis (cytomegalovirus), granular vaginitis (*Ureaplasma* infection), necrotic vaginitis and vulvitis in cows and ewes, and dourine (*Trypanosoma equiperdum*) in equidae.

*Trauma* of the vagina and vulva occurs frequently in connection with difficult parturition in all species and is generally less serious than uterine injuries. Laceration of the vagina and vulva may also follow vaginal prolapse, robust service from a large bull or even a malicious act by a human being. It may, however, be followed by sepsis, gangrene and peritonitis.

### Tumours of the uterus, vagina and vulva

Squamous cell carcinoma of uterus (cows and mares); adenocarcinoma of the endometrium and cervix (cows, mares, rabbits); fibropapilloma of the vulva (cows) and a transmissible form in the prepuce of boars; diffuse and nodular forms of lymphosarcoma of uterus and vagina (all species, especially cows); leiomyoma and leiomyosarcoma of uterus (cattle and sheep).

*Polyps* may occasionally occur in the endometrium of cattle as sessile, spherical non-neoplastic structures.

## Mammary glands

*Mastitis*, or inflammation of the udder, is a common condition in all species, especially cows, and is caused by a wide variety of bacteria (streptococci, staphylococci, *E. coli, Corynebacterium, Pseudomonas, Mycoplasma, Klebsiella, Cryptococcus, Proteus, Citrobacter, Actinomyces (Corynebacterium) pyogenes, Fusobacterium, Bacteroides, Myco. tuberculosis*), *Pasteurella haemolytica* (ewes), *Corynebacterium pseudotuberculosis* (ewes), etc.; fungi (*Aspergillus, Trichosporon*); and yeasts (*Candida, Neoformans*).

In the cow the commonest form of *mastitis* is caused by *Str. agalactiae* and is essentially a catarrh of the milk ducts which is mostly chronic in nature and unaccompanied by systemic disturbance but can sometimes be acute. Lesions include interstitial oedema, fibrosis (diffuse or nodular) causing induration of one or more quarters, swollen glandular tissue and stringy clots in the reduced milk secretion. Resolution may occur but progressive fibrosis leads to atrophy of the quarter(s). *Staphylococcal mastitis* is more severe, even peracute, and may eventually result in moist gangrene with the teat or quarter assuming a bluish or blackish colour. Adjacent lymphatics are dilated, the supramammary, iliac and lumbar lymph nodes are enlarged and oedema is evident in the vicinity of the udder. Secretion is reduced and is brownish in colour or blood-stained.

Bovine mastitis due to *A. pyogenes* (summer mastitis) is associated with a severe toxaemia, which may be fatal. It is essentially a severe suppurative mastitis which progresses to necrosis.

*Tuberculosis* of the cow's udder is haematogenous in origin and second in prevalence to pulmonary TB. Usually chronic in form, it may affect one or more quarters, most often hind quarters. It occurs in three main forms – chronic organ tuberculosis (most common), caseous TB mastitis and disseminated miliary tuberculosis. In *chronic organ TB* the mammary tissue is indurated, lobulated, reddish-white in colour and when cut, projects above the organ surface. Caseation usually occurs with collection of exudate in the sinuses but the supramammary lymph node is unaffected. The *caseous* form shows as large yellowish, cheese-like areas surrounded by hyperaemic zones. *Miliary TB mastitis* takes the form of numerous typical caseous or calcified nodules, about 1 cm in size, which project above the surface when the glandular tissue is cut.

Mastitis in *sheep* can occur in a peracute, gangrenous form due to *Staph. aureus* with less severe cases being associated with the same organism and other staphylococci, streptococci, *E. coli*, *C. pyogenes* and *Past. haemolytica*.

*Contagious agalactia* (CA) in the *ewe* and *goat* due to *Mycoplasma agalactiae* is not unlike bovine summer mastitis; the udder is swollen and hot, milk secretion thick and yellowish and sometimes contains pus and/or blood. One or both glands are indurated with fibrosis, brownish-black in colour and later atrophied. Abortion, arthritis and conjunctivitis may complicate the disease. Other forms of mastitis (catarrhal, suppurative and gangrenous) are common in the ewe. Although the udder is removed in dressing, portions of the supramammary lymph nodes usually remain *in situ* and should be removed. Enlargement with oedema of these nodes is present in acute forms along with oedematous infiltration of the external abdominal wall.

Abnormalities of the udder of the ewe are a common cause for culling. A survey of the mammary glands of 1650 culled ewes in southern England revealed gross lesions in 211 (12.8%), of which 77% were abscesses (Madel, 1981). Earlier surveys confirmed this high incidence of abscesses in the substance and on the surface of the udder, obviously the sequelae of mastitis.

Mastitis in the *sow* may be caused by *Staph. aureus* or *Actinomyces bovis* and is granulomatous in type and chronic affecting one or more glands; the type due to *E. coli* is oedematous with a scanty serous or blood-stained secretion containing clots of fibrin.

*'Seedy belly'*, a form of *melanosis* in the udders of sows, takes the form of round, black spots in the mammary tissue.

**Tumours of the mammary glands** Adenoma and adenocarcinoma are relatively rare.

## Testes

One or both testes may be absent *(agenesis)*, reduced in size (hypoplasia), undescended (*cryptorchidism*) or associated with female organs, e.g. ovaries (*hermaphroditism*) in all species. Incomplete descent of the testes (*cryptorchidism*, rig, ridgling) is most common in the horse and is usually unilateral, the undescended small, indurated testicle being found in the peritoneal cavity at any point during its descent from near the kidney to the internal inguinal ring.

Testicular inflammation (*orchitis*) and *degeneration* can occur during the course of several toxaemic diseases, e.g. brucellosis, trypanosomiasis, anaplasmosis, babesiosis, ionising radiations, noxious metals and plants, deficiency diseases, hormonal factors, etc. In the early stages of orchitis the testes are enlarged and oedematous but later become smaller owing to degenerative changes in the parenchyma. Fibrosis and calcinosis may be final results of degeneration.

*Epididymitis* (inflammation of the epididymis) in the bull is probably more common than orchitis, infection usually resulting by extension from the upper genitourinary tract. Various microorganisms are involved – *Brucella, Actinobacillus seminis, Actinomyces pyogenes, E. coli, Streptococcus* spp. *Mycoplasma, Corynebacterium pseudotuberculosis,* etc. The organ becomes enlarged and may assume a nodular appearance, with abscess formation a frequent occurrence. Epididymitis is not uncommon in rams, in which the epididymis is swollen irregularly, the causal organism often being *Actinobacillus seminis.*

The *spermatic cord* may be acutely or chronically-inflamed and is most common in horses, pigs and cattle, being caused by staphylococci. The chronic form (*schirrhous cord* or botryomycosis) appears as a granulation mass with numerous tiny abscesses, fistulae and foul-smelling exudate. The condition is not uncommon in castrated pigs. Granulomata of the spermatic cord may be caused by aberrant larvae of *Strongylus* spp.

### Penis and prepuce

Developmental abnormalities include hypoplasia and aplasia of associated structures.

*Balanitis* (inflammation of the penis) and posthitis (inflammation of the prepuce) occur in most species as a result of specific diseases such as dourine due to *Trypanosoma equiperdum* and *equine coital exanthema* (equine herpesvirus-3) in the stallion, bovine herpesvirus-1 in the bull, and in male goats. The abundance of commensal microorganisms in the prepuce (*Corynebacterium renale, A. pyogenes, Pseudomonas aeruginosa, Mycoplasma* spp., *E. coli*, streptococci, *Proteus*, chlamydia, protozoa and fungi) is often responsible for local inflammatory changes which include hyperaemia, sepsis, necrosis and ulceration with varying forms of exudates (serous, catarrhal and purulent). Ulcerative balanitis and posthitis are often seen in rams and wethers, one venereal form being associated with vulvovaginitis in ewes.

The penis and prepuce are liable to injury and rupture. Injury may be the cause of *paraphimosis* – inability to retract the penis in the stallion due to its swollen condition or a constriction of the preputial orifice.

**Tumours of the penis and prepuce** Fibropapilloma (bull), squamous cell carcinoma (horse, bull) and squamous papilloma, lymphosarcoma, haemangioma (all species).

*Judgement of conditions of the reproductive system*

**Total condemnation** Acute septic, necrotic or diphtheritic metritis with circulatory disturbance. Presence of putrefied fetus with systemic effects. Septic, necrotic or gangrenous mastitis with sytemic effects. Retained placenta with systemic changes. Dystocia with acute metritis and vaginitis. Prolapse, torsion and rupture of uterus with peritonitis and fever. Septic and gangrenous mastitis with general signs Malignant neoplasms with extensive metastases.

**Approved as fit for food with disposal of affected part:** All chronic and localised conditions without systemic effects and satisfactory carcase condition, subject, where necessary, to results of laboratory examination.

*N.B.* (1) *Because of the prevalence of subclinical mastitis in the bovine, it is recommended that all udders be rejected for food.* (2) *In cases of* Brucella *reactors and suspects, uteri, vaginas, vulvas and udders should not be incised or handled with bare hands. Appropriate instruments should be used in dressing operations along with suitable arm and face protection for careful disposal.*

## SKELETAL SYSTEM

### Bone

*Terms*

- *Diaphysis* – shaft of long bone containing medullary cavity.
- *Epiphysis* – wide end of long bone.
- *Epiphyseal cartilage (physis)*, plate, disc – thin growth area between epiphysis and diaphysis which later ossifies.
- *Metaphysis* – part of shaft beside epiphyseal disc containing growth zone and new bone.
- *Articular cartilage* – layer of hyaline cartilage covering epiphyses and forming articular surface of joint.

Genetic and developmental defects, systemic and metabolic disease, malnutrition, and endocrine imbalances may lead to bone deformities such as angular distortions in limbs, rickets, osteomalacia, osteopetrosis, osteoporosis, chondrodysplasia, osteodystrophia fibrosa etc. Some deformities are unlikely to be encountered at meat inspection since they occur in fetuses dying at or soon after birth.

Bone is also liable to injury (*fractures* being a common reason for casualty slaughter) and infection (osteitis, osteomyelitis, spondylitis, arthritis).

Variations of length, shape and thickness occur in the *physis* (part of bone involved in the lengthening of long bones), in the shape and density of the *epiphysis* (end of bone adjacent to articular cartilage) and in the *articular cartilage* itself. Limb deformities affect all species, especially horses and cattle. In foals the lower limbs (carpus, tarsus and fetlocks) are most commonly involved. Changes related to the cartilages may be associated with osteochondrosis.

*Rickets* is a disease of *young* animals in which there is defective mineralisation of growing bones (Plate 2, Fig. 12). The corresponding condition in *adult* animals is *osteomalacia*. The main function of vitamin D (which also acts as a hormone) is to maintain adequate plasma levels of calcium and phosphate in conjunction with parathyroid hormone. Both diseases are associated with a deficiency, impaired metabolism or malabsorption of vitamin D and phosphorus leading to failure of mineralisation (calcification) of bones, which become abnormally soft. Rickets is characterised by softening, swelling and curvature of the weight-bearing bones and widening of the epiphyseal plates at joints. The costochondral junctions are swollen forming the so-called *'rickety rosary'* and advanced cases may show deformity of the spine, pelvis and skull. It is characteristic of rickets and osteomalacia that the ends of affected bones are easily cut by a knife. Rachitic young pigs may exhibit little more than swelling of the joints and button-like rib enlargements, but the condition is usually associated with emaciation.

Rickets in chicks is often caused by dietary deficiencies (vitamin D, phosphate, calcium) and toxicities (hypervitaminosis A, mycotoxins).

*Osteomalacia* (softening of bones) due to phosphorus deficiency develops in grazing animals in areas devoid of this mineral in the soil, e.g. South Africa and northern Australia. Cattle, and less commonly, sheep and pigs, are affected and crave phosphorus-rich substances, even bones. Long bones, ribs and pelvis become liable to fracture and distortions of the skeleton are evident. A deficiency of vitamin D in grass and fodder can also lead to osteomalacia, especially in sheep, in the same regions and even in the UK. In the early stages the animal may be well-nourished, but progression involves muscular atrophy with serous infiltration of the intermuscular connective tissue.

*Osteoarthritis* is one of several degenerative, non-inflammatory diseases which are more common in horses (spavin, ringbone, navicular disease, curb) than in the other food animals. These have various causes – nutritional, hereditary, developmental, traumatic, possibly autoimmune – with some unknown. Pigs, cattle and sheep are less prone to osteoarthritis, which mainly affects the hip and stifle joints. The articular cartilage becomes degenerated, bone is transformed into an enlarged ivory-like mass and the joint capsule becomes fibrosed and calcified. *Osteophytes* (bony outgrowths) are common in the affected joint.

*Osteitis* and *osteomyelitis* (inflammation involving the medullary cavity) are not uncommon in cattle. These terms are often used synonymously. Some cases are traumatic in origin, e.g. a contaminated fracture, and some haematogenous from a pyogenic focus. All are caused by bacteria (staphylococci, streptococci, *Fusobacterium necrophorum, E. coli, A. pyogenes,* salmonella spp., *Brucella suis,* etc.). Examples are atrophic rhinitis (q.v.), poll evil and fistulous withers in horses, and bacterial polyarthritis. There is cloudy exudate, dilated vascular sinusoids in marrow spaces and later pus formation and bone necrosis. A sequestrum of dead bone may form with new bone round it. Pus eventually tracks to the surface via a sinus.

*Osteochondrosis (dyschondroplasia)* is an abnormality of growth of cartilage of unknown origin which occurs in pigs, horses, turkeys, fowls and young bulls. The bones most commonly affected are the humerus, ulna, scapula and thoracic and lumbar vertebrae. The lesions may appear as an incomplete or complete separation of articular cartilage from the underlying bone (osteochondritis dissecans), or conical cores of articular cartilage may project inwards into the metaphysis. Loose plaques of cartilage may break into small granules and disappear or larger plaques ossify. Fibrocartilage eventually fills the defect.

*Osteodystrophia fibrosa* occurs in all the food animals and is caused by oversecretion of parathyroid hormone leading to a deficiency of calcium and/or vitamin D with excess phosphate. Bone is replaced by fibrous tissue, resulting in thickening and distortion of bones of the head and in advanced cases those of the body with liability to injury and fracture.

*Osteogenesis imperfecta* (*paperbone disease*) is a rare inherited condition seen mostly in Charolais and Holstein calves and lambs. The neonates are stunted and their bones very thin and brittle and liable to fracture.

*Osteopetrosis* or *marble bone disease* occurs in the rabbit, horse, sheep, ox and pig. The disease is inherited and is sometimes seen in Hereford, Holstein, Simmental and Aberdeen-Angus calves. Affected neonates are stunted and possess overshot jaws, protruding tongue and sloping forehead. Long bones are shorter than normal and, like those of the head, vertebrae and others, are compact, dense and fragile.

*Osteoporosis* is a lesion in which there is a resorption of bone tissue in part or all of the skeleton giving bones a cancellated appearance and making them light and fragile. It may be due to malnutrition, deficiency of calcium, phosphorus or vitamin A, endocrine dysfunction, senility or disuse. It occurs on rare occasions as a complication in avian leukosis complex.

The most common specific infection of bone occurs in *actinomycosis* in cattle (q.v.). Other infections of bone include tuberculosis, brucellosis, coccidiodomycosis and abscesses associated with pyaemia (q.v.). In brucellosis, abscess formation takes place, especially in calves and pigs, in which exostoses may develop. The lesions of coccidiodomycosis resemble those of bovine TB and appear as greyish granulomatous nodules in bone marrow with or without pus.

*Presternal calcification* or *putty brisket* is occasionally encountered in the cushion of the bovine brisket and less frequently in sheep. Repeated trauma is usually the cause. The lesion is essentially a fat necrosis and is manifested by irregular putty-like masses in the presternal fat, the necrotic tissue eventually becoming calcareous.

*Parasitic infections* of bone are rare, although hydatid cysts may occur, distinguished from tuberculosis by the absence of involvement of the associated lymph nodes.

*Xanthosis* occasionally occurs as a pigmentation of bone in young cattle and pigs.

*Skeletal disorders* are fairly common in all classes of *poultry* and include rickets/osteomalacia, twisted leg, crooked toes, splay legs, ruptured achilles tendons, scoliosis (lateral deviation of the vertebral column), and tibial dyschondroplasia (q.v.), spondylolisthesis (subluxation of a deformed 4th thoracic vertebra with compression of the spinal cord).

*Fractures* are a frequent cause of emergency slaughter in all classes of food animals. Recent cases display considerable blood clotting and gelatinous infiltration around the fracture with congestion of the adjacent lymph node. Old fractures which have healed by callus formation are common in the ribs of cattle, sheep and pigs.

**Tumours of bone and cartilage** Bone tumours may be primary or secondary arising as malignant metastases from other sites such as the lung, mammary gland and skin. Benign tumours include osteoma, chondroma, fibroma, the equivalent malignant forms being osteosarcoma, chondrosarcoma and fibrosarcoma. All are relatively uncommon in the food animals.

## Joints

*Arthritis*, or inflammation of the joint, synovial membrane and articular surfaces, usually involves periarticular tissues. It may be infectious (from a penetrating wound, extension of infection from a nearby focus or blood-borne) or non-infectious. One form of the latter is typified by *gout* in which sodium urate crystals are deposited in the synovial fluid and tendon sheaths, which occurs in articular gout in poultry.

The condition may be acute or chronic, septic or non-septic and fibrinous and may affect one or several joints (polyarthritis) (q.v.). Bacteria involved include streptococci (all species), *Actinomyces pyogenes* (cattle, pigs) *E. rhusiopathiae* (pigs, sheep), *Actinobacillus suis* (pigs), *E. coli* (pigs, cattle, sheep), *Chlamydia* spp. (sheep), *Haemophilus* spp. (sheep, pigs), *C. pseudotuberculosis* (sheep), *Salmonella* spp. (pigs, horses), *B. abortus* (cattle), and *Mycoplasma* spp. (cattle, sheep).

Arthritis is a very common cause of partial and total condemnation, especially in pigs. A survey of 51 843 pig carcases in Australia examined in an abattoir revealed arthritis in 554 (1.07%). Total rejection was necessary in 147 (0.28%) and partial rejection in 407 (0.79%). The joints most frequently involved were the stifle, tarsus, carpus and elbow. Partial condemnation was higher in the 16–55 kg dressed weight range than in the heavier carcases. It was suggested that undetected arthritic lesions, possibly containing *E. rhusiopathiae*, were finding their way to the consumer (Cross and Edwards, 1981).

In *non-septic* arthritis (other than gout) the synovial fluid is opaque, sometimes blood-tinged, and there is a proliferation of synovial villi which gives the synovial membrane an appearance of being covered with a red pile. Some forms of polyarthritis may be non-septic.

*Fibrinous* arthritis of bacterial origin is hyperaemic and oedematous in type. The synovial fluid is increased in amount and turbid. In later stages the villi are greatly enlarged and show granulation tissue. Healing may occur by cessation of the inflammatory process or by fibrosis.

*Septic* arthritis in a single joint may be due to a penetrating wound or part of a specific septicaemic disease, e.g. tick pyaemia, joint ill, melioidosis and polyarthritis. The disease also occurs in calves as a complication of omphalophlebitis and in cows as a sequel to septic metritis. Affected joints are swollen and the synovial membrane is oedematous and thickened. The synovial fluid is increased in amount, turbid and, in later stages, purulent. Ulceration of the synovial lining takes place and the adjacent tendon sheaths are infiltrated with serum. Longer-standing cases show erosion of articular cartilage which may become completely detached from the epiphysis. Further progression may lead to purulent osteomyelitis with complete destruction of the epiphysis.

*Septic omphalophlebitis* or *navel ill*, especially in calves and piglets, is most frequently caused by pyogenic organisms, although at times by *Salmonella* spp. and *F. necrophorum*. The infection is acquired after birth, usually by the umbilicus which is hard and swollen with borders infiltrated with a serosanguineous or purulent fluid. A large abscess may sometimes be found in the abdominal wall near the umbilicus. Alternatively, abscesses may occur in the substance of the liver. The umbilical vein in places is filled with blood clot which is partially or completely transformed into a dirty red, foul-smelling mass. If the inflammation has extended to the peritoneum, adhesions may be found between the intestine, omentum and liver.

A common cause of emergency slaughter in the cow is *luxation of the hip joint* which, if accompanied by rupture of the round ligament, can result in severe bruising in the surrounding tissues. This deep bruising may require a special incision to detect it. A less severe condition in the heavy bovine may occur during hoisting to an overhead rail.

*Bursitis*, or inflammation of a bursa (a small sac containing clear fluid inserted under ligaments and tendons near joints to avoid friction) occurs mostly at the elbow ('capped elbow'), knee ('capped knee'), hock ('capped hock'), shoulder or hip mainly in horses and cattle.

A *hygroma* is an undue accumulation of fluid in a bursa, sac or cyst. Poll evil and fistulous withers in horses are forms of bacterial infection (*B. abortus*, *Streptococcus zooepidemicus*, *Actinomyces bovis*, etc.) and parasitic (*Onchocerca cervicalis*) involvement of the supra-atlantal bursa.

Most cases of bursitis are initially caused by trauma. There is an increase in clear serous fluid, which in infected cases becomes purulent, this occurring especially in poll evil and fistulous withers with the formation of granulation tissue and a tendency to fistulate to the exterior.

**Tumours of joints** Sarcoma and synovioma of the synovial membrane are rare.

### *Judgement of diseases of bone and joints*

**Total condemnation** Fractures, with infection and general effects. Gangrenous/suppurative osteomyelitis. Arthritis – acute infectious, purulent or fibrinous. Generalised tumours. Septic omphalophlebitis.

**Approval as fit with seizure of affected part** Fracture, uncomplicated. Localised osteomyelitis. Pigmentation. Chronic non-infectious arthritis. Presternal calcification. Osteofluorosis. Bursitis. Hygroma. Osteoporosis. Localised xanthosis. Actinomycosis. Localised parasitic infestations. Localised tumours.

## MUSCULAR SYSTEM

Various *congenital deformities* of muscle and tendons occur in all species, some being associated with defects in the spinal cord and motor nerves. They include one or more crooked joints (arthrogryposis), contracture and rigidity of joints, splayleg, diaphragmatic clefts, muscular hypoplasia and hyperplasia, muscular dystrophy and muscular steatosis.

*Atrophy* of muscle may be due to severe malnutrition, senility, disuse, denervation, ischaemia, injury to motor nerves and pressure, e.g. from tumours. Wasting of the shoulder and foreleg muscles of cattle and sheep is often due to radial nerve paralysis.

*Hypertrophy* of individual muscle fibres occurs in overactivity and, with *hyperplasia* (increase in the total number of fibres), involves an increase in muscle size. The latter is seen in the quest for increased productivity of meat in all the food animals. In cattle the so-called, but erroneous, 'double muscle' effect occurs in many breeds, the Belgian Blue being a typical distortion, as is the increase in breast muscle in some turkey breeds.

(Atrophy, hypertrophy and hyperplasia are forms of myopathy which are diseases of skeletal muscle excluding those of inflammatory and neural origin.)

### Myositis

Inflammation of muscle may be part of a specific disease, e.g. eosinophilic myositis, bluetongue, toxoplasmosis, foot-and-mouth disease, clostridial infections (blackleg, braxy, malignant oedema) (q.v.). It may also occur as a local lesion in which *abscesses* are formed in the muscle due to *Haemophilus* spp., *Actinobacillus* spp., *Actinomyces pyogenes, C. pseudotuberculosis*, streptococci and staphylococci. These abscesses are normally due to non-sterile inoculations and penetrating wounds.

*Actinobacillosis* commonly affects the masseter and tongue muscles with normal tissue being replaced by varying amounts of fibrous tissue interspersed with the typical nodular lesions (q.v.).

### Parasitic diseases of muscle

*Eosinophilic myositis* is a relatively rare condition occurring mainly in cattle, with sheep less often affected. Individual muscles or groups of muscles are affected with well-defined greenish, brown-green or grey-green focal stripes or patches which become whitish on exposure to air. The greenish colour is due to the presence of eosinophils which accumulate in and between the muscle fibres, causing them to necrotise. Lesions may also be present in the myocardium and even throughout the whole musculature. In chronic cases there is excess connective tissue formation which replaces degenerated muscle fibres. There is now good reason to associate this form of myositis with degenerating *Sarcocystis* spp. since remnants of these sporozoan parasites are found in the centre of the lesions.

*Sarcocystis* spp. have dogs, foxes, wolves and other carnivores as definitive hosts from which sporocysts are liberated in the faeces. Sporocysts ingested by the intermediate hosts release sporozoites in the intestine to invade many forms of tissues. The sporozoites develop in the endothelium of blood vessels into schizonts, the second or third generation of which encyst in striated muscle fibres and produce bradyzoites some three months after infection. The cycle is completed when the infested flesh is consumed by a definitive host.

Sarcocysts in cattle: *S. cruzi, S. bovifelis, S. hominis.*

Sarcocysts in sheep: *S. tenella, S. ovicanis.*

Sarcocysts in pigs: *S. porcifelis, S. miescheriana, S. porcifelis.*

Sarcocysts in horses: *S. bertrami, S. fayeri.*

*Toxoplasma gondii* (q.v.) and *Neospora* spp. (q.v.) may occasionally be seen in muscle.

*Onchocerca gobsoni, O. gutturosa* and *O. lienalis* (q.v.) are common in Australia and North America in the tendons, e.g. ligamentum nuchae (*O. gutturosa*) and connective tissues of cattle.

*Cysticercosis* is due to *C. bovis (T. saginata), C. cellulosae (T. solium)* (q.v.).

*Trichinellosis* is due to *Trichinella spiralis* (q.v.)

In severe infestations, *hydatid cysts* and *cysts of Multiceps multiceps* may be found in muscles.

All parasitic infestations of muscle show a marked tendency to degenerate and become calcified; greenish foci or calcareous nodules are almost certainly of parasitic origin.

*Interstitial myositis* or muscular fibrosis, is usually seen in imported hindquarters of beef but may also occur in home-bred stock. The normal muscular tissue is replaced by bands of white fibrous connective tissue, the lesion being usually localised in the round of beef but sometimes occurring in the shoulder and lumbar muscles. The probable cause is trauma.

*Roeckl's granuloma (nodular necrosis)* is occasionally found in cattle of various ages. It is characterised by greyish-yellow nodules (walnut to golf ball in size) of a firm elastic consistency, encased in fibrous tissue in the muscles and under the skin of the tail, neck, shoulder, back, croup and limbs. They are usually fairly superficial – not deeper than 2.5 cm – but can also be found in the viscera, the liver, lungs, testes and lymph nodes in particular. No specific cause has been found.

## Myodegeneration

Muscles may undergo *degeneration*, being seen in severe toxaemic cases, while hyaline degeneration occurs in haemoglobinaemia in horses and in milk fever in cows. Hyaline changes appear as pale muscle somewhat resembling the flesh of fish. The condition may also affect the diaphragm, abdominal and intercostal muscles in pigs, the affected muscles being so watery in nature that they can be easily penetrated.

Nutritional myodegeneration involving the ventral serratus muscles has been recorded in young Friesian cattle turned out to pasture in the spring. These muscles, the main attachment of the scapula to the thoracic wall, ruptured as a result of degeneration, causing the chest to drop and the scapulas to protrude above the thoracic spine, the so-called *'flying scapulas'* (Gunning and Walters, 1994).

*White muscle disease* (*WMD*), *nutritional myopathy, stiff lamb disease, enzootic muscular dystrophy* of calves and lambs is an important myodegeneration associated with an inadequate intake of selenium (q.v.). It may also occur in goats, foals, deer, rabbits and poultry.

A form of myopathy, similar to WMD, has been noted in cattle and horses which have undergone moderate physical stress during transport, the animals showing acute stiffness, the lesions at post-mortem resembling those of WMD.

See also porcine stress syndrome and dark, firm dry (DFD) muscle.

*Calcification*, and even *ossification*, may follow degenerative changes and various injuries.

*'Yellow fat' disease (nutritional steatitis, nutritional panniculitis)* is a form of myodegeneration which occurs in piglets and foals. It is associated with an excess of unsaturated fatty acids and deficiency of vitamin E and other antioxidants in the diet as represented by the feeding of fish and fish offal which has become rancid. *Ceroid* pigment is deposited in the adipose tissue which is coloured greyish, the fat itself being soft and possessing a fishy odour. The muscle degeneration is accompanied by gastric ulceration and degenerative changes in the liver.

*Muscle injuries* are extremely common, most often occurring from external trauma and probably constituting the most common reason for casualty slaughter. In addition to a degenerative cause, muscle, especially the diaphragm, can *rupture* during energetic exercise or following myositis, the muscle bulging at the end opposite to the rupture. *Hernias* occur when the muscle protrudes through the overlying fascia.

## Muscular haemorrhages or splashing

Haemorrhages associated with slaughter may be seen in various locations, e.g. large intestine of sheep, endocardium of calves and beneath the splenic capsule of cattle, but those of most interest to the meat inspector occur in skeletal muscles. Here they appear as dark-coloured streaks somewhat resembling brush marks or as a collection of dark red spots varying in size from being scarcely visible to as large as 30 mm.

The muscular portion of the diaphragm is probably the area most frequently affected. Splashing may also be evident on the inner aspect of the thoracic or abdominal wall and, in cattle, on the neck and the longissimus dorsi muscle. In the pig it may be found in any muscle but most often in the hip, thigh, loin, diaphragm and shoulder. At times the lymph nodes draining tissues affected with splashing are suffused with blood. The frequency of blood splash in pigs is sometimes related to their close confinement in sties with little exercise. Such a situation also results in muscles heavily infiltrated with fat and disposed to rupture.

Much research has been carried out on the cause of blood splashing and its prevention.

The main factors involved are thought to be undue delay between stunning and bleeding and the increased blood pressure arising from violent muscle contractions at stunning. Blood pressure is likely to be raised by a long journey or pre-slaughter stress and it is noteworthy that the incidence of splashing is lower in animals that have been rested. Hot weather and excitement before slaughter may also be implicated.

The rise in arterial blood pressure following stunning is immediately caused by vasoconstriction but this effect does not occur in the capillaries, which are virtually passive tubes, their diameter being controlled by the state of tone of the blood vessels supplying them. When the arterioles are constricted the capillaries contain relatively little blood, but when the stimulus which causes vasoconstriction ceases, e.g. when the tongs are removed from the head in electrical stunning, the arterioles immediately dilate and blood rushes into the capillaries. The capillaries, their walls already weakened by anoxia, permit the passage of blood into the surrounding tissues, possibly by rupture or diapedesis.

The higher the blood pressure the more severe will be the impingement of blood on the capillary wall when vasodilatation occurs. Any factor, such as excitement, that elevates the blood pressure prior to slaughter predisposes to splashing. Conversely, any procedure which rapidly reduces the blood pressure following stunning, e.g. immediate bleeding, will reduce the occurrence of splashing.

The UK Meat Research Institute at Bristol has assessed the overall incidence of blood splash in sheep at 10%. Its occurrence has increased with the introduction of electrical stunning. A study of 2700 lambs showed that electrical stunning (either at 90 V and 50 Hz or 130 V and 1500 Hz) produced a much higher frequency of muscular haemorrhages than captive bolt stunning.

In addition to stunning techniques, it is likely that other factors such as diet may be involved. *Anticoagulant compounds* such as coumarins in certain pastures may be responsible for prolonging the blood-clotting time as well as making the capillaries more fragile and liable to rupture (Winstanley, 1981).

For *rigor mortis* see Chapter 2.

## Downer syndrome

This is a neuromuscular-skeletal paralysis with recumbency and inability to rise which occurs most often in the cow but can affect all other species. It develops as a result of various factors – injury to bone, muscles, joints, nerves, fractures, dislocations, etc., or as a sequel to a metabolic disorder such as milk fever or gross tetany in the cow, in which it is most common. It may also follow acute mastitis and dystocia but the term is usually applied to *parturient paresis* cases.

The condition occurs in heavy animals when a limb is flexed under the body, the weight of the animal creating ischaemia in certain muscles after prolonged recumbency. Although the syndrome is seen most often in hindlimbs, forelimbs may be involved.

Downer syndrome is a very common reason for casualty slaughter and one which presents great difficulty in judgement for reasons of condition, oedema, injuries, presence/absence of antibiotic residues etc.

**Lesions** Pressure on the affected limb leads to muscle ischaemia due to the collapse of veins and arteries. The affected muscles are swollen and oedematous and the area in contact with the floor shows superficial sores and muscle blanching. Continued pressure causes infarction of the muscles, which become dark in colour and haemorrhagic, these changes being more severe in the depths of the muscles. In very prolonged cases scar tissue may be evident as irregular patches in the muscle tissue.

## Bruising

A *bruise* is caused by the release of blood from ruptured vessels into surrounding tissue. Bruises may occur on or in any part of the animal body but the vast majority in cattle involve the hip area (loin damage), in pigs the ham area, and in sheep the hindleg. Bruising may be slight, causing little or no trimming, or so extensive that the whole carcase must be condemned.

In the USA an estimated $61 million is lost each year due to bruising and it appears to be increasing. A considerable proportion of the huge loss is attributable to poor transportation, especially by contractors. The rough handling that causes bruising can also reduce carcase weight, tenderness, colour and flavour.

In Australia the relative susceptibility of cattle of different sexes was assessed in five trials (Yeh *et al.*, 1978). It was found that bruising was more serious in cows than in steers based on the amount of meat trimmed from carcases. The extent of bruising in cows, but not in steers, increased with longer transportation.

Two recent surveys in the UK (McNally and Harris, 1992) showed that of a total of over 16 000 carcases, animals from live auctions had more bruising and more meat rejected for bruising than animals from dealers and farms. The proportion of carcases with *stick markings* was higher in market cattle (2.5%) than in cattle from farms (0.9%). The amount of bruising was much higher in animals which were stick-marked (35%) than in the whole population surveyed (6.5%). Young bulls had the lowest percentage of bruising and the least amount of meat rejected of all the categories of animals surveyed. There was less 'important' bruising in animals travelling less than 50 miles from markets, but over 50 miles the amount of important bruising did not increase. However, the incidence of all bruising increased with the distance travelled and with the time the animal spent in the lairage. More than half the carcases surveyed (59%) had some degree of bruising caused by pre-slaughter handling. The areas most frequently bruised were the butt and hip, loin, shoulder/foreleg and neck, hindleg and flank/brisket. The number of carcases with an ultimate pH (pHu) of over 5.8 and the average pHu of the muscle increased with the amount of carcase bruising. The average weight of meat rejected from each carcase was 0.308 kg from the most valuable parts of the carcases. At a wholesale value of £2 per kg this loss due to bruising was estimated at £616 per 1000 cattle slaughtered. If the survey at this particular plant were representative of the whole UK meat industry, the total losses from the 2.8 million cattle slaughtered annually would amount to approximately £1.7 million.

However, it was found that the loss from down-grading was 1.75 times greater than the loss due to trimmed bruised tissue (Grandin, 1980). If this figure were to apply to the British meat industry, the overall annual loss would be £4.5 million.

Besides the actual loss of meat, the act of trimming is time-consuming, adds to meat inspectors' duties and interrupts the operation of the meat plant. A very serious animal welfare situation is also involved.

In addition to muscle and fat damage, the act of bruising can also damage hides, fleeces and skins, the problem being all too common in horned and mixed stock.

Defects in flooring (rough surfaces, jagged edges, uneven slats, etc.) in vehicles, byres and even meat plant lairages are responsible for many injuries, especially to limbs but also to other parts of the body. Pigs in particular are affected, some even developing shoulder abscesses.

A troublesome condition in hams, incorrectly termed *ham bruise*, is a haemorrhagic area seen at the inner aspect of the ham anterior to the head of the femur. It is caused by escaped blood-stained fluid from the hip joint as a result of tearing of the round ligament and rupture of the joint capsule, and is brought about largely during shackling and hoisting of the pig to the overhead rail for bleeding. A similar condition occurs in cattle.

### *Age of bruises*

This can with some accuracy be gauged visually; for the first few hours bruises are red and haemorrhagic; at 24 h they are dark coloured, becoming watery up to 38 h; after 3 days bruises have a rusty appearance and are soapy to the touch.

The *bilirubin test* for bruise age has not justified initial claims. The test depends on a colour reaction between Fouchet's reagent and bilirubin, the breakdown product of haemoglobin from the haemorrhage. There is no useful colour change with early bruises; older ones can be seen visually without a test.

Another test for bruise age is available in kit form. It measures the circulating blood levels of two enzymes (glutamic-oxaloacetic transaminase) (GOT) and creatine phosphokinase (CPK), which are released from damaged muscle tissue.

The most accurate method of dating bruises comes from forensic medicine. This depends on the recognition of *haemosiderin*, a breakdown product of haemoglobin and particular cell types. It is, however, unsuitable for large numbers of samples and requires experienced personnel.

## Injection abscesses

Necrosis, abscesses or localised areas of oedema may be observed as a result of subcutaneous, intramuscular or intravenous *injections* of drugs, antibiotics and hormones. If injection sites are evident at post-mortem inspection, it is advisable to obtain samples of muscle, body fluids or blood for the presence of illegal substances. Common sites for *injection damage* are the prescapular region of the neck, the shoulder and gluteal muscle groups. In cattle, *hormone implants* may be found in the subcutaneous muscle, especially on the mid-line of the back between the shoulders, at the root of the tail and in the region of the triceps of the foreleg. In fact, almost anywhere but the ear.

**'Wet carcase syndrome'**

This condition has been observed in lambs in South Africa and is responsible for significant condemnations (Brock, 1983). Affected animals are of the non-wool type and come from regions where supplementary feeding with concentrates is necessary. Lesions in the form of layers of slimy translucent jelly-like encapsulated material occur over the buttocks, briskets and flanks. Unlike oedematous carcases, however, the renal, sternal and mesenteric fat is normal. A similar condition is said to exist in the Sudan and France.

**Porcine stress syndrome** (PSS, malignant hyperthermia, back muscle necrosis, transport death, enzootische herztod) (see also Chapter 2)

Malignant hyperthermia occurs worldwide, being most common in those breeds of pigs (Piétrain, Poland China, Hampshire, Landrace and crosses) selected for heavy muscling and leanness with short legs. PSS results from a hereditable defect in which there is an inability to maintain homeostasis (the maintenance of the body's internal equilibrium in response to external and internal changes), stress causing an excessive stimulation of β-adrenergic receptors with rapid depletion of ATP, glycolysis of muscle and the production of localised or generalised amounts of lactic acid in muscle.

Any factors calculated to induce stress in susceptible pigs may bring on acute dyspnoea, tachycardia, hyperthermia and, possibly, rapid onset of death. These stressors include adverse transport conditions, fighting, overcrowding, fatigue, high temperatures and humidity. The mixing of different social groups of pigs may also predispose to PSS. The condition is also recognised in man and dogs.

Susceptible live pigs can be recognised by brief exposure to the anaesthetic halothane, the animals developing rigidity of limbs which can be reversed by stopping the anaesthesia and by cooling with cold water or ice. The exact action of the halothane in not known.

**Lesions** PSE describes accurately the appearance of affected skeletal muscle, which are pale, soft and exudative. Rigor mortis develops very rapidly with a pH of 5.8 or lower. The muscles most often involved are those of the loin, back, shoulder and thigh and these may show haemorrhages. The myocardium may be very pale in colour. Usually there is pulmonary oedema, hydropericardium, hydrothorax and congestion of the liver.

*Tumours of muscle*

These are relatively rare, although neoplasms of supporting tissues, e.g. fibromas, are fairly common. The most common tumour of muscle is metastatic lymphosarcoma (malignant lymphoma). Rhabdomyoma and rhabdomyosarcoma are respectively benign and malignant tumours which may occasionally be seen.

*Judgement of diseases of the muscular system*

**Total condemnation** Generalised bruising. Malignant tumours. Multiple tumours. Generalised wet carcase syndrome. Generalised sarcocystosis. Trichinellosis.

**Approved as fit with seizure of affected part** Localised bruising. Calcareous deposits. Localised tumour formation. PSS. DFD. Localised wet carcase syndrome. Injection and other abscesses. Muscular haemorrhages. Yellow fat disease. Myodegeneration. Localised sarcocystosis. Roeckel's granuloma. Localised parasitic cysts. Interstitial myositis. Muscle atrophy. Actinobacillosis. Localised congenital deformities.

## NERVOUS SYSTEM

*Encephalitis* is an inflammation of the brain; *meningitis* is an inflammation of the meninges (*pachymeningitis* when dura mater is inflamed and *leptomeningitis* when the pia arachnoid is involved). *Myelitis* is an inflammation of the spinal cord and *choroiditis* when the choroid plexus (which secretes the cerebrospinal fluid) is affected. Various combinations of these terms occur depending on the parts of the CNS involved, e.g. encephalomyelitis (brain and spinal cord), meningoencephalitis (meninges and brain).

*Brain and spinal cord abscesses:* Infection of the brain may occur via the blood, peripheral nerves, from adjacent infected structures in the skull/sinuses/vertebral column or directly by trauma. Infection includes the various pyogenic organisms (*Actinomyces pyogenes, Str. pneumoniae, Past. haemolytica, P. multocida, Listeria monocytogenes, Haemophilus somnus, E. rhusiopathiae, Pseudomonas aeruginosa*), all of which can produce abscesses.

They occur mostly in pigs (usually as a result of tail biting) and in sheep (often from careless docking methods) and are usually small in size, faintly yellowish in colour and placed between the dura mater and the bone. Pressure is often exerted on the CNS and spinal cord, resulting in nervous symptoms and paralysis.

*Listeriosis* causes an encephalitis in adult ruminants, pigs and sometimes in calves and lambs. Although responsible for abscessation in the liver, heart and other organs, there are no gross lesions in the brain but on occasions meninges may show microabscess formation.

*Leptomeningitis* is nearly always purulent in type and like cerebral abscesses is usually haematogenous in origin.

*Tuberculous meningitis* in the bovine is an example of haematogenous infection of congenital origin and is usually encountered in young cattle up to 1½ years old. Tuberculous abscesses may be found in the lumbar vertebrae of pigs.

*Specific diseases* which may affect the CNS include listeriosis, Aujeszky's disease, rabies, bovine malignant catarrh, infectious bovine meningoencephalitis, classic swine fever, African swine fever, enzootic ataxia, border disease, louping ill, scrapie, bovine spongiform encephalopathy (BSE).

Certain metabolic affections of the live animal are associated with symptoms of nervous derangement, necessitating casualty slaughter. Hypomagnesaemic tetany, parturient paresis (milk fever) and ketosis in cows, pregnancy toxaemia in ewes and eclampsia in sows – the so-called 'production diseases' – come into this category. Apart from a fatty liver in ketosis and pregnancy toxaemia, bruising and subcutaneous extravasations of blood, there are few significant lesions.

**Congenital defects** These are relatively common in all the food animals because of the susceptibility of the CNS to teratogens and because of its fundamental position in embryogenesis. Some of the abnormalities recorded have been shown to be due to the action of certain viruses, e.g. Rift Valley fever, Bluetongue, Border disease, and classic swine fever. Abnormalities in the size, shape and structure of the brain as well as aplasia and hypoplasia of the brain and spinal cord occur. Hydrocephalus is an excess of fluid in the cranial cavity, either in the ventricles or the arachnoid space or both and may be associated with an enlargement of the cranium.

The so-called *Dandy–Walker syndrome* affects sheep, calves and dogs and comprises hydrocephalus, cystic enlargement of the roof of the posterior aspect of the 4th ventricle and agenesis or hypoplasia of the cerebellar vermis. This rare congenital brain and skull malformation was recorded in a total of 34 lambs from 222 ewes in three apparently unrelated flocks of Suffolk sheep in England and Scotland in 1992 (Pritchard *et al.*, 1992).

*Syringomyelia* is a rare inherited condition of the spinal cord in which the central canal is distended with fluid, with necrosis of the adjoining nerve tissue.

**Degenerative changes** The brain and spinal cord are susceptible to various poisons acquired in the feed or via metabolic disturbances. Examples of poisons are lead, nitrate/nitrite, fluoroacetate and sodium chloride, while ketosis in cows and pregnancy toxaemia in ewes can result in convulsions and neuronal degeneration.

Necrosis of brain tissue is termed *encephalomalacia* and *myelomalacia* when the spinal cord is affected, the term malacia meaning softening. Such changes are seen in enterotoxaemia in lambs and mulberry heart disease in pigs and in various forms of injury.

**Tumours** Most neoplasms of the CNS in the food animals are secondary and are of a wide variety, some being congenital in origin. They can arise from nerve tissue (glioma, meningioma, astrocytoma, sarcoma, neurofibroma, Schwann cell tumour, medulloblastoma, ganglioneuroma) or vascular tissue (haemangioma, meningioma).

**Pigmentation** Blue-black deposits of *melanin* are frequently evident on the spinal cord and meninges of calves and older cattle and are normal if localised.

**Parasitic diseases** Various cysticerci (*C. bovis* (cattle), *C. cellulosae* (pig), *C. tenuicollis* (sheep)) may be found occasionally in the brain, but whether this is a normal predilection site or not is difficult to say. However, *Coenurus cerebralis* is quite common in the brains of sheep, and less commonly in cattle, suggesting that this is a site to the parasite's liking. Immature worms of *Setaria* spp. may occur in the CNS of horses, sheep and goats, while *Stephanurus dentatus* (q.v.) is often found encysted in the meninges of pigs. The first stage larvae of *Hypoderma bovis* use the spinal canal and its epidural fat as a resting stage and can regularly be found there. Because of their proximity to the brain in the frontal sinuses, the young larvae of *Oestrus ovis* are frequently found in the CNS of sheep.

**Injuries** Fractures of the vertebral column may nip or sever the spinal cord, causing paralysis, a condition which may be encountered in bulls. Lesser forms of injury may result in localised necrosis of the spinal cord due to vascular damage. The brain and spinal cord may suffer injury from various forms of trauma, some of which may result in concussion or even immediate death. All forms of injury are liable to secondary infection.

Cows may suffer mechanical damage to spinal nerves from accidents, parturition or mating sufficient to produce posterior paralysis.

### *Judgement of diseases of the nervous system*

**Total condemnation** Brain abscesses associated with pyaemia. Acute encephalitis and meningitis. CNS lesions associated with specific infective disease. Malignant tumours. Multiple tumours. Abnormal behaviour and signs of infection. (Downer syndrome with signs of acute disease.)

**Approved as fit with seizure of affected part:** Localised brain or spinal cord abscess. Chronic encephalitis, meningitis without fever, etc. Abnormal behaviour without fever, etc.

## ORGANS OF SPECIAL SENSE

While it is unlikely that most lesions of the eye and ear *per se* will be of consequence in the judgement of carcases, some relating to the eye are of importance in making an overall diagnosis besides being of value to the livestock producer in the feedback of disease information.

### Eye

The state of the conjunctiva, cornea, lens and eyelids is important in the diagnosis of certain specific diseases. It is important to note evidence of a discharge from the eyes, inflammation/pigmentation/pallor of the conjunctivae and membrana nictitans, oedema and abnormal movements of the eyelids, corneal opacity and ulceration and cataract of the lens, since these may denote certain systemic disease particularly those associated with anaemia and icterus, keratoconjunctivitis (cattle, sheep and goats), mycoplasmosis (*M. bovoculi*), photosensitisation and neoplasia, especially squamous cell carcinoma while eyelid and eyeball movement can sometimes detect lesions of the CNS.

Emaciation is associated with a retraction of the eyeballs in their sockets.

The condition and position of the membrana nictitans (third eyelid) is important since it may indicate tetanus and encephalitis if prominent and inflamed.

Oedema of the eyelids is usually diagnostic of oedema disease in pigs and of photosensitisation in sheep and other species in which it is usually accompanied by oedema of the ears, muzzle and face.

Anaemia is shown by pallor of the conjunctivae and other mucosae and may be caused by extensive haemorrhage (haemorrhagic anaemia) or by extensive destruction of RBCs (haemolytic anaemia). Petechial haemorrhages in the conjunctivae may also occur in cases of haemolytic anaemia.

Jaundice or icterus is indicated by a yellow discoloration of the conjunctivae and may signal obstructive jaundice, hepatocellular jaundice or haemolytic jaundice (cf. haemolytic anaemia).

*Blepharitis* (inflammation of the eyelids) may be a local infection, part of a generalised dermatitis, or the result of irritants.

*Conjunctivitis* (inflammation of the conjunctivae) may be a local infection or part of a serious disease, e.g. chlamydial conjunctivitis in sheep and goats (*Chlamydia psittaci*).

*Keratitis* is an inflammation of the cornea and may be a local infection, part of a systemic disease, or due to parasitic infection, e.g. infectious keratoconjunctivitis (contagious ophthalmia) (q.v.).

*Ophthalmia* is a term applied to severe inflammatory changes in the eye which may be localised or part of a general disease, e.g. contagious ophthalmia. Periodic ophthalmia (equine uveitis, moon blindness) is a disease of uncertain origin (leptospirae, *Onchocerca cervicalis*) in which there is blindness due to major changes in the eyes.

*Parasitic infections* include infectious keratoconjunctivitis (q.v.), periodic ophthalmia and thelaziasis, a common condition in all species of food animals, especially in North America, caused by various genera of *Thelazia* spp. eye worms. *Dirofilaria immitis*, *Toxocara* spp., *Onchocerca cervicalis*, *Setaria* spp. and cysticerci (pigs) may also cause severe ophthalmia.

*Tumours* of the eyes include squamous cell carcinoma, the most important bovine tumour in North America (occurring mostly in Herefords) and responsible for significant condemnation rates in meat plants. Horses may also be affected, the tumour occurring in the eyelids, membrana nictitans and limbus (edge of the cornea).

Eye neoplasms may be either primary or secondary, occurring as metastases from other sites. Less common forms include melanoma and adenoma.

## Ear

Like the eye, the ear may be affected with primary conditions such as parasitic diseases, e.g. mange mites, ticks, ringworm, or be associated with generalised disease.

*Necrosis* of the pinna may be due to various bacteria involved in septicaemia, e.g. blue ear disease, *Borrelia* spp. infection, ergot poisoning, parasites such as sarcoptic mites and cannibalism in pigs. It may also be a sequel to photosensitisation, both primary and secondary. The use of some types of ear tags is currently causing severe infection, especially in cattle and sheep.

The most common *tumours* are squamous cell carcinoma, adenoma, chondroma in cattle and sarcoid in horses.

### *Judgement of diseases of the eyes and ears*

**Total condemnation** Eye and ear lesions as part of specific infective disease with fever, etc. Malignant tumours with metastases. Multiple benign tumours. Blue ear disease. Ergot poisoning. Secondary photosensitisation with icterus, etc.

**Partial condemnation/seizure of head less tongue** Localised eye and ear conditions. Primary photosensitisation.

## REFERENCES


Biss, M. E., Hathaway S. C., Purchase, R. W. and Wilkinson, B. H. P. (1993) *Vet. Rec.* **132**, 548.

Bogin, E., Avidar, Y., Merom, M., Soback, S. and Brenner, G. (1988) *J. Comp. Pathol.* **98**, 337.

Bowie, J. (1993) *Vet. Rec.* **131**, 255.

Bradley, R. and Duffell, S. J. (1982) *J. Comp. Pathol.* **92**, 85–97.

Bradley, R. and Duffell, S. J. (1982) *Vet. Rec.* **102**, 269–270.

Bremner, A. S. (1994) *Vet. Rec.* **136**, 622.

Brock, R. M. (1983) *Vet. Rec.* **20**, 118.

Brock, R. M. (1983) *Vet. Rec.* **118**, 56.

Buchanan and Crawshaw (1995) *Vet. Rec.* **136**, 640.

Carr, J. and Walton, J. R. (1993) *Vet. Rec.* **132**, 575–577.

Codex Alimentarius Commission. Alinorm 93/16A.

Cross, G. M. and Edwards, M. J. (1981) *Aust. Vet. J.* **57**, 153.

Doxey, D. L. and Scott, P. R. (1983) *Vet. Rec.* **113**, 112.

Duffell, S. J. and Edwardson, R. (1978) *Vet. Rec.* **102**, 269–270.

Elbers, A. R. W. *et al.* (1995) *Vet. Rec.* **137**, 290–293.

Evans, D. G. and Pratt, J. H. (1978) *Br. Vet. J.* **134**, 476.

Flesja, K. I. and Ulvesaeter, H. O. (1980) *Acta Vet. Scand.* **74**, Supp. 74.

Gezon, H. M. *et al.* (1991) *J. Amer. Vet. Med. Assoc.* **198**, 257–263.

Grandin, T. (1980) *Int. J. Study Anim. Prob.* **1**, 121.

Green, L. E., Wyatt, J. M. and Morgan, K. L. (1992) *Vet. Rec.* **130**, 121–122.

Gunning, R. F. and Walters, R. J. W. (1994) *Vet. Rec.* **135**, 433–434.

Hartley, P. E., Wilesmith, J. W. and Bradley, R. (1988) *Vet. Rec.* **123**, 173–175.
Hayward, A. H. S. and Baker-Smith, J. (1978) *Vet. Rec.* **102**, 96–97.
Head, K. W. (1990) *In Practice* (March), 68–76.
Herenda, D. and Dukes, T. W. (1988) *Canad. Vet. J.* **29**, 730.
Jackson, P. G. G. (1993) *In Practice* (May) 119–127; (July) 193–196.
Jones, J. E. T. (1980) *Res. Vet. Sci.* **28**, 281.
Lamont, M. H., Hunt, B. and Mercer, R. (1984) *Vet. Rec.* **115**, 22.
Madel, A. J. (1981) *Vet. Rec.* **109**, 362–363.
McNally, P. W. and Harris, P. D. (1992) *Vet. Rec.* **138**, 126–128.
Monaghan, M. L. M. and Hannan, J. (1983) *Vet. Rec.* **113**, 55.
Monaghan, M. L. M. (1982) *Irish Vet. J.* **36**, 88.
Obwolo, M. J. and Lawson, G. (1992) *Vet. Rec.* **130**, 122–123.
Poulson, J. S. D. (1976) *Vet. Rec.* **98**, 149.
Pritchard, J. *et al.* (1992) *Vet. Rec.* **135**, 163–164.
Welchman, D. de B. and Baust, G. N. (1987) *Vet. Rec.* **121**, 586–590.
Wells, G. H., Hebert, C. N. and Robins, B. C. (1980) *Vet. Rec.* **106**, 532
Winstanley, M. (1981) *Meat Magazine* (May) 12–13.
Yeh, E., Anderson, B., Jones, P. N. and Shaw, F. D. (1978) *Vet. Rec.* **103**, 117.
Yogaratnam, V. (1995) *Vet. Rec.* **138**, 215.

# Chapter 17
# Infectious Diseases

*Infection* is an invasion of body tissues with microorganisms which multiply and cause cell damage with the production of toxins, and, usually, a high temperature and an antigen–antibody response.

*Infectious diseases* (bacterial, viral, fungal, protozoal and parasitic) are responsible for most losses in the food animals throughout the world and are, therefore, of great economic importance. Viral diseases, in particular, are capable of affecting large numbers of animals and spreading very rapidly. Along with certain bacterial disease they are endemic (present at all times) in some countries.

Control measures include accurate diagnosis, detailed epidemiological and laboratory investigations, quarantine and movement control, treatment or slaughter of affected stock, burial/burning of affected carcases, cleansing and disinfection of premises, proper disposal of contaminated materials, including feed, water, wildlife, etc., vaccination of susceptible animals and sound husbandry measures, including the breeding of resistant livestock.

*Emphasis will be placed on those conditions most likely to be encountered at meat inspection.* These are most likely to be chronic in nature, although acute cases, even dead and moribund animals, are sometimes presented. So the inspectors responsible for ante-mortem examination must be on the alert for untoward conditions, even notifiable diseases, delivered as casualty animals, especially in those countries where veterinary certification is lax. Indeed, the abattoir has often been the place where notifiable disease was first recognised.

*Each disease will be described under the headings: identification* **(I)**, *occurrence* **(O)**, *infectious agent* **(IA)**, *reservoir* **(R)**, *mode of transmission* **(MT)**, *clinical findings* **(CF)**, *pathology* **(P)**, *diagnosis* **(D)** *and judgement* **(J)**.

*Pathology* (lesions, necropsy findings) will be treated in some detail in order to assist the meat inspector in diagnosis.

## Judgement

Authority is given in some countries, e.g. the USA and Canada, to condemn on ante-mortem examination. These cases include those dead on arrival and moribund animals and all conditions requiring total carcase condemnation at post-mortem inspection. In the USA all cases of CNS disorders, rabies, various poisonings (metal, fluorine, pesticide, etc.) and diseases and conditions requiring further observation or treatment are totally condemned.

Eventual judgement of carcase meat and offal is based on all the accumulated evidence – the history of the animal, clinical signs, post-mortem lesions and any laboratory results. Decisions on post-mortem inspection, like systems of inspection, vary in different countries. For example, while only three categories of decisions are allowed in the United Kingdom – (a) *fit for human consumption*, (b) *totally unfit for human consumption and* (c) *partially condemned* – other countries adopt extra categories: *utilisation of heat treatment and freezing for infected and contaminated meat, the use of inferior meat fit for human consumption, and the approval of meat as fit for human consumption but restricted in distribution*, all three categories being under official supervision.

The following *judgement* symbols (Disposition Codes) are used, with modifications, according to the Codex Alimentarius Commission Report on Meat Hygiene, Rome. 1993:

*Ante-mortem:*

T Totally condemn.

R Retain for rest and treatment.

S Treat as suspect.

*Post-mortem:*

A Approve as fit for human consumption.

T Totally unfit for human consumption.

D Partially condemn.

K Conditionally approve as fit for human consumption (Kh, heat treatment. Kf, freezing or heat treatment).

I Meat showing minor deviations from normal but fit for human consumption.

L Approved as fit for human consumption with distribution restricted to limited areas.

... Not applicable, e.g. in total condemnation the columns referring to D are not applicable.

In some countries approval for human consumption may be given subject to restriction of distribution to limited areas, e.g. meat from animals derived from an area under quarantine because of an outbreak of contagious disease *provided there is no risk to human health.*

# BACTERIAL DISEASE

## ACTINOMYCOSIS ('LUMPY JAW') ACTINOBACILLOSIS ('WOODEN TONGUE')

**I. (Identification)** Both diseases are chronic, suppurative conditions in which granulomatous lesions are formed in bone (actinomycosis) or soft tissues (actinobacillosis). They occur infrequently and sporadically, usually being encountered as single cases though several animals may be involved at any one time. Cattle, pigs and sheep are most commonly affected with horses and man less so.

**O. (Occurrence)** Worldwide in distribution.

**IA. (Infectious agents)** Different species of *Actinomyces* and *Actinobacillus* are involved in the production of these granulomas (probably in association with pyogenic and other bacteria) and have been isolated from various other conditions.

- *Actinomyces bovis* – Actinomycosis (cattle), udder actinomycosis (sows) and fistulous withers and poll evil (horses).
- *Actinobacillus lignieresi* – Actinobacillosis (cattle and sheep)
- *Actinomyces actinoides* – Secondary invader in enzootic pneumonia (calves) and seminal vesiculitis (bulls).
- *Actinobacillus equuli* – Peritonitis (horses), diarrhoea (calves).
- *Actinobacillus suis* – Septicaemia and arthritis (young pigs).
- *Actinobacillus seminis* – Epididymitis (rams), septicaemia, synovitis and abscessation (young lambs).

Human actinomycosis is usually caused by *A. israelii*, *A naeslundii*, *A. meyeri* and *A. propionicus*.

All *Actinomyces* and *Actinobacillus* spp. are Gram-positive, non-acid-fast, anaerobic/ microaerophilic organisms which are branched rods with a tendency to mycelial growth (mass of thread-like process or hyphae) in young cultures.

*Nocardia* spp., especially *Nocardia madurae*, can also cause granulomatous and suppurative lesions in man (madura foot) and animals. *Staph. aureus* has been incriminated in causing cases of udder actinomycosis in the cow and sow.

**R. (Reservoir)** *A. bovis* and *A. lignieresi* are normal inhabitants of the mouth, the latter also occurring in the bovine rumen.

**MT. (Mode of transmission)** The bacteria gain entrance through wounds caused either by teeth defects or sharp objects like barley awns or foreign bodies.

**CF. (Clinical findings)** Actinomycosis – enlargement of mandible or maxilla, at first painless but later painful, with presence of lesions described below. Salivation, chronic indigestion, bloat, diarrhoea, depraved appetite and loss of condition are found in both conditions.

**P. (Pathology)** *Actinomycosis* – in *cattle* the lesion confined to the mandible or maxilla, especially the former, which becomes inflamed (osteomyelitis), rarefied and thickened (*'lumpy jaw'*). The bone assumes a honeycombed appearance on section. In later stages the thickened bone is evident from the exterior. The swellings eventually break through the skin and discharge a sticky, honey-like fluid containing fine, firm yellowish-white granules.

Extension to nearby tissues may occur, e.g. muscles of the throat, although this is often difficult to differentiate from actinobacillosis. The two conditions may co-exist. Rarely, there may be extension via the bloodstream to other organs, the most common lesions involving the oesophagus and the reticulum. Interference with prehension and mastication with digestive upset and diarrhoea in the extensive form occur with eventual loss of condition.

In *pigs* extensive granulomatous nodules may occur on the skin and udder. Wounds due to fighting and the teeth of sucking piglets are the probable means of entry. In the sow's udder a more common lesion takes the form of a firm fibrous tumour containing several abscesses affecting part or all of the udder. Less commonly, indurated ulcers form on the skin surface.

In *man* actinomycosis may occur in the jaw, thorax or abdomen (liver), the lesions taking the form of indurated fibrous areas containing pus. These may form sinuses which reach the surface. There is no evidence that actinomycosis in man is acquired from animals, the species of organisms being specific for man. *A. israelii* has been isolated from carried teeth, tonsils and vaginal secretions.

*Actinobacillosis* – in *cattle* the tongue is swollen and firm especially at its base. Ulcers and granulomas appear at the side of the tongue along with lymphadenitis of the submaxillary, parotid, retropharyngeal and occasionally, mediastinal lymph nodes. Nodules may rupture to the surface and discharge a yellowish-green pus containing granular '*sulphur bodies*'.

In the bovine rumen and reticulum lesions take the form of raised plaques on the mucosa with fibrous thickening of the stomach wall. These plaques may ulcerate with extension of the process to the liver, oesophagus, diaphragm, peritoneum and lungs. On the peritoneum, usually the left side, cauliflower-like fibrous nodules containing minute yellowish foci appear, while in the liver the lesions are circular and may be as large as 5 cm in diameter. In the lungs, where the lesion can reach a huge size, the smaller ones are irregular in shape without pus while the older and larger lesions contain a yellowish-green pus. Incision of these older lesions reveals a marbled appearance due to the presence of a greenish-black pigment.

In cattle, sessile fibrous tumours may occur on the skin.

In *sheep*, lesions up to 8 cm in diameter occur on the nose, face and lower jaw but the tongue is not usually affected. There is an associated lymphadenitis, the cranial and cervical lymph nodes being enlarged. These fibrous nodules rupture and discharge through several openings a thick yellowish-green pus containing fine yellowish granules. As in cattle, extension may occur to stomachs and peritoneum.

**D. (Diagnosis)** A yellowish sulphur granule should be crushed between two microscope slides and fixed. Stain one slide with Gram's stain and another with modified Ziehl–Neelsen stain. With Gram the organisms appear as a Gram-positive central filamentous mass surrounded by a Gram-negative zone of radiating clubs which represent deposited lipoid material. With Z–N stain the clubs are acid-fast and the mycelial mass non-acid-fast (also Culture, serology).

**J. (Judgement)**

Carcase: Lesions confined, e.g., to head, A. Extensive lesions, T.

Viscera: Lesions confined, e.g., to head, A. Extensive lesions, T.

Diseased or affected parts/organs: D.

Approval (A) is subject to satisfactory condition of carcase with no evidence of anaemia or degenerative changes.

If head is condemned, tongue is also condemned.

## ANTHRAX

(Malignant pustule, Splenic fever, Malignant oedema, Woolsorters' disease, Ragpickers' disease, Milzbrand, Charbon.)

**I.** A usually acute or peracute, septicaemic infective *zoonosis* which may occur in a chronic form, especially in the pig. Although normally fatal, recovery sometimes occurs, particularly in the pig. While usually sporadic in temperate countries, anthrax can occur as serious outbreaks in tropical and subtropical countries with high rainfall, e.g. an outbreak in Western Province in Zambia in 1947 in which 156 cattle and about 100 wildebeest died (Tuchili *et al.*,

1993). The disease also affects other wildlife such as elephant, hippopotami, buffalo, lechwe, impala and zebra. All domestic animals are susceptible, although goats and horses are less commonly affected.

Notifiable disease (UK).

**O.** Worldwide in distribution but probably more common in African, Asian and European countries. The organism is often restricted to certain soils – 'anthrax belts' where it is enzootic (present constantly in a location). A serious outbreak occurred in Victoria, Australia in January 1997 with over 140 deaths in cattle and three in sheep on 59 properties. Vaccination of cattle and sheep in the affected areas was carried out.

**IA.** *Bacillus anthracis*, a Gram-positive encapsulated, spore-forming, non-motile rod 4–8 μm × 1–1.5 μm. A facultative anaerobe, it is one of the largest of the pathogenic bacteria and very resistant in its spore form. Spores, which are formed in the presence of sufficient oxygen, can resist heat for long periods (dry heat at 140°C for 1–3 h and moist heat at 100°C for 5–10 min). Spores never occur in tissues, only when the bacteria are shed, e.g. from nose, mouth and anus of affected animal and when grown on artificial media.

A new variant of the anthrax toxin which is totally resistant to antibiotics has been developed in Russia, a sinister production in the field of biological warfare.

**R.** Animals, as listed above. The spores of anthrax can survive for as long as 3 years or more. There is evidence that *B. anthracis* can multiply in the soil under favourable conditions of temperature, pH and nutrients and thus be responsible for serious outbreaks in both domestic and wild animals, especially in tropical and subtropical countries.

**MT.** Infection occurs through ingestion, inhalation or via the skin. Ingestion of contaminated water and food, e.g. meat, bone meal or other foods and soil, is a common mode of transmission. Inhalation anthrax is due to the inhalation of spores. Skin infection is due to contact with the tissues of affected animals, contaminated materials (hair, wool, hides, skins, etc., and products made from them). Biting flies which have fed on anthrax carcases have been incriminated. Some forms of wildlife, e.g. vultures and various other predators, may act as carriers of infection.

**CF.** *Peracute* form: cattle and sheep – animal is usually found dead without any premonitory symptoms. Rigor mortis is absent or incomplete. Dark, tarry-like blood which does not clot is evident at mouth, anus, nostrils and vulva.

*Acute* form: Usually lasts about 48 h. Fever, depression, very high temperature (ca. 107°C), rapid respiration, anorexia, congested mucosae, diarrhoea or dysentery and possible abortion.

In *pigs* and horses there is fever, anorexia, listlessness with oedema of throat, face, neck and abdomen with petechial haemorrhages on the skin. Dysentery may be present with bloody froth at the nostrils.

*It must always be remembered that antibiotic therapy may mask the symptoms of anthrax and other diseases.*

**P.** *The possibility of anthrax in all cases of sudden or rapid onset of death should be excluded by the examination of a blood smear before any attempt at post-mortem is made. If there is reason to suspect anthrax the carcase must not be opened. The opening of a carcase with discharge of blood creates widespread sporulation with disinfection problems.*

Ecchymoses throughout the body tissues. Engorgement of superficial veins of skin and muscle giving the carcase a fiery red colour. Blood-stained fluid in body cavities. Very enlarged soft spleen (may be absent in sheep). Dark tarry non-clotting blood. Haemorrhagic enteritis. Cloudy swelling of heart, liver and kidneys. Rapid decomposition. Bloat. In horses and pigs gelatinous material in subcutaneous swellings with enlargement of local lymph nodes. In *pigs* a local intestinal form has been recognised in which the lymph nodes of the head and mesentery undergo necrosis, the degenerated material becoming surrounded with fibrous material, enlargement and engorgement of some lymph nodes with a dark grey appearance and necrotic foci evident in others.

**D.** Diagnosis is confirmed by the examination of a smear of peripheral blood, oedematous fluid or lymph node where the organisms are difficult to demonstrate in the circulating blood, e.g. in horses and pigs. Blood is best carefully collected from an ear vein to avoid unnecessary contamination and sporulation. In cases of malignant pustule in man, a swab is taken from one of the vesicles or alternatively fluid is collected in a capillary tube which is then sealed.

Smears stained by McFadyean's methylene blue show the anthrax bacilli as large blue organisms surrounded by purple capsular material – McFadyean's reaction.

Fluorescent and monoclonal antibody techniques as well as animal passage (mice, guinea pigs or rabbits) and culture may be necessary to identify *B. anthracis*, especially in difficult cases, e.g. where antibiotic treatment has been used in the live animal.

**J.**

Carcase: T.
Viscera: T.
(Included are affected and in-contact animals and all contaminated meat and offal.)

The meat from anthrax carcases is dangerous to man and other animals. Carcases must not be opened. The complete carcase must be destroyed along with *all* contaminated material.

### Anthrax in man

The disease occurs most commonly in fellmongers, woolsorters, knackermen, personnel involved in the preparation of meat and bone products, veterinarians, abattoir and farm workers.

Infection normally occurs through the skin which comes directly or indirectly in contact with infected tissues, blood and contaminated materials such as hair, wool, hides or products such as brushes, drums, etc., contaminated bone meal and soil. Biting flies may also transmit the disease.

Inhalation of spores is also a mode of infection leading to fulminating pneumonia. Intestinal and otopharyngeal anthrax are due to the ingestion of infected material, e.g. meat but not milk, resulting in acute gastroenteritis and dysentery.

*Cutaneous anthrax* takes the form of a localised pimple which develops rapidly in 2–3 days into a dry, black adherent scab surrounded by a circle of purplish vesicles. This is the typical anthrax sore – *malignant pustule* – which is neither malignant or pustular. It is usually about 2–3 cm in diameter but may be as large as 6–7 cm or only pinhead in size, in which case it is surrounded by extensive oedema. Anthrax sores may be acquired by scratching an itchy part with infected fingers.

*Symptoms* in man include high temperature, rigors, headache, lack of appetite and nausea.

Untreated cases may die in 2–3 days. Rapid diagnosis and treatment (penicillin, tetracyclines, erythromycin, chloramphenicol) are effective in most cases.

Human cases are notified to the Local Health Authority in most countries. The patient is isolated with disinfectant precautions regarding discharges from lesions and articles soiled by them. Source of infection and in-contacts, exposure to animals, etc., is investigated.

### Procedure when anthrax is detected

In Britain, as in most countries, anthrax is a *notifiable* disease under the Anthrax Order 1991, which requires notification by the owner or veterinary surgeon to the local Divisional Veterinary Officer or local police of the existence or suspected existence of the disease.

In Britain confirmation of the existence of anthrax may only be made by the Ministry of Agriculture.

Steps must then be taken to dispose of the carcase by burning or deep burial along with disinfection. Opening or moving of carcases is prohibited.

Natural orifices should be packed with tow or cotton wool and the animal's head covered with sacking. Discharged blood should be absorbed with sawdust, earth or peat, all being eventually destroyed by burning.

The detection of anthrax during dressing represents a very serious situation – all further dressing and slaughter should be stopped and the affected and contiguous carcases, offal and blood condemned.

All equipment, e.g. knives, steels, saws, shovels, etc., involved in the handling of infected material must either be destroyed by burning or thoroughly disinfected (e.g. hot 5% sodium hydroxide, 10% formaldehyde).

## ATROPHIC RHINITIS (turbinate atrophy of pigs)

**I.** A disease usually of young pigs characterised by inflammatory changes of the nasal mucosa and sneezing followed by atrophy of the turbinate bones and deformity of the face.

**O.** The disease occurs mainly in intensive pig rearing areas and is especially common in mid-western USA.

**IA.** *Bordetella bronchiseptica*, a small ovoid to rod-shaped Gram-negative bacillus along with toxigenic strains of *Pasteurella multocida*, a small Gram-negative, capsulated non-motile bacillus which exhibits bipolar staining when stained with methylene blue. It is possible that genetic, nutritional and other husbandry factors are also involved.

**R.** Both organisms are commonly found in commercial herds of pigs and at least *B. bronchiseptica* may be harboured by dogs, cats, rodents and other forms of wildlife.

**MT.** By direct and indirect contact, especially through droplet infection.

**CF.** Sneezing, coughing, lachrymation, mucopurulent discharge from nostrils. Respiratory distress in later stages with difficulty in prehension and mastication. Loss of condition. Distortion of face.

**P.** Varying degrees of softening/atrophy of turbinate bones with deviation of nasal septum.

**D.** Diagnosis is confirmed by examining a cross-section of the skull at the level of the second premolar teeth where typical lesions are best seen.

**J.**

Carcase and viscera:

No nasal discharge, condition good, A.
Nasal discharge, local lesions, D.
Systemic effects, e.g. abscessation, T.
Affected parts: head, D.

**BRUCELLOSIS** (undulant fever, contagious abortion, Bang's disease, Malta fever, Mediterranean fever)

**I.** A specific contagious disease of major importance of cattle, goats, pigs, sheep, and occasionally horses and man. The disease has also been recorded in bison, deer, elk, moose, other wild animals and dogs. The disease is associated with abortion, retained placenta and sterility in the female and infection of the accessory sex glands with infertility in the male.

Notifiable disease (UK).

**O.** Brucellosis is a *zoonosis* of major importance in most countries of the world.

**IA.** *Brucella abortus*, a very small almost coccal-like Gram-negative bacillus which is aerobic (but can only grow in the presence of 5–10% $CO_2$), non-motile, non-capsulated and non-sporing.

Cattle: *B. abortus* and less commonly *B. melitensis* and *B. suis*.

Pigs: *B. suis*.

Sheep: *B. melitensis*. *B. ovis* causes orchitis and epididymitis.

Goats: *B. melitensis* and less commonly *B. abortus*.

Horses: *B. abortus* and *B. suis*.

**O.** Worldwide, especially in Mediterranean countries, North and East Africa, India, Asia, Mexico and Central and South America. Many countries have made great progress towards eradication.

**R.** Animals listed above, except the dog, which not considered to be a natural reservoir.

**MT.** Direct and indirect contact with infected uterine discharges, blood, fetuses and fetal membranes. Mechanical vectors probably play a part in the transmission of infection. Large numbers of bacteria are present in infected cattle during abortion. Water, milk and feedingstuffs are often contaminated.

Infection takes place by ingestion, inhalation and through the skin and mucous membranes. Venereal transmission from infected bulls is said to be rare but infection has occurred in cows through the use of infected semen by AI.

**CF.** Brucella organisms have an affinity for the pregnant uterus, udder and the accessory male sex glands, lymph nodes and joints. Clinical findings include late abortions (after fifth month of pregnancy in cattle) with stillborn calves, kids and lambs, retained placentas and lowered milk yield. Orchitis and epididymitis occur in males.

**P.** Lesions are rarely diagnostic. The *placenta* is usually oedematous with cotyledons dull and granular in early stages. Later stages appear as yellowish granular necrotic plaques on the fetal cotyledons with the remainder opaque and leathery in appearance. A sticky, brownish, odourless exudate like soft caramel is present on the surface of the placenta.

The fetus is oedematous with blood-stained fluid in the body cavities, focal necrosis and granuloma in various organs, broncho-pneumonia and sometimes meningitis.

The mammary gland and supramammary lymph nodes usually harbour the bacilli and may be indurated and diffusely inflamed.

In males the scrotum is enlarged and indurated. A thickened tunica vaginalis due to fibrous tissue formation may compress or replace the testes.

There may be necrosis of the contents with rupture to the surface. Epididymitis, especially involving the tail, with oedema and fibrosis, are evident.

In *sows*, firm yellowish-white nodules, sometimes possessing a caseous centre, appear on the uterine mucosa, lymph nodes, liver, spleen and kidneys. Large abscesses are sometimes present in the same organs and in the testes and epididymis.

**D.** While symptoms and lesions may indicate the possibility of brucellosis, they are not diagnostic.

*B. abortus* can be recovered most easily from the aborted fetus (stomach and lungs) and also from the placenta, blood, milk, vaginal mucus.

Serology tests (agglutination, complement fixation, ELISA, Rose Bengal, milk ring) are used for antibody detection.

**J. Brucellosis in man (undulant fever)**

*Human infection with B. abortus* or *B. melitensis* is an occupational disease affecting people working with livestock – farm workers, veterinarians and abattoir personnel. (In the USA some 50% of cases of human brucellosis – due to *B. suis* – occur in abattoir workers.)

It may be acquired by drinking infected milk from cows, goats and sheep. There is, however, no evidence that eating infected meat can cause the disease in man. Isolated cases have been associated with dog carriers of the bacillus.

It is an acute or chronic condition characterised by continuous or intermittent fever and various symptoms such as headache, sweating, weakness, anorexia, chills, depression, nausea, body, joint and muscle pains and polyuria. The condition may last for some days or as long as a year or more.

Enlargement of various lymph nodes, especially the cervical and axillary, may be evident with an enlarged spleen and liver.

Complications such as osteoarthritis, osteomyelitis, meningitis, orchitis and epididymitis may occur. Recovery is usual but various disabilities may ensue.

*Action to be taken in meat plant*

While attention to personal hygiene, sterilisation of equipment, etc., is of paramount importance for all abattoir staff, it is essential where brucellosis cases and brucella reactors are handled.

In Britain brucellosis is now prescribed as an *industrial disease*. Most cases in the UK are associated with bovine infection.

It is essential that staff are adequately alerted about the entry of infected and reactor stock.

*Great care has to be taken when handling and dressing known brucella cases.* Hooks should be used to handle uteri and udders, which must not be incised. All uteri and udders from affected and reactor animals must be condemned.

Face masks to cover nose and mouth, goggles to protect the eyes, use of barrier cream and arm-length gloves are advocated, although this protection may render dressing difficult and prolonged.

It is advisable that reactor animals are not crowded into a single plant but dispersed over several premises.

**J.** *Cattle:*

Carcase, A.
Viscera, A.
Diseased organs, e.g. udder, uteri, lymph nodes, testes, seminal vesicles, etc., D.

If *B. melitensis* is suspected, T or Kh, depending on prevalence and as economically feasible, is advocated.

*Pigs*

Carcase: T.
Viscera: T.
If T is not economically feasible Kh, but with mammary glands, genital organs and associated lymph nodes: D.

## CAMPYLOBACTERIOSIS (see also Chapters 14 and 17)

The microorganisms *Campylobacter* and *Mycoplasma* have since 1977 assumed importance as causes of disease, although their exact significance is doubtful in some instances where they are associated with other bacteria and/or viruses. In these cases it is difficult to ascertain the true pathogen.

Some *Campylobacter* spp. were formerly classified in the genus *Vibrio*. They are Gram-negative, facultatively anaerobic, motile, thermophilic, oxidase-positive small rods resembling vibrios in morphology and motility. Vibrios are typically comma-shaped and possess polar flagella.

*Campylobacter* spp. are *zoonotic* organisms since they can cause gastroenteritis in man (q.v.), this being the most common form of food poisoning in man, although not as severe as salmonellosis.

They are widely distributed in nature and can be found in the intestines of healthy livestock, poultry and wild animals.

Among the diseases associated with *Campylobacter* infection are the following:

- Gastrointestinal campylobacteriosis (calves, sheep, mink, ferrets, dogs, cats) – *C. jejuni* or *C. coli*.
- Bovine genital campylobacteriosis – *C. fetus* subsp. *venerealis*.
- Ovine genital campylobacteriosis – *C. fetus* subsp. *fetus* or *jejuni*.
- Abortions and infertility in cattle – *C. fetus* subsp. *venerealis*.
- Avian infectious hepatitis – *C. fetus* var. *jejuni* (q.v.).

### Gastrointestinal campylobacteriosis

**I.** An acute bacterial *zoonotic* gastroenteritis of variable severity occurring in a wide variety of hosts – calves, sheep, pigs, goats, poultry, mink, man (in which it is the commonest form of food poisoning), dogs, cats and wild animals and birds.

**O.** Worldwide. The organisms can be isolated from the intestines of normal animals and man.

**IA.** *Campylobacter jejuni* and *C. coli* are thin Gram-negative, curved rods resembling vibrios which are motile, microaerophilic and possess a terminal flagellum.

**R.** See **I** and **O**. As with many intestinal pathogens, e.g. *Salmonella* spp., asymptomatic carrier animals are often responsible for causing outbreaks of the disease.

**MT.** Infection is acquired through the ingestion of contaminated food and water. The consumption of raw and undercooked poultry and other meat products is a common mode of infection for man and animals such as mink and ferrets.

**CF.** Watery diarrhoea which may contain mucus and/or blood. Anorexia. Depression. Loss of condition when disease is prolonged. Late abortion has been recorded in cattle and goats. Recovery is spontaneous in most cases.

**P.** Varying degrees of enteritis, sometimes haemorrhagic, especially in the jejunum, ileum and colon. The associated mesenteric lymph nodes are enlarged and oedematous and the intestinal mucosa thickened.

**D.** The disease is confirmed by microaerophilic (10% $CO_2$) culture of faeces when distinctive colonies are formed. Dark field or phase-contrast microscopy. Serological techniques to determine antibody titres.

**J.** Carcase and viscera, T.

## CASEOUS LYMPHADENITIS (CLA) (Figs 17.1 and 17.2)

**I.** A chronic contagious disease of sheep and goats, and less commonly horses, cattle, pigs, poultry, water buffalo and other wild ruminants in which abscesses are formed in lymph nodes and sometimes in internal organs. Human beings, particularly shearers, are occasionally affected.

**O.** Worldwide, especially where there are large populations of sheep and goats – Australia, New Zealand, North and South America, Middle East, Europe (Spain, France, Netherlands, Italy, Romania, Norway, Switzerland, Germany), and South Africa. Britain was free until cases were discovered in imported goats in the late 1980s.

According to veterinary staff at the Scottish Agricultural College, St Boswells, caseous

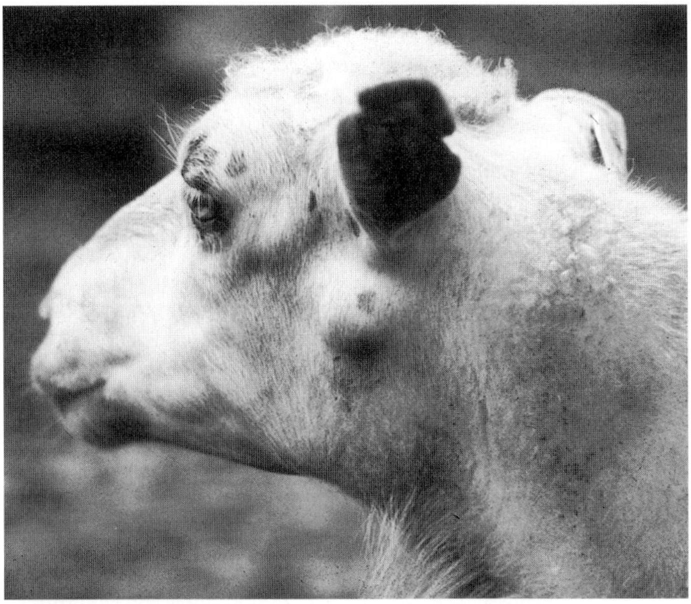

**Fig. 17.1** Caseous lymphadenitis in the head of a sheep. (By courtesy of Dr B. E. C. Shreuder)

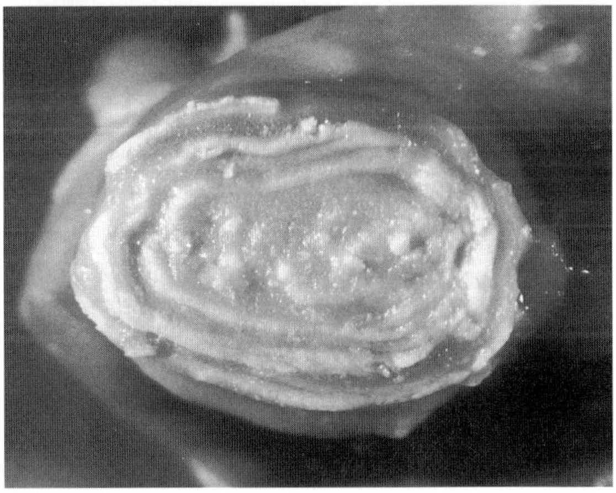

**Fig. 17.2** Caseous lymphadenitis abscess showing laminations. (By courtesy of Dr B. E C. Shreuder)

lymphadenitis is spreading rapidly among sheep in Northumberland and the Scottish Borders. Shearing time poses the highest risk for spread, cuts becoming infected with the causal organisms to produce skin abscesses and internal infection. Slaughter of affected animals is being advised.

The disease is of considerable economic importance, being responsible for condemnations – as high as 1% at meat inspection. Hides and fleeces are also reduced in value.

**IA.** *Corynebacterium pseudotuberculosis* (*ovis*), a small pleomorphic, Gram-positive, non-motile, aerobic/facultative anaerobic, non-sporing and non-capsulate rod found in soil and materials contaminated with pus. The organisms, which appear like Chinese lettering in suitable smears, show a characteristic barred appearance with certain stains, darker-staining metachromatic (volutin) granules being visible in the protoplasm of the bacteria. It is capable of surviving in hay for months. This organism also causes contagious acne and chronic pectoral and midline abscesses in horses.

**R.** Infected animals, soils and contaminated materials.

**MT.** Via skin wounds, including shearing, docking and castration wounds, through contamination with purulent material from ruptured abscesses in infected animals. The organism is capable of gaining entry through unbroken skin. Carrier animals are responsible for introducing infection into herds. Infection is spread through contaminated equipment (dipping baths and dips, handling and feeding appliances, hay, soil, etc.).

**CF.** Little evidence of clinical disease except some loss of condition in the more common lymph node form apart from visible abscesses. Infertility is often present. The more severe visceral type in which abscesses occur, for example, in lungs, liver, kidney, brain and spinal cord can lead to emaciation and death.

**P.** Enlargement of one or more of the superficial lymph nodes, especially of the head or neck. These abscesses, which may also occur at the point of entry, are painless and slow to develop. Some loss of condition occurs in the superficial form but emaciation (*'thin ewe syndrome'*) is evident where internal abscesses develop. Caseous bronchopneumonia, abortion, arthritis, neurological signs (when CNS abscesses occur), paraplegia, orchitis and mastitis may be manifested.

The typical abscess in CLA is discrete and contains a greenish-yellow or white thick, dry pus. In sheep the abscess often assumes a laminated or 'onion-ring' form in cross-section, with caseous exudate or pus surrounded by layers of fibrous tissue. The nature of the abscess depends on its age. In early stages only pin-point foci are apparent. In goats the exudate in the abscess is usually paste-like.

**D.** Diagnosis is based on clinical signs and the isolation of *C. pseudotuberculosis* from pus. The condition must be differentiated from other conditions caused by pyogenic organisms.

**J.** Carcase: A, T or D depending on extent of infection and carcase condition.

Viscera: A, T or D.

Some countries, notably Canada, resort to *total condemnation* of carcase and viscera where there is:

1 Systemic generalisation and/or associated systemic effects irrespective of the size and number of lesions.
2 Poor condition with marked involvement of either the body and visceral lymph nodes.
3 Good carcase condition with marked involvement of the body and visceral lymph nodes.
4 Carcases affected to a lesser extent may be approved subject to removal and condemnation of all affected parts.

## CLOSTRIDIAL DISEASES

These are usually acute or peracute toxaemias caused by members of the genus *Clostridium*, which are large, Gram-positive, spore-bearing rod-shaped bacilli. The organisms are normal saprophytes (living on dead and decomposing plant and animal matter) in soil and the intestines of animals and man.

The spores of clostridia are spherical or oval and may occupy a central, subterminal or terminal position in the bacterial cells.

Clostridial diseases are among the most serious occurring in animals and man, producing potent exotoxins (q.v.) which may (1) be elaborated in the intestine, e.g. entertotoxaemia, (2) preformed in the food and then ingested, e.g. botulism, or (3) formed in the tissues, e.g. blackleg, malignant oedema.

Fortunately, clostridial diseases occur sporadically, often being confined to certain districts, even particular fields.

Except for mild cases and tetanus, it is unlikely that many clostridial diseases will be encountered at meat inspection since in most there is a rapid onset of death. *Apparently healthy animals presented for slaughter following an outbreak of botulism, however, must be regarded with great suspicion since it is likely there is circulating botulinum toxin in these animals.*

### Bacillary haemoglobinuria

**I.** An acute highly fatal toxaemia of cattle, and less commonly, sheep, pigs and dogs in which there is high fever, jaundice, haemoglobinuria and necrotic infarcts in the liver.

**O.** North America, especially on the west coast, Canada, Mexico, Chile, Venezuela, Turkey, Australia and New Zealand. Cases have also been recorded in Britain and Ireland.

**IA.** *Clostridium haemolyticum* (*Cl. novyi* Type D). This organism can persist in contaminated soil and carcases for long periods, besides being a normal commensal of the gut.

**R.** See **IA**.

**MT.** Via ingestion of contaminated material.

**CF.** Disease is of short duration and animals may be found dead. If found alive – fever, depression, abdominal pain, suspension of rumination, dysentery, shallow respirations, jaundice and urine dark red.

**P.** Rapid onset of rigor mortis. Anaemia. Often oedema of subcutaneous tissues with blood-stained fluid in body cavities. Haemorrhagic enteritis with bloody contents. Raised anaemic infarcts in liver. Kidneys pale and friable and showing petechial haemorrhages.

**D.** Presence of haemoglobin in urine and especially anaemic infarct in liver are diagnostic.

Diagnosis is confirmed by culture (although the organism is difficult to culture) and agglutination test.

**J.** Carcase and viscera: T.

### Bighead in rams

**I.** An acute infectious disease of young rams in which there is oedema of the head and neck.

**O.** Worldwide where sheep are kept.

**IA.** *Clostridium novyi*, and on occasions *Cl. sordelli* and *Cl. chauvoei*.

**R.** As for clostridia in general.

**MT.** The organisms gain entrance to the subcutaneous tissues through wounds in the skin usually caused by fighting.

**CF.** There is a non-haemorrhagic, non-gaseous swelling of the head, face and neck.

**P** and **D.** As for **CF**.

Diagnosis is confirmed by isolation of *Cl. novyi*.

It is important to distinguish the disease from a similar 'Bighead' condition in sheep – photosensitisation caused by the ingestion of certain plants containing photodynamic substances, e.g. St John's wort, buckwheat, bog asphodel.

**J.** Carcase and viscera: Depends on the extent of the lesions, T or D.

Infection localised to head and neck, and condition good, D.

Since the disease responds to antibiotics, e.g. penicillin, it may be advisable in some cases to delay slaughter and hold for treatment at ante-mortem inspection.

### Blackleg

**I.** An acute, highly fatal, toxaemic disease of sheep and cattle characterised by oedematous swellings, especially in the skeletal and cardiac musculature. Usually animals in good condition are affected.

**O.** Worldwide. The disease tends to occur in particular areas, even fields, and has been associated with soil disturbance, e.g. after excavations and flooding. The presence of the spores is indicative of previous blackleg cases.

**IA.** *Clostridium chauvoei.*

**R.** The organism is a normal inhabitant of soil where it can exist for years in a sporing form.

**MT.** In sheep *Cl. chauvoei* usually gains entrance to the tissues through wounds including those caused by shearing, docking, castration, fighting and barbed wire, etc. The disease in sheep can occur after lambing. In cattle there is often no history of wounds and it probably enters the body via the alimentary tract after being ingested.

**CF.** The affected animal is often found dead. If alive, there is depression, anorexia, high temperature and oedema with crepitation of the affected part, which is painful and hot to the touch at first but later becomes cold and insensitive. There is lameness if a leg is involved. Almost any muscular part of the body can show lesions – brisket, shoulder, chest, back, neck, etc. – but in some cases the heart, tongue and diaphragm alone show the typical lesions.

**P.** The affected parts show dark red, spongy tissue with bubbles of gas, blood-stained fluid and a rancid odour. The lesion varies greatly in size and may be so small as to be overlooked. Blood-stained fluid and fibrin are present in the body cavities.

**D.** The acuteness of the condition and the typical lesions are suggestive of blackleg. Diagnosis can be confirmed by the culture of the organism and serology. Fluorescent-antibody technique in which the organism is stained with a dye, e.g. fluorescein isothiocyanate, which fluoresces when exposed to UV light.

**J.** Carcase and viscera: T.

### Braxy (bradsot)

**I.** An acute, infectious disease of sheep characterised by toxaemia, abomasitis and a high death rate.

**O.** The condition appears to be restricted to the British Isles (especially Scotland, Wales and Ireland), Denmark, Norway, Iceland and Australia.

**IA.** *Clostridium septicum*, the cause of malignant oedema.

**R.** The organism is a normal inhabitant of the sheep's intestinal tract and is also found in the soil.

**MT.** The disease occurs most commonly in mid-winter when snow, ice and frost abound. The organism is believed to gain entrance through the ingestion of frosted grass or other feed which predisposes the abomasal mucosa to infection.

**CF.** Anorexia, depression, fever and recumbency in animals found alive.

**P.** Inflammation, oedema, necrosis and ulceration of the abomasal wall with some enteritis and subepithelial haemorrhages in the intestinal wall.

**D.** Diagnosis is based on the necropsy findings. *Cl. septicum* can be detected in smears from the abomasal wall and cultured from blood.

*Because of the rapid onset of decomposition in sheep carcases post-mortem examinations of sheep must be carried out shortly after death if an accurate diagnosis is to be made.*

**J.** Carcase and viscera: T.

### Enterotoxaemia

Included under this heading are several forms of enterotoxaemia caused by different types of *Clostridium perfringens:*

| | *Cl. perfringens* |
|---|---|
| Lamb dysentery: | Type B |
| Struck in sheep: | Type C |
| Pulpy kidney of ruminants: | Type D |
| Necrotic haemorrhagic enteritis (calves): | Type E |
| Focal symmetrical encephalomalacia | Type D |

Enterotoxaemia due to *Cl. perfringens* Type C also occurs in calves, goats, pigs and foals. *Cl. perfringens* Type A has been isolated in cases of haemorrhagic enteritis in cattle, sheep and horses.

**I.** An acute or peracute infective disease in which there is toxaemia, fever, enteritis and high mortality.

As with all clostridial diseases, potent exotoxins are elaborated which act both locally in the tissues and centrally on the CNS and cardiovascular system.

**O.** The various entertoxaemias are worldwide in distribution.

**IA.** *Clostridium perfringens*, a normal commensal of the alimentary tract found also in soil.

**R.** See **IA**. Spores are capable of survival for years in soils. The exact predisposing factors are not known, although enterotoxaemia occurs most commonly in well-nourished animals.

**MT.** By ingestion of contaminated feed and soil. The spores germinate and proliferate in the wall of the intestine, liberating various exotoxins to produce haemorrhage, inflammation, necrosis, etc., in different organs.

**CF.** Dullness, depression, toxaemia and diarrhoea. As with most cases of acute illness, the animal separates from the rest of the flock. Acute cases may show convulsions with opisthotonus (spasm of head and neck, which are bent backwards). Muscle tremors and staggering gait.

**P.** *Pulpy kidney:* A characteristic lesion is the presence of soft pulpy kidneys. A small stream of water on a kidney dissolves the soft parenchymatous tissue leaving only the fibrous matrix.

Increased pericardial fluid. Petechiae in epi- and endocardium. Pulmonary oedema. Enteritis, which may be haemorrhagic and ulcerative. Brain lesions – oedema, haemorrhages and liquefaction.

*Struck, lamb dysentery, haemorrhagic necrotic enteritis:* Apart from the pulpy kidney lesions, these conditions are very similar to Type D in relation to lesions.

**D.** This is based on the type and distribution of the lesions. Smears from intestinal contents show large numbers of *Cl. perfringens*. Culture of organism. Serology (neutralisation of toxin with specific antiserum).

**J.** Carcase and viscera: T.

## Infectious necrotic hepatitis (black disease)

**I.** An acute infectious disease of sheep and less commonly cattle, pigs and horses.

**O.** Worldwide, especially in Australia, New Zealand, British Isles, USA and Europe.

**IA.** *Clostridium novyi* Type B. (Not all strains are pathogenic).

**R.** Intestines of animals and soil. Normal animals act as carriers.

**MT.** Ingestion of contaminated feed, grass and soil.

**CF.** Clinical findings in sheep resemble those in Types B, C and D infections without, however, the intestinal complications.

**P.** Black disease is due to a combination of *Cl. novyi* infection and liver damage caused by immature fluke infestation. On occasions liver damage caused by *Cysticercus tenuicollis* may be responsible.

Black disease gets its name from the very dark appearance of the inside of the skin due to engorgement of blood vessels. Subcutaneous oedema is present. The liver is congested and presents typical lesions of yellowish-grey necrosis about 1–5 cm in diameter surrounded by a red hyperaemic zone. Excess straw-coloured fluid is present in the pericardial sac and peritoneal and thoracic cavities. Haemorrhages show on the epicardium and endocardium.

**D.** A firm diagnosis can only be made by laboratory examination although the liver lesions and the presence of immature liver flukes (no adult flukes are present) should be a strong indication of black disease.

**J.** Carcase and viscera: T.

## Focal symmetrical encephalomalacia

**I.** An atypical form of enterotoxaemia of sheep and less often calves in which neurological signs are exhibited.

**O.** Sporadic occurrence throughout the world, especially New Zealand and South Africa.

**IA.** *Clostridium perfringens* Type D.

**R.** As for other clostridia.

**MT.** By ingestion of contaminated grass and feed.

**CF.** Many cases are found dead. If alive, there are nervous symptoms somewhat resembling those of listeriosis but without circling movements – incoordination, head pressing, blindness, convulsions, episthotonus.

**P.** Lesions occur solely in the brain – softening with haemorrhage in the thalamus and cerebellum.

**D.** Based mainly on clinical findings and lesions. The toxin of *Cl. perfringens* can be detected by a toxin neutralisation test.

**J.** Carcase and viscera: T.

## Malignant oedema

**I.** An acute toxaemic disease of animals including cattle, sheep, goats, pigs, horses and reindeer. The condition also occurs in man.

**O.** Worldwide.

**IA.** Various organisms of the genus *Clostridium* – *Cl. septicum, Cl. chauvoei, Cl. perfringens, Cl. novyi, Cl. sordelli, Cl. fallax.*

**R.** All of these organisms are found in the soil and in intestinal contents.

**MT.** Infection occurs through wounds with contaminated material, soil, etc. Wounds in animals have many causes – accidents, fighting, castration, docking, aseptic injection techniques, especially intramuscular injection. The disease may also arise at parturition.

**CF.** Toxaemia, anorexia, fever, depression, muscle tremors, lameness with rapid onset of death. Soft painful swellings are evident in the subcutaneous tissues.

**P.** Infection with the various clostridia show differences of pathological change. Affected areas (subcutis and interconnective tissues of muscle) show a blood-stained oedema which varies in consistency from being thin and yellowish to a thick gelatinous material with a sweetish odour. The affected muscles are dark in colour. Crepitation due to gas formation is usually absent in spite of the name. The overlying skin becomes stretched and dark in colour. Blood-stained serous fluid is normally present in the body cavities with haemorrhages evident under serous membranes.

**D.** The typical lesions point to malignant oedema. It is differentiated from blackleg because of absence of muscle involvement and from anthrax in pigs by restriction of oedema to the throat region.

Diagnosis is confirmed by laboratory methods – fluorescent antibody staining, etc.

**J.** Carcase and viscera: T.

### Botulism (lamziekte, limberneck, western duck disease) (see also Chapter 14)

**I.** A rapidly fatal intoxication in which preformed toxin in the feed is ingested to produce motor paralysis mainly in cattle, sheep, horses, mink, poultry, various wild animals, wildfowl and human beings.

**O.** Sporadic outbreaks of botulism occur worldwide. Bovine botulism appears to be most common in South Africa where it is associated with a phosphorus-deficient diet. In the western United States of America the disease has caused enormous losses in poultry, up to one million or more yearly.

A major outbreak (McLoughlin *et al.*, 1988) has been recorded in Northern Ireland in which 80 animals in a beef herd of 150 were affected with 68 deaths. In England botulism occurred in grazing cattle on three adjacent farms. Two heifers in a group of 10 died following feeding with ensiled poultry litter (Hogg *et al.*, 1990). In England in 1994 botulism was suspected when 150 of 550 fattening cattle (1–2 years old) died or were euthanased. Laboratory examinations could not confirm the diagnosis, this being based on clinical evidence.

**IA.** Some eight strains of *Clostridium botulinum* exist, differentiated according to the serological specificity of its neurotoxin: A, B, Ca, C, D, E, F and G. These toxins are among the most potent poisons known.

Type Ca is most common in poultry, pheasants and wildfowl; Type C in cattle, sheep, horses and mink; Type D in cattle; Types A, B and E are most common in man, in whom Types F and G occur on rare occasions. Type E is usually associated with outbreaks in fish, seafoods and meat from marine animals.

**R.** The source of infection is invariably decomposed carcases or decaying vegetable material (grass, silage, grain). Chicken manure used as feed or fertiliser, poultry litter used for bedding or ensiled as feed and poultry waste imperfectly dried as a feed supplement are important causes of botulism in livestock.

**MT.** The neurotoxin elaborated in the feed is ingested.

**CF.** Peracute cases in cattle and sheep die without premonitory symptoms. In less acute forms there is muscular paralysis, disturbed vision, difficulty in chewing and swallowing, salivation and general weakness. Death occurs in 1–4 days. Milder cases are occasionally encountered in which there is restlessness, anorexia, lack of thirst, incoordination, difficult respiration, roaring and recumbency.

**P.** Lesions are non-specific. There may be endocardial and epicardial haemorrhages in the heart and similar haemorrhages in the cerebrum and cerebellum.

**D.** The presence of foreign material in the stomach, abomasum or rumen may be suggestive of botulism, as is the characteristic motor paralysis. It is often difficult, however, to distinguish botulism from other conditions in which nervous symptoms are displayed, e.g. rabies, encephalomyelitis of equines, parturient paresis in cattle, hypocalcaemia, scrapie and louping ill in sheep.

The toxin can be demonstrated in filtrates from stomach contents and suspect feed by mouse inoculation.

**J.** Carcase and viscera: T.

### Tetanus (lockjaw)

**I.** A usually fatal toxaemia of virtually all mammals in which tetany (tonic spasm of muscles), hyperaesthesia (increased sensitivity to stimuli) and convulsions are present. Horses are the most sensitive animals while birds and cats appear to be resistant.

**O.** The disease occurs sporadically worldwide, especially in intensively cultivated areas.

**IA.** *Clostridium tetani.* Found in soils and intestinal tracts of animals. The organism forms spherical spores which appear terminally in the organisms. Under specific anaerobic conditions with necrosis at the point of entry, a very potent neurotoxin travels along motor nerves to the CNS, the organisms remaining at the initial site, where they multiply.

**R.** See **IA**.

**MT.** Via deep puncture wounds, e.g. those caused by nails in the feet of horses or caused by careless shearing, castration, docking or injection operations. Infection may also enter through wounds in the buccal mucosa.

**CF.** The incubation period varies from one week to several months, the longer incubation period usually being associated with milder symptoms.

Symptoms in the horse include muscular stiffness, muscle tremors and spasm, incoordination, sweating, increased heart and respiratory rates and congested mucous membranes. Muscle spasm affecting the masseter muscles cause difficulty in prehension, mastication and swallowing (the so-called '*lockjaw*'), while spasm of the back and neck muscles produce extension of the head and neck – opisthotonus and the so-called 'sawhorse' posture. The nictitating membrane of the eye is prolapsed. The tail is stiff and extended, the ears are pricked and the animal becomes very excitable, responding to even minor stimuli. Bloat is apparent in cattle with rumenal contractions.

Severe cases end fatally with marked tetanic spasm (prolonged muscular spasm without intervening relaxation), respiratory and cardiac arrest.

**P.** There are usually no significant post-mortem lesions, although necrosis of the spermatic cord may be evident where castration has been involved. Often in cases of long incubation periods the initial wounds have healed on the surface.

**D.** Distinctive clinical signs especially spasm of the jaw muscles and the prolapsed third eyelid are usually adequate for an accurate diagnosis. However, the differential diagnosis may be difficult as tetanus can be confused with conditions such as lactation tetany, enzootic muscular dystrophy, various forms of meningitis, BSE, strychnine poisoning, etc.

The organism may be cultured from the causal wound, if detected.

**J.** Cases of tetanus, especially in lambs, have in the past been presented as casualties at meat plants. They represent one of many conditions where total condemnation on ante-mortem inspection is fully warranted.

Ante-mortem: T.

Post-mortem: Carcase and viscera: T.

## COLIBACILLOSIS (DIARRHOEA, SCOURS, GASTROENTERITIS, SEPTICAEMIA NEONATORUM)

The causes of diarrhoea in the *newly-born animal* are many and varied and include enterotoxigenic strains of *E. coli*, *Salmonella* spp., *Chlamydia* spp., *Cl. perfringens*, *Campylobacter*, *Yersinia*, *Shigella*, *Cryptosporidium* and *Providentia* acting alone or in combination. Various viruses are also incriminated, e.g. rotavirus, coronavirus, enterovirus, adenovirus and herpesvirus, which also act in unison with different bacteria. Initial errors in husbandry are important predisposing factors in the causation of diarrhoea in young stock.

**I.** An extremely common infectious disease of calves, piglets, lambs, kids, foals and probably all young mammals, characterised by diarrhoea and dehydration with rapid onset of death (1–4 days) in the septicaemic form and a longer period of illness in the more common enterotoxigenic type.

**O.** Worldwide, causing great economic losses.

**IA.** Various strains of *Escherichia coli* which vary in virulence, and antigenic structure (O, H, K, L, A and B), some being extremely virulent, e.g. K99, F17, O157.H7 (a verotoxigenic bacillus which has recently been responsible for food poisoning in man) and those producing the EDP (edema disease principle).

*E. coli* is a Gram-negative, motile, non-sporing bacillus.

**R.** *E. coli* is widely distributed in the environment and in the intestines of animals (domestic and wild) and man.

**MT.** By the ingestion of food and water contaminated with the faeces of affected animals.

Factors predisposing to infection include lack of colostrum and its immunoglobulins (responsible for septicaemic colibacillosis but not the enterotoxigenic type), excessive feeding of milk, use of inadequate milk replacers, and poor standards of housing, hygiene and stockmanship.

**CF.** *Septicaemic colibacillosis:* Acute illness with depression, weakness, anorexia, initial high fever, dehydration, diarrhoea and death in 1–4 days.

*Enterotoxigenic colibacillosis:* Profuse watery to pasty white, foul-smelling diarrhoea which may contain mucus and/or blood clots, depression, temperature normal and later subnormal, cold clammy skin and recumbency. Death may occur in 12–24 h.

**P.** Gastroenteritis which varies in extent and severity. Subserous and submucosal haemorrhages may be present along with pneumonia, arthritis, omphalophlebitis, peritonitis and meningitis.

**D.** Differentiation of the various causal organisms is difficult in the enteric type of colibacillosis in which mixed infections may occur. Laboratory diagnosis is based on the use of specialised techniques to detect *E. coli* as well as viruses, cryptosporodia, etc., in faecal samples.

**J.** Carcase and viscera: T.

### Bowel oedema (*E. coli* enterotoxaemia, oedema disease, bowel oedema, gut oedema)

**I.** An acute, highly fatal enterotoxaemia of *weaner and growing pigs* characterised by oedema of the subcutaneous and subserosal tissues.

**O.** Worldwide, where modern pig husbandry is practised.

**IA.** Haemolytic *E. coli* which produce the oedema disease principle (EDP) – mainly O138.K81, O139.K82, O141.K85 strains. (Hemolysis refers to rupture of red blood cells with release of haemoglobin.)

**R.** Intestines of pigs and soil.

**MT.** By ingestion of contaminated food and water. Special environmental conditions are necessary for oedema disease to appear. The condition mainly affects pigs in good condition subjected to various stressors, e.g. rapid changes in diet, especially at weaning, changes to new pens, transportation, immunisation and chilling. Genetic factors may be involved, although there is no correlation with breed.

**CF.** Sudden death may occur without any premonitory symptoms. Incoordination, anorexia, ataxia, knucklng of fetlocks, oedema of eyelids and face, altered squeal, constipation, paralysis and recumbency with death usually within 24 h.

**P.** Oedema with serogelatinous fluid in various sites – subcutaneous especially of eyelids and face, stomach wall (cardiac gland region), mesocolon and sometimes larynx. Stomach is usually full of feed. Pleural, peritoneal and pericardial cavities may contain excess serous amber-coloured fluid with strands of fibrin. Focal malacia (softening) of brainstem may be present.

**D.** Based on epidemiology, sudden onset of symptoms in susceptible animals and typical lesions. Diagnosis is confirmed by culture from small intestine and colon.

**J.**

Carcase: A, provided condition is good and other abnormalities absent.

Viscera: T (stomach and intestines).

### Coliform gastroenteritis (enteric colibacillosis, post-weaning diarrhoea)

**I.** An acute infectious toxaemic disease of *weaner* pigs associated with gastroenteritis, lack of growth, dehydration, diarrhoea and much economic loss.

**O.** Worldwide.

**IA.** Certain pathogenic strains of *E. coli* which produce enterotoxins and also have the ability to adhere to the mucosal cells of the small intestine – K88, 987P, K99, F41 and certain O groups.

**R.** Intestines of pigs.

**MT.** By ingestion of contaminated food and water. The disease is precipitated by errors in husbandry – dietary changes, poor housing conditions, poor sanitation standards, low temperatures, etc.

**CF.** Watery diarrhoea, unthriftiness in later stages of disease, dehydration, pink skin discoloration, normal temperature. Deaths usually occur in 7–10 days.

**P.** Cutaneous erythema, dehydration, gastritis with dilated small intestine containing yellowish mucoid fluid, sometimes haemorrhagic, oedema in the spiral coils of the colon.

**D.** Depends on consideration of husbandry methods, age incidence, lesions, etc. Isolation of *E. coli* of above strains confirms diagnosis.

Disease must be distinguished from salmonellosis, coccidiosis and viral conditions.

**J.**

Carcase: A. Provided condition is good with no evidence of fever, etc.

T, if carcase is fevered and/or emaciated.

Viscera: T (stomach and intestines).

## CONTAGIOUS BOVINE AND CAPRINE PLEUROPNEUMONIA (CBPP AND CCPP) (Plate 1, Fig. 6)

**I.** A very contagious pneumonia and pleurisy of cattle and goats in which typical lesions in the lungs are displayed.

Notifiable disease (UK).

**O.** These diseases are endemic in Africa, Asia, Middle East, Italy, Russia, Poland, Spain and Portugal, especially NW Portugal, where 270 outbreaks of CBPP occurred in the first quarter of 1993. In Italy there were 34 outbreaks of CBPP in 1992 and 10 during 1993. The disease (CBPP) was eradicated from Great Britain in 1898, from the USA in 1892 and South Africa in 1916.

**IA.** *Mycoplasma mycoides* var. *mycoides SC* causes CBPP and *mycoplasma* strain 38 is responsible for CCPP. These are tiny, mutant, pleomorphic bacteria which do not form normal cell walls. As L-forms they are delicate and friable but can multiply in suitable environments, unlike protoplasts which also have no cell walls.

**R.** Saprophytic types of mycoplasmas can be isolated from soil, sewage, etc., and parasitic forms from plants and animals, mainly cattle and goats.

Infection in cattle usually arises from an affected or an asymptomatic carrier animal. The organisms can remain infective for long periods in urine and other discharges.

**MT.** Inhalation of infective droplets.

**CF.** The disease may be either acute or chronic. Acute forms show high fever, rapid respiration, anorexia, depression, coughing with arched back and extended head, with death from fibrinous pneumonia/pleurisy in several days to 3–4 weeks. Chronic cases show symptoms of less intensity with apparent recovery after weeks or months.

**P.** The post-mortem lesions, apart from varying loss of condition, are typical, diagnostic and confined to the thoracic cavity. They take the form of fibrous thickening with serous effusion of the pleura and interlobular lung septa – the classical *'marbled lung'*. Pulmonary lobules show either the red or grey hepatisation of pneumonia. Pleural adhesions are commonly present and there may be clear yellowish fluid in the pleural cavity.

**D.** Based on clinical findings and especially the typical lung lesions. Diagnosis can be confirmed by dark field microscopy of smears from the lungs or pleural effusion, complement fixation, immunofluorescence and histopathology.

**J.**

Carcase: A, provided condition is satisfactory.

Viscera (lungs and pleurae): D.

Carcase and viscera: T, where emaciation is present.

*Mycoplasmas*, on occasions with different forms of viruses, *Pasteurellae*, etc., can also be involved in the causation of bovine respiratory disease (BRD) (q.v.). They also are implicated in contagious agalactia of goats and sheep, mycoplasmal arthritis in cattle and pigs, enzootic pneumonia in pigs, vulvovaginitis and keratoconjunctivitis (pink eye) in cattle, sheep and goats, although the main cause of the latter is *Moraxella bovis* (q.v.).

### Mycoplasmal arthritis in cattle

**I.** A benign to severe infectious disease of young cattle (6–8 months).

**O.** USA and Canada (in feedlots), Europe and British Isles.

**IA.** *Mycoplasma agalactiae* var. *bovis.*

**R.** Mycoplasmas can be isolated from the respiratory and genital tracts of normal, affected and recovered animals.

**MT.** The organisms probably gain entrance to the bloodstream (bacteraemia) from the respiratory and genital sites during periods of stress and are conveyed to the joints.

**CF.** Lameness, inappetence, fever in more acute cases and loss of condition. Enlargement of leg joints. Mortality rates vary from 5% to 50%.

**P.** Affected joints show varying degrees of change from an increase in synovial fluid with some inflammation of cartilage to a severe purulent synovitis with erosion of cartilage and granulation tissue formation. There is usually an associated tenosynovitis.

**D.** Based on lesions, history of outbreak, etc., and confirmed by culture of *Myco. agalactiae.*

**J.** Carcase: D. If evidence of fever is present, T.

### Mycoplasmal arthritis in pigs

**I.** A fairly benign syndrome in piglets and growing pigs with usually low morbidity and mortality.

**IA.** *Mycoplasma hyorhinis* and *M. hyosynoviae.* Occurrence, reservoir, mode of transmission and diagnosis resemble those in cattle.

**CF.** Similar to symptoms in cattle except that there are usually respiratory symptoms in the older pigs.

**P.** Joint lesions as in cattle. Evidence of pleurisy, pericarditis and peritonitis with fibrous adhesions in the chest cavity.

**J.** Carcase: A. If fever present, T.

### Mycoplasmal (enzootic) pneumonia in pigs (EP)

**I.** A chronic, usually mild infectious disease of weaning and growing pigs in which pneumonia, lack of growth and feed conversion feature. The disease is associated with huge economic loss.

**O.** Most areas of the world, especially in intensive units.

**IA.** *Mycoplasma hyopneumoniae*, a host-specific organism. The term *'virus pneumonia'* was applied to this disease before the actual cause was known.

**R.** As for *Myco. agalactiae.*

**MT.** Direct and indirect contact between pigs via respiratory tract. Airborne infection is known to occur. Certain stressors can precipitate the disease, e.g. poor housing conditions, substandard hygiene, mixing of pigs, and climatic conditions, especially at weaning.

**CF.** Such is the infectious nature of the disease that all pigs in a herd may be affected. The disease is most typical when it first appears. A dry, hacking cough is the most common sign, noticeable when pigs are aroused and at feeding time. There is usually no fever. Loss of condition is evident in later stages.

**P.** The lesions of mycoplasmal pneumonia are the most common encountered on meat inspection in pigs and may account for 75% or more of a herd, especially during the winter months in northern climates. They take the form of pneumonia and pleurisy – greyish or purplish areas of consolidation affecting mainly the apical and cardiac lobes of the lungs. The bronchial and mediastinal lymph nodes are enlarged. There may be a fibrinous pericarditis and pleurisy and catarrhal exudate in the bronchi and bronchioles.

**D.** The clinical findings along with the typical lesions are adequate for a diagnosis which is confirmed by fluorescent antibody staining of lung smears and complement fixation tests.

**J.** Carcase and viscera: A, provided condition is satisfactory and fever absent. Condition poor and/or fever: T.

Trimming of thoracic cavity may be necessary.

### Contagious agalactia of sheep and goats

**I.** A subacute or chronic disease of sheep and goats associated with mastitis, arthritis and ophthalmia and fairly high mortality (10–20 per cent).

**O.** Worldwide, but occurring most commonly in Mediterranean countries.

**IA.** *Mycoplasma agalactia*, *Myco. mycoides*, *Myco. putrefaciens Myco. capricolum*, *M. putrefaciens* and *M. capricolum* are the causes of mastitis in small ruminants, especially goats.

**R.** As for CBPP and CGPP.

**MT.** Probably the intramammary route from infected milk, contaminated equipment, milkers' hands, etc. Carrier animals are common, the organisms being found in the milk and in ears.

**CF.** The condition occurs at or shortly after parturition. Fever. Inappetence. Acute mastitis with thick yellowish milk. Enlarged supramammary glands. Milk secretion may cease. Atrophy of udder tissue may occur. Polyarthritis is common but keratoconjunctivitis less so. Abortion on occasions.

**P.** See CF.

**D.** Isolation of organisms from milk and blood. Culture of organisms. Serology – complement fixation, indirect haemagglutination and ELISA tests.

**J.** Carcase and viscera: A, provided condition satisfactory and no general signs.

Diseased organs: D (udder and associated lymph nodes).

### Contagious vulvo-vaginitis of cattle, sheep and goats

**I.** An acute or chronic infectious disease in which there is granular vulvovaginitis and infertility.

**O.** Worldwide.

**IA.** *Mycoplasma agalactiae* is said to be involved but its exact importance is uncertain. Other organisms may act in unison with *M. agalactiae*.

**R.** Affected and carrier animals, organism being found in the external genital tract.

**MT.** Via vulva/vagina.

**CF.** Granular and nodular inflammation of the external genital tract. Similar lesions may occur on the penis of the bull.

**P.** See CF.

**D.** Based on type of lesions and isolation of *Myco. agalactiae* alone or in combination with other bacteria.

**J.** Carcase and viscera: A, provided condition is good with no general signs.

Affected organs: D (vagina and vulva).

## BOVINE FARCY (BOVINE NOCARDIOSIS, MYCOTIC LYMPHANGITIS)

**I.** A chronic infection of cattle characterised by purulent, granular and nodular lesions in the superficial lymphatics and lymph nodes. The disease also occurs in horses, sheep, goats, dogs, cats and birds.

**O.** The disease appears to be mainly confined to tropical and subtropical countries, especially the West Indies and East and Central Africa.

**IA.** The main bacterium involved is *Nocardia farcinicus* which is related to *Actinomyces* (q.v.). Unlike the genus *Actinomyces*, the *Nocardia* are aerobic organisms and some are acid-fast. Other bacteria incriminated are *Mycobacterium farcinogenes* and *Myco. senegalese*.

A few species are pathogenic to man, e.g. *N. asteroides*, which causes chronic granular lesions in the lungs similar to TB, and *N. madurae*, one of the causative agents of Madura foot or mycetoma, a chronic granulomatous disease of the human foot encountered in south India and Africa.

**R.** The *Nocardia* are soil saprophytes and are found in infective discharges.

**MT.** Via skin wounds.

**CF.** Firm nodular lesions along lymphatic tracts and in associated lymph nodes. These rupture and discharge thick greyish or yellowish pus through sinuses or ulcers. The lesions resemble those of farcy in horses and actinobacillosis but are entirely distinct. The lymphatic tracts are enlarged and surrounded by cellulitis. The most typical lesions are found in the lower limbs, neck and shoulder but may involve any part of the body. The lungs, however, may be affected in complicated cases and mastitis may occur. In severe mastitis cases the udder may rupture.

Unless the disease is complicated there are generally no symptoms. But fever, inappetence, lameness, loss of condition and respiratory distress may be present.

**P.** See **CF.** The lesions take the form of firm granulomatous nodules resembling those of actinobacillosis but sulphur granules are absent.

**D.** Smears of pus, sputum, milk or tissue stained by Gram's stain show the typical branching filaments and bacillary forms of *Nocardia*.

**J.**

Carcase and viscera: A, where lesions are localised and general signs absent.

Affected parts: D.

Carcase and viscera: T. Fever and other complications present and/or poor condition.

## CONTAGIOUS BOVINE PYELONEPHRITIS

**I.** A sporadic inflammatory infection of the bovine urinary tract (kidneys, ureters and bladder). The condition sometimes occurs in sheep.

**O.** Worldwide, but appears to be more common in Europe, N. America, Israel and Australia.

**IA.** *Corynebacterium renale*, alone or in mixed infections with other organisms. *E. coli*, *Cl. pyogenes* and various streptococci and staphylococci may cause similar lesions. The bacterium is also responsible for enzootic posthitis in sheep (q.v.).

The bacterium is a Gram-positive, aerobic, non-sporing rod which forms palisades or 'Chinese characters' in culture, resembling *Erysipelothrix* and *Listeria*. The genus *Corynebacterium* gets its name from the club-shaped appearance of the ends of the bacilli.

**R.** The bacilli appear to be normal commensals on skin and in genital and respiratory tracts. Carrier animals are a common source of infection.

**MT.** Direct and indirect contact with contaminated materials such as bedding, cloths, brushes, etc.

**CF.** Restlessness, colic, tail switching, possible fever, straining to urinate, frequent passage of blood-stained urine, gradual loss of condition.

**P.** Very thickened ureters with haemorrhagic and ulcerated mucosae; enlarged haemorrhagic kidneys with evidence of pus and blood in calyces; bladder wall oedematous and sometimes ulcerated with necrotic debris in the bladder.

**D.** The lesions are fairly conclusive. Sporadic nature of disease assists in diagnosis. Important to differentiate from leptospirosis, bacillary haemoglobinuria, etc.

Stained smears of urine sediment will show the characteristic bacilli.

**J.**

Carcase and viscera: T, in cases of poor condition and systemic changes.

Carcase and viscera: A, no systemic effect and condition good.

Affected parts: D.

## CYSTITIS AND PYELONEPHRITIS

**I.** An infective disease of the urinary tract of sows, and sometimes boars, which is similar to the bovine condition but on occasions is peracute and can lead to sudden death.

**IA.** *Corynebacterium (Eubacterium) suis*. The occurrence, reservoir, mode of transmission and clinical findings are similar to the bovine disease.

**P.** The bladder wall is oedematous and congested and may show ulceration in places, while interstitial nephritis is present in the kidneys.

**D.** Based on fairly typical clinical signs and post-mortem lesions. Culture of the offending organism confirms the diagnosis.

Differential diagnosis: the condition must be differentiated from kidney worm infestation (*Stephanurus dentatus*) and other causes of haemoglobinuria.

**J.** As far contagious bovine pyelonephritis.

## DERMATOPHILOSIS (CUTANEOUS STREPTOTRICHOSIS, LUMPY WOOL, STRAWBERRY FOOT ROT)

**I.** An infectious dermatitis of the epidermis characterised by exudation and scab formation in cattle (cutaneous streptotrichosis), sheep (lumpy wool, 'mycotic dermatitis', strawberry foot rot), goats, horses and less commonly pigs and man.

**O.** The disease is encountered worldwide but is more common in tropical and subtropical countries.

**IA.** *Dermatophilus congolensis*, a Gram-positive, facultative anaerobe, non-acid-fast bacillus which appears as filamentous, branching hyphae like *Actinomyces* and flagellated, containing motile zoospores.

**R.** The organism exists as a saprophyte in the soil and in carrier and affected animals in the epidermis of the skin.

**MT.** Via skin wounds and abrasions. Certain factors are most important in predisposing to the disease. These include moisture (the disease is most common during rainy seasons), high temperatures and the wounds caused by various ectoparasites such as ticks and biting flies and by shearing, castration, etc.

**CF.** Infection in susceptible skin begins with the action of the zoospores, which later germinate to produce branched hyphae. Acute inflammation of the superficial layers of the skin results and spreads to other areas. These acute lesions heal in 2–3 weeks but may progress to produce the chronic form of the dermatitis in which thick, horny scabs are formed which adhere to the wool and hair staples.

The areas of skin most commonly affected are the head, neck and dorsal surface of the body.

*Strawberry foot rot* (proliferative dermatitis) in sheep is an infection of the lower limbs, from knee to coronet, with *D. congolensis*. Brown scabs appear which, when removed, reveal a raw, bleeding, granuloma surrounded by an ulcer. The disease, if severe and prolonged, causes considerable loss of body weight.

Strawberry foot rot has been recorded only in the British Isles and Australia.

**P.** See **CF**.

**D.** Diagnosis is largely based on the appearance of the lesions and confirmed by smears from scabs, culture of the organism and fluorescent antibody and ELISA tests. Differential diagnoses include ulcerative dermatosis in sheep, contagious ecthyma ('orf') in sheep and goats, ringworm and lumpy skin disease in cattle.

**J.** Carcase and viscera: A, provided condition is satisfactory.

## ENZOOTIC BALANOPOSTHITIS (SHEATH ROT, PIZZLE ROT)

**I.** A contagious infection of sheep and goats, and sometimes cattle, in which ulcers appear on the prepuce and less commonly on the vulva.

**O.** Australia, South America and USA mainly, where Merino sheep and Angora goats are affected. The outbreaks are often severe with high mortality.

**IA.** *Corynebacterium renale*, which also causes contagious bovine pyelonephritis (q.v.).

**R.** The organism can be found in normal animals (prepuce of rams and some bulls and the vulva of ewes and goats).

**MT.** As for contagious bovine pyelonephritis. The disease is associated with the feeding of high-protein diets. Flies may play a part in transmission.

**CF.** Brownish scab formation of prepuce and vulva with ultimate haemorrhagic ulceration and fibrosis. Condition may extend to occlusion of prepuce and vulva with vagina involvement. Difficulty in urination. Restlessness. Kicking at belly. Uraemia, toxaemia and septicaemia (q.v.) often ensue. Spontaneous recovery sometimes takes place.

**P.** See **CF**.

**D.** Lesions are fairly characteristic. Differential diagnosis: the viral diseases, ulcerative dermatosis of sheep and pustular vulvovaginitis of cattle.

**J.**

Carcase and viscera: A, provided condition good and no general signs.

Affected organs: D.

Carcase and viscera: T, in cases of uraemia, toxaemia, septicaemia.

## ERYSIPELAS (SWINE)

**I.** An acute or chronic infectious disease of pigs in which skin, lesions, high fever and sometimes septicaemia, occur in the acute form and proliferative lesions in chronic cases.

**O.** Common in most areas of the world.

**IA.** *Erysipelothrix rhusiopathiae* (insidiosa), a Gram-positive, non-motile, non-capsulated, microaerophilic, straight or slightly curved, slender rod which resembles *Listeria monocytogenes* but which is feebly motile.

*E. rhusiopathiae* is also responsible for arthritis (polyarthritis) in sheep and cattle, post-dipping lameness in sheep and acute septicaemia in turkeys, ducks and geese (q.v.).

*Erysipeloid* in man is a localised zoonotic skin infection caused by *E. rhusiopathiae*, often accompanied by arthritis, in persons handling animals (farmers, meat and fish plant workers), poultry, meat, reptiles and freshwater fish and shellfish.

As with animals, the infection is acquired through cuts and abrasions. After an incubation period of 2–7 days a red, painful, oedematous lesion appears on the skin, commonly on the hands, legs and face, and occurring more often in women than men. This lesion often has a raised border.

Patients are fevered owing to a bacteraemia which rarely extends to a septicaemia and arthritis, especially of the fingers, may be present. Other constitutional symptoms such as inappetence and depression may occur depending on the severity of the condition. Most cases, however, remain as a mild skin infection.

Erysipeloid responds well to penicillin and erythromycin, but recurrences may take place.

The condition is prevented by ensuring high standards of personal hygiene and care in the handling of animals, especially pigs, carcase meat, poultry and fish.

**R.** *E. rhusiopathiae* is very widely distributed in nature, in soils, fish and other forms of wildlife. Pigs and other livestock may act as carriers, the organism existing in the tonsils, other lymphoid tissues and intestinal tract.

In the soil it can exist as a saprophyte for a year or more and this accounts for the sporadic outbreaks of the disease which in Britain occur mainly in the warmer summer months. Its persistence in soil depends on many factors such as temperature, pH and the presence of other organisms.

Although the bacillus is easily destroyed by water at 100°C and by disinfectants such as caustic soda and the hypochlorites in a few minutes, it is resistant to formaldehyde and phenol and can remain viable for long periods in buried carcases, dried blood, frozen and chilled carcases (10 months) and salted and smoked meat (3–4 months).

**MT.** Soil contaminated with the faeces of affected animals and birds. Direct and indirect contact with affected, in-contact, and carrier animals which discharge the bacteria in their faeces, urine, saliva and nasal secretions. Flies are known to play a part in the transference of infection. Infection probably takes place by ingestion and also through skin wounds.

Contaminated materials such as bedding, soil, feed and water serve as media for indirect transmission of infection.

Infection has been reported via surface water contaminated by rodents and sewage from meat plants and from fish meal used in feed.

As with many diseases, predisposing factors such as poor housing, low standards of hygiene and inefficient husbandry methods act as stressors in causing the disease, which seems to be more prevalent in recently farrowed sows. It is possible that genetic factors play a role, as does the actual virulence of the organisms.

**CF.** The disease occurs in *four* main forms – acute septicaemia, subacute skin form, chronic arthritis and vegetative endocarditis. While the acute and subacute types are dramatic and frequently lead to death, the chronic forms are by far the most important economically. Clinical signs are classified as acute, subacute and chronic manifestations. There may be a subclinical form in which no symptoms are evident but which develops into chronic swine erysipelas.

*Acute swine erysipelas* begins with a *bacteraemia* (the temporary presence of bacteria in the bloodstream) in which the organisms may be quickly eliminated with the sole development of temporary localised skin lesions which quickly disappear without septicaemia occurring. In this case either the animal is partly immune or the bacteria are of low virulence. More typically, the bacteria are virulent and/or the pig lacks immunity and the case quickly develops into a generalised infection *(septicaemia)*.

Clinical signs appear suddenly and some pigs may be found dead. Other pigs show very high temperatures (104–109°F), stiffness of gait with evident leg pain; difficulty in lying down; shifting from one foot to another; recumbency; depression; inappetence; constipation sometimes followed by diarrhoea, and resentment and squealing when disturbed. Abortion may occur in sows which also may develop agalactia.

*Skin lesions* vary from generalised erythema with purplish discoloration of the ears, snout and belly to light pink or purple diamond- or quadrangular-shaped raised, firm weals on any part of the body but most commonly seen on the back and sides. Necrosis of the skin lesions may occur, with sloughing of the affected parts. Fatal SE is usually associated with livid dark red or purplish lesions affecting ears, belly, thighs, tail and jowls, whereas light pink lesions normally lead to recovery. Healing of the skin changes takes weeks owing to secondary infection.

*Subacute SE*: The symptoms are less severe – pigs may still feed; temperature is lower; skin lesions few in number; no evidence of leg stiffness and quick recovery.

*Chronic SE*: This may follow either acute or subacute SE and is manifested mainly by signs of arthritis and sometimes cardiac insufficiency.

There is enlargement and stiffness of joints with lameness and disinclination to move. In those cases which progress to valvular endocarditis (seen most often in young adult or mature pigs), death may occur from embolism at times of undue exertion. Dyspnoea (difficult or laboured breathing) is evident especially after exertion. Feeding usually continues but there is progressive loss of condition.

In all forms of SE the type and severity of symptoms and the outcome largely depend on early diagnosis and the initiation of effective treatment with penicillin.

**P.** All the changes produced by *E. rhusiopathiae* are non-suppurative in type, unless complicated by secondary invaders.

The diamond or rhomboid skin lesions are characteristic of SE but not the various other changes. These skin lesions sometimes only become evident in the carcase after scalding.

*Acute SE:* In addition to the 'diamonds' there may be oedema and congestion of the lungs, petechial haemorrhages on the epicardium and myocardium, especially in the left atrium. Varying degrees of gastritis are common, from a mild catarrhal to a haemorrhagic type. The liver is congested, as is the spleen, which may also be enlarged. The kidneys show petechiae in the cortex and the bladder is usually congested. Lymph nodes are enlarged and congested and may be haemorrhagic.

*Chronic SE:* The main finding is a chronic non-suppurative arthritis affecting mainly the stifle, hock, elbow and carpal joints. On occasions the spine is affected. Some granulation tissue with erosion of the articular surfaces may be present along with serosanguinous fluid containing fibrin in the synovial cavities. The joint capsule is thickened and its synovial membrane is hyperaemic. Changes in the joints may be so advanced with fibrous tissue formation as to cause ankylosis.

The *vegetative endocarditis* cases show wart-like growths which contain the bacilli in large numbers. These are present on the heart valves, usually the mitral valve. Mitral stenosis normally gives rise to compensatory enlargement of the heart. Emboli from these cardiac vegetations may give rise to infarcts, which are usually observed in the kidneys.

**D.** The typical *'diamond'* skin changes are diagnostic of acute SE but less obvious lesions along with arthritis and endocarditis make for difficulty in diagnosis. Acute SE usually responds to treatment with penicillin within 24 h which supports a tentative diagnosis.

At post-mortem *E. rhusiopathiae* can be detected in stained smears from blood, heart, joints, kidneys, liver, etc., and cultured on enriched media.

*Serology*: Agglutination, complement fixation and immunofluorescence tests have been used but may not always be specific and sensitive.

**J.** Judgement in cases of SE is notoriously difficult because of the various categories involved and the situation regarding ante-mortem inspection, antibiotic residues and the results of microbiological examination.

*Ante-mortem*: Acute and subacute SE: R, retain for treatment. Slaughter to be delayed until after treatment and recovery.

*Post-mortem*:

1 Acute and subacute SE: Carcase, T.
2 Chronic SE: Carcase, A. (Arthritic/cardiac lesions localised, condition satisfactory and no systemic effect. No hazard to consumers.)
3 Chronic SE: Carcase, T. (Arthritis widespread and/or condition poor with systemic effects.)
4 Chronic SE: Carcase, A. (Cardiac lesions mild, condition good, no systemic effects, no hazard to consumers.)

An alternative judgement for (2) and (4) above in some instances would be heat treatment (Hh) with condemnation of affected parts.

### Polyarthritis in sheep and cattle

In *lambs E. rhusiopathiae* infection is responsible for arthritis which commonly affects the knee, elbow, stifle and hock joints. Although the condition may be acute in type, it is usually chronic and may also affect calves and kids. Infection takes place through skin wounds, very often following docking and castration, but it can also occur via the navel.

Affected joints are swollen, painful and hot to the touch, but non-suppurative. Septicaemia is transient in the acute form and the animal usually recovers in 2–3 weeks, although death is sometimes a feature in very acute cases. However, the more common sequel is a chronic arthritis when the bacteria lodge in the joints. In adult sheep a valvular endocarditis may be present along with necrotic skin lesions. (Valvular endocarditis in sheep may be also caused by *Streptococcus faecalis*.)

The condition must be differentiated from the arthritis of joint ill due to streptococci, muscular dystrophy (q.v.) and other forms of lameness.

In *cattle* erysipelas is rare, but polyarthritis has been recorded with evidence of abscesses in the lungs and liver.

*Post-dipping lameness in sheep* is associated with the fact that sheep dips through continued use become contaminated with various bacteria including *E. rhusiopathiae*. Infection takes place through skin abrasions, especially on the hoof and fetlock, these areas becoming hot and painful.

While deaths may occur in all these erysipelas conditions, loss of condition is the more common sequel.

*Judgement* in cases of polyarthritis and post-dipping lameness can be more lenient than in typical SE provided carcase condition is satisfactory, since these are essentially chronic diseases.

## GLANDERS (FARCY, MALLEUS)

**I.** An acute or chronic, highly fatal, contagious disease of solipeds (horses, asses and mules) manifested by ulcerating nodules in the upper respiratory tract, lungs and skin. A *zoonosis*, the disease may occur in man, in whom it is generally fatal. Cases have occurred rarely in sheep and goats. Cats and dogs may be infected by eating infected meat.

Notifiable disease (UK).

**O.** Glanders, at one time widespread throughout the world, has been eradicated from many countries by test and slaughter programmes and no longer occurs in the western hemisphere. The disease was eradicated from Britain and Denmark in 1928, N. Ireland (1913), France (1959), Germany (1955), Sweden (1943), Switzerland (1937), Russia (1940), Austria and Portugal (1952) and Spain (1956). S. Africa has had no cases since 1945, the USA since 1956, Japan since 1935 and Australia since 1891. Glanders has never been recorded in New Zealand.

Glanders is now restricted to exceptional outbreaks in Turkey, Syria, India, Burma, Afghanistan and China.

**IA.** *Pseudomonas (Malleomyces) mallei*, a Gram-negative, aerobic, flagellated bacillus which is a true parasite unable to survive for longer than 6 weeks in the absence of its specific animal host. The organism is fairly easily destroyed by light, heat and most disinfectants.

**R.** The organism is present in the exudates from respiratory and skin lesions of infected and carrier animals.

**MT.** Infection usually takes place by the ingestion of food and water contaminated by nasal discharges.

**CF.** In the *acute* form of glanders there is high fever (temperature 106°C) due to a septicaemia, coughing, respiratory distress with a nasal discharge, at first serous and later purulent and blood-stained. Nodules (about 1 cm in diameter) appear in the nasal passages and on the lower legs and abdomen. Death from septicaemia usually occurs within a few days following a rapid loss of weight.

The symptoms in the *chronic* form of glanders are related to the specific lesions which develop in the various sites – nasal passages, lungs or skin – although there may be combinations of all three. Chronic cases are ill for several months, the outcome being either death or apparent recovery to become carriers.

In the *nasal* form, granulomatous nodules develop on the nasal septum and the lower parts of the turbinate bones. These nodules, which resemble tubercles, become ulcerated and later heal with star-shaped scar tissue. The nodules are usually discrete but some may coalesce. The submaxillary lymph nodes are enlarged and oedematous.

In the *pulmonary form* of glanders, small pea-sized tubercle-like nodules with caseous or calcified centres are formed in the lungs. There is usually an accompanying bronchopneumonia caused by breakdown of the nodules with discharge of infective pus. The bronchial and mediastinal lymph nodes are normally involved and nodules and ulcers may be present in the larynx and trachea. Old nodules, which sometimes may be found in the liver and spleen, often develop a fibrous capsule.

The *cutaneous* form of glanders (*'farcy'*) shows nodules along the lymphatics, especially of the lower limbs. They degenerate to form ulcers with the discharge of a thick, viscous pus. The associated lymphatics become tortuous and indurated and local lymph nodes are enlarged and oedematous and eventually discharge a similar type of pus.

**P.** See **CF.**

**D.** Diagnosis is confirmed by the *mallein test* (injection of 0.1 ml of mallein intradermally into the lower eyelid with reading in 24 h). Positive reaction is marked oedema of eyelid with purulent conjunctivitis. Also indirect haemagglutination and conglutinin complement absorption tests.

The condition must be distinguished from epizootic lymphangitis (q.v.) and melioidosis (q.v.).

**J.**

Ante-mortem: T. Glanders cases should not be admitted to meat plants.

Post-mortem: Carcase and viscera, T.

Glanders in *man* is a rare occurrence – veterinarians, horse butchers and laboratory workers being usually affected. Symptoms include fever, malaise, muscle pains, pneumonia and pleurisy and usually death within 3 weeks. The lesions are similar to those occurring in equidae.

Glanders is a *notifiable* diseases in most countries with a test and slaughter programme.

## HAEMOPHILOSIS

**I.** An infectious, often fatal, disease of cattle in which meningitis and encephalitis are the main manifestations but which is also associated with pneumonia, pleurisy, myocarditis, arthritis, mastitis and infertility.

**O.** Worldwide, but most common in North America (in feedlot animals), Europe and Australia.

**IA.** *Haemophilus somnus*, a small, Gram-negative, non-motile, non-sporing, microaerophilic coccobacillus which requires special X and V factors for growth.

**R.** The organism appears to be a commensal in the respiratory tract and is present in the urine and vaginal discharges of infected animals.

**MT.** Exact mode of transmission is unknown but is probably by inhalation.

**CF.** There is a very high temperature (up to 108°C), depression, inappetence, blindness, opisthotonos (head and tail bent upwards and backwards), incoordination, nystagmus (involuntary movement of eyeballs in unison), circling, hyperaesthesia, paralysis and coma in 1–2 days. On occasions animals may be found dead. Less severe forms of the disease show mastitis, otitis, endometritis, myocarditis, pneumonia, arthritis, abortion and infertility.

**P.** The main form of the disease shows haemorrhagic infarcts and fibrinous meningitis in the brain and spinal cord. Other lesions in the less acute forms of haemophilosis are consistent with the clinical findings.

**D.** Diagnosis is based on **CF** along with isolation and culture of *H. somnus*. Histopathology of brain tissue.

Differential diagnoses include rabies, Aujeszky's disease, lead poisoning, polioencephalomalacia, listeriosis.

**J.** Only the less acute forms of haemophilosis are likely to be encountered at meat inspection.

Carcase and viscera: T.

Other species of haemophilus are responsible for causing disease: *Glasser's disease (infectious polyarthritis of young pigs)* is due to *H. suis* (parasuis); *Septicaemia complex of sheep* is due to *Haemophilus agni*, and *Pleuropneumonia of pigs* is caused by *H. (Actinobacillus) pleuropneumoniae.*

## INFECTIOUS KERATOCONJUNCTIVITIS (INFECTIOUS OPHTHALMIA, BLIGHT, PINK EYE)

**I.** An acute, non-fatal, infectious disease of cattle, sheep and goats characterised by conjunctivitis, lachrymation, photophobia, spasm of the circular muscle of the eyelid and corneal opacity and ulceration.

**O.** Worldwide.

**IA.** *Moraxella bovis*, either alone or in mixed infections with *Mycoplasma*, *Neisseria*, *Rickettsia*, *Chlamydia* and certain viruses, e.g. IBR virus.

*Mor. bovis* is a Gram-negative, strictly aerobic, non-flagellated short rod or coccus which varies greatly in virulence.

**R.** Carrier animals, in which the organisms exist in the nostrils.

**MT.** Via the conjunctiva by direct and indirect contact with materials contaminated with the ocular and nasal discharges of affected and carrier animals. Various species of flies, especially those which tend to favour the orbital regions, play an important part as vectors in causing infection.

**CF.** See **I**. The disease occurs most often during the summer and autumn when flies are active. Susceptibility among livestock varies greatly, Zebu cattle being very resistant. Bright sunlight, pollen, dust, grass seeds, etc., are predisposing agents.

There may be a mild to moderate fever in some cases, with inappetence and a fall in milk yield, but most cases recover in a few weeks time with no untoward effects or some opacity in one or both eyes. The degree of eye damage varies greatly depending on susceptibility. On occasions, small ulcers appear on the cornea without opacity.

**P.** See **CF**.

**D.** The condition must be distinguished from conjunctivitis due to trauma, foreign bodies, parasites, etc. Similar symptoms are seen in other diseases such as bovine malignant catarrh (q.v.), infectious bovine keratoconjunctivitis (q.v.), mucosal disease (q.v.) and keratitis due to various pathogens.

**J.**

Ante-mortem: R.

Post-mortem: Carcase and viscera, A.

## LEPTOSPIROSIS (WEIL'S DISEASE, HAEMORRHAGIC JAUNDICE, SWINE HERD FEVER, MUD FEVER, CANICOLA FEVER)

**I.** A group of contagious diseases of all farm livestock and man which vary in severity and are characterised by septicaemia, fever, haemoglobinuria, jaundice, infertility and abortion in most animals. Weil's disease in human beings is an important *zoonosis*.

**O.** Worldwide. The disease is endemic in some countries where it is more important as a zoonosis than a clinical disease in livestock. Some serotypes are restricted geographically.

**IA.** Pathogenic *leptospires*, which belong to the single species *Leptospira interrogans complex*, which itself is subdivided into over 200 serovars (serotypes) arranged in 23 serogroups.

Leptospires belong to the order Spirochaetales which are Gram-negative, elongated and slender (6–20 µm × 0.1 µm), very motile, aerobic, non-sporing bacilli occurring as loops or tight coils.

The most common leptospires occur as follows:

*Cattle: L. interrogans*, serovars *hardjo*, *pomona* and *grippotyphosa*. *Canicola* and *icterohaemorrhagiae* have also been isolated.

*Pigs:* serovars *pomona*, *bratislava*, *grippotyphosa*, *canicola* and *icterohaemorrhagiae*.

*Sheep:* serovars *pomona*, *hardjo*, *grippotyphosa*.

*Horses:* serovar *bratislava*.

*Dogs:* serovars *canicola*, *icterohaemorrhagiae*, *grippotyphosa*, *pomona*.

*Brown rat:* serovar *icterohaemorrhagiae*.

Serovars *pomona* and *grippotyphosa* are commonly found in wild animals.

**R.** Domestic and wild animals, reptiles and amphibians. Affected and shedder animals are responsible for introducing infection. Wild animals acting as carriers include badgers, deer, raccoons, skunks, opossums, foxes, squirrels, rats, mice and other rodents. Saprophytic, non-pathogenic strains of leptospires also occur, being abundant in water, even in domestic water supplies. In Victoria, Australia, a survey of kidney samples from 218 cattle revealed leptospires in 18 (8.3%), all being identified as *L. hardjo*.

**MT.** The portal of entry of *Leptospira* species is usually through wounds or abrasions in the skin or through mucous membranes (usually conjunctiva, nares and vagina). *In utero* infection has been recorded and the disease has been transmitted by coitus in cattle. Urine is a common source and, less commonly, contaminated feed and water. Urine can be infective for long periods after an animal has apparently recovered.

**CF.** Some leptospires are pathogenic for certain animals (although they can cause disease in any mammals) while others are found in accidental hosts in which, however, they are capable of producing septicaemia and acute disease.

The disease occurs in acute, subacute and chronic forms, the symptoms being fairly similar in all animals.

*Acute* leptospirosis is manifested by septicaemia, high fever, icterus, haemoglobinuria, anorexia, anaemia, loss of milk yield, respiratory distress and listlessness. Abortion with stillbirths and retention of the placenta, infertility and mastitis with thick, yellowish, blood-tinged milk are common in cows. Mortality in general ranges from 5% to 15%, the higher rates occurring in calves, which are more susceptible.

In the *subacute* form the symptoms are milder and jaundice may be absent.

Abortion and stillbirths may be the only sign evident in the chronic form, in which symptoms are often so mild as to be overlooked. This is the type most common in pigs and is rarely fatal.

**P.** In addition to the symptoms listed in the clinical findings, there are haemorrhages under mucous membranes, abomasal ulceration and mucosal haemorrhages, and petechiae in the epicardium and lymph nodes in the more severe forms. The urine is a dark port-wine colour. The most significant lesion in chronic leptospirosis is in the kidneys, which have a mottled appearance owing to the presence of numerous small red or white infarcts in the cortex.

**D.** Diagnosis is confirmed by demonstration of the organism in urine; culture from blood, milk or urine; animal (guinea pig) inoculation; microscopic agglutination and ELISA tests.

Leptospirosis must be distinguished from brucellosis, babesiosis, anaplasmosis, brucellosis, bacillary haemoglobinuria in cattle, erysipelas in sows and chronic copper poisoning in sheep.

**J.**

Acute leptospirosis: Carcase and viscera, T.

Chronic leptospirosis: Carcase and viscera, A. Affected organs (kidneys), D.

Leptospirosis in *man* (*Weil's disease*) has a wide range of symptoms – haemolytic anaemia, jaundice, muscular pains, headache, conjunctivitis, vomiting, mental confusion and sometimes meningitis. The death rate is low but increases with advancing age.

The disease is an occupational hazard, occurring among sewer workers, farmers, veterinarians, abattoir personnel, fish workers and all persons exposed to river, canal and lake water contaminated with the urine of infected domestic and wild animals. The disease is easily treated with penicillin G and amoxycillin.

## LISTERIOSIS (LISTERELLOSIS, MONONUCLEOSIS, CIRCLING DISEASE)

**I.** A sporadic infectious disease affecting a wide range of animals, especially cattle, sheep, goats, sometimes horses and pigs, birds and man, characterised by encephalitis/meningoencephalitis and/or septicaemia, abortion and sometimes enteritis in ewes.

**O.** The disease occurs throughout the world but is more common in temperate climates – USA, British Isles, Europe, Australia and New Zealand – where it has a winter–spring prevalence.

Listeriosis is notifiable in several countries – Cuba, Salvador, Bahamas, Bermuda, Israel, Malaysia, Bulgaria, Czechoslovakia, Finland, Latvia, Sweden and Ukraine.

**IA.** *Listeria monocytogenes*, a Gram-positive, microaerophilic, non-sporing, flagellated (but only weakly motile) coccobacillus which grows well under a wide range of temperatures, even down to 4°C. *L. monocytogenes* resembles *E. rhusiopathiae* which, however, is non-motile. *L. ivanovii* is another pathogen but many listeriae are non-pathogenic, e.g. *L. innocua*, *L. seeligeri*.

*L. monocytogenes* is probably present more widely in carrier animals than is generally realised. Examination of brain smears from apparently normal sheep showed the presence of the organisms in 5% of them (Gracey 1961, unpublished data). The exciting conditions which enable such organisms to multiply and become pathogenic are as yet unknown.

**R.** The organism is very widely distributed in nature. Soil, rotting vegetation, feedingstuffs, faeces, surface water, sewage sludge, plants and even insects harbour *L. monocytogenes*. It is a normal commensal in the intestines of animals and man.

As with many diseases, there are important predisposing factors such as poor standards of hygiene, low levels of nutrition, overcrowding, severe climatic conditions (e.g. from warm to extremely cold and wet), pregnancy and parturition.

The increased use of *poor-quality silage* has been held responsible for outbreaks of listeriosis in cattle and sheep as well as nutritional deficiencies (reduction of voluntary food intake, loss of body weight, ketosis, reduced milk yield and infertility), fungal diseases, bacilli (especially *B. licheniformis* abortion), and botulism.

Poor-quality silage is classified as silage which is poorly fermented, has a pH of 5.0 and over, often contains soil, moulds and fungi and has aerobic/microaerophilic conditions. Under these conditions, *L. monocytogenes* multiplies rapidly within the silage. Good-quality silage requires rapid and efficient lactic acid fermentation, low pH, high dry matter content, strict anaerobic conditions and freedom from soil. Big bale silage is believed to be more responsible for multiplication of *Listeria* than clamp silage since low pH, anaerobic conditions and freedom from moulds and fungi are more difficult to achieve owing to the entry of air through air holes and broken bales.

**MT.** Ingestion and inhalation of contaminated materials are the usual routes of infection, which may also occur via the conjunctiva. It is possible that small wounds in the buccal mucosa may be a portal of entry.

**CF.** Predilection sites for *Listeria* appear to be the intestinal wall, brain (medulla oblongata) and uterus/placenta, and organisms localise in these sites from the appropriate portals of entry.

The most common manifestations of listeriosis are encephalitis or meningoencephalitis, septicaemia and abortion, but they rarely occur together.

*Encephalitis* affects all ages and both sexes and is exhibited by a rapid onset and usually death in 2 days in sheep (up to 14 days in cattle). Although recovery may take place, there is always permanent brain damage. Affected animals separate from the flock or herd, show incoordination and ataxia, push the head against stationary objects, crowd into corners and walk in circles, always in the same direction. Salivation, nasal discharge, anorexia, conjunctivitis, strabismus (squint) and blindness with pus in the anterior chamber of the eyes are commonly observed. Paralysis of the face and throat, with difficulty in the prehension of food and slow mastication and swallowing may be evident. Paralysis and recumbency eventually take place and death due to respiratory failure. Mortality may be as high as 90%.

*Abortion* usually occurs in late pregnancy without any premonitory signs. While fetuses normally die *in utero*, stillbirths and neonatal deaths are not uncommon. In some cases in sheep, septicaemia accompanies abortion with death on occasions.

*Septicaemia* appears to be more common in young calves and lambs than adults. In pigs it is seen in piglets under 1 month of age. In all cases it terminates rapidly.

*Enteritis* as an entity in listeriosis seems to be on the increase. Indeed, it is possible that the clinical manifestations of listeriosis are changing, at least in the UK.

**P.** In encephalitis, apart from congestion of the meninges, there are no gross lesions. Histological examination is necessary to show the microabscesses in the brain (pons and medulla) and spinal cord. In the septicaemic form tiny, yellowish, discrete necrotic foci may be found in any organ but especially in the liver, spleen, heart, lymph nodes, adrenal glands and lungs. Similar lesions may also occur in aborted fetuses, which are usually oedematous and autolysed and have blood-tinged fluid in the serous cavities.

**D.** At ante-mortem, listeriosis may be confused with many other diseases showing neurological signs – BSE, acetonaemia, sporadic encephalomyelitis, lead poisoning, brain abscess, rabies, and with pregnancy toxaemia, brain abscess, gid, otitis media in sheep. Other causes of abortion, e.g. brucellosis, must also be borne in mind in all species.

At post-mortem the appearance of numerous discrete necrotic foci in the septicaemic form and in fetuses is very suggestive of listeriosis. Diagnosis is confirmed by isolation of *L. monocytogenes* from brain, cerebrospinal fluid, blood, fetus and placenta in particular. Culture on enriched selective media is necessary to distinguish the organism from other diphtheroid bacteria. Immunofluorescence is of value but not serology.

**J.** Carcase and viscera: T.

**Human listeriosis** Infection results from the ingestion of contaminated food – unpasteurised milk, cheese (usually soft cheese), vegetables and other forms of food. Inhalation of the organism is also a possibility. Skin lesions may result from direct contact with infected animals and contaminated materials. Neonatal infection occurs *in utero* from an infected mother.

Symptoms are very similar to those in animals. A mild infection may only show influenza-like signs but the meningoencephalitis type is manifested by fever, intense headache, nausea, vomiting, delirium and coma. Endocarditis and liver necrotic foci may be present, along with internal and cutaneous abscesses. Fatality may reach 30% in adults and in new-born infants.

Susceptibility is greatest in the newborn, the elderly and immunocompromised individuals.

Pregnant women, elderly persons and the immunocompromised must avoid contact with infective materials, aborted fetuses and known infected persons. Pregnant women should not assist with lambing/calving or even be present at such events. Only pasteurised foods, especially soft cheeses, should be consumed.

Cases should be reported to the Local Health Authority, an obligatory requirement in several US states and some countries.

## MELIOIDOSIS (PSEUDO-GLANDERS, RODENT GLANDERS, WHITMORE'S DISEASE)

**I.** An uncommon bacterial disease mainly of rodents but also occurring in a wide range of farm livestock (sheep, goats, pigs, horses, cattle and dogs) and wild animals, including primates, and man. Lesions take the form of suppurative or caseous changes in lymph nodes and viscera resembling those of glanders.

**O.** Although originally thought to be restricted to tropical and subtropical countries – Mexico, S. America, Brunei/Darussalam, Iran, Malaysia and Singapore – the disease has been recorded in Australia, Papua New Guinea, New Caledonia and France and is a notifiable disease in New Zealand.

**IA.** *Pseudomonas (Malleomyces) pseudomallei*, a Gram-negative, oval-shaped motile (with polar flagella) aerobic bacillus.

**R.** The organisms are very widely distributed in nature, where they can survive as saprophytes for long periods in soil and water, although they are easily destroyed by heat and the usual disinfectants. *P. pseudomallei* is found in the faeces and discharges of infected animals. Rodents and other wild species act as reservoirs.

**MT.** Ingestion of contaminated food and water, through skin wounds and by inhalation.

**CF.** Clinical signs vary according to the body part involved. In sheep there is fever due to septic pneumonia, coughing, anorexia, listlessness, weight loss, ocular and nasal discharges (when the nasal bones become ulcerated). Arthritis with lameness may be present as well as mastitis and encephalitis. Most cases are chronic, especially in pigs and goats, with frequent recoveries, but acute encephalitis cases with death within one week sometimes occur. Cases of encephalitis show the usual signs of incoordination, blindness, abnormal gait, head deviation, etc.

**P.** Abscesses with thick greenish pus or caseous material in most organs, especially the lungs. Pneumonia. Microabscesses in brain.

**D.** Culture of the organism from infective material, abscesses, etc., on the usual media. Agglutination test. Differential diagnoses: glanders and strangles (q.v.) in horses.

**J.** Carcase and viscera: T.

**Human melioidosis** Symptoms in man vary from virtually no signs to a rapidly fatal septicaemia which, however, is uncommon. Agricultural workers are mainly affected. Many of these have antibodies to *P. pseudomallei* without clinical disease. Symptoms in clinical cases include respiratory distress, coughing, fever, chest pain, osteomyelitis and skin abscesses.

Preventive measures are mainly directed towards the prevention of wounds and their contamination, and avoidance of ingestion of contaminated water and dust.

## NECROBACILLOSIS

**I.** A complex of several usually chronic diseases in which necrotic lesions are formed in different parts of the animal body by bacteria of the *Fusobacterium* genus. Included are foot rot of cattle, sheep, goats and pigs, foot abscess of sheep, interdigital dermatitis of sheep, necrotic rhinitis of pigs, oral/laryngeal necrobacillosis and focal necrosis of the liver of cattle and sheep.

**O.** Worldwide in distribution, except arid and semi-arid areas.

**IA.** *Fusobacterium* spp. especially *F. (Sphaerophorus) necrophorum*, a large (up to 10 μm long) Gram-negative, anaerobic, non-sporing, non-motile beaded bacillus which is frequently found as a commensal in the mouth, intestine or genital tract of many animals and man. It can act as a secondary invader in mixed infections as well as being the primary cause of disease, even to producing septicaemia.

**R.** See **IA**. The organism also exists in soil and water.

**MT.** Via wounds and abrasions in skin, mouth, intestinal and genital tracts from discharges from infected and carrier animals. Predisposing factors which reduce the integrity of skin and mucous membranes, e.g. wet conditions, badly laid concrete and stony surfaces, play an important part in infection.

### Foot rot of cattle (pododermatitis, interdigital necrobacillosis)

**I.** An infectious disease of the feet of cattle caused by *F. necrophorum* acting in conjunction with *Bacteroides nodosus* and *Bacteroides melaninogenicus*, associated with severe lameness and loss of condition. It is the most common form of lameness in cattle, in which it is of great economic importance.

**CF.** Sudden onset of severe lameness usually in one foot (especially a hind foot), which becomes oedematous owing to a fissure in the interdigital cleft which becomes necrotic with a foul-smelling discharge. This may progress to a purulent arthritis and tenosynovitis. There is fever, reduced milk yield and loss of condition in longstanding cases.

**P.** See **CF**.

**D.** Based on the typical lesions in which there is no foreign body.

**J.** Foot rot cases are frequently presented as casualties.

Carcase and viscera: A, provided condition is satisfactory and general signs are absent.

*Infectious foot rot of sheep and goats* is associated with invasion of the interdigital skin of the feet by *Bacteroides nodosus*, either alone or in association with *F. necrophorum*. It is common in feet with overgrown claws, especially fore feet, and has the same predisposing factors as the bovine condition. The hoof matrix becomes infected and partially detached from the digit. Affected feet have a characteristic odour. Severe lameness and loss of condition ensue.

*Foot rot in pigs* is usually the result of infection with *F. necrophorum* associated with *Corynebacterium pyogenes* and various staphylococci. *Foot abscess of sheep (septic laminits)* may affect either the toe or the heel of the foot, which becomes painful and hot due to purulent inflammation. The causes are the same as in foot rot in pigs.

*Interdigital dermatitis (scald)* in sheep is generally less severe than foot rot in that there is no separation of hoof. As with foot rot, almost the whole flock may be affected and all four feet. The skin of the cleft is red and swollen and suppuration may extend to deeper tissues.

*Necrotic stomatitis and rhinitis in pigs: F. necrophorum* is commonly isolated from necrotic lesions on the skin, mouth, tongue and nares of pigs of all ages. As with many conditions, mixed infections occur with *C. pyogenes*, streptococci, staphylococci, spirochaetes and *E. coli.* Necrotic rhinitis begins with ulceration of the nasal and turbinate bones, which later become necrotic with swelling and deformity of the face and a foul-smelling nasal discharge, the swelling of the face distinguishing it from atrophic rhinitis.

## Oral/pharyngeal/laryngeal necrobacillosis

**I.** An infectious, highly fatal disease, mainly of calves, but also occurring less commonly in sheep, in which ulceration and necrotic diphtheritic membranes are formed in the mouth, pharynx or larynx.

**O.** Worldwide, especially under intensive conditions.

**IA.** *Fusobacterium necrophorum.*

**R** and **MT.** See under Necrobacillosis.

**CF.** Oral necrobacillosis (necrotic stomatitis) – Fever, inappetence, depression, salivation, dyspnoea, fetid breath with difficulty in prehension and chewing. Well-defined ulcers with central necrotic material are present in the buccal mucosa.

*Pharyngeal/laryngeal necrobacillosis (calf diphtheria)* differs only from the oral form in the siting of the necrotic ulcers, which are present in the pharynx and larynx and may involve the vocal cords. Severe cases may extend to complete occlusion of the laryngeal opening. These organs are oedematous and there is a blood-stained purulent discharge. Lesions in both instances may extend to the lungs to cause a septic pneumonia and death from toxaemia.

**P.** See **CF**.

**D.** Clinical signs and lesions are usually sufficient to establish a diagnosis. Stained smears and culture of organism from necrotic ulcers.

## Focal necrosis of liver in cattle and sheep

**MT.** *Fusobacterium necrophorum* is a normal inhabitant of the rumen microflora and gains entrance to the liver following inflammatory changes and wounds in the rumen or through the navel via the umbilical vein. Feedlot cattle are commonly affected, as are barley-beef animals. High levels of carbohydrates in the feed appear to predispose to the disease.

**CF.** Most animals show no clinical signs but severe cases exhibit loss of weight and a few animals may die suddenly from peritonitis and toxaemia due to the rupture of one or more large abscesses. In such cases there is evidence of colic or vague digestive disorder.

**P.** The term *'liver abscesses'* is a misnomer since most of the early lesions are circumscribed areas of coagulative necrosis, although older lesions (one month) may be true abscesses. They are a fairly common finding at meat inspection – up to almost 100% in some feedlots in the USA. A figure of 22% of barley-beef animals has been recorded in the UK. The lesions are usually pale yellowish in colour, about 2–5 cm in diameter. The actual number in a liver varies greatly but a number between 5 and 8 is common.

A complication which sometimes occurs is erosion and perforation of the wall of the posterior vena cava with sudden death from septicaemia in an otherwise healthy animal.

The term *'sawdust livers'* encountered commonly in young fattening cattle in the USA relates to livers containing several minute yellowish foci of necrosis (1–2 mm in diameter). They are collections of liver epithelial cells undergoing coagulative necrosis along with white blood cells (lymphocytes and neutrophils). Although their exact nature is unknown, it is considered that they may represent the beginning of telangiectasis or abscesses alongside of which they often exist.

**J.** (*Hepatic necrobacillosis*)

Carcase and viscera: A, provided no general signs present and condition good.

Affected part (liver): D.

## PARATUBERCULOSIS (JÖHNE'S DISEASE)

**I.** A chronic, infectious disease of cattle, sheep, goats, deer and wild ruminants in which there is persistent diarrhoea, loss of weight and eventual death.

**O.** Worldwide. The disease, however, appears to be more common in certain countries, being enzootic in cattle in the United Kingdom, France, Denmark, Colombia, Ecuador, Mexico, Bangladesh, Australia and New Zealand, and of high occurrence in Puerto Rico. A recent survey in south-west England showed the proportion of farms affected with Johne's disease to be 1.0% and the cumulative incidence on these farms to be 1.9% per year (Cetinkaya *et al.*, 1994). In Greece it is enzootic in sheep and goats. Several countries – Ireland, N. Ireland, Sweden, Ukraine, Australia, New Zealand, USA and others – have made Johne's disease a notifiable disease.

**IA.** *Mycobacterium paratuberculosis* (*johnei*). Like *Myco. bovis* and *Myco. tuberculosis*, it is an acid-fast, usually stumpy, non-motile, non-sporing, aerobic bacillus which often appears in clumps. This *'acid-fastness'* is related to the presence of a waxy material in the cell wall which makes the mycobacteria difficult to stain. However, staining with hot carbol fuchsin allows the stain to penetrate but it is retained despite efforts to remove it with acid or alcohol. Three major strains of *Myco. paratuberculosis* exist – one bovine and two sheep strains, one of which is a yellowish pigmented one – in addition to several variants.

**R.** The organism is very resistant and can survive for over one year in soil and faeces, although it is susceptible to sunlight and drying. The organism is shed in the faeces of infected and clinically normal carrier animals.

**MT.** By the ingestion of contaminated food and water. The bacteria enter the mucosa of the small intestine and the mesenteric, retropharyngeal lymph nodes and tonsils.

**CF.** Infection takes place early in life (usually under 1 month of age in cattle), calves acquiring infection soon after birth. As with probably all disease, predisposing factors play an important part in producing clinical disease. Breed is believed to be important, the disease being more common in Jersey, Guernsey and Shorthorn cattle in the UK. At one period in Northern Ireland, Johne's disease was most common in Ayrshire cattle and in Blackface sheep but was not encountered in other sheep breeds.

The incubation period in cattle is long, probably not less than 2 years. Symptoms include loss of condition which extends to emaciation, reduced milk yield, intermittent or continuous watery 'hose-pipe' diarrhoea, dehydration and weakness which warrants culling. Although appetite is usually maintained and temperature is normal, there is an increased thirst. Coat colour is lost and oedema may develop in the intermandibular space. In sheep and goats diarrhoea is not as serious as in cattle, the faeces being only soft. Emaciation is the main feature in these species.

**P.** In *cattle* and *goats* changes may be minimal in the early stages. Well-developed lesions are characteristic and are present in the small intestine, caecum and beginning of the colon in all species. The wall of the intestine is grossly thickened, with the mucous membrane assuming a corrugated appearance – it looks almost like the surface of the cerebrum. The mesenteric and ileo-caecal lymph nodes are enlarged and oedematous and the ileo-caecal valve is inflamed and oedematous.

*Sheep* usually show a deep yellow pigmentation of the intestinal wall, which may be thickened but not corrugated. The associated lymph nodes present oedema and enlargement.

**D.** The characteristic lesions, loss of condition, diarrhoea and chronic nature of the disease are reasonably diagnostic. Differential diagnoses include salmonellosis, coccidiosis, parasitic gastroenteritis and chronic molybdenum poisoning.

The organism can be demonstrated in stained smears from faecal and lymph node samples, which can also be cultured in special media. Serological tests (complement fixation, agar gel immunodiffusion, ELISA).

**J.**

Carcase and viscera: A, provided condition is satisfactory and no systemic or degenerative changes evident. Affected organs: Intestines and mesentery, D.

## PASTEURELLOSIS

Bacteria of the genus *Pasteurella* are involved, either as direct causes or as secondary invaders in many animal diseases. Direct cause diseases include the following:

*Pasteurella multocida*

- Haemorrhagic septicaemia of cattle.
- Meningoencephalitis of cattle.
- Pneumonic pasteurellosis of pigs, sheep and goats.
- Lymphadenitis in lambs.
- Septicaemia of horses and donkeys.
- Abscesses in rabbits (q.v.).
- Genital infection of rabbits (q.v.).
- Rhinitis (snuffles) and bronchopneumonia of rabbits (q.v.).

*Pasteurella haemolytica*

- Pneumonic pasteurellosis of cattle (shipping fever).
- Pneumonic pasteurellosis of sheep and goats.
- Pneumonic pasteurellosis of pigs.
- Meningoencephalitis of calves.
- Meningoencephalitis of horses, donkeys and mules.

*Past. anatipestifer* is the causative agent in duck septicaemia (q.v.).

The pasteurellae are small, oval, facultatively anaerobic, capsulate, non-motile, Gram-negative bacilli which show bipolar staining with methylene blue. They are very virulent, especially *Past. multocida*, for animals and birds and can be carried by apparently normal animals and birds.

### Haemorrhagic septicaemia (HS, barbone)

(Plate 3, Fig. 14)

**I.** A septicaemic pasteurellosis of cattle and water buffalo, the latter being the most susceptible. On occasions deer, bison, camels, yaks, horses and pigs have been affected.

**O.** The disease is mainly confined to tropical and subtropical countries. In Africa it has a high incidence in Gambia, Mali, Niger, Sudan, East Timor and Tanzania. In S. America it is enzootic in Colombia, Costa Rica, Dominican Republic, Panama, Venezuela and Argentina. Although at one time most common in South and East Asia, it now appears to be confined to Nepal (high incidence), Pakistan (enzootic), Vietnam, Saudi Arabia, Sri Lanka and Mongolia. There is a low sporadic occurrence in Spain, Portugal, Greece and Latvia.

**IA.** *Pasteurella multocida*, serotypes 6:B and 6:E, the latter causing HS in Africa and 6:B elsewhere.

**R.** The organism is found in affected and carrier animals (upper respiratory tract and pharynx).

**MT.** By ingestion of contaminated food and water.

**CF.** Acute or peracute illness almost always resulting in death in less than one day. Some animals may be found dead. High fever, dullness, respiratory distress, salivation and nasal discharge. Oedematous swellings on throat, neck, head and brisket with congested mucosae showing numerous petechiae.

**P.** In addition to CF lesions, petechial haemorrhages are distributed throughout the body, especially under serous membranes. Oedema of lungs, retropharyngeal and cervical lymph nodes. Blood-stained fluid in thoracic and abdominal cavities and in pericardial sac.

**D.** Rapid course of disease, high fever, earlier history (especially if no vaccination) and lesions are indicated of haemorrhagic septicaemia. Differential diagnoses include rinderpest, salmonellosis and anthrax.

Isolation of organism from blood and organs. Serology – indirect haemagglutination, coagglutination, immunodiffusion.

**J.** It is unlikely that cases of HS will be presented for slaughter, nor should they be.

Carcase and viscera: T.

**Meningoencephalitis of cattle** due to *P. multocida* and the same disease caused by *P. haemolytica* present clinical signs similar to all cases in which the brain and meninges are affected with inflammatory change – incoordination, ataxia, fever, depression (opisthotonos), blindness, delirium, seizures, progressive paresis, coma.

The causes of meningoencephalitis are legion and include many other bacteria and viruses, fungi, worm parasites, protozoa and chemical agents.

*Judgement* in meningencephalitis due to Pasteurellae is the same as that for HS.

### Pneumonic pasteurellosis of pigs

**I.** An acute septicaemic or chronic infectious disease of pigs characterised by sudden death in the septicaemic form and acute or chronic bronchopneumonia.

**IA.** *Pasteurella multocida*, usually in association with other organisms such as *Mycoplasma hyopneumoniae* and *Actinobacillus pleuropneumoniae*.

Occurrence, reservoir, mode of transmission, clinical signs and diagnosis are similar to those in other respiratory diseases.

**P.** Acute, septicaemic and chronic cases show the relevant changes of bronchopneumonia, the acute cases with marked fibrinous bronchopneumonia while chronic ones reveal abscess formation in the lungs and sometimes pericarditis.

**J.**

Carcase and viscera: T, acute, septicaemic cases.

Carcase and viscera: A, no general changes and condition good.

Affected parts and organs: D, heart, lungs and pleurae.

**Lymphadenitis of lambs** caused by *Pasteurella multocida* differs from caseous lymphadenitis (CLA) due to *Corynebacterium pseudotuberculosis* in being more acute and the lymph nodes (submaxillary, cervical, prescapular, cranial), although swollen, do not contain the caseous material seen in CLA.

**J.** Judgement warrants total condemnation because of the fevered carcase.

**Septicaemia of equidae** caused by *P. multocida* has a sudden onset and a rapid course and is unlikely to be encountered at meat inspection. *Judgement* merits total condemnation.

### Pneumonic pasteurellosis of cattle (shipping fever, transit fever)

**I.** A severe infectious respiratory disease of cattle in which acute fibrinous bronchopneumonia and toxaemia occur following long-distance transportation causing huge economic losses.

**O.** Worldwide. The disease is common in temperate countries, especially the USA, Canada and Europe.

**IA.** *Pasteurella haemolytica*, alone or sometimes in combination with *P. multocida*. They can act in combination with viruses, mycoplasmas, etc.

**R.** Both organisms are normal inhabitants of the upper respiratory tract. Affected, recovered and carrier animals also act as sources of infection.

**MT.** By inhalation. Spread of the disease is more common under crowded conditions.

**CF.** Shipping fever is more common in young cattle (up to 2 years of age) but can affect adult animals. It frequently occurs in animals which have undergone long journeys. Young cattle recently conveyed to feedlots or markets are very susceptible and often develop the disease within a few hours of arrival. In some instances clinical signs do not appear for several weeks. The stress associated with transport plays a part but other stressors such as overcrowding, poor ventilation, prolonged holding without feed and water, sudden weather changes, mixing of stock from different sources and stressful handling are important factors in causing the disease.

Clinical signs include depression, fever, inappetence, dyspnoea, nasal discharge with mucopurulent material and coughing. Some 50% of stock may be affected, with up to 10% mortality after some weeks or months. Condition is lost as the disease progresses.

**P.** Fibrinous bronchopneumonia mainly affecting the anterior and ventral portions of the lungs. Serofibrinous exudate which may become necrotic in later stages is present between lung lobules. There may be pleural and pericardial adhesions. Catarrhal bronchitis and bronchiolitis are usually present.

**D.** The circumstances surrounding the outbreak, the lesions and the clinical signs are usually adequate for a diagnosis. Early treatment normally brings a good response.

**J.** Slaughter should be delayed until treatment is completed.

Acute pneumonic pasteurellosis: Carcase and viscera, T.

Recovered cases of shipping fever: Carcase and viscera, A.

Affected organs (lungs, heart): D.

### Pneumonic pasteurellosis ('enzootic pneumonia') of sheep and goats

**I.** An infectious respiratory disease of sheep and goats which can occur in an acute septicaemic form or as a more chronic entity. A systemic type of pasteurellosis occurs in lambs up to one year of age.

**O.** In countries with temperate climates – Europe, USA, Canada, Australia and New Zealand.

**IA.** *Pasteurella haemolytica*. Biotype A strains cause septicaemia and the more chronic form of pasteurellosis while biotype B strains are responsible for the peracute systemic disease.

**R** and **MT.** As for shipping fever in cattle.

**CF.** *Pneumonic pasteurellosis*: All ages of sheep may be affected. The predisposing factors are very similar to those for cattle. Animals may be found dead while others show respiratory distress, mucopurulent discharge, fever, inappetence and coughing.

*Septicaemic pasteurellosis*: Occurs primarily in young lambs and kids. Onset and progression is very rapid. Both pneumonic and septicaemic types may be present in a flock at the same time.

*Systemic pasteurellosis*: Affected animals are usually found dead. Those found alive are listless, show dyspnoea and a frothy discharge from the mouth.

*Past. haemolytica* has been recorded as a cause of mastitis in ewes.

**P.** Lesions vary according to the type of disease. In the *acute* and *septicaemic* forms there is lobar pneumonia affecting the apical and cardiac lobes of the oedematous lungs with a fibrinous exudate in the pleural and pericardial cavity. Petechiae and ecchymoses are present throughout the carcase.

The *systemic* form shows no evidence of pneumonia but there is haemorrhagic abomasitis with ulceration and petechiation of the visceral peritoneum and parietal pleura. Ulceration may also be present in the pharynx and larynx. The kidneys may present changes similar to those of pulpy kidney.

**J.**

Acute septicaemia and systemic forms: Carcase and viscera: T.

Chronic pasteurellosis: Carcase and viscera, A or Kh.

Affected organs: D.

## SALMONELLOSIS (PARATYPHOID) (see also Chapter 14)

**I.** A contagious *zoonotic* disease of great economic importance affecting all farm animals, poultry and man occurring either as a peracute septicaemia, acute enteritis or chronic enteritis.

**O.** Worldwide. The disease is more prevalent where intensive livestock husbandry methods are practised and where animals are imported into farms.

Infection rates vary greatly in different parts of the world and in different species, but figures as high as 15% have been recorded in healthy dairy cattle (with higher isolations in calves) and as high as 54% in pigs kept intensively. In the USA 45 (75%) of 60 herds with an average of 584 cows showed that at least one cow had recently been exposed to salmonellae when milk samples were tested. Up to 50% of healthy horses have been shown to be salmonella carriers.

In the UK in 1992 there was a general decline in the number of isolations of salmonellae in cattle, sheep and poultry. In the latter species this reduction was probably due to the implementation of government Codes of Practice for the control of salmonella in the production of final feed for livestock, controls on salmonella contamination in processed animal protein and alterations in the composition of compound poultry feed.

Isolations of salmonellae from *pig carcases* have shown varying levels: 7.3% in Northern Ireland; 9.9% in England (Nottingham *et al.*, 1972); 27.0% in Australia 1970; 44.8.% in USA (Gustafson *et al.*, 1976), the materials used being mainly faeces or caecal contents. *Pig products* (sausages) have also shown high isolations: 28.0% in USA (Surkiewicz *et al.* 1972) and 29.7% in England (Roberts *et al.*, 1975).

Even higher isolations are being recorded in poultry. In Scotland a survey of 480 fresh and frozen poultry carcases gave 215 positive salmonella isolations, an incidence rate of 45%. Each carcase was rinsed in a sterile polythene bag with 300 ml of sterile buffered peptone water (pre-enrichment broth).

A survey by the Consumers Association in Britain in October 1994 showed that three out of five poultry carcases contained food poisoning bacteria and of 160 raw chicken samples examined salmonellae were present in 36% of them. Portugal had the worst record, with 48% of samples contaminated with salmonellae, while Norway came out best with only 1% contaminated followed by Greece with 4%.

A 1994 survey of poultry carcases in Northern Ireland revealed an incidence of 5%, this lower incidence being occasioned by the institution of strict control measures.

In Britain the Zoonoses Order 1989 requires statutory isolation of salmonellae from all the food animals and poultry as well as horses, deer and pigeons to be reported. An *isolation* is defined as 'the reported identification of salmonella from an animal or group of animals, an animal carcase, animal feed, or from animal products or surroundings which can be specifically related to identifiable animals'.

Details of total salmonella isolations and the main serotypes isolated from cattle, calves, sheep, poultry and animal feed in Great Britain during the period 1986–92 are given in Chapter 14.

**IA.** Members of the genus *Salmonella*, of which there are now over 2000 serotypes. Only a relatively small number, however, are responsible for clinical disease in animals and man. Division and subdivision of the genus is made on the basis of their antigenic analysis, most strains possessing two or more somatic (O) antigens and one or more flagellar (H) antigens. Like most microorganisms they vary greatly in virulence between different serotypes and even in individual serotypes.

Salmonellae are Gram-negative, motile, non-capsulate, facultative anaerobes which form small rods (less than 0.5 µm), either straight or curved.

Virulence depends on the presence of cell toxins (cytotoxin, enterotoxin, lipopolysaccharide) as well as the action of flagella. Most salmonellae are intracellular parasites.

There is a wide variation in the incidence of the various serotypes from country to country. While *S. typhimurium* and *S. enteritidis* are probably the most common serotypes isolated, an increasing number of exotic types, e.g. *S. indiana*, *S. seftenberg*, *S. hadar*, *S. taksony* are being encountered. Some salmonellae are host-specific, e.g. *S. pullorum* and *S. gallinarum* (both non-food-poisoning organisms) for poultry, *S. cholerae-suis* for pigs and *S. typhi* and *S. paratyphi* for human beings. But the pattern of serotypes in any one locality can change in a very short time. The all-too-frequent occurrence of antibiotic resistance has further complicated the picture. The extensive use of antibiotics in animal feeds and in the treatment of animal and human disease has created strains of resistant bacteria which have become widely disseminated and are transferable between animals and man.

**R.** While infected, carrier and shedder animals and birds can be regarded as the main sources of infection, salmonellae are also found in wild animals and birds, including cold-blooded species. Pets such as tortoises, terrapins, turtles, dogs, cats and human beings are also incriminated although humans are rare as chronic carriers.

The organisms exist in water, although they do not multiply there but can grow well in foods of high $a_w$ (water activity); pH values of 4.0 and below inhibit their multiplication in foods (also restricted by the presence of lactobacilli). Although they may not grow in certain foods, they can survive to cause illness. They are fairly easily killed by heat (above 70°C) but are fairly sensitive to beta- and gamma-irradiation and pasteurisation. Salmonellae can persist in dried faeces and dust for years.

Like all Gram-negative organisms – *Escherichia*, *Pseudomonas*, *Shigella*, *Yersinia*, *Campylobacter*, *Vibrio*, etc., *Salmonella* spp. are more sensitive to freezing than Gram-positive bacteria such as *Clostridium*, *Bacillus*, *Staphylococcus*, *Streptococcus* and *Lactobacillus*.

The *epidemiology* of salmonellosis is very complex and not all the various factors determining the occurrence and frequency of the disease are known. Among the culprits are intensive systems of husbandry, especially those combined with failure to batch bought-in animals; lack of routine cleansing and disinfection procedures; overcrowding; inadequate facilities for handling slurry; the application of fresh slurry directly to pasture with immediate grazing by livestock; careless disposal of carcases, fetuses and placentas; bad housing designs; contamination of feedingstuffs and water supplies with faecal material; inadequate control of rodents and other pests; unsatisfactory storage of feedingstuffs; feedingstuffs of low biological value; inadequate nutrition.

Breeding programmes which are designed to promote production (of milk and meat) to the total exclusion of disease resistance are believed to play a significant part in causing salmonellosis and other diseases.

Other predisposing factors include deprivation of food and of colostrum in the newborn animal; long-distance transport; recent parturition; intercurrent disease, e.g. internal parasitism, especially liver fluke disease; the administration of certain drugs; prolonged exercise; rough handling; mixing of different groups; chilling; internal parasitism. In fact any stressful situation may generate salmonellosis, especially in the young animal and those with low resistance. The frequency with which young calves are transported to markets is a notorious cause of salmonellosis. The disease can also occur in animals which have been subjected to prolonged surgical techniques.

**MT.** The usual route of infection is by the *ingestion* of contaminated food and water. Infected, carrier and shedder animals excrete the organisms in the faeces, which contaminate the environment in a multiplicity of ways – via premises, vehicles, equipment, personnel (including those with unhygienic habits and infected and chronic carrier personnel), feed, milk, water supplies, pasture, streams, rivers, etc. The feeding of milk contaminated with salmonellae to calves has been responsible for outbreaks, as have fresh and processed meats and animal and plant products used as feedingstuffs. Infected human and animal sewage spread on pasture is a further means of infection, which can also be mediated by rodents and birds.

Salmonella organisms may also be transmitted via the airborne route.

**CF.** Once salmonellae gain entrance to the animal body, a *carrier* or clinical state ensues. Animals acting as carriers may be *active* carriers, with the organisms being regularly or intermittently passed in the faeces, or *latent* carriers in which the organisms remain in the tonsils and/or lymph nodes, with the faeces salmonella-free. *Passive* carriers are those that acquire infection (without subsequent invasion) which disappears in a salmonella-free environment. All types of carriers can become clinical cases when stressed.

Salmonellae cause clinical infection (most common in cattle) by invading the cells of the intestinal mucosa, especially of the ileum and caecum, where they multiply, their various toxins causing enteritis. If resistance is low, the organisms spread beyond the gut and mesenteric lymph nodes to invade the bloodstream. A bacteraemia or a severe septicaemia may result, depending on bacterial virulence and body resistance. Salmonellosis occurs in four main forms – septicaemia, enteritis, abortion and carrier.

**Septicaemia** This is most common in young animals – calves, piglets, foals and lambs. Illness is very acute with high fever, depression and death usually within 1–2 days. Young pigs often show a purplish discoloration of the skin, the ears and abdomen being mainly affected. Scab formation and subcutaneous petechiation may also be present.

**Enteritis** Inflammation of the intestine may be acute, subacute or chronic.

*Acute enteritis* (most common in adults) is accompanied by fever and inappetence with putrid, watery diarrhoea or dysentery which may contain mucus or fibrin or even shreds of mucous membrane. Colic is evident, straining to defaecate (tenesmus) and dehydration. The death rate may reach 100%. Abortion is common in cows and arthritis in calves which survive this acute stage, while others may develop pneumonia and encephalitis with eventual death, these symptoms being also common in pigs.

*Subacute enteritis* assumes a milder form with less severe diarrhoea and fever and a greater chance of recovery. Abortion, however, may be prevalent in cows and ewes.

*Chronic* enteritis – a common form in cattle and pigs – is manifested by intermittent fever, diarrhoea of reduced amount but with changes similar to the acute and subacute forms, inappetence and severe loss of condition. Abortion is common in cows, in which gangrene of the extremities (ears, tail, lower limbs) may occur as complications. Animals recovering from all forms of salmonellosis inevitably become carriers.

**P.** *Septicaemic form*: Apart from submucosal and subserous haemorrhages there may be no other changes.

*Acute enteritis*: Inflammation of the small and large intestine – mucoid or haemorrhagic. Oedema of the spiral colon and caecum, especially in pigs. Mesenteric lymph nodes enlarged, haemorrhagic and oedematous. Submucosal petechiation. Intestinal contents resemble respective types of diarrhoea. There may be fatty degeneration of the liver with thickening of the wall of the gall bladder. Petechiae may be present under the epicardium.

A fairly constant finding in pigs is fine petechiation of the kidney (*'turkey egg kidney'*) along with lung congestion or consolidation.

*Chronic enteritis*: The caecum and colon show focal (in cattle) or diffuse (in pigs) necrosis with greyish-yellow adherent material covering a red, roughened, granular mucosa. Mesenteric lymph nodes, spiral colon and caecum are oedematous and swollen. Pneumonia may be present in all species.

In *pigs* the necrosis may take the form of so-called *'button'* ulcers which are raised, discrete areas in the caecum. (Some contend that these ulcers are caused by the swine fever virus.) The spleen is enlarged and rectal stricture caused by prolonged scarring of its wall due to chronic enteritis is evident.

**D.** Diagnosis is often difficult since salmonellosis presents symptoms similar to many other conditions. *Cattle*: enteric colibacillosis, coccidiosis, cryptosporidiosis, paratuberculosis, parasitic gastroenteritis, bovine viral diarrhoea, infectious bovine rhinotracheitis, etc., arsenic and molybdenum poisoning, etc. *Pigs*: colibacillosis, swine dysentery, swine fever, classical swine fever, swine dysentery, pasteurellosis, septicaemic swine erysipelas, etc. *Sheep*: coccidiosis, pasteurellosis, colibacillosis, parasitic gastroenteritis, campylobacteriosis, etc.

Diagnosis is confirmed on laboratory examination of faeces, tissues, feed, etc. by culture of the organism using selective media because of the large number of other bacteria present, especially in faeces.

**J.** Carcase and viscera: T.

## SWINE DYSENTERY (HAEMORRHAGIC DYSENTERY, BLOODY SCOURS, 'VIBRIONIC DYSENTERY', SD)

**I.** A common contagious disease of pigs in which there is haemorrhagic or mucoid inflammation of the large intestine.

**O.** Common in most pig-producing countries, especially the USA, Canada, Europe, Australia and New Zealand.

**IA.** *Treponema hyodysenteriae*, a spirochaete (elongated, loosely-coiled, motile but with no flagella), Gram-negative, anaerobic, haemolytic) bacillus 6–8.5 μm in length. It is possible that other bacteria and viruses in the pig intestine may contribute in causing swine dysentery. (*T. pallidum* is the cause of syphilis in man.)

**R.** Faeces of affected, recovered and carrier pigs. It is possible that rodents may be sources of infection.

**MT.** By ingestion of contaminated food and water and by direct and indirect contact, e.g. via contaminated clothing of attendants.

**CF.** The disease is common in pigs of 15–70 kg liveweight but can affect all ages.

*Treponema hyodysenteriae* proliferates rapidly in the intestine and produces its inflammatory effects on the mucosa by means of two toxins, haemolysin and lipopolysasccharide (LPS).

Symptoms include diarrhoea which at first is grey and soft, later becoming watery with mucus, blood and fibrinous exudate. In chronic forms of the disease the faeces contain dark blood (*'bloody or black scours'*). Affected pigs show fever, anorexia, dehydration with increased thirst, weakness, incoordination and marked loss of weight with prolonged disease.

**P.** Lesions are mostly confined to the large intestine (caecum, spiral colon and rectum), although some congestion may be present in the stomach.

In the *acute* stages of the disease there is hyperaemia and oedema of the large intestine wall and swelling of the mesenteric lymph nodes. The mucous membrane is covered with flecks of mucus, blood and fibrin.

More *chronic* stages show yellowish necrotic debris overlying a red, granular mucosa.

**D.** Clinical signs and post-mortem findings are usually adequate for a tentative diagnosis, which is confirmed by isolation of *T. hyodysenteriae* in smears and anaerobic culture.
Differential diagnoses: as for salmonellosis.

**J.**
Acute swine dysentery: Carcase and viscera, T.
Chronic swine dysentery: Carcase, A.
Affected organs: D, provided no systemic changes present and condition satisfactory.

## TICK PYAEMIA (ENZOOTIC STAPHYLOCOCCOSIS)

**I.** An endemic bacterial disease of lambs (2 weeks up to 3 months of age) characterised by septicaemia or bacteraemia with the development of pyaemic abscesses mainly in joints but which can occur in any organ.

**O.** The disease appears to be restricted to the British Isles.

**IA.** *Staphylococcus aureus*, a small, spherical, mainly aerobic, non-motile Gram-positive organism (0.7–1 μm in diameter) which is a common commensal of the skin and nasopharynx of man and animals but has to be regarded as a potential pathogen.
It is a pyogenic, i.e. pus-producing, organism having the ability to cause abscesses, pustules and infections in accidental or surgical wounds. Much of this pathogenicity is its ability to produce coagulase, a thrombin-like enzyme, which coats the coccus with protective fibrin, and deoxyribonuclease (DNase), another aggressin which assists to make the organism more virulent.

**R.** Affected and carrier sheep.

**MT.** Tick pyaemia is associated with the activity of the tick *Ixodes ricinus*, and the agent of tick-borne fever, *Cytocetes phagocytophila* (q.v.). This particular agent reduces the defences of the animal by, for example, causing a leukopenia following the puncture of the skin by the three-host tick. Infection may also occur via the umbilicus.

**CF.** A septicaemia or bacteraemia ensues, the former rapidly leading to death while the latter results in lameness with stiff, swollen and painful joints due to the formation of abscesses. Some lambs exhibit nervous signs while others become paraplegic. There is rapid loss of condition.

**P.** Abscesses are commonly found in the enlarged joints, liver, lungs, heart, kidneys, brain and spinal cord. These abscesses, which contain a greenish-yellow pus, may also be found in the skin and vertebral column.

**D.** The clinical signs along with the lesions and the presence of *Ixodes ricinus* ticks are presumptive of tick pyaemia. Isolation of the causal organism confirms the diagnosis.
Differential diagnoses include tick-borne fever, joint ill, erysipelothrix infection.
The organism, *Staphylococcus aureus*, is also involved in the causation of ulcerative dermatitis in sheep, pyoderma in horses, and chronic mastitis in cows.
A related organism, *Staphylocccus hyicus*, causes *exudative epidermitis in pigs ('greasy pig disease')* an acute generalised eczematous inflammation of the skin which occurs worldwide and is especially serious in younger pigs, older animals being more resistant.
Affected pigs show intense reddening of the skin which becomes thickened and encrusted with exudate of serum. Sometimes vesicles appear which become infected and burst. Erosions of the coronary band of the feet are common. Affected pigs have a high temperature with inappetence. The mortality rate in young pigs may be as high as 90%.
It is unlikely that acute cases will be presented for slaughter, but older more chronic cases probably merit total condemnation because of emaciation.

**J.** Tick pyaemia and Exud. epidermitis: T.

## TUBERCULOSIS (TB) (see also Chapter 16)

**I.** A usually chronic, debilitating, but sometimes acute, infectious disease of all vertebrates, birds and man characterised by the development of tubercles in any part of the body. Zoonosis.

**O.** Animal tuberculosis is now rare in developed countries which have instituted eradication programmes, although breakdowns still occur and the organisms continue to be occasionally detected at meat inspection. In Britain many of the younger meat inspectors have not encountered a TB lesion, although the disease is now (1998) spreading in the south-west of England, being associated with infection in badgers, and has subsequently appeared in the north and east.

Germany was declared free of bovine tuberculosis in December 1996. Annual testing is no longer required, the disease being monitored by the meat hygiene authorities. It is estimated that Germany will save about DM 10 million annually in control costs.

In developing countries, especially in Africa, the picture is very different. In the Côte d'Ivoire in 1992 50% of all totally condemned bovine carcases and 10% of totally condemned sheep and goat carcases were due to tuberculosis. Isolation rates in Morocco in 1992 were 30% for *M. bovis* and 9.7% for *M. tuberculosis*. Recently reported prevalence in cattle in Somalia was 4.54–10.20%. Some 44 African countries recognise the presence of bovine TB in their herds (WHO/FAO/OIE, 1993), with high occurrences in Benin, Gambia, Mali, Niger, Sudan and Tanzania. Bovine TB appears to be less of a problem in the Americas and Asia. Although *M. tuberculosis* is the most frequent cause of human TB, some cases are due to the bovine strain, making bovine TB a *zoonosis* of great public health significance.

Animal tuberculosis is most common in cattle, pigs and goats and less so in sheep and horses. Goats are very susceptible, especially if kept in the vicinity of affected cattle, and sheep – although previously thought to be resistant – may also develop the disease but to a lesser extent.

Wildlife may also be affected with tuberculosis. In New Zealand it was diagnosed in 36 of 53 (68%) of bush tail possums as well as in stoats and hares.

**IA.** There are three main types of tubercle bacilli – human (*Mycobacterium tuberculosis*), bovine (*Mycobacterium bovis*) and avian (*Mycobacterium avium*). All three types can produce disease in species other than their own. However, *M. tuberculosis* mostly affects man, only on rare occasions causing disease in dogs, parrots and non-human primates. Most cases of infection in animals caused by *M. tuberculosis* are of minor importance and easily overcome.

*M. bovis* can affect most vertebrates, including man.

*M. avium* (of which only two serovars – 1 and 2 – are pathogenic) is the only strain pathogenic for birds but can also cause TB in most vertebrates and some cold-blooded species.

Organisms of the genus *Mycobacterium* (which includes *M. leprae*, the cause of leprosy in man and *M. intracellulare* and *M. scrofulaceum*, (pathogens for pigs) are acid-fast (q.v.), Gram-positive, non-motile, non-sporing, non-capsulate, aerobic bacilli which occur as slender, curved or straight rods (3 µm × 0.3 µm), often appearing singly, as pairs or in bundles.

Only a few members of the mycobacteria are pathogenic, the majority existing as saprophytes in soil, water and plant life.

The organisms are fairly resistant: *M. bovis* can remain viable for over 2 years in frozen carcases and for months in pickled meat. Decomposition does not affect viability – virulent tubercle bacilli have been discovered in decomposed bovine lung after 167 days, in decomposed bovine carcases after several years and in tuberculous poultry carcases buried 2½ metres deep for 27 months.

**R.** Affected, subclinical and carrier animals excrete the organisms in sputum, faeces, milk, urine, uterine and vaginal material and discharges from open lymph nodes. Mycobacteria have been isolated from the tonsils and lymph nodes of apparently normal pigs and can easily escape detection in all species at meat inspection, which in most countries is a solely visual procedure.

Human beings, although primarily responsible for infecting other human beings, are occasionally responsible for the disease in animals, as are cats, dogs and goats. Wildlife, e.g. badgers and possums, also makes a contribution to the maintenance of infection. In the south-west of England in 1983, 11.4% of badger carcases contained viable *M. bovis*, a lower incidence being found in foxes and rats. Wild birds, e.g. starlings, harbouring *M. avium*, have been incriminated as a source of infection in pigs.

**MT.** Infection is most commonly developed through inhalation (90% of bovine cases) or the ingestion of contaminated food, especially milk, and water. Inhalation is the common route in housed stock where the opportunity for the spread of tuberculosis from animal to animal is greatest. The feeding of infected milk and dairy products to young animals and to children is a common means of acquiring the disease. The feeding of untreated swill and abattoir offal to pigs has caused the disease as has the use of improperly cooked offal from a poultry plant.

Tuberculosis may also on occasions be set up via coitus from infected uterine discharges or infected semen.

Direct invasion through mucous membranes or broken skin may be rare routes of infection. Where TB lesions are confined to a prescapular or precrural lymph node, however, infection may be attributed to a skin route.

**CF:** Clinical signs depend on the nature and locations of the lesions but in some situations, e.g. miliary tuberculosis and extensive caseous lesions in the spleen, liver and lungs, premonitory symptoms may be entirely absent.

*Cattle:* Pulmonary involvement in *advanced* cases is associated with a typical intermittent, moist cough with the head held low and tongue extended, great loss of condition, sluggishness, fast and difficult breathing, anorexia and usually rough coat. Enlargement of the retropharyngeal lymph nodes produces a typical snoring sound with difficulty in swallowing.

Tuberculous meningitis is evidenced by disturbances of behaviour – excitability, mania and sometimes blindness.

TB mastitis takes the form of induration and enlargement of the udder, especially its upper part, along with similar changes in the supramammary lymph nodes, and sometimes the precrural and iliac nodes. Such changes are only found in the more acute caseating breakdown type of TB mastitis, which is of vital importance for public health.

Tuberculous enteritis is associated with diarrhoea but is a rare occurrence as is TB metritis. This latter results in either infertility or abortion (the calf being affected with generalised TB). In tubercular orchitis in the bull the testes are enlarged and indurated but painless.

*Sheep and goats*: Symptoms in the pulmonary form resemble those in cattle.

*Pigs*: Early TB lesions in pigs are usually confined to the retropharyngeal, submaxillary and mesenteric lymph nodes. Generalisation is not common but may occur with the bovine type and less commonly the avian bacilli and present signs similar to those in cattle. Joint lesions due to TB may be present and should meningitis ensue nervous symptoms become evident. On occasions infected superficial lymph nodes may rupture to the exterior.

*Horses*. Symptoms similar to those in cattle with pulmonary TB may occur but a common sign is neck stiffness due to TB of the cervical vertebrae.

**Pathogenesis and lesions** All types of the tubercle bacilli are able to produce progressive disease, this ability being ascribed in part to the complex lipids in the bacterial cell walls. Their virulence, however, is a complex entity, and may also be associated with the action of toxic lipids and factors released by bacteria which inactivate body defence mechanisms. Concurrent deficiencies in mononuclear function may also contribute to the spread of infection.

Tuberculosis spreads in the animal body in two stages – primary complex and post-primary dissemination. When tubercle bacilli first gain entrance to the body they create a *primary focus*. This lesion usually occurs in the *lung* (most often in cattle, pigs, man) or *intestine* (most often in poultry). In cattle it is commonly found on the upper border of the lung and may be so small as to be overlooked, with the only obvious lesion being present in the retropharyngeal lymph nodes (or the mesenteric lymph node if infection occurs by ingestion). Lymphatic drainage from this primary focus leads to the formation of secondary tiny yellowish-white caseous lesions in the associated lymph node(s). Tissue reaction to the invading and multiplying bacilli takes the form of a proliferation of epithelioid and giant cells with necrosis and caseation or calcification and the formation of connective tissue creating a tumour-like granulomatous nodule or '*tubercle*'. The combination of the primary focus and adjacent lymph node lesion is known as the '*primary complex*'.

A typical *tubercle* is a firm, hard nodule, whitish or yellowish-white in colour and about 1–2 cm in diameter. This can become larger owing to the combination of two or more adjacent tubercles. Section reveals a necrotic, caseous (cheesy) or calcified centre, depending on the age of the lesion. A grating feeling is experienced on section when calcification is present. If body resistance is high, the tubercle becomes reduced in size and encapsulated by fibrous tissue. If healing does not take place, secondary infection usually occurs followed by suppuration or liquefaction necrosis and cavitation. In calcified tubercles, virulent bacilli may be found but are usually few in number and undergoing degeneration. Typical tubercles are not always formed in tuberculous infection – a fibrinous or fibrinopurulent exudate may be the only evidence in rapidly fatal situations, e.g. tuberculous meningitis, and in immuno-compromised animals.

If body resistance is low, this first stage of spread is followed by the *second stage – post-primary dissemination* – when spread to other organs takes place by contiguity, e.g. from lung to pleura, by the lymphatic system or by the systemic circulation. The number and extent of secondary, generalised lesions are related to the number and virulence of circulating bacilli. Secondary infection of the intestine may also follow a pulmonary lesion when virulent organisms are coughed up and then swallowed. Pulmonary lesions may also give rise to a suppurative bronchopneumonia.

Entry of bacilli into the systemic circulation can take place by a tubercle eroding the wall of an artery or vein or breaking down the lymphatic barrier in a lymph node. (In *man* infection has been known to cause rupture of the aorta.) Large numbers of bacilli are disseminated into the systemic circulation and lodge in capillaries of remote organs (lungs, kidneys, spleen, liver, bones, etc.), giving rise to the millet-sized lesions of rapidly fatal *miliary tuberculosis*.

More often, however, generalisation results in *'breakdown'* tuberculous lesions occurring as caseous masses in the uterus, kidneys, lungs, pleura, lymph nodes, etc. These are large, dry, cheesy areas interspersed with small haemorrhages which in lymph nodes often take the form of radiating lines of caseation – the so-called *stellate caseation* in which calcification is absent. Such changes are indicative of complete absence of body resistance.

The *judgement* of tuberculous carcases depends on the *number and disposition* of the lesions as well as their *character*, whether acute or chronic, the overall picture being an indication of the success or failure of tissue reaction. Much the same can be said for all disease conditions.

Traditional meat inspection procedures were largely based on the pathology of bovine tuberculosis as elucidated by the German veterinarian Robert von Ostertag, who published his *Handbuch der Fleischbeschan für Tierartze, Arzte und Richter in 1872*. However, the elimination of bovine tuberculosis in many countries with the introduction of so-called *'production diseases'* with emphasis on the health status of the live animal has significantly altered the situation regarding post-mortem examination and the need for lymph node incision with its inevitable risk of contamination.

## Reactions in different species

The nature of the reaction to tubercle bacilli by the animal body depends on several factors – the virulence of the organisms; the type of the TB bacilli (bovine, avian or human); the defensive ability of the animal, including that produced by a previous assault and the species of the animal itself.

Moderately pathogenic organisms are fairly easily destroyed by macrophages (epithelioid, endothelioid, reticuloendothelial cells) with giant cell and granulation tissue reaction, while very virulent bacilli produce an exudative tissue reaction and usually generalisation.

**Cattle, sheep and goats** TB is fairly rare in sheep and goats and resembles that in cattle when caused by the bovine bacillus. *M. avium* may be responsible for disseminated tuberculosis.

Calcification is usually prominent, especially in lymph nodes. Lesions may be either cellular (if resistance is high) or exudative (if resistance is low). In *cattle* tubercles on the pleura and peritoneum are fairly common – the so-called *'grapes'* or *'pearl disease'*. These are normally 0.5–1.0 cm in diameter and on section show caseous and calcified centres under a thickened pleural membrane.

Tubercles may occur in any lymph node, especially the retropharyngeal, submaxillary, bronchial, mediastinal and mesenteric nodes.

TB lesions may be found in the bovine vagina in the form of tubercles or ulcers.

## Affections of specific organs

### *Lungs*

In cattle the primary focus is usually on the upper border of a main lobe appearing as a rounded nodule or tubercle beneath the pleura. This may heal by fibrosis or progress by caseation and liquefaction of the lung tissue.

Progression takes the form of greyish or yellowish areas of caseous bronchopneumonia which tend to be circumscribed by serous infiltration into the interlobular septa, the infiltrate eventually becoming fibrosed to localise the lesion. Should localisation not occur, however, these caseous lesions may coalesce to create even larger areas in the lung tissue.

Discrete encapsulated and calcified foci with similar lesions in bronchial and mediastinal lymph nodes may occur.

*Miliary tuberculosis* is manifested by the presence of numerous small tubercles widely distributed throughout the lungs, which are enlarged and oedematous, and is the result of haematogenous spread.

In *pigs* the lung lesions assume a fatty appearance without lymph node involvement and are usually devoid of caseation, calcification or fibrosis.

### *Pleurae*

Tuberculous pleurisy occurs following a primary lung infection via lymphatic drainage or by direct rupture of a pulmonary lesion or thoracic lymph node.

In *cattle* early stages show as soft, velvety, red granulations. The typical chronic stages of *'grapes'* or *'pearl disease'* appear as large numbers of shiny grey nodules (tubercles) which on section have caseous or calcified centres overlaid with very thickened fibrous pleural membranes.

In *pigs* serous membranes are rarely affected but assume the form of tiny, scattered discrete nodules which penetrate to the subpleural tissue.

### *Peritoneum*

Uncommon in cattle and other animals. Changes similar to the pleural lesions occur when infection arises from a liver lesion or congenitally.

### *Alimentary tract*

Primary infection with lesions in the intestinal tract is relatively rare but ulcers in the tonsils, tongue and intestine may occur, the latter resulting from the breakdown of lung lesions and swallowing of bacilli. Infection of the tongue results in enlargement and induration with caseous lymphadenitis in the retropharyngeal and parotid lymph nodes. Occasionally, nodules may occur in the small intestine, especially the ileum, and these coalesce to produce ulcers covered with greyish mucopurulent material.

### *Pericardium*

Tuberculous pericarditis is always a sequel to TB pleurisy. Early stages are in the form of red, velvety granulations near the base of the heart which appear as caseous areas encasing the heart in later stages. Extensions to the myocardium and endocardium are rare.

### *Liver*

The liver and the hepatic nodes may become infected from a primary intestinal infection via the lymph from the duodenum, by secondary infection from the intestine when bacilli are swallowed (via the mesenteric lymph nodes and portal venules), by the bloodstream or congenitally via the umbilical vein.

In *pigs* the tubercles due to the bovine strain are very tiny, being no larger than a pinhead, and are caseated or calcified and encapsulated. In avian infection yellowish-grey tubercles of a productive type form and resemble small metastatic tumours, e.g. lymphosarcoma or parasitic spots.

### *Spleen*

Tuberculosis of the spleen may be haematogenous in origin, an extension from a tuberculous peritonitis, or (in calves) of congenital origin.

In the calf and pig lesions are more common in the spleen substance, while adult cattle more often exhibit surface lesions.

### *Kidneys*

Infection occurs via the bloodstream. In *cattle* small discrete greyish-white nodules are usually confined to a few lobes but may be scattered throughout the kidney parenchyma. Coalescence of these small foci can result in larger areas of caseation from which infection of the ureter and bladder may ensue.

*Bones and joints*

Bacilli may disseminate from a primary focus by the bloodstream to the vertebrae and ends of long bones. This can occur early in life and infection may develop then or months, even years, later.

In *cattle* TB is most often seen in vertebrae and ribs and less often in the spongy tissue of the epiphyses of bones and the sternum. (The reverse appears to be the situation in *man* in whom the weight-bearing bones are most often involved.)

*Cavitation* or *caries* of the bone occurs with destruction and rarefaction of bone tissue and the formation of yellowish granulation tissue. Extension of the process may take place through the epiphysis into the joint capsule – TB arthritis – which most commonly affects the knee, hock and stifle.

In *pigs* lesions may be found in the vertebrae, especially the lumbar, and the ischiopubic symphysis.

*Female genitalia*

**Cattle** The vagina, uterus and ovaries may become affected by haematogenous spread, by contiguity from an infected peritoneum or from coitus from an infected bull (penis, epididymis, testis). Rarely, treatment for infertility has introduced the disease.

Tuberculous *vaginitis* shows as nodules or ulcers in the vagina. Tuberculous *metritis* is evidenced by either small pin-head yellowish foci or larger, fleshy, translucent lesions in the endometrium. Older lesions appear as pea-sized nodules in the submucous tissues. The endometrium becomes thickened and thrown into folds, the disease process eventually involving all the layers of the uterus and the peritoneum.

TB metritis is normally bilateral and usually originates in the region of the bifurcation of the cornua.

Affected *ovaries* have an uneven appearance with caseous, calcareous or purulent nodules, while the fallopian tubes are invariably involved, showing numerous greyish-white granulations.

*Udder*

In *cattle*, infection may arise by haematogenous spread, by lymphatic route from an abdominal lesion or by the teat canal through the introduction of infected equipment.

The lesion may be an acute caseating one of one or more quarters with enlargement of the associated supramammary and iliac lymph nodes. If a forequarter is affected, the precrural node on that side may be involved. In chronic tuberculosis mastitis, lesions are absent in the supramammary lymph nodes. The udder is enlarged and indurated in both forms.

*Male genitalia*

Haematogenous in origin, tuberculous *orchitis* involves first of all the epididymis and afterwards the testis, in which tubercles appear with great enlargement of the organ.

*Muscle*

Lesions of tuberculosis are rarely encountered in muscle. If found, for example, in the tongue or myocardium, they usually result from contiguity with other infected organs such as joints, serous membranes or bones.

*Central nervous system*

Tuberculous meningoencephalitis most commonly develops in the primary infection stage via the bloodstream and occurs most often in calves and young cattle. Caseous foci may be found in the brain and extend to the meninges. Tuberculous lesions in the vertebrae may, by contiguity, produce meningitis of the spinal cord.

*Other organs*

Tuberculous lesions of the adrenal body, prostate gland, thyroid gland, eye or pancreas are usually indicative of a generalised systemic infection, although the pancreas may become infected by contiguity with a TB liver.

**D.** Accurate diagnosis in the live animal is only possible in advanced cases in cattle. Reliance has to be placed in the tuberculin skin test (single intradermal test (SID), Stormont test, short thermal test, comparative test, etc.). Immunity to tuberculosis is cell-mediated and depends largely on interaction between sensitised T lymphocytes and macrophages.

The *tuberculin test* is based on the phenomenon of *acquired hypersensitivity* which occurs when the body encounters a foreign substance. When the host again meets the same antigen (q.v.) a vigorous reaction takes place, the reaction varying in degree from minor tissue damage to severe illness and even death. There are four types of hypersensitivity depending on the form of mechanism involved. Type I is the anaphylactic type or immediate hypersensitivity reaction. Cell-mediated or delayed-type reactions are classified as Type IV, in which the hypersensitivity reaction to the skin test is delayed, taking some 48–72 h to reach its maximum response in which there is oedema and induration at the site of introduction of the antigen (tuberculin).

Most countries now use a standard purified-protein-derivative (PPD) tuberculin for the routine testing of animals in disease eradication programmes. The tuberculin is prepared from cultures of *M. bovis* and *M. tuberculosis* grown on special media. In the SID test in cattle, 0.05 ml of tuberculin is injected into the skin, usually of the neck but sometimes the anal or caudal fold and the reaction is read 2–3 days later, pre- and post-injection skin measurements being made using calipers.

Smears of sputum, milk and discharges stained by the *Ziehl–Neelsen method* are employed in the live animal, and material from lesions in the carcase which can also be used for culture.

## Differential diagnosis

Tuberculosis may be confused with many other diseases, especially those of pulmonary origin – lung abscess, contagious bovine pleuropneumonia, aspiration pneumonia, coccidioidmycosis, mucormycosis, Johne's disease, actinobacillosis, actinomycosis and lymphosarcoma.

Some parasitic infestations (*Ascaris*, *Cysticercus tenuicollis*, *Fasciola*, hydatid cysts, *Muellerius*, *Metastrongylus*, etc.) give rise to lesions which on occasions resemble tubercles, in particular if calcification is present.

Many lesions in pigs resemble TB, especially those occurring in the submaxillary nodes. These take the form of small, yellowish necrotic foci surrounded by a connective-tissue capsule which are easily expressed on incision or pressure, leaving smooth cavities. These lesions are caused by *Corynebacterium pyogenes*.

The chronic nature of the disease and its similarity to many other infections makes clinical diagnosis difficult except perhaps for the fulminating pulmonary form in cattle with its typical chronic cough. Clinical diagnosis is normally only possible in the later stages of the disease.

*Widespread lesions involving lungs, liver, spleen and associated lymph nodes have been found in the carcases of cattle in good condition reacting to the tuberculin test, the live animals having shown no premonitory symptoms.*

Lesions that bear a close resemblance to tuberculosis but are caused by *Brucella suis* have been reported in the vertebrae of *pigs* in the USA. These foci appear as greyish-white abscesses and are usually found in the lumbosacral region but sometimes in the carcase lymph nodes; they usually originate in the intervertebral spaces and extend to the vertebral bodies. In some cases of *Br. suis* infection, lesions are confined to the spleen.

*Mesothelioma* of the bovine pleura and peritoneum may assume a grape-like form superficially resembling tubercles.

### *Parasitic infections*

Certain parasites in the food animals give rise to cheesy, sometimes calcareous, necrotic foci in various tissues, especially where the parasite dies and undergoes degeneration.

The liver of the horse may show nodular or serpentine, caseous or calcareous foci due to the larvae of some types of *strongyles*. In other animals TB-like lesions may be found in the liver caused by invasion of *Ascaris* larvae or, especially in sheep, the wandering larvae of lung strongyles. Irregularly distributed nodules and serpentine-like burrows which are common in the substance and on the surface of sheep livers, are most likely to be produced by the immature forms of *Fasciola hepatica*, *Ascaris* spp. or *Cysticercus tenuicollis*. The former may also give rise to tuberculous-like changes in the liver of pigs, these foci taking the form of white spherical nodules, usually situated superficially and composed of a thick connective-tissue capsule with brownish or yellowish semi-solid contents.

*Hydatid cysts* in the liver and lungs may degenerate to form a cheesy mass encapsulated in connective tissue; multilocular cysts in particular may bear a resemblance to TB, but the laminated cuticular membrane is still present even after the cyst has degenerated and can be readily picked up with a pair of forceps. In most parasitic infections microscopical examination of the caseous mass will usually reveal some residual portion of the causal parasite, e.g. hooklets or calcareous corpuscles from a tapeworm.

The subpleural tissue of *sheep* lungs frequently shows grey, sharply delimited nodules caused by lungworms of the genus *Muellerius*. In the *pig*, the larvae of the lungworm *Metastrongylus apri (elongatus)* or *M. pudendotectus* may appear as glistening, translucent nodules beneath the lung pleura and sometimes in the lung substance; these foci are common in young pigs and are often discrete, though sometimes aggregated or in long chains with no associated lymph node changes.

### *Other types of mycobacteria*

While *M. bovis*, *M. tuberculosis* and *M. avium* are the classic mycobacteria, other types exist, some of which can cause disease in animals and interfere with the interpretation of the tuberculin test, especially to avian tuberculin. *M. paratuberculosis (M. jöhnei)*, the cause of Jöhne's disease in ruminants. A major bacterium is *Mycobacterium leprae*, the cause of leprosy in man, who is affected with hypopigmented macules and nodules on the skin and mucous membranes in addition to damage and enlargement of peripheral nerves.

Other less important forms include *M. fortuitum*, *M. scrofulaceum*, *M. intracellulare*, *M. chelonei*, *M. phlei*, *M. smegmatis*, *M. aquae*, *M. marinum* and *M. kansasii*.

Most of the tuberculous-like, non-progressive lesions are encountered in pigs, in which *M. intracellulare* causes a lymphadenitis of mesenteric lymph nodes, which tend to become calcified, and *M. fortuitum* causes a chronic arthritis. *M. smegmatis* has been isolated from TB-like lesions in porcine lymph nodes. *M. aquae* is associated with nodular teat lesions in cows. *M. scrofulaceum* produces TB-like lesions in cattle and dogs. *M. marinum* causes tuberculous lesions in fish and man. *M. chelonei*, *M. phlei* and *M. fortuitum* produce cutaneous TB-like lesions in cats and dogs. *M. kansasii* is responsible for cervical lymphadenitis and pneumonia in human beings and skin TB in cattle.

### *'Skin tuberculosis'*

This misnamed condition is important in connection with TB eradication schemes since a proportion of affected animals react to the several tuberculin tests, especially to avian tuberculin. The number of cases is said to be increasing in Great Britain, although probably not more than 50% of clinical cases of 'skin tuberculosis' give a reaction to mammalian tuberculin.

The path of infection is probably via the skin, since cattle lose their sensitivity when the lesions are removed surgically.

The lesions are indurated, painless, subcutaneous nodules, varying in size from being just noticeable up to the size of a hen's egg. Most are about 1–2 cm in diameter, occurring singly or in chain formation, usually following the course of a lymphatic vessel. They are attached to the skin and are most commonly found on the limbs, especially the fetlock, forearm, hock and less frequently, the chest wall and shoulder. They have also been recorded in the prescapular, popliteal and submaxillary lymph nodes and the connective tissue surrounding the sheath of the metatarsus but are considered to be extensions of the typical skin forms.

The *nodules* consist of a fibrous wall, commonly enclosing a caseocalcareous centre but in other cases a thick, yellow glutinous pus, a dried material resembling powdered maize or dried flake-like pellicles. Microscopically, the lesions are indistinguishable from tuberculous nodules, and although acid-fast bacilli (not pathogenic mycobacteria) can nearly always be detected, they cannot be grown on ordinary culture media nor are they pathogenic for guinea pigs.

Various bacteria have been isolated, but the organism considered the main cause is *Mycobacterium kansasii*.

**Differential diagnosis** The condition must be distinguished from ulcerative lymphangitis and cattle farcy. These conditions, however, involve thickening of the associated lymphatics with chronic ulceration and discharge of pus.

**Judgement of 'skin TB'** The condition is of no importance in meat inspection since the nodules are removed with the skin.

## Judgement of tuberculosis

The character of the lesions, whether acute or chronic, their extent and disposition, localisation or generalisation, carcase condition (although if good, total condemnation may be warranted on occasions) must all be taken into consideration.

## Routine post-mortem procedures and judgements

These vary to some extent in different countries.

GREAT BRITAIN

*Routine post-mortem inspection for tuberculosis*

Under the Fresh Meat (Hygiene and Inspection) Regulations 1995, Schedule 10, Part VIII, it is prescribed that:

Where an inspector or OVS has reason to suspect that any part of the carcase or offal of any animal is infected with tuberculosis, he shall, in addition to carrying out the provisions of the preceding Parts of this Schedule —

(a) in the case of any carcase, require the carcase to be split, examine the vertebrae, ribs, sternum, spinal cord and, if he considers it necessary, the brain, and if a lesion of a kidney is visible or suspected, incise the kidney;

(b) in the case of the carcase of any *bovine* animal, soliped or farmed deer, examine in detail (i.e. examine by making deep multiple incisions into lymph nodes) the following lymph nodes (being lymph nodes not already examined), namely, the superficial inguinal, prepectoral, presternal, suprasternal, xiphoid, subdorsal, intercostal, prescapular, iliac, sublumbar, ischiatic, precrural and popliteal, those lymph nodes which are least likely to show infection being examined first; and

(c) in the case of the carcase of any *swine*, examine in detail the following lymph nodes (being lymph nodes not already examined) namely, the superficial inguinal, cervical, prepectoral, prescapular, subdorsal, iliac, precrural, and, if he considers it necessary, the popliteal.

*Code of judgement. Indications of unfitness for human consumption. Part IX*

1. (1). If upon inspection of any carcase an inspector or OVS is satisfied that the animal was suffering from *tuberculosis (generalised) or tuberculosis with emaciation*, he shall *condemn the whole carcase and all the offal and blood* removed or collected therefrom as being unfit for human consumption.

*Indications of generalised TB or TB with emaciation*

(a) Miliary tuberculosis of both lungs with evidence of TB elsewhere.

(b) Multiple and actively progressive lesions of TB.

(c) Widespread TB infection of the lymph nodes of the carcase.

(d) Diffuse acute lesions of TB of both the pleura and peritoneum associated with an enlarged or tuberculous lymph node of the carcase.

(e) Active or recent lesions present in the substance of any two of the following: spleen, kidney, udder, uterus, ovary, testicle, brain and spinal cord or their membranes, in addition to TB lesions in the respiratory and digestive tracts.

(f) In the case of a calf, congenital tuberculosis.

*Indications of localised tuberculosis*

(1) Where an inspector or OVS is satisfied that *a carcase of offal is affected with tuberculosis other than generalised tuberculosis or tuberculosis with emaciation*, he shall reject the following parts of the carcase and offal as unfit for human consumption:

(a) any part of the carcase infected with localised tuberculosis and any other part contiguous thereto;

(b) the head, including the tongue, when tuberculosis exists in any lymph node associated with the head or tongue, save that where in a particular lymph node or nodes the lesion is small and inactive and the lymph node is not enlarged, he may regard the head and tongue, or both, as fit for human consumption after the removal of the affected lymph node or nodes and the surrounding tissue;

(c) any organ or viscera when tuberculosis exists in the substance, or on the surface thereof, or in any lymph node associated therewith.

(2) An inspector or OVS shall reject any part of a carcase and any offal or blood contaminated with tuberculosis material as unfit for human consumption.

### Canada

Food Production and Inspection Branch, Meat and Poultry Products Division

The following instructions apply to *ruminants*, *pigs* and *horses*.

NOTE. The following disposition applies to the carcases of animals presented as part of the regular kill. When lesions similar to those caused by *M. bovis* are detected in carcases of animals from premises being depopulated because of tuberculosis, their carcases shall be condemned regardless of extent of infection.

Entry of the tubercular organism, and organisms which produce granulomatous lesions similar to those caused by *M. bovis,* is most common via the respiratory or digestive tract. Evidence of infection, therefore, is expected in three primary areas – the lymph nodes of the head, the lymph nodes of the lungs and the mesenteric lymph nodes. When granulomatous lesions similar to those caused by *M. bovis* are detected in more than one of these primary sites, the other body lymph nodes shall be incised and examined for lesions.

Disposition of affected carcases reflects both the location and extent of lesions detected.

Affected carcases shall be condemned if:

(i) lesions are detected in one or more primary sites and one or more body lymph nodes; or

(ii) lesions are detected in any other organ, e.g. lungs, liver, spleen.

When carcases are affected to a lesser extent, the affected lymph node and the corresponding portion of the carcase shall be condemned, e.g. head and tongue, lungs or intestines and stomach(s).

The term '*granulomatous lymphadenitis*' shall be used to report the condemnation of carcases and portions.

In cases where *swine* carcases are condemned for granulomatous lymphadenitis, typical lesions shall be sent to ADRI (Nepean) for examination. Use of the Bovine Tuberculosis Kit is permitted to allow shipment of specimens in both formalin and borate. Specimens are not required from carcases affected to a lesser extent.

*Swine* carcases with mandibular and mesenteric lymph nodes affected which are subsequently approved, must be 'held' and stamped four times on each side with the letter 'T'. Carcases so stamped shall be held on a designated rail in the cooler.

The cutting of such carcases shall be done under the direct supervision of an inspector, at the end of the pork cutting operations. The cuts may either be sold or processed for domestic trade only (the export of such meat is prohibited). Containers of such cuts and trimmings shall be stamped with the letter 'T'. The veterinarian in charge may approve alternative procedures which ensure that these products are not exported.

Needle-point and rubber stamps bearing the letter 'T' (at least 5 cm in height) have been issued.

### Codex Alimentarius Commission

Food and Agriculture Organization of the United Nations. World Health Organization. Alinorm 93/16A

#### *Section VI. Post-mortem procedures*

Para 58. *(a) in all animals in which a systemic or generalised disease is suspected, in all animals positive to the tuberculin test, in all animals in which lesions suggestive of tuberculosis are found at post-mortem inspection*, and in all horses reacting to the mallein test, the main carcase lymph nodes (being the precrural, popliteal, anal, superficial inguinal, ischiatic, internal and external iliac, lumbar, renal, sternal, prepectoral, prescapular and atlantal nodes), as well as the lymph nodes of the head and viscera, should be incised and examined.

#### *Section IX. Recommended final judgement in cases of tuberculosis*

*Judgement symbols*

A – Approved as *fit* for human consumption.

T – Totally *unfit* for human consumption.

D – Designates organs or parts *unfit* for human consumption.

K – Conditionally approved as *fit* for human consumption. (Kh – heat treatment; Kf – freezing or heat treatment.)

I – Meat showing minor deviations from normal but *fit* for human consumption.

L – Approved as *fit* for consumption, with limited distribution.

... – Not applicable, e.g. in cases of T, the columns referring to partial condemnation are not applicable. (Meat from animals affected in any way by tuberculosis is excluded from international trade.)

Cattle and buffaloes

(i) *Carcase and viscera:* Cases of residual infection or reinfection where an eradication scheme has terminated (including reactors without lesions: ***T***)

(ii) During final stages of an eradication scheme and where natural prevalence is low:

- Reactor without lesions: ***Kh***. Lungs and udder: ***D***. Alternatively *L* or *A*, but excluded from international trade.
- One organ only affected and no miliary lesions: ***Kh***. Lungs and udder: ***D***. Provided chronic conditions such as anaemia, cachexia, emaciation, loathsome appearance, degeneration of organs and oedema are absent.
- More than one organ affected or miliary lesions in one organ: ***T***

(iii) During early stages of an eradication scheme and in high prevalence areas:

- Reactor without lesions: ***L***. Lungs, udder: ***D***. ***A*** instead of ***L*** if ***L*** not economically feasible, but excluded from international trade.
- One organ only affected and no miliary lesions: ***Kh***. Lungs, udder. ***D***. Provided chronic conditions, etc., absent.
- More than one organ affected but no signs of generalisation of recent haematogenous spread: ***Kh***. Lungs, udder: ***D***. ***T*** if economically feasible and chronic conditions, etc., absent.
- Generalisation: ***T***

Pigs

*Carcase and viscera*:

(i) Localized in throat or mesenteric lymph nodes (bovine or avian type): *Kh*. Parts of carcase ***D***. Organs ***D***. Intestines ***D***. However, *T* in areas where bovine TB eradication scheme is concluded or in final stages, or at any time if of bovine type. Alternatively to *Kh heat treatment at 77°C* if not found beyond one primary site.

(ii) Avian type confined to submaxillary glands: ***A***. Parts of carcase: ***D***. Head: ***D***.

(iii) Extensive lesions in lymph nodes or other organs affected:

Small ruminants and horses: ***T***.

## TULARAEMIA (RABBIT FEVER, FRANCIS DISEASE, DEERFLY FEVER, O'HARA'S DISEASE)

**I.** A highly contagious *zoonosis* affecting mainly wild animals (jack and cottontail rabbits, hares, beavers, muskrats, voles, mice, birds, reptiles and fish) but which may also infect domestic animals (usually sheep, pigs, horses and less commonly calves and dogs) and man.

**O.** The disease appears to be confined mostly to the northern hemisphere, having been recorded in Czechoslovakia, France, Norway, Sweden, British Isles, USA, Canada, China and Japan.

**IA.** *Francisella (Pasteurella) tularensis*, a small Gram-negative, non-sporing, encapsulated, non-motile coccobacillus.

**R.** Various forms of wildlife (see above), affected and carrier animals, hard ticks, deerflies and mosquitoes.

**MT.** The organism is capable of being transmitted in several ways – by inoculation through the skin or conjunctiva, e.g. from bites of ticks and flies or from handling or dressing infected carcases; by ingestion of contaminated food, e.g. insufficiently cooked rabbit and hare or contaminated water; by inhalation of dust from contaminated hay, soil or grain and occasionally by the bites of infected animals.

**CF.** *Animals:* Symptoms associated with septicaemia are evident – high temperature, anorexia, lethargy, stiffness, dyspnoea, progressive loss of weight, coughing, diarrhoea and recumbency with death in a few days to 2 weeks. Cases usually develop in the spring when ticks are active.

*Man:* Incubation period is usually 3 days. Symptoms vary greatly from formation of a painful, indurated swelling at the site of inoculation which usually ulcerates with lymphadenitis in the regional lymph node to pneumonia or a condition resembling typhoid with pharyngitis, abdominal pain, diarrhoea and vomiting. Widespread involvement of lymph nodes usually results in death.

**P.** The skins of sheep are often infested with large numbers of ticks. Most consistent lesions are tiny whitish foci of miliary necrosis in the liver, spleen and lymph nodes, these organs being very enlarged. On occasion larger areas of necrosis may develop. The presence of ticks on the skin may be associated with areas of congestion and necrosis under the skin with enlargement and congestion of the regional lymph nodes.

Pigs develop pneumonia with abscesses in the submaxillary and parotid lymph nodes.

Great care is required in the handling of carcases in endemic areas and in the laboratory with infected material.

**D.** Symptoms of septicaemia along with gross lesions and the presence of ticks suggest tularaemia. Diagnosis is confirmed by culture of the organism from lesions, by indirect fluorescent antibody or tube agglutination test.

*Differential diagnoses* include other septicaemic diseases, acute pneumonia, tick borne fever, etc.

**J.** Carcase and viscera: T.

### YERSINIOSIS (PSEUDOTUBERCULOSIS)

**I.** A usually self-limiting acute bacterial *zoonosis* which occasionally causes disease in animals and man.

**O.** Worldwide, especially in Scandinavia, Canada, Australia and New Zealand.

**IA.** *Yersinia pseudotuberculosis*, *Y. enterocolitica* and *Y. pestis*. These are short, oval, capsulate, non-motile Gram-negative bacilli which exhibit bipolar staining with methylene blue and other dyes.

*Y. pestis* is the cause of *bubonic plague* (the Black Death of the Middle Ages) which is still endemic in many countries. Transfer of infection to man occurs when an infected rat flea *(Xenopsylla cheopis)* or other rodent aspirates human blood and then regurgitates the bacilli into the puncture wound, causing septicaemia, enlargement of regional lymph nodes, often in the groin, and sometimes pneumonia (pneumonic plague.)

**R.** Many types of wildlife, especially rodents and birds, which show no sign of disease, harbour the organisms in their intestines. Infected and carrier animals, including sick puppies and kittens, also act as sources of infection. The organisms are known to inhabit the tonsils of pigs, making undercooked pork a potential source of infection for man. Pigs so infected usually show no signs of disease.

**MT.** By ingestion of contaminated food and water and by contact with infected animals or people.

**CF.** Clinical signs vary according to the species of organism and animal involved. *Y. pseudotuberculosis* can cause enterocolitis, abortion, mastitis, pneumonia, lymphangitis and abscesses in ruminants as well as epididymitis and orchitis in rams. Subclinical cases are, however, common. As with many diseases, the presence of predisposing factors plays a vital role in causing the disease.

*Y. enterocolitica* appears to be a less common cause of disease in animals than *Y. pseudotuberculosis* but can be responsible for enterocolitis and abortion in sheep.

In *man* both organisms have been recognised in recent years as the causal agents of gastroenteritis (especially in children), mesenteric lymphadenitis, fever, headache, pharyngitis, anorexia, arthritis, abscess formation in the liver and spleen and even osteomyelitis and septicaemia.

**P.** Common findings are microabscesses with ulceration and thickening of the intestinal wall. Affected animals usually great loss of condition. See also **CF.**

**D.** A positive diagnosis can only be made by an efficient microbiological investigation.

*Differential diagnoses* include all those conditions in which gastroenteritis is manifested.

**J.** Carcase and viscera: T.

## VIRAL DISEASES

### AFRICAN HORSE SICKNESS (AHS)

**I.** A peracute, subacute or mild febrile disease of equidae, transmitted by insects and characterised by oedematous and respiratory, changes.

**O.** Until 1943 when the first cases were recorded in Egypt by the Royal Army Veterinary Corps, the disease was restricted to Africa south of the Sahara. Since then it has spread throughout the Middle East and reached Afghanistan, Pakistan and India in 1960. Cases have been recorded in Spain (last occurrence 1990) and Portugal (last occurrence 1989), having apparently reached there from North Africa.

**IA.** An *orbivirus* of the family Reoviridae.

**R.** Affected horses, mules and donkeys and insect carriers. It is probable that an unknown reservoir, possibly some form of wildlife, also exists.

**MT.** The disease is transmitted during warm, wet weather by the bites of various bloodsucking flies and insects, e.g. midges of the genus *Culicoides*, mosquitoes (*Aedes aegypti, Anopheles stephensi* and *Culex pipiens*) and possibly ticks.

**CF.** Symptoms vary according to the virulence of the virus. The *mild* form exhibits only fever and malaise for a few days.

The *subacute cardiac or oedematous* (Dikkop) form is manifested by oedema of the supraorbital fossae (which may extend to the head, eyelids, lips, shoulders and brisket), fever, conjunctivitis, cyanosis of tongue and gums, dyspnoea, restlessness and some loss of appetite. Mortality is less than 50%.

In the *peracute or respiratory form* (Dunkop) there is severe respiratory distress, colic, intense conjunctivitis, dyspnoea, spasmodic coughing often accompanied by a frothy, yellowish, nasal discharge and rapid onset of death.

**P.** Lesions vary according to the severity of the disease and include pulmonary oedema (especially of the interlobular septa); oedema of the intestinal wall and congestion of the liver in the peracute form of AHS, while the cardiac form exhibits hydropericardium with petechiae and ecchymoses in the epicardium and endocardium; subcutaneous oedema especially of the head and neck. Myocarditis, haemorrhagic gastritis and petechiation of the ventral surface of the tongue and of the peritoneum, may also be present.

**D.** Clinical signs are fairly typical of the cardiac (subacute or 'Dikkop') form but less so of the peracute and mild forms.

Laboratory investigation is necessary to confirm diagnosis. This includes isolation of and typing of the virus by mouse inoculation, cell culture, complement fixation, virus neutralisation and haemagglutination-inhibition tests.

*Differential diagnoses* include babesiosis, purpura haemorrhagica and equine infectious anaemia.

**J.**

Carcase and viscera: In clinical cases, T.
Reactor animals: L.

## AFRICAN SWINE FEVER (WARTHOG DISEASE, AFRICAN PIG DISEASE, ASF)

**I.** A highly contagious, febrile, viral disease which represents a more virulent form of swine fever (hog cholera, HC) and characterised by the presence of multiple haemorrhages and high mortality.

Notifiable disease (UK).

**O.** The disease was confined to Africa until 1957 when it appeared in Portugal and in 1960 in Spain. A total of 65 outbreaks (86 in Italy and 13 in Spain) were confirmed in the European Community in 1996. The last cases in France occurred in 1974, in Malta in 1978, in Cuba in 1980 and Belgium in 1985. Cases have also appeared in Brazil, Haiti and the Dominican Republic. ASF is currently enzootic in Angola, Zaire, Zambia, Cameroon, and Guinea Bissau and of high occurrence in Malawi.

**IA.** A DNA virus of the family Iridoviridae. Although the clinical signs and pathology resemble those of swine fever, the latter is caused by a different virus (pestivirus, family Togaviridae).

**R.** The natural hosts are wild swine – warthogs, bush pigs and giant forest hogs, carrier domestic pigs and argasid (*Ornithodoros* spp.) ticks which also act as vectors.

**MT.** By ingestion (e.g. by the feeding of uncooked infected pork) and inhalation of materials contaminated with the secretions, including urine, of infected pigs.

**CF.** High fever, inappetence, listlessness, incoordination, diarrhoea, dyspnoea and cyanosis. Pregnant sows may abort. With virulent forms of the virus mortality may reach 100%.

**P.** *Peracute* cases may show no significant changes. *Less severe* cases exhibit petechial haemorrhages in the submucous and subserosal tissues, lymph nodes, heart, ileo-caecal valve, larynx, bladder and renal cortex. There is excess fluid in the pericardial, pleural and peritoneal cavities and ecchymoses are present on the skin of the abdomen and legs. The spleen is usually enlarged. More *chronic* cases may exhibit ulcers in the caecum and colon (but are less common than in SF) with nodular infarcts in the liver and spleen.

**D.** The disease is easily confused with swine fever and can only be confirmed by laboratory examination – fluorescent antibody staining, ELISA test, indirect immunofluorescence, radioimmunoassay, haemadsorption, etc.

*Differential diagnoses* include swine fever and acute swine erysipelas.

ASF is a notifiable disease in most countries.

**J.** Carcase and viscera: T.

## AUJESZKY'S DISEASE (PSEUDORABIES, MAD ITCH, INFECTIOUS BULBAR PARALYSIS)

**I.** A highly fatal, contagious disease of pigs and rodents and less commonly cattle, sheep, goats, dogs and cats which affects primarily the CNS with nervous symptoms (incoordination, tremors, pruritus, convulsions), especially in older pigs, being prominent.

Notifiable disease (UK).

**O.** Widespread throughout the world, causing serious economic losses, especially in the USA. Aujeszky's disease is currently subject to eradication programmes (test and slaughter of infected pigs) in several countries – GB and USA (commenced 1983), N. Ireland (commenced 1994) – and vaccination (New Zealand North Island) using gene-deleted 'marker' vaccines.

**IA.** A porcine herpesvirus-1 which is present in saliva and nasal discharges and may persist in pigs for life. It has an affinity for ganglion neurons in infected animals and is sensitive to heat, sodium hypochlorite, formaldehyde, lime and phenol.

**R.** Infected and carrier pigs.

**MT.** By inhalation or via skin abrasions through direct and indirect contact with infected pigs and contaminated materials such as feed, water, bedding, floors, etc. The virus infects the upper respiratory passages and travels along the cranial nerves to the brain. A viraemia results, with virus reaching all parts of the body.

**CF.** The main symptoms of Aujeszky's disease are fever, depression, anorexia and convulsions. Virulence of the virus, age of pig and route of exposure determine the mortality rate, which is highest in piglets. Other signs include muscular spasms, pruritus, blindness, vomiting, incoordination and loss of weight. Sneezing with nasal discharge and coughing are common symptoms in older pigs which also show head pressing, opisthotonos (head and tail bent upwards and abdomen downwards), constipation and prostration, coma and death.

Illness in young pigs may be as short as 24–48 h, while older pigs have a longer period of sickness and may even survive after 6 weeks.

Cattle, sheep, dogs and cats exhibit similar clinical signs, with pruritus and various nervous manifestations being prominent.

**P.** The primary lesions are in the brain, which shows congestion of the meninges and excess cerebrospinal fluid. There is rhinitis, pharyngitis, tonsilitis, tracheitis and oesophagitis with petechiation of lymph nodes and kidneys. On occasions small necrotic foci are present in the liver and spleen.

**D.** History, clinical signs and post-mortem lesions provide a tentative diagnosis.

Confirmation of diagnosis is based on the isolation of virus in culture, virus neutralisation, immunofluorescence, ELISA, complement fixation and indirect haemagglutination tests, etc.

*Differential diagnoses* include transmissible gastroenteritis, leptospirosis, influenza, viral encephalomyelitis (Teschen disease), encephalomyocarditis, *E. coli* septicaemia, swine erysipelas, Glasser's disease, hypoglycaemia in young pigs, etc.

**J.** Diseased pigs: Much depends on the severity and extent of the lesions and the condition of the carcase.

Carcase and viscera: T, A or Kh.

Parts of carcase and organs (brain, spinal cord): D if conditionally approved for human consumption with heat treatment (Kh).

## BLUE-EARED PIG DISEASE (PORCINE REPRODUCTIVE AND RESPIRATORY SYNDROME, PRRS)

**I.** A usually mild 'new' contagious disease affecting pigs of all ages in which influenza-like symptoms, abortions and stillbirths, and sometimes cyanosis of extremities are evident.

**O.** The disease first appeared in the USA, Canada and Europe in 1987, after which Germany (1990), Netherlands, Denmark, Spain, British Isles and Myanmar reported cases.

Since its introduction into England in 1991 the disease has assumed a much milder form and controls operating under the Blue-eared Pig Order 1991 were revoked in November 1992; the disease is no longer notifiable. All EC member states have taken similar action.

It is reported (1999) that some 240 of Northern Ireland's pig herds are infected by Blue-Ear disease. Testing showed 8% of 450 herds to be positive for PRRS raising fears that a high number may be infected which may warrant a test and slaughter programme. To date no reactors have been reported in the Republic of Ireland. In Denmark the US PRRS vaccine caused devastation, with abortions in about one-third of the initial 1000 herds vaccinated.

**IA.** A new virus, the *Lelystad agent*, named after its discovery at the Central Veterinary Laboratory, Lelystad, Netherlands. The ingestion of *fumonisin*, a mycotoxin, has been incriminated in the USA as a possible vehicle for the introduction of the virus.

**R.** Affected and carrier pigs and their secretions and stillbirths.

**MT.** Probably by inhalation and ingestion of contaminated materials (airborne spread of the disease was suspected in Germany).

**CF.** Symptoms vary from outbreak to outbreak; not all affected pigs show blue ears. Fever, inappetence, reduced growth rate, diarrhoea, abortions and stillbirths (generally occurring in late pregnancy), respiratory distress (dyspnoea, hyperpnoea) and cyanosis of extremities especially ears, teats, abdomen and vulva are among the signs demonstrated.

**P.** Pneumonia, which may be lobar or bronchial in type.

**D.** A definite diagnosis can only be made by serological tests.

*Differential diagnoses* include porcine encephalomyocarditis, swine fever, leptospirosis, Aujeszky's disease and all causes of abortion in sows.

**J.** Carcase and viscera: T or A, depending on extent of pathological changes and condition of carcase.

## BLUETONGUE

**I.** A non-contagious, insect-borne disease of sheep, and less commonly cattle, goats, camels and antelopes in which there is intense congestion of the buccal/nasal mucosa and coronary bands of the feet with severe lameness.

Notifiable disease (UK).

**O.** The disease appears to be confined to Africa, USA (where it is enzootic), Middle East, and parts of Asia. Many countries report serological evidence of infection but no clinical cases, e.g. in North and South America.

**IA.** An orbivirus of the family Reoviridae.

**R.** Affected and carrier sheep, cattle, goats, camels and wild ruminants.

**MT.** Transmission occurs by insect vectors, e.g. biting midges of the *Culicoides* spp. and mosquitoes.

**CF.** Sheep of all ages are susceptible except those from immune ewes. After an incubation period of 1–2 weeks during wet weather, affected animals develop fever, anorexia, depression and dyspnoea. The dental pad, buccal and nasal mucosae become inflamed and then ulcerated and there is a watery, afterwards bloody, discharge from the nose. The tongue is swollen and, less often, cyanosed while the lips are swollen and bleed easily. Oedema of the face, ears and submaxillary region sometimes occurs. Other signs include pneumonia, conjunctivitis, lameness and torticollis.

**P.** See **CF**. The superficial changes are accompanied by gelatinous oedema of the subcutaneous tissues with petechiation and sometimes degeneration of skeletal muscles.

**D.** Symptoms are suggestive of a tentative diagnosis. Confirmation requires isolation and identification of the virus (fluorescent antibody, serum neutralisation tests, etc.).

Bluetongue must be distinguished from foot-and-mouth disease, contagious pustular dermatitis, photosensitisation, vesicular stomatitis, malignant catarrhal fever, etc.

**J.** Carcase and viscera: T. Reactor animals: A.

## BOVINE MALIGNANT CATARRH (MALIGNANT CATARRHAL FEVER, MALIGNANT HEAD CATARRH, CATARRHAL FEVER, BMC)

**I.** An acute and peracute infectious, viral disease of cattle, deer, buffaloes and wild ruminants (and sometimes sheep and pigs) characterised by nasal and eye lesions, stomatitis, gastroenteritis and usually high mortality.

**O.** Worldwide, but occurring most often in Africa. In most countries, BMC has a low sporadic prevalence.

**IA.** Two distinct viruses – an alcelaphine herpesvirus (carried by species of the family Alcelaphinae of antelopes, mostly wildebeest and hartebeest) and a sheep-associated BMC virus, probably a herpesvirus. Although the latter infects sheep it does not cause clinical disease.

**R.** Infected and carrier cattle, wildebeest, hartebeest and other wild ruminants and sheep and their fomites (fomes) – inanimate objects and materials on which disease-producing organisms are conveyed such as bedding, faeces, etc.

**MF.** Probably by ingestion.

**CF.** *Peracute* (alimentary) form – high fever, hyperaesthesia (increased sensitivity to external stimuli), gastroenteritis, diarrhoea, dyspnoea and convulsions with rapid onset of death.

*Acute* (*head and eye*) *form*: This is the most common type and is accompanied by fever, anorexia, depression, mucopurulent nasal and eye discharges, conjunctivitis, oedema of eyelids, salivation, necrosis of skin of nostrils, teats, vulva and scrotum. Lymph nodes are usually enlarged and haemorrhagic. Nervous symptoms are usually present – incoordination, leg weakness, muscular tremors, head-pushing and paralysis. Death usually occurs in 1–7 days.

*Chronic form*: Mild fever with recovery in 7–10 days.

**P.** Virtually all organs in the body are affected. In addition to the lesions in **CF** above, the following changes may be found: inflammation extending to erosion of the buccal, nasal, pharyngeal, oesophageal, gastric and intestinal mucosa, blood-stained intestinal contents; enlarged liver showing degeneration changes; generalised lymphadenitis and petechial haemorrhages in the brain and meninges.

**D.** Accurate diagnosis is only possible using histopathology and virology – ELISA, indirect immunofluorescence and virus neutralisation tests.

*Differential diagnoses*: rinderpest, bluetongue, East Coast fever, infectious bovine rhinotracheitis, etc.

**J.**

Carcase and viscera: T, where general signs of fever, toxaemia, etc., exist.

Carcase: I and viscera: D, provided general changes absent.

## BOVINE PAPULAR STOMATITIS

**I.** A benign, contagious, viral condition of young cattle in which papules (small raised firm nodules 0.5–1 cm in diameter) appear on the buccal mucosa, muzzle and inside the nostrils.

**O.** The disease occurs in Europe, USA, Canada, New Zealand, Australia and Africa as a sporadic entity.

**IA.** Parapoxvirus.

**R.** The secretions, especially the saliva of infected and carrier animals.

**MT.** Via minute wounds and abrasions in the buccal and nasal mucosae.

**CF.** Frequently no general signs are evident but slight fever, anorexia, some weight loss and salivation may be present on occasion. The papules usually heal in a few days, although sometimes successive crops of papules may develop.

**P.** See **CF**. The papules are round and dark red in colour. Some may coalesce to form larger areas with a roughened surface.

**D.** The disease is only important because of its possible confusion with other forms of bovine stomatitis, e.g. foot-and-mouth disease, vesicular stomatitis, bovine erosive stomatitis (a zoonosis), etc.

The lesions suggest a diagnosis of papular stomatitis, which can be confirmed by a virus neutralisation test, electron microscopy and cell culture.

**J.** Carcase and viscera: A. Head and tongue: D.

## BOVINE SPONGIFORM ENCEPHALOPATHY (BSE, PRION DISEASE, 'MAD COW DISEASE')

**I.** A progressively fatal, non-inflammatory, nervous disease of cattle which is one of a group of transmissible spongiform encephalopathies (TSEs) occurring in animals – scrapie in sheep and goats (to which BSE is closely related), transmissible mink encephalopathy (TME), chronic wasting disease (CWD) of mule deer and Rocky Mountain elk and the human diseases of Creutzfeld–Jakob disease, Gerstmann–Straussler–Scheinker syndrome and Kuru.

Notifiable disease (UK). Zoonosis.

BSE is regarded by some as a distinct entity from scrapie, but may not be so.

To date (November 1998) spongiform encephalopathy has also been recorded in 19 captive wild animals in eight zoological collections in the British Isles – 6 greater kudu, 8 cheetah, 2 ocelot, 6 eland, 3 puma, 1 gemsbok, 1 nyala, 2 Arabian oryx and 1 scimitar-horned oryx, 1 tiger, 1 bison and 2 ankole cows.

TSE has been recorded in 85 domestic cats in Britain and the disease has been successfully transmitted experimentally to cattle, sheep, goats, pigs, mink, mice, marmosets and macaques.

A spongiform encephalopathy disease closely resembling BSE has been reported in three ostriches (*Struthio camelus*) in zoos in Germany. The first incident occurred in 1986 in a female weighing 150 kg, the others in a younger hen of 80 kg and a juvenile male weighing 60 kg. All birds showed symptoms of ataxia and incoordination. The birds were fed on an omnivorous diet which included meat from casualty slaughtered cattle. It was not determined, however, whether contaminated feed was the source of the infection. At this time Germany was officially free of scrapie and BSE. Spongiform degeneration of the medulla oblongata was evident. Since no material was available for examination for the presence of scrapie-associated fibrils or mouse-transmission studies, a diagnosis of BSE could not be established nor could the possibility of an environmental toxaemia or a dietary deficiency be ruled out.

All these diseases have common features – long incubation period (commonly 3–5 years in cattle), only adult animals showing clinical signs, long clinical course, transmissibility, similar neurological brain changes and probably a common feed source.

*Creutzfeld–Jakob disease* (subacute spongiform encephalopathy, CJD) affects adult human beings of either sex in mid-life and is characterised by progressive dementia and myoclonic seizures (rhythmic contractions of muscle groups), cerebellar ataxia, disorientation, hyperaesthesia, loss of speech and blindness. It occurs worldwide and the incidence is usually given as one in a million, but this probably represents an underdiagnosis. In addition to the sporadic form there is a familial form – 15% of CJD cases in Israelis of Libyan origin. Little is known about the method of transmission but human-to-human methods with deaths in all cases have occurred – via corneal grafts, contaminated brain electrodes and the use in children of growth hormone derived from human pituitary glands. The infectious agent (prion, slow virus), the histopathology and the abnormal fibrils appear to be similar to the scrapie and BSE findings. While CT (computer tomography), MRI (magnetic resonance imaging) and EEG assist in diagnosis, CJD, like scrapie and BSE, can only be confirmed at present by histopathology.

The *Gerstmann–Straussler–Scheinker syndrome* is a variant of CJD and is usually familial in origin. It is attended by varying symptoms including dementia, memory loss, intellectual decline and cerebellar ataxia. There is amyloid plaque deposition in the brain (which may to some extent differentiate it from BSE, scrapie and CJD) and has been diagnosed in a family with presenile dementia by prion protein gene analysis (Collinge *et al.*, 1990). The authors state that because of the underdiagnosis of CJD and GSS, previous epidemiological studies may have underestimated their prevalence, a fact which may be of significance in the possible transmission of BSE.

*Kuru* is a similar progressive neurological disorder which was once prevalent (up to the early 1960s) in the Fore natives of the New Guinea highlands. Affecting mainly women and children it was associated with ritual cannibalistic practices associated with the care of the dead, whose brains containing the infective agent were consumed. Affected persons showed cerebellar ataxia and helpless incapacity, with death usually within 1 year.

The custom of mortuary feasting, in which females and children ate the brain and other internal organs of a dead relative while the men would mainly eat meat, ended some 40 years ago. No one born after 1959 has contracted kuru disease, but odd cases of kuru still occur because of the very long incubation period.

**O.** BSE was first identified at the Central Veterinary Laboratory, Weybridge, England in November 1986 (Wilesmith *et al.*, 1988). However, it is possible that the disease was inapparent and endemic before this date and that this situation may also apply to countries other than Great Britain. The possibility exists that it may have been confused with other diseases such as listeriosis, acute metabolic diseases, lead poisoning, polioencephalomalacia, cerebro-spinal abscess, tremorogenic mycotoxins, etc.

The current worldwide distribution of reported cases of BSE is shown in Table 17.1.

The sixth case recorded in Germany was believed to have been imported from Switzerland. Germany has had no homebred cases of BSE to date.

**Table 17.1** Number of cases of BSE in the UK and other countries. June 1998.

| Country | Date of last report | Total cases |
|---|---|---|
| **UK** | | |
| Great Britain | Jan 1999 | 171 391 |
| Northern Ireland | Dec 1998 | 1783 |
| Guernsey | Jan 1999 | 677 |
| Isle of Man | Jan 1999 | 431 |
| Jersey | Dec 1998 | 141 |
| Alderney | June 1995 | 2 |
| **Other countries** | | |
| Republic of Ireland | Jan 1999 | 345 |
| Switzerland | Dec 1998 | 282 |
| Portugal | Jan 1999 | 195 |
| France | Jan 1999 | 50 |
| Germany | Jan 1999 | 6 |
| Belgium | Jan 1999 | 7 |
| Netherlands | Jan 1999 | 4 |
| Italy | Jan 1999 | 2 |
| Oman | Feb 1994 | 2 |
| Luxembourg | Jan 1999 | 1 |
| Denmark | Jan 1999 | 1 |
| Falklands | Feb 1994 | 1 |
| Canada | Feb 1994 | 1 |

Source: BSE Progress Report. Dec. 1998. MAFF.

It is likely that these cases arose from the consumption of infected animal feed and/or the importation of infected cattle from Britain. In view of the latter trade it is also probable that there has been serious underreporting of BSE cases in Europe.

It is known that France imported considerable amounts of meat and bone meal from Britain, some of which may have been re-exported. But the possibility exists that some of the BSE cases confirmed outside Britain may also have been due to the existence of endemic scrapie (or 'avirulent' endemic BSE).

The fact remains that the exact incidence of many diseases in animals and man is not known because of the existence of subclinical infection and the fact that relatively few histopathological examinations are performed. Brain lesions similar to those associated with scrapie have been encountered in sheep found dead without any premonitory symptoms (Clark, Dawson and Scott, 1994).

Since November 1986 the disease in Great Britain has developed into a major epizootic with 173 391 (N. Ireland 1783) cases occurring over 30 000 in Great Britain up to January 1999. 30.9% of herds with adult breeding cattle, 49.8% of dairy herds and 12.5% of beef suckler herds have experienced at least one case of BSE. Of the total 30 000 herds, 39% have had only one confirmed case while 75% have had four or fewer.

Out of an adult cattle population of some 4.5 million in Great Britain the current annual incidence is 7.5 cases per 1000. Up until 7 February 1977, 31 497 cases (N. Ireland 182) were confirmed in animals born after the ruminant feed ban (July 1988). Most of these animals were born immediately after the feed ban was introduced and were fed feedingstuff containing ruminant protein already in the feed chain and being used up despite the ban. The very long incubation period means that further cases will be confirmed in such animals. However, it is fully expected that cases will reduce significantly and eventually cease from this common-source epidemic.

BSE has been of great economic importance, especially in the British Isles, because of the high cost of detection, control measures and compensation involved. This does not apply, however, to individual herds where the in-herd incidence is low. The occurrence of BSE has been accompanied by extensive, and often misguided, media involvement in Britain, with consumer concern about the safety of beef for human food. The fact that little is known about the pathogenesis of the disease (on which comprehensive research is currently being conducted) has fuelled these fears.

Since all the evidence pointed to the fact that BSE was caused by the ingestion of feedingstuff containing infected protein, a ban on the use of ruminant-derived protein in ruminant feedingstuffs was introduced by the Ministry of Agriculture, Fisheries and Food in July 1988. The feed ban refers to The Bovine Offal (Prohibition) Regulations 1989 which prohibit the use of 'specified bovine offal' (brain, spinal cord, thymus, tonsils, spleen and intestine (from duodenum to rectum) in ruminant feedingstuffs. These specified bovine offals (SBO) now termed specified risk material (SRM) were also banned in human food in 1989 (1990 in Scotland).

The feed ban, as predicted, has markedly reduced the number of suspected cases now being reported, these being significantly less than in the years 1991–1996. Between 1 January 1996 and 26 June 1997 the number of reported cases was 22% below that for the same period in 1997 and 65% lower than the same period in 1996. In addition, fewer young animals are being affected.

It is confidently expected that, while some cases of BSE will be confirmed in cattle exposed to infected feed and born shortly after the feed ban because of the prolonged incubation period, the overall number of cases will continue to drop and eventually cease to occur. At least the feed ban has prevented some 50 000 cases which would otherwise have occurred.

**IA.** The exact nature of the causal agent is not yet known. It has been variously described as a *'slow virus'*, a *prion* (a minute infectious pathogen which contains a form of protein resistant to procedures that hydrolyse nucleic acids), a *virin* (a tiny microorganism devoid of nucleic acid and associated with cellular protein) and a *filamentous virus.* That it is infectious in nature there is no doubt since both crude and purified extracts from the brain and other tissues of infected cattle can reproduce the disease in a wide range of animals (see above).

Although infectious in form, it does not produce any immune response in the animal, which makes the development of a suitable diagnostic test difficult.

The infective agent is an extremely resistant entity having the ability to endure extreme physical and chemical conditions. Some strains of the agent (more than 15 have been identified) can resist boiling while others retain some infectivity after heating for 1 h at 121°C or at 240°C for 1 min. High-temperature autoclaving is necessary to totally destroy it. The processes normally used to inactivate infectious agents have little effect on it, e.g. detergents and disinfectants at normal concentrations, organic solvents, concentrated salt solution and UV and ionising radiation.

Rapid freezing and exposure to ether and 20% formalin do not inactivate the scrapie agent.

The BSE infective agents can be detected in the brain, spinal cord, retina, tonsils, spleen and intestines but not in muscle and milk. In all the transmissible spongiform encephalopathies (TSEs) these agents are abnormal, distorted prions (PrP), which are minute glycosylated protein molecules devoid of nucleic acid. They are also protease-resistant, i.e. they are not broken down into amino acids during digestion. Different species of animals have brain cell prion proteins of different compositions.

Distorted prions in the brain are able to deform normal prions. Over a long period of time the resultant process of spongiosis, gliosis and neuronal death is due, it is believed, to the depletion of normal brain prions rather than the deposition of distorted prions.

It has been suggested that organophosphorus compounds used for killing migrating warble larvae have caused BSE by altering the prion protein to become an infectious agent. This concept, however, by an individual organic farmer in Somerset, England, has been dismissed by most experts. However, studies on the possible connection are being carried out at the Institute of Psychiatry in London.

The concept that BSE is an autoimmune disease and not an infection – put forward by Ebringer and colleagues in London – is also dismissed because of the non-infectivity of these conditions.

For decontamination purposes it has been recommended that high concentrations of sodium hypochlorite, and possibly molar sodium hydroxide, are the most effective chemicals against the unconventional transmissible agents of BSE and scrapie (Taylor, 1989).

**R.** The SRMs (especially brain and spinal cord) of infected and carrier animals.

**MT.** All the evidence suggests that BSE was acquired through the ingestion of feedingstuff containing the infective agent, making it an extended common-source epidemic.

Changes in the rendering process of inedible meat and offal were made in the late 1970s and early 1980s, presumably for economic reasons. The hydrocarbon fat solvent extraction process was abandoned and lower rendering temperatures were adopted, resulting in the scrapie agent (or an existing agent of BSE) not being destroyed in the meat and bone meal. Some of this material was exported to Europe and Ireland where it was probably responsible for further cases.

The situation was also accompanied by a huge increase in the sheep population in which the subclinical incidence of scrapie is much greater than realised, the long incubation period revealing only a relatively few clinical cases.

Unlike scrapie, which appears to run in families, BSE does not appear to be simply inherited. But the possibility exists that the susceptibility of individual animals to BSE is inherited. (Wijeratne and Curnow, 1990).

It is known that the agents of BSE can also be transmitted via the conjunctiva, broken skin and nasal mucosa. *Extreme care is therefore necessary in handling all suspect animals, carcases and tissues.*

**CF.** Symptoms vary greatly in type and severity. They are insidious in onset, become progressively pronounced over a period of 1–6 months or so.

Since the disease is essentially a CNS involvement, the clinical signs are associated with disturbances in behaviour and posture and may vary from day to day. The most commonly reported signs are apprehension, hyperaesthesia and locomotor ataxia. Although appetite is usually retained, there is progressive loss of condition and milk yield.

Some animals are reluctant to move while others display changes of gait with a characteristic high-stepping action of the forelegs accompanied by hindquarter incoordination, swaying gait and difficulty in turning.

Many animals exhibit aggression – to other cattle and to human beings – by butting activity. Some resent handling by drawing the head away and kicking violently. Increased noise tends to produce exaggerated reactions with startled looks, ear twitching and muscle tremors.

While aggression is a common sign, some cows may tend to avoid other cattle. There may be excessive licking of the coat with rubbing and scratching, but pruritus, which is common in scrapie, is not a feature. Nose licking and hip movements in response to stroking are sometimes observed.

Animals in later stages of BSE show increased weakness and loss of weight with stumbling, falling and inability to rise. Affected animals are normally slaughtered under the government eradication scheme before death ensues.

**P.** Lesions are confined to the central nervous systems. Apart from loss of condition there are no gross pathological changes.

The major changes are in the brainstem (pons, medulla oblongata and midbrain) which connects the cerebral hemispheres to the spinal cord. These take the form of microscopical degenerative changes in the grey matter with discrete round or oval vacuoles or microcavities and BSE-associated fibrils (SAFs) and accumulation of prion protein (PrP). (Plate l, Fig. 3.) (See also Infective Agent.)

Statutory diagnosis in Great Britain is achieved by examination of the brainstem obtained through the foramen magnum, which obviates the need for total brain extraction.

**D.** The clinical signs, especially their progressive nature and whether they display certain characteristic locomotor disturbances, may be of value in making a tentative diagnosis of BSE. But hypomagnesaemia and nervous ketosis (usually of short duration and confirmed by clinical chemistry), listeriosis, lead poisoning, sporadic encephalomyelitis, rabies, downer cow syndrome, cerebrospinal abscess, etc., have to be borne in mind.

Positive diagnosis can only be made by detailed histopathology.

**J.** Carcase and viscera: T.

All suspect BSE cases must be treated in accordance with government regulations.

(It has been recommended as an additional public health precaution that mechanically-recovered meat should not be used for human consumption.)

### New variant-CJD (nvCJD)

Although there had been no scientific evidence linking BSE and CJD in man, the occurrence of 14 clinical cases of variant-CJD during 1994–96 prompted a reassessment of the situation. These cases exhibited unusual features – younger average age and different clinical symptoms, EEG brain activity and pathology (Collinge *et al.*, 1996a).

The Spongiform Encephalopathy Advisory Committee (SEAC) in March 1996 conjectured that 'on current data and in the absence of any credible alternative the most likely explanation at present is that these cases are linked to exposure to BSE before the introduction of the SBO ban in 1989'. The CJD Surveillance Unit (CJDSU) also reported in a similar fashion. Since these reports were issued, 35 cases have been confirmed in the UK (December 1998).

More recent work by Collinge and his team (Collinge *et al.*, 1996b), has shown that the physicochemical 'signature' or marker of prions in patients dying of nvCJD, after transmission to mice, matches that of prions in BSE, in cats with naturally transmitted BSE and in mice and macaque monkeys experimentally-infected with BSE but not with prions in humans with acquired or sporadic CJD. This work, besides providing a rapid result, also holds out the prospect of an ante-mortem test for CJD and nvCJD and possibly BSE.

According to experts at the London School of Hygiene and Tropical Medicine and the National CJD Surveillance Unit in Edinburgh, there remains the potential for a UK epidemic of nvCJD even though the link between BSE and nvCJD has yet to be proved. If BSE is linked to CJD, the best-case scenario was assessed at 75 cases, assuming a 100% effective SBM ban and a mean incubation period of 10 years. The worst-case scenario was estimated to be 80 000 cases of CJD if the specified bovine material ban was only 90% effective and the incubation period is 25 years. If the incubation period is longer, there could even be more cases.

*Control measures*

Control measures have been directed towards the protection of both animal and human health.

1 The elimination of the causal agent by banning the feeding of ruminant-derived protein to ruminants.
2 The slaughter and proper disposal of all clinical cases of BSE.
3 The specified risk material ban, which removes all tissues containing the causal agent in animals incubating the disease.

*Specified risk material* refers to the head (including the brain but excluding the tongue), spinal cord, spleen, thymus, tonsils and intestines of a bovine animal 6 months or over which has died or been slaughtered in the United Kingdom. For animals less than 6 months of age SBM includes the thymus and intestines only where an animal less than 2 months of age has been slaughtered for human consumption in the UK or, if over 2 months old, where it has died or been slaughtered, in the UK.

The SBM (No. 3) Order 1996 required specified solid waste recovered from any part of the drainage system in slaughterhouses handling bovines or other premises processing bovine carcases where SBM is handled, to be disposed of as SBM.

**BSE checks** In Great Britain these are carried out on the slaughter and disposal of animals, rendering plants, storage and transport of SBM, etc., mainly by the State Veterinary Service and the Meat Hygiene Service. The Environment Agency, Health and Safety Executive, local authority EHOs and trading standards officers are also involved.

## Bovine offals (prohibition) regulations 1989

In addition to the controls listed above, these Regulations also stipulated that whatever the source of SBO (meat plants or farms), the methods of identification, control and ultimate disposal remained the same.

Once removed from the slaughtered animal after dressing, the SBO must either be sterilised, thoroughly denatured or stained with a specified dyestuff and subsequently removed, under permit from a local authority, to rendering plants, collection centres (for onward transfer to a rendering plant) on excepted premises such as a hospital, medical or veterinary school (where SBO may only be used for instructional, research or diagnostic purposes).

Handling at rendering plants is designed to ensure that SBO is kept separate at all times from other material that is intended to be used, after processing, for use in feedstuffs for non-ruminant animals. After rendering, the meal derived from SBO remains under official control and may only be moved from the site of production under authority of a movement permit to a specified destination – burial in a licensed landfill site or incineration.

The SRM Order 1997 and the SRM Regs. 1997 supplement the above controls which are now EU-wide.

## Precautions to be taken by persons handling known or suspected cases of BSE

Although the Southwood report stated that BSE was unlikely to affect man, the UK Ministry of Agriculture in January 1990 issued *Guidelines for Veterinary Surgeons handling known or suspected cases of BSE*, much of which also applies to abattoir personnel.

### *1. Initial examination of suspect cases*

Extra care must always be taken when handling a BSE suspect. Isolate the animal away from noise. Avoid handling in places where an excited cow could trap anyone. Handle firmly but quietly. Arrange for the animal to be restrained safely, preferably in a crush. When examining the oral cavity, wear plastic or latex gloves and carefully wash off any traces of saliva from protective clothing. Dispose of gloves by incineration. Beware when examining the udder – BSE cases can kick out violently and repeatedly. Examination of the head may be resented. Notify the Divisional Veterinary Officer immediately BSE is suspected. Note that milk from a BSE suspect placed under restriction by the Ministry may only be fed to its own calf.

### *2. Venepuncture*

When blood samples have to be taken for differential diagnosis, use vacutainers rather than syringes and dispose of needles carefully into an appropriate safe container. Apply rigorous standards of hygiene to the handling of all samples. Blood splashes should be thoroughly removed.

### *3. Calvings, cleansings and caesarian sections*

If it behaves like scrapie, the BSE agent may be present in the placenta and/or fetal fluids of affected cows. Washable protective clothing and armlength gloves should be worn when calving a BSE suspect, either naturally or by caesarian section, or if cleansing is needed. If available, a face mask should also be used. Placentae should be disposed of with the minimum of handling and disposal should preferably be by incineration, but careful burial is an acceptable alternative. This is, in fact, a condition of the Restrictive Notice (Form A) served on BSE suspects by the Divisional Veterinary Officer.

### *4. Post-mortem examinations*

Note that post-mortem examinations of suspects are not normally permitted. Where

## CHRONOLOGY OF BSE

**1732.** First record of scrapie in sheep.

**Late 1970/early 1980.** Changes made in rendering techniques.

**Apr. 1985.** First suspect cases of BSE.

**Nov. 1986.** BSE identified as a new disease entity.

**Apr. 1988.** Southwood Committee appointed.

**June 1988.** BSE made a notifiable disease in England, Scotland and Wales.

**July 1988.** Government ban on the feeding of ruminant-derived to ruminants.

**Aug. 1988.** Compulsory slaughter for BSE-suspect animals with 50% compensation.

**Dec. 1988.** Government bans use of milk from BSE suspects other than for feeding to cow's own calf. Duration of ruminant feed ban extended.

**Jan. 1989.** First BSE case reported in Ireland.

**Feb. 1989.** Southwood report published – risk of transmission to man 'remote and theoretical'. Tyrrell Committee set up to establish R&D requirements.

**Nov. 1989.** Ban on use of 'specified offals' – brain, spinal cord, spleen, thymus, tonsils and intestines (SBOs) – in human food (England, Wales). Original regulation referred to bovines over 6 months of age; later extended to include thymus and intestines of younger cattle. Case numbers exceed 9000 (200 weekly in GB; 50% in SW England). 32 cases in N. Ireland and 15 in Republic of Ireland.

**Jan. 1990.** Tyrrell Report published. Government to spend £12 million on BSE research in next 3 years. SBO ban for human food (Scotland).

**Feb. 1990.** Compensation increased to 100% for suspect animals.

**Sept. 1990.** Ban on use of SBO in any animal and bird feed with export of such feed to Third Countries stopped by rendering industry.

**Oct. 1990.** Introduction of improved cattle records so that offspring of confirmed cases can be identified.

**July 1991.** Ban on export of SBO feed to Third Countries.

**Nov. 1991.** Ban on use of SBO meat and bone meal for fertilisers.

**Mar. 1992.** Bovine Offal Prohibition (Amendment) Regs 1992 prohibited use of the head after the skull is opened and removal of the brain except in an area free from any food intended for human consumption.
Tyrrell Committee satisfied with current control measures.

**May 1992.** EC Commission decision prohibits Community trade in bovine embryos derived from BSE confirmed or suspect dams or those born after 18.7.88.

**July 1993.** 100 000th confirmed case of BSE in Great Britain announced.

**June 1994.** Commission Decision 94/381 prohibited feeding of mammalian protein in Community other than in Denmark. EC Decision 94/382 approved alternative heat treatment for processing animal waste.

**July 1994.** Commission Decision 94/474 required bone-in beef for export to be derived from cattle certified not to have been on holdings where BSE was confirmed in the previous 6 years.

**Nov. 1994.** Bovine Offal (Prohibition) (AM) Regs 1994 extended ban on use of some SBO in human food to calves under 6 months of age slaughtered for human consumption.

Spongiform Encephalopathy (Misc. AM) Order 1994 extended ban on use of SBOs in animal feed, banned use of mammalian protein in ruminant feedingstuffs and made notifiable laboratory suspicion of TSEs in species other than cattle, sheep and goats.

**Dec. 1994.** Beef from cattle born after 1 January 1992 excluded from certification requirement.

**Mar. 1995.** Restriction lifted on use of milk, gelatin, amino acids, dicalcium phosphate, dried plasma and other blood products from mammalian tissues in feedingstuffs for ruminants.

Portugal reported first case of BSE in 1995 – in a 6-year old cow born in Portugal. Mode of infection unknown. Portugal had 6 cases in 1994.

**Apr. 1995.** The Meat Hygiene Service (MHS) was established in Great Britain (1.4.95) taking over responsibility from local authorities for hygiene, inspection and welfare requirements in licensed meat premises in Britain.

**May 1995.** The number of reported cases of BSE in Great Britain was 45.3% lower than in the same period in 1994 and 56.2% lower compared with 1993. There was a continued downturn in the incidence of BSE in 5-year old and younger animals.

The numbers of confirmed BSE cases born after the introduction of the ruminant feed ban on 18 July 1998, by year of birth, were 9983 (1988), 7858 (1989), 1589 (1990), 116 (1991) and 1 (1992).

**July 1995.** Commission Decision 95/287 repealed earlier Decisions regarding certification – animals less than 2½ years old at slaughter now exempted. A 100% check on age declarations and holding freedom from BSE was demanded along with removal of lymph nodes from boneless beef during cutting.

Export certification requirement introduced – beef from cattle less than 2½ years old at slaughter now exempted.

**Aug. 1995.** Specified Bovine Offal Order 1995 made tighter; controls on record keeping and dedicated lines for rendering plants processing SBO; prohibited removal of brains and eyes – whole skull to be disposed of as SBO; prohibited removal of spinal cord except in slaughterhouses.

(Up to 1 July 1998, 36 657 cases of BSE had been confirmed in Great Britain after the feed ban, suggesting 'some continued leakage of infective material into animal feed'. 'Some fine tuning of controls and processing plants was needed to prevent potentially infected material finding its way into cattle feed'.)

**Oct. 1995.** Fourth case of variant CJD reported in under 3 years; renewed speculation over the possible transmission of BSE to man. Investigations by CJDSU in Edinburgh showed that the incidence of CJD in Britain was not significantly different from other European countries where there is no reported BSE. The CJD Unit failed to find any increased incidence in veterinary surgeons or abattoir workers.

**Dec. 1995.** GB Government Chief Medical Officer, Sir Kenneth Calman, stated that there was no scientific evidence that BSE could be transmitted to humans or that eating beef caused CJD. 'All the studies to date on transmission have shown that beef is safe. There is no epidemiological evidence of transmission from beef to humans or of transmission when muscle (meat) from cattle clinically affected with BSE is injected into mice.'

Scientists investigating possible links between BSE and beef sold to consumers said there could be a 'species barrier' which prevents humans developing BSE. Professor J. Collinge said he was reassured by the findings of experiments in genetically engineered mice which indicated that the disease did not react with a protein which triggers CJD. The research, however, was not yet finalised and would continue for another 6 months.

SBO (AM) Order 1995 prohibited use of bovine vertebral column in manufacture of mechanically recovered meat (MRM) and some other products for human consumption and the use of bovine MRM from vertebral column in food for humans. All plants producing bovine (MRM) to be registered. Export of bovine MRM derived from vertebral column prohibited to other EC Member States and to Third Countries for human consumption.

**Jan. 1996.** Eire: All cattle taken from herds in which a BSE animal was found to undergo post-mortem histopathology before being allowed into the human food chain. Policy in Eire was to destroy the whole herd if a BSE animal was detected.

German Parliament decided to ban all imports of UK beef but this action was branded illegal by Britain and the European Commission, which gave the German government one month to end the ban on British beef.

**Mar. 1996.** British Secretary of State for Health, Mr Stephen Dorrell, announced that a new form of CJD had been identified in 10 people who had recently died of the disease. The SEAC advised that, although there was no direct evidence of a link with BSE, in the absence of any credible alternative, the most likely explanation was that the cases were linked to exposure to BSE before the introduction of the SBO ban in 1989.

British government set out proposals for the selective culling of cattle in order to accelerate the decline in the number of BSE cases and to meet the conditions for a phased lifting of the EU ban on the export of cattle, beef and beef products agreed by European heads of government at the recent summit in Florence. The scheme would be targeted on animals likely to have had access to the same feed as confirmed BSE cases. The scheme was declared unscientific and unjustified by the British Veterinary Association, scientists and farmers.

Commission Decision 96/239 prohibited export from the UK of live bovines, semen and embryos, meat and products from bovine animals slaughtered in the UK, materials for use in medicinal, cosmetic and pharmaceutical products and meat and bone meal (MBM).

The Beef (Emergency Control) Order 1996 prohibited sale for human consumption of meat from bovines showing more than 2 permanent incisors.

The BSE (Amendment) Order 1996 prohibited sale or supply of mammalian MBM or any feedingstuff containing mammalian MBM for feeding to farm animals, horses and farmed fish.

Specified Bovine Material Order 1996 replaced SBO Order 1995 and required the whole head of all cattle over 6 months, except uncontaminated tongues, to be treated in the same way as 'SBO'.

**Apr. 1996.** Scheme for compulsory deboning replaced by scheme to slaughter all animals over the age of 30 months.

Use of Cattle Identification Documents approved.

Derestriction of meat derived from animals slaughtered in certain Third Countries where no cases of BSE were recorded.

Use of MBM as, or in, fertiliser for use on agricultural land prohibited.

Fresh Meat (Hygiene and Inspection) (AM) Regs 1996 allowed slaughterhouses to slaughter all cattle over 30 months and calves under 10 days of age with strict separation of meat.

**May 1996.** SBM (No. 2) Order required SBM to be removed from carcases and handled separately, as for animals under 30 months. The carcase meat must be dyed a different colour from SBM.

Cold storage of carcases and rendered material before incineration would mean slaughtering capacity would rise to 30 000 a week in Great Britain.

The Dutch government planned to destroy 64 000 young cattle although no cases of BSE had been reported in Holland even in animals imported from Britain. The action was described in veterinary circles as 'emotional and political'.

**June 1996.** Concern was expressed that some stocks of MBM were still held on farms and feed mills which could be incorporated into animal feed. The amount eventually transpired to be 10 500 tonnes, with 9500 tonnes at feed mills. This material was collected to be safely disposed of along with effective cleansing of premises. It is now an offence to have MBM or animal feed containing MBM on farms, feed mills and feed merchants' premises.

**July 1996.** Commission Decision 96/449/EC approved alternative heat treatment systems for processing animal waste in order to inactivate the infective agent.

**Aug. 1996.** Preliminary results of a 7-year MAFF experiment on the possible maternal transmission of BSE indicated that the disease could pass from dam to calf but at a low level. The SEAC concluded that the rate under field conditions would be 1%. The actual route of transmission was not determined.

UK Government launched its *Beef Assurance Scheme* for specialist grass-reared beef herds (established for 4 years) which have not been affected by BSE or been in contact with MBM. Animals born in registered herds would be permitted under strict conditions to be sold for slaughter for human consumption up to the age of 42 months. A report 'Transmission dynamics and epidemiology of BSE in British cattle' by Professor R.M. Anderson and colleagues in Oxford concluded that the BSE epidemic was 'well past its peak', in 'rapid decline' and 'likely to fade close to extinction by the year 2001 even in the absence of a targeted cull'.

Trading Standards Officers discovered evidence of adulteration of lamb mince with beef in Manchester. Some 62% of minced lamb and pork samples contained beef, some more than 20% beef. The discovery, conducted in 50 stores, followed similar checks in west London where 6 out of 10 packets of lamb mince tested contained more than 2% beef. Two samples from a supermarket chain had a beef content of 10%. Accidental contamination of mincing machines due to inadequate cleaning was discounted by officials because of the high levels.

**Sept. 1996.** An official cover-up of the BSE situation in Europe by the European Commission was reported with the start of an enquiry by the European Parliament into the handling of the 1996 beef panic. The UK Government submitted a proposal to the EU for a *Certified Herds Scheme* which would certify animals under 30 months of age from herds free from BSE as suitable for export. The scheme would be of special benefit to Northern Ireland, which has a low incidence of BSE and an efficient cattle traceability system.

*Mechanically-recovered meat (MRM).* Use of MRM is banned in minced meat but may be used for human consumption from the bones of cattle, sheep, pigs and poultry, except the backbone of cattle. The production of MRM is controlled by the Food Safety (General Food Hygiene) Regs 1995 which require the registration and inspection of premises, analysis of any potential food safety hazards and assessment of methods used by producers.

Heads of Sheep and Goats Order 1996 came into effect and banned the sale for human consumption of sheep and goats heads (excluding the tongue) except from animals born, reared and slaughtered in Australia or New Zealand.

**Oct. 1996.** A report in *Nature* by Professor J. Collinge and colleagues at the Imperial College School of Medicine showed a link of BSE with the new variant CJD (nvCJD). A molecular marker which distinguished nvCJD from other forms of the disease and which is also found in BSE cases and in BSE experimentally transmitted to other species. The results are believed to be 'consistent with the hypothesis that nvCJD results from transmission to humans'. They also suggested that the work identifying the molecular marker could be used in the differential diagnosis of nvCJD and may allow strain typing in various animals to determine if BSE has also been transmitted naturally to these species.

**Nov. 1996.** Scientific Meeting at Wellcome Trust Centre for the Epidemiology of Infectious Diseases, University of Oxford: BSE reported to be virtually eliminated from younger British cattle and epidemic estimated to be over by mid-1988. Individual ages of cattle over 30 months that were slaughtered had not been recorded, making attainment of Florence Agreement in June 1996 uncertain. The incidence of scrapie should be determined and the EU advised to eradicate the disease as a long-term objective. Strains of sheep resistant to scrapie can be bred. Studies being conducted to determine if BSE can be transferred back into sheep.

The need for a diagnostic test in subclinical cases was stressed. The CJDSU in Edinburgh predicted that hundreds of Britons would die each year from the new variant CJD (linked to BSE) with the peak occurring in about 7 years' time.

A new brain disease in cattle – idiopathic brainstem neuronal chromatolysis (IBNC) – has to date killed over 100 cattle. First discovered in 1989, three years after BSE was first reported, it has mainly affected beef cattle in Scotland aged between 6 and 12 years of age.

A 50.7 m ecu research programme into the TSEs was launched by the European Commission.

Switzerland decided to subsidise the slaughter of 230 000 cows born after 1 December 1990 to restore the confidence of consumers.

**Dec. 1996.** UK Government announced the slaughter of up to 128,000 more cattle deemed most at risk from BSE to conform to the Florence Agreement and asked to have the EU ban on British beef and beef products lifted. The European Union farm ministers, however, said it could be a long time before the ban was lifted.

The US Government proposed a wide-ranging ban on the use of tissues from cattle, sheep and goats in animal feed as a precaution against an outbreak of BSE. The continued use of blood, milk and gelatin would be permitted. If approved, the ban would codify a voluntary ban already being observed by the US meat industry.

Norway announced details of an intensive research programme on the pathology and epidemiology of scrapie and its implications for human health.

**Jan. 1997.** Hill *et al.* (1997) studied PrP in human tonsillar tissue obtained at necropsy and were able to confirm nvCJD by Western blot analysis, the findings being the same as those from the brain of the same patient (a 35-year-old woman). This work may well pave the way for the early clinical diagnosis of CJD, nvCJD, scrapie and BSE using tonsillar tissue obtained under local anaesthesia.

A Rhode Island hen which has been showing unusual nervous symptoms on a farm on the Surrey–Kent border in England where six cows developed BSE is to be humanely destroyed and its brain examined for evidence of BSE by Dr Harash Narang. Although tests carried out by the UK Ministry of Agriculture in 1990 showed no evidence of poultry susceptibility to BSE, a spongiform encephalopathy has been recorded in ostriches in Germany (see above).

The Republic of Ireland recorded 74 cases of BSE in 1996 compared with 16 in 1995. In 1997, 11 new cases have been confirmed. This marked increase in incidence has caused concern about exports and has prompted an investigation by EU officials.

In Germany 15 000 cattle, including 2052 imported from Britain and 3074 from Switzerland were to be slaughtered following the occurrence of a case of BSE in a cow born in Germany. Four previous cases were associated with imported animals.

In 1997 (up to 11 February) there were 858 cases of BSE (1 in Germany; 1 in France; 3 in Portugal; 14 in Ireland and 839 in the UK).

The 20th Commission Directive 97/1/EC banned the sale of cosmetic products containing material derived from the brains, spinal cords and eyes of cows, sheep and goats giving legal effect to the situation already existing in the cosmetics industry. The ban is provisional and will be reviewed in the light of new knowledge.

The draft of the European Parliament's Inquiry Committee into BSE was published and revealed numerous misdemeanours and failures in the handling of the BSE crisis by both the European Commission and the British Government.

*EC revised proposal on Specified Risk Materials (SRM)* In order to achieve a common level of basic controls on SRM throughout the Community the following SRM would be banned from human and animal food: (1) The *head* (including the *brain* and *eyes* but excluding the tongue) and *spinal cord* of cattle over 12 months of age and sheep and goats over 12 months of age or which have a permanent incisor tooth erupted from the gum; (2) the *spleen* of all sheep and goats; (3) vertebral column from cattle, sheep and goats banned from use in MRM. Strict controls (similar to those in place for disposal of SBM in the UK to be applied to the disposal of SRM; and equivalent SRM controls to apply to imports from third countries.

This Proposal differs from existing British controls in cattle in terms of tissues covered and the age of the animal but goes beyond them for sheep and goats in including the spinal cord and spleen.

In Germany 15 000 cattle (imports from Britain and Switzerland) are to be slaughtered following the occurrence of a case of BSE in a Galloway calf born to a cow imported from Scotland.

It has been suggested that organophosphorus compounds used for killing migrating warble larvae have caused BSE by altering the prion protein to become an infectious agent (see text).

**Feb. 1997.** Two proteins belonging to the group 14-3-3 have been detected in the cerebrospinal fluid (CSF) of CJD patients which are absent from normal individuals and those suffering from other dementing diseases (Harrington *et al.*, 1996). These proteins are thought to originate from pathological neuronal tissue.

The first case of BSE in a cow in Holland is recorded. All close relatives of the animal along with 110 cows are slaughtered.

Lamb and pork mince sold by UK supermarkets and butchers is shown to contain as much as 30% beef on occasions. Some of these samples had been labelled 'beef free'.

**Mar. 1997.** The European Union Scientific Veterinary Committee confirmed that British milk is safe to drink, a finding endorsed by the World Health Organization which concluded that there is no evidence that BSE can be passed on through milk.

Poland confirmed the existence of 51 cases of BSE – 29 of them in 1996. Main source of infection is thought to be MBM imported from the UK during 1988–89. (MBM from the UK was exported widely in EU and non-EU countries.)

Total number of BSE cases in the UK in 1996 was 6871, a reduction of 53% from 14 471 in 1995. A total of 1.18 million cattle have been slaughtered under the UK's over 30-month scheme by January 1997.

British government submits proposal for a Certified Cattle Herds Scheme to EU in attempt to get ban on beef exports lifted for herds which had no association with BSE, all preconditions for a phased lifting of the ban having been met. These include a selective slaughter of cattle most likely to have been exposed to contaminated feed; the introduction of a passport system to record movements; removal of all MBM from farms and feedmills; implementation of a scheme for the slaughter and disposal of cattle over 30 months of age; tightening of controls in abattoirs to ensure complete removal of SBM.

Examination of brain sections from an 11-year old Labrador dog in Oslo, Norway, which showed symptoms of incoordination and seizure, revealed changes in common with SE. Confirmation is sought from the Institute of Animal Health Neuropathogenesis Unit in Edinburgh. In Norway SBM was removed from the animal food chain in 1990. This investigation recalls tests in the UK in 1991 on the brains of 400 hounds, which showed some fibril abnormalities but which were inconclusive owing to spoilage changes in the brain tissues.

European Parliament adopted a report from its Committee of Enquiry into BSE criticising Britain's handling of the BSE crisis and accused the EU of giving priority to the beef market rather than human health. Many final recommendations also made.

SBM Order 1997 revokes and replaces SBM (No. 3) Order 1996 as follows. SBM tallow and derivatives must not be used in cosmetic, medical and pharmaceutical products or in feed. Their use in technical products may be permitted subject to plant approval and end-use of product guaranteed.

More stringent staining provisions are laid down – stains to remain visible over whole surface of SBM until either incinerated or rendered.

Enforcement is given stronger legal base.

*The role of water companies* providing sewerage services for domestic, industrial and commercial customers: SEAC recommends that appropriate containment and control measures are introduced for discharges from premises handling SBM. WSCs and MAFF to work closely together to ensure implementation of recommendations and operational practices.

*Tallow production*: The Bovine Products (Production and Dispatch) Regulations 1997 require all UK tallow for food, feed, pharmaceutical, medical and cosmetic use to be manufactured to export standards in registered premises, bovine vertebral column to be supplied to registered renderers separate from other raw materials and manufacturers using UK-manufactured tallow for above uses to use only tallow produced in a registered plant.

Scientists at the Institute of Grassland Research, Aberystwyth, Wales report that a urine test for the early diagnosis of BSE may be available within 18 months.

A drug, IDX, has been developed at the Instituto Nazionale Neurologico Carla Besta, Milan, which prevents the development of amyloid and prion protein deposits in Alzheimer's disease, Creutzfeld–Jacob disease and BSE. Too toxic as yet for clinical use in patients, IDX is being regarded as a prototype for the development of safer alternatives.

The current lack of knowledge of many aspects of BSE is exemplified by a second call from the EU Commission for BSE research funding, the priorities being possible transfer to man, transmission mechanisms of prion diseases and the prevention and treatment of TSEs.

**Apr. 1997.** European Commission reports that many Member States have not taken adequate steps to detect BSE or to prevent its further spread. The number of expected cases of BSE in continental Europe is estimated at several thousand, yet only a few hundred have been officially reported. Deficiencies in Europe include poor surveillance systems; farmers not always compensated in full for declaring cases acting as a disincentive; feed labelled as MBM-free often found to contain as much as 5% owing probably to cross-contamination in feed mills; rendering plants not converting to batch-processing at 130°C and 3 bars pressure for at least 20 min.

EU calls for laboratory examination of all suspect BSE cases, complete record keeping, better training and a reference laboratory to ensure uniform application of standardised procedures.

New EU heat treatment rules for SBM are 130°C at 3 bar pressure for at least 20 min, based on scientific research on the survival of the BSE agent in mice carried out in mid-1990s.

Case for the early lifting of the ban on the export of beef in Northern Ireland is made by a Committee of MPs in London because of its lower incidence compared with the rest of the UK.

EU informs Britain that it must meet conditions (set in June 1996) for ensuring freedom of gelatin from BSE if export trade of gelatin is to be restored.

Latest case (fifteenth in 1997) of BSE in Switzerland believed to be result of maternal transmission since infected dam was born after the ban on feed containing SBM.

Final results of MAFF's 7-year cohort study to determine maternal transmission indicate the risk to be less than 10% according to SEAC. However, variation in genetic susceptibility to BSE following feed-borne exposure may be an additional factor in the aetiology of the disease. Further research on the mechanism of direct maternal transmission and on genetic factors recommended by SEAC. Current control measures to protect the public considered adequate by SEAC, who advise UK government to consider the possibility of a cull of calves from BSE-affected mothers and its effects.

**May 1997.** UK Ministry of Agriculture uncertain of numbers of BSE cases buried in landfill tips in England between 1988 and 1991.

UK Environment Agency is currently investigating the geology and hydrology of six landfill sites in England to determine whether BSE infection is leaching into watercourses and/or contaminating topsoil. Preliminary results suggest that contamination is minimal due to microbial activity which, however, is very slow. BSE-prion emissions of MBM incinerated in power stations are also to be assessed by the Environment Agency. Although it has been suggested that the BSE prion can survive temperatures up to 1100°C this is now considered improbable. Certain amino acids can, however, survive power station high temperatures.

European Commission planned to introduce Specific Risk Materials (SRM) and clarified terms of the export ban, especially in relation to raw bovine materials, e.g. gelatin.

SEAC advised that SRM controls be extended to imported meat despite absence of Community measures.

**June 1997.** The Commission's Scientific Veterinary Committee commented on the UK proposal to set up an export certified scheme as a step towards lifting the export ban.

The UK government reminded farmers about compulsory registration of cattle under the cattle passport scheme.

**July 1997.** Agriculture Council accepted the European Commission proposals on SRM (Commission Decision 97/534/EC).

UK selective cull – animals in groups of 10 or less to be valued by one valuer instead of two in order to speed up the cull.

Setting up of new computerised cattle tracing system – British Cattle Movement Service – announced. System to be operational during 1998.

The UK Bovine Products (Production and Despatch) Regulations 1997 revoked earlier legislation on emergency measures to protect against BSE.

**Sept. 1997.** The UK Fresh Meat (Hygiene and Inspection) (Amendment) Regulations 1997 removed provision for the slaughter of private kill animals, ensuring full meat inspection for all red-meat animals.

Definition of 'animal by-products'. Category of 'meat from a bovine animal slaughtered for human consumption and subsequently to be from an animal over 30 months of age' added to definition.

**Oct. 1997.** UK proposal for export of meat and meat products from cattle born after 1 August 1996 and proposal for compulsory slaughter of offspring born on or after 1 August 1996 to affected BSE dams submitted to European Commission.

SEAC satisfied with UK measures on the safety of beef following review of human blood and blood products.

**Nov. 1997.** European Commission to visit Northern Ireland to examine their computerised system for tracing animals, which has been in force for some 10 years.

Final report on BSE endorsed by European Parliament (19 November).

**Dec. 1997.** UK government announced measures to require the deboning of all beef from cattle of over 6 months of age before sale (Beef Bones Regulations 1997).

UK government announced Public Enquiry into BSE to be conducted by Lord Justice Phillips.

**Jan. 1998.** Existing SBM Order replaced by The Specified Risk Material Order 1997 in UK, providing further controls on specified risk material.

**Mar. 1998.** UK BSE Enquiry. Public hearings commenced.

European Commission Agriculture Council allowed export of beef and beef products from Northern Ireland under Export Certified Herd Scheme and laid down new conditions for the export of tallow from UK cattle and gelatin from non-UK cattle.

**Apr. 1998.** Previous cattle identification orders revoked by The Cattle Identification Regulations 1998: cattle born after 1 January 1998 to have a MAFF-approved eartag and a cattle passport. The system will come into force on 28 September 1998 and will include a register of cattle, compulsory cattle tagging and a history of the animals until their death. New system will only affect animals born after 28 September 1998.

**May 1998.** Controls on exports of meat, meat products and 'preparations' from UK strengthened by The Bovines and Bovine Products (Trade) Regulations 1998.
Validity of export ban on UK beef upheld by EC.

**June 1998.** Ban lifted on the export of certified beef herds from Northern Ireland.
Switzerland confirmed fifth case of BSE of 1998 (in a 7-year-old cow). Total number of cases of BSE in Switzerland in 1997 was 38.

**July 1998.** First case of BSE in Liechtenstein is reported.
The UK National Audit Office announced the cost of BSE from 20 March 1996 (when the link between BSE and nvCJD was reported) to be £2.5 million. By the year 2000 it was expected to cost £l billion more.
New legislation requiring the compulsory slaughter of scrapie-affected sheep and goats is announced for England, Scotland and Wales following advice from SEAC and Decision (8/272/EC) of the European Commission. Controls on scrapie-affected animals will be enhanced and research work furthered.

**Aug. 1998.** France confirmed three further cases of BSE. All affected animals and associated herds destroyed in line with government policy.
EU's Calf Processing Aid Scheme to cease in the UK after November 1998. 1.2 million calves were slaughtered under the scheme in the UK from April 1996.

**Sept. 1998.** UK Cattle Tracing System launched: (Cattle Database Regs. 1998).

**Oct. 1998.** SRM (AM) Regs. 1998 enabled carcases of sheep over 12 months without spinal cords removed to be sent to France, subject to certain conditions. Scientific Steering Committee confirmed safety of bones and of hydrolysed proteins from bovine hides.

**Nov. 1998.** Postal survey on incidence of scrapie commenced in UK.

**Jan. 1999** Cattle Identification (AM) Regs. 1998 required one tag to be applied within 36h of birth and second tag within 30 days. BSE Offspring Slaughter Regs. 1998 implemented compulsory cull of offspring born on or after 1 Aug. 1996 to BSE cases confirmed before 25 Nov. 1998.

In the UK the number of reported cases of BSE between 1 January and 26 June was 22% lower than in the same period in 1997 and 65% lower than in the same period in 1996.

About 80 suspect cases per week are being reported in the UK compared with 1000 per week during the peak of the epidemic in 1993.

These figures indicate that the feed ban is affecting the course of the disease in the manner predicted. By 2001 the disease will decline to insignificant levels.

*BSE in the European Union:* There were 2382 reported outbreaks of BSE during 1998 (up to 27 August 1998): 3 in Belgium, 9 in France, 51 in Portugal, 37 in the Republic of Ireland and 2281 in the UK.

required for insurance or other purposes, it should be under carefully controlled conditions which have been agreed with the Divisional Veterinary Officer. Extreme care must always be taken when carrying out post-mortem examinations, particularly to avoid puncture wounds. Protective clothing must be worn at all times, including thick rubber gloves and, preferably, face masks. Instruments must be sharp and in good condition and must be thoroughly washed and disinfected after use.

Sodium hypochlorite freshly diluted 1:5 with water yields a solution containing 2% available chlorine and should be used to wash down contaminated areas. In view of the caustic nature of sodium hypochlorite, it should be stored and used with care.

*5. Accidents*

Care should be taken to avoid puncture wounds and cuts. Accidental injuries should immediately be washed thoroughly in running water and further first aid treatments rendered as appropriate to the type of injury. Existing cuts and abrasions should be covered with waterproof dressings.

### Precautions to be taken by meat plant personnel engaged in the slaughter and dressing of carcases where BSE is known to exist

The UK Health and Safety Executive has issued the following advice:

> In the UK cows suffering from BSE are now slaughtered and their carcases taken for disposal.
>
> While it is very unlikely that BSE will affect human health, it is important to take reasonable precautions in handling the carcases of these animals.
>
> The precautions suggested here will also protect you from other diseases of cattle known to affect man.
>
> So when handling BSE carcases:

- cover cuts and abrasions with waterproof dressings before work starts;
- wear protective clothing including gloves;
- avoid cuts and puncture wounds during work;
- use eye protection if there is risk of splashing;
- wash your hands before eating, drinking and smoking;
- wash down contaminated areas with detergent and water;
- rinse protective clothing free of debris after use and wash with water and detergent.

REPORT ALL ACCIDENTS TO YOUR EMPLOYER

Because of the very long incubation period it follows that there is a large number of subclinical carriers of the BSE and scrapie agents, which no one can recognise, the above precautions should be supplemented by the following in all cattle and sheep dressing:

- Do not pith cattle. Provided stunning and shackling are efficiently performed, pithing is unnecessary, besides creating another possible infection hazard.
- Do not remove spinal cords by hand, thereby risking cuts. If carcase splitting is uneven use a chine saw to remove the spinal cord.
- Do not remove brains (bovine or ovine) by any method from skulls. Handle only head meat and tongues.
- Face masks, gloves and saw guards should be used at the carcase-splitting point.
- All tools, especially carcase-splitting saws and captive bolt pistols, should be frequently and thoroughly sterilised.
- Carcase-splitting saws and captive bolt pistols should be provided with splash guards. (There should be immediate research into effective non-penetrative stunning.)
- Adopt a high standard of personal hygiene, washing hands and arms frequently using antibacterial soap.

### Advisory notes for farmers. UK Ministry of Agriculture, Fisheries and Food (MAFF) and Health and Safety Executive (HSE)

> All suspect cases of BSE must be reported immediately to the Ministry of Agriculture (Divisional Veterinary Officer).
>
> A Restrictive Notice (Form A) is served on all suspect BSE cases and this restricts movement. Form B lifts restriction when BSE is excluded.
>
> If BSE is confirmed a Notice of Intention to Slaughter (Form C) is served and slaughter and proper disposal arranged as soon as possible.

### *Handling of suspect BSE animals*

Since some BSE suspects become aggressive, hypersensitive and difficult to handle, MAFF/HSE have issued the following advice:

- Handle the animal quietly.
- Isolate it on a quiet loose-box on straw.
- Handle it firmly but quietly, always allowing a route of escape for the handler in case the animal becomes aggressive; take particular care in handling the head and udder as they can be headshy and violent kickers.

### *Treatments*

Whenever animals have to be treated on farm, whether or not BSE, the following advice reduces the risk of spreading diseases from animal to animal, and from animal to handler:

- For injections, use new needles each time.
- If treating several animals without using up all the medicine in the bottle, place one needle in the bottle and use another for injecting the stock. This prevents contamination of medicines that will be kept in store.
- Dispose of used needles safely in a strong container. Puncture wounds are frequently caused by leaving needles lying around where they can injure stock or their handlers.
- Accidental injuries should immediately be washed thoroughly in running water before giving appropriate first aid treatment. Existing cuts and abrasions should be covered with waterproof dressings. Blood splashes from animals under treatment should be washed off thoroughly.

### *Hygiene*

Always follow simple hygiene practices when handling all animals, whether or not they are BSE suspects; although there is no evidence that humans can be infected with BSE there are a number of diseases where this is possible.

### *Breeding*

Experiments are being carried out to determine whether BSE can be transmitted from dam to calf, but results may not be available for several years. If you wish to obtain advice on breeding from the offspring of cows affected with BSE, you should consult your veterinary surgeon.

### *Calving*

There will be few cases in which it is necessary for a suspect cow to calve. As soon as a veterinary officer is certain that an animal is affected with BSE, Form C will be served and slaughter arranged. Slaughter will *not* be postponed to allow a cow to calve normally, and you are strongly advised not to attempt to have a calf delivered prematurely by caesarian section.

Suspect animals which do calve must be housed whilst calving and for 72 hours afterwards. An isolation box for calving must be approved by a veterinary officer beforehand, and must, after calving, be disinfected with chlorine-based disinfectant diluted to give 2% active chlorine.

If calving has to be assisted, wear washable protective clothing and arm-length gloves. Always avoid direct handling of placenta (cleansings). If unable to do so, wear gloves. This is sound advice when dealing with cattle, whether or not they are BSE suspects. For disposal of cleansings, the preferred method is by incineration, but careful burial is an acceptable alternative. For suspects under Ministry Restrictions this is in fact a legal requirement.

## Future research

A wide-ranging research programme is being conducted on several aspects of bovine in the UK spongiform encephalopathy including the following:

- Epidemiology
- Study of tissues showing infectivity
- Vertical transmission from dam to calf
- Embryo transfer
- Development of diagnostic tests.
- Effectiveness of statutory controls to be monitored
- Evidence of TSEs in other species to be monitored
- Mechanism of BSE infection, etc.

## BOVINE VIRAL DIARRHOEA (BVD), MUCOSAL DISEASE COMPLEX (MD)

**I.** An infectious, febrile disease of cattle (mostly 6–24 months), deer, buffaloes and wild ruminants in which the lesions are confined to the alimentary tract.

**O.** Occurs throughout the world. Although infection is common BVD is usually mild or subclinical in type with few deaths but occasionally serious illness with high mortality takes place.

**IA.** A pestivirus of the family Togaviridae which is related to the viruses of classical swine fever and border disease, all of which have the ability to cross the placenta and invade the fetus.

**R.** Infected and carrier animals. Fetuses infected early in gestation with a cytopathic strain of the virus eventually become major sources of infection.

**MT.** Direct and indirect contact with faeces, nasal discharges, saliva, urine, uterine discharges following abortion, semen and milk in addition to congenital infection.

**CF.** BVD may affect cattle of all ages but is most common and most serious in 6–24-month-old animals, while young calves are rarely affected.

In the *mild* form there is slight fever, inappetence and some diarrhoea, with recovery in a few days. *Acute* mucosal disease is manifested by fever, salivation, depression, anorexia, dehydration and the voiding of profuse watery, evil-smelling faeces which may contain mucus, blood and strands of fibrin – the signs of a haemorrhagic enteritis. Death may take place in 1 week. In *chronic* BVD there is intermittent diarrhoea, progressive loss of weight, rough coat, bloat, hoof ulcerations and deformities and erosive skin lesions.

**P.** The main lesions are seen in the acute form – erosion and ulceration of the buccal mucosa, tongue and muzzle. These erosions may extend to the oesophagus, forestomachs, abomasum and intestine. Congestion of the nasal passages with a mucopurulent discharge and lymphoid tissue necrosis, especially of the intestine, may be present.

**D.** History, clinical signs and post-mortem lesions may assist in diagnosis but this can only be confirmed by virus isolation, immunological and histopathological investigations.

*Differential diagnoses*: foot-and-mouth disease, rinderpest, bovine malignant catarrh, winter dysentery, Jöhne's disease, parasitic gastroenteritis, salmonellosis, molybdenum and arsenic poisoning.

**J.**

Carcase and viscera: T. Acute cases with fever, general changes, T.

## CONTAGIOUS ECTHYMA (CONTAGIOUS PUSTULAR DERMATITIS, SORE MOUTH, ORF)

**I.** A very infectious viral disease of sheep and goats in which pustules and scabs ('scabby mouth') develop on the muzzle, lips and teats. It also occurs in musk ox, caribou, buffalo, camels and other wild ruminants and has been recorded in dogs which have had access to infected carcases. It is a *zoonosis* since the disease can affect man (q.v.) (see Occupational Infections and Injuries).

**O.** Occurs throughout the world, affecting mostly young animals.

**I.** A parapoxvirus of the family Poxviridae which is related to the viruses of pseudo-cowpox, goatpox and bovine papular stomatitis. The virus is very resistant to desiccation and can remain viable in scabs for years. It spreads rapidly within susceptible animals.

**R.** Affected and carrier animals, carcases, wool and contaminated equipment and materials.

**MT.** Via cuts and abrasions in the skin.

**CF.** *'Orf'* occurs most commonly in young lambs (2–6 months of age) in the spring in temperate climates when lambs are at grass. Mortality rates are normally low (5–15%), these being due to complications, probably pneumonia.

The primary lesion, a papule, develops on the skin of the lips at the corner of the mouth and soon becomes a vesicle, and then a pustule, with the formation of adherent scabs covering painful areas of ulceration and granulation. The papule, vesicle and pustule stages are, however, rarely noticed. Spread to the nostrils and sometimes to the mucosa of the mouth below the incisor teeth then follows.

The scabs become confluent and fissured and attempts at removal are resented by the animal. Sucking and grazing are made virtually impossible and the animal becomes unthrifty.

There is often transfer of infection from the mouths of lambs to the udders of ewes.

On occasion, lesions develop on the coronets and interdigital clefts of the feet, causing lameness, and on the ears.

Secondary infection with *Sphaerophorus necrophorus* and other organisms is a frequent occurrence.

In severe cases a viraemia occurs with systemic invasion leading to gastroenteritis and pneumonia.

**P.** See **CF**. In some instances ulcers in the nasal passages, upper respiratory tract and alimentary tract represent additional lesions.

**D.** Lesions, especially of the lips and mouth, are fairly typical. Foot lesions, however, may be confused with dermatophilosis (cutaneous streptotrichosis, strawberry foot rot) which can co-exist with 'orf'.

Other *differential diagnoses* include bluetongue, mycotic dermatitis, facial eczema and ulcerative dermatosis of sheep. The latter is a viral condition in which raw, granulating ulcers appear on the lips, feet, legs, vulva and penis. Scab formation is not normally present and the granulomas assume cauliflower-like shapes.

**J.**

Carcase and viscera: A, provided condition is satisfactory and no systemic changes are evident.

Head: D.

## CRIMEA-CONGO HAEMORRHAGIC FEVER (CCHF, CONGO VIRUS DISEASE)

**I.** A very severe, often fatal disease primarily of *man* but which can also occur in a less severe form in a wide range of domestic (especially cattle and goats) and wild animals and birds (zoonosis). Following an incubation period of about 1 week the disease is characterised (in man) by marked haemorrhagic fever. **Zoonosis.**

**O.** Africa (especially the Congo and Nigeria), USSR, Middle East, West Pakistan, India and southern China.

**IA.** A nairovirus, serogroup Crimean-Congo, named after the Nairobi Sheep disease and related to three other viruses known to infect man – Dugbe virus, Ganjam virus and Hazara virus.

**R.** Infected and carrier animals, birds and ticks.

**MT.** The virus is transmitted in Africa mainly by *Hyalomma* ticks, especially *H. anatolicum* and *H. plumbeum plumbeum*, the latter being more involved with infections in wild animals and birds. *Amblyomma* and *Boophilus* ticks are also known vectors in Africa while *Ornithodoros* and *Amblyomma* transmit infection in west Pakistan, India, Russia and the Middle East. The link between Africa, Russia and Asia is attributed to migrating birds, many of which are unaffected by the virus.

**CF.** The main clinical signs in animals and birds are fever, anorexia and depression with some degree of haemorrhage from the natural orifices.

In *man* the onset is sudden with usually continuous fever, headache, vomiting, back pain, photophobia, joint pains and bleeding from all natural orifices and under the skin. Mortality is usually 15–30% but may be as high as 80%. Nervous symptoms may be present.

**P.** Haemorrhagic inflammation of virtually all body systems.

**D.** Isolation of the virus in sucking mice. ELISA test. Tissue culture.

**J.** Total condemnation in animals and birds.

The European Union banned (November 1996) imports of ostrich meat and live birds from South Africa following an outbreak of Congo Fever in meat plant workers in Oudtshoorn in Western Cape Province. Sixteen workers were affected and one woman died. The infection is said to be more virulent in ostriches than in other animals and birds. The South African authorities are currently assessing the risks of this *zoonosis* to human health.

The EU imports some 800 tonnes of ostrich meat annually from South Africa.

## ENZOOTIC BOVINE LEUKOSIS (EBL, BOVINE VIRAL LEUKOSIS, BOVINE LYMPHOSARCOMA, MALIGNANT LYMPHOMA, LEUKAEMIA, LYMPHOMATOSIS, RETICULUM CELL SARCOMA, LYMPHOCYTOMA)

(The terms above have been used at various times for the same disease and are virtually synonymous).

**I.** A highly fatal, neoplastic condition of cattle in which there is a malignant proliferation of the leukocyte-forming tissues in almost any part of the animal body.

Leukocytes are colourless blood corpuscles whose chief function is to protect the body against invasion by microorganisms. They include granulocytes (basophils, eosinophils, neutrophils), non-granulocytes (lymphocytes, monocytes) and thrombocytes (platelets).

Notifiable disease (UK). Under Council Directive 64/432 'Animal health problems affecting intra-community trade in bovine animals and swine' cattle exported to another Member State must come from EBL-tested herds.

**O.** EBL has been reported in Europe, Africa, Asia, North and South America, Australia and New Zealand. It is enzootic in many countries in South America and Europe and of high occurrence in Latvia. Serological surveys have shown various levels of reactors, from none to 100%. Infection with the virus does not necessarily mean that animals will develop clinical disease, a situation which applies in many viral and bacterial diseases. Other factors are involved in the precipitation of disease, an important one being genetic predisposition.

Enzootic bovine leukosis is of economic importance in those countries in which it occurs because of the culling of affected animals, reduction in body weight and milk yield, infertility, meat plant condemnations and the cost of eradication programmes.

A national testing programme for EBL was commenced in Britain in 1992 using blood and milk samples. The milk testing procedure using bulk samples has not been sensitive enough to comply with EU regulations. Future testing will rely on milk samples from individual cows and a blood sample from all other cattle. The overall prevalence is very low.

The EBL eradication programme in Sweden is due to be completed in 1997 and will mark the end of a successful campaign commenced in 1989. Sweden will be declared EBL-free one year later in accordance with EU regulations.

**IA.** The bovine leukaemia virus (BLV), a C-type retrovirus which causes a chronic B-cell proliferative disease in cattle. B lymphocytes are involved in humoral immunity mechanisms in the production of antibodies. When activated by an antigen – in this case the BLV virus – proliferation of the cell results.

The virus in EBL is present in lymphocytes, lymphoid tumours, blood and milk but rarely in saliva, nasal secretions or semen except when contaminated by blood or tissue exudates. It can be intermittently excreted in urine.

The virus, which does not persist for long outside the animal's body, is readily destroyed by detergents and disinfectants at normal concentrations and by pasteurisation of milk at 74°C for 17 s or 60°C for 30s.

**R.** Infected and carrier cattle and discharged blood from these animals.

**MT.** Transmission of the disease takes place by the transfer of lymphocytes from affected cattle. This normally requires close animal contact, the presence of a wound or abrasion and/or the use of infected surgical and other instruments, e.g. hypodermic syringes, tattooing instruments, dehorning saws and gouges. The use of vaccines inadvertently containing BVL virus has been known to produce the disease. Bloodsucking insects such as ticks, horse and stable flies may play a part in transmission.

Congenital infection takes place in less than 10% of calves born to seropositive dams.

**CF.** Once the virus gains access to the animal's bloodstream it remains permanently. The animal becomes seropositive in 1 to 3 months after infection but only some 30% develop a lymphocytosis. In spite of the presence of virus, relatively few animals become clinical cases, the average annual rate of infected animals showing tumours being about 0.3%. Not all animals become infected probably because of innate genetic resistance.

At least four forms of EBR are recognised. *Enzootic EBR* is a disease of adult cattle in which tumours develop in various sites in the body, symptoms varying according to the sites involved. After an incubation period of some 4–5 years, these include loss of condition, anaemia, inappetence and enlargement of superficial lymph nodes, which are softish but non-painful to the touch. There is a rapid onset of death (2–3 weeks).

Tumours in the alimentary tract may be accompanied by bloat and chronic diarrhoea, the dark-coloured faeces being due to the presence of blood pigments arising from ulceration and haemorrhage. Enlargement of the retropharyngeal nodes give rise to snoring and difficult breathing. Heart lesions may show oedema of the brisket and jugular vein engorgement with extreme weakness.

Nervous symptoms in the form of posterior paresis, incoordination, fetlock knuckling and recumbency attend cases where the central nervous system is involved. If lymphosarcoma develops in the orbital fossae, protrusion of the eye occurs.

*Skin leukosis* occurs in young adults and is non-fatal. Superficial flat tumours develop which regress after a few weeks.

*Thymic leukosis* affects calves of 6–18 months and is characterised by a huge enlargement of the thymic region due to virtual replacement of the gland by lymphosarcoma. Local oedema and dyspnoea are also evident.

*Calf lymphosarcoma* is seen in calves under 1 year of age and is manifested by weakness, depression, inappetence, fever, paraplegia and death in a few weeks due to widespread tumour formation.

**P.** Lymphosarcomas are probably the most common forms of tumour encountered in the food animals. They occur as resilient white or slightly yellowish, textured masses of tumours by metastasis in reticuloendothelial tissue anywhere in the body. These masses vary in size and shape and may occur as large bodies, small discrete tumours or fine streaks.

The kidneys, spleen, lymph nodes, liver and thymus are especially involved in the young animal. In the older animal the heart is often affected, especially the right atrium. One or more discrete masses may be found in the heart but some infiltrate among the muscle fibres, giving the appearance of whitish streaks. The abomasum and intestine are frequently affected with ulceration, especially in the abomasum.

Nervous system involvement takes the form of thickening of the peripheral nerves and the meninges.

Lymphosarcoma may be encountered in the uterus and cervix of the cow.

Lymph node leukosis appears as a gross enlargement of the node in which there is both normal lymphoid and neoplastic tissue, differentiated by colour, the neoplastic tissue being whiter in colour than the normal lymphoid. Discrete foci of yellowish necrosis may be found in the neoplastic zone.

**D.** The presence of multiple superficial lymph node enlargement makes a diagnosis of enzootic leukosis in the adult reasonably safe. But other forms of the disease are difficult to diagnose and may be confused with bovine tuberculosis (especially where retropharyngeal lymph nodes are affected causing snoring), Jöhne's disease, bovine viral diarrhoea, cerebrospinal abscess and actinobacillosis.

While a negative test suffices to rule out EBL, a seropositive test does not necessarily indicate EBL. Only histopathology of neoplastic tissues can confirm a diagnosis of EBL.

**J.**

Carcase and viscera: T, in cases of widespread lesions. A, where lesions are restricted, with D, Kh if economically feasible.

Reactor animals: A.

Since enzootic bovine leukosis is a *notifiable disease* in Britain, all cases in bovines showing swollen, painless lymph nodes and lymphocytosis must be reported to the Ministry of Agriculture for histopathological examination. If lymphosarcoma is diagnosed, the Ministry will arrange for a veterinary examination of the herd of origin, which will be placed under restriction until the results of serological tests are known. Positive cases of EBL are slaughtered.

## EQUINE ENCEPHALOMYELITIS (EQUINE ENCEPHALITIS)

**I.** An infectious viral disease of horses, mules and donkeys transmitted by biting insects, and manifested by signs of nervous derangement, paralysis and moderate to high mortality.

**O.** The disease appears to be mostly confined to south and north America, where it is of low sporadic occurrence in Argentina, Brazil and USA but enzootic in Guyana. Venezuela had its last case in 1991. Canada has recorded cases but is now free following a vaccination programme.

*Borna disease* (an encephalomyelitis of equidae caused by an unclassified RNA virus) is reported to be of exceptional occurrence in the former GDR.

*Japanese encephalitis*, transmitted by mosquitoes, is primarily a disease of human beings which can infect horses and pigs causing abortions and stillbirths in the latter. Cattle, sheep and goats can also be subclinically infected.

**IA.** An alphavirus of the family Togaviridae of which there are three strains (eastern, western and Venezuelan). A subtype of the Venezuelan virus can infect man, causing a zoonosis of significant public health importance.

**R.** Infected and carrier horses along with a bird (domestic and wild) and rodent-mosquito cycle.

**MT.** Equine encephalomyelitis is transmitted by the bites of insects – mosquitoes, bugs, lice and mites.

**CF.** Clinical cases occur during the summer months when biting insects are active. There is fever, depression, inappetence, hyperaethesia, impaired vision, difficulty in swallowing, head pressing, circling, inability to prehend food, drooping lower lip, paralysis and death often in 3 days.

**P.** Apart from changes associated with fever, there are no gross lesions.

**D.** The seasonal occurrence of the disease, its localisation and the presence of nervous symptoms point to a tentative diagnosis of encephalomyelitis. Confirmation is made by serology – virus neutralisation, haemagglutination inhibition and complement fixation tests.

*Differential diagnoses* – rabies, degenerative myeloencephalopathy, botulism, verminous encephalitis, cerebrospinal abscess, chemical and plant poisonings.

**J.**

Carcase and viscera: Clinical cases, T.
Reactors, L.
Brain and medulla: D.

## EQUINE INFECTIOUS ANAEMIA (EIA, SWAMP FEVER)

**I.** An acute or chronic infectious viral disease of equidae in which anaemia (temporary or permanent) occurs with usually low mortality.

**O.** EIA appears in sporadic form worldwide but is most common in south America, where it is enzootic in some countries. USA, Mexico and Canada have low sporadic outbreaks as has Australia. It was last reported in Great Britain in 1976, in Spain (1983) and in Sweden (1989).

**IA.** A lentivirus of the family Retroviridae, related to the human HIV virus. Although easily destroyed by drying it is resistant to boiling for 15 min but readily inactivated by the usual disinfectants.

**R.** Infected and carrier horses and biting flies (mosquitoes, deer flies and stable flies).

**MT.** Via the bites of biting flies, use of contaminated surgical instruments and needles intrauterine, and by the ingestion of infected milk by foals.

**CF.** EIA is prevalent during warm periods when biting flies are active. When the virus gains access to the bloodstream, a viraemia occurs and persists in infected WBCs of infected horses for life. Red blood cells and macrophages are destroyed and blood vessel walls and nerves are damaged.

Intermittent fever, inappetence, depression, weakness, loss of condition and jaundice are evident along with ventral abdominal oedema. Mucous membranes become pallid and show petechial haemorrhages especially in the mouth and conjunctivae. Pregnant mares may abort. Recovery often takes place but some animals become weaker and die.

**P.** In addition to the lesions given in **CF** there is enlargement of the spleen and liver and associated lymph nodes. All tissues are pale in colour and loss of condition is marked. Clotting in blood vessels is prominent in most cases.

**D.** Clinical signs of anaemia and seasonal occurrence point to EIA, which is confirmed by the immunodiffusion or 'Coggins' test.

*Differential diagnoses* include babesiosis, purpura haemorrhagica, leptospirosis, phenothiazine poisoning.

**J.**

Carcase and viscera: Clinical cases, T.
Reactors: A, provided no systemic changes present and condition is good.

## EPHEMERAL FEVER (THREE-DAY SICKNESS)

**I.** An infectious viral disease of cattle and water buffalo transmitted by biting insects, probably mosquitoes and sandflies. Subclinical cases occur in wild ruminants, e.g. deer, wildebeest, waterbuck and cape buffalo.

**O.** Africa, Asia, Australia and East Indies.

**IA.** A rhabdovirus.

**R.** Infected animals. The virus does not persist in recovered animals.

**MT.** The disease is transmitted solely by the action of biting insects.

**CF.** As with all insect-borne diseases, ephemeral fever occurs during the warm summer months when biting insects are active. Symptoms vary but include inappetence, fever, depression, lachrymation, nasal discharge, dyspnoea, muscular stiffness, decreased milk yield and recumbency. Abortion occurs in a few cases. Recovery in a few days is the usual outcome and mortality rates are very low.

**P.** Polyserositis involving the pleural, peritoneal and joint surfaces, and pulmonary oedema with collapsed lungs.

**D.** Based entirely on clinical signs and the short duration of the illness.

**J.** Carcase and viscera: T or A depending on severity of changes. Kh may be utilised in certain areas.

## EPIZOOTIC HAEMORRHAGIC DISEASE OF DEER

**I.** An acute, viral disease of deer, especially white-tailed deer, transmitted by biting insects and characterised by haemorrhagic and necrotic changes in the alimentary and respiratory tracts and heart. The disease closely resembles bluetongue.

Notifiable disease (UK). A definite threat to British deer exists.

**O.** The disease at present appears to be confined to North America.

**IA.** Epizootic haemorrhagic disease virus (EHDV) of the Orbivirus group related to the bluetongue virus (BTV).

**R.** Infected and carrier deer.

**MT.** Biting insects of the species *Culicoides* (a variety of biting midges).

**CF.** Fever, depression, inappetence, conjunctivitis, mucopurulent nasal discharge, inflammation of the coronary bands of the feet with lameness and usually death in 2–4 days. The tongue is swollen and cyanotic, making swallowing difficult, and cyanosis with oedema is present in the submandibular tissues. Morbidity may be as high as 90% and mortality 60%.

**P.** The lesions resemble those of bluetongue. There is widespread hyperaemia, oedema and petechiation, often with necrosis of the mucosae of the respiratory and alimentary tracts accompanied by fibrinous thrombosis of small blood vessels. Petechiae may also be present in the myocardium.

**D.** The rapid clinical course and fairly specific lesions are suggestive of epizootic haemorrhagic disease.

Diagnosis is confirmed by serology, tissue culture, etc.

**J.** Carcase and viscera: T.

## EQUINE INFLUENZA

**I.** An acute, highly infectious and contagious febrile disease of equidae in which bronchiolitis and sometimes pneumonia and pleurisy occur.

**O.** Most countries of the world have reported cases.

**IA.** An orthomyxovirus of two distinct strains and several subtypes, all varying in virulence.

**R.** Infected animals and their fomites. It is not known whether a carrier state exists.

**MT.** By inhalation of aerosol deposition into the upper respiratory passages directly from infected animals and contaminated materials.

**CF.** After a short incubation period (1–3 days), clinical signs include fever, coughing, nasal discharge (at first serous but later mucopurulent), lachrymation, depression, anorexia, dyspnoea and weakness. Head lymph nodes are enlarged and limb stiffness with laminitis often ensue. Mild cases usually recover in 2–3 weeks but more seriously affected animals may be ill for several months. The mortality rate (highest in younger animals) is normally low.

**P.** Bronchiolitis, pneumonia, pleurisy and sometimes perivasculitis (inflammation of the tissues surrounding blood vessels) and myocarditis (in fatal cases). Serous/mucopurulent discharge in upper respiratory tract.

**D.** Clinical signs are presumptive of equine influenza especially when movements of horses are involved.

*Differential diagnoses* include equine viral arteritis, strangles, equine viral rhinopneumonitis and other respiratory infections.

**J.** Carcase and viscera: A, provided no systemic signs are present. T or Kh if febrile changes are evident.

Animals in acute stages of the disease (as for all febrile conditions) should not be presented for slaughter – *delayed slaughter* should be undertaken.

### Equine viral rhinopneumonitis

Caused by a herpesvirus, this occurs throughout the world but is not now present in Australia (last case 1990), Spain (last case 1989), Czechoslovakia and Bulgaria (last cases 1989). It presents clinical signs and lesions similar to, but more intense than, equine influenza and warrants similar, but more severe, action.

## EQUINE VIRAL ARTERITIS (EVA, EQUINE TYPHOID, EPIZOOTIC CELLULITIS, PINKEYE)

**I.** An acute, infectious, viral disease of equidae characterised by fever, inflammatory and degenerative changes in blood vessels, especially small arteries and venules and muscle cells with abortion in mares.

**O.** Some sporadic outbreaks of EVA have occurred in the USA, Canada, Europe (especially Denmark, where it appears to be enzootic, Netherlands and Sweden). Serological evidence without clinical cases is reported from most EU Member States, Australia and New Zealand.

Statutory control is planned in Britain in the event of further outbreaks. It has been recommended that all entire colts and stallions imported into Britain should all be tested for EVA.

**IA.** An arterovirus of the family Togaviridae.

**R.** Infected horses and carrier stallions. The virus is plentiful in aborted fetuses.

**MT.** Via the respiratory, digestive and venereal routes.

**CF.** Fever, conjunctivitis, lachrymation, spasm of the orbital muscle of the eyelid, photophobia, inappetence, periorbital oedema, seropurulent nasal discharge, respiratory distress, muscle and joint pain, skin rash, colic, diarrhoea and jaundice. Ventral and preputial oedema may be evident in stallions. Abortion in mares is not uncommon, often with partly autolysed fetuses. Many animals display few clinical signs. Symptoms are more severe in young, old and debilitated animals.

**P.** In addition to the lesions mentioned under **CF**, systemic changes in the form of respiratory congestion and petechiation, swelling and necrosis of vascular walls, especially of the smaller arteries and venules, are present.

There is also subcutaneous oedema with petechiation, mostly of the limbs and abdomen, excess fluid in the body cavities, pulmonary oedema, enteritis and splenic infarcts.

**D.** Diagnosis can only be confirmed by virus isolation since the disease may be confused with equine influenza, African horse sickness, Garth virus infection, leptospirosis, equine rhinopneumonitis and salmonellosis.

**J.** Carcase and viscera: T, clinical cases.
Reactor animals: A.

## FOOT-AND-MOUTH DISEASE (FMD, APHTHOUS FEVER)

**I.** An acute, highly contagious viral disease of all cloven-footed animals (domestic and wild) in which fever and vesicular epithelial desquamation appears in the mouth and on the feet and teats. FMD also affects hedgehogs, voles, moles and rats.

FMD infection is rare in *man*, taking the form of a mild fever with mouth dryness and small vesicles in the mouth, lips, tongue and fingers at the base of the nail.

Notifiable disease (UK and most countries).

**O.** Foot-and-mouth disease has occurred in most countries of the world but many are now free, apart from occasional outbreaks, as a result of control programmes.

However, freedom over some years is frequently followed by a recurrence; for example, Greece experienced 95 outbreaks in 1994 having been free of FMD since 1984. Similarly, in 1993, Italy had 57 outbreaks, the previous cases occurring in 1989. Japan has not had an outbreak since 1908 and Australia since 1871, while FMD has never occurred in New Zealand. USA has not had any outbreaks since 1929 and Canada since 1952. In 1996 there were 39 reported outbreaks in the European Union – all in Greece

In Argentina, Brazil, Colombia, Paraguay, Peru and Bolivia on the other hand, FMD is enzootic as it is in many countries in Asia where Bhutan and Myanmar have high occurrences. Several African countries (Nigeria, Ghana, Cameroon, Ethiopia, Tanzania) have enzootic prevalences, while Swaziland has been free of FMD since 1969.

**IA.** An aphthovirus of the family Picornaviridae of which there are seven major serotypes (A, O, C, SAT (Southern African Territories) 1, SAT 2, SAT 3 and Asia 1) and several subtypes.

The virus is able to survive for several months outside the animal body, especially under low-temperature and dry conditions. In bone marrow it can remain infective for 76 days, but decomposition reduces this to 30 days.

High or low pH rapidly inactivates the virus, as do strong sunlight and high temperatures.

It is susceptible to acid conditions and in muscle is inactivated in 2 days by lactic acid. In chilled infected carcases the virus remains infective for 2 months and for 100 days in frozen infected ones. On muscle fascia and fat stored at 1°C it will survive for 14 days, and on frozen muscle fascia and fat for 21 days. Commercial refrigeration of imported meat in the past has played an important part in maintaining the infectivity of the virus. The greatest danger is undoubtedly infection from meat scraps and bones of infected animals and uncooked swill containing infective material. Contaminated biological products such as vaccines have also been responsible for outbreaks of FMD.

Foot-and-mouth virus is not destroyed by pasteurisation temperatures since it is protected by milk fat and cells. The virus can also survive for considerable periods in skins and hides which have been salted or disinfected.

FMDV is fairly easily destroyed by the usual disinfectants, alkali being the most effective. Disinfectants such as phenol and mercuric chloride (bichloride of mercury) which coagulate protein, are much less effective since the virus lacks a lipid-containing envelope. A 4% solution of sodium carbonate (washing soda) or 2% caustic soda is recommended, while 5% formalin is of value in the disinfection of stacks of hay and straw.

**R.** Infected and carrier animals and their fomites. Although pigs are not generally regarded as carriers, sheep and goats along with wild fauna act as reservoirs for the virus, as may certain insects such as ticks.

**MT.** The primary methods of transmission of infection are by inhalation and ingestion.

Direct contact between animals and indirect contact through the medium of contaminated materials are involved in the spread between pigs and from pigs to cattle. Airborne infection undoubtedly plays an important part in causing outbreaks, the migration of birds being incriminated in introducing infection from Europe to Britain.

The movement of animals, people (via their clothing and even nasal mucosa) and infected inanimate objects plays a major part in spreading the disease, since FMDV can survive for long periods in temperate and subtropical conditions. It is known that wind can transport the virus almost 200 miles, so that birds may not necessarily have been involved in some outbreaks in Britain coincident with outbreaks in northern Europe.

On gaining entry to the body, the virus lodges in the nasopharynx, where it persists. From there it enters the bloodstream, causing a viraemia which leads to the virus appearing in all tissues of the body, being present in urine, milk, saliva, semen and faeces as well as vesicles.

**CF.** Because of its high infectivity, loss of production of meat and milk, losses in young stock, interference with livestock movements, cost of control, etc., FMD creates huge economic losses even though it does not cause a high mortality.

Cattle and pigs are the most susceptible animals while sheep and goats are relatively resistant. Very young animals are most severely affected, the death rate in piglets and young calves often being very high.

After an incubation period of 2–14 days a fever develops, at the end of which vesicles appear and the temperature falls. The virus is capable of penetrating intact mucosa and is probably assisted by abrasions and cuts.

Vesicles are most commonly found on the buccal mucosa, tongue, muzzle, udder (which develops mastitis), teats and the snout of pigs. The animal becomes dull, with lack of appetite and cessation of rumination. Prehension of food, chewing and swallowing become difficult and a peculiar smacking sound is occasionally heard when the mouth is opened. Salivation is prominent in the bovine (but not in pigs, sheep and goats), the flow of saliva becoming thick and glairy and hanging from the commissures of the mouth.

The mouth lesions have a whitish appearance, measure up to 5 cm in diameter and contain a straw-coloured fluid. These eventually rupture within 48 h, leaving red, painful erosions and ragged portions of epithelium.

Coincident with the mouth lesions is evidence of lameness, the animal often lifting a foot and shaking it as though to dislodge a foreign body. The lameness is due to the development of vesicles in the interdigital cleft, on the heel, on the dewclaws and around the coronet. One or more feet may be affected.

In sheep and goats the vesicles are much smaller in size, disappear more quickly and may be absent from the mouth. A disinclination to move is a common finding in all classes of animals once foot lesions develop.

Pigs are most often affected by foot lesions rather than mouth lesions, although vesicles may occur on the snout, inside the nares and in sows on the udder around the nipples. Pregnant sows may abort with either stillbirths or piglets which die in a few days, the latter showing no vesiculation and death being due to myocarditis. Abortion may also take place in cattle, with subsequent infertility.

In sheep, goats and pigs it is common for the claw of the foot to be gradually shed with the formation of new horn underneath, a process known as *'thimbling'*.

In all species secondary bacterial infection tends to develop after vesicle eruption, especially in the feet.

All species lose condition, but adult resistant animals usually resume feeding in 3–4 days, with the mouth and foot lesions healing rapidly.

**P.** In addition to the superficial lesions mentioned under **CF**, similar vesicles may develop in the oesophagus, trachea, bronchi, stomach and intestine. Haemorrhages may be present on the epicardium in young calves, lambs, piglets and kids. The myocardium may assume a striped appearance due to the development of small, greyish foci of varying size, this being due to hyaline degeneration and necrosis of muscle fibres along with a lymphocytic infiltration – the so-called *'tiger heart'*. Similar changes may be found in skeletal muscles.

**D.** The fact that the clinical signs of FMD are virtually indistinguishable from vesicular stomatitis of cattle, swine and horses, vesicular exanthema of swine, swine vesicular disease and other ill-defined vesicular diseases makes an accurate diagnosis of FMD difficult.

While a tentative diagnosis may be made, reliance has to be placed on serological tests – complement fixation, ELISA, virus neutralisation, agar-gel precipitation, etc.

**J.** Carcase and viscera: T, diseased animals and contacts, in countries normally free of FMD.

> In other countries or areas judgement must be in accordance with current animal health requirements and consistent with effective public health protection. Particular attention must be paid to secondary bacterial infections and general findings. Sanitary measures must comply with national animal health policy. (Codex Alimentarius Commission, Alinorm 93/16A, 1993)

In those countries where slaughter of contacts is practised, but destruction is not economically feasible, diseased carcases are totally condemned and *in-contacts* conditionally approved, subject to heat treatment.

In countries where a slaughter policy is not practised because of economics, recovered animals and in-contacts 60 days after the last case are passed for human consumption after deboning and condemnation of the oesophagus, udder, testes, pharynx and bones.

Diseased carcases are totally condemned or subjected to heat treatment.

## INFECTIOUS BOVINE RHINOTRACHEITIS (IBR, RED NOSE)

**I.** A very infectious viral disease of cattle in which upper respiratory and genital infections and sometimes encephalitis are present. Many wild ruminants are seropositive to the virus and a mild form may affect them.

**O.** IBR has been reported in all four continents, being enzootic in Canada, USA and many south American and European countries including Great Britain. The disease has a high incidence in New Zealand.

**IA.** A bovine herpesvirus 1 (BHV-1) which is related to the virus causing infectious pustular vulvovaginitis and balanoposthitis in bulls.

**R.** Infected and carrier cattle and wild ruminants.

**MT.** Via the respiratory and genital tracts.

**CF.** In the *respiratory form* there is fever, inappetence, depression, conjunctivitis, lachrymation, coughing, dyspnoea and a nasal discharge, at first serous and becoming purulent later. Bronchopneumonia is a common feature, as is abortion in late pregnancy. (Abortion may accompany either form of the disease.) There is intense hyperaemia of the nasal passages (*'red nose'*) and buccal mucosa.

In the *genital form* there is vaginitis with papule formation and then ulceration and vaginal discharge. Infection may extend to the uterus, causing a septic metritis. Similar lesions occur on the penis and prepuce of bulls.

Encephalitis, or, more strictly, meningitis, in the young animal is evidenced by incoordination, ataxia, paralysis, excitement and death.

Mild cases usually recover in 2 weeks but deaths may occur in bronchopneumonia and cases complicated by secondary bacterial infection.

**P.** In addition to the changes noted under **CF**, there are petechiae or ecchymoses and/or focal areas of necrosis in the nasal passages, sinuses, pharynx, larynx and trachea. In young animals these changes may extend to the forestomachs, with white necrotic foci evident in the liver, spleen, kidney and visceral lymph nodes. If bronchopneumonia is present there may be desquamation of columnar epithelium. Meningitis shows as an intense hyperaemia of the meninges.

**D.** The lesions in uncomplicated cases are suggestive of IBR. The disease must be distinguished from bovine virus diarrhoea, bovine malignant catarrh and calf diphtheria.

**J.** Carcase and viscera: T, systemic changes present. A, systemic changes absent and condition good.

## JAPANESE B ENCEPHALITIS (JE)

**I.** An acute inflammatory viral encephalitis of *man* which can be transmitted to horses, cattle, sheep and pigs.

It is one of a group of arthropod-borne encephalitic diseases which can affect man – Eastern and Western equine encephalitis, California encephalitis, Australian encephalitis, St. Louis encephalitis, Rocio encephalitis, etc. – each having specific viruses.

**O.** At present the disease is confined to Asia, where it occurs sporadically in Korea. It has been eradicated from Japan (1985), Singapore (1988) and Indonesia (1989). It has never been reported in Africa, north and south America, Europe or Oceania, although it has been reported rarely in man in some of the Pacific islands.

**IA.** A group B flavivirus.

**R.** There is a wide range of hosts including man, pigs, rodents, birds, amphibians, bats and mosquito adults and eggs.

**MT.** Via the bite of infective mosquitoes, *Culex tritaeniorhynchus* and *C. vishnui*. These mosquitoes play an important part in maintaining a constant human–mosquito–pig cycle.

**CF.** Clinical signs in acute cases in horses include fever, lassitude, inappetence, jaundice, incoordination, ataxia, blindness, hyperaesthesia, muscle tremors. Mild cases, which are the most numerous, recover in a few days, but severe cases take longer and a few end fatally.

In pigs there is encephalitis and abortion with stillbirths in sows.

In all species of domestic animals JE may be asymptomatic, especially in cattle, sheep and goats.

**D.** The differentiation of the various forms of encephalitis and encephalomyelitis is probably the most difficult task presented to the clinician. Accurate diagnosis requires the use of laboratory procedures – virus neutralisation, ELISA, mouse inoculation tests.

**J.** Carcase and viscera:

Horses: Clinical cases, T Reactors, L or Kh and D (blood).

Pigs: L or Kh and D (blood, brain, genital organs).

## LUMPY SKIN DISEASE (LSD) (Plate 1, Fig. 1)

**I.** A highly infectious viral disease of cattle in which round, firm nodules appear on the skin and sometimes in the nares, turbinate bones, mouth, muzzle and the mucosae of the respiratory, alimentary and genital tracts.

Notifiable disease (UK).

**O.** At present lumpy skin disease appears to be confined to Africa, except for Lebanon where it is known to exist although the distribution and occurrence are unknown. Lumpy skin disease is enzootic in Rwanda and Zambia and of high occurrence in Réunion and Tanzania. Israel, Congo and Côte d'Ivoire had their last cases in 1989 and Egypt and Sudan in 1990.

**IA.** A capripoxvirus, the Neethling poxvirus, which is related to the virus of sheep and goat pox.

**R.** Infected and carrier animals and probably buffaloes. Native breeds like the Zebu cattle are more resistant than European breeds and probably also act as carriers.

**MT.** Infection is probably transmitted by biting insects, mainly mosquitoes and midges, although the disease has apparently occurred where insects have been absent. Contact spread is also probable since saliva, nasal and lachrymal discharges, semen and milk contain the virus.

**CF.** The nodules are raised, round, circumscribed (1–4 cm in diameter), firm and painful. Most disappear quickly but those which persist remain as hard nodules for years or develop yellowish or greyish necrotic centres with sloughing of the overlying skin. The regional lymph nodes are enlarged and oedema is present on the ventral abdomen, udder and legs.

General symptoms vary from peracute to mild, even inapparent. Fever, depression, inappetence, rhinitis, conjunctivitis and lachrymation are evident. Severely affected animals quickly lose condition. The mortality is usually low – less than 2%, with morbidity 5–50%.

Losses are occasioned by reduced body weight and milk yield and hide damage.

**P.** See **I** and **CF**.

**D.** The type of skin lesions and their sudden appearance makes the diagnosis relatively easy, but lumpy skin disease has to be differentiated from pseudo-lumpy skin disease due to a herpes-virus, rinderpest, bluetongue, pox and contagious ecthyma.

**J.** Carcase and viscera: T, where systemic changes are present. A or Kh, absence of general signs and condition good.

## NAIROBI SHEEP DISEASE (NSD)

**I.** An infectious highly fatal, viral disease of sheep and goats transmitted by ticks and characterised by dysentery and abortion in pregnant ewes.

Man can be affected with a mild form of the disease.

**O.** Although the disease has occurred in Kenya, Rwanda, Burundi, Zaire and Somalia, Tanzania and Uganda, recent information indicates that it is now confined to Somalia.

**IA.** A bunyavirus of the genus Nairovirus.

**R.** Infected and carrier sheep, goats, wild ruminants and certain ticks.

**MT.** The virus is transmitted by the ticks *Rhipicephalus appendiculatus*, *R. pulchellus* and *Amblyomma variegatum*, all stages of which can be infective.

**CF.** After an incubation period of 1–2 weeks, fever develops with mucopurulent, blood-stained nasal discharge, depression, inappetence and dysentery. Pregnant animals may abort. Mortality may be as high as 90% in sheep but goats are more resistant.

**P.** Haemorrhagic gastroenteritis, especially severe in the caecum and colon, enlargement of abdominal lymphoid tissues (spleen, lymph nodes, Peyers patches, etc.) and petechiation of endocardium and epicardium.

**D.** Symptoms and lesions are suggestive of Nairobi disease but it must be differentiated from heartwater by isolation of the virus (immunodiffusion test, mouse inoculation, hamster kidney cell culture, etc.).

**J.** Carcase and viscera: T, severe clinical disease. Kh and D, no systemic changes and carcase, drug and bacteria-free.

## OVINE ENCEPHALOMYELITIS (LOUPING ILL)

**I.** An acute viral disease of the central nervous system of sheep transmitted by ticks.

The disease also occasionally affects goats, cattle, pigs, horses, deer, dogs and man.

**O.** Originally thought to be confined to southern Scotland, Louping Ill has now been confirmed in England, Ireland, Norway, Spain, Bulgaria and Turkey.

**IA.** A virus of the Flaviviridae family closely related to a group of viruses transmitted by ticks and primarily associated with human encephalitis.

**R.** Infected and carrier sheep, horses, grouse and ticks (in salivary glands), the latter having the ability to carry the virus to the following year.

**MT.** Infection is transmitted by the bite of the nymphal and adult stages of the three-host tick *Ixodes ricinus*, which is most commonly found on rough hill pastures. Infection can also be spread by contaminated equipment, e.g. hypodermic needles, and possibly by droplet infection.

**CF.** Louping ill occurs mainly in the spring and autumn when ticks are active. After inoculation by an infected tick, the virus replicates in lymphoid tissues and produces a viraemia which lasts up to a week. High fever ensues but CNS signs only appear after the virus enters the brain. These take the form of depression, muscular tremors, twitching lips and nostrils, ataxia with a jerky gait, head pressing, torticollis, hyperaesthesia, convulsions, collapse and death in a few days. Mild cases may recover but others, especially young lambs, may die suddenly without showing nervous symptoms.

**P.** No gross changes are evident. Pneumonia may be present as a complication. Histopathological examination of the brain reveals a non-suppurative polioencephalomyelitis.

**D.** The seasonal occurrence of the disease, the nervous symptoms and the presence of ticks on rough upland pastures point to louping ill.

Confirmation of diagnosis can only be confirmed by laboratory methods – virus isolation, mouse inoculation, serum neutralisation, etc., are necessary since histopathological changes are not specific for louping ill.

**J.** Carcase and viscera: A and D, provided no general changes present. T or Kh, provided condition good, drug and bacteria-free.

## OVINE PROGRESSIVE PNEUMONIA (MAEDI, MAEDI-VISNA, LA BOUHITE, GRAFF–REINERT DISEASE, LAIKIPIA LUNG DISEASE)

**I.** A chronic, viral disease of sheep and goats manifested by progressive pneumonia, arthritis, mastitis (*maedi* syndrome) and on occasions, acute encephalomyelitis (*visna* syndrome).

**O.** Maedi and maedi-visna are limited to Canada (where they are of high occurrence), Europe and South Africa, where they were first recorded, along with the USA. It is of low sporadic occurrence in many European countries but was eradicated from Iceland in 1965 and no longer occurs in the USA. Asian countries, South America and Oceania are currently free of the disease.

Caprine arthritis-encephalitis of goats is caused by a similar retrovirus and exhibits symptoms similar to those of maedi-visna.

**IA.** Retroviruses of the family Lentovirinae which persist in WBCs and are able to produce proliferation in lungs, joints, udder, brain and lymphoid tissues.

**R.** Infected and carrier sheep.

**MT.** By ingestion of colostrum containing the virus, by inhalation of aerosol droplets or by intrauterine transmission.

**CF.** The incubation period is long and may extend to several years, the disease being uncommon in animals less than 2 years of age.

In the *maedi* syndrome there is a progressive loss of condition with listlessness, dyspnoea, coughing with copious bronchial exudate and non-inflammatory mastitis.

The *visna* syndrome is distinguished by the appearance of nervous symptoms in the form of ataxia, muscle tremors, paresis and eventual paralysis. Arthritis is also present.

Except in very young lambs and kids, the development of symptoms is slow and progressive.

**P.** The lungs exhibit pneumonia with marked consolidation and hyperplasia of interlobular tissues and are very firm and heavy. The associated lymph nodes (bronchial, mediastinal and retropharyngeal) are enlarged and oedematous and lymphoid hyperplasia of tissues other than the lymph nodes is evident in the thoracic cavity.

The mastitis is of a non-inflammatory type, the udder being very indurated.

The CNS lesions take the form of an encephalomyelitis which apart from some superficial inflammation, requires histopathology for diagnosis.

**D.** The progressive nature of the disease, clinical signs and PM lesions may point to maedi-visna but laboratory procedures – complement fixation, agar gel immunodiffusion and ELISA tests – and histopathology are necessary for an accurate diagnosis.

**J.** Carcase and viscera: T or A, depending on extent of lesions and condition of carcase.

## PAPILLOMATOSIS (WARTS)

**I.** A viral disease of cattle and horses (and less commonly sheep, goats, deer, dogs, birds, fish, and man) in which papillomas or warts develop as benign tumours on the skin of any part of the body but mostly the head, neck, shoulders, back, abdomen, vulva, penis and prepuce.

**O.** Worldwide.

**IA.** Papillomaviruses, of which several distinct types have been identified, all responsible for different types of warts and all host-specific. In cattle there are five types and in man up to 20.

**R.** Infected animals, clinical and subclinical, and possibly insects.

**MT.** The virus gains entry to the epidermis through cuts and abrasions by direct and indirect contact with infected animals and their fomites. On occasions infection has been introduced through the use of infected equipment, e.g. tattooing and dehorning instruments, metal ear tags, etc. The actual warts themselves are infectious by contact.

**CF.** The type, site and duration of the warts depend on the specific virus involved. All are actual outgrowths of the epidermis.

Papillomas vary in size from tiny, diffuse elevations to large pedunculated growths. Shape also varies, some being flattened while others are elongated and some cauliflower-like in appearance. The small forms, common in horses, tend to be multiple and the large fibropapillomas, usually found in cattle, single in occurrence. All are self-limiting with recovery usually within 6 months. Some, however, especially those in the urinary (e.g. bladder), genital and gastrointestinal tracts (which are often associated with bracken poisoning), may persist for long periods, causing great loss of condition. Such cases, along with warts on the penis and in the vulva and vagina, justify casualty slaughter.

In horses, warts are usually numerous and small in size and affect all ages, while cattle tend to have single larger forms. Sheep, goats and pigs are less commonly affected, but warts may occur on the udder and teats of goats and may progress to malignant squamous cell carcinomas.

Although papillomas are usually sporadic entities, outbreaks have occurred where large numbers of cattle – even up to 75% – may be involved in a herd.

**P.** See **CF**. The actual warts in the early stages are round and smooth but become rough and keratinised later. They actually consist of a very thickened stratum spinosum of the epidermis in which fibrous tissue occurs, especially in cattle.

**D.** Diagnosis is fairly straightforward except in equidae where the lesions may be confused with *sarcoid*, the most common form of neoplasm in this species. Equine sarcoids possess some malignancy and may be present anywhere on the body but are most common on the penis and limbs. They may be wart-like, fibroblastic, simulating granulation tissue and sessile or flat.

**J.** Papillomatosis is of little meat hygiene significance except when complications occur with the internal forms and when condition is lost in severe and long-standing cases. The value of hides and skins is reduced.

Carcase and viscera: A, provided no systemic changes and condition good, or I and D.

## PESTE DES PETITS RUMINANTS (PPR, PEST OF SMALL RUMINANTS, GOAT PLAGUE, KATA)

**I.** An acute or subacute viral disease of goats and sheep and some wild ruminants, resembling rinderpest and characterised by necrotic stomatitis, gastroenteritis and pneumonia.

Notifiable disease (UK).

**O.** The disease at present is confined to Africa (where it is of low sporadic occurrence in many countries but has a high prevalence in Ghana and Senegal) and the Middle East (Lebanon, Oman and United Arab Emirates).

**IA.** A morbillivirus of the family Paramyxoviridae which has an affinity for lymphoid tissue and the epithelium of the gastrointestinal tract. It is related to the morbillivirus of rinderpest.

**R.** Infected goats and sheep and wild ruminants and their excretions, secretions and fomites. A carrier state does not exist but subclinical cases may spread the disease during the incubation period.

**MT.** By inhalation, and via the conjunctiva and buccal mucosa. Direct and indirect contact with the reservoir of infection.

**CF.** Clinical signs, which are usually subacute in sheep, include fever, depression, anorexia, nasal discharge, at first serous, later becoming mucopurulent, catarrhal conjunctivitis with matting of the eyelids and profuse diarrhoea which may be mucoid and blood-stained. A secondary pneumonia with coughing often develops. Abortion is common in pregnant animals. Emaciation is prominent in long-standing cases. Death may take place in 1–2 weeks.

**P.** Stomatitis with shallow necrotic lesions inside lower lip, under surface of tongue and on cheeks and gums. The hard palate and pharynx may also show lesions. Similar erosions occur in the forestomachs, small and large intestine, even extending to the rectum, Peyer's patches being severely affected. The ileo-caecal junction and the rectum often show characteristic '*zebra stripes*' due to congestion of the folds of the mucosa.

There is lymphadenitis of the retropharyngeal and mesenteric lymph nodes and the spleen is often enlarged.

A lobar pneumonia affecting the cardiac and apical lobes, particularly on the right side is present. Should complications develop, this pneumonia becomes bronchopneumonic in type.

**D.** A presumptive diagnosis is based on clinical signs, history (especially where new stock have been recently introduced) but virus isolation and identification by complement fixation, agar-gel precipitin or virus-neutralising tests are necessary to distinguish PPR from contagious caprine pleuropneumonia, contagious ecthyma, heartwater, coccidiosis, pasteurellosis and rinderpest.

**J.** Carcase and viscera: T or A or Kh with D depending on systemic changes and carcase condition.

## POX DISEASES (VARIOLAE)

**I.** Peracute, acute, subacute or benign highly contagious viral diseases of animals (excluding dogs), non-human primates, birds and man characterised by typical vesicular eruptions on the skin (and mucous membranes in sheep and goat pox).

The lesions commence as *macules* (discoloured spots) which progress to *papules* (small, solid, circumscribed elevations), then *vesicles* (small sacs containing fluid) and finally *pustules*, which erupt forming crusts.

The pox diseases affect many different species of animals and man (smallpox or variola major and alastrim or variola minor) – sheep and goats (Plate 2, Fig. 11), cows, horses, pigs, camels, rabbits and poultry.

Sheeppox and goatpox are serious and often fatal conditions in which infection is transmitted by inhalation, by direct contact and possibly by biting insects. The other pox diseases are benign in nature, immunologically distinct from sheeppox and goatpox and spread by direct contact only.

## SHEEPPOX AND GOATPOX

Notifiable diseases (UK).

**O.** These diseases are at present confined to Africa, Middle East and parts of Asia. They have a high occurrence in Gambia, Mali, Niger and Senegal and are enzootic in Ethiopia, Iran, Lebanon, Turkey, Yemen, Pakistan and Afghanistan. Mongolia had its last case in 1977 and China in 1989. Europe appears to be free at present.

An outbreak of sheep and goatpox occurred in Greece in 1994.

**IA.** Capripoxviruses of the family Poxviridae. The sheeppox virus (SPV) affects only sheep while the goatpox virus (SGPV) affects both sheep and goats, the two viruses being antigenically distinct.

**R.** Infected animals and their fomites.

**MT.** See above under **I**.

**CF.** The incubation period is about 4–14 days, after which there is severe systemic reaction with fever, depression, inappetence, mucopurulent discharges from nose and eyes and salivation, with up to 80% mortality in the acute form. The lesions described above may be found on any part of the body but most commonly on the muzzle, ears and parts devoid of wool and hair. A benign form of the disease exhibits only skin lesions and without systemic disturbance. As fever regresses, the pustules become covered with exudate and finally scabs which darken in colour and are very irritant, making the animal scratch intensely. Star-shaped scar formation takes place after scabs are shed.

The condition in goats is more severe than that in sheep.

**P.** In addition to the skin lesions described above, changes may also occur in the form of white pocks in soft viscera and lungs. On mucous membranes the lesions are ulcerated and a haemorrhagic enteritis may be present in severe cases.

**D.** The skin lesions associated with systemic changes are strongly suggestive of sheeppox and goatpox.

*Differential diagnoses* include contagious pustular dermatitis, bluetongue, mange, cutaneous streptothricosis.

**J.** Carcase and viscera: T or Kh or L with D depending on presence/absence of systemic changes, body condition.

Recovered cases: A and D.

In Britain carcases intended for human consumption may be removed from an infected place only if they are certified free from sheeppox/goatpox and after the skin has been removed; an affected carcase must be burned or buried in a manner similar to one affected with FMD.

## COWPOX (VACCINIA, VARIOLOVACCINIA)

Cowpox is a rare, mild contagious disease of dairy cows in which lesions appear on the udder, teats and sometimes the perineum, thighs, vulva and mouth. Calves may show lesions on the lips and mouth and bulls on the scrotum. A sporadic infection, it may affect virtually all animals in a herd.

The causal cowpox virus is related antigenically to the smallpox virus and is identical to that causing horsepox.

Cowpox has only been reported in western Europe and is becoming less common. Infection is spread during milking and milkers may acquire infection on the hands and arms and sometimes the face, along with mild fever and lymphadenitis.

## PSEUDO-COWPOX (MILKER'S NODULE, PARAVACCINIA)

This is a very common, benign condition occurring worldwide caused by a parapoxvirus which is related to that of bovine papular stomatitis and contagious ecthyma.

Lesions begin as small papules or vesicles on the udder and teats of dairy cows. Scab formation quickly develops, with granulation tissue under the scabs. This heals from the centre, producing a circular ring of small scabs which persists for several months.

Spread through the herd is slower than in cowpox and, as with the latter, milkers' hands may be infected with itchy, red nodules which heal spontaneously in a few weeks.

## SWINEPOX

In this disease, typical pox lesions appear on the abdomen, sometimes the sides of the body, and may actually involve the whole body surface. Unlike the other pox conditions, the lesions rarely proceed beyond the vesicle stage, but scabs do form with eventual healing.

The cause is a suipoxvirus of the family Poxviridae.

The disease occurs in the USA, especially in the mid-west, where 1–5% of pig herds may be affected at any one time, especially during the summer months. It also occurs in South America (Chile, Uruguay) and some African countries.

Transmission is by contact with infected animals, by wounds and by the bites of the pig louse, *Haematopinus suis*.

## HORSEPOX

A very rare, benign pox disease of horses which at the moment appears to be confined to Panama and Mozambique.

Two forms of the disease are recognised – a *buccal* form in which typical pox lesions appear in the mouth, pharynx, nostrils and larynx and a *leg* form in which the pasterns and fetlocks are affected. Lameness along with fever and salivation may be present, but the condition is usually self-limiting and clears up in a month or so.

### Judgement of cowpox, horsepox and swinepox

Carcase and viscera: A or L with D.

## PULMONARY ADENOMATOSIS (DRIVING DISEASE, JAAGSIEKTE, OVINE PULMONARY CARCINOMA)

**I.** A contagious, viral, usually fatal, disease of adult sheep, and less commonly goats, in which chronic pneumonia with adenocarcinoma are manifested.

**O.** Jaagsiekte occurs throughout the world except Australia and New Zealand. It is enzootic in Peru and of low sporadic occurrence in many European countries including the United Kingdom. Iceland had its last case in 1952, Yemen in 1968, Uruguay in 1982, Romania in 1987 and Spain in 1990.

**IA.** Probably a retrovirus.

**R.** Infected and carrier sheep and goats.

**MT.** Natural transmission is by the respiratory route.

**CF.** The incubation period is long (1–3 years), resulting in clinical signs occurring when sheep are 3–4 years of age.

Respiratory involvement appears as increasing dyspnoea and a watery nasal discharge which is accompanied by marked loss of condition. Fever is absent and there is no loss of appetite. Death, from congestive heart failure or coincident pasteurellosis, usually ensues in 2–5 months.

**P.** Lesions are confined to the thoracic cavity. In addition to lobar pneumonia, the enlarged lungs exhibit firm, greyish areas of neoplastic tissue (adenocarcinoma). Some of these may be small, discrete foci while others are extensive lesions, all demarcated from the lung tissue. The trachea and bronchioles contain large amounts of white, frothy fluid and the mediastinal and bronchial lymph nodes are enlarged and may contain metastases of the tumour.

**D.** The clinical signs in adult sheep, and especially the lesions, are indicative of pulmonary adenomatosis.

*Differential diagnoses* include maedi-visna and pasteurellosis.

Diagnosis is confirmed by histopathological examination of the neoplastic tissue, there being at present no available serological tests.

**J.** Carcase and viscera: T or A or L with D.

## RABIES (HYDROPHOBIA, LYSSA)

**I.** An acute, fatal viral infection of all warm-blooded animals and man transmitted by the saliva via bites of rabid animals and characterised by nervous symptoms and ascending paralysis.

Notifiable disease in all countries.

Rabies occurs throughout the world, with an estimated 30 000 human deaths per annum. It is enzootic in animals in many African, Asian and South American countries and of high occurrence in Angola, Mali, Senegal, Tanzania, Uganda, Bolivia, Ecuador, Guatemala, India, Pakistan, Mexico, Bhutan, Cambodia and Yemen. The disease is enzootic in the eastern and southern states of the USA.

Many countries in all four continents are now free of rabies as a result of successful eradication measures. Australia had its last case in 1867, Republic of Ireland in 1903, N. Ireland in 1923 and Britain in 1970.

Rabies has never been reported in many countries, many of them island communities, which possess rigid quarantine regulations. Included are New Zealand, Mauritius, Bahamas, Bermuda, Jamaica, St Vincent Grenadines, Cyprus, Finland, Greece, Sweden, Eire, Singapore, Iceland, Isle of Man, Fiji, Hawaii Oceania and Norway.

Other regulations, in addition to *quarantine*, proposed by WHO for *control of dogs* include notification of suspected cases; destruction of infected animals, those bitten by rabid or suspect dogs and unvaccinated animals; leashing and muzzling; control of movement; control of stray dogs; mass immunisation and dog registration.

On the other hand, rabies has become a serious threat in Europe where it has spread westward, mainly by infected red foxes (300–400 cases annually) in wooded areas, and is now a problem in France, Germany, Austria, Czechoslovakia, Estonia, Hungary, Latvia, Poland and Lithuania. The migration of foxes has also been responsible for the spread of rabies southward in Canada, where wolves, skunks and bats also act as reservoirs, while in the USA skunks, racoons and coyotes spread the disease. The jackal is a common reservoir in the Middle East.

In addition to foxes, vampire, frugivorous and insectivorous bats have been responsible for causing bovine rabies in Mexico, Central and South America and in South Africa mongooses have a high incidence of rabies. In recent years rabies virus has been isolated from insectivorous bats in Denmark and Germany. In May 1996 a Daubenton's bat (*Myotis daubentoni*) which had bitten two women in Newhaven, England, was found to be infected with the rabies virus (lyssavirus 2, ELB 2). As a precaution, prophylactic treatment (immunoglobulin injected into the wound followed by six subcutaneous injections of vaccine in the upper arm) was given to the women. The case was regarded as an isolated one, the bat probably having flown across the English Channel, although this species of bat can be found in the United Kingdom. Bat rabies is endemic in France, Germany, Denmark, Holland and Spain and has caused two deaths in humans, the most recent being in Finland in 1985.

A UK Ministry of Agriculture surveillance programme since 1987 in which 2000 bats were tested for rabies virus gave negative reactions in all of them.

In the second quarter (April to June) of 1996, WHO reported 2035 cases of rabies in Europe (including non-EU countries), of which 1373 (67.5%) were in wild animals and 660 (32.4%) in domestic animals.

The *wild animals* included 1151 foxes, 53 raccoon dogs, 19 badgers, 31 roe deer, 33 reindeer, 24 pine martens, 14 stone martens, 9 polecats, 5 hares, 5 bats, 4 squirrels, 2 black rats, 2 musk vats, 2 wolves and a single case in a lynx, aretic fox, ferret, red deer, wild boar and hedgehog.

The *domestic animals* included 298 dogs, 144 cats, 158 bovines, 28 sheep, 24 horses, 1 donkey, 2 pigs and 5 goats (35 of the dog cases occurred in Turkey). Four cases of bat rabies occurred in Germany and one in England (see above).

It is remarkable that, with numerous wild and domestic animal cases in Europe, few human cases occur. There were, however, two human cases in the Russian Federation and one in Germany (imported from Sri Lanka).

**IA.** A rhabdovirus of the genus Lyssavirus, of which there are four serotypes, serotype 1 being responsible for classical animal and human rabies. Serotypes 2, 3 and 4 are antigenically related but rarely cause serious infection. Serotype 4 has been identified in European bats.

Rabies virus resembles that of vesicular stomatitis. It is one of the largest viruses, being 75–80 nm in width and up to 180 nm long.

**R.** See **O**. The predominant animal species responsible for maintaining the virus varies in different parts of the world. Canine or urban rabies is transmitted by dogs, while sylvatic rabies is a disease of wild carnivores and bats, with sporadic spillover into dogs, cats and domestic animals.

Mass oral rabies vaccination, using attenuated live virus vaccines in baits such as chicken heads, fish meal, polymer, etc., and directed mainly at foxes and other wild carnivores, was introduced in Europe (1978) by WHO and followed by Canada and USA. The European programme covers 300 000 km$^2$ in ten countries – Austria, Belgium, Czech Republic, France, Germany, Italy, Poland, Slovakia, Slovenia and Switzerland. Manual distribution at predetermined points is now mainly practised, although small helicopters are used in some countries. The programme is showing success and is constantly the subject of research.

In 1986 the world's first controlled field trials of rabies vaccines contained in baits for free-roaming dogs was launched. These dogs cannot easily be immunised by injection.

It is confidently hoped that by using all these strategies rabies will be eliminated from most European countries within the next few years. Many types of rabies vaccine are now available for the different species – (Human Diploid Cell Rabies Vaccine (HDCV) and Rabies Vaccine, Adsorbed (RVA)), both inactivated vaccines, for human beings and inactivated oral SAG2, SAD B19, RV675, etc., vaccines for dogs. In some endemic areas, e.g. Central and South America vaccination of cattle is practised to protect against infection by vampire bats.

**MT.** Rabies is almost always transmitted by the bite of an infected animal via the saliva, which contains large amounts of the virus. Less commonly, the virus may gain entrance through abrasions and cuts on the skin and buccal mucosa. Inhalation is also a possibility in certain instances, e.g. bat-infested caves.

Multiplication of the virus occurs at the site of inoculation (in muscle or mucous cells), after which it travels via the peripheral nerves to the spinal cord and then the brain.

**CF.** The *incubation period* is very variable, in some cases being as short as 21 days and others as long as 6 months and longer. (A 6-month quarantine cannot be relied upon to give protection since rabies occurred in two dogs in quarantine in Britain (1970) following an incubation period believed to be 7–9 months.) Most cases of canine rabies are said to develop within 3–12 weeks.

In all species, two forms of rabies are recognised – paralytic and furious – which follow a short prodromal period.

In the *paralytic form*, clinical signs include incoordination, paralysis of the throat, inability to swallow, salivation, drooping of lower jaw, straining to defaecate and urinate, eventual total body paralysis, coma and death in a few hours.

The *furious form* of rabies – the so-called 'mad-dog syndrome' – is manifested by mania and aggression after a period of melancholy which lasts one or two days. Symptoms are very variable, especially in animals other than dogs and cats. Anxiety, alertness, hyperaesthesia and aggression are prominent. Dogs will attack other animals, people and moving objects, wander, and chew and swallow foreign objects, even the wire of cages to the extent of breaking teeth. Natural fear is lost. Muscular seizures and incoordination ensue with eventual paralysis after one or two days of mania with death in a few hours.

Cattle tend to bellow hoarsely, become dangerous and will pursue and attack human beings and other animals and sometimes show sexual excitement.

Horses and mules have been observed to display symptoms simulating spasmodic colic, incoordination, hyperaesthesia, lower jaw rigidity, biting at the near knee, throwing the body forcibly down on the off side but no aggression, biting or kicking (Gracey, unpublished). Some cases, however, bite and kick viciously.

Pigs are inclined to be aggressive and excitable and exhibit salivation, convulsions and paralysis but, like horses, can display many different signs.

Affected cats and foxes are aggressive and attack and scratch viciously. Foxes and skunks will attack large animals like cattle and have been known to invade houses and attack human beings.

**P.** Apart from self-inflicted wounds and the presence of foreign bodies in the stomach, especially in dogs and cats, there are no gross lesions. The lesions of rabies are microscopic and limited to the CNS, where they may be indiscernible except for some meningeal and cerebral congestion.

Microscopic examination shows some diffuse encephalitis in the form of perivascular cuffing, necrosis of neurons and the presence of cytoplasmic inclusion bodies (Negri bodies), especially in the hippocampus, brainstem and gasserian ganglia.

**D.** Diagnosis of clinical signs, especially in the early stages, is frequently very difficult as rabies can be confused with many other nervous diseases such as lactation tetany, polioencephalomalacia, lead poisoning, listeriosis, louping ill, enterotoxaemia, Aujeszky's disease, Teschen disease, Glasser's disease, African swine fever and various forms of meningitis.

A common early symptom in the dog is an inability to swallow, giving the impression of an obstruction in the throat or between the teeth or of tenderness in the mouth.

Since human beings may be exposed to infection, it is vital that an accurate diagnosis is made as quickly as possible. The importance of an accurate diagnosis cannot be overstressed because of the risk of human exposure and the necessity for prophylactic treatment which, in itself, is psychologically very traumatic.

If the animal is rabid, it will die. The brain is then carefully removed using rubber gloves and goggles and placed in ice. If a delay is anticipated, half of the brain should be put in 10% formalin and half in 50% glycerine.

## Tests

The simplest test is the demonstration of typical Negri inclusion bodies following the staining of impression smears or sections of brain tissue (especially of the hippocampus of the dog and Purkinje cells in herbivores) with Sellers.

Mouse inoculation tests may be used where Negri bodies cannot be demonstrated in some cases.

The fluorescent antibody test using fresh, frozen or glycerolated brain or salivary tissue is now the diagnostic method of choice.

**J.** Carcase and viscera: T.

(It has been recommended (Codex Alimentarius Commission, Alinorm 9316A) that the carcases of food animals slaughtered within 48 h of being bitten can be approved (L) as fit for human consumption and condemnation of the bite area with surroundings and distribution restricted to limited areas. Special precautions are to be taken to prevent occupational hazards. Alternatively, slaughter may be delayed during an extended quarantine period to permit confirmation.)

## Control

Various measures are in force in different countries depending on factors such as rabies-free status, geographical position (e.g. whether an island), threat posed from rabies-endemic areas, convention, etc.

*European Union*: Dogs, cats and other pets travelling from rabies-free countries to other countries, rabies-free or not, have no restrictions. Pets from other countries require prior vaccination (within 30 days and 1 year).

*Norway and Sweden*: Previous strict quarantine regulations are now replaced by a 'passport' system: Microchip or tattoo identification of dogs and cats; effective vaccination; residence in a EU/EFTA country for the preceding 12 months; at least 4 months after vaccination, a blood sample must show an antibody titre (REFIT) of at least 0.5 i.u/ml which for animals previously immunised can be measured 1 month after vaccination; quarantine for all animals failing tests and those from non-EU/EFTA countries not rabies-free.

The Norwegian and Swedish system (which is said to operate very efficiently) is currently being advocated by some authorities to replace the present UK regulations, which require 6 months' quarantine with vaccination on entry and revaccination after 14 days.

## RIFT VALLEY FEVER (INFECTIOUS ENZOOTIC HEPATITIS OF CATTLE AND SHEEP, RVF)

**I.** An acute, infectious, viral disease of ruminants (mostly sheep) and man transmitted by mosquitoes in which focal hepatic necrosis is a prominent feature.

Notifiable disease (UK).

**O.** The disease is confined to Africa at present but, being an insect-borne entity, has a potential for spread outside this continent. Rift Valley fever occurs in several central African countries. It appeared for the first time in West Africa in 1987 and stimulated much research on epidemiology, surveillance, diagnostics and animal and human vaccine production.

RVF was recognised in Egypt in 1993 in animals and human beings after an absence of 12 years. In this outbreak in the Aswan Governate an abnormally high number of abortions occurred in cattle and water buffalo. Only ocular forms of RVF in man were reported, but of 676 humans tested, 41 (6.1%) were positive for RVFV-specific IgM.

**IA.** A phlebovirus of the family Bunyaviridae which can remain viable for a considerable time in the eggs of the mosquito *Aedes lineatopinnus* and possibly other biting flies. The virus is easily inactivated by acid conditions.

**R.** Primary vertebrate reservoirs are not known but may be various wild ruminants, the virus being supported by various species of biting flies and rodents.

**MT.** Several species of mosquitoes of the genera *Aedes* and *Culex* and possibly midges of the genus *Culicoides* and sandflies (*Phlebotomus* spp.).

Infection in man occurs through skin abrasions and by inhalation from infected animals, their excretions and secretions and fomites.

**CF.** The disease occurs during warm, wet weather when biting insects are active. Symptoms include rapid onset, high fever, leukopenia, inappetence, depression, incoordination, collapse and death in 1–2 days in young animals, which may suffer up to 90% mortality. Adult animals appear to be more resistant, with symptoms less severe and the death rate lower. Pregnant animals abort. Abortion and diarrhoea may be the only signs present in adults, in which infection may pass unnoticed.

In man an influenza-like fever develops with myalgia, arthralgia, headache, chills and ocular lesions in which retinal haemorrhage takes place.

**P.** The characteristic lesion is a focal necrosis of the liver, large diffuse, greyish lesions being present in lambs and discrete foci in adult animals. The liver is enlarged and yellowish or brownish in colour and shows haemorrhages in the parenchyma, haemorrhages being also present on the body serous surfaces, heart and skin.

**D.** Rift valley fever should be suspected during warm, wet weather where mortality rates are high in young animals (under 1 week), with abortions and stillbirths in adults and all showing characteristic liver changes. Mild fevers in stockmen, veterinarians, etc., assist in the diagnosis.

Diagnosis is confirmed by virus isolation and identification using mice or cell cultures. Histopathology of liver sections may be performed to identify cell necrosis and acidophilic inclusion bodies. Differential diagnoses include bluetongue, ephemeral fever, Nairobi sheep disease and Wesselbron disease. The latter affects sheep and wild ruminants and is caused by a flavivirus transmitted by culicine mosquitoes. It presents much the same symptoms and lesions as RVF and can only effectively be distinguished by serology.

**J.** Carcase and viscera: T. A and D with condemnation of liver and blood. Reactors only.

## RINDERPEST (CATTLE PLAGUE)

**I.** A peracute to mild, highly contagious, viral disease of all cloven-footed animals, domestic and wild.

Notifiable disease (UK).

**O.** Cattle plague, at one time a terrible scourge of livestock in Africa, south America, Asia and Europe, is now confined to Africa (Djibouti, Ethiopia and Uganda), Asia (India and Sri Lanka) and the Middle East (Saudi Arabia, Oman and Yemen), where it still causes epizootics.

Europe is completely free and much of the New World has never experienced the disease. Effective control measures (movement control, quarantine, disease surveillance, prevention of feeding of uncooked swill, vaccination, etc.) have dramatically eradicated the disease in many countries – as long ago as 1770 in Sweden, 1772 in Denmark, 1870 in Holland, 1875 in Switzerland and 1877 in the United Kingdom.

**IA.** A morbillivirus of the family Paramyxoviridae with many strains and degrees of virulence. It is related to the virus of peste des petits ruminants, canine distemper and human measles.

The virus is not very resistant and cannot survive for long outside the host. It is rapidly inactivated by sunlight and heat, being inactivated in dried secretions in 24–28 h and in salted raw hides in 48 h. At temperatures of 25.5°C and over it does not persist in muscle and offal for longer than 10 days but can remain viable for 1 year in frozen and chilled carcases. The greatest danger arises from lymphoid tissues such as bone marrow and lymph nodes where virus concentration is highest.

**R.** Infected animals, domestic and wild. A carrier state apparently does not exist.

**MT.** The virus is present in all excretions and secretions and is transmitted by ingestion or inhalation. Since the virus does not survive for long outside the body, close contact between animals is required for infection to take place. Contaminated food and water are other vehicles of infection but insects do not appear to be involved.

Following entry via the nasopharynx, the virus multiplies first in the retropharyngeal lymph nodes and tonsillar tissue and then spreads by a viraemia to the lymphoid tissues of the gastrointestinal and respiratory tracts, causing extensive tissue damage.

**CF.** Susceptibility varies greatly among the various species of animals – high in African buffalo, wild pigs, antelopes, giraffes, Ankole cattle, Channel Island and other introduced breeds; moderate in wildebeest and zebu and mild in gazelles, domestic pigs, sheep and goats.

Following an incubation period of 3–15 days, clinical cases may be peracute, acute, subacute or subclinical. Peracute cases exhibit sudden onset of fever, collapse and death in a few days.

*Acute* cases show the more typical signs of fever, depression, inappetence, ocular and nasal discharges, at first serous but later mucopurulent, congested mucosae, dyspnoea, dehydration and bloody/mucoid diarrhoea. The mucosal lesions are evident in the mouth, dental pad, undersurface of tongue, hard palate, lips, vulva and vagina and take the form of small necrotic pinpoint foci which enlarge and coalesce with desquamation of the epithelium, leaving red, shallow erosions. Pregnant animals abort. Most cases die in 1–2 weeks. Morbidity may be as high as 100% and mortality 90% in severe outbreaks.

*Subacute* cases occur in animals with innate resistance where the disease is endemic, acutely affected animals being found in places originally free of the disease. These subacute cases show mild fever, transient diarrhoea, dyspnoea and skin lesions in the form of macules/papules/scab formation on the udder, perineum and scrotum. Most subacute cases recover.

**P.** Lesions vary according to the severity of the disease.

Most carcases are dehydrated and emaciated, especially where the disease has persisted for some time. Lesions are mostly limited to the alimentary tract from the mouth and pharynx to the anus.

The buccal mucosa is congested and covered with soft, greyish, necrotic plaques which look like sprinkled bran. These plaques often coalesce into a soft, cheesy mass which sloughs, leaving erosions with ragged edges.

The necrotic process is also evident in the abomasum (which may also show petechiae) and intestine along with a haemorrhagic mucosa. Where the transverse furrows alone are inflamed or petechiated, the mucous membrane presents a typical *'tiger skin'* appearance. Similar haemorrhagic/necrotic changes affect the vagina, vulva and prepuce. The turbinate bones and nasal septa are congested and covered with a thick, tenacious mucopurulent discharge. Epicardial and endocardial haemorrhages are often present in peracute cases.

**D.** Rinderpest is suspected where recent animal movements have occurred and where fever and a highly infectious disease has occurred with erosive alimentary changes.

Confirmation of diagnosis is based on isolation and identification of the virus and identification of specific antigens.

*Differential diagnoses* include haemorrhagic septicaemia, FMD, bovine malignant catarrh, bovine virus diarrhoea, bluetongue, Nairobi sheep disease and peste des petits ruminants.

**J.** Carcase and viscera: T. L and D, subacute cases in endemic areas. Without general carcase changes. Distribution limited to areas affected by outbreak and covered by vaccination, Kh if economically feasible.

## SCRAPIE (RIDA, TREMBLANTE DU MOUTON) (Plate 1, Fig. 2)

**I.** A progressive, non-febrile, fatal disease of the CNS of adult sheep and goats characterised by a long incubation period, pruritus and abnormal gait.

It is one of the so-called transmissible spongiform encephalopathies similar to bovine spongiform encephalopathy (BSE) (q.v.), transmissible mink encephalopathy (TME), chronic wasting disease of mule deer and elk and Creutzfeld–Jakob disease, Gerstmann–Straussler–Scheinker syndrome and Kuru of man.

**O.** Scrapie is now limited to Europe (UK, Ireland, Belgium, Czechoslovakia, Iceland, Norway), Cyprus, Canada and USA. Except for South Africa (last case 1972), it has not occurred in Africa or in Asia (except for Cyprus and Japan). Only sporadic cases occur, but early slaughter probably reduces the actual number of cases because of the very extended incubation period. *The fact that scrapie has been diagnosed in sheep found dead without premonitory symptoms also indicates that the true incidence is higher than generally thought.*

In 1992 the USA established a voluntary flock certification programme with four different categories of certified scrapie-free stock, a measure which should materially assist in eradication of the disease, which occurs almost exclusively in pure-bred sheep, especially Suffolks.

In June 1992 a case was diagnosed in Norway, following which a stamping-out policy and movement control was adopted.

The largest sheep-raising countries of the world, Australia and New Zealand, had their last cases of scrapie in 1952 and 1954, respectively.

**IA.** See also BSE. The causal microorganism, an 'unconventional virus', does not produce any kind of immune response in the host, either in natural or experimental infection. Over 15 strains of the 'slow virus' have been identified.

In the brain it produces distinctive fibrils, termed scrapie-associated fibrils (SAF), which contain an amyloid protein, an abnormal substance deposited between cells in many body tissues in several clinical disorders of animals and man (see **I** above). Amyloid protein also occurs in the senile plaques of the cortex in human patients suffering from Alzheimer's disease, the most common of the senile dementias.

Scrapie, BSE, CJD and Kuru can be experimentally transmitted to susceptible host species. Some 20 stable strains of the scrapie agent have been identified. Based on clinical signs, two main types of scrapie are recognised. Type 1, which causes sheep to lose their wool, is the most common type and when inoculated into cattle causes clinical disease without equivalent BSE brain lesions. Type 2 is the rarer form of scrapie, occurring as a trembling ataxia similar to the symptoms of typical BSE and to variant-CJD. Type 2 is the form of scrapie most likely to have infected cattle and man.

The nature of the scrapie agent is controversial. It multiplies very slowly with a long incubation period and takes the form of tubulofilamentous particles (nemaviruses, NVP) and scrapie-associated fibrils as ultrastructural markers, while PrP (protease-resistant protein) is a protein marker. Nemaviruses are specific to all the SEs.

**R.** Infected sheep, goats, placentae, fetal fluids, pastures and possibly fomites.

**MT.** Natural transmission occurs by contagion, contact and maternally – vertical and horizontal transmission. Virus in placentas and fetal fluids is thought to be the source of infection for both newborn lambs and other sheep. The young animal is the most susceptible to infection.

In sheep, and possibly also in goats, scrapie tends to run in families. However, while host genetic variation occurs in both natural and experimental scrapie in sheep, this is not the case in BSE. Differences in susceptibility occur in different breeds, families and individuals and these are related to the genetic make-up of the sheep and to a single gene termed *Sip* (scrapie incubation period).

Recent work (Hunter *et al.*, 1997) has shown that scrapie is not solely a spontaneous genetic disease, i.e. dependent on the PrP genotype alone, but requires an additional exogenous factor such as an infectious agent, or possibly a toxic agent. This work stemmed from a study of Cheviot and Suffolk sheep of UK, Australian and New Zealand origin. Scrapie-associated PrP alleles were present in the sheep from all three countries even though Australia and New Zealand are free of scrapie. These countries possess strict quarantine regulations – only sheep from low-risk regions are imported and are quarantined off-shore for 3 years. If healthy, the progeny are introduced into the national flock by embryo transfer. If scrapie occurs in quarantine, all the animals are slaughtered.

Suffolk sheep coding QQ171 are highly susceptible to scrapie while coding RR171 animals are resistant. Gene testing of all sheep breeds should enable the development of a pool of scrapie-resistant stock.

**CF.** The incubation period is long and extends from 3 months to 5 years or more. Clinical signs also continue for 6 months or so and include changes in behaviour, with the animals becoming excitable, even aggressive, with fine muscular tremors appearing on the head and neck. Pruritus is prominent, the animal biting and rubbing the skin, especially over the rump, shoulders and chest. Wool is lost over large areas, the animal looking like a sheep scab case. A loss of weight takes place, although appetite is lost only in the later stages of the disease. The head is elevated and characteristic nibbling movements are made with the lips. Hyperaesthesia is present, the animal reacting abnormally to external stimuli of noise, sudden movement, etc.

There is incoordination of gait and head carriage, weakness which progresses to emaciation and collapse with sternal or lateral recumbency and death.

In the UK, sheep and goats showing clinical signs of scrapie must by law be slaughtered with compensation paid to owners.

**P.** Except for loss of wool and condition and abrasions caused by rubbing and biting, there are no gross lesions.

*Microscopic changes* are confined to the CNS and take the form of vacuoles in the grey matter and neurons with hypertrophy of astrocytes (supporting cells of ectodermal origin in the CNS). Amyloid-like fibrils termed scrapie-associated fibrils (SAF) are present and considered to be diagnostic. They consist of a prion protein and are believed to be associated with the length of incubation period and in susceptibility.

**D.** The clinical signs, age incidence and flock history point to scrapie. Diagnosis is confirmed by histopathological examination of brain tissue, especially the medulla.

**J.** Carcase and viscera: Clinical cases: T. Contacts, offspring and ancestors: L.

## SWINE FEVER (SF), CLASSICAL SWINE FEVER (CSF), HOG CHOLERA

**I.** A highly contagious, febrile, viral disease of pigs of all ages occurring as a peracute, acute, chronic or subclinical entity.

Notifiable disease UK and most countries.

**O.** Worldwide in distribution, having first appeared in the USA. Except for Madagascar, Guinea Bissau and South Africa, most countries in Africa have not experienced classical swine fever. It is common in South America and Asia, where it is enzootic in occurrence. Canada had its last case in 1963 and the USA in 1976. Australia and New Zealand have not encountered classical swine fever, which has been eradicated in many countries through efficient control measures – quarantine, slaughter, vaccination.

There were 55 outbreaks of CSF in the European Union in 1966 (49 in Italy, 4 in Germany and 2 in Austria).

**IA.** A pestivirus of the family Togaviridae which possesses strains of varying virulence and antigenicity.

The virus is destroyed in the carcase within 1 or 2 days by post-mortem muscular acidity, but in carcases of animals slaughtered in the incubative stage and immediately chilled, the bone marrow may remain infective for 3–6 months or more. It survives in frozen pork for 5 years and at least 27 days in bacon that has been pickled, dried and smoked, salting having a preservative action on the virus.

The virus is fairly easily destroyed by the usual disinfectants at standard concentrations, e.g. 2% sodium hydroxide, 5% phenol, and by drying.

In pig houses the virus remains infective in faeces, bedding, etc., for several weeks.

**R.** Infected and carrier pigs.

**MT.** The main route is by ingestion. A common source of infection is unprocessed or inadequately processed swill containing infected meat scraps. Since all excretions and secretions are infective, the disease can be spread by direct and indirect means – clothing, boots, equipment, animal and human vectors, unsterilised syringes and needles and even birds, flies and mosquitoes.

**CF.** The incubation period is usually short (5–10 days). On gaining entry to the animal body the virus multiplies in the tonsils, thereafter spreading by a viraemia to involve lymphatic tissues. The blood vascular system (WBCs and blood vessel endothelia) are also involved in the spread of the virus in the body, as is the bone marrow and spleen.

Affected pigs show fever, lethargy, inappetence, diarrhoea, dyspnoea, conjunctivitis, often with matting of the eyelids, reddening of the skin, especially of the abdomen, and nervous symptoms such as circling, incoordination, muscle tremors and convulsions.

Morbidity may be as high as 100% and mortality in young pigs, in particular, may be as high.

**P.** Peracute cases may show no lesions. Acute cases exhibit widespread petechiae (rarely ecchymoses) on the skin, larynx, bladder, kidney (*'turkey egg kidney'*), brain, lymph nodes and ileo-caecal junction. The gall bladder may show infarcts.

The typical *'button'* ulcers, which used to be common at the ileo-caecal junction and were probably the result of secondary salmonella infection, are now rarely seen.

Encephalitis of a non-suppurative type is considered diagnostic of SF. Enteritis is a common finding, as is congestion of the liver and lungs.

In chronic SF there is a necrotic enteritis of the large intestine accompanied by enteritis of the small intestine and pneumonia.

Where abortion has taken place, fetuses are frequently mummified, oedematous, malformed or resorbed. Petechial haemorrhages are common in fetuses.

**D.** While the clinical signs and post-mortem lesions may indicate SF, an accurate diagnosis can only be made by laboratory examination – immunofluorescence, ELISA, and histopathology of brain tissue.

*Differential diagnoses* include African swine fever, enzootic pneumonia, salmonellosis, swine erysipelas, pasteurellosis, mulberry heart disease, purpura haemorrhagica and leptospirosis.

**J.** Carcase and viscera: T, acutely diseased carcases, or Kh and D. Also for in-contacts.

## SWINE INFLUENZA (PIG FLU, HOG FLU, FERKELGRIPPE)

**I.** An acute, highly contagious, febrile, viral disease of pigs in which prominent respiratory symptoms are evident.

**O.** Swine influenza occurs in many parts of the world – the USA, where it first appeared in 1918, Canada, Europe, South America, Japan and eastern Asia. Except for Kenya, it does not appear to be common in Africa.

**IA.** Swine influenza virus (SIV) is a type A influenza virus of the RNA orthomyxovirus group. There are several different antigenic strains. While pigs are the principal hosts of SIV, humans may also be infected, but the disease apparently does not spread in man. Influenza viral infections also occur naturally in horses, mink, seals and birds. Animal reservoirs are suspected as sources of new human influenza virus subtypes, recombination taking place between the pig and human strains.

**R.** Infected and carrier pigs.

**MT.** By inhalation, the virus multiplying in the bronchial epithelium eventually producing congestion and atelectasis (collapse) of the lungs and profuse bronchial and tracheal exudate.

**CF.** Clinical signs, which appear suddenly, include high fever (up to 108°C), dyspnoea, sneezing, coughing, inappetence, mucoid oronasal discharge, weakness, loss of weight and prostration. The death rate is usually low (less than 5%), but morbidity may be as high as 100%.

**P.** Lesions are mainly confined to the chest cavity. The lungs are collapsed and show purplish-red areas of pneumonia and of emphysema, especially of the apical and cardiac lobes. Severe pulmonary oedema may on occasion affect the lungs. Mucoid or mucopurulent exudate is present in all the air passages, which are congested. The cervical, bronchial and mediastinal lymph nodes are oedematous.

Changes may also be present in the abdominal cavity as gastritis, enteritis of the large intestine and enlargement of the spleen.

Overall the changes are similar to those of enzootic pneumonia caused by *Mycoplasma hyopneumoniae* (q.v.).

**D.** Confirmation of diagnosis can only be made by isolation of the virus or demonstration of the specific antibody by haemagglutination-inhibition, etc.

*Differential diagnoses* are similar to those for classical swine fever, especially enzootic pneumonia.

**J.** Carcase and viscera: T, A or Kh, depending on degree/extent of body changes and condition.

## SWINE VESICULAR DISEASE (SVD)

**I.** A mild, self-limiting disease of pigs in which vesicles, indistinguishable from those of FMD, vesicular exanthema of swine (VES) and vesicular stomatitis (VS), appear in the mouth and on the feet.

Notifiable disease in UK.

**O.** SVD was first recorded in Italy in 1966, since when it has appeared in many European countries, Hong Kong and Japan. Africa has been free, as has South America except for Bolivia, where the last case occurred in 1991.

Several countries have eradicated SVD – Poland (1972), Switzerland and Japan (1975), Malta (1978), Austria and Greece (1979), Britain (1982), France (1983) and Germany (1985) – but the disease still persists in Italy, Holland and Hong Kong.

There were 5 reported cases of SVD in the European Union in 1996, all in Italy.

**IA.** An enterovirus of the family Picornaviridae, which includes the human coxsackie viruses which cause similar lesions in man – enteroviral vesicular pharyngitis, enteroviral vesicular stomatitis with exanthem and enteroviral lymphonodular pharyngitis.

As with many viruses, there is variation in virulence with the different strains.

SVD virus is very resistant to the actions of heat, cold and disinfectants, requiring low and high levels of pH and heating to 68°C to destroy it. It can survive in frozen pork products indefinitely.

**R.** Infected and carrier pigs.

**MT.** Infection occurs by direct and indirect contact via abrasions on the skin and probably also by ingestion. The virus is present in all secretions and excretions and especially in vesicular fluid. As with FMD, a common method by which infection is acquired is the feeding of swill containing infected material derived from slaughtered infected pigs. Intermediate means of transmission include human and animal vectors, vehicles, contaminated equipment, clothing, etc.

**CF.** Symptoms are usually mild, with morbidity high and mortality low. Slight fever and inappetence accompany the lameness caused by the foot lesions and the salivation which occurs in some cases. The foot vesicles occur most often on the coronary bands of the claws and the supernumerary digits, especially at the heels. Shedding of the horn of the claws may take place as in FMD. The mouth lesions are evident on the lips, snout and tongue and other vesicles may be present on the legs and abdomen. The vesicles appear first of all as raised, whitish macules which become darker in colour and eventually rupture leaving a small ulcer. In many cases symptoms may be so mild as to go unnoticed. Recovery usually follows in 2–3 weeks.

**P.** See **CF.**

**D.** Diagnosis is based on the examination of skin samples or vesicle fluid by complement fixation, ELISA, serum neutralisation, or agar-gel diffusion.

**J.** Carcase and viscera: A or Kh and D (head, feet, intestines) depending on severity and extent of lesions.

## TRANSMISSIBLE GASTROENTERITIS (TGE)

**I.** A prevalent highly infectious, viral disease of pigs of all ages characterised by diarrhoea, dehydration, vomiting and high mortality.

**O.** The disease appears to be mainly confined to the northern hemisphere. It is uncommon in Africa, being only recorded in Cameroon and Zaire. It is enzootic in the USA, Bolivia, Costa Rica and France. A number of European countries have successfully eradicated TGE, including Spain, Latvia, Lithuania, Holland and Romania. The disease does not occur in Australia, New Zealand and the rest of Oceania.

**IA.** A coronavirus which has an affinity for epithelial cells, especially of the small intestine where it causes villous atrophy. Although resistant to low temperatures, TGEV is easily destroyed by drying, sunlight, boiling and the action of the usual disinfectants.

**R.** Infected and carrier pigs.

**MT.** Probably by ingestion and inhalation. Direct and indirect spread, including aerosol transmission, can occur.

Vehicles of infection are similar to those operating for FMD, SVD, etc., the feeding of unsterilised swill and human and animal vectors, transport vehicles, dogs, cats, rats, birds and flies being involved in the transfer of the virus.

**CF.** Following entry of the virus into the body, it multiplies in the respiratory and intestinal tracts.

The *incubation period* is short (1–2 days) and is followed by profuse watery, fetid diarrhoea (yellowish-green in colour), slight fever, inappetence, vomiting (the vomitus being a yellowish foam), thirst, depression and dehydration. Young pigs are more likely to succumb than older animals and their mortality may reach 100%. Older pigs exhibit less severe symptoms and generally recover in about 1 week.

**P.** There is carcase dehydration with greenish or yellowish watery contents in a thin-walled translucent small intestine (SI) due to the destruction of the intestinal villi. Gastritis may be evident along with enteritis, especially where secondary pathogens operate.

**D.** Clinical signs and the characteristic SI picture are suggestive of TGE. Confirmation of diagnosis depends on immunofluorescent antibody examination, demonstration of TGE viral antigen, histopathology, etc.

**J.** Carcase and viscera: T, or Kh and D if economically feasible.

## VESICULAR EXANTHEMA OF SWINE (VES, SAN MIGUEL SEA LION VIRUS DISEASE)

**I.** An acute, highly infectious, viral disease of pigs in which vesicles are formed in the mouth, on the snout and tongue, and on the soles, coronary bands, interdigital clefts of the claws of the feet.

The lesions are very similar to those of FMD, swine vesicular disease and vesicular stomatitis.

**O.** The disease appears to be restricted to the USA and the state of California (where it was eradicated in 1959), Hawaii and Iceland.

**IA.** A calcivirus which may also affect cattle, horses, mink, fish, snakes, marine mammals, primates and man. The San Miguel sea lion virus is indistinguishable from VESV.

**R, MT, CF, P, D and J.** As for swine vesicular disease.

## VESICULAR STOMATITIS

**I.** A highly contagious, febrile, viral disease of cattle, horses and pigs, and less commonly, sheep and goats, in which vesicles similar to those in FMD, SVD and VES are formed.

Notifiable disease UK.

**O.** Vesicular stomatitis is restricted to the New World – North and South America – where it is enzootic in Mexico, Colombia and Nicaragua. The USA has been free from 1980 and Canada from 1949, and in recent years Argentina, Belize, Bolivia, and Brazil have successfully eradicated the disease.

**IA.** A vesiculovirus of the family Rhabdoviridae which also infects many forms of wildlife – deer, raccoons, bobcats, monkeys, rodents and cold-blooded animals.

**R.** Infected and carrier animals, including wildlife forms and biting insects and frogs.

**MT.** By ingestion through direct and indirect contact with contaminated food, pasture and water. Sandflies and mosquitoes are also involved in the transmission of the virus to susceptible hosts.

**CF.** The disease occurs during the warm season when biting insects are active. After a short incubation period (2–8 days), vesicles form in the mouth, on the dorsum of the tongue, dental pad, hard palate, gums, lips, angles of the mouth and muzzle. These appear as blanched, raised swellings, some of which may undergo necrosis. The teats of cattle and the feet of pigs may be affected.

**P.** See **CF.** There are no significant internal changes.

**D.** Differentiation from FMD in particular is of importance. This is achieved by the use of complement fixation, ELISA, virus neutralisation, mouse passage, etc.

Differentiation from FMD in horses is simple since horses are not susceptible to foot-and-mouth disease.

**J.** Carcase and viscera: As for VES.

**Viral papular stomatitis**, probably of viral origin, may occur in *cattle*, mostly young stock, as a mild condition without general symptoms. Small, reddish papules are present in the nostrils, muzzle and buccal mucosa and disappear in about 1 week.

**Viral papular dermatitis** is a mild *equine* disease caused by unidentified viruses in which firm papules form on the skin which disappear in 1 week leaving a dry crust.

## VIRAL ENCEPHALOMYELITIS OF PIGS (PORCINE POLIOMYELITIS, TESCHEN DISEASE, TALFAN DISEASE)

**I.** An acute or subacute viral disease of pigs, analogous to human poliomyelitis, in which nervous symptoms predominate.

**O.** Teschen disease was first reported in Czechoslovakia in 1929, where it was restricted to certain areas. Since then many European, and a few African and South American countries, have encountered outbreaks but few have been recorded in Asia or Oceania. Many European countries have succeeded in eradicating the disease – Switzerland (1940), Romania (1954), Germany (1957), Poland (1967), Czechoslovakia (1973), Austria (1980) and Latvia (1982).

The disease now appears to be confined to the Ukraine, Madagascar and Guyana. Overall there has been a marked decline in incidence.

In 1992, viral encephalomyelitis was diagnosed serologically in Northern Ireland in pigs without clinical signs, the disease being never suspected or recorded.

**IA.** An enterovirus of the family Picornaviridae of several different antigenic strains varying in virulence, all capable of causing encephalomyelitis in pigs. The Teschen strain is a virulent form whereas Talfan (first described in England in 1957) and other strains are less pathogenic.

**R.** Infected and carrier pigs.

**MT.** By ingestion and inhalation.

**CF.** Following an *incubation period* of 7–21 days, symptoms in Teschen disease include fever, lassitude, anorexia and nervous disturbance manifested by seizures, incoordination, circling, stiffness, knuckling of fetlocks, opisthotonus, nystagmus (rhythmic movement of both eyeballs in unison), paralysis, coma and death within a few days of onset.

Clinical signs in Talfan and related conditions are less severe and consist of ataxia (muscular incoordination) and paresis (slight paralysis), usually with recovery but with loss of weight.

**P.** Gross lesions are confined to the medulla and cerebrum, which show an encephalomyelitis, and the body cavities, where there is pleurisy, pericarditis and peritonitis.

**D.** While the clinical signs and the post-mortem lesions may suggest encephalomyelitis, laboratory procedures (complement fixation, virus neutralisation) are necessary to establish an accurate diagnosis.

*Differential diagnoses* include listeriosis, Aujeszky's disease, rabies, classical swine fever, African swine fever, oedema disease, pasteurellosis and lead poisoning.

**J.** Carcase and viscera: T or Kh and D (brain, spinal cord, alimentary tract).

## DISEASES CAUSED BY RICKETTSIAE

*Rickettsiae* are tiny (0.3 μm × 4.0 μm) rod-shaped, pleomorphic, Gram-negative, obligate intracellular parasites in certain arthropods, mainly mites, fleas, lice and ticks, in which they cause no disease, but when transmitted to a vertebrate host are capable of causing extremely serious plagues in animals and man.

Like the bacteria, they contain RNA and DNA, glucosamine and muramic acid in their cell walls and enzymes for metabolic activity, and have the ability to reproduce by binary fission. Fortunately, they are unstable outside the cell walls of the host, except *Coxiella burnetii*, and are sensitive to antibiotics and disinfectants.

The family Rickettsiaceae comprises several genera including *Rickettsia*, *Coxiella*, *Anaplasma*, *Ehrlichia*, *Coxiella burnetii*, the cause of Q fever, is Gram-positive, unlike the rickettsiae.

The rickettsiae have a very wide range of hosts in nature in both domestic and wild animals and birds.

They are the causal agents of the diseases listed in Table 17.2.

## ANAPLASMOSIS (GALL SICKNESS)

**I.** An acute, subacute or chronic non-contagious disease of cattle, sheep, goats and wild ungulates associated with fever, anaemia, jaundice and emaciation.

**O.** Anaplasmosis has a wide distribution in tropical and subtropical countries with a slight extension into temperate zones. Most African and South American countries experience the disease and in some of them anaplasmosis has a high occurrence – Lesotho, Uganda, Guyana and Puerto Rico. It is exceptional in the USA and Mexico but does not occur in Canada. Many Asian countries are affected but to a

**Table 17.2** Diseases caused by rickettsiae with their vectors and hosts.

| Disease | Organism | Vector | Host |
|---|---|---|---|
| Typhus group | *R. prowazeki* | Body louse | Man |
| | *R. mooseri* | Rat flea | Rats |
| Spotted fever group | *R. rickettsi* | Tick | Small wild mammals dogs, birds |
| | *R. siberica* | Tick | Wild animals, birds |
| | *R. conorii* | Tick | Small wild mammals, dogs |
| | *R. akari* | Mite | House mouse |
| | *R. australis* | Tick | Bush rodents |
| Scrub typhus | *R. tsutsugamushi* | Mite | Small wild rodents, birds |
| Trench fever | *Rochalimaea quintata* | Body louse | Man |
| Anaplasmosis | *Anaplasma* spp. | Tick, fly | Cattle |
| Bovine petechial fever | *Ehrlichia ondiri* | (Tick) | Cattle |
| Eperythrozoonosis | *Eperythrozoonosis* spp. | Lice and biting flies | Cattle, sheep, pigs, llamas |
| Equine erlichiosis | *E. risticii* | (Tick or fly) | |
| Contagious ophthalmia | *R. conjunctivae* | Fly | Sheep and goats |
| Heartwater (Cowdriosis) | *R. ruminantium* | Tick | Cattle, sheep, goats, wild ruminants |
| Q fever | *Coxiella burnetii* | Tick | Man, goats, cattle, sheep |
| Tick-borne fever | *R. bovina* | Tick | Sheep, cattle, goats, deer |
| | *R. ovina* | | |

lesser degree than Africa and South America. Japan had its last case in 1991. The disease is enzootic in Australia, but New Zealand is free.

In Europe, anaplasmosis has an exceptional occurrence in the Ukraine, Albania, Bulgaria, Portugal and Spain. Romania eradicated the disease in 1991.

**IA.** The causal agent, *Anaplasma marginale* (*A. ovis* in sheep and goats), is an obligate intraerythrocytic parasite which invades red blood cells and reproduces by binary fission within the RBC into 2–8 round initial bodies (0.2–0.5 µm in diameter) which then leave to infect other RBCs. Some 15% of red blood cells have to be infected and destroyed before clinical disease becomes apparent.

**R.** Infected and subclinical carriers, domestic and wild.

**MT.** The source of infection is the blood of an affected animal. This is transmitted by the bite of a tick or blood-sucking fly. The main ticks involved are members of the genera *Ixodes*, *Boophilus*, *Dermacentor*, *Rhipicephalus*, *Haemaphysalis*, *Hyalomma* and *Argas*. The flies belong to the family Tabanidae, which includes the stable, horse and deer flies and are predators on vertebrates.

Anaplasmosis can also be spread by mechanical means – vaccination, dehorning, ear tagging, castration and bleeding, operations.

**CF.** Clinical signs (which are more severe in the older animal) include fever, depression, inappetence, anaemia, dehydration, jaundice and weight loss. Peracute cases may die within 2 days, but gradual recovery usually ensues in those animals which are resistant and which survive the RBC destruction.

**P.** Gross changes are those associated with anaemia, dehydration and jaundice. The spleen is enlarged and soft and the enlarged liver has a mahogany or deep orange colour. Body fat, viscera and conjunctivae are yellowish or orange in colour. Lymph nodes are enlarged and oedematous and the gall bladder is distended with bile. The blood is thin and watery and the heart shows petechial haemorrhages while the lungs are pale and oedematous and the kidneys congested. The alimentary tract may show patches of haemorrhage and oedema.

**D.** A tentative diagnosis of anaplasmosis may be made on clinical signs, history, presence of insect vectors, etc., and confirmed on examination of a blood smear stained with Giemsa, when the initial bodies will be detected in the RBCs. However, these can be confused with the Jolly bodies of circulating immature blood cells in cases of anaemia or with babesias or trypanosomes.

Complement fixation, agglutination, indirect fluorescent antibody and a DNA probe can be used. A convenient rapid card agglutination test is now in use in the USA.

**J.** Carcase and viscera: T.

## BOVINE PETECHIAL FEVER (ONDIRI DISEASE)

**I.** A non-contagious rickettsiosis of domestic and wild ruminants in which numerous petechial haemorrhages are present on mucous membranes.

**O.** The disease appears to be confined to the highlands of East Africa, mainly Kenya.

**IA.** *Ehrlichia ondiri*, a rickettsia which is related to the causal organisms of tick-borne fever, *R. bovina* and *R. ovina.*

The organism is pleomorphic and 1.5–5 µm in diameter and possesses a rippled cell wall, a plasma membrane and a nucleoid. It multiplies initially in the spleen and parasitises granulocytes (WBCs containing granules) and less commonly monocytes.

**R.** Infected and carrier animals. The carrier state exists for many months.

**MT.** It is possible that a tick, biting insect or mite is involved, but the actual vector has not been determined.

**CF.** Symptoms vary from being inapparent to peracute, acute and subacute. Included in the severe forms are fever, depression, inappetence, agalactia, petechiation of mucous membranes and death within 3 days.

As with many blood parasite diseases, fluctuations of fever occur with disappearance and reappearance of petechiae with the onset of fever. A nasal discharge, which may be blood-stained, is present and there may be exophthalmia with marked protrusion of an eyeball – the so-called '*poached egg eye*' – along with oedema of the conjunctiva. Dysentery is a usual feature. Death in 20% of cases is due to a profound anaemia.

**P.** Submucosal and subserosal haemorrhages are numerous and ecchymoses are present in the heart, coronary vessels, upper respiratory tract, bladder and alimentary tract. Lymph nodes are enlarged and oedematous but the spleen may or may not be swollen. All changes are associated with destruction of the RBCs.

**D.** History of the outbreak, its occurrence on high scrub land and the fairly typical PM lesions may suggest bovine petechial fever, but confirmation can only be made by detection of *E. ondiri* in blood smears stained with Giemsa, by electron microscopy, and by animal inoculation.

*Differential diagnoses* include heartwater, babesiosis, anaplasmosis, acute trypanosomiasis and theileriasis and arsenic poisoning.

**J.** Carcase and viscera: T.

## CONTAGIOUS OPHTHALMIA OF CATTLE, SHEEP AND GOATS (INFECTIOUS KERATOCONJUNCTIVITIS, PINKEYE)

(See under Infectious Keratoconjunctivitis caused by *Moraxella bovis*.)

## EPERYTHROZOONOSIS

**I.** A usually subclinical or acute, febrile, haemolytic rickettsial disease of pigs, cattle, sheep, goats, llamas, mule deer and elk characterised by anaemia and icterus.

**O.** The disease has been reported in all six continents. Serological evidence indicates that subclinical infection is high in many countries – 16.9% in sheep in Australia and 15% in pigs in the USA.

**IA.** *Eperythrozoonosis* spp. The causal agent in pigs is *Eperythrozoonosis suis*, in sheep *E. ovis* and in cattle *E. wenyonii*. The parasites appear to be host-specific.

The organisms are intracellular parasites of red blood cells, although sometimes they are seen in the plasma. They are mostly coccoid in shape with an average diameter of 0.8–1 μm. Rod-shaped and ring forms are also observed on occasions. They may occur singly or there may be as many as five in one RBC. Although described as intracellular, the parasites infect the membrane of the red blood cells, rupturing them and releasing the contents to produce anaemia, haemoglobinuria and jaundice in clinical cases. Parasitised red blood cells are removed from the bloodstream by the spleen.

**R.** Infected and carrier animals.

**MT.** In pigs eperythrozoonosis is transmitted by lice and biting flies. Transplacental transmission can also occur. In cattle the responsible vectors are the mosquitoes *Aedes camptorhynchus* and *Culex annulirostris*.

The use of infected surgical instruments and needles is also a possible means of infection transfer.

**CF.** As with all haemolytic diseases, there is fever, inappetence, malaise, anaemia with skin and conjunctival pallor, jaundice and loss of weight. Examination of the pinna of the ear in severe cases reveals the absence of the network of small blood vessels with jaundice when light is transmitted through the ear. Icterus usually disappears in about 1 week and the pinna blood vessel network becomes evident, with the ear assuming a normal pink colour.

New-born piglets are frequently anaemic and weak and sows often develop infertility.

In cattle similar signs occur and stiffness of movement with oedema of the udder (with agalactia) and hindlimbs may be evident in acute cases. The subclinical picture, however, is very common as it is in sheep. Secondary infection is not uncommon in all species and it may be that such a situation is required for the clinical picture of anaemia, haemoglobinuria, etc., to develop. Stress also probably plays an important part in the haemolytic syndrome.

**P.** Carcases are anaemic, jaundiced and lacking in condition in severe cases.

**D.** Diagnosis is made by demonstrating large numbers of ricksettiae in blood smears stained by the Giemsa method. The organisms may be present on the surface of the RBCs, surrounding the platelets or in the plasma.

**J.** Carcase and viscera: A, T or Kh and D, depending on the severity of the disease, carcase condition, etc.

## EQUINE EHRLICHIOSIS (EQUINE MONOCYTIC EHRLICHIOSIS, POTOMAC HORSE FEVER, EQUINE EHRLICHIAL COLITIS)

**I.** An infectious, non-contagious rickettsial, febrile disease of *horses* characterised by depression, colic, watery diarrhoea, jaundice, ataxia and limb oedema.

**O.** Equine ehrlichiosis is restricted in occurrence to the United States (northern states) and Canada. It was first diagnosed in 1984 in horses near the Potomac River in Maryland and Virginia.

**IA.** *Ehrlichia equi (risticii)*, which parasitises monocytes, macrophages and the epithelial cells of the intestinal tract.

*E. equi* resembles the rickettsiae of tick-borne fever and bovine petechial fever. It invades neutrophils, and sometimes eosinophils, and appears in them as one or more morulae or inclusion bodies. These are coccoid or coccobacillary, pleomorphic organisms (1–5 µm in diameter) which stain bluish-grey in blood smears with Giemsa stain.

**R.** Infected and carrier horses and possibly ticks, biting flies, dogs and foxes.

**MT.** The exact mode of transmission and the vector are not known but the occurrence of the disease near rivers suggests a tick or some form of biting fly.

**CF.** Symptoms vary according to the virulence of the organism and the susceptibility, resistance and age of the host.

Clinical signs may be inapparent and overlooked, but in the typical disease there is fever, anorexia, depression, icterus, reluctance to move, ataxia, colic and diarrhoea with dehydration. Oedema is present in the lower limbs and ventral abdomen and visible mucous membranes are petechiated. Laminitis may occur as a complication. The mortality rate is in the region of 10%.

**P.** The action of the rickettsiae on epithelia is demonstrated in the alimentary tract, where the caecum and colon are congested and display areas of necrotic erosion and ulceration. The contents of the alimentary tract are watery and the mesenteric lymph nodes are swollen and oedematous. Oedema, with petechiae and ecchymoses, pervades the ventral abdominal wall, lower limbs and subfascia.

**D.** A firm diagnosis can only be made by demonstration of the cytoplasmic inclusion bodies in blood smears. An indirect fluorescent antibody test may be used.

*Differential diagnoses*: Various forms of colitis, salmonellosis, equine viral encephalitis, equine infectious anaemia, purpura haemorrhagica, viral arteritis and certain poisonings, plant and chemical.

**J.** Carcase and viscera: T, A or Kh, depending on severity of lesions.

## HEARTWATER (COWDRIOSIS)

**I.** An infectious, non-contagious, tick-borne, rickettsial disease of cattle, sheep, goats and wild ruminants in which there are high fever and nervous symptoms.

**O.** Heartwater appears to be confined at the moment to Africa (south of the Sahara where it is enzootic in Botswana, Mozambique, South Africa and especially Tanzania) and South America where it is limited to Antigua and St Vincent Grenadin. The disease has not been reported in Asia, Europe or Oceania.

**IA.** *Cowdria ruminantium*, an intracellular rickettsia which parasitises reticuloendothelial and vascular endothelial cells, in which it multiplies by binary fission to produce morulae or colonies in the cytoplasm. Rupture of the cells allows the rickettsial morulae access to the blood and lymph streams, making them infective.

*C. ruminantium* possesses several different strains of varying antigenicity and virulence between which there is only partial protection. It is a fragile organism which is easily destroyed outside the animal body. It can, however, remain viable for 3 years in the larval stages of ticks.

Smears from vascular intima or brain tissue stained by Giemsa or May–Grunwald show the morulae as bluish-purple or reddish-purple chromatic granules (up to several hundred on one cell).

**R.** Affected and recovered animals, domestic and wild, and several stages of three-host ticks.

**MT.** Heartwater is transmitted by three-host bont ticks of the genus *Amblyomma*. Although infection is transmitted from one stage to the next in the tick cycle, there is no transovarian infection.

**CF.** Symptoms vary according to the severity of the disease – peracute, acute, subacute or inapparent.

*Peracute* cases exhibit high fever, collapse and die in convulsions in 1–2 days. In the typical acute cases there is fever and inappetence with nervous signs in the form of circling, high-stepping gait, ataxia, standing with legs apart and head bowed, blinking of eyelids, apparent blindness, hyperaesthesia, chewing movements, convulsions, prostration and death in 2 weeks.

Mortality varies from 100% in peracute cases with much lower death rates in *acute* and *subacute* cases, many of which recover.

**P.** The multiplication of cowdria in the reticuloendothelial and epithelial cells with their ultimate destruction results in vascular permeability, haemorrhages and oedema. Oedema is evident as hydrothorax, hydropericardium and hydroperitoneum. Pulmonary oedema is also present, along with enlarged and oedematous lymph nodes. The spleen is enlarged and subserosal petechiae and ecchymoses are present in the body cavities.

**D.** Diagnosis, based on history, clinical signs and post-mortem findings, enzootic prevalence, etc., is fairly straightforward in acute cases.

Confirmation is made by detection of *C. ruminantium* by Giemsa staining of lymph node samples aspirated by needle biopsy or brain grey matter. Antibody detection may be carried out using an indirect FA test.

**J.** Carcase and viscera: T, R, A or Kh, depending on severity and extent of lesions and if economically feasible.

## Q FEVER (QUERY FEVER, ABATTOIR FEVER, PNEUMO-RICKETTSIOSIS)

**I.** A usually mild, febrile rickettsial disease which can occasionally cause abortion in sheep and goats and influenza-like symptoms in human beings, making it a true *zoonosis*. The disease in livestock and in man is frequently asymptomatic.

**O.** The disease has a worldwide distribution but only occurs sporadically and then in low incidence. Few Asian countries appear to experience Q fever, which seems to be more common in the USA, Canada and European countries, this being probably due to superior investigative procedures. The incidence in animals and man is probably far greater than recorded because of the mildness of many cases, limited clinical suspicion and lack of testing laboratories.

A survey in Ontario, Canada (Lang, 1988), revealed a high dairy cattle serological incidence of 67%, with 20% of dairy goats and 4% of sheep being positive. Although sheep are generally regarded as the main source of infection, this finding would appear to cast doubt on this assertion.

**IA.** *Coxiella burnetii*. Unlike other rickettsiae, *C. burnetii* is fairly stable outside the body and relatively resistant to many disinfectants. It can remain viable in soil and contaminated materials such as bedding, wool and dust for many months, even years. Pasteurisation effectively kills the organism.

The organism has the ability to localise in the uterus, placenta, mammary gland and supramammary lymph nodes, thereby providing a source of infection at subsequent parturitions.

**R.** The organism has a wide distribution in nature and cycles, as do many other pathogens, in domestic and wild animals and their arthropod vectors. Bandicoots and some species of wild rodents can act as natural reservoirs. Many infected domestic animals, including cats and dogs, are usually asymptomatic but can shed numerous organisms at parturition.

**MT.** Two main methods of transmission exist: (1) between wild animals and their arthropod vectors, mainly ticks; and (2) dissemination of the organism by direct and indirect means without arthropod involvement between domestic animals and from them to man. Tick transmission, however, may be involved in domestic animal and human infection, but only rarely.

The main sources of disease for animals and human beings are infected placentas, fetal fluids, uterine discharges and milk.

Infection of animals and man arises from these sources by direct contact, in the form of aerosols (which can be inhaled) or by the ingestion of contaminated food such as raw milk and water. The most important source of infection for man is probably airborne transmission of dust particles containing active coxiellae as well as the handling of infected carcases. Dust particles can be carried considerable distances downwind.

Direct transmission by blood and bone marrow transfusion has been reported in man.

**CF.** Abortion with anorexia in sheep and goats in late pregnancy has occurred on occasions in severe infections. According to recent reports, cattle can also experience abortion and infertility. Infection in animals and man, however, is usually subclinical, but a mild, febrile condition simulating influenza can occur in man.

**P.** There are no gross lesions.

**D.** Accurate diagnosis depends on the use of complement fixation, agglutination and immunofluorescence test and microscopy of stained tissues.

**J.** Carcase and viscera: T, A or Kh and D (udder, uterus).

### Q fever in man

The disease affects those individuals handling affected animals and carcases – farmers, veterinarians, meat and rendering plant workers, dairy workers, wool sorters and laboratory personnel.

After an incubation period of 2–4 weeks, fever develops with chills, headache, weakness, myalgia, malaise and sweating. Considerable variation in symptoms occurs and there may be none at all even though the patient is positive serologically.

Pneumonia with coughing, pericarditis, vegetative endocarditis and hepatitis have been reported in some instances, but mortality rates are generally low except in the patients with endocarditis.

## TICK-BORNE FEVER (TBF)

**I.** A mild, febrile, rickettsial, tick-borne disease of ruminants (cattle, sheep, goats, deer and sometimes horses) manifested by leukopenia (reduction in the number of white blood cells), and increased susceptibility to secondary infections.

**O.** TBF has been identified in Europe (British Isles, Norway, Sweden, Finland, Spain), India and Africa.

**IA.** *Cytoecetes* (*Ehrlichia*) *phagocytophila*, formerly *Rickettsia phagocytophila*. A rickettsia of uncertain classification, it parasitises the cytoplasms of leukocytes, especially granulocytes and monocytes, in which it appears as clusters (morulae) of pleomorphic bodies (0.5–2.0 µm in diameter) each possessing a rippled cell wall, ribosome-like granules and a nucleoid (cf. *Ehrlichia ondiri*).

**R.** Infected and carrier animals and ticks, especially the nymphal and adult stages.

**MT.** In temperate regions the three-host hard tick *Ixodes ricinus* is responsible for transmission of *C. phagocytophila* to susceptible hosts but in tropical and subtropical countries *Rhipicephalus*, *Amblyomma* and *Hyalomma* spp. are the vectors.

Ticks are mainly active during the spring months, but secondary activity can occur in the autumn.

**CF.** The incubation period is 1–2 weeks, following which there is high fever, agalactia, inappetence, dullness, loss of weight and late abortion in pregnant animals. Young stock are more severely affected.

The action of the parasites on the leukocytes produces a marked reduction in blood granulocytes and monocytes and increased susceptibility to other diseases such as tick pyaemia and tick-borne virus encephalitis.

**P.** Hydropericardium, splenomegaly, sub-endocardial haemorrhages and petechiae in the intestinal mucosa and thymus.

**D.** A tentative diagnosis is made on the basis of clinical signs, tick activity and PM lesions.

Diagnosis is confirmed by detection of inclusion bodies in blood smears stained by Giemsa or Leishman. Serology is performed by indirect immunofluorescence.

**J.** Carcase and viscera: T, A or Kh.

## DISEASES CAUSED BY FUNGI (MYCOSES)

The fungi along with the yeasts, moulds, mildews, smuts, rusts and mushrooms belong to the order Mycota. They lack chlorophyll and are now grouped with the protozoa and most algae as Eumycetes.

They are ubiquitous in nature and most are of great benefit to man, being responsible, along with bacteria, for the disintegration of organic matter and the release of valuable carbon, oxygen, nitrogen and phosphorus into the soil or atmosphere. They are necessary in the making of bread, cheese, wine and beer and are used in the production of some organic acids, enzymes, vitamins and antibiotics. They are also used as food in the form of mushrooms, truffles and morels.

A typical *fungus* grows as long filaments or hyphae which branch to form a large network or mycelium. They reproduce by forming spores which are disseminated into the atmosphere, eventually germinate and develop into hyphae and mycelia.

Reproduction, as opposed to growth, occurs by sexual and asexual methods.

While most fungi are beneficial to man, a few are able to cause disease in crops, animals and man, while others destroy foods, including meat.

## ASPERGILLOSIS

**I.** A mainly respiratory, and sometimes generalised, fungal disease of virtually all domestic animals, poultry and many wild species characterised by pneumonia, placentitis and abortion in cattle, horses and pigs and by pneumonia in poultry (q.v.).

Humans can be affected with several species of *Aspergillus*, notably *A. fumigatus*, *A. niger* and *A. flavus*, which give rise to pneumonic aspergillosis with sometimes thrombosis and infarction of blood vessels. They are also responsible for otomycosis, a fungal infection of the outer auditory meatus and canal.

**O.** Aspergillosis occurs throughout the world, *A. fumigatus* being ubiquitous.

**IA.** *Aspergillus* spp. of fungi, especially *A. fumigatus*.

**CF.** In cattle, sheep and pigs aspergillosis may occur as a pneumonia with fever, anorexia, dyspnoea, nasal discharge and coughing or as a placentitis with late abortion and stillbirths.

Horses develop lesions in the guttural pouches with epistaxis (nose bleeding) and difficulty in swallowing. Extension of infection to the brain results in blindness and locomotor disturbances.

Poultry are affected with brooder pneumonia (pneumomycosis) (q.v.).

**P.** In cattle, in the respiratory form, lobar pneumonia, without atelectasis, is present and there may also be yellowish, caseous nodules or plaques or granulomatous lesions resembling tuberculosis. In abortion cases the uterine wall is dark red or brownish in colour and very thickened and leathery and may show areas of necrotic erosion with a yellowish-grey desquamated pseudo-membrane. Fetal membranes are retained and show corresponding lesions, while fetuses are sometimes affected with skin lesions resembling ringworm.

Equine lesions take the form of necrotic inflammation of thickened guttural pouches.

**D.** Diagnosis requires demonstration of the branching hyphae in the lesions and the use of ELISA, agar gel double diffusion and immunofluorescence tests.

**J.** Carcase and viscera: A, provided condition is satisfactory and no secondary lesions are present.

## COCCIDIOIDOMYCOSIS (COCCIDIOIDAL GRANULOMA, DESERT FEVER)

**I.** A usually mild, chronic, dust-borne, fungal infection occurring in many species of animals but often fatal in man, characterised by granulomatous lesions resembling TB in the lungs and associated lymph nodes.

**O.** North and South America.

**IA.** *Coccidioides immitis*, a dimorphic fungus which grows in soil as a saprophytic mould. The parasitic form grows as spherules (spherical cells) which reproduce by the formation of endospores.

**R.** Soil, dust and many species of domestic and wild animals (coyotes, desert rodents, chinchillas, etc.).

**MT.** By inhalation of infective arthroconidia and sometimes via skin abrasions.

**CF.** Cattle and dogs are most often affected, with pigs, sheep and horses less so. After an incubation period of 2–4 weeks, clinical signs include loss of weight, fluctuating temperature, dyspnoea, coughing, wheezing, colic, leg oedema and superficial abscesses.

**P.** Lesions are usually confined to the lungs but may be disseminated to other body organs such as the liver, spleen and intestinal tract. They take the form of granulomatous nodules which contain yellowish pus or calcified material often mistaken for tuberculosis. The associated lymph nodes – bronchial, mediastinal and retropharyngeal – are also affected, and mesenteric nodes when infection involves the abdominal organs.

**D.** Diagnosis is confirmed by demonstration of the spherules in tissues, pus and giant cells as fairly large bodies (20–200 µm).

An intradermal skin test using an extract of the fungus, coocidioidin, indicates exposure to the fungus in positive cases.

Precipitin and complement fixation tests may also be used.

**J.** Carcase and viscera: T or A and D.

Care is essential in handling meat and offal because of the hazards for man.

### Coccidioidomycosis in man

The disease is systemic following the respiratory infection and is frequently fatal. It occurs in all ages, but most often in younger females after dust storms. Symptoms resemble those of influenza – fever, chills, muscular pains, coughing and sometimes chest pain – in the primary infection. Healing of the lesions (pyogranulomas) may then take place with recovery of the patient, but organ dissemination may ensue with fatal results.

## CRYPTOCOCCOSIS (BLASTOMYCOSIS, TORULOSIS)

**I.** A systemic fungal disease which may affect horses, cattle, sheep, goats and man, causing respiratory and sometimes nervous and skin conditions. The disease is probably most common in dogs and cats.

**O.** Sporadic cases occur throughout the world.

**IA.** *Cryptococcus neoformans*, a yeast which is widespread in nature and can grow as a saprophyte in soil. It is frequently isolated from pigeon droppings and nests and on occasions from human faeces and skin.

Yeasts are unicellular fungi which reproduce by budding. *C. neoformans* is spherical in shape and measures 5–20 µm in diameter but, unlike other fungi, does not normally form a mycelium. It stains positive with Gram's stain.

**R.** Bird faeces are the main source of *C. neoformans*, although birds are not susceptible to infection. It may also be found in soil and dust.

**MT.** Infection occurs by the inhalation of dust and also via skin wounds.

**CF.** Respiratory symptoms include anorexia, coughing, sneezing and oculonasal discharge, while CNS involvement is shown by ataxia, hyperaesthesia, stiffness, circling and sometimes blindness.

Skin lesions take the form of nodules and ulcers accompanied by local oedema.

General signs usually accompany mastitis in which affected quarters are swollen and indurated with reduction of milk supply, the milk being thickened and greyish-white or watery with flakes. *C. neoformans* is the most serious fungal cause of mastitis, and can persist for months and result in total cessation of lactation.

**P.** Lesions are common in the thoracic cavity, upper respiratory tract and mouth in the form of granulomas, abscesses and ulcers. Such changes may extend as metastases to other organs in the body. Like coccidioidomycoses, they tend to resemble tuberculosis in the ruminant. Lymphadenitis may be evident with slimy cut surfaces. The lesions in mastitis are essentially granulomatous. The CNS changes show as thickened meninges with translucent material resembling oedema.

See also **CF**.

**D.** The encapsulated organism can be identified in stained H&E preparations and by fluorescent antibody technique.

**J.** Carcase and viscera: A with D (lungs, udder), Kh or T, depending on overall findings.

## EPIZOOTIC LYMPHANGITIS (EL, CLASSICAL HISTOPLASMOSIS, PSEUDO-GLANDERS) (Plate 2, Fig. 8)

**I.** A chronic, contagious, disease of horses and mules (rarely donkeys) and more rarely cattle, in which there is lymphangitis and lymphadenitis with the formation of skin nodules, abscesses and ulcers emitting a thick, yellowish, viscid pus. Natural infection also occurs in dogs, cats, rodents, bats and man.

**O.** Epizootic lymphangitis is now confined to some countries in Africa (Benin, Ethiopia, Gambia, Guinea Bissau, Nigeria, Togo and South Africa), South America (Dominican Republic) and Asia (Mongolia). It has never been recorded in Oceania or in North America.

Many countries have succeeded in eradicating EL – Britain and Eire (1906), Romania (1918), Denmark (1945), Israel (1951), Albania (1953), Spain (1973), and Kuwait and Lebanon (1986).

**IA.** *Histoplasma capsulatum*, a dimorphic saprophytic fungus found in soil contaminated with the droppings of birds and animals in many subtropical parts of the world. It forms a mycelium with microconidia and macroconidia in soil and a yeast form in animal and human tissues.

**R.** Soil, especially that with a high organic content, e.g. in the vicinity of poultry houses, carrier animals, domestic and wild, including brown bats and flies.

**MT.** Infection arises through abrasions in the skin and possibly by the action of biting flies. The inhalation of airborne spores or conidia appears to be the usual mode of transmission in man. Since EL lesions can on occasion be found in internal organs in animals, the possibility of inhalation as a mode of infection in animals cannot be discounted. Animal-to-animal or man-to-man transmission does not occur except by inoculation of infected tissue.

Contaminated bedding, saddlery, grooming tools, etc. can act as sources of infection.

**CF.** On entry, the spores invade the subcutaneous tissues and infect the superficial lymphatics and nodes, creating nodules which ulcerate and exude thick, viscid, yellowish pus. The ulcers have a tendency to close with the formation of scabs and reopen at intervals. The nodules are pyogranulomas possessing a thickened fibrous capsule. The local superficial lymphatic vessels are enlarged and stand out below the skin. The regional lymph nodes are enlarged and firm and may also ulcerate and discharge pus. The skin overlying the infected lymphatics is thickened and adherent to the lymph channels and the whole limb may be grossly enlarged. Some 2–3 months are required for the abscesses and ulcers to regress and heal, leaving a scar.

Sometimes the larger lymph nodes are infected to the extent that they become an abscess with all the lymphoid tissue destroyed. The abscess bursts through the skin, creating a granulating fistula which takes weeks to heal.

These lesions are found most often on the lower limbs and shoulders but may occur on almost any part of the body.

Sometimes, similar lesions may be found on the lips and nasal septum and in the lungs as a septic pneumonia. Conjunctivitis and keratitis may also occur in some cases.

**P.** See **CF.**

**D.** The lesions are fairly typical in endemic areas but must be distinguished from the more acute ulcerative lymphangitis caused by *Corynebacterium pseudotuberculosis*, glanders due to *Pseudomonas mallei* (q.v.), sporotrichosis due to the fungus *Sporothrichum schenckii* and bovine farcy caused by *Mycobacterium farcinogenes*.

The mallein test serves to differentiate between EL and glanders and identification of the causal organism, *Histoplasma capsulatum*, confirms epizootic lymphangitis.

**J.** Carcase and viscera: A, T or Kh with D (limbs, lungs, etc.), depending on extent of lesions and carcase condition.

## MONILIASIS (CANDIDIASIS, CANDIDOSIS, CANDIDAMYCOSIS, THRUSH)

**I.** A fungal infection of animals, birds and man caused by members of the mycelial yeast *Candida albicans* and closely related species.

**P.** These fungi are common inhabitants of the alimentary tract, to which they are normally confined as an infection, although extensions may take place to other organs such as the lungs, kidneys, heart, liver, placenta, udder and skin.

The disease is of most importance in poultry but also occurs in calves and piglets in which plaques of soft, yellowish-white pseudo-membrane overlying a red granulomatous area are found on the back of the tongue, oesophagus and stomach.

Affected animals show anorexia, profuse diarrhoea and dehydration.

**J.** Carcase and viscera: A, T or Kh, depending on extent of lesions and carcase condition.

## MUCORMYCOSIS (ZYGOMYCOSIS)

**I.** A contagious fungal infection of various species of animals (cattle, pigs, sheep, goats, horses, dogs, cats and certain wild animals) caused by members of the order Mucorales – *Mucor*, *Absidia*, *Mortierella* and *Rhizopus*.

**MT.** The mode of infection is by ingestion and also inhalation of spores in mouldy hay and feedingstuffs.

**P.** Lesions are in the form of granulomas in the intestinal wall and mesenteric lymph nodes. These caseous or calacareous nodular lesions, white or yellow in colour, may also be found in the liver, lungs and kidneys, especially in cattle and pigs. In some instances round, shallow ulcers occur in the forestomachs of cattle and intestinal tract of pigs and are sometimes associated with the use of prolonged antibiotic therapy.

**J.** Carcase and viscera: As for moniliasis.

## DERMATOPHILOSIS (MYCOTIC DERMATITIS, CUTANEOUS STREPTOTRICHOSIS, LUMPY WOOL DISEASE, STRAWBERRY FOOTROT)

**I.** An infection of the epidermis of cattle, sheep and goats, and less commonly horses, pigs and occasionally man. An ulcerative exudative dermatitis occurs with brownish crust formation, loss of hair, and granulation tissue formation (sheep) and from time to time general signs.

The disease in sheep is termed mycotic dermatitis when the body is involved but not the limbs, and strawberry foot rot when the lower limbs are affected.

**O.** Dermatophilosis occurs on all six continents but appears to be most common in Africa, South America and Oceania. It is enzootic in Chad, Comoros, South Africa and Zimbabwe and of high occurrence in Gambia. In South America, Antigua, Barbuda and St Lucia have a high occurrence. It is enzootic in Australia, New Zealand and Fiji and of sporadic occurrence in several European countries.

The disease was first reported in the USA in 1961, but that country is now free of the dermatophilosis.

Several countries have managed to eradicate the disease, including Guatemala (1985), Papua New Guinea (1987), Solomon Islands (1988) and Israel and Northern Ireland (1991).

**IA.** *Dermatophilus congolensis*, a Gram-positive, non-acid-fast facultative anaerobic euactinomycete which differs from the other actinomycetes in having two stages of growth – one of motile flagellated rods which reproduce by budding and the other of aggregates of non-motile coccoid cells which reproduce by cell fission.

**R.** The main source of infection is probably resistant carrier animals which have a few active lesions. The organism does not remain alive for long outside the animal body except in recently discarded scabs, in which it can survive for several months. The possibility that ticks and other biting insects can spread the infection may make these vectors a reservoir.

**MT.** The disease is most common during warm, wet weather of high humidity when the natural resistance of the skin tends to be reduced and also when biting insects are prevalent.

Infection occurs through minor abrasions in the skin. Operations such as shearing, dipping and use of instruments are also involved in causing infection as are the activities of ticks and biting flies.

**CF.** The zoospores germinate to produce hyphae which penetrate the skin at susceptible points and spread in all directions. An exudative inflammatory reaction results, with the matting of hair and wool by brownish crusts. These lesions vary in size from 1 cm in diameter to confluent lesions covering large areas of the body.

The lesions are most common on the back, sides, shoulders and head but may involve other parts. Calves are often affected on the muzzle, with subsequent spread to the head and neck.

The disease in sheep takes two forms: that already described, and a proliferative dermatitis (*'strawberry foot rot'*) which affects the lower limbs from the knee or hock to the carpus, especially on the coronets and heels. Here the lesions appear as dome-shaped growths covered with brown scabs below which is a granulating cauliflower-like mass which tends to bleed.

Young lambs may succumb in severe infections, but in most cases healing takes place in 3 weeks or so.

**P.** See **CF.** On occasion a secondary pneumonia may ensue.

**D.** Diagnosis is confirmed by demonstration of the organism in scrapings.

*Differential diagnoses* include lumpy skin disease, fleece rot, ulcerative dermatosis in sheep, contagious ecthyma ('orf'), etc.

**J.** As for Moniliasis.

## RHINOSPORIDIOSIS

**I.** A chronic, benign disease of the nasal mucosa and skin of cattle, horses, dogs, aquatic birds and man caused by the fungus *Rhinosporidium seeberi.*

**P.** Soft, pinkish, polypoid growths with granulomatous surfaces develop in the upper nasal passages, and sometimes the mouth and vagina. There is a blood-stained mucoid nasal discharge and dyspnoea. Granulomatous-like lesions also form on the skin.

**J.** Carcase and viscera: As for moniliasis, but judgement can be more lenient.

## RINGWORM (DERMAPHYTOSIS, DERMAMYCOSIS, TRICHOPHYTOSIS, MICROSPOROSIS, TINEA (MAN))

**I.** An infection by dermatophytes (fungi causing skin and hair infections) of the keratinised tissues (skin, hair, nails) of animals and man characterised by pityriasis (formation of greyish-white scales) and alopecia on thickened skin.

**O.** Worldwide in distribution, especially where animals are closely housed. It is usually a self-limiting condition occurring during the winter months in temperate regions in cattle and clearing up once livestock experience the spring sunshine, which may point to the importance of the animal's nutritional status and especially its vitamin D status.

**IA.** A variety of different fungi affecting both animals and man, some species occurring in several different animal hosts.

Two main genera are responsible for ringworm in animals – *Trichophyton* and *Microsporum.*

The following represent the most common dermatophytes in farm animals:

Cattle: *Trichophyton verrucosum, Tr. mentagrophytes, Tr. magninii.*

Horses: *Tr. equinum, Tr. mentagrophytes, Tr. verrucosum, Tr. quinckeanum, Microsporum equinum, M. gypseum*

Pigs: *Tr. mentagrophytes, Tr. verrucosum, Tr. rubrum, M. equinum, M. canis, M. nanum*

Sheep: *Tr. verrucosum, Tr. quinckeanum, Tr. mentagrophytes, Tr. gypseum, M. canis*

Goats: *Tr. verrucosum.*

*Man* (in whom the disease is termed tinea) is infected by members of the genera Trichophyton, Microsporum and Epidermophyton, notably *Tr. mentagrophytes, Tr. verrucosum, Tr. tonsurans, Tr. schoenleinii, M. andouinii* and *Epidermophyton floccosum.*

The dermatophytes are either saprophytes in the soil where they break down keratinised tissues of dead animals or pathogens acting on the skin of animals and man. They can be passed from animals to animals, man to man (rarely), animals to man and from soil to man. The disease they cause is thus a true *zoonosis.*

The spores are very resistant and can survive for months in dry, cool conditions although the usual disinfectants and heat easily destroy them.

Their structure consists of a mycelium of hyphae and arthrospores (formed by segmentation of the hyphae) and grow in the keratinised layers of the skin, on and inside hair shafts and in nails (in man). Under conditions of warmth, humidity, slightly alkaline pH and CO tension, the spores attack the outer layers of the skin (stratum corneum) and hairs producing autolysis and exudation which dries to form greyish-white flakes or crusts.

**R.** Infected and carrier animals, including dogs and cats, man and soil.

**MT.** Direct contact with infected animals is the usual mode of transmission, but infection may also be caused by indirect contact with bedding, harness, saddlery, grooming kits, clothing, etc.

**CF.** In cattle (the species most commonly affected) ringworm is more common in the younger animal. The lesions are roughly circular in outline, 3 cm in diameter and raised above the surrounding skin. The hair in the infected area breaks off, leaving thick, round, sharply circumscribed, greyish-white areas some 3 cm in diameter. Coalescence of lesions may take place to involve large areas of the skin. Commonly a reddish ring (where spores are actively creating inflammation) may be evident at the periphery of the hairless greyish centre. The usual sites in cattle are the head and neck, but lesions may occur on any part of the body. There is no evidence of pruritus.

Slight differences in lesion type are manifested in the different animal species, but scaling and alopecia are common in all of them.

Spores may be present on the skin and hair without apparent infection, a fact which emphasises the need for high standards of personal hygiene in all meat plant staff, especially those directly concerned with the handling of the live animal, the early stages of its stunning and slaughter and the handling of hides.

Staff must be alerted to the presence of all zoonoses encountered at ante-mortem inspection.

**P.** See **CF.**

**D.** The lesions are fairly characteristic but can be confused with mycotic dermatitis and dermatophilosis in cattle and pityriasis rosea and exudative dermatitis in pigs.

Diagnosis may be confirmed with the use of Wood's lamp, the direct demonstration of hyphae and spores in skin scrapings and hairs, and by culture.

**J.** Carcase and viscera: A, provided condition is satisfactory.

## SPOROTRICHOSIS

**I.** An uncommon, chronic, contagious disease of equidae and less commonly in cattle, camels, dogs, cats and man in which pyogranulomas and ulcers develop in animals on the limbs and sometimes on the head and thorax, with or without lymphangitis and lymphadenitis.

**O.** The disease has been reported in the USA, India and Europe.

**IA.** *Sporothrix schenckii*, a dimorphic Gram-positive fungus which lives as a saprophyte in organic matter in the soil, animal faeces and vegetable matter. In the body or culture at 37°C it is in the form of a spherical or rod-shaped yeast $3 \times 10\,\mu m$ in size. Filamentous forms with lateral hyphae and asexual single-walled conidia are formed at 22°C.

**R.** Soil and infected and carrier animals.

**MT.** The pathogenic spores (conidia) gain entrance to the body through skin abrasions or wounds, infection being conveyed by direct contact with infected animals or indirectly through contaminated materials such as bedding, saddlery, harness, grooming equipment, etc.

**CT.** Small, firm, elevated crusted nodules devoid of hair appear along the tracts of the lymphatic vessels, mainly on the lower limbs but also on the head and thorax. These eventually ulcerate and discharge a thick, creamy pus. The lymphatic vessels are inflamed and the associated lymph nodes are enlarged. On occasions these pyogranulomas may become generalised and involve thoracic and abdominal viscera.

**P.** See **CF.**

**D.** Sporotrichosis is very similar to epizootic lymphangitis, from which it can be differentiated by microscopical examination of pus/tissues to detect the round rod-shaped single spores within macrophages or by culture.

Other *differential diagnoses* include glanders, ulcerative lymphangitis and maduromycosis.

**J.** Carcase and viscera: A, T or Kh, depending on extent of lesions and carcase condition.

## DISEASES CAUSED BY PROTOZOA

The Protozoa are generally regarded as the lowest form of animal life, being unicellular microorganisms with a protoplasm differentiated into cytoplasm and nucleus. They vary greatly in size (2–100 µm) and shape, some, like the amoebae, possessing pseudopodia, while others are flagellated like *Giardia* and *Trichomonas* or ciliated like *Balantidium*.

*Reproduction* may be *asexual* by binary fission or schizogony in which there are successive divisions of the nucleus and cytoplasm to produce as many as 40 000 merozoites. *Sexual* reproduction also occurs in some species, e.g. Sporozoa where male and female gametes are formed which on union give rise to a zygote from which large numbers of sporozoites are produced.

Altogether there are some 30 000 species of Protozoa, most of whom are free-living, with only about 20 genera of pathogenic forms. Many species are saprophytic and some actually ingest bacteria. Some of the pathogenic forms, however, are able to inflict major plagues on animals and man, e.g. the genus *Plasmodium* responsible for malaria is estimated to cause the death of one million children yearly.

The classification of the phylum Protozoa (parasitic and non-parasitic) is very complicated, but the parasitic forms in animals and man can be placed in four main groups:

1 Superclass Mastigophora (Flagellates): Movement by flagella. Asexual reproduction by binary fission. Parasites of the intestine and genitourinary tract., e.g. *Giardia, Leishmania, Trichomonas, Trypanosoma.*
2 Subphylum Sporozoa: Babesia, malaria and allied parasites. Movement by gliding, sometimes by pseudopodia. Asexual and sexual life cycle. Reproduction by schizogony. Majority produce spores. Parasites of tissues, e.g. *Besnoitia, Coccidia, Eimeria, Neospora, Plasmodium, Sarcocystis, Toxoplasma.*
3 Subphylum Ciliophora (Ciliates): Movement by cilia. Asexual and sexual reproduction. Parasites of the gut but also invade tissues, e.g. *Balantidium.*
4 Superclass Sarcodina (Amoebae): Movement by pseudopodia. Asexual reproduction by binary fission. Some free-living. Parasites of the intestine but also invade tissues, e.g. *Babesia, Entamoeba, Theileria.*

Pathogenic effects are exerted in many different ways, for example, *Babesia* and *Plasmodium* are parasites of red blood cells, which are ruptured releasing the contents (plus results of reproduction) to cause haemoglobinuria. There is also interference with the kallikrein system (a body system of proteolytic enzymes produced by certain WBCs and platelets) which results in increased vascular dilatation and permeability to cause haemoglobinaemia, anaemia and anoxia, leading all too frequently to prostration and death. Other Protozoa, e.g. *Coccidia* act by invading and destroying the mucosal cells of the intestine producing intense diarrhoea, emaciation and often death.

### AMOEBIASIS

**I.** An acute or chronic protozoal infection of man and, less commonly, animals in which there is fever and haemorrhagic, ulcerative colitis.

**O.** Mainly West Africa, SE Asia, Natal, Mexico and South America and less commonly Europe and North America.

**IA.** *Entamoeba histolytica* is primarily a parasite of man but on occasion can infect animals. It can exist as a commensal in the intestine (surveys have shown up to 50% of people in tropical in countries harbouring the parasite) but can cause severe haemorrhagic enteritis. Other less pathogenic amoebae are *Ent. gingivalis, Ent. coli* and *Ent. hartmanni.*

**R.** The organisms are ubiquitous in tropical and subtropical regions.

**MT.** By ingestion of cysts in contaminated food and water.

**CF.** The cysts establish themselves in the mucosal crypts of the intestine, penetrate the submucosa and form abscesses which rupture the mucosa, creating ulcers with necrotic centres. In acute cases a severe dysentery develops which may resolve or progress to a chronic form. There is loss of weight, anorexia, dehydration and tenesmus. In the chronic form the diarrhoea may be constant or intermittent.

**P.** See **CF**. On occasion the amoebae may enter other organs such as the genitalia and skin.

**D.** Diagnosis depends on demonstrating *Ent. histolytica* trophozoites in faecal or tissue smears.

**J.** Carcase and viscera: Acute cases: T. Chronic cases, T, A or Kh.

## BABESIOSIS (PIROPLASMOSIS, REDWATER, TEXAS FEVER, CATTLE TICK FEVER)

**I.** A group of tick-borne diseases of cattle, water buffaloes, sheep, pigs and horses characterised by fever, anaemia, icterus, haemoglobinaemia and haemoglobinuria.

**O.** Babesiosis appears to occur worldwide, especially in tropical and subtropical countries. The USA and Canada are free at present. It is of enzootic occurrence in many countries including Albania, Sweden, Greece and N. Ireland, but last cases were recorded in Solomon Islands in 1929, Latvia in 1988, New Caledonia in 1988 and in 1989 in Mauritius, Yemen, Haiti and Yugoslavia. Both vectors and disease have been eradicated from the USA and Canada. Babesiosis is endemic in Australia but absent from New Zealand.

The occurrence of babesiosis is related to the distribution and activity of the various tick and biting fly vectors. The ticks involved include the genera *Ixodes* (*I. ricinus*, *I. persulcatus*), *Boophilus* (*B. annulatus*, *B. microplus*), *Haemaphysalis* (*H. punctata*), *Rhipicephalus* (*R. bursa*, *R. sanguineus*), *Dermacentor* and *Hyalomma*. *Boophilus microplus* is the tick vector in Australia and *B. decoloratus* in Africa.

Ticks abound in the permanent grass and bushes of rough low-lying ground and do not travel far on the ground. This means that babesiosis tends to be limited to such districts or fields.

*Ixodes ricinus* differs from the American tick, *Boophilus annulatus*, which transmits Texas fever, in that it is a three-host tick, leaving its host at each of its stages of development. It attaches itself to cattle during the larval, nymphal and adult stages and on each occasion sucks the blood of the host and becomes engorged. *Boophilus annulatus*, on the other hand, is a one-host tick and the various stages of its development take place on the one bovine host.

In areas in Zimbabwe where guinea fowl are protected, these birds have multiplied and, by consuming ticks, have virtually eliminated tick-borne disease, a beneficial effect which can be compared with the use of ducks and geese to consume *Limnaea truncatula* to control liver fluke.

**IA.** Several different babesia are involved in the different animal species as follows:

Cattle: *Babesia bovis*, *B. bigemina*, *B. berbera*, *B. argentina*, *B. major*, *B. divergens*

Water buffaloes: *B. bovis*, *B. bigemina*

Sheep and goats: *B. ovis*, *B. motasi*

Pigs: *B. trautmanni*, *B. perroncitoi*

Horses: *B. equi*, *B. caballi.*

*B. bovis* and *B. bigemina* are normally confined to tropical and subtropical countries, while *B. divergens* and *B. major* occur in temperate regions. In NW Europe the main parasite is *B. divergens*, *B. bovis* and *B. major* being of lesser importance.

A serological survey in cattle in N. Ireland (Taylor *et al.*, 1982) showed that the mean prevalence of *B. divergens* was 31.8%, the overall annual cost in terms of deaths, production loses and veterinary treatment being of the order of £250 000. It was found that the disease was mainly confined to the three counties of Armagh, Fermanagh and Tyrone.

**R.** Infected and carrier animals, domestic and wild, in addition to ticks and, less commonly, certain biting flies. The various protozoa pass part of their life cycle in the tick vectors, although *B. bovis* is only found in the larval stage of *B. microplus*. Transovarian transmission of infection occurs in ticks, the parasite passing through the egg to the next generation.

**MT.** Infection is transmitted from infected animals mainly by ticks, blood being transferred from an infected to a susceptible animal. When ticks feed on animals, the parasites in the tick's saliva pass into the bloodstream. It is also possible that contaminated needles and instruments play a part in the transmission of infection. Infection is more easily transmitted by certain species, e.g. *B. bigemina* and *B. equi*.

Once transference of infection occurs, multiplication of protozoa by binary fission begins in the RBCs in either the peripheral or visceral blood vessels. Haemolysis of the erythrocytes occurs, with release of haemoglobin into the plasma. There is also an accompanying vasodilatation and permeability of blood vessels through activation of the kallikrein system, which can lead to circulatory collapse and shock due to oxygen and nutrient insufficiency, $CO_2$ and waste products build-up, anaemia, jaundice, etc.

**CF.** *Babesia* infections assume several different forms depending on the virulence of the organism, resistance of the host, etc. The infection may be peracute, acute, chronic or inapparent.

After an incubation period of 2–3 weeks, in typical acute cases there is fever, inappetence, cessation of rumination in ruminants, malaise, anaemia, jaundice and haemoglobinuria with dark red to brown urine. Some cases display nervous symptoms when the CNS is affected, with incoordination, mania, convulsions, coma and death. Abortion may occur in pregnant animals.

In horses colic is often apparent with oedema of the fetlocks, head and ventral abdomen, but clinical anaemia is not evident.

Affected animals can remain carriers for months, even years, after recovery.

**P.** The lesions are typical of all conditions where red cell destruction by intraerythrocyte parasites occurs. Acute cases show jaundice, enlargement of the spleen, which is soft and pulpy, and enlargement of the liver, which is dark brown in colour. The gall bladder is distended with thick, dark-coloured granular bile. The enlarged kidneys are also very dark, even black in colour, and this coloration is often seen in animals which have long recovered from babesiosis. There is subcutaneous and intramuscular oedema with yellow, gelatinous fat and thin, watery blood. Clotting of the blood is characteristic in cattle and horses which have died of the disease.

Subendocardial and subepicardial ecchymoses are usually present in the heart. Loss of condition is evident in the carcase.

Cattle which have recovered from attacks of babesiosis are occasionally encountered at meat inspection. Such carcases show a typical light orange colour of the superficial fat. Further examination will often reveal very dark, even black coloured kidneys with some evidence of anaemia.

**D.** The post-mortem lesions encountered in an endemic area at a time of tick activity (spring and autumn) are suggestive of babesia. Confirmation, however, must be made by the examination of Giemsa- or Leishman-stained smears (absolute alcohol fixed) from the peripheral blood in the live animal. Similar smears may also be made at post-mortem. The protozoa can also be demonstrated in the kidney.

The organisms usually appear singly in the RBCs as pear-shaped bodies seldom exceeding 1.5 μm in length. Two may be found with their pointed ends in contact, the angle between the two organisms being obtuse. Sometimes the parasites occur singly as rounded or, less commonly, rod-shaped or lanceolate bodies, 1–2 μm in diameter.

Resort may also be made to serological tests such as complement fixation, indirect haemagglutination and indirect fluorescent antibody, especially the last.

**J.** Carcase and viscera: A, T, or Kh and D, depending on degree and extent of lesions and carcase condition.

## BALANTIDIOSIS (BALANTIDIASIS, BALANTIDIAL DYSENTERY)

**I.** A protozoan infection of the caecum and large intestine, mainly of pigs (the main host), higher primates, sometimes man and rarely dogs and rats in which there is enteritis, anaemia, diarrhoea and poor growth.

Zoonosis.

**O.** Worldwide in distribution.

**IA.** *Balantidium coli*, an actively mobile protozoan parasite, the vegetative forms of which are 30–150 μm in length and 25–125 μm wide. It is ellipsoidal in shape and possesses longitudinal spiral rows of cilia over the whole body. The cytoplasm contains a kidney-shaped macronucleus and a smaller micronucleus along with several food vacuoles.

The parasite is a commensal in the large intestine, where it feeds on *Ascarops* (nematode) eggs, starch, bacteria and ingesta. It may invade the mucosa to produce enteritis and ulceration with haemorrhage but normally there is little change in the mucous membrane.

*B. coli* produces yellowish-green cysts which are spherical or oval in shape and about 45–65 µm in diameter. The cysts are very resistant organisms, much more so than the trophozoites, which are the adult, active, motile stage of *B. coli*.

*B. coli* reproduces in the large intestine by binary fission. Conjugation, i.e. the temporary union of two individuals to transfer genetic material, may also take place.

**R.** Pigs, rats and other animals, especially primates.

**MT.** Via the ingestion of cysts in foods and water contaminated with pig faeces. Sows' faeces are the main source of infection for piglets.

**CF.** Usually only anaemia, enteritis, anorexia, diarrhoea (which may be blood-stained) and poor growth are evident. But severe infections can result in serious haemorrhage and death when intestinal ulceration occurs.

In man, in which the disease is very acute, there is severe colitis with desquamation of the intestinal mucosa and watery diarrhoea. In debilitated individuals the disease can be fatal.

**P.** See **CF**.

**D.** Diagnosis is based on the clinical signs, post-mortem changes and the demonstration of large numbers of trophozoites or cysts of *Balantidium coli* in faeces, mucosal scrapings or intestinal contents.

**J.** Carcase and viscera: Depends on degree of infection and carcase condition. Usually A or T and D (intestine).

## BESNOITIOSIS

**I.** A sporozoan disease of cattle, horses, burros, goats, cats, reindeer and certain forms of wildlife in which there is severe inflammation of the skin, subcutis and blood vessels.

**O.** Besnoitiosis has been reported in Africa, Europe, Soviet Union, Asia and South America.

**IA.** Besnoitia are *Toxoplasma*-like organisms which form large, thick-walled cysts full of bradyzoites in endothelial, histiocytes and other cells.

Several forms of the parasite are known to cause disease – *Besnoitia besnoiti* in cattle, *B. bennetti* in horses and burros and *B. tarandi* in reindeer.

**R.** Domestic and wild cats (in which the organism is *B. wallacei*) are believed to be the definitive hosts. The reservoir also includes infected and carrier animals and wildlife.

**MT.** Infection probably takes place by ingestion (cat faeces are a common source of infection) and also by the bites of flies. Mechanical transmission via syringes is also possible.

**CF.** An initial fever is followed by inappetence, malaise, increased respiratory rate, rhinitis, swelling of superficial lymph nodes, anasarca, photophobia, lachrymation, nasal discharge and orchitis. Severe dermatitis develops with thickening and induration of the skin, which becomes wrinkled, especially on the shoulders, neck and hindquarters. Affected parts of the skin become hairless and portions of the superficial layers are shed. Pregnant animals are liable to abort and affected bulls become sterile. Animals which are severely affected become emaciated. The mortality rate is in the region of 10%.

**P.** In addition to the skin changes, there are widespread lesions in the blood vascular and muscular (skeletal and cardiac) systems. There is extensive perivasculitis and myopathy due to the presence of cysts, which are also present in the scleral conjunctiva and nasal mucosa. Fine seed-like granules can be felt in the subcutis.

**D.** Diagnosis depends on the demonstration of the spindle-shaped bradyzoites in affected tissues, especially skin biopsy smears and scleral conjunctiva.

**J.** Carcase and viscera: A and D, localised lesions with no systemic effect. T, widespread lesions or systemic effect.

## COCCIDIOSIS (RED DYSENTERY IN CATTLE)

**I.** A usually acute, but sometimes chronic, contagious protozoan disease of all domestic animals, especially rabbits and poultry, characterised by haemorrhagic enteritis and dysentery in the acute form.

**O.** Coccidiosis occurs worldwide, the disease in poultry being of high occurrence in many countries and causing severe economic losses. The close confinement of poultry and other animal species provides an ideal environment for infection to develop and be maintained.

**IA.** Coccidia of the genera *Eimeria*, *Isospora* and *Cystoisospora*. All coccidia are host-specific and cross-immunity does not exist between the different species.

The coccidia are sporozoan parasites which, in the form of merozoites, invade and destroy the epithelial cells of the intestine.

**Life cycle of coccidia** The life cycle is complex and slight differences exist between the different species. For example, *Eimeria*, *Isospora* and *Cystoisospora* typically require only one host in which to complete their life cycle, but *Cystoisospora* can utilise an intermediate host and the number of sporocysts and sporozoites produced also varies.

Infection takes place when *oocysts* (present in the faeces of infected animals) are ingested. Under suitable conditions of oxygen, temperature, moisture and available nutrients, etc., the oocysts sporulate with the production of *sporozoites* within secondary cysts (*sporocysts*). In *Eimeria* spp. the sporulated oocyst has 4 sporocysts, each with 2 sporozoites, while the sporulated oocysts of *Isospora* and *Cystoisospora* spp. have 2 sporocysts, each with 4 sporozoites.

In the small intestine (posterior half) the sporozoites leave the sporocyst and invade the mucosa of the villi and the epithelial cells of other organs, e.g. liver, where they develop into multinucleated *schizonts*, each nucleus of which becomes a *merozoite*. The merozoites (of which there can be hundreds or thousands) are liberated when the cell is ruptured and invade cells in the large intestine to repeat the whole process. After a few generations of asexual reproduction, merozoites develop into either *macrogametes* (female) or *microgametes* (male) to begin the sexual aspect of the coccidial cycle.

The microgametes can be regarded as the spermatozoa of the higher animals. When released into the lumen of the intestine, they penetrate the intestinal cells containing the macrogametes and fertilise them, producing *zygotes* which become *oocysts*. When mature, the oocysts are liberated from the intestinal cells and are passed out in the faeces.

The cells of the host are destroyed by the production of shizonts and gametes and the release of oocysts. Each oocyst, with the vast increase in subsequent progeny, has the capacity to destroy hundreds or thousands of individual intestinal cells. Subsequent cell damage is caused by secondary bacterial infection.

*Hosts of coccidia* are as follows:

Cattle: *Eimeria zuernii*, *E. bovis*, *E. ellipsoidalis*, *E. canadensis*, *E. pellita*, *E. subspherica*, *E. alabamensis*, *Isospora absaica*

Sheep and goats: *E. arloingi*, *E. faurei*, *E. ahsata*, *E. ovinoidalis*, *E. ovina E. parva*, *E. pallida*, *E. crandallis*, *E. granulosa*, *E. marsica*

Pigs: *E. debliecki*, *E. scabra*, *E. porci*, *E. scrofae*, *E. perminuta*, *E. polita*, *E. cerdowis*, *E. spinosa*, *E. romaniae*, *I. suis*

Horses: *E. leuckarti*.

(The above list is by no means complete.)

**R.** Clinically affected and carrier animals.

**MT.** By the ingestion of food and water contaminated with oocyst-containing faeces or the licking of a coat contaminated with faeces.

**CF.** Coccidiosis is more prevalent under conditions of overcrowding, poor nutrition, unhygienic conditions, stressful situations such as transportation, weaning, sudden changes of feed, inclement weather, etc.

The destruction of the epithelial cells in the villi of the intestine, which can extend to the submucosa, is accompanied by haemorrhage into the lumen, catarrhal inflammation and diarrhoea or dysentery.

The incubation period varies in the different species from 2–4 weeks in cattle to 2–3 weeks in sheep and 1 week in pigs.

Coccidiosis is mostly a disease of younger animals – usually under 1 year old in cattle and horses and under 6 months of age in sheep, goats and pigs.

The severity of symptoms depends largely on the degree of infection, the species of coccidia, isospora, etc., involved, the form of husbandry, the factors listed above, and the susceptibility of the animal.

In addition to the diarrhoea, there may be whole blood, mucus and portions of sloughed mucosa in the faeces. Animals lose weight, with a rough hair coat, hindquarters are soiled with faeces, and exhibit weakness, inappetence and dehydration. In light infestations, however, there may be watery faeces with little or no blood and the animal showing no significant signs of ill-health.

During the acute period in cattle, many animals die. Those which survive take a long time to recover body weight.

Central nervous symptoms have been described in some instances in cattle.

**P.** Haemorrhagic enteritis with the presence of blood-stained contents in the intestine is the most significant finding. The mucosa may be ulcerated with portions sloughed off. The mucosa of the whole intestine from caecum to rectum is thickened and may even be formed in ridges. Less severe infections may show only a catarrhal inflammation of the intestinal mucosa.

Small whitish cysts may be visible on the tips of the intestinal villi, especially in the ileum.

Anaemia and loss of condition are evident in more severe cases.

**D.** The demonstration of numbers of *oocysts* in the faeces is diagnostic. It may be necessary to examine several faecal samples because of the many factors involved in the coccidial life cycle, stage of infection, number of infective oocysts ingested, method of examination, etc.

**J.** Carcase and viscera: A, T, or Kh and D, depending on carcase condition.

## CRYPTOSPORIDIOSIS

**I.** A self-limiting acute or chronic protozoan zoonotic disease of cattle, sheep, pigs, humans, some forms of wildlife and less commonly horses, dogs and cats in which there is loss of weight and diarrhoea.

**O.** The disease has an occurrence on all six continents in a wide variety of hosts.

A monoclonal antibody technique was used in a US nationwide survey of 7369 faecal samples taken from calves on 1103 farms. Oocysts of cryptosporidia were found on 652 (59.1%) of the farms and in the faecal samples from 1648 (22.4%). About 50% of the calves (1–3 weeks old) had oocysts in their faecal samples. The prevalence of cryptosporidiosis was highest during the summer months and farms with more than 100 milking cows and those where the cows did not calve in individual boxes were significantly more likely to have calves with cryptosporidia (Garber *et al.*, 1994). Other studies have revealed the presence of *Cryptosporidium* oocysts in 5% of piglets.

In some instances the organisms have been isolated from clinically healthy animals, a fact which lends some doubt as to the real pathogenicity of *Cryptosporidium* at least under certain conditions.

The organism has also been isolated from human faecal specimens in some 50 countries, the prevalence varying from less than 1–4.5% in developed countries to 3–20% in developing regions.

**IA.** The coccidian protozoan parasites *Cryptosporidium parvum* and *C. muris*. Both have been successfully transmitted experimentally to a wide variety of mammals including cattle, pigs, sheep, goats, cats, dogs and mice, thus making *Cryptosporidia* non-host-specific parasites unlike the *Coccidia*, which are host-specific.

The life history has both asexual and sexual cycles of reproduction. Unlike *Eimeria* and *Isospora*, however, *Cryptosporidium* oocysts can sporulate in the intestine and are immediately infective when passed in the faeces, whereas the former two genera only sporulate when they have been passed from the host.

Although intracellular parasites like *Eimeria* and *Isospora*, *Cryptosporidia* are extracytoplasmic in that the organism is fused with the cytoplasm of the epithelial cells, all being enclosed by host membranes.

The oocysts of *Cryptosporidium* possess very thick walls which make them resistant to many environmental influences. They can remain infective for months under suitable conditions of moisture and temperature. They are more easily destroyed under dry conditions and the usual disinfectants in normal concentrations are effective against them.

**R.** Since the organism can cross species barriers, the reservoir of infection includes a wide range of domestic and wild animals as well as man himself.

**MT.** By the faecal–oral route, either directly from animal to animal or man or vice versa or indirectly via fomites.

**CF.** Cryptosporidiosis is essentially a disease of the young animal. Organisms are usually shed within 5 days of infection and continue to be shed for about 2 weeks. The clinical signs include anorexia, loss of weight, diarrhoea, some dehydration and tenesmus.

Symptoms resemble those of other diseases in which enteritis is the major entity. The diarrhoea, although persistent, is self-limiting. The mortality rate varies greatly but is generally in the region of 5%.

**P.** Affected carcases are dehydrated and anaemic. The distal small intestine is hyperaemic with yellowish contents. There is severe villous atrophy due to the presence of large numbers of the parasite (trophozoites and schizonts).

**D.** Diagnosis is confirmed by demonstration of the oocysts in mucosal scrapings or faecal samples (flotation in sucrose or zinc sulphate). The oocysts are much smaller than *Eimeria* and *Isospora*, being in the case of *C. parvum* less than 5 μm in diameter. *C. muris* is slightly larger (less than 6 μm in diameter).

The acid-fast technique of staining may be used, when *Cryptosporidium* oocysts stain red, while yeasts, which are about the same size, stain blue or green with the counterstain.

Cryptosporidiosis must be distinguished from many other diarrhoeic diseases including coccidiosis, salmonellosis, coronavirus and rotavirus infections.

**J.** As for coccidiosis.

## GIARDIASIS (LAMBLIASIS)

**I.** A usually chronic or inapparent zoonotic infection of most domestic animals, especially cattle and sheep, birds and man in which the main symptom is continuous or intermittent diarrhoea or steatorrhoea.

**O.** Worldwide in distribution, most cases occurring in tropical and subtropical countries as a silent inapparent condition.

**IA.** *Giardia intestinalis*, *G. duodenalis*, *G. lamblia* and *Lamblia intestinalis*.

The *Giardia* are pear-shaped binucleate protozoa possessing eight flagella. The ventral surface of the trophozoitc (which is released from the ingested cyst) is concave and arranged as a sucker for attachment to the intestinal mucosa of the host. The trophozoites are 9–21 μm long, 5–15 μm wide and 2–4 μm thick.

The organism would appear to act as a commensal in the intestine of animals and man, only acting as an opportunist parasite under ill-defined conditions of host susceptibility.

The term zooanthroponosis has been suggested for giardiasis and for those diseases (amoediasis, cryptosporidiosis, etc.) which are maintained in nature by lower vertebrates.

**R.** Infected and carrier animals, birds and man and many forms of wildlife.

**MT.** By the faecal–oral route. The ingested cysts release the flagellated trophozoites in the intestine, where they adhere to the villi of the mucosa.

**CF.** The disease is most common in cattle, sheep, human beings, dogs and cats and less common in horses and pigs. Young animals and children are most often affected.

The main symptoms in active cases are diarrhoea and loss of weight. In some instances there is steatorrhoea in which excess fat is present in the faeces due to malabsorption initiated by the adherent trophozoites. In these cases the faeces are pale in colour, greasy and malodorous, the situation which obtains in human beings.

**P.** There are usually no gross lesions in the intestine, although a mild enteritis may be present.

**D.** Diagnosis is made by demonstrating the trophozoites in intestinal scrapings or the cysts (averaging 10 μm × 15 μm) in faeces. For the latter the zinc sulphate centrifugal flotation method is used.

**J.** Carcase and viscera: A, T, or Kh and D, depending on carcase condition.

## NEOSPOROSIS

**I.** A protozoan infection of cattle associated with neonatal paresis, encephalitis and abortion.

**O.** The disease has been reported in North America, Australia, Japan, South Africa, United Kingdom and the Netherlands.

**IA.** Species of *Neospora*. Although *Neospora caninum* (the cause of paresis and mortality in young dogs) is known to cause abortion in cattle under experimental conditions, it is not certain whether this organism is the cause in all instances. *Neospora* species isolated from cases of bovine abortion in the USA were immunologically indistinguishable from *N. caninum*, but the exact relationship with *N. caninum* was not clear.

**R.** Infected and carrier cattle and dogs.

**MT.** The exact mode of transmission is not known. It may, however, occur by the placenta, which is the route in dogs. Since only the asexual stages of the life cycle are known, many aspects of *Neospora* spp. infection are not clear. In the past, the organisms have been confused with *Toxoplasma gondii*.

**CF.** Affected animals show neonatal paresis, encephalomyelitis and abortion with stillbirths.

**P.** Fetuses exhibit a gliosis in the CNS (an excess of astroglia, neuroglial cells of ectodermal origin). There is also some degree of placentitis.

**D.** Diagnosis can only be confirmed with certainty by immunohistochemical identification of the organisms in fetal tissue.

**J.** Carcase and viscera: A, providing condition is adequate.

## SARCOCYSTOSIS (SARCOSPORIDIOSIS)

**I.** A usually subclinical sporozoan disease of cattle, pigs, sheep, goats, horses, birds, dogs, cats, man and wild carnivores, rodents and reptiles characterised mainly by a cystic invasion of most tissues of the body (mainly skeletal muscle and nervous tissue) but which on occasions is associated with severe clinical signs and death.

**O.** Probably worldwide. Most reports of sarcosporidiosis have come from Canada, USA, England, Iceland, Norway and Australia.

Sarcocystosis was at one time common in swill-fed pigs in the USA, with an incidence of 75% in some areas compared with 5% in grain-fed pigs. The incidence, however, has reduced significantly with the compulsory boiling of swill before use. Although at one time recorded in 20–30% of pigs in Denmark, it is now rarely encountered.

In South Africa 0.01% of cattle and 0.04% of pigs are condemned because of sarcocystosis.

In Australia records of the Bureau of Animal Health in 1973 showed that of 17.4 million sheep slaughtered 0.27% were infested with *Sarcocystis* spp. In the same country there have been high rejection rates, even up to 100%, due to sarcocystosis, many of the sheep having originated from irrigation areas. Microcysts of *S. hominis* and *S. tenella* (which can only be detected microscopically) were found in 90.3% of young sheep (less than 15 months of age) and in 96.1% of adult sheep, which had macrocysts in 13.4%. (Seneviratna and Ford, 1980).

*Sarcocystis bertrami* (*equicanis*) has been detected in oesophageal samples from 62% of 394 horses and ponies at an abattoir in Cheshire, England (Edwards, 1982). The prevalence was greater in older animals and in females.

**IA.** Sporozoan parasites of the genus *Sarcocystis* are recorded in more than 50 species of mammals and birds, all being host-specific.

*Sarcocystis* spp. develop in two-host cycles, the definitive or final (predator) hosts being dogs, cats and wild carnivores – foxes, wolves, raccoons, coyotes, etc. – while the farm livestock are intermediate hosts or prey hosts. Only the prey hosts are harmed, the organisms rarely causing disease in the predator hosts.

Some of the more common *Sarcocystis* spp. occurring in farm animals are as follows:

- Cattle: *S. cruzi* (cattle–dog, fox, etc.), *S. hirsuta* (*S. bovifelis*) (cattle–cat), *S. hominis* (cattle–man)
- Sheep: *S. tenella* (sheep–dog, fox, etc.), *S. arieticanis* (sheep–dog, fox, etc.), *S. gigantea* (sheep–cat), *S. medusiformis* (sheep-cat)
- Goats: *S. capracanis* (goat–dog), *S. hircicanis* (goat–dog), *S. moulei* (goat–cat)
- Pigs: *S. miescheriana* (pig–dog, fox, etc.), *S. suihominis* (pig–man), *S. porcifelis* (pig–cat)
- Horses: *S. bertrami* (horse–dog), *S. neurona* (unknown).

**Life cycle** The predator or scavenger host becomes infected by eating flesh containing infective sarcocysts, which are shed as *sporocysts* or sporulated oocysts in the faeces after 1 week. The intermediate or prey host then ingests these sporocysts in contaminated food and water and in the small intestine *sporozoites* are released by the action of digestive enzymes and bile. The sporozoites penetrate the intestinal mucosa and enter arterioles in the wall and lymph nodes. Each sporozoite then divides by multiple fission into first generation *schizonts*. Numerous *merozoites* are liberated from each schizont, enter the bloodstream and develop into second-generation schizonts in the capillary endothelium throughout the animal body. Merozoites liberated from second-generation schizonts circulate in the bloodstream in mononuclear cells or extracellularly. Merozoites from second and third generations penetrate muscle cells and neurons and glial cells in the brain, where they encyst. These tissue cysts contain one or two parasite forms (*metrocytes*) each of which divides to produce an infective cyst some 2–3 months after initial ingestion.

Although many sporocysts are small, some are large enough to be recognised at meat inspection. (Average size of *S. cruzi* is 16.3 μm by 10.8 μm.)

**R.** All infected and carrier species listed above.

**MT.** Animals become infected through eating foodstuffs and pasture contaminated with the sporocysts from dogs, foxes, etc., which acquire infection from eating infected meat and offal.

**CF.** Although sarcocysts have not been regarded in the past as pathogenic, recent experience has shown that they can produce disease. Their importance is being increasingly recognised. For example, the chronic condition Dalmeny disease, in which there is emaciation, submandibular oedema and exophthalmia, is now believed to be a bovine sarcocystosis. In most instances, however, sarcocystosis is subclinical. The species of *Sarcocystis* largely determines the severity of the disease.

Severely affected *cattle* show fever, anorexia, loss of condition and milk yield, muscle spasms, diarrhoea, hyperaesthesia, weakness, anaemia and sometimes death. Abortion occurs in some cases.

Other species of livestock display similar symptoms. Sarcocystosis in *sheep*, however, is frequently seen as an encephalomyelitis with weakness, ataxia, hyperaesthesia and paresis while still maintaining appetite and alertness. Cases of lymphadenopathy, non-suppurative interstitial pneumonia and encephalitis have also been recorded.

The incidence of *Sarcocystosis* is higher in the older animal and in stall-fed cattle and pigs fed on swill.

In *horses* there is a tendency for nervous symptoms to develop owing to the presence of sarcocysts in the brain and spinal cord.

*Humans* can act as intermediate hosts and have been infected with *S. suihominis* by eating uncooked pork and with *S. hominis* from uncooked beef. Symptoms in man include transient nausea, diarrhoea and abdominal pain.

**P.** Schizonts are distributed throughout the body in endothelial cells, being especially common in striated muscle, heart, brain, liver, lung and kidneys.

In muscle the cysts lie within or between individual muscle fibres and have a characteristic cigar-shape known as *Miescher's bodies*, sacs or tubules (4.5 μm × 0.35 μm). The larger cysts may lie loose in the perimuscular connective tissue and are globular, oval or bean-shaped. Although the size of the cyst is determined by its age and the host species, its basic structure remains the same, namely a cell which may be striated and consists partly of sarcolemma, a cavity which may or may not be subdivided by septa, and contents that are viscous or gelatinous and opaque to milky white or yellowish in colour. The cyst contains sporoblasts along the periphery and varying numbers of sickle-shaped nucleated sporozoites known as *Rainey's corpuscles*.

In cattle sarcocysts are found chiefly in active muscles such as the tongue, masseter muscles, heart and diaphragm. Slight infestations found in the masseter muscles at post-mortem tend to disappear during overnight chilling. On occasions, the muscle lesions may be concentrated in foci varying from 3 or 4 spots to a solid greenish area about 10 cm in diameter.

Only larger cysts are visible to the naked eye, appearing as light grey dots on cross-section and spindle-shaped on longitudinal section. Small cysts are only visible when degeneration and calcification occur.

Lesions of focal *eosinophilic myositis*, characterised by spindle-shaped greenish areas which may coalesce to form lesions several centimetres in diameter, may be caused by degenerating or decomposing sarcocysts, but similar lesions occur without any apparent connection with *Sarcocystis*. The two conditions may co-exist. It has also been shown that other parasitic organisms and allergic reactions focused on muscle may elicit eosinophilic myositis. A connection between sarcocystosis and eosinophilic myositis has, therefore, not been proved.

There is a wide variation in pathological findings in sarcocystosis, from few gross lesions apart from multiple areas of pallor in heavily infested muscle, to widespread petechial and ecchymotic haemorrhages and hepatitis, glomerulitis and retinitis in encephalomyelitis cases in sheep. Erosions and ulcerations in the mouth and oesophagus have been described in cattle.

In the pig the muscles of the abdominal wall, diaphragm and the masticatory and skeletal muscles are most often affected.

Lesions designated as *'sarcocysts'* are sometimes encountered in the shoulder muscle (*m. triceps brachii*) incision during routine inspection of bovine carcases in Africa, these lesions being of a light green iridescent coloration or forming streaky greyish-white areas elongated along the course of the muscle fibres. Sometimes the lesions are widely distributed throughout the carcase musculature without evidence of sarcosporidiosis. The lesion is essentially a focal eosinophilic myositis and may be an allergic manifestation to an unidentified parasite.

**D.** Diagnosis depends on an accurate evaluation of the herd/flock and its association with dogs, along with the clinical signs listed above, detection of humoral antibodies and histopathological examination of a wide range of organs, including kidney, liver, spleen, muscle, spinal cord and lymph nodes.

**J.** Carcase and viscera: A, T, or Kh and D, depending on the degree of infestation and carcase condition.

## THEILERIOSIS

**I.** A group of protozoan tick-borne infections of cattle, sheep, goats and wild ruminants, e.g. blue wildebeest, eland and siberian roe, in which there is fever, lymphadenopathy, leukopenia, anaemia and often high mortality.

Theileriosis includes East Coast fever, Corridor disease, tropical theileriosis or Mediterranean Coast fever and benign bovine theileriosis.

Members of the genus *Theileria* and *Babesia*, having similar life cycles, are sometimes termed *piroplasms* and their diseases piroplasmosis. While both parasites attack RBCs, *Theileria* spp. utilise both red and white blood cells to complete their life cycle in the mammalian host.

**Life cycle of *Theileria parva* in the bovine:** The infective uninuclear *sporozoites* (1.5 µm in diameter) are transmitted in the saliva of infected ticks, e.g. *Rhipicephalus appendiculatus* when its nymphal and adult stages feed on the susceptible mammalian host. In the lymphocytes, lymphoblasts and lymph nodes the sporozoites replicate into several multinucleated *macroschizonts* (*Koch's blue bodies*). After a series of macroschizont replications *microschizonts* containing numerous nuclear particles or 'cocci' (up to 120) are formed. When the cell ruptures, they are freed as *micromerozoites* and enter red blood cells to form the characteristic piroplasms which represent the end-form of the infection in the bovine.

In the *nymphal ticks*, merozoites are liberated in the tick gut from the red blood cells by lysis and develop into several sexual forms of *microgametes* and *macrogametes*. From these 'male' and 'female' forms, *zygotes* are produced, which increase in size to form motile *ookinetes* which pass to the salivary gland. In the salivary gland, sporogony occurs with the production of numerous infective *sporozoites*.

The various stages of development of the parasite pass through the larval, nymphal and adult forms of the ticks, but there is no transovarian transmission.

## EAST COAST FEVER (ECF)

**I.** An acute, non-contagious, protozoan tick-borne disease of cattle, water buffalo and certain wild ruminants characterised by high fever, lymphadenopathy, leukopenia, anaemia, emaciation and high mortality.

(*Corridor disease* is a form of East Coast fever which occurs primarily in buffaloes but can be transmitted to cattle. It is caused by *T. lawrencei (bovis)* and is transmitted by the tick *Rhipicephalus zambiensis.*)

**O.** As the name implies, ECF is mainly confined to East and Central Africa, being of especially high occurrence in Sudan and Zambia. Namibia had its last case in 1986, Central African Republic in 1986 and Nigeria in 1990. The disease has been eradicated from South Africa, Swaziland, Mozambique and Zimbabwe.

**IA.** *Theileria parva,* a sporozoan parasite whose merozoite forms (1.5 μm × 0.5–1 μm) in red blood cells are comma, rod, round, ring or annular-shaped. With Romanowsky stains they appear as a blue cytoplasm with a red chromatin granule at one end. In lymphocytes, and occasionally in lymph nodes and the spleen, where they are actively multiplying, they become larger, circular or irregularly-shaped bodies (schizonts or Koch's blue bodies) up to 12 μm in diameter.

There are three subtypes of *Theileria parva*: *T. parva parva,* transmitted between cattle; *T. parva lawrencei,* transmitted from buffalo to cattle; and the feebly pathogenic *T. parva bovis,* which is transmitted between cattle.

**R.** Infected animals and the larval, nymphal and adult stages of the vector ticks, only the latter two being capable of transmitting infection. Carrier status is believed to be rare in East Coast fever but recovered cases of Corridor disease (benign form of ECF) can act as carriers. Water buffaloes and wild bovidae can sustain the tick population but not the parasite.

**MT.** The main vector tick is *Rhipicephalus appendiculatus,* but other species of *Rhipicephalus* as well as species of *Hyalomma* are probably also involved. Adults and nymphs of *R. appendiculatus* can remain alive on the ground for over a year without feeding, but *T. parva* infection in the ticks only remains infective for about 9 months.

Once an infected nymph or adult tick feeds to engorgement it loses its infection completely.

Infection is transmitted by the nymphal and adult stages of the ticks, the infective sporozoites being injected into the ruminant host when the ticks engorge on it.

**CF.** Many factors are involved in the degree of virulence of the disease – immune status of the animal (e.g. buffaloes and zebu cattle and young animals are less susceptible), level of tick infestation, origin of tick population, level of infective dose, strain of organism, etc.

An initial sign is enlargement of the lymph nodes in the region of the tick bite (in 1–2 weeks after tick attachment).

In the acute form of ECF there is high fever, depression, anorexia, lymphadenopathy, lachrymation, nasal discharge, diarrhoea and/or dysentery, emaciation, weakness, prostration and death in 7–10 days in severe cases. In some instances there is CNS involvement with circling (*'turning sickness'*), convulsions, head pressing and muscular tremors. A few animals show blepharospasm (spasm of the orbital muscle of the eye) and keratitis.

Most of the clinical signs are associated with the tremendous damage to the reticuloendothelial system.

**P.** The principal pathological features are emaciation, lymph node enlargement, marked pulmonary oedema and hyperaemia along with hydrothorax and hydropericardium. The lung interlobular septa are well-defined and the bronchi and trachea are full of frothy exudate. Ecchymotic haemorrhages are evident on the serosal and mucosal surfaces of many organs. The liver is often slightly enlarged and shows mottled grey areas. The thymus, lymph nodes, abomasum and intestines may exhibit necrosis and ulceration.

Sometimes the lymph nodes are oedematous and haemorrhagic and show areas of necrosis.

**D.** Diagnosis is based on clinical signs and the demonstration of schizonts in lymph node biopsy smears and piroplasms in blood smears.

The complement fixation test and especially the indirect fluorescent antibody test can be used to detect infection with *T. parva.*

*Differential diagnoses*: babesiosis, anaplasmosis, trypanosomiasis.

**J.** Carcase and viscera: T, A, or Kh and D, according to severity of lesions and carcase condition.

## MEDITERRANEAN COAST FEVER (TROPICAL THEILERIOSIS)

**I.** A non-contagious tick-borne protozoan disease of cattle and water buffalo characterised by fever, lymphadenopathy, emaciation, anaemia and icterus.

**O.** The disease occurs in the Middle East from Morocco to Egypt and Iran (enzootic both countries), Iraq, Kuwait and Yemen. Portugal, Russia and Greece have a low sporadic occurrence and Great Britain an exceptionally low one. It would appear to have been eradicated from Japan and Malaysia but is important in the Far East, notably in Bhutan. Australia and New Caledonia are sporadically affected, but there is only serological evidence without clinical signs in New Zealand.

**IA.** *Theileria annulata* (*T. dispar*) is the usual organism involved in the Middle East, but *T. orientalis* (transmitted by *Haemaphysalis* spp. ticks) is active in Russia, Asia and the Far East.

**R.** Water buffaloes and infected ticks.

**MT.** The tick vectors are species of the genus *Hyalomma*.

**CF.** Fever, inappetence, malaise, oculonasal discharge, diarrhoea and dysentery following early constipation, loss of condition, enlargement of peripheral lymph nodes, anaemia and jaundice. Mild, subacute, acute and chronic forms of the disease may occur.

Different strains of organisms vary in pathogenicity, some strains of *T. annulata* causing mortality rates of up to 90%.

**P.** Pallor of mucous and serous surfaces with widespread petechiation which is also present on the epicardium and endocardium. The liver is enlarged and brownish in colour and the spleen is swollen and pulpy. Lymph nodes are enlarged, hyperaemic and oedematous. The lungs show oedema and congestion, while mucosal erosion and ulceration is common in the abomasum.

**D.** As for East Coast fever.

**J.** As for East Coast fever.

## BENIGN THEILERIOSIS OF CATTLE, SHEEP AND GOATS

**I.** A non-contagious, protozoan disease of cattle, buffaloes, sheep and goats in which the mild clinical signs are malaise, fever, anaemia and lymphadenopathy.

**O.** Middle East, South Africa, Kenya, Korea, India and Australia.

**IA.** Cattle: *Theileria mutans*, only small numbers of which are present as schizonts and sporozoites.

Sheep and goats: *T. ovis*.

**R.** Recovered animals and infected ticks.

**MT.** Cattle: Transmission is effected by the tick *Rhipicephalus appendiculatus*, *R. evertsi*, *Amblyomma variegatum* and others.

Sheep and goats: *Rhipicephalus bursa* and *R. evertsi*.

**CF.** Mild fever, malaise and low degrees of anaemia and lymphadenopathy.

**P.** Slight anaemia and slight enlargement of lymph nodes. In more acute cases lesions resemble those due *to T. parva*.

**D.** As for East Coast fever.

**J.** As for East Coast fever.

*Malignant theileriosis* occurs in sheep and goats, in which there is severe damage to the lymphatic system, with high fever, jaundice, anaemia and a mortality which may reach 100%.

Malignant theileriosis is caused by *Theileria hirci*, which is similar in morphology and distribution to *T. annulata*, the cause of Mediterranean Coast fever.

The post-mortem findings, diagnosis and judgement are similar to those for East Coast fever.

## TRICHOMONIASIS

**I.** A non-febrile, contagious, venereal, protozoal disease of cattle associated with early fetal death, abortion and infertility in cows and bulls.

**O.** Worldwide.

**IA.** *Trichomonas foetus*, a pear-shaped flagellated protozoan (10–25 μm × 5–15 μm) possessing three flagella of the same length as the organism body at the rounded anterior end and one flagellum at the pointed posterior end. An undulating membrane runs the length of the body and a prominent nucleus and axostyle are present.

The organism multiplies by longitudinal fission, there being no sexual development.

*T. foetus* commonly occurs as a commensal in the genital tracts of the cow and the bull, where it may cause no abnormality but on occasions leads to early fetal death (2–4 months after conception), abortion, post-coital pyometra and urethritis in the bull.

Trichomoniasis also occurs in fowls, turkeys and other birds, *T. gallinae* being the cause of '*oral canker*' in which yellowish necrotic lesions appear in the mouth, crop and oesophagus.

Three species of *Trichomonas* are found in man: *T. vaginalis* in the genitourinary tract, *T. hominis* in the caecum; and *T. tenax* in the mouth.

**R.** Infected and carrier animals.

**MT.** By coitus, an infected bull being a constant source unless properly treated. Artificial insemination may also be involved on occasions with the use of contaminated AI pipettes and artificial vaginas.

**CF.** At one time regarded as a serious cause of bovine abortion and infertility, trichomoniasis is now of minor importance mainly because of the widespread use of artificial insemination.

The parasite localises in the vagina, uterus and oviduct and initially does not interfere with conception. But later a vaginitis and endometritis with a mucopurulent discharge develops and leads to early fetal death, placentitis and abortion followed by repeat breeding and delayed calving. Pyometra results from death and maceration of the fetus.

Trichomoniasis is self-limiting in the female, infection being cleared after one normal oestrus following a normal parturition.

In the bull, trichomoniasis is usually asymptomatic. The parasite invades the epithelium of the penis, prepuce and anterior urethra.

**P.** See **CF**.

**D.** Based on history and clinical signs along with the examination of fetal fluid, placental fluid, uterine exudate, samples of smegma from bull.

**J.** Carcase and viscera: A and D, provided carcase condition satisfactory.

## TOXOPLASMOSIS (see also Chapter 14)

**I.** A usually latent or asymptomatic protozoan disease of most animals, birds and man but which in *systemic form* can cause abortion with stillbirths in ewes and encephalitis, pneumonia and neonatal mortality in all species of livestock.

Its occurrence in man, in whom it produces fever, mononucleosis, lymphadenopathy, lymphocytosis, even myocarditis and death, make it an important *zoonosis.*

**O.** Toxoplasmosis occurs worldwide, being of special importance in Africa, where it is of high occurrence in Angola, in North and South America (enzootic in the USA and Costa Rica) and Europe (enzootic in Great Britain and Northern Ireland). In Northern Ireland and New Zealand the disease is widespread in sheep.

Asian countries appear to be less seriously affected. Several countries, notably, Belize (1983), St Vincent Grenadin (1991), Oman (1991), Namibia (1990) and Singapore (1988) have managed to eradicate toxoplasmosis.

Seroprevalence surveys have shown high rates of infection (as high as 25% or more in pigs, goats, sheep and cattle) in many different countries.

**IA.** *Toxoplasma gondii,* a sporozoan intracellular parasite whose trophozoites are crescent-shape and 6 μm × 3 μm in size. The organism was first isolated in 1908 in a North African rodent, the gundi. Its exact role in disease, however, was not recognised until 1939, one reason being that great differences in virulence exist between different strains of the organism.

It occurs in a wide range of mammalian, including man, and avian hosts (intermediate hosts) and its entire complex *life cycle*, which has asexual and sexual stages, takes place mainly in members of the cat family, which are the definitive hosts. Two main cycles are recognised – an *enteroepithelial cycle* in *cats* and an *extraintestinal cycle* which takes place mainly in *non-felines* but can also occur in cats.

The *enteroepithelial cycle* is similar to that of other coccidia and consists of several multiplication stages in the mucosal cells of the small intestine with the production of *gamonts* and *oocysts*. Oocysts are shed in the faeces some 15 days after infection.

The *extraintestinal cycle* takes place mainly in non-felines, e.g. rodents, and consists of the development of *tachyzoites* (rapidly multiplying stages) in many different tissue cells (fibroblasts, liver, reticular and heart cells, etc.) and *bradyzoites* (slowly multiplying stages) in the brain, heart and skeletal muscle.

Cats acquire infection in two ways, by carnivorism (of mice, rats, birds, etc.) and by eating infected meat.

**R.** Although it has been shown that up to 65% of cats may be serologically positive to *Toxoplasma*, only 1% of infected cats shed oocysts at any one time. However, on these occasions, which may be coincident with carnivorism, several millions of oocysts are passed in the faeces. The feral cat is more prone to infection than the domestic cat, and young cats are more susceptible than older ones. Predation probably plays an important part in facilitating transmission. It is also likely that certain wild animals and birds, in which the organism is passed through successive generations, act as reservoirs, all these factors together making for a widespread availability of oocysts, which are very resistant organisms.

**MT.** Farm livestock acquire infection through the ingestion of oocysts from infected cats in contaminated food and water. It is possible that pigs can be infected by eating infected carrion (dead rodents, piglets, etc.).

Congenital infection has been reported and is of significance in man.

**CF.** *Toxoplasma gondii* is an intracellular parasite which has a predilection for reticuloendothelial and central nervous system cells. Multiplication of sporozoites or bradyzoites in intestinal cells results in their destruction and the liberation of numerous organisms into the bloodstream to reach other parts of the body.

Most infections are usually subclinical and clinical cases are not common. But sporadic cases, and even epidemics, can occur. Clinical signs vary according to the body system attacked, the species of animal, its age, sex and whether pregnant or not. When they do happen, they may be acute (more common in the younger animal) and include fever, inappetence, malaise, dyspnoea, diarrhoea, jaundice and nervous signs (ataxia, convulsions, muscular tremors, teeth grinding). Abortion and fetal death are common in sheep and less so in pigs and cattle.

**P.** Granulomata, which may undergo necrosis, are characteristic of toxoplasmosis and are found in the lungs, heart muscle and CNS. Pneumonia, focal necrosis of the liver, kidneys and spleen, hydrothorax, ascites, lymphadenitis, necrotic enteritis, nephritis, metritis, placentitis and vaginitis may also be evident.

**D.** The lesions, epidemiology and clinical signs are suggestive of toxoplasmosis but must be supported by isolation of *T. gondii*, its demonstration in tissue sections, and serology (complement fixation, indirect fluorescent antibody, indirect haemagglutination and Sabin–Feldman dye tests).

**J.** Carcase and viscera: Clinical cases: T. Reactors, A and D.

## TRYPANOSOMIASIS

**I.** A group of diseases of animals and man caused by protozoan trypanosomes transmitted by biting flies or bugs (except for dourine, which is transmitted by coitus) characterised by intermittent fever, anaemia, loss of condition and frequent high mortality.

**O.** Trypanosomiasis is of most serious consequence in Africa south of the Sahara, especially in Guinea Bissau, Mali, Niger, Uganda and Tanzania, where it is of high occurrence. Asia and South America are affected to a less degree and the disease has been eradicated from several countries – Japan (1987), Mexico (1988), Oman, Pakistan and Papua New Guinea (1991).

The distribution of trypanosomiasis corresponds with that of its insect vectors, except in the case of dourine.

**IA.** *Trypanosomes* are undulating, thread-like cells (15–30 μm × 3 μm) possessing a central *nucleus* and a *kinetoplast* with a *flagellum* attached to the body by an *undulating membrane*. The kinetoplast is an accessory body which is found in some Protozoa, contains DNA and replicates independently. There is also a granular *blepharoplast* or basal granule from which the *axoneme* arises, the axoneme representing the spine of the flagellum. The overall shape of the organism and the position of its contents vary in the different species and in its four stages of development.

The *epimastigote stage* occurs mainly in arthropods but also in a few vertebrates. Multiplication takes place in gut of *arthropods* (tsetse flies, etc.) to form the infective (*trypomastigote stage*) in the salivary glands of arthropods. Infection is transmitted when the arthropod ingests blood from the host. In some cases trypomastigotes accumulate in the hindgut of the arthropod and are passed out in the faeces to cause infection by contaminating the skin and/or wounds.

A *promastigote stage* in the form of a round body without an undulating membrane occurs in arthropods, while an *amastigote stage* is found in arthropods and vertebrates.

Those trypanosomes which produce infective stages in the salivary gland of the arthropod belong to the *Salivaria* group and those in which infective stages are formed in the gut and passed out in the faeces belong to the *Stercoraria* group. Most pathogenic trypanosomes belong to the Salivaria group – including *Trypanosoma vivax, T. congolense, T. evansi, T. suis, T. brucei, T. rhodiense, T. uniforme, T. simiae, T. gambiense, T. equinum* and *T. equiperdum*. An exception is *T. cruzi*, the cause of Chagas' disease, which belongs to the Stercoraria group.

Trypanosomes are closely related to the *Leishmania* which are found in man, canidae and rodents.

They are parasitic mainly in the blood and lymph of vertebrates and invertebrates, although some invade tissue cells in the former.

Most species spend part of their life cycle in the intestines of insects with the adult stage occurring in the vertebrate host.

Pathogenic infections caused by trypanosomes are as follows:

Tsetse fly-transmitted African trypanosomiasis (nagana): Caused by *T. congolense, T. vivax, T. brucei, T. simiae, T. uniforme* and *T. suis*

Surra: *T. evansi*

Dourine: *T. equiperdum*

Chagas' disease: *T. cruzi*

Sleeping sickness in man: *T. gambiense* and *T. rhodesiense*

## Tsetse fly-transmitted African trypanosomiasis (nagana)

**I.** An acute, peracute or chronic disease of all species of domestic animals and certain forms of wildlife (warthog, duiker, bush pig, eland, buffalo, etc.) in which there is intermittent parasitaemia, fever, anaemia, loss of condition, infertility and frequent high mortality.

**O.** Nagana is limited to those regions of Africa where the tsetse fly (*Glossina* spp.) is found, between latitudes 14° N and 29° S. Some 23 species of tsetse flies are known to be capable of transmitting infection, but there are three main species involved – *Glossina morsitans* (found in savannah areas), *Glossina palpalis* (inhabiting land round rivers and lakes) and *G. fusca* (occurring in high forest areas). Occurrence of the disease also varies according to the distribution of the different trypanosomes.

The presence of tsetse flies is not necessary for the maintenance of *T. vivax* and this trypanosome has been isolated in South America (Colombia, Guyana, Panama, Suriname and Venezuela).

Control measures (directed at the tsetse fly, the use of prophylactic treatment and resistant stock) have reduced the incidence of trypanosomiasis.

**IA.** See above.

**R.** Carrier animals in the chronic state and numerous wild animals as well as tsetse flies.

**MT.** Tsetse flies become infected when they feed on an infected animal host. Such infected flies then inoculate the animal when they feed on its blood. Other biting flies are also involved since trypanosomiasis occurs where tsetse flies have been eliminated. When the trypanosomes are taken up by the tsetse fly, their life cycle undergoes a further development in the proboscis of the fly. This normally takes 7 days in the case of *T. vivax*, 2 weeks for *T. congolense* and 3 or more weeks for *T. brucei*. Mature infective parasites, termed metacyclic trypanosomes, colonise the salivary glands and mouth parts of the tsetse, transfer of infection being thus made a simple task. Once infected, tsetse flies remain so for life.

Other biting flies (*Tabanidae* spp., horse flies; *Stomoxyinae* spp., stable flies; and *Hippoboscidae* spp., forest flies) are capable of infecting animals since trypanosomiasis occurs where tsetse flies have been eliminated.

In this instance transmission is mechanical and non-cyclical when the flies feed on more than one host within a short time.

On entry into the animal's bloodstream the organisms divide by binary fission. *T. congolense* attaches to endothelial cells and localises in capillaries and arterioles. *T. brucei* and *T. vivax* invade tissue cells and damage different organs.

**CF.** Many different clinical signs are apparent depending on the species and strain of trypanosome involved, the degree of dose, the breed and age of the animal and its management, etc.

In the *acute* cases, after an incubation period of 1–3 weeks there is intermittent fever (coincident with the parasitaemia), dullness, inappetence, loss of condition, ocular discharge, anaemia and lymphadenitis. Small localised swellings (*chancres*) appear at the site of inoculation. *T. vivax* is especially virulent for cattle, *T. brucei* for horses and dogs and *T. simiae* for pigs.

The mortality rate in acute and peracute cases may be as high as 80% in cattle and even higher in pigs.

*Chronic* trypanosomiasis occurs as an intermittent fever with progressive loss of condition, anaemia, lymphadenitis, photophobia, debility, lachrymation, and oedema of the limbs, ventral abdomen, scrotum and vulva.

Animals which recover may take weeks or months to regain initial weight.

**P.** Anaemia, lymphadenitis, anasarca, emaciation, enlargement of the liver and spleen, widespread mucosal and serosal petechial haemorrhages, pulmonary congestion and varying degrees of enteritis. Subcutaneous oedema, hydropericardium and hydrothorax are evident in chronic cases, especially in horses and dogs infected with *T. brucei.* Necrosis is evident in many organs in cases of *T. brucei* infection – heart, skeletal muscles, brain and serosal membranes.

**D.** Diagnosis is based on clinical signs, geographical incidence of the disease and the detection of trypanosomes in blood smears or lymph node biopsies stained by Giemsa or Leishman's stain.

Serology (fluorescent antibody, ELISA, capillary agglutination, etc.) may be necessary to confirm diagnosis.

**J.** Carcase and viscera: T, A, or Kh and D, depending on extent of lesions and carcase condition.

## Surra

**I.** An acute, subacute or chronic trypanosomiasis of horses and camels in which fever, oedema, emaciation and frequent high mortality are manifested. Dogs may also suffer infection.

In endemic regions cattle and buffalo may be affected subclinically with odd acute cases simulating anthrax.

**O.** Surra has a limited occurrence in Africa (Ethiopia, Niger and Sudan (high occurrence)), India, Indonesia, Mongolia, Myanmar and Panama. Several countries have managed to eradicate the disease – Oman (1990), Iran (1991), Philippines, (1988), Yemen (1989), Bolivia and Colombia (1990).

**IA.** *T. evansi* and the closely related *T. equiperdum*. (Some regard these two species as one – *T. evansi*.)

**R.** Infected and carrier horses and camels and biting flies. The carrier rate in wild animals is believed to be low.

**MT.** Mechanical transmission of *T. evansi/T. equiperdum* is performed by biting flies of the genera *Tabanus*, *Stomoxys* and *Haematopota*. It is also claimed that vampire bats may be involved in transmitting infection. Dogs and other carnivores can be infected by eating the meat of infected animals.

**CF.** Clinical signs in the more severe cases include fever, progressive emaciation, anaemia, oedema of lower limbs, ventral abdomen, chest wall, prepuce and scrotum, and paralysis. Death may take place in a few days to several months. Chronic cases show mild symptoms which may persist for months and even years.

**P.** Post-mortem lesions are ill-defined but resemble those associated with *T. brucei* infection. Skin necrosis may occur over the oedematous areas. There is anaemia, ascites and hydrothorax with petechiae on serosal surfaces and in the liver and kidney.

**D.** As for nagana.

**J.** As for nagana.

## Dourine

**I.** A usually chronic venereal infection of horses and donkeys caused by the trypanosome *T. equiperdum* and transmitted by coitus.

**O.** Dourine apparently only occurs in southern Africa: Botswana (enzootic form), with low sporadic occurrence in Benin, Ethiopia, Lesotho, Namibia and South Africa. Most European countries managed to eradicate dourine in the 1950s and 1960s, while Israel had its last case in 1952, Canada in 1921, USA in 1934, Mexico in 1973 and Syria in 1960. The United Kingdom, Sweden, Norway, Iceland and Oceania never experienced the disease.

**R.** Carrier breeding equidae.

**MT.** At coitus. Infected stallions can infect numerous mares.

**CF.** Fever, mucopurulent discharge from prepuce/vagina, oedema of the genitalia, udder and ventral abdomen in the more acute form. Characteristic plaques (2–10 cm in diameter) may appear on the skin in later stages. Chronic dourine displays great loss of condition and progressive paralysis. Mortality is high (50–70%) in untreated cases.

**P.** Anaemia and emaciation with oedema of the subcutaneous tissues in the areas listed above and hydrothorax, hydropericardium and ascites. The urogenital tract shows inflammatory changes.

**D.** Clinical signs along with history make diagnosis reasonably straightforward. Trypanosomes, however, can be demonstrated in urethral and vaginal discharges after centrifugation. Complement fixation is only of value in areas where *T. evansi* and *T. brucei* do not exist because they exhibit common antigens.

**J.** As for nagana and surra. Chronic cases probably merit more lenient judgement.

### Chagas' disease (American trypanosomiasis)

**I.** A disease of domestic and wild animals and man transmitted by blood-sucking bugs in which cardiac complications are prominent.

**O.** The disease is confined to the western hemisphere, being distributed in Central and South America, Mexico and the southern states of the USA.

**IA.** *Trypanosoma (Schizotrypanum) cruzi*, a trypanosome with a prominent kinetoplast and a poorly developed flagellum which is lost when the parasite enters cardiac muscle cells. The flagellum is regained when multiplication to form a '*pseudocyst*' takes place.

**R.** The organism is found in numerous wild animals, especially armadillos, opossums, wood rats and mice, all of which act as reservoir hosts along with infected and carrier domestic animals, especially dogs, cats and pigs and infected bugs.

**MT.** Chagas' disease is transmitted by blood-sucking bugs of the *Reduviidae* family. Trypanosomes in blood ingested by bugs multiply as epimastigotes in the bug's hind-gut and are passed out in the faeces, defaecation occurring during feeding.

Animals and man are infected when bug faeces contaminate skin wounds and abrasions, conjunctiva and mucous membranes.

Transmission can also occur in human beings through the transfusion of blood from infected donors, in which case the incubation period is long (30–40 days).

**CT.** The incubation period is 1–2 weeks after the vector bite. In the acute form there is fever, anaemia, progressive emaciation and oedema. Death is often due to myocardial degeneration. Chronic cases may persist for years and show few, if any, symptoms, although some may demonstrate cardiac disorders with death occurring due to heart failure.

In humans acute Chagas' disease usually occurs in children, who show malaise, fever, lymphadenopathy and hepatosplenomegaly with oedema of the eyelids and at the site of infection. The chronic form in man takes place in later life and often involves myocarditis and meningoencephalitis. In some instances infection is subclinical.

**P.** Inflammation and subcutaneous oedema at the site of infection, oedema of eyelids, degenerative changes in heart and other organs, enlargement of liver and spleen and lymphadenopathy.

**D.** *Acute cases*: Demonstration of trypanosomes in blood and lesion smears stained by Leishman's or Giemsa stains after centrifugation.

*Chronic cases*: Serological tests (complement fixation, immunofluorescence and haemag-glutination). Xenodiagnosis (feeding clean bugs on the suspect animal and demonstrating the parasite in bug faeces 6–8 weeks later) may be utilised.

**J.** Carcase and viscera: T.

### Sleeping sickness or African trypanosomiasis

In man this is caused by *T. gambiense* and *T. rhodesiense* and transmitted by the bites of infected tsetse flies (*Glossina* spp.). On occasions infection can occur mechanically on the proboscis of other biting flies, e.g. horse flies.

The disease is confined to central Africa, its occurrence corresponding to the distribution of the tsetse fly. Wild animals, especially bushbuck, antelopes, cattle and man act as reservoir hosts.

Clinical signs in acute cases include fever, anaemia, lymphadenopathy (which is painless), headache, insomnia, oedema, skin rash and loss of weight and sometimes CNS symptoms in later stages. Sleeping sickness is usually fatal without treatment.

## DISEASES CAUSED BY ALGAE

*Algae* are primitive plant-like organisms containing chlorophyll which live mostly in stagnant water and include the scums of ponds, the stains of rocks and tree trunks and the seaweeds. They vary in size from being microscopic (3 µm) and unicellular to the large multicellular seaweeds 60 metres or more in length.

Except for the blue-green forms (*Cyanophyta*), which resemble the bacteria in structure, all algae possess a nucleus, mitochondria and a chloroplast membrane and are classed as eukaryotes, as opposed to prokaryotes which lack these structures.

Although most forms are responsible for providing food for aquatic life and for supplying oxygen to the atmosphere, there are some species which are extremely toxic for animals, birds, fish and man. Certain larger algae are a source of human food, additives, etc., and some may be developed and utilised for the feeding of livestock.

Like the bacteria and viruses, toxic algae produce exotoxins which are secreted into water and endotoxins which either have to be ingested by the animal or released for ingestion when the organism dies. Algal toxin production is at its optimum at about 25°C.

Strains of the genera *Microcystis, Anabena, Aphanizomenon, Chlorella, Nodularia, Oscillatoria* and others have been known to cause *poisoning* and deaths in livestock drinking water from stagnant ponds and lakes. Of the *blue-green algae* the three most common toxin-producing species are *Microcystis aeruginosa*, which produces an endotoxin termed micocystin; *Anabena flos-aqua* (exogenous neurotoxin); and *Aphanizomenon flos-aqua* (endogenous neurotoxin).

The toxin derived from *M. aeruginosa* is a cyclic decapeptide (the *'fast death factor'*), and that from *Aphanizomenon* is a *saxitoxin*. Blue-green algae can also produce lipopolysaccharides which can produce severe skin irritation and oral blisters. Some manufacture a photodynamic pigment, *phyocyan*, which can cause photosensitisation in animals and man.

*Anabena flos-aqua* is believed to be the cause of the most severe forms of algal poisoning, which can result in death from respiratory paralysis.

Algal poisoning usually occurs during periods of dense bloom growths of blue-green algae at times of high temperature, drought, shallow water with high organic content, etc.

Algal poisoning has been recorded in cattle, sheep, pigs, horses, fowls, turkeys, dogs and various forms of wildlife.

**O.** Algal poisoning occurs worldwide.

**IA.** Strains of *Microcystis, Anabena, Aphanizomenon, Chlorella, Nodularia, Oscillatoria* and others.

**MT.** By ingestion and occasionally by direct action on skin.

**CF.** The onset is rapid and appears within 1 h of ingestion of the toxin. Death may occur in 1 h.

Symptoms include intense abdominal pain, vomiting, anorexia, muscular tremors, dyspnoea, salivation, diarrhoea, prostration and convulsions. Photosensitisation occurs with *Microcystis*.

**P.** This varies according to the type of toxin ingested. In peracute cases there is sudden death without any gross lesions, while other cases are more chronic in nature.

Lesions range from congestion of the CNS with pulmonary oedema hydroperitoneum and hydrothorax in acute cases to hepatic necrosis, haemorrhagic gastroenteritis, widespread petechiation, visceral congestion, ascites, icterus and photosensitisation.

*Chlorellosis* is an infection of mammals caused by the ingestion of the chlorophyll-containing algae of the genus *Chlorella*, which has been recorded in cattle, sheep, beaver and man. It has been encountered in sheep during meat inspection in Sudan, when the post-mortem findings included a grossly enlarged liver and hepatic lymph nodes with ecchymoses and delineation of the hepatic lobules with bright green pigment, giving the liver a honeycomb appearance (Zakia *et al.*, 1989).

**D.** Diagnosis is based on the history of the incident(s), the presence of dense algae blooms, clinical signs, PM findings, and histopathological examination of liver to show centrilobular hepatic necrosis in *Microcystis* poisoning.

Samples of algae and stomach contents are collected for toxicological examination.

**J.** Carcase and viscera: T.

## REFERENCES


Anderson, R. M. *et al.* (1996) *Nature* **382**, 779.

Cetinkaya, B., Eqan, K. and Morgan, K. L. (1994). *Vet. Rec.* **134**, 494–497.

Clark, A. M., Dawson, M. and Scott, A. C. (1994) *Vet. Rec.* **134**, 650–651.

Coleman, J. D. *et al.* (1994) *NZ Vet. J.* **42**, 128–132.

Collinge, J. (1990) *The Lancet* **336**, 7–9.

Collinge, J. *et al.* (1995) *Nature* **378**, 779.

Collinge, J. *et al.* (1996a) *The Lancet* **348**, 56.

Collinge, J. *et al.* (1996b) *Nature* **383**, 685–690.

Curnow, R. N. and Hau, C. M. (1996) *Vet. Rec.* **138**, 407–408.

Edwards, G. T. (1982) *Vet. Rec.* **119**, 511.

Foster, J. D. *et al.* (1996) *Vet. Rec.* **138**, 546–548.

Garber, L. P. *et al.* (1994) *J. Am. Vet. Med. Assoc.* **205**, 86.

Gustafson, R. H. *et al.* (1976) *Proc. Int. Pig. Vet. Soc. Cong.*, M2.

Harrington, M. G. *et al.* (1996) *N. Engl. J. Med.* **315**, 279.

Heatherington, W. (1987) *Meat Hygienist* (March), 17, 18.

Henderson, J. A., Graham, D. A. and Stewart, D. (1995) *Vet. Rec.* **136**, 555–557.

Hill, A. W. *et al.* (1997) *The Lancet*, **349**, 99–100.

Hogg, R. A., White, V. J. and Smith, G. R. (1990) *Vet. Rec.* **126**, 476–479.

Hunter, N. *et al.* (1997) *Nature* **386**, 137.

Lang, G. H. (1988) *Vet. Rec.* **123**, 582–583.

Luria, S. E. and Darnell, J. C. (1967) *General Virology*, 2nd edn.

MAFF. Quarterly Report. (1990) *Vet. Rec.* **127**, 416.

McCaughey, W. J. *et al.* (1970) *Vet. Rec.* **86**, 422–424.

McIntyre, D. (1996) *Vet. Rec.* **135**, 338.

McLoughlin, M. F. *et al.* (1988) *Vet. Rec.* **122**, 579–581.

Morrison, P., Stanton, R. and Pilatti, R. (1986) *Aust. Vet. J.* **65**, 97.

Nottingham, P. M. *et al.* (1972) *NZ J. Agric.* **15**, 279–283.

Okolo, M. I. O. (1988) *Vet. Rec.* **122**, 939.

Riley, M. G. I. (1970) *Aust. Vet. J.* **46**, 40–43.

Roberts, D. *et al.* (1975) *J. Hyg.* **75**, 173–184.

Seneviratna, P. and Ford, G. (1980) *Meat Hygienist* (May/June), 21–24.

Shreuder, B. E. C. and Straub, O. C. (1997) *Vet. Rec.* **139**, 575.

Shreuder, B. E. C. *et al.* (1996) *Nature* **381**, 563.

Sticht-Groh, R. (1982) *Vet. Rec.* **110**, 104–106.

Suarez, D. L. *et al.* (1993) *J. Virol.* **67**, 5051.

Surkiewicz, T. *et al.* (1972) *Appl. Microbiol.* **23**, 575–520.

Taylor, D. M. *et al.* (1982) *Br. Vet. J.* **138**, 384.

Taylor, D. M. (1989) *Vet. Rec.* **24**, 291–292.

Taylor, D. M. *et al.* (1996a) *Vet. Rec.* **138**, 160–161.

Taylor, D. M. *et al.* (1996b) *J. Gen. Virol.* **77**, 1595–1599.

Taylor, S. M. *et al.* (1988) *Br. Vet. J.* **138**, 384.

Tuchili, L. M. *et al.* (1993) *Vet. Rec.* **132**, 487.

Van der Maatan, M. J. *et al.* (1972) *J. Natl. Cancer Inst.* **449**, 1649.

Von Ostertag, R. (1872) *Handbuch der Fleischbeschan für Tierartze, Artze und Richter.*

Wijeratne, W. V. S. and Curnow, R. N. (1990) *Vet. Rec.* **126**, 5–8.

Wilesmith, J. W. *et al.* (1988) *Vet. Rec.* **123**, 638.

WHO/FAO/OIE (1993) *Animal Health Yearbook*, Geneva: WHO.

Zakia, A. M., Osheik, A. A. and Halima, M. O. (1989) *Vet. Rec.* **125**, 625–626.

# Chapter 18
# Diseases Caused by Helminth and Arthropod Parasites

A *parasite* is usually defined as an organism that lives on another organism (the host), derives nutriment from it, but confers no benefit in return.

However, it would probably be more accurate to regard *parasitism* as a state in which the parasite is metabolically dependent on the host since not all parasites are pathogenic; some indeed are beneficial, for example, the forms of protozoa called *Ciliata* which inhabit the rumen of ruminants and which, along with yeasts and bacteria, form the microflora which digests cellulose, ferments carbohydrates to volatile fatty acids and converts nitrogenous substances to ammonia, amino acids and protein. This seems to be consistent with the Greek derivation *parasitos*, originally 'fellow guest' later '*parasite*'; para = (beside) + *sitos*, grain, food. On the other hand, parasites such as *Fasciola hepatica* are very pathogenic organisms and are responsible for huge losses in cattle and sheep.

Parasites, strictly speaking, include single-celled and multicelled organisms – bacteria, fungi, yeasts, protozoa and even viruses.

The most common use of the word 'parasite' refers to the multicellular helminths (worms), arachnids (ticks, mites, lice, etc.) and arthropods (insects) and it is the parasitic forms of these organisms which will be treated here.

Although parasites of various forms can cause deaths in food animals, in many cases (e.g. with helminths), their deleterious effects are more insidious, causing digestive or respiratory disturbance, retardation of growth and loss of body weight, meat and wool. Indeed parasitic worms, in combination with malnutrition, are probably the greatest single factor influencing livestock production today.

Parasites affect the animal host in several ways:

1 By *sucking blood and fluids*, producing anaemia, e.g. *Haemonchus contortus* in sheep and blood-sucking flies and ticks.

2 By *competing for food*, especially where a specific entity is involved, e.g. the competition for vitamin $B_{12}$ by *Diphyllobothrium latum*. This may lead to a depraved appetite and reduced food intake or an increased passage of food through the digestive tract.

3 By *mechanical injury* of the host's tissues, e.g. liver cirrhosis due to *Fasciola hepatica* and *Ascaris suum* caused by the migration of larval stages through the parenchyma; the use of destructive organs of attachment, e.g. spines or teeth; pressure due to increasing size, e.g. hydatid cysts, blockage of ducts and blood vessels to produce infarction (*Strongylus*), of lymphatics causing oedema *(Filaria)* and of the intestinal canal to produce rupture and necrosis (ascarids).

Damage to the intestinal epithelium and often the underlying submucosa is caused by several parasites, notably the oocysts of *Coccidia*.

Mechanical injury may permit the entry of pathogenic bacteria, e.g. Black disease in sheep is finally caused by *Clostridium novyi (oedematiens)* inhabiting the areas of the liver damaged by young migrating flukes.

In some instances there is an increased proliferation of epithelium, e.g. an aneurysm caused by *Strongylus*, and of lymphoid tissue, e.g. in leishmaniasis. Tissue damage may also be due to the immunological response of the host, being evident in cases of dermatitis in man due to schistosomes and oedema brought about by *Dictyocaulus viviparus* in the lungs of cattle.

4 By the continued *excretion of toxic products*. The systematic changes associated with chronic fascioliasis of sheep and cattle are attributed by some authorities to the action of toxins secreted by the parasites. It is more likely, however, that these changes are caused by a combination of factors.

The most important parasites in meat hygiene are those transmissible to man through the consumption of infected meat and offal, e.g. *Cysticercus bovis*, *C. cellulosae*, *Trichinella spiralis*. Other parasites, though not transmissible to man, may render the flesh repugnant and therefore unmarketable, e.g. extensive muscular sarcosporidiosis.

The parasitic helminths and arthropods of importance in meat inspection may be classified as follows:

Nemathelminthes – Nematodes (round worms)

Platyhelminthes – Cestodes (flatworms) and Trematodes (flukes)

Protozoa

Arthropoda (joint-footed organisms) – insects, lice, mites, bugs, linguatula

# HELMINTH (WORM) PARASITES

The helminths (*nematodes* or roundworms, *cestodes* or flatworms and *trematodes* or flukes) constitute a large class of both parasitic and non-parasitic forms. Included in these phyla are organisms such as earthworms that are beneficial but which may act as intermediate hosts of parasitic helminths and leeches.

The helminths are probably of more importance in those areas where agriculture is more intensive and where large numbers of animals are concentrated together. But since the nutritional status of the animal is of vital importance in parasitism, especially the gastrointestinal pulmonary forms, nutritional deficiency is also of consequence in poorly developed countries.

Many different factors determine the incidence of helminthiasis – stocking rates at pasture, type, strain and number of individual grasses, short ley or permanent pasture, fertilisation methods, drainage, access to swampy areas, life cycle of the parasite and its control, immune status of the animals, grazing management, handling of faecal contamination, use of anthelmintics, use of clean and safe grazing systems, etc.

Strategic and tactical treatments with anthelmintics are important measures in the control of parasitic diseases. They must be used alongside the measures listed above and care must be taken to ensure correct dosage with usage at the proper time otherwise anthelmintic resistance may result.

Control by vaccination is limited to lungworm infestation in cattle, sheep and goats.

**Nematodes** or **roundworms** are elongated, unsegmented, cylindrical in shape with both ends pointed. They possess a *mouth* which usually possesses two or three lips, an *alimentary canal* which runs the length of the body, and a terminal *anus*. In most cases the sexes are separate and the life cycle may be direct or indirect (including an intermediate host, e.g. an earthworm in the case of *Metastrongylus elongatus*). *Males*, which are normally smaller than the females have a *testis*, a *vas deferens*, sometimes a *seminal vesicle* and an *ejaculatory duct* which opens into the *cloaca* at the tail. *Females* possess an extensive *uterus* (which may be subdivide), *vagina*, *vulva*, *oviduct* and *seminal receptacle* in which spermatozoa are stored and where fertilisation takes place.

Egg shape and size vary in the different species and are important entities in diagnosis. Several thousand eggs may be produced by one female in one day. Eggs are produced by division of the original egg cell, each eventually forming a larva which may undergo several stages before becoming infective for the definitive host.

**Cestodes** or **tapeworms** are segmented, flat, hermaphrodite worms which may be small (1 mm) or very long (15 m or more). Some 3000 species, free-living and parasitic, are known to occur worldwide. The parasitic forms are internal parasites affecting the alimentary canal and liver of all vertebrates, including fish and man. Some tapeworms involve a single host while others require one or two intermediate hosts as well as a final, or definitive, host to complete their life cycle.

At the anterior end is a *scolex* or *head*. The scolex usually possesses four suckers which sometimes are armed with hooks. It is joined to the rest of the body or *strobila* by a short *neck*. The strobila consists of several segments or *proglottids*, each of which contains one or two sets of reproductive organs (male and female). These proglottids are formed from the neck and when gravid contain hundreds of eggs.

Respiratory, skeletal and circulatory systems are absent and there is no coelom or body cavity. But a primitive nervous system and sense organs exist in the scolex. The *female organs* consist of one or two *ovaries*, *uterus*, *vagina*, *seminal receptacle* and *vitellaria* or *yolk gland*.

The *male organs*, which develop first, comprise a large number of *testes*, a *vas deferens* and a *cirrus* or *penis*. Female and male *genital pores* lie close together on the ventral or lateral side of the proglottid.

Self-fertilisation usually occurs, although cross-fertilisation takes place in some species.

The *life cycle* of the parasitic cestodes is very complex and is indirect in that it involves several larval stages (*metacestodes*) in other intermediate hosts, which may be either vertebrate or invertebrate.

Ripe segments are excreted from the intestine, either singly or in small groups. While the segments (containing eggs) survive for only a few days, the contained *oncospheres* can survive on pasture for months, even at temperatures as low as 0°C. Desiccation is the main factor in the inactivation of cestode oncospheres.

When passed from the animal host, eggs may or may not contain embryos. If *embryonated* an egg contains an *oncosphere* within the external embryonic envelope (there are four in all) and is armed with six hooks. The *embryophore* develops from the inner envelope and assumes different forms and subsequent activities in the various tapeworms.

On hatching in the intestine of the host, the oncosphere is liberated, penetrates the intestinal mucosa and migrates in the bloodstream to its predilection site in the body where it forms a *cyst* or *bladderworm* (*metacestode* or *larval stage*). When the infected flesh of the intermediate host is eaten, the metacestode is transferred to the definitive host.

The *metacestodes* of the parasitic cestodes encountered in meat inspection are as follows:

*Cysticercus:* Possesses an outer membrane and scolex invaginated into vesicle containing fluid. When eaten this cyst gives rise to one tapeworm – *T. saginata*, *T. solium*, *T. pisiformis*, *T. serialis*, *T. hydatigena*, *T. ovis*.

*Coenurus:* A large bladder containing fluid and several invaginated scolices each of which when ingested gives rise to a single tapeworm – *T. multiceps*.

*Cysticercoid:* A non-invaginated scolex withdrawn into a small vesicle – *Thysanosoma actinoides*, *Moniezia expansa*.

*Hydatid:* A large bladder holding fluid-containing cysts termed brood capsules which develop scolices – *Echinococcus granulosus*.

*Plerocercoid:* Solid, elongated body with a scolex which develops from the procercoid in the second intermediate host – *Diphyllobothrium latum*.

*Strobilocercus:* A single scolex, non-invaginated, attached to a bladder by a segmented strobila. *T. taeniaeformis*.

**Trematodes** or **flukes** are mostly flattened, leaf-like worms which vary in size from 5 mm to 100 mm. A few, like the amphistomes, have thick, fleshy bodies while the *schistosomes* or *blood flukes* are long and worm-like. The 6000 or so species occur worldwide and are parasitic in a wide range of animals, fish, turtles, crustaceans and in man, in whom they cause schistosomiasis (blood fluke infestation). Some act as external parasites (ectoparasites) while others are endoparasites infesting internal organs.

The fluke body is covered with a *cuticle* on which are muscular *suckers*, *spines* and *hooks* for attachment. Both sides of the fluke body are similar.

A *mouth* at the anterior end or on the ventral surface leads into a *pharynx* after which there is a branched *digestive system* but usually no anus. The digestive system, however, is followed by an *excretory system* which possesses a posterior opening. There is no circulatory system but a rudimentary *nervous system* typically consists of two anterior ganglia and three pairs of long nerve cords.

Most species are hermaphrodite, i.e. male and female organs occur in the same fluke. The *male* organs normally comprise two single, lobed or branched *testes*, two *vasa deferentia* and a *terminal cirrus* and *genital pore*. *Female* organs include a lobed *ovary*, *oviduct*, *receptaculum seminis*, paired *vitelline gland*, *ootype*, *uterus* and *genital pore*.

*Life cycles* may be direct or indirect. The parasitic forms belong to the latter and require one, two or more *intermediate hosts* to complete the life cycle.

Eggs are excreted in the faeces of the host animal and pass through five larval stages – *miracidium*, *sporocyst*, *redia*, *cercaria* and *metacercaria*.

In the case of *Fasciola hepatica*, the intermediate host is a mud snail, *Limnaea truncatula*, into whose respiratory cavity the *miracidium* enters and is transformed into an oblong sac, the *sporocyst*. In the next 2–4 weeks the sporocyst gives rise to 6–8 *rediae*, which are elongated structures containing a sac-like intestine. In a further 4–6 weeks each redia becomes actively motile, migrates to the liver of the snail and eventually forms 15–20 *cercariae* which have an oral and ventral sucker, a long tail and bifurcated intestine. Millions of cercariae can be produced from a single miracidium. The cercariae escape from the rediae, leave the snail and find their way to a grass stalk or aquatic plant, completing a period of 6–10 weeks development in the snail.

The cercariae may float on the surface of the water or attach themselves to a blade of grass and become encysted by the excretion of an adhesive substance, to appear like grains of sand. This encysted form undergoes further development into a *metacarceria*, which is the infective form. The period from egg to cercaria takes 2–4 months and cercariae can remain infective in waterlogged areas for up to 12 months and in hay for several weeks.

When ingested by ruminants, the cysts are dissolved in the intestine and the metacercariae migrate to their predilection site, the liver, in the bile ducts of which they reach their adult stage.

## GASTROINTESTINAL PARASITES OF RUMINANTS

Parasitic gastroenteritis is responsible for great economic losses (deaths and poor growth) in sheep (in which wool is also lost), cattle and goats. Many of the cases of emaciation and oedema encountered in these species at meat inspection are probably a combination of roundworm infestation accompanied by malnutrition, especially if there is no evidence of concurrent disease. It often co-exists with lungworm infestation.

### Parasitic gastroenteritis of cattle

**I.** An infestation of the various parts of the alimentary canal of young cattle with roundworms and associated with ill-thrift and often profuse, watery diarrhoea and deaths.

**O.** Most are worldwide in occurrence, especially where livestock are kept intensively. *Bunostomum phlebotomum*, the most important hookworm of cattle, however, is a serious pathogen in Africa, Australia and the USA and *Bunostomum trigonocephalum*, which infests sheep, goats and deer, also prefers warmer climates. *Mecistocirrus digitatus*, found in the abomasum of cattle, sheep, goats, the stomach of pigs and sometimes man, occurs in the Far East and Central America. While many trichostrongyles are found in cattle and sheep in Europe, others such as *T. falculatus* and *T. rugatus* occur in Africa and Australia and *T. orientalis* in Asia and the Middle East.

*Parasitic gastroenteritis in cattle and sheep, associated as it is with profuse diarrhoea, is an all-too-common cause of carcase-dressing problems in meat plants.*

**IA.** The most common nematodes in cattle and their main sites are as follows (SI, small intestine):

| | |
|---|---|
| *Haemonchus placei* (barber's pole worm) | Abomasum |
| *Ostertagia ostertagi* | Abomasum |
| *Trichostrongylus axei* (small stomach worm) | Abomasum |
| *T. colubriformis, T. longispicularis* | SI |
| *Mecistocirrus digitatus* | Abomasum |
| *Bunostomum phlebotomum* (hookworm) | SI |
| *Agriostomum vryburgi* (hookworm) | SI |
| *Chabertia ovina* | SI and colon |
| *Cooperia punctata, C. oncophora, C. pectinata* | SI |
| *Nematodirus spathiger, N. battus, N. helvetianus* | SI |
| *Nematodirus filicollis, N. abnormalis* | SI |
| *Oesophagostomum radiatum* | SI, caecum, colon |
| *Strongyloides papillosus* | SI |
| *Toxocara vitulorum* | SI |
| *Trichuris ovis, T. discolor, T. globulosa* (whipworm) | Caecum |
| *Gongylonema verrucosum* | Rumen |
| *Gongylonema pulchrum* | Oesophagus |

*Haemonchus placei* (barber's pole worm, large stomach worm, wire worm) and *Mecistocirrus digitatus* are parasites in tropical areas, the remainder preferring more temperate regions.

Although infestations of *Trichostrongylus, Ostertagia, Cooperia, Namatodirus* and *Haemonchus* can be regarded as specific diseases they often occur as mixed infestations, sometimes with other species of worms. Usually, however, one particular species predominates.

**R.** Young cattle are the principal sources of these particular nematodes. Eggs and preparasitic forms can survive under optimal conditions of temperature (~18–24°C) and moisture for several weeks. In the case of *Nematodirus* the larvae develop slowly within the eggs until the infective third larval stage and only hatch after rain to produce heavy infections on pasture. *Nematodirus* eggs are very resistant and are able to overwinter and produce large numbers of larvae to infect calves the next season and are able to survive from one year to the next. *Haemonchus placei* can also become dormant over the winter and resume development when suitable conditions prevail in the spring. The eggs and larvae of many nematodes can survive reasonable winter conditions. *Ostertagia*, for example, can remain viable for 18 months or more.

Egg production by the females of many of the nematodes is very prolific. In the case of *Haemonchus contortus*, the female can lay as many as 10 000 eggs a day for several months, causing extensive contamination of pasture, foodstuffs and water. Desiccation, however, is the enemy of the progeny of most nematodes.

Thus reservoir infection is a combination of infected and carrier animals as well as voided eggs and larvae.

**MT.** Ingestion of infective larvae on pasture, food and water. The hookworm (*Bunostomum*) species, however, in addition to being ingested can penetrate the skin from where they migrate to the lungs. Skin penetration by infective larvae occurs in *Strongyloides* infection which may also arise through the consumption of milk. Subsequent life cycles, predilection sites and organ damage vary in the different species.

In the case of *Trichostrongylus, Ostertagia, Cooperia* and *Nematodirus* the ingested third-stage larvae undergo several moults in the mucosa and finally becoming an adult worm. The period from ingestion of infective larvae to development of adult worm is about 3 weeks, *Nematodirus* requiring 4 weeks. Where hypobioisis (inhibited development) occurs, several months are required for adult worms to develop.

**CF.** Young cattle are most often affected, although adult animals which have not previously experienced been exposed, may suffer severe infestations.

Clinical signs of helminthiasis include persistent watery diarrhoea (often dark green or yellowish in colour), weight loss, weakness, rough coat and anorexia. In *Haemonchus* infection there is a severe anaemia and oedema of the lower jaw (bottle jaw) and ventral abdomen. Oedema may also be seen in *Ostertagia* and *Trichostrongylus* infections. Similar signs are also evident in *Trichuris* and *Strongyloides* infections.

In *hookworm* infections, penetrations of the skin by larvae produces uneasiness, stamping and licking of feet. There is initial constipation followed by attacks of diarrhoea and colic. Severe infestations cause pallor of the mucosae, anasarca, submandibular and ventral abdominal oedema, weakness and death in a few days.

Infection with *Oesophagostomum* spp. (nodular worm disease, pimply gut) produces severe fetid diarrhoea, which may alternate with constipation, anorexia, anaemia and emaciation. Intestinal nodules may be palpated *per rectum*.

**P.** In *Trichostrongylus, Ostertagia, Cooperia* and *Nematodirus* infections there may be no apparent lesions apart from some loss of condition, anaemia, dehydration and evidence of scouring. More severe cases, however, reveal a villous atrophy and catarrhal inflammation in the abomasum and duodenum. In ostertagiasis the mucosa assumes a morocco-leather appearance with umbilicated nodules.

*Haemonchus* infection results in a severe anaemia, all the mucous membranes and the conjunctiva being very pale. Anasarca (generalised subcutaneous oedema) is present. The abomasal mucosa may show congestion, blood clots and small ulcerations with blood-stained contents caused by the attachment of the adult worms.

The most diagnostic lesions occur in *Oesophagostomum* spp. infestations, in which there is a catarrhal enteritis with a thickened mucous membrane. Nodules of varying sizes (some up to 6 mm in diameter) containing greenish or yellowish-brown caseous or partly calcified material are present in the ileum and colon in cases of repeated infection.

The skin-penetrating larvae of *Strongyloides* spp. damage the skin of the lower limbs, causing lesions resembling early foot rot.

The larger adult worms of *Haemonchus*, *Bunostomum*, *Oesophagostomum*, *Trichuris* and *Chabertia* are clearly visible at post-mortem examination, but the smaller worms of *Trichostrongylus*, *Cooperia*, *Ostertagia* and *Nematodirus* are more difficult to detect, their presence being shown by their movement in the ingesta.

Total worm counts are sometimes taken as measures of the degree of infestation. For cattle, counts of 2000 or less as regarded as light burdens while counts of over 10 000 are heavy. But reliance must not be placed on light total worm or egg counts, especially the latter. Much depends on the species of worm involved and the nutritional status of the animal.

### Parasitic gastroenteritis of sheep and goats

In general the infective agents, pathogenesis, clinical signs, and post-mortem findings, etc., resemble those in cattle (q.v.).

The most important nematodes and their main predilection sites in the alimentary tract of sheep and goats are as follows:

- Abomasum – *Haemonchus contortus; Ostertagia circumcincta, O. trifurcata; Trichopstrongylus axei; Mecistocirrus digitatus*
- Oesophagus – *Gongylonema pulchrum*
- Small intestine – *Trichostrongylus colubriformis, T. longispicularis, T. capricola, T. rugatus, T. probolurus; Bunostomum trigonocephalum; Gaigeria pachyscelis, Cooperia curticei, C. punctata, C. oncophora; Nematodirus spathiger, N. battus, N. filicollis, N. abnormalis; Oesophagostomum columbianum, O. venulosum, O. asperum, O. radiatum, O. multifoliatum, O. okapi, O. walkeri; Strongyloides papillosus; Toxocara (Neoascaris) vitulorum; Trichuris ovis*
- Rumen – *Gongylonema verrucosum, G. monnigi*

*Haemonchus* is most prevalent in tropical and subtropical regions, while *Ostertagia* and *T. axei* are more common in temperate zones where rainfall is greater.

*Gaigeria pachyscelis* occurs in Africa and India, while *Agriostomum pachyscelis* is prevalent in Southern Asia and South Africa.

As with cattle, infection with most alimentary helminths is most severe in the young animal, weaner lambs and yearlings being most commonly affected. In general the same clinical signs of depression, anorexia, weakness, diarrhoea, lack of growth with anaemia in some infestations.

The effects of many helminth infections, in addition to the production of anaemia in many cases, are the impairment of gastric digestion and the non-utilisation of metabolisable energy and protein, these losses occurring across the damaged abomasal mucosa.

*Trichostrongylus* and *Ostertagia* infections in lambs are similar to those in cattle in relation to clinical signs and post-mortem findings, which occur as villous atrophy of the mucous membrane of the abomasum and upper duodenum, which is often affected with fibrinocatarrhal gastritis.

*Haemonchosis* may be peracute or chronic, the peracute cases resulting in rapid onset of death due to profound anaemia and anasarca. Death may actually be so sudden as to exclude premonitory symptoms. Anaemia is also present in chronic haemonchosis in which there is also progressive emaciation.

*Bunostomum* and *Gaigeria* spp., being hookworms, are potent bloodsuckers, especially the latter, and require only a relatively small number (~100) to cause clinical disease. Ingestion and skin penetration are the modes of transmission.

The adult worms of *Chabertia ovina* cause inflammation, petechial haemorrhages, and ulceration in some instances, of the colon, resulting in anaemia and ill-thrift.

*Oesophagostomum* spp. are parasites in the small and large intestine of cattle, sheep, pigs (q.v.) and primates.

The worms are referred to as nodular worms since several species cause nodule formation in the intestinal wall: *O. columbianum* and *O. radiatum*. *O. venulosum*, which occurs in the colon, however, rarely produces this effect and is relatively harmless.

*O. columbianum* is a serious pathogen in sheep, goats, camels and wild antelopes, in which it occurs in the small and large intestine. It is worldwide in distribution but more common in tropical and subtropical regions. It does not occur in Britain. The adult worms are stout white worms with a curved body at the anterior end. The male is 8–16 mm and the female 10–21 mm long.

**Life cycle** Eggs are passed in the faeces and reach the infective stage in 1 week. When ingested, the infective larvae lose their sheath and bore into the intestinal wall creating cysts. Two further moults take place and the larvae return to the lumen of the gut where they moult again to become adults.

**Lesions** Lambs and adult sheep experiencing first infection develop localised inflammation and eventually greyish-white fibrous nodules round the larvae in the wall of the intestine. These nodules vary in size from a pinhead to a pea and produce distinct elevations of the mucosa. Caseation and calcification of nodules take place, resulting either in the death of the parasites or their evacuation of the nodules through a small orifice. Penetration of the bowel wall may occur and result in peritonitis and death. The intestinal wall becomes thickened and covered with mucus. Repeated infections may result in extensive involvement of the whole small intestine with secondary infection of the nodules causing abscesses containing greenish or yellowish pus.

Such severe lesions result in diarrhoea, and sometimes dysentery, weakness, anorexia, anaemia, loss of wool and progressive emaciation due to malabsorption and interference with digestion. Severe cases often result in death.

*O. radiatum* is found in the colon of cattle, zebu and water buffalo and produces lesions similar to those of *O. columbianum*.

*Nematodirus* infection is a very serious disease in lambs in some parts of the world, notably the UK, New Zealand, Australia and the USA. The ability of the very resistant eggs to overwinter and to hatch under very moist conditions when large numbers of larvae are produced are serious drawbacks to its control. A mild enteritis is usually present but this may be acute in more severe infestations.

Infection with *Strongyloides* spp. resembles that of *Trichostrongylus*. The mode of transmission is similar to that of *Bunostomum* and *Gaigeria* in that it can occur by either ingestion or skin penetration. In lambs there is anorexia, loss of condition, anaemia, dermatitis (due to the penetrating larvae) and lameness when the feet are involved. Most cases of *Strongyloides* infection, however, are usually mild, with lambs recovering quickly.

*Toxocara vitulorum* occurs in the small intestine of cattle, zebu and buffalo and is a serious problem in parts of Africa, India, Philippines and Sri Lanka. The ingestion of embryonated eggs is followed by larvae passing through the intestinal wall and being distributed to various organs, including the mammary gland, by the bloodstream. In the cow these larvae remain dormant until late pregnancy, when they migrate to the placenta and amniotic fluid, the fetus being infected by ingestion of larvae. Calves may also be infected by the consumption of infected milk. Adult worms are produced in the small intestine of calves.

Clinical signs in more serious infections include diarrhoea with fetid faeces, steatorrhoea, colic, emaciation and often death.

Lambs are occasionally affected with *Trichuris* whipworms which inhabit the caecum. Large numbers are generally required in order to produce lesions and clinical signs which resemble those of helminthiasis in general. The species is so called because the adult worms (2–5 cm long) have a long and very slender anterior part while the posterior portion is shorter and much thicker. In addition to cattle and sheep, dogs and pigs can be affected.

### Diagnosis of gastroenteritis in ruminants

The *differential diagnoses* include numerous conditions in which emaciation and diarrhoea occur such as Jöhne's disease, coccidiosis, salmonellosis, chronic fascioliasis, secondary copper, cobalt or molybdenum deficiency, viral diarrhoea, verminous pneumonia, shipping fever, trypanosomiasis, babesiosis, anaplasmosis, East Coast Fever, etc.

A presumptive diagnosis is based on clinical signs, epidemiology, season of occurrence, weather conditions, post-mortem findings, etc. The level of nutrition, stocking rates and other factors related to grazing are important as is the response to the use of broad-spectrum anthelmintics.

Laboratory examinations include faecal egg and total worm counts. The actual significance of results depends on the species of helminths present and the particular host involved. While as few as 100 *Haemonchus contortus* worms can cause clinical disease in lambs, it requires as many as 5000–10 000 *Ostertagia* worms. Differentiation of the various ova is a task for a specialised laboratory. Serological diagnosis using enzyme-linked immunosorbent assay

(ELISA) is utilised in some quarters for specific nematodes such as *Ostertagia* and *Cooperia*.

### Judgement of parasitic gastroenteritis in ruminants

This depends on the degree of emaciation, anaemia and oedema in the carcase as well as the extent of organ degeneration. Emaciation associated with oedema is probably one of the most difficult conditions with which the meat inspector has to contend, especially where conditional approval/heat treatment is practised.

Carcase and viscera: A, T or Kh and D.

## INTERNAL PARASITISM OF PIGS

**I.** An infection of roundworms inhabiting the stomach and intestine (small and large) of pigs resulting in varying signs of loss of appetite, anaemia, lack of growth (due to reduced feed conversion and organ damage) and diarrhoea.

Internal parasites in pigs continue to cause much economic loss, which has been estimated at up to $3 per pig in the USA because of loss of weight and meat plant condemnations. A considerable number of affected organs such as livers (*'milk spots'*), intestines (*'pimply gut'*), stomachs (parasitic gastritis) and kidneys (*Stephanurus dentatus* infection) are rejected.

The occurrence of the serious zoonosis *trichinosis* in many parts of the world lends further prominence to porcine helminthiasis.

The factors which influence the prevalence of helminthiasis in pigs are much the same as those for cattle and sheep: overcrowding, lack of hygiene, housing defects, soil type and drainage and climate.

Although there had been a general decline in the incidence of ascariasis in pigs in Northern Ireland, recent studies there have shown that the disease is on the increase, this being blamed on inadequate cleansing and disinfection of premises.

**O.** Helminthiasis in pigs occurs throughout the world.

**IA.** The principal roundworms occurring in pigs are as follows:

Oesophagus, tongue and oral cavity – *Gongylonema pulchrum*

Stomach – *Ascarops strongylina, A. dentata; Hyostrongylus rubidus* (red stomach worm); *Physocephalus sexalatus, P. cristata; Simondsia paradoxa*

Small intestine – *Ascaris suum; Globocephalus* spp.; *Macracanthorhynchus hirudinaceus* (thorny-headed worm); *Oesophagostomum dentatum, O. brevicaudum, O. georgianum; O. granatensis, O. quadrispinulatum; Strongyloides ransomi; Trichinella spiralis*

Large intestine – *Metastrongylus elongatus (M. apri), M. pudendotectus, M. salmi; Oesophagostomum dentatum, O. brevicaudum, O. georgianum, O. quadrispinulatum, O. granatensis; Trichuris suis*

**R.** Infected and carrier pigs and intermediate hosts, e.g. earthworms, dung beetles, cockroaches, in indirect life cycles.

### *Gongylonema pulchrum* (gullet worm)

This tiny worm (males 30–62 mm, females 80–145 mm) may be found coiled in the stratified squamous epithelium of the oesophagus and stomach, not only of the pig but also of cattle, sheep, goats and horses. It apparently does not cause any pathological changes. The eggs are ingested by cockroaches.

### *Ascarops strongylina* and *Physocephalus sexalatus*

These worms are found in swine in the USA, East Asia and Australia. They have indirect life cycles with intermediate hosts in dung beetles.

Both worms are capable of causing atrophy of the glandular epithelium of the stomach with chronic catarrhal gastritis and sometimes superficial ulceration.

### *Hyostrongylus rubidus* (red stomach worm)

This is a small, filiform red coloured worm 0.5–1.25 cm long. It is very common in pigs in Britain, Germany and North and South America.

The worms appear as tiny red streaks in the gastric mucosa, where they cause nodules and a catarrhal or diphtheritic inflammation with mucoid or sometimes dry, adherent deposits up to 4 cm in size surrounded by a bright red zone of mucosa.

The *life cycle* is direct, eggs hatching in 1–2 days and third-stage larvae ingested by pigs. These migrate to the stomach and enter the gastric glands of the cardiac and fundic regions where L4 larvae develop on the mucosa in a further 2–3 days, adult worms emerging in 2–3 weeks post-infection.

### *Simondsia paradoxa*

This worm occurs in pigs in Europe and Asia and is responsible for nodules on the stomach and chronic gastritis.

### *Ascaris suum*

A survey in the North of England (Pattison *et al.*, 1980) recorded an incidence of 10% in pork and bacon pigs and sows, which was lower than the infestations due to *Hyostrongylus rubidus* (28.5%) and *Oesophagostomum* spp. (85%).

Recent surveys in Northern Ireland have shown that *A. suum* has increased in prevalence, this probably being accounted for by the high resistance of the eggs combined with the absence of effective cleansing and disinfection procedures.

*Ascaris suum* is the largest of the gastrointestinal parasites of pigs, smooth and yellowish-white in colour with the larger females 20–40 cm × 5 mm in size and the thinner males 15–25 cm × 3 mm. Males have a hook-shaped posterior end surrounded by spicules. There is a short head with three smooth lips arranged around the mouth, each lip bearing a row of minute denticles.

**Life cycle** *A. suum* lives for some 55 weeks, during which the female lays up to 1.4–2 million eggs daily. The fertilised eggs (zygotes) are passed in the faeces and develop to the infective stage (after a first moult) in 14 days. There is some doubt as to whether the second- or third-stage larva is the infective one.

The larvated eggs, which possess thick shells, are extremely resistant and can survive for as long as 4 years. Desiccation and direct sunlight, however, can kill them in a few weeks. Earthworms and dung beetles probably act as reservoirs of infection for larvated eggs.

After ingestion (in food contaminated with faeces) the outer envelopes of the eggs is digested by the host's small intestinal juices. The larvae are freed and penetrate the bowel wall, causing small haemorrhages in the duodenum and jejunum, and are conveyed to the liver by the portal vein. Many pass rapidly through the liver, forcing their way through the liver capillaries, but some are arrested and, by their irritation, give rise to chronic focal interstitial hepatitis. Early lesions are haemorrhagic but later become ill-defined whitish foci in the parenchyma and on the surface (*'milk spots'*). These attain their maximum size in 2 weeks after infection. The change from a haemorrhagic appearance to a whitish one is associated with an infiltration of leukocytes and the formation of collagen in the interlobular septa.

In the liver the L2 larvae moult to become L3 larvae. These leave the liver via the hepatic vein and posterior vena cava to reach the heart and subsequently the lungs. Some may lodge in the kidneys and other organs, where they cause haemorrhage and necrosis, but most of the L3 larvae break out of the lung capillaries into the lung alveoli and moult to become L4 larvae. These migrate up the bronchioles, bronchi, trachea and larynx to the pharynx and are then swallowed, finally reaching the small intestine, where they grow rapidly and moult to become stage 5 larvae and eventually adult male and female worms some 35–60 days after infection. Egg laying begins 7–14 days later.

The passage of *ascaris* larvae through the lungs causes considerable systemic disturbance ('thumps') manifested by fever, coughing, dyspnoea and symptoms resembling pneumonia. This is due to the destruction of lung alveoli, resulting in haemorrhage, and sometimes oedema and emphysema, by the migrating larvae. Should re-infection occur, ulcers with perivascular cuffing may develop in the oesophageal and gastric mucosae, a possible manifestation of an immune response.

Pigs up to 4–5 months of age are most severely affected. On occasions diarrhoea, pot belly and unthriftiness occur.

In recent years it has been suggested that migrating larvae of *A. suum* have caused necrotic lesions in lambs' livers resulting in high condemnation rates (Mitchell and Linklater, 1980; Gibson and Lanning, 1981; Borland *et al.*, 1980; Crooks, 1980). While *A. suum* has been definitely encountered in naturally infected lambs, experimental work has shown that only tiny liver lesions (up to 2 mm in diameter) are produced (Brown *et al.*, 1984).

*Judgement of ascariasis in pigs*

Carcase and viscera: A and D, provided condition is adequate.

Livers affected with *'milk spot'* are unfit for human consumption and are utilised as inedible by-products or utilised for pharmaceutical purposes subject to negative residue tests.

## *Globocephalus* spp.

*Globocephalus longemucronatus* (males 5 mm and females 8 mm long) and *G. somoensis* are found in the small intestine of pigs in Africa, Far East and North and South America, and along with other species are capable of causing anaemia in severely affected animals.

## *Macracanthorhynchus hirudinaceus* (thorny-headed worm of pigs)

The adult worms are long and flat with males up to 10 mm in length and females as long as 40 mm or more. The worm is found in the small intestine of the pig, mainly the jejunum, and sometimes in man. Superficially the worm resembles *Ascaris*, being a thick, cylindrical white worm, but it increases in width towards its anterior end where it possesses a thorny proboscis composed of five or six rows of backwardly curving hooks. There is no intestinal canal, food being absorbed directly through the body surface.

It is common in Europe, Belorussia, North and South America and Australia.

**Life cycle** The eggs are passed in the faeces and are ingested by the intermediate hosts, *dung* and *water beetles*. The eggs hatch when ingested by the larvae of these beetles and encyst in their body cavities. Pigs are infected when they ingest the adult beetles or the infective grubs. The larvae are freed and develop into adult worms in the intestine.

**Lesions** The parasite attaches itself to the mucosa and bores deeply into the intestinal wall creating inflammation (*'strawberry mark'*) and a granuloma and sometimes perforation and ulcers with heaped-up edges. Peritonitis may ensue with rapid onset of death.

### Judgement

Affected intestines are unfit for use as sausage casings.

Dropsy and emaciation of the carcase may occur in severely infected cases, justifying total condemnation. Most cases, however, are mild infections warranting approval of the carcase with rejection of the small intestine.

## *Oesophagostomum* spp.

The *Oesophagostomum* spp. occur in the caecum and large intestine of pigs and have a life cycle similar to that of the species occurring in ruminants.

*Oesophagostomum dentatum*, probably the most serious pathogen in pigs, is found worldwide, but the other species are restricted to southern USA and Puerto Rico.

Pigs become infected through eating contaminated food. It is possible that rodents, sandflies and midges may act as carriers of infection.

**Lesions** resemble in general those found in cattle and sheep and are found especially in the caecum and anterior colon. The walls of these parts become oedematous due to extensive lymphatic thrombosis and may develop a localised fibronecrotic membrane. Secondary infection with *Salmonella, Vibrio* and *Balantidium* may ensue.

### Judgement

As for Ascaris.
Intestines: Usually T.

## *Strongyloides ransomi*

*Strongyloides ransomi* is an intestinal threadworm (male 0.80–0.90 mm and female 1.0–1.5 mm long) which occurs in the anterior small intestine of the pig. It is worldwide in distribution.

**Life cycle** Both parasitic and free-living forma of *Strongyloides* spp. can occur, unlike all other nematodes. Reproduction is asexual, eggs being developed without fertilisation by the male (parthenogenesis). These are passed in the faeces and hatch in 12–18 h and the parasitic forms become infective (L3) in 2–3 days.

Infection of the host occurs by either ingestion or penetration of the skin. Those entering via the skin migrate to the lungs in the blood. Transmission of infection may also occur in neonatal pigs via the colostrum.

More severe infections result in diarhoea, anaemia, anorexia, emaciation and sometimes death.

**Lesions** Focal inflammation with pus formation may be evident at the site of penetration of the larvae. Erosion of the intestinal mucosa and a catarrhal enteritis may be present along with local haemorrhages in the lungs caused by laval migration.

### Judgement

Judgement depends on the degree of infection, which may be so severe as to justify total condemnation due to emaciation and anaemia. In milder infections, carcases may be passed with rejection of affected lungs and intestines.

## *Stephanurus dentatus* (kidney worm of pigs)

Stephanuriasis occurs mainly in pigs kept outdoors in tropical and subtropical countries but is now decreasing in incidence owing to sanitary control measures.

The adult male worms are 2–4 cm long and the females 3–5 cm.

**Life cycle** From cysts in the kidneys, ureters and perirenal fat, eggs are passed out in the urine from the adult worms. They hatch and reach infective stage in 3–5 days. *Earthworms* serve as transfer hosts, infection of pigs occurring when the earthworms are ingested. Transdermal infection may occur.

Infective larvae migrate from the small intestine via the mesenteric lymph nodes and portal vessels to the liver and some to the lungs, bronchial lymph nodes, spleen and pancreas. After 2–4 months they break through the liver capsule into the peritoneal cavity and migrate to the kidney, ureters, perirenal and mesenteric fat depots.

**Lesions** In percutaneous infection there are subcutaneous nodules with oedema and enlargement of the associated lymph nodes.

The liver is enlarged and cirrhotic and shows tracts, nodules and scars (probably healed abscesses). Ascites and peritonitis may accompany the hepatic cirrhosis. The portal vein may show fibrinous tracts. The ureters are thickened and may even be obliterated. Fat round the kidneys and ureters is honeycombed with many chambers containing a creamy, greenish fluid and numerous parasites. Obliteration of the ureters may produce hydronephrosis, with conversion of the kidneys into fibrous sacs distended with urine. The walls of these sacs may contain purulent cysts containing adult worms.

**Symptoms** Most affected pigs display few, if any, *symptoms* except in severe infections when there may be posterior paralysis (due to spinal cord involvement), anorexia and loss of weight.

**Diagnosis** Post-mortem changes are diagnostic.

### Judgement

Carcase and viscera: A, T, or Kh and D (affected organs).

## Trichinellosis (Trichinosis, Trichiniasis)

**I.** A parasitic disease of great public health importance in which the larvae of the small roundworm (*Trichinella spiralis*) of pigs, rats, man and other mammals migrate to and encyst in the musculature, causing severe illness, even death, in heavy infections in man but usually only subclinical infection in domestic and wild animals.

Zoonosis.

**O.** The Animal Health Yearbook of 1992 gives the incidences of trichinosis in pigs as follows:

*Exceptional occurrence*: Norway (all carcases tested at meat plant), Sweden.

*Low sporadic occurrence*: Austria, Bulgaria, Finland, Latvia, Poland, Romania, Yugoslavia, Ukraine, Argentina, Egypt, Mexico, USA, Hong Kong, Myanmar.

*Enzootic occurrence*: Costa Rica, Lebanon.

Several countries have eradicated the disease, notably Denmark (1930), Uruguay (1932), Portugal (1951), New Zealand (1974), Hungary (1975), Britain (1977), N. Ireland (1979) and Canada (1986, where trichinoscopic examinations of some 79 000 pigs and horses are performed annually).

**IA.** *Trichinella spiralis*, a small roundworm (male 1.5 mm, female 3.5 mm long, possessing a slender body and a round unarmed mouth. The male has a pair of flaps on either side of the cloaca (Fig. 18.1).

There are *four species* differentiated according to their infectivity: *Trichinella spiralis*, the main zoonotic form occurring in pigs, rats, mice, man and many mammals; *T. pseudospiralis* (infects

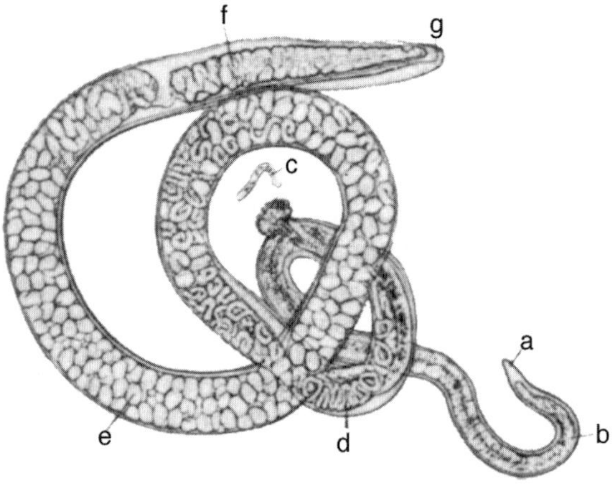


**Fig. 18.1** Adult female *Trichinella spiralis*: a, oral opening; b, oesophgus; c, newborn larva just expelled from vulva; d, larvae in anterior portion of uterus; c, fertilised and developing ova; f, ovary; g, rectum, ×100. (By courtesy of Dr S. E. Gould)

birds and mammals but does not produce a muscle cyst – has been found in Tasmania, Eastern Europe and India); *T. nativa* (Canada, USSR, Arctica); and *T. nelsoni* (Africa and Europe). All four species occur in wild carnivores. All four species occur initially in the small intestine of the hosts.

**R.** Swine, rats, mice, dogs, cats and numerous wild animals including fox, wolf, raccoon. bear, polar bear, wild boar, hyaena, jackal, lion and leopard.

**Life cycle** When encysted muscle larvae are ingested, they are liberated in the small intestine by the digestive juices and undergo four moults to reach the adult stage in 4 days. Copulation occurs, after which the males die and the females penetrate into the mucosa, where eggs hatch in the uterus to produce 500–1000 larvae during 2–6 weeks.

The *larvae* (each 0.1 mm long) reach the bloodstream by way of the mesenteric lymph stream, thoracic duct and the posterior vena cava to reach all parts of the body. The larvae encyst primarily in the voluntary skeletal muscles, especially those poor in glycogen – diaphragm, tongue, larynx, eye and the intercostal and masticatory muscles.

Penetrating the capillary walls, the larvae enter the muscle sarcolemma 7–8 days after infected meat is ingested. They increase greatly in size and are about 0.5–1.0 × 0.25 mm in size at 14 days after infection; they coil up within the muscle fibre in a typical spiral form, cease to grow and become surrounded by a capsule, the process being completed in 4–5 weeks.

In addition to dilating the sarcolemmal sheath, the larvae cause the muscle fibre to lose its cross-striation, the fibre degenerating to form a granular mass while the muscle nuclei increase in size and number along with an increase in the number of mitochondria.

The final *muscle cyst* is lemon-shaped with its long axis parallel to the muscle fibres. It is not readily detected until 2–3 months have elapsed and is only really evident at 6–8 months. The poles of the cyst become infiltrated with fat globules and later with lime salts. Calcification in the pig may begin at 5 months after infection and be complete in 9 months but the parasite can remain viable if the process does not involve the actual worm. Even calcified trichinae in man have been known to remain alive for 31 years and for 12 years in pigs.

### *Location of* Trichinella *cysts*

The *predilection sites* vary according to the host species. In pigs the skeletal muscles liable to invasion are those concerned with respiration and are, in order of frequency, the pillars of the diaphragm, the costal area of the diaphragm, the muscles of the tongue and larynx and the abdominal and intercostal muscles. The frequency of infestation of these muscles may be associated with their constant activity and consequent abundant blood supply.

Most larvae are found near the tendons and beneath the sarcolemmal sheath where there is greatest resistance to their passage through the capillaries. In rodents the muscles of mastication are most often affected.

**MT.** Infection results from the consumption of raw or undercooked flesh of animals containing viable encysted larvae. In relation to human beings, the usual meats are pork and pork products and beefburgers containing raw pork, but other meats such as bear, polar bear, wild boar and walrus have been implicated in epidemics. Outbreaks of trichinosis in man have also been associated with the consumption of horse flesh.

The prevalence of trichinosis in pigs has been shown by American studies to be higher in those animals fed on meat plant offal (0.5%) compared with pigs fed on grain (0.125%). Trichinosis in the pig is, therefore, most likely to be acquired from the flesh of another pig via raw or unboiled garbage. The rat probably obtains the infection from a similar source and also via cannibalism.

Animal hosts remain infective for months and meat from such animals stays dangerous for considerable periods unless properly cooked or frozen. A temperature of at least 77°C (171°F) to reach all parts of the meat is required to destroy all larvae. A freezing temperature of – 15°C (+5°F) for 30 days or –25°C (–13°F) or lower for 10 days is necessary to make the meat safe. Thicker pieces of pork must be held at the lower temperature for at least 20 days. It is stressed that these temperatures will not kill the *T. nativa* arctic strains found in walrus and bear meat.

**CF.** In *domestic* and *wild animals* most infections go undiagnosed. The intestinal worms may create a degree of enteritis which may be marked in severe infections, with diarrhoea. Larvae in muscle may give rise to fever, stiffness, muscle pain, dyspnoea, facial oedema and hoarseness. Very severe infections can result in death due to failure of the respiratory muscles.

In *man* the incubation period is usually 1–2 weeks after ingestion of infected meat. Clinical signs vary greatly and range from inapparent infection to a fulminating, fatal disease. There is muscle pain and oedema of upper eyelids in the early stages, sometimes followed by conjunctival and retinal haemorrhages and photophobia. Remittent fever, weakness, anorexia, sweating, chills, diarrhoea and prostration develop with cardiac and respiratory complications, death being finally due to myocardial failure in either the first or second weeks or between the fourth and eighth weeks.

**P.** See life cycle and location of cysts.

**D.** Naked-eye examination of pork carcases cannot be regarded as reliable for the detection of trichinosis because, although cysts are just visible after they have undergone calcification, this does not occur until after 8 months, sometimes one year. Several immunodiagnostic tests have been used to diagnose trichinosis – complement fixation, haemagglutination, flocculation, intradermal and enzyme-linked immunosorbent assay (ELISA). The latter is highly sensitive in detecting antibodies to *T. spiralis* in the mass screening of pigs.

In Great Britain, currently free of trichinosis, The Fresh Meat Hygiene and Inspection Regulations 1995, Schedule 10, require that 'fresh meat from horses shall be examined for trichinellosis and shall be rejected as unfit for human consumption if so affected; an OVS or an inspector shall examine fresh meat from swine for trichinellosis and shall reject as unfit for human consumption fresh meat so affected; and fresh meat from swine not examined for trichinellosis shall be subjected to cold treatment in accordance with Annex 1 to Directive 77/96/EEC'.

Pending agreement between EU Member States about the granting of derogations, all pig meat which is consigned to Germany and Denmark must either be subjected to a specified treatment, e.g. cold treatment or, examined and found to be free from trichinellosis.

Such examinations or treatments may have to be carried out on pig meat exported to countries outside the European Union but only if the importing Third Country so requires.

Directive 77/96/EEC of 21 December 1976 as amended (and Directive 94/59/EEC of 2 December 1994) 'on the examination for trichinae (*Trichinella spiralis*) upon importation from third countries of fresh meat derived from domestic swine' specifies that the examination of such meat must: (1) Be made under the supervision of an official veterinary surgeon (Article 2.1) Be carried out in accordance with one of the methods provided for in Annex 1 (Article 2.2). (2) Be undertaken in a slaughterhouse approved in the exporting country or in the importing country at an approved inspection post (Articles 2.3 and 2.5). (3) Take place before the approved system of health marking (Article 2.4). (4) Be health marked in the approved manner (Article 2.6). (5) Involve an approved method of freezing in lieu of examination in the exporting country (Articles 3.1, 3.2 and 3.3 and Annex IV). (6) Be carried out in authorised laboratories and by qualified personnel and in approved boning, cutting and freezing premises (Article IV and Annex IV).

### *Quality control procedures in approved laboratories*

These may either involve running controls in tandem with standard procedures – a costly procedure – or the use of control indicators to determine whether the acid-digestion methods are within satisfactory limits. The digestion of the blue indicator and the retention of the red indicator establishes that the process is within satisfactory limits. Other approved QC testing methods may be used.

## APPROVED LABORATORY METHODS FOR THE EXAMINATION FOR TRICHINAE (ANNEX 1)

### METHODS FOR PIG MEAT

1. *Examination of pig meat using a trichinoscope:*

The following samples are required:

In the case of whole carcases, at least one specimen the size of a hazelnut must be taken from each of the diaphragm pillars at the transition of the sinewy part. If there is only one diaphragm pillar, one specimen the size of two hazelnuts is to be taken. In the absence of both diaphragm pillars, two specimens approximately the size of a hazelnut are to be taken from one of the following sites:

- the rib part or the breastbone part of the diaphragm;
- the lingual muscle;
- the jaw muscle; or
- the abdominal muscles.

(Samples are normally taken during or after post-mortem inspection. They must be correlated with the carcases or cuts of meat from which they came.)

If the samples above cannot be taken, three other pieces of meat the size of a hazelnut containing little fat should be taken from each cut of meat from points as near as possible to bones or tendons.

The trichinoscopic examination must be carried out in such a manner that each preparation is scanned slowly and carefully. If the trichinoscopic examination reveals suspect areas, the nature of which cannot be definitely ascertained even with the most powerful magnification of the trichinoscope, these must be checked by microscope.

The microscopic examination should be carried out in such a manner that each preparation is scanned slowly and carefully at a magnification of 30 to 40 ×.

In the case of an uncertain result, the examination must be continued on a further number of specimens and slide preparations, if necessary with the aid of higher magnifications, until the required information is obtained. The trichinoscopic examination must be carried out for at least three minutes.

The trichinoscopic examination must be carried out for at least six minutes in the case of substitute specimens taken from the rib part or breastbone part of the diaphragm pillars, the lingual muscle or the jaw muscle or the abdominal muscles.

The minimum time fixed for the examination does not include the time necessary for sample taking and for making the preparations.

As a general rule, the trichinoscope examiner should not inspect more than 840 pieces a day, though by way of exception he may inspect up to 1050.

The trichinoscope cannot be used for the examination of horse meat.

2. *Examination of pig meat by the artificial digestion method*

The following samples are required:

In the case of whole carcases a sample of at least 20 g (3/4 oz) must be taken from a diaphragm pillar at the transition of the sinewy part. In the absence of diaphragm pillars a specimen of at least 20 g must be taken from one of the sites listed under (1) above.

If the samples above cannot be taken, another piece of meat of approx. 20 g and containing as little fat as possible should be taken where possible from a site near to bones or tendons.

3. *Pig meat for examination by the artificial digestion of collective samples*

4. *Pig meat for examination by the mechanically-assisted pooled sample digestion method/sedimentation technique*

5. *Pig meat for examination by the mechanically-assisted pooled sample digestion method/on filter isolation technique*

6. *Pig meat for examination by the magnetic stirrer method for pooled sample digestion*

7. *Pig meat for examination by the automatic digestion method for pooled samples of up to 35 g*

For methods 3–7 the following samples are required:

In the case of whole carcases, a specimen approx. 2 g should be taken from a pillar of the diaphragm at the transition of the sinewy part.

In the absence of diaphragm pillars a specimen of at least 2 g should be taken from one of the following:

- rib part or the breastbone part of the diaphragm;
- the lingual muscle;
- the jaw muscle; or
- the abdominal muscles.

If the above samples cannot be taken, a sample of approx. 2 g and containing as little fat as possible should be taken from a site as near as possible to bones or tendons.

METHODS FOR HORSE MEAT

8. *Examination of horse meat by the artificial digestion of collective samples.*
9. *Examination of horse meat by the mechanically-assisted pooled sample digestion method/sedimentation technique.*
10. *Examination of horse meat by the mechanically-assisted pooled sample digestion method/on filter isolation technique.*
11. *Examination of horse meat by the magnetic stirrer method for pooled sample digestion.*
12. *Examination of horse meat by the automatic digestion method for pooled samples of up to 35 g.*

For methods 8–12 the following samples are required: A specimen of at least 10 g is to be taken from the lingual muscle or the jaw muscle. In the absence of these a specimen of the same size with no fat or connective tissue attached must be taken from the pillar of the diaphragm at the transition of the sinewy part.

*Details of the apparatus and techniques of examination for* trichinae *are given in Annex 1 of Directive 94/59/EEC – 3rd Amendment.*

*Despatch of samples to approved laboratories*

Samples should be despatched to the approved laboratory as soon as possible after taking. They should not be batched together without the agreement of the veterinary supervisor or other designated person in the laboratory.

*Holding meat pending receipt of results*

It is essential that carcases and cuts of meat are kept under secure control until the results of the laboratory examinations are notified. This is particularly important if the oval or square health mark has been applied to the carcases or the cuts of meat labelled accordingly. Such carcases and cuts of meat need not be kept in the detained area of the abattoir.

*Post-mortem judgement and application of the trichinellosis health mark*

If *trichinae* larvae or eggs have been or are suspected of having been isolated from samples originating in pigs or horses, in any approved laboratory, then the veterinarian responsible for supervising that laboratory or other authorised person must notify the local DVO (Divisional Veterinary Officer) of that finding. If notification is received that the laboratory examination has proved positive or suspicious, it is essential that carcases or cuts of meat are detained pending confirmation of the disease or otherwise. Other carcases which have come from the same holding must be detained pending further sampling. The local DVO must be advised accordingly.

*If trichinellosis is confirmed* then the *whole carcase* must be considered *unfit for human consumption* and dealt with accordingly.

MARKING OF MEAT WHICH HAS BEEN EXAMINED FOR *TRICHINAE* (ANNEX III OF DIRECTIVE 77/96/EEC (AS AMENDED)

**1.** Marking of the meat must be carried out under the responsibility of the official veterinarian. For this purpose, he shall keep and maintain:

- the instruments intended for marking which he may hand over to the assistant staff only at the time of marking and for the length of time required for this purpose,
- the tags mentioned in para. 5. These tags shall be given to the assistant staff at the time when they must be used and in the required number.

**2.** The mark must be round with a diameter of 2.5 cm. The following information must appear on the mark in perfectly legible characters:

- towards the centre the capital 'T' with arms 1 cm long and 0.2 cm wide,

- under the letter 'T' one of the following sets of initials; CEE, EEG, EWG, EOF, or EEC. The letters must be 0.4 cm high.

3. Carcases must be marked in ink or hot-branded on the inside of the thighs, in accordance with para. 2.

4. Heads must be marked in ink or hot-branded with a mark meeting the requirements of para. 2.

With the exception of cuts exempt from health marking by virtue of Annex B, Chapter X(43) of Council Directive 72/462/EEC, those taken in cutting plants in accordance with the rules must, where they bear no stamp, be marked in accordance with para. 2 before the health mark is affixed.

The label provided for in the second subparagraph of the above-mentioned para. 43 must comply with the conditions of para. 6 below.

5. Marking may also be effected by means of a round tag. This tag, to be affixed to each piece or to each carcase must not be reusable, must be made of strong materials and must meet all hygiene requirements. The following information must appear on the stamp seals in perfectly legible characters:

   - towards the centre of the capital letter 'T',
   - under the letter 'T' one of the following sets of initials: CEE, EEG, EWG, EOF or EEC. The letters must be 0.2 cm high.

6. The label provided for in Annex B, Chapter X(44) of the Directive mentioned in para. 4 above must, in addition to the health mark, bear a clearly legible mark identical to that provided for in para. 2.

## FREEZING OF MEAT (ANNEX IV)

### *Method 1*

1. Meat brought in already frozen must be kept in this condition.
2. The technical equipment and energy supply of the refrigerating room must be such as to ensure that the temperature referred to under para. 6 is reached very rapidly and maintained in all parts of the room and of the meat.
3. Insulated packaging should be removed before freezing, except for meat which has already reached throughout the temperature referred to under para. 6 when it is brought into the refrigeration room.
4. Consignments in the refrigeration room must be kept separately and under lock.
5. The date and time when each consignment is brought into the refrigeration room must be recorded.
6. The temperature in the refrigeration room must be at least -25°C. It should be measured with calibrated thermo-electric instruments and continuously recorded. It may not be measured directly in the cold air flow. The instruments must be kept under lock. The charts must include the relevant numbers from the meat inspection register on importation and the date and time of the commencement and completion of freezing, and must be retained for one year after compilation.
7. Meat with a diameter or thickness of up to 25 cm must be frozen for at least 240 consecutive hours, and meat with a diameter or thickness of between 25 and 50 cm must be frozen for at least 480 consecutive hours. This freezing process may not be applied to meat which has a larger diameter or is thicker.

   The freezing time shall be calculated from the point when the temperature referred to in para. 6 is reached in the freezing room.

### *Method 2*

The general provisions of paras 1 to 5 of Method 1 shall be complied with, and the following time–temperature combinations applied:

1. Meat with a diameter or thickness of up to 15 cm must be frozen according to one of the following time–temperature combinations:

   - 20 days at – 15°C
   - 10 days at – 23°C
   - 6 days at – 29°C

2. Meat with a diameter or thickness of between 15 cm and 50 cm must be frozen according to one of the following time–temperature combinations:
   - 30 days at – 15°C
   - 20 days at – 25°C
   - 12 days at – 29°C

The temperature of the refrigeration room must be no higher than the level of the selected inactivation temperature. It should be measured with calibrated thermoelectric instruments and continuously recorded. It may not be measured directly in the cold air flow. The instruments must be kept under lock. The charts must include the relevant numbers from the meat inspection register on importation and the date and time of the commencement and completion of freezing, and must be retained for one year after compilation.

*Method 3*

Control of the temperature at the centre of the meat pieces.

1. The following time–temperature combinations shall be applied where the temperature is controlled at the centre of the meat pieces and the conditions in paras 2 to 6 are fulfilled:
   - 106 hours at – 18°C
   - 82 hours at – 21°C
   - 63 hours at – 23.5°C
   - 48 hours at – 26°C
   - 35 hours at – 29°C
   - 22 hours at – 32°C
   - 8 hours at – 35°C
   - 1/2 hour at – 37°C
2. Meat brought in already frozen must be kept in this condition.
3. Consignments in the refrigeration room must be kept separately and under lock.
4. The date and time when each consignment is brought into the refrigeration room must be recorded.
5. The technical equipment and energy supply of the refrigeration room must be such as to ensure that the temperature referred to under para 1 is reached very rapidly and maintained in all parts of the meat.
6. The temperature should be measured with calibrated thermoelecric instruments and continuously recorded. The probe of the thermometer has to be placed at the centre of a calibrated piece of meat of a size no smaller than the thickest piece of meat to be frozen. The calibrated piece of meat should be placed at the least favourable site in the freezing room, not close to the cooling instruments or directly in the cold air flow. The instruments must be kept under lock. The charts must include the relevant numbers from the meat inspection register on importation and the date and time of the commencement and completion of freezing, and must be retained for one year after compilation.

INSPECTION AND FREEZING OF HORSE MEAT (ANNEX V)

1. *Inspection*

The inspection of horse meat has to be performed according to a digestion method in Annex 1 with the following modifications:

- Specimens of at least 10 g to be taken from the lingual muscle or the jaw muscle. In the absence of lingual muscle or jaw muscle a specimen of the same size to be taken from a pillar of the diaphragm at the transition of the sinewy part. The muscle should be clean of connective tissue and fat.
- A 5 g sample is digested for inspection if the artificial digestion of collective samples according to Annex 1, Nos III to VII is applied. For each digest, the total weight of muscle under examination must not exceed 100 g for Methods III, IV, V and VI in Annex 1 or 35 g for Method VII in Annex 1.
- In the case of a positive result a further 10 g specimen must be taken for a subsequent independent examination.

2. *Freezing of horse meat*

To kill *trichinae* by freezing, horse meat must undergo cold treatment in accordance with one of the methods described in Annex IV.

(The above tests are being replaced by immunodiagnosis with the ELISA test.)

*Control of trichinellosis*

Since treatment of affected animals is impractical, control measures must be directed at preventing the ingestion of viable *Trichinella* cysts in muscle by animals or man. Treatment of affected human beings is carried out with thiabendazole for the intestinal worms and mebendazole for the muscle cysts.

The examination of meat for viable trichinae as outlined above is effective in preventing infection in humans in those countries where trichinellosis exists. This, however, must be combined with other measures such as the hygienic management of livestock, the effective control of rodents, the proper cooking (at least 30 min at 100°C) of swill fed to pigs, and the prevention of access to carcases, including wildlife carcases, e.g. those of walrus, bear, seal, wild boar and other wild animals.

It is equally important that the public be educated to properly cook fresh pork and pork products and meat from wild animals which have not been processed by heating, curing or freezing to kill trichinae, so that all parts of the meat reach a temperature of at least 77°C (171°F) or until the meat changes colour from pink to grey.

Pork should be ground in a separate grinder or the grinder thoroughly cleaned before and after use with other meats.

Adopt the freezing temperatures outlined in Directive 94/59/EEC. These temperatures, however, will not kill the cold-resistant Arctic strains of *Trichinella spiralis nativa* found in wild animals and sometimes in pigs.

Expose the meat to low level gamma irradiation.

### *Metastrongylus elongatus (M. apri), M. pudendotectus, M. salmi*

*Metastrongylus* spp. of worms, of which *M. elongatus* is the most common, are found in pigs (domestic and wild) and occasionally sheep, cattle, deer and other ruminants and occasionally man. They occur in the bronchi and bronchioles and in natural infections there may be one, two or all three species involved. The worms are slender in shape and white in colour, males up to 25 mm in length and females up to 60 mm.

**O.** *M. elongatus* and *M. pudendotectus* – worldwide. *M. salmi* is confined to S. Africa, S.E. Asia, S. America and USA.

**Life cycle** This is an *indirect* one involving *earthworms* as intermediate hosts. Eggs are laid in the lungs, coughed up and swallowed. Earthworms ingest either hatched or unhatched eggs. The larvae develop in the blood vessels of the oesophagus and proventriculus of the earthworms. When infective (at 0.50 mm) after two moults as L3 larvae they are ingested by pigs, in which they penetrate the small intestinal wall and enter the mesenteric lymph nodes where they moult. The L4 larvae are conveyed to the right heart and then the lungs, where they become adults after another moult, egg laying commencing at about 24 days post-infection.

**CF.** Most cases appear to be asymptomatic but severe infections may cause dyspnoea, anorexia, poor feed conversion, loss of weight and infrequent coughing.

**P.** There may be no gross changes but bronchitis, bronchiolitis and pneumonia, especially of the diaphragmatic lobes may be evident and sometimes atalectasis. Nodular lesions produced by discarded cuticles and less than 2.5 cm in diameter may be apparent in the lung substance or under the visceral pleura.

**D.** Post-mortem examination reveals the presence of adult worms when the diaphragmatic lobes are incised at the posteroventral border and the bronchioles are squeezed.

The typical thick-shelled larvated eggs can be demonstrated in the faeces. Immunofluorescence may be used in serodiagnosis.

**J.** Carcase and viscera: Usually A and D (lungs).

### *Oesophagostomum dentatum, O. brevicaudum, O. quadrispinulatum, O. georgianum*

*Oesophagostomum* spp. infect the caecum and large intestine of pigs, *O. dentatum* occurring throughout the world while *O. brevicaudum* and *O. georgianum* are found in the USA, India and Central America and *O. quadrispinulatum* infects pigs in North and South America, Europe and the Philippines.

**MT.** Pigs acquire infection through the ingestion of L3 infective larvae on contaminated pasture or feed. It is possible that infected larvae may be carried by adult sandflies or owl flies or by infected rodents which are eaten by pigs.

**CF.** Cases are usually asymptomatic but some loss of weight gain and diarrhoea may occur in more severe infections.

**P.** As in ruminants, the main lesions are greyish-white nodules (2–8 mm in diameter) in the caecum and large intestine caused by encapsulated larvae in the muscularis mucosae (*'pimply gut'* or *'nodular pig disease'*). These nodules normally contain yellowish-black necrotic material in the older nodules.

Petechiation may be present at the point of entry of the larvae and there may be oedema of the intestinal wall arising form thrombosis of the lymphatics.

**D.** Faecal examination of eggs may be carried out, but the eggs of *Oesophagostomum* spp. are similar to those of *Hyostrongylus.* Differentiation is made by larval culture.

**J.** Carcase and viscera: Usually A and D (intestines).

### *Trichuris suis*

The *Trichuris* spp. are usually termed *'whipworms'* because the anterior part is very long and slender while the posterior part is very much thicker.

*Trichuris suis* infects pigs, wild boars, monkeys and humans throughout the world and occurs in the caecum, colon and human appendix.

The adult male worm is 3–4 cm and the female 6–8 cm.

**O.** Worldwide.

**Life cycle** The barrel-shaped eggs containing L1 larvae are passed in the faeces and become infective in 3 weeks. When ingested by pigs, they hatch in the small intestine and caecum, penetrate the mucosa and enter the cells of the crypts where they undergo four moults to become adults in 6–7 weeks after infection.

**MT.** Ingestion of embryonated eggs on pasture or in feed.

**CF.** In itself *T. suis* is probably not a serious parasite but it can cause enough damage in younger pigs (2–6 months of age) for secondary bacterial invaders to become established and cause a catarrhal enteritis and dysentery. Some workers describe nodule formation, intestinal oedema and necrotic erosion of the mucosa.

In severe infections there is anorexia, weakness, anaemia, emaciation, dysentery, dehydration and loss of weight.

**P.** See **CF**.

**D.** Based on clinical signs, post-mortem findings and demonstration of typical eggs in faeces.

**J.** Carcase and viscera: Usually A and D (intestines).

## MISCELLANEOUS NEMATODE INFECTIONS

### *Onchocerciasis* (worm nodule disease)

**I.** A parasitic infection of cattle, water buffalo, zebu, goats and horses caused by filarial worms of the *Onchocerca* spp. in which nodules containing microfilariae are found in the connective tissue in various parts of the body.

**O.** The disease is of great economic importance in Australasia, Malay Peninsula, S. Africa, USA and Central America but possibly less so in Europe. Documentation, however, is poor in many countries.

In the USA infection rates of 59% of horses were recorded in surveys in Kentucky, 77% in Ohio and 37% in Michigan. In France Collobert *et al.* (1995) examined the ligamentum nuchae and umbilical skin of 368 horses and found only 4 (1.09%) affected. In two separate investigations in England, incidences of 14% and 23% were recorded, but no lesions in 105 horses examined in the the Republic of Ireland (Mellor, 1973).

**IA.** At least 15 species of *Onchocerca* are known, most of which are capable of causing nodules in various sites in animals.

The main species are as follows:

*O. gibsoni* – produces nodules in the brisket and hind limbs of cattle and zebu.

*O. gutturosa* – ligamentum nuchae, scapular cartilage, hip, shoulder and stifle of cattle and buffalo.

*O. armillata* – the aorta of cattle, buffalo, sheep and goats.

*O. ochengi* – flanks, ventral abdomen, udder and scrotum of cattle.

*O. lienalis* – gastrosplenic ligament, spleen capsule and xiphoid process area of cattle.

*O. cervicalis* – ligamentum nuchae of horses and mules causing poll evil, fistulous withers, dermatitis and uveitis.

*O. reticulata* – flexor tendons and suspensory ligament of horses, mules and donkeys.

All the *Onchocerca* worms are essentially parasites of connective tissue.

The most important of the *Onchocerca* parasites, *O. gibsoni*, is a long, slender filariform worm, the males of which are 30–50 mm long and the females 140–200 mm or more long. The larvae or microfilariae (260 μm) are found chiefly in the briskets of cattle.

Its developmental cycle involves a midge, *Culicoides pungens* (*nubeculosus*).

*Lesions of* O. gibsoni (Plate 4, Fig. 19)

The worm nodules or '*worm nests*' are found in the briskets, in the ligaments at the junction of the ribs and the costal cartilages, usually between the second and tenth ribs and on the external aspect of the stifle and other parts of the hind limbs.

In the early stages the affected ligaments appear thickened and dotted with haemorrhagic spots which may become caseous or calcified. Later the parasite becomes encased in yellow swellings the size of a pigeon's egg or larger. These consist of an outer wall of white fibrous tissue with a centre composed of a soft, spongy network in which one or two microfilariae of *O. gibsoni* are intimately entangled. These tumours may be flattened or irregular in shape, and are found in the subcutaneous connective tissue or in the connective tissue between the muscles. They never involve the muscular tissue itself.

Lesions that are markedly fibrous generally contain numerous larvae, but nodules in which the connective-tissue reaction is slight are usually sterile; the central spongy area, however, shows little variation in diameter, even in nodules of different size.

Those microfilariae which occur in the *ligamentum nuchae* are present in tunnels and nodules in the connective tissue. Although they were in the past believed to be associated with poll evil and fistulous withers in equidae, this is now known to be incorrect.

The microfilariae of *O. armillata* produce thickening of the *aortic wall* with the formation of nodules and tunnels.

**CF.** Clinical signs are normally absent in cases of onchocerciasis but occasionally lameness may be noted where nodules occur on flexor tendons, etc., of equidae. Periodic ophthalmia, blindness and epileptiform fits have been associated with infection due to *O. armillata.*

**D.** By detection of adult worms in the ligamentum nuchae, brisket, gastrosplenic ligament, etc., at post-mortem. Alternatively, a skin biopsy (6 mm) is taken from the usual superficial predilection sites (brisket, ear, umbilicus, etc.) and macerated in warm normal saline solution and incubated for 6 h. Microfilariae, if present, appear in the deposit. They may be stained with New Methylene Blue after removal of skin pieces.

**J.** *Judgement of onchocerciasis due to* O. gibsoni: In Australian meat inspection the superficial fascia on the lateral aspect of the stifle joint is incised and a hook and thin-bladed knife inserted to remove as much connective tissue as possible. The cavity is then palpated to ensure that all nodules have been removed and the incision closed by a metal pin which is removed after chilling.

Briskets and plates are removed from forequarters of beef to be exported to Britain and examined by incisions into the intermuscular tissue; those free of nodules are utilised locally for canning. Removal of the brisket and plate is not considered necessary for the Eastern trade.

The other forms of onchocerciasis usually warrant only the rejection of affected parts.

## Strongylosis (strongylidosis) of equidae (redworm infestation)

**I.** An infestation of the caecum and colon of horses, asses and mules with large strongyle worms (blood worms, red worms, palisade worms, sclerostomes) associated with anaemia, colic, debility and sometimes verminous arteritis.

**O.** Worldwide in occurrence.

**IA.** The most common strongyle worms are *Strongylus vulgaris* (the common or double-toothed strongyle), *S. edentatus* (the toothless strongyle) and *S. equinus* (the triple-toothed strongyle). These are large, firm, dark-grey worms which bear several leaf crowns at their anterior end (hence the name *'palisade' worms*) and in the intestine suck blood (hence the name *'red worms'*) by means of well-developed buccal capsules with teeth in the buccal cavity.

*S. vulgaris* is the smallest of the three, being about 15 mm long in the male and 22 mm in the female, *S. edentatus* and *S. equinus* being twice as long.

**Life cycle** The life cycle of *S. vulgaris* is direct. Its thin-shelled eggs are passed in the faeces and under favourable conditions reach the infective third-stage larva in 1–2 weeks. When ingested, these infective larvae penetrate the intestinal wall and become L4 larvae in 8 days after infection. These enter the submucosal arterioles and migrate to the cranial mesenteric artery, where after 14 days they cause thrombi and aneurysms. In about 5 days the L4 larvae migrate back to the caecum and colon to become L5 larvae in 3 months PI. In the lumen of the intestine eggs are laid after 7 months.

**MT.** Via the faecal–oral route.

**CF.** The worms are active feeders, ingesting plugs of mucosa and blood to produce anaemia, enteritis, diarrhoea, weakness and loss of condition.

*S. vulgaris* causes damage to the anterior mesenteric artery and its branches (thrombus formation and aneurysms) with interference of blood flow to the large intestine. Colic, torsion of the large intestine, intussusception and even rupture of the bowel may ensue. Detachment of thrombi from the arteries and arterioles may result in sudden death from occlusion of a coronary artery or pulmonary embolism and right ventricular failure.

Thrombosis of the iliac artery may result in hindleg lameness.

**P.** In addition to the lesions listed under **CF**, *Strongylus* spp. adult worms can cause haemorrhagic ulcers which may coalesce to form large areas of desquamating epithelium. While the arterial lesions due to *S. vulgaris* usually affect the *cranial mesenteric artery*, any part of the arterial system may be damaged by endarteritis, thickening of the arterial wall and thrombus formation (verminous arteritis). Verminous aneurysms are less common and occur as dilated and sacculated segments of the artery whose wall may be either thick or thin.

Other lesions include infarction of the kidney due to occlusion of the renal artery by an embolus.

*S. edentatus* has been associated with subserous nodules (3 mm high and 5 mm wide) in the small and large intestine. At first these are bright-red in colour but later become yellowish-brown. They contain a central caseous core, oedema, connective tissue, red and white blood cells and sometimes a degenerated larva.

**D.** Diagnosis is based on the demonstration of eggs in the faeces. In the case of mixed infections, the individual infective larvae are identified after faecal culture.

Verminous arteritis of the cranial mesenteric artery may be diagnosed *per rectum* in the live animal, appearing as an enlargement at the root of the mesentery.

**J.** Carcase and viscera: Normally A and D (affected intestines and arteries), provided condition is adequate.

## Mixed nematode infections in horses

Infections of large strongyles are often mixed and combined with those of 'small strongyles' such as *Triodontophorus* spp., e.g. *T. tenuicollis*, *Cyathostomum* spp., *Oesophagodontus* spp., *Cylicostephanus* spp., etc. (all of which are bloodsuckers) and other round worms.

The small stomach worm of horses, *Trichostrongylus axei* (also found in ruminants), may occur in mixed infections. In a dominant infection it causes a chronic catarrhal gastritis which may extend to nodular areas of thickened mucosa with erosions and ulcerations involving, on occasions, the whole glandular stomach lining.

Adult worms of the *Habronema* spp. (6–25 mm in length) produce large fibrous nodules (up to 10 cm in diameter) in the stomach wall of horses. These nodules contain necrotic material and large numbers of worms. On occasion they rupture to cause a fatal peritonitis.

The life cycles of *H. muscae*, *H. megastoma* and *H. microstoma* are indirect, the eggs or larvae being ingested by the maggots of house (*Musca domestica*) or stable flies (*Stomoxys calcitrans*), horses acquiring infection through eating the adult flies containing the infective larvae or the actual larvae which have emerged from the flies. In addition to the nodules, the *Habronema* spp. cause a catarrhal gastritis and abundant mucus formation.

*Oxyuris equi*, a pinworm (male 10 mm long and females up to 150 mm), is found mainly in the large intestine (caecum and colon), where the egg-laying females produce yellowish or white crusty masses round the anus and cause pruritus, restlessness, tail and buttock rubbing and often loss of condition.

The equine ascarid, *Parascaris equorum*, is a large, thick worm, up to 30 cm long, which may also infect cattle. Its life cycle is similar to that of *A. suum*. Foals are mainly affected, but adult horses may occasionally acquire infection. The migrating larvae cause respiratory symptoms (coughing, dyspnoea, etc.) in addition to loss of condition, colic and anorexia.

The *diagnosis and judgement* of these mixed infections follow the same lines as for the *Strongylus* spp.

## MISCELLANEOUS NEMATODE INFECTIONS

### *Chabertiasis*

Chabertiasis is an infection of the colon of sheep, goats, cattle and other ruminants with the nematode *Chabertia ovina*. A mucoid enteritis with oedema and punctiform haemorrhages in the intestinal wall are produced, resulting in dysentery, anaemia and loss of condition. Cattle appear to be fairly resistant to infection, the disease usually being asymptomatic.

### *Elaeophoriasis (filarial dermatitis of sheep, sorehead, clear-eyed blindness)*

Elaeophoriasis is responsible for a chronic disease in sheep, mule deer and black-tailed deer in the USA in which it causes dermatitis, arteritis, blindness, keratitis and rhinitis. The causal nematode is *Elaeophora schneideri*, which has intermediate hosts in several horse flies. The arteritis involves the common carotid, internal maxillary and leptomeningeal arteries in which there is inflammation and fibrosis of the arterial wall with thrombosis. The filarial dermatitis occurs on the face and feet takes the form of a granulomatous inflammation due to lesions in the supplying arteries made by adult parasites.

Filarial dermatitis may also be caused by *Parafilaria multipapillosa*, *P. bovicola* and *Stephanofilaria* spp. *Parafilaria multipapillosa* occurs in horses in Africa, South America, Europe and the Far East and causes focal skin haemorrhages (*'bleeding spots'*) on the forequarters which bleed for some time and then dry and clot, matting the hair. *P. bovicola* and *Stephanofilaria* spp., on the other hand, are found in cattle and produce similar lesions. Chambers (1991) recorded the overall incidence of lesions in cattle caused by *Parafilaria bovicola* in Zimbabwe to be 4.4%, with the highest prevalence in bulls (17.36%).

### *Gnathostomiasis*

Gnathostomiasis is an infection of the stomach of pigs in Europe and Asia in which adult worms are found in the stomach, causing gastritis, and the liver, causing hepatitis. The main parasite is *Gnathostoma hispidum*, which has an intermediate host in freshwater crustaceans or water fleas, *Cyclops* spp. Human infection by *G. spinigerum* acquired by eating raw or undercooked fish results in subcutaneous abscesses and tunnels and sometimes meningitis due to invasion of the eye and brain.

### *Neurofilariasis*

Neurofilariasis is an infection of the brain, spinal cord and lungs of sheep and deer in Europe, Canada and New Zealand with nematodes of the genus *Elaphostrongylus*, especially *E. tenuis*. The life cycle is indirect, involving several snails and slugs. Affected animals show lameness, incoordination, circling, blindness and paralysis.

### *Rhabditiasis*

Rhabditiasis has been recorded in cattle and horses but is most common in the dog. It is caused by the nematode *Rhabditis (Pelodera) strongyloides*, which invades the skin of the neck, flanks, ventral abdomen and udder, causing thickening and wrinkling with scurfing and pustule formation. The pustules contain thick yellowish caseous material and larvae or adult worms.

*Thelaziasis (eyeworm disease)*

Worms of the *Thelazia* spp., e.g. *T. gulosa, T. rhodesii, T. alfortensis* and *T. skrjabini* infest the conjunctival sac of cattle in the USA to produce conjunctivitis, keratitis, photophobia and corneal ulceration. The parasite in horses is *T. lacrymalis* and that in sheep is *T. californiensis*. Many other animals, including pigs, goats, deer, camels, dogs, rabbits, birds and man are hosts to the various species of *Thelazia*. The parasites have an indirect life cycle, various species of muscid flies (e.g. *Musca autumnalis*) acting as intermediate hosts.

A survey in France (Collobert *et al.*, 1995) found 10.3% of horses examined to be infected by *Thelazia lacrimalis*, animals of 6 months to 2 years being most frequently involved.

## Verminous bronchitis/pneumonia of ruminants

**I.** A parasitic infection of the lower respiratory tract, chiefly of young cattle, resulting in bronchitis and/or pneumonia.

**O.** Verminous bronchitis/pneumonia occurs in many countries of the world, especially in temperate regions.

**IA.** The cattle lungworm *Dictyocaulus viviparus* is responsible for the disease in cattle ('hoose or 'husk') and deer, while *D. filaria, Protostrongylus rufescens* and *Muellerius capillaris* (probably the most common lung parasite in sheep and goats) are the parasites in the latter animals. (*Dictyocaulus arnfeldi* is the parasitic nematode causing the disease in horses, mules and donkeys.)

The adult worms, *D. viviparus* and *D. filaria*, are about 5 cm (male) and 7 cm (female) long. Both life cycles are similar and are direct. Larvated eggs are laid by the females in the bronchi and the L1 larvae are coughed up and swallowed. (Hatching may also occur in the intestine.) These L1 larvae are passed in the faeces and reach the infective stage (L3 larvae) in 1 week.

The infective larvae are ingested by the hosts and, in the intestine, penetrate the wall and enter the mesenteric lymph nodes and undergo two further moults to become male and female worms. These enter the lymph and the blood vessels and reach the lungs, where they penetrate the capillary walls and enter the alveoli. Maturation takes place when the larvae reach the bronchioles and bronchi about 1 month post-infection (PI) for *D. viviparus*, 5 weeks PI for *D. filaria* and 4 months PI for *D. arnfeldi*.

*Protostrongylus rufescens* is a slender, reddish worm (male 20 mm and the female 30 mm long) which requires a snail intermediate host before becoming infective. The definitive host is infected by eating the snails.

The life cycle of *Muellerius capillaris* involves a snail or slug intermediate host into which the larvae penetrate for further development.

**R.** Infected animals and pastures and snails and slugs for *P. rufescens* and *M. capillaris*.

**MT.** Faecal–oral route.

**CF.** *Muellerius capillaris* and *Protostrongylus rufescens*, although responsible for some lung lesions, are not generally thought to cause clinical signs unless the infestation is very severe.

In the case of *Dictyocaulus* and *Protostrongylus* infections, there is bronchitis, coughing with abundant, clear, frothy mucus, anorexia and weight loss. Complications such as interstitial emphysema, pulmonary oedema and secondary infection and pneumonia often ensue to cause death.

**P.** See **CF**. There is considerable damage to the respiratory epithelium in the bronchioles and bronchi, which are blocked with frothy exudate. Lung lobules may show consolidation and the alveolar epithelium haemorrhages and hyaline membrane development.

Section of the trachea, bronchi and bronchioles shows a greenish, frothy exudate containing numerous worms, which may be so numerous as to occlude the lumens. The bronchial mucosa is oedematous and may show haemorrhagic streaks and patchy pneumonia with the edges of the lungs consolidated.

Numerous shot-like foci, the size of a millet seed to a pea, and yellowish or yellowish-brown in colour, are evident in the lungs at a later stage of infection.

Changes in sheep due to *Muellerius capillaris* are in the form of greyish-green, fibrous, sub-pleural nodules up to 2 cm in diameter in which there are eosinophils, eggs and perhaps a dead worm. These nodules may calcify. In goats there is a diffuse infection quite distinct from the nodular formation seen in sheep.

**D.** Diagnosis is based on clinical signs, epidemiology, post-mortem findings and the demonstration of first-stage larvae and eggs in faecal samples. Larvae are not present in prepatent, post-patent or early stages of infection and examination of bronchial mucus smears may be necessary to confirm a diagnosis.

**J.** Carcase and viscera: A – Kh, or T and D (lungs).

## CESTODES OR TAPEWORMS

Some 3000 species of tapeworms occur in virtually all forms of invertebrates and vertebrates including fish and man. They vary greatly in length, ranging from the tiny *Echinococcus granulosus* (6 mm) to 12 m or more, e.g. *Diphyllobothrium latum.*

All tapeworms are flattened, elongated worms devoid of an alimentary canal and a body cavity, partly digested food being absorbed through their integument.

Some tapeworms attack a single host while others require one or two intermediate hosts and a final, definitive, host to complete their life cycle.

They are bilaterally-symmetrical worms, both sides being similar. Each adult worm possesses a globular *scolex* or head and an unsegmented, thin *neck* followed by a wider *strobila* consisting of a number of wider and larger *proglottids* or segments which vary from three to many hundreds (one *Taenia saginata* tapeworm in a woman measured 90 feet!). The posteriorly-placed proglottids are gravid and contain fertile eggs. The head usually has four circular *suckers* for attachment to the intestinal wall but some, e.g. *Diphyllobothrium latum* possesses two elongated grooves (bothria) instead of suckers. In some cestodes hooks or hooklets are present on the suckers which are then said to be armed. These hooks are placed centrally to the suckers around a contractile organ termed the *rostellum.* Most of the tapeworms found in herbivores, however, are unarmed.

There is a rudimentary excretory system of flame cells and efferent canals and a central nervous system in the scolex consisting of a nerve ring and two ganglia from which several nerve cords run posteriorly.

Most tapeworms are hermaphrodite, each proglottid containing one or two sets of male and female organs. The *male organs* consist of a number of *testes*, united by ducts and leading to a *vas deferens*, along with a *seminal vesicle* and a *cirrus* or *penis*. The *female organs* comprise *ovaries, oviduct, uterus* and *vagina.* The ducts of both male and female organs open at a common *genital pore* which is usually situated at the lateral margin of the proglottid.

After fertilisation the *ova* are passed from the host in ripe segments usually in small groups in the faeces. At this stage they may or may not contain *onchospheres* (embryos with three pairs of hooks). Several envelopes are acquired by each egg, the main one and most resistant one being termed the embryophore. The stage when the embryophore contains an onchosphere is called a *coracidium.* Although the actual segments can survive for only a few days, the eggs are more resistant – under favourable conditions the eggs of *Taenia saginata* can survive on pastures for 6 months while those of *Echinococcus granulosus* can remain viable for over one year, resisting temperatures as low as 0°C for 4 months. Sunlight and desiccation are the main factors in the inactivation of *Taenia* eggs.

On hatching (which occurs in the intestine of the intermediate host in *Taenia* tapeworms) the released onchosphere penetrates into the intestinal wall by means of its hooklets and reaches its predilection site by the bloodstream. At the predilection site the onchosphere forms a *metacestode, cyst* or *bladderworm* which is the larval or immature form of the tapeworm.

The metacestode or cyst stage is transferred to the definitive host on ingestion of the infected intermediate host.

*Metacestodes* of parasitic cestodes in animals and man assume several different forms:

*Coenurus:* A very large vesicle or bladder containing clear fluid with numerous invaginated scolices attached to its wall., e.g. *Taenia multiceps.*

*Cysticercoid:* A single scolex non-vaginated withdrawn into a small vesicle without fluid, e.g. *D. caninum.*

*Cysticercus:* A single scolex invaginated into a large fluid-containing vesicle or bladder, e.g. *Taenia saginata.*

*Hydatid:* A large bladder containing fluid and smaller cysts termed brood capsules in which scolices develop, e.g. *Echinococcus granulosus.*

*Plerocercoid:* An elongated metacestode with an adult scolex, e.g. *D. latum.*

*Strobilocercus:* A single, uninvaginated scolex attached to a bladder by a long strobila, e.g. *T. taeniaeformis.*

The importance of cestodes in animals is associated with the presence of metacestodes in suitable hosts where they may be injurious or even fatal, e.g. *Multiceps multiceps* in sheep and hydatid disease in man. Adult worms in the intestine rarely cause problems in animals apart from some irritation, unless in very severe infections when they may exert deleterious effects due to obstruction as well as diarrhoea and unthriftiness due to appropriation of nourishment and the excretion of toxic substances. Armed tapeworms, however, may give rise to inflammation of the intestinal mucosa.

Young animals are more susceptible to tapeworm infestation, which is believed to make the animals more prone to fly-strike.

*Thyanosoma actinioides* causes inflammatory changes in the bile ducts of sheep and is responsible for considerable losses due to condemnations.

## Tapeworms of cattle, sheep and goats

*Moniezia expansa* is probably the most common tapeworm of ruminants throughout the world, but *M. benedini* and *Thyanosoma actinioides* ('fringed tapeworm') are occasionally found.

In the western parts of USA and Canada some 40–50% of sheep are infested with *M. expansa* and *T. actinioides.*

*M. expansa* has a small scolex with four prominent suckers without rostellum and hooks. It can attain a length of 6 metres.

The gravid segments of *M. expansa* are passed out in the faeces on to pasture. From them the eggs escape and are ingested by free-living, non-parasitic oribatid mites of the genus *Galumna* and others. The onchosphere or hexacanth embryo is released in the arthropod's intestine and burrows into its body cavity, where it develops into a cysticercoid in 3–6 months depending on environmental conditions. (These oribatid mites also act as intermediate hosts for other tapeworms, e.g. *Anoplocephala, Paranoplocephala, Avitellina* spp.) The intermediate hosts in the case of *T. actinioides* are psocids or book lice.

Each cysticercoid develops into a single tapeworm when the mite is eaten by the final, definitive, ruminant host.

## Tapeworms of horses, asses and mules

The main cestodes in equidae are *Anoplocephala magna* (Plate 3, Fig. 17), *A. perfoliata* and *Paranoplocephala mammilana,* which occur mainly in the small intestine and more rarely in the stomach.

The life cycles are similar to that of *M. expansa,* oribatid mites acting as intermediate hosts.

*A. perfoliata* is probably the most common of the horse tapeworms and occurs throughout the world.

A survey in the Republic of Ireland showed that of 363 horses examined 51% had *A. perfoliata* attached to the mucosa of the ileo-caecal junction and/or to the caecal mucosa. The lesions recorded included intestinal congestion, diphtheresis, ulceration, mucosal thickening and fibroplasia. Age, breed and source of origin did not influence the degree of infestation and no clinical signs were reported before slaughter, but these may have been overlooked since body condition was adversely affected because of the high burdens of tapeworms and other helminths (Fogarty *et al.*, 1994).

### Judgement of M. expansa and Anoplocephala

Carcase A. if condition good. Intestines D.

## Tapeworms of the dog

These tapeworms are a most important group, not only in meat inspection but also in the causation of *hydatid disease* in animals and man.

Seven tapeworms, which also occur in wild carnivores, e.g. foxes, wolves, coyotes, jackals and dingos, are included in this group – *Echinococcus granulosus, E. multilocularis, Taenia hydatigena, T. multiceps, T. ovis, T. pisiformis* and *T. serialis. T. pisiformis* is occasionally found in the cat.

There are many other tapeworms occurring in dogs, cats, wild carnivores and rodents but which do not produce lesions in the food animals, e.g. *Dipylidium caninum* (probably the most common tapeworm in dogs throughout the world), *T. taeniaeformis* (cats and wild carnivores), *T. krabbei* (dogs and wild carnivores), *T. crassiceps* (wild carnivores) and *Mesocestoides* spp.

### *Diphyllobthrium latum*

This tapeworm occurs in the small intestine of dogs, cats, man, polar bear and other sea mammals and causes lesions in the musculature of several freshwater fish, which act as intermediate hosts.

The adult worms are yellowish-grey in colour and may reach 20–25 m in length and 2–3 cm in width. The worm is composed of some 3000–4000 proglottids with an oval or club-shaped unarmed head 2.5 mm long. Two slit-like bothria (grooves) are present on the head which has no suckers. There is a rosette-shaped uterus situated centrally in each segment.

*D. latum* is common round the lakes of Italy, Switzerland and Germany, Central Europe, Poland, Finland, Russia, Far East, USA and Canada. There is a high incidence among Eskimos.

The *life cycle* of *D. latum* involves two intermediate hosts. Coracidia from the hatched eggs are ingested by minute *crustaceans* such as *Cyclops strenuus* and *Eudiaptomus gracilis* in which a first larval stage or procercoid develops. These in turn are ingested by the second intermediate hosts, freshwater fish such as pike, turbot, perch, etc., in which a plerocercoid is formed. Human beings acquire infection through eating raw, inadequately cooked or pickled fish or which contain infective plerocercoids. The practices of eating sliced raw fish, common in countries like Japan and Finland and of consuming raw pike roe in Russia and Jewish gefullte fisch provide an opportunity for infection.

In man, diphyllobothriasis is usually a benign infection resulting in little discomfort, but on occasions there may be vague abdominal pain, anaemia (due to $B_{12}$ deficiency), diarrhoea alternating with constipation, dizziness and urticaria. Some of these symptoms may be due to toxins produced by the worms. Intestinal obstruction caused by heavy infestations is rare, as is the vomiting up of worms.

*Diagnosis* is based mainly on epidemiology and the demonstration of typical operculated *D. latum* eggs in the faeces.

#### Judgement

Infected fish. T.

### *Spirometra mansoni* and *S. mansonoides*

These occur in dogs, cats and raccoons in the Orient (Japan, China, Vietnam, Korea) and have a morphology similar to that of *D. latum*.

They possess two *intermediate hosts* (*freshwater crustaceans* of the genus *Cyclops*) in which a procercoid is formed. When these minute crustaceans are eaten by the *second intermediate hosts* (water snakes and other amphibia as well as mammals, including pigs, poultry, and man) plerocercoids (spargana) develop. The life cycle is completed when the definitive hosts (dogs, cats, raccoons) eat the various amphibia.

Man can be infected by consuming either first or second intermediate hosts. Pork, poultry and snakes are important sources of infection. The drinking of untreated water containing infected *Cyclops* spp. can give rise to *sparganosis*.

Infection in man is a disease of rural people, many of whom have strange eating habits. When ingested, the larvae penetrate the abdominal wall and reach various sites in the subcutaneous or muscular tissues of the abdominal wall, limbs, heart, brain, spinal canal, scrotum, etc., where inflammation and haemorrhage occur and sometimes secondary infection with ulceration and necrosis.

*Diagnosis* is usually based on the history of eating raw suspect foods, detection of a migrating mass of larvae and the recovery of worms at surgery.

#### Judgement

Infected meats. T.

## HYDATID DISEASE

### *Echinococcus granulosus*

#### *Occurrence of hydatid disease*

Hydatidosis due to *E. granulosus* is a serious *zoonosis* occurring throughout the world in which man is an accidental intermediate host.

Enzootic areas in Africa are Botswana, Cape Verde, Mozambique, Namibia, Somalia and Tunisia, while there is a high occurrence in Morocco. In South America, Brazil, Chile and Uruguay have enzootic incidences, the last country having prevalences of 63% in cattle, 35% in sheep and 31% in pigs. In Asia the disease is important in Bangladesh, Iran, Lebanon and Syria, while in Greece, Albania and Yugoslavia it is enzootic.

Some countries have instituted national hydatid control schemes and several have managed to eradicate the disease, notably Cyprus (1985), Korea (1989), Kuwait (1986), New Zealand and Tasmania. Hydatid disease has been eradicated from cattle in Iceland and is now only of exceptional occurrence in sheep.

There is a low sporadic occurrence in Great Britain – 0.86% in sheep in 1960, which rose to 2.5% in 1977, the highest incidence being in Wales where it was up to 50% in some localities (Edwards, 1982). Highly successful control schemes have reduced these figures significantly.

It is now known that there are strains of *E. granulosus* with different host specificities. For example, no cases of horse infection have been recorded in New Zealand, where hydatid disease is endemic, whereas in the United Kingdom and parts of Europe horses are frequently infected. The horse strain apparently does not infect man, unlike the sheep strain.

The *epidemiology* of hydatidosis varies from one country to another and so control measures appropriate in one are not necessarily of value in another.

**R.** The incidence of echinococcal infection in an area can be determined from its level in the *dog*. A taeniacide such as praziquantel is administered to a representative sample of canines and the faeces are examined for *E. granulosus* worms. It is valuable also to examine foxes, wolves, coyotes and other wild carnivores and then to investigate the management and feeding of dogs to determine how the cycle of infection is maintained. Where dogs are highly domesticated, fed on prepared foods and have no access to farmland, there is rarely a problem of hydatid disease.

Where, however, sheepdogs can eat sheep carcases – a common occurrence in Wales and elsewhere – the cycle of infection is readily maintained, the more so if the dogs receive little protein in their diet at home and are not kept under control. In New Zealand, prior to the introduction of control measures, up to 25% of dogs were affected in certain areas, but the incidence now is less than 1%.

**IA.** *E. granulosus* is one of the smallest of the tapeworms, the adult worms being about 3–9 mm long composed of an armed scolex with 30–36 hooklets arranged in two rows and usually three or four proglottids.

**Life cycle** Up to 30 000 adult *E. granulosus* may be found in the small intestine of the dog, but the usual number is about 35. Eggs from the adult worms are passed out in the faeces and the infective onchospheres, when ingested by an ungulate, penetrate the intestinal wall and reach the *liver* (by the portal vein) or lungs and other organs (via the lymphatic system) to form *metacestodes, echinococci* or *hydatid cysts* (Plate 3, Fig. 18).

It has been demonstrated in New Zealand that the eggs of *E. granulosus* can be spread up to 10 km by blowflies, dispersion being greatest in winter. The possibility of birds being involved – as they undoubtedly are in relation to *T. saginata* – needs to be investigated (Torgerson, 1992).

The shape of the hydatid cyst is controlled to some extent by the organ in which it grows. When uninfluenced by pressure, it is oval or spherical, but in the liver, especially in sheep, it may assume an irregular shape because of the presence of the bile ducts. In bone, it follows the structure of the bony tissue and grows into the small crevices and channels.

The size of hydatid cysts in animals varies from that of a marble to a small football but they are usually about the size of a goose egg. They develop slowly, their longevity probably being limited by that of their host. Cysts in the liver and lungs grow very slowly. Early forms appearing as white nodules, as yet containing no fluid, may be seen in the liver 4 weeks after ripe eggs are ingested, while after another 4 weeks the cysts are 2.5 mm in size and contain fluid. In 6 months hydatid cysts are 15–20 mm in diameter and only then do they produce scolices and brood capsules and become infective. An average-sized hydatid cyst may contain as many as 2 million protoscolices.

In time, many hydatid cysts show degenerative changes, becoming smaller with the fluid being replaced by caseous material, which may calcify. Such changes are frequent in sheep and horses.

The hydatid cysts develop slowly, taking months to increase in size to 5–10 cm although some, especially in man, may reach 50 cm in diameter. They are usually unilocular, although often multilocular in sheep, and contain clear or slightly turbid fluid inside the germinal layer of the thick outer membrane.

*Brood capsules*, which are infective, hollow or bladder-like structures, become attached to the germinal layer by a short pedicle or stalk and develop 5–20 protoscolices or tapeworm heads about 5 months after infection. The brood capsules may detach themselves from the germinal layer to form hydatid sand. Occasionally, hydatid cysts do not form brood capsules and protoscolices and are sterile.

Hydatid infection of the *liver* is always associated with a marked fibrous tissue reaction which may be up to 13 mm thick. Affected livers are enlarged in proportion to the number and size of the cysts. Bovine livers of 91–113 kg and pig livers of 50 kg have been recorded. Such livers, being markedly cirrhotic, usually cause ascites.

### *Types of hydatid cysts*

There are two varieties of cysts. The *unilocular*, which is the cystic stage of *E. granulosus*, is the more common form in the food animals. Although older unilocular cysts may sometimes form daughter cysts, the parent cysts becoming distended with tense, spherical, small cysts of various sizes, this is simply a growth from of *E. granulosus* though in cattle it is often classified as multilocular.

The *multilocular* type originates from the tapeworm *E. multilocularis*. Cattle may sometimes harbour this alveolar cyst, which occurs only in certain parts of southern Germany, Switzerland and the Austrian Alps.

Sometimes *daughter cysts* are formed within or outside the parent cyst (when ruptured) either from shreds of detached germinal layer, from brood capsules or from protoscolices.

**R.** Definitive hosts are dogs, wolves, dingos, coyotes, jackals and other Canidae infected with adult worms in the small intestine. The intermediate stage (metacestode or hydatid cyst) occurs in a wide variety of ungulates – sheep, cattle, horses and pigs and man.

**MT.** The definitive carnivore host is infected when it eats the protoscolices. In the small intestine they evaginate and become attached to the mucosa of the intestinal villi. Eggs are able to survive for several months on pasture. Carnivores become infected by eating viscera containing hydatid cysts. The sheep–dog cycle is important in many areas, e.g. Great Britain, while in other regions the dog–cattle, dog–horse, dog–camel, dog–pig, dog–moose or dog–kangaroo cycle predominates. In man infection usually occurs by hand-to-mouth transfer of tapeworm eggs from dog faeces and via contaminated food and water.

### *Incidence of cysts in organs*

In sheep the lungs are affected as often as the liver, the commonest form being the fertile unilocular cyst. In the ox the lung is involved more frequently than the liver, usually with the small unilocular sterile cyst, though larger cysts occasionally occur. In pigs and horses the liver is the most frequent site of infection.

## ***Echinococcus multilocularis*** (Fig. 18.2)

**O.** Distribution is limited to the northern hemisphere – Europe, Russia, Japan, Alaska, Canada and the northern states of the USA.

**IA.** *E. multilocularis* is smaller than *E. granulosus*, being about 1.5–4.5 mm long. Other minor differences in morphology are present in addition to the multilocular cysts in the different intermediate hosts.

**Life cycle** See *E. granulosus*.

**R.** The adult tapeworms are found in foxes, wolves, dogs, coyotes, jackals and cats, the *intermediate hosts* being shrews, field mice, voles, lemmings, ground squirrels, etc., and sometimes man (who is an abnormal host). The food animals are not affected.

**MT.** By the ingestion of infective eggs in carnivore and small rodent faeces. Faecally soiled food, including fruit and vegetables, is a common source of infection for man.

**P.** The multilocular cysts are usually found in the liver and less commonly in the brain and lungs of the intermediate hosts (rarely in man).

## ***Echinococcus vogeli***

**IA.** The adult worm is about the same size as *E. granulosus*. It possesses up to to 36 large and small rostellar hooks on the scolex which distinguish it from the other *Echinococcus* spp.

**O.** Cases of polycystic hydatid disease in man due to *E. vogeli* have been recorded in Central and Southern America (Ecuador, Colombia, Brazil, Venezuela and Panama).

**R.** The main *definitive hosts* are bush dogs and domestic dogs, the principal intermediate hosts

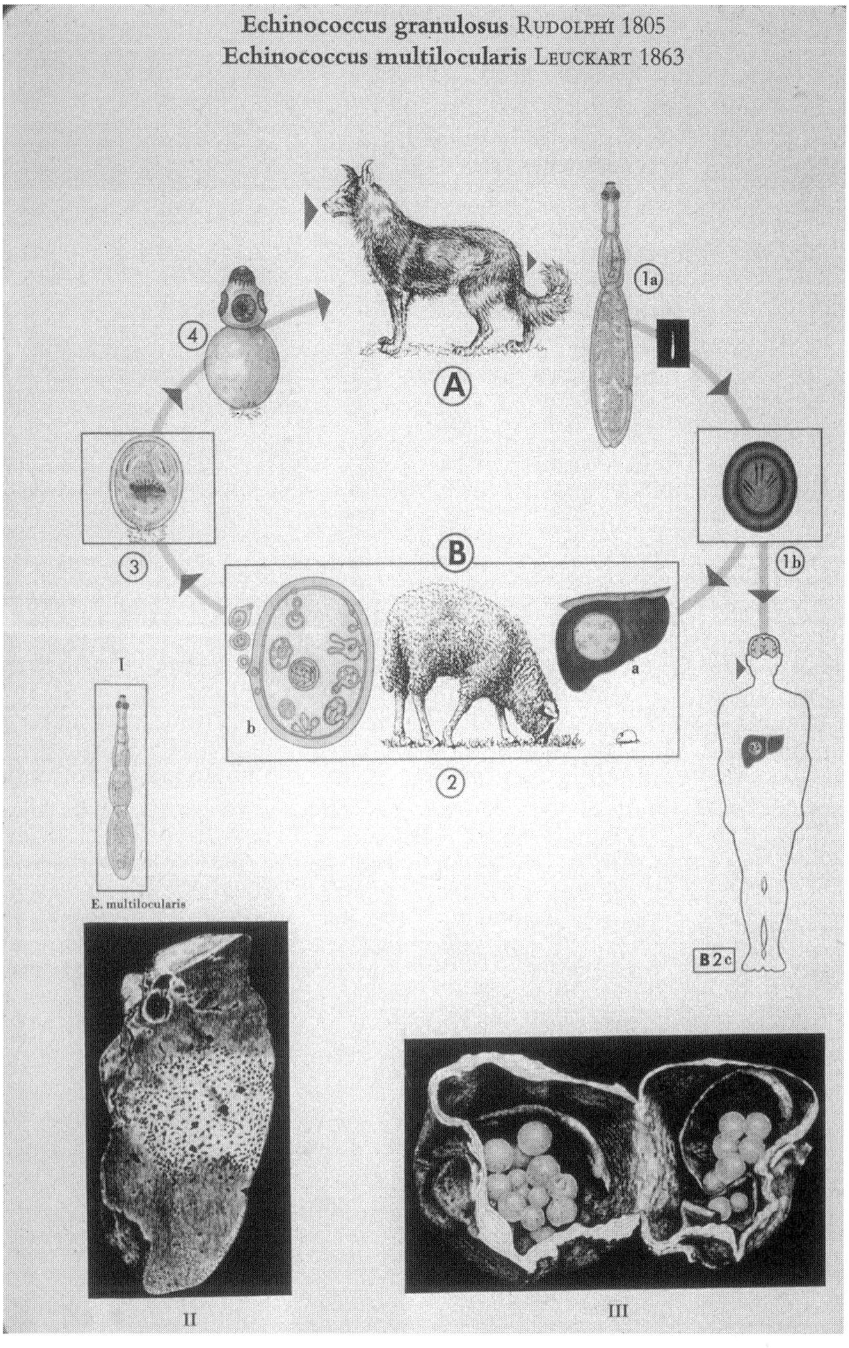


**Fig. 18.2** Life cycle of *Echinococcus multilocularis*. (Courtesy of Prof. A. T. Trees.)

being pacas and spiny rats. Domestic hunting dogs act as serious sources of human infection.

**MT.** Via the faecal–oral route.

**P.** The hydatid cyst is a polycystic one and is unique in that the germinal membrane proliferates externally to form new cysts and internally to create numerous microcysts by means of septa. Brood capsules with numerous protoscolices are produced in the microcysts.

*Hydatid disease in man*

The incidence of human hydatid disease (associated mainly with *E. granulosus* infection) is closely related to the prevalence of the disease in domestic animals and is highest where there is a large dog and sheep population.

In England an average of 3.5 people die each year from unilocular echinococcosis, the fatality rate in Wales being 3.5 and in Scotland 1.0. Since the disease is not notifiable, the exact incidence is not known. Serological surveys in Wales in 1978 gave up to 30% of asymptomatic young farmers (Clarkson, 1978).

The average annual incidence of hospital-diagnosed hydatid disease during 1974–1983 was 0.4 per 100 000 people in Wales and 0.02 per 100 000 in England. Within Wales, the county of Powys had the highest incidence (7 per 100 000 people). Although the prevalence has declined, there is still a need for intensive control measures (Palmer and Biffin, 1987).

As noted above, infection in man is acquired through the ingestion of ova from the dog tapeworm. Contamination of the hairs of the dog's coat with ova from faeces is probably the most common source of infection. Dogs may also transfer ova from the anus to humans by licking. In Lebanon it was shown that the relative risk of hydatid infection was over 20 times greater in dog owners than in persons without dogs and that Lebanon Christians were affected with hydatid disease twice as often as Lebanon Moslems, who are enjoined to wash their hands seven times after touching a dog.

Another less common source of human infection is the hand-to-mouth transfer of tapeworm eggs following the handling of fleeces of sheep contaminated by sheepdog faeces.

Rats, mice and cockroaches avidly consume proglottids in dog faeces and eliminate the proglottids within 24 h. The ova remain viable in this faecal matter for 3–4 months and the ingestion by man of food such as watercress, lettuce, etc., contaminated by these pests may account for a number of human hydatidosis cases. The rarity of the disease in the USA is related to the fact that dogs are not used to herd sheep, all stray dogs are shot and sheep are confined by dog-proof and wolf-proof fencing. In addition, the sheep population in the USA is relatively low.

Cases of *human infection* in Britain show the average distribution of cysts to be liver 65% (Fig. 18.3), lungs 10%, kidneys 7%, other abdominal organs 8%, cranial cavity 7% and bones 2%. Of 1802 patients in an Australian Hydatid Survey, the following distribution was recorded: liver 3%, lungs 25%, muscle 25%, bone 3% and kidney 2%.

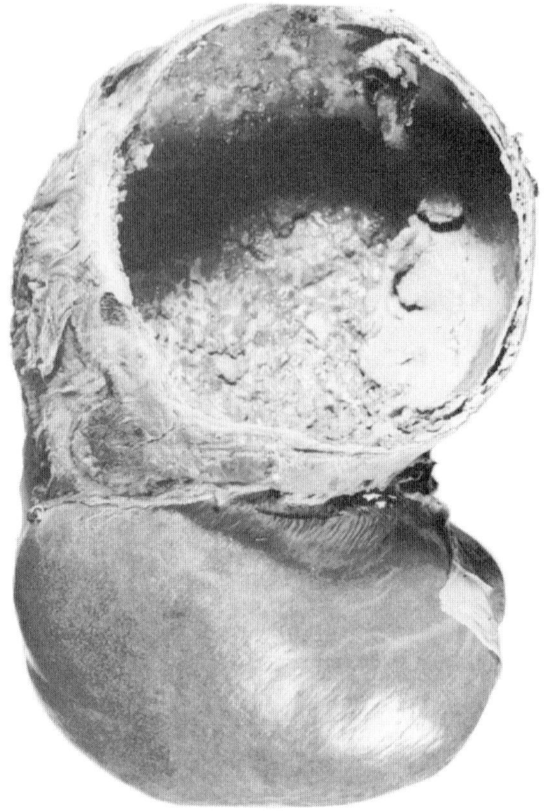

**Fig. 18.3** Large hydatid cyst (diameter 15 cm) in right lobe of human liver. A fibrous capsule, partly calcified, surrounds the 1 mm thick acellular cyst wall inside which is the cellular germinal lining. (By courtesy of the Editor, *Ulster Medical Journal*)

**CF.** *Clinical signs in animals*: There are generally few, if any, clinical signs associated with the presence of cysts in animals despite quite severe levels of infection. If, however, a large cyst is present in the liver ascites may result due to hepatic cirrhosis. Adult worms in the dog rarely cause problems except some enteritis in heavy infestations.

*Clinical signs in man*: Symptoms in humans are related to the severity of the infection and the site and size of the cysts (Fig. 18.3). Usually both liver (especially the right lobe) and lungs are affected, but cysts may be found in almost any organ in the body, even in the pulmonary artery and the inferior vena cava. Many cases, however, are asymptomatic and in some cases cyst growth is arrested with calcification. Some are picked up at post-mortem and others during chest X-rays, CT scanning and sonography for unrelated conditions.

In pulmonary cases there is often coughing, with or without haemoptysis (spitting of blood) with coughing up of membrane from a ruptured cyst. Liver lesions are sometimes painful and cranial cysts produce nervous symptoms. On occasions cysts rupture to become secondarily infected and/or cause fatal anaphylaxis.

**D**. *Diagnosis in animals*: In the food animals diagnosis is normally made *post mortem*. Confirmation of diagnosis is made at PM or by the demonstration of adult *E. granulosus* worms in the faeces of dogs purged with praziquantel or other taeniacide.

**D.** *Diagnosis in humans*: In human medicine, X-rays, computerised tomography and ultrasound are used as aids to diagnosis. Immunodiagnosis – immunoelectrophoresis (IEP) (the most specific test), complement fixation, latex agglutination, indirect haemagglutination, radioimmunoassay and ELISA – are among the tests used.

**J.** Carcase and viscera: A or T and D (affected organs), depending on carcase condition.

### *Control of hydatidosis*

Some of the most successful disease eradication programmes have been associated with hydatid disease (see Occurrence). It is significant that Iceland in the nineteenth century had the world's highest incidence in man, with a quarter to one-third of all autopsies showing evidence of the disease. Today it is free of hydatidosis and several other countries are in the process of being added to the list.

In New Zealand hydatid disease in both animals and man was a major public health problem prior to the introduction of a control campaign in 1959. This required the registration of all dogs and their periodic examination for infestation by three-monthly treatment with effective vermifuges. Other measures included the destruction of organs containing hydatid cysts and the prevention of access of dogs to raw offal (on pasture and in meat plants), these two measures being the most important in interrupting the life cycle of the parasite and lowering the incidence of the disease in animals and man.

The above measures must be combined with an educational programme to raise the level of awareness of the public, especially farmers, in relation to responsible dog ownership, with literature, media and school programmes. In Bulgaria an educational programme reduced the dog population from 1.5 million in 1960 to 75 000 in 1970 and lowered the incidence of the adult *E. granulosus* worm in dogs from about 60% to 14%.

It is vital that carcases of dead animals, especially sheep, are properly, and immediately, disposed of by deep burial or incineration as is the control of environmental contamination by dog faeces. The latter is also of importance in the control of toxocariasis.

The control of stray dogs is considered essential.

Efficient meat inspection procedures with effective control of rejected meat and offal are a prerequisite in hydatid control.

### *Taenia hydatigena (T. marginata)*

**IA.** The largest of the *dog* tapeworms, *T. hydatigena* is 0.7–5 m long and possesses four round suckers and a double row of 26–44 hooklets. The proglottids number about 400 with the more posterior and sexually mature ones being oblong in shape (5 mm wide).

The adult tapeworm occurs in the small intestine of dogs, wolves, coyotes, lynx and other wild carnivores and the intermediate stage (*Cysticercus tenuicollis*) in sheep, cattle and wild ruminants (rarely pigs, hares and rodents).

**Life cycle** Eggs in the faeces of the definitive host are ingested by ruminants and hatch in the small intestine, liberating the onchospheres. These penetrate the mucosa and reach the liver via the portal vessels. In the liver parenchyma they migrate for up to 4 weeks, causing serpentine haemorrhagic tracts especially near the thin edge. At first these tracts are dark red in colour but soon become brown or green and finally whitish due to fibrosis.

Some of the developing cysticerci or bladderworms pierce the liver capsule and migrate in the peritoneal cavity, become attached to the greater omentum, mesentery and visceral surface of the abdominal organs, especially the liver, where they reach maturity in 5–8 weeks after infection. Mature bladderworms (*C. tenuicollis*) vary in size but are commonly 2–6 cm round or elongated structures with a single scolex invaginated into a long neck. Those parasites that fail to reach the surface rarely grow bigger than a pea, rapidly degenerate and undergo calcification, appearing as whitish cauliflower-shaped foci. Severe infections may result in hepatitis.

**O.** *T. hydatigena* has a worldwide distribution, especially in farm dogs with access to sheep carcases.

**R.** Domestic dogs (rarely cats) and wild carnivores for adult worms and domestic and wild ruminants for cysticerci.

**MT.** Intermediate hosts by ingestion of eggs in contaminated food and water and definitive hosts by eating flesh containing cysticerci.

**CF.** Adult cestodes in dogs and other carnivores seldom cause trouble but heavy infestations may result in diarrhoea and unthriftiness in young animals especially if associated with roundworms.

Sheep in Britain are commonly affected with cysticerci but rarely show any symptoms except in severe cases in young lambs, which may lose body weight and even die suddenly where there is extensive liver damage with hepatitis (Livesey *et al.*, 1981).

**P.** See *Life cycle.*

**D.** Usually based on post-mortem findings which show the typical *C. tenuicollis* bladderworms. Since the ova of *Taenia* and *Echinococcus* spp. are similar, it is necessary to demonstrate the adult worms in affected dogs (see *E. granulosus*).

Some liver lesions due to *C. tenuicollis* may be confused with tuberculosis in cattle and pigs. However, the parasitic forms do not involve the portal lymph nodes and the degenerated material within the cyst is readily removed, leaving a white, folded membrane which is the cyst wall.

*C. tenuicollis* in the liver can be distinguished from the hydatid cyst by its subserous position and the presence of a single scolex and long, thin neck. *Ascaris* spp. cause small, discrete, pale foci in lambs' livers.

Histopathology may be necessary in cases where lesions are confined to the liver.

**J.** Most cases of *C. tenuicollis* infection are readily dealt with. Where only a few bladderworms are adherent to serosal surfaces, these only require removal.

In cases where the omentum and/or mesentery is extensively affected, these should be condemned.

Livers affected with extensive haemorrhagic or degenerated tract formation merit condemnation.

The rare cases in which oedema and emaciation occur warrant total rejection of the carcase and viscera.

Heavy condemnations of lambs' livers due to migrating *T. hydatigena* occur in many parts of the world, especially New Zealand, Australia and the United Kingdom, where it probably represents the chief cause of condemnation. A recent Meat and Livestock Commission survey in England showed an incidence of 8% in 70 000 slaughter lambs. At certain times of the year, especially midsummer, the incidence may be very much higher, one meat plant in SW England estimating that it lost £1100 ($1375) a week due to liver rejections because of *C. tenuicollis* infestation.

### *T. multiceps*

**O.** *T. multiceps* occurs throughout the world.

**IA.** Originally termed *Multiceps multiceps*, this tapeworm is 40–100 cm long and possesses 22–32 large hooklets and four suckers on a small scolex.

The adult worm occurs in dogs, foxes, jackals and other wild carnivores and sometimes man. A coenurus or bladderworm occurs in sheep, goats and other ungulates such as deer, chamois and antelopes, hares, horses and less commonly cattle all of which act as intermediate hosts. Man sometimes develops the coenurus.

**Life cycle** Eggs passed out in carnivore faeces are ingested by the intermediate hosts, usually from pasture. The contained onchospheres hatch in the small intestine, penetrate the mucosa and reach the systemic circulation via the liver, where many are arrested and die. The developing larvae have a predilection for the brain and spinal cord (which they reach in 8–14 days post-infection) but may also reach other organs.

In the CNS the maturing larva at first migrates, causing reddish or yellowish-grey purulent tracts, and then develop into a large, round, fluid-containing bladderworm or coenurus (*Coenurus cerebralis*, Plate 3, Fig. 16). This varies in size from a pea to a hen's egg or larger and is composed of a thin transparent wall on the inner side of which are up to 400 or 500 small, white, irregularly grouped spots, each of which represents an invaginated larval tapeworm head. The coenurus is infective after 6–8 months post infection. In the brain there is usually only one large cyst, which is found most often on the convexity of the cerebrum and occasionally in the cerebellum, at the base of the brain or even in the spinal cord, especially in the lumbar region where it becomes elongated in shape.

Infective larvae which become arrested in other organs degenerate and either disappear or become encapsulated foci 1–4 mm in diameter containing a greenish pus-like material which later becomes calcified. On rare occasions viable cysts have been recorded in the intermuscular tissues of sheep and goats.

**R.** Dogs and other carnivores for the adult tapeworms, and a wide variety of ungulates as intermediate hosts for infective bladderworms.

**MT.** By the ingestion of ripe segments and eggs passed in the faeces of carnivores, usually through grass or water contaminated with infected dog faeces. Dogs and other carnivores acquire infection through eating infected carcases, frequently sheep carcases, which contain the infective metacestodes.

**CF.** The infection in sheep (coenurosis, coenuriasis, sturdy, circling disease, gid, or turnsick) occurs most often in 1-year-old sheep and occasionally in goats and cattle, especially calves. Horses and other herbivores appear to be fairly resistant.

In some 20% of cases there are symptoms of meningoencephalitis with nervousness and excitability. This primary acute stage is followed by a latent period of 4–6 months, which is succeeded by the chronic phase associated with the growth of the cyst and pressure atrophy of the brain substance. Affected animals may squint, hold the head to one side, stagger or turn in circles, always circling to the side on which the cyst is located in the brain. Such animals are sometimes termed 'pivoters'. Blindness and hypermetria may be evident. Sometimes the head is held high with a jerky gait. In advanced cases there is anorexia and loss of weight. In some instances there may be actual pressure atrophy of the frontal bone of the skull, providing a site for surgical excision of the cyst which is often successful and is justified in valuable animals.

Cysts located in the lumbar region are often responsible for paralysis.

**P.** See *Life cycle*.

**D.** Coenurosis is usually diagnosed on clinical signs. Demonstration of *T. multiceps* proglottids in dog faeces. Post-mortem findings. The disease has to be differentiated from other neurological conditions such as listeriosis.

**J.** In the early stages of coenurosis it is only necessary to condemn the head. Advanced cases justify total condemnation because of emaciation.

Carcase and viscera: A and D or T.

### *Taenia ovis*

**O.** *Taenia ovis*, formerly known as *T. coenurus*, occurs worldwide, especially in Europe, North America, New Zealand and Australia, where the feral cat also harbours the adult worm.

The infection in sheep is not very common – in 1988 in the USA the FSIS reported only 387 cases in 5 million sheep slaughtered. In the past a considerable amount of Australian boned mutton was refused entry to the USA because of *C. ovis*, but its incidence now is virtually nil.

*C. ovis* in sheep in the United Kingdom is only occasionally encountered, its incidence in 1960 being 0.2%.

**IA.** Adult tapeworms are 1–2 cm long and possess a small head with up to 32–38 large hooks on the rostellum. They are found in dogs and wild carnivores and less commonly in cats. The cystic stage (*Cysticercus ovis*) occurs in the *intermediate hosts* – sheep and goats.

**Life cycle** Mature proglottids are shed in dogs' faeces and eggs are ingested at pasture by sheep and goats. In the small intestine of the intermediate hosts the onchosphere is liberated, penetrates the mucosa and eventually reaches the systemic circulation via the portal system and liver.

The predilection sites for these developing onchospheres are cardiac and skeletal muscles, especially the heart, diaphragm and masseter muscles. The cysticercus measures 3–9.5 mm in size and is ovoid in shape. It reaches these predilection sites after some 3 months development from the ovum.

**R.** Dogs and wild carnivores (less commonly cats) for adult worms and sheep and goats for the infective metacestodes.

**MT.** As for *T. hydatigena*.

**CF.** Adult worms in dogs rarely produce clinical signs unless in very heavy infestations, when unthriftiness and diarrhoea may be evident.

There is no record of illness in sheep and goats affected with cysticerci.

**P.** The cysticerci are essentially parasites of the intermuscular connective tissues. In the heart they are found under the epicardium and in the diaphragm under its pleural covering. They may also be found in the masseter muscles, tongue, oesophagus and flank.

Cysts in the heart tend to degenerate early and may show well-marked degeneration in less than 3 months after infection. In later stages, degenerating cysts appear as greenish blood-stained material which eventually calcifies.

Typical *C. ovis* cysts are easily recognised during meat inspection and are readily distinguished from *C. bovis*, being much larger with marked tissue reaction, making them stand out from the surrounding tissue, at least in the heart.

**D.** Demonstration of specific proglottids in dog faeces. Post-mortem findings.

**J.** United States regulations prescribe that if the total number of cysts in muscle and heart does not exceed 5, the cysts may be removed and the carcase passed, otherwise the carcase must be condemned.

The use of ultrasound and X-rays for deepseated lesions is being studied in some countries.

Generalised cases of *C. ovis* are rare, at least in the United Kingdom where usually only the heart is affected.

Carcase and viscera: A and D or T, depending on local or generalised infection, carcase condition, etc.

### *Taenia pisiformis*

**O.** *T. pisiformis* is found throughout the world.

**IA.** Formerly known as *T. serrata*, this tapeworm measures 15–60 cm, even up to 2 m, in length and 5–6 mm maximum in width. There are some 4000 proglottids, the posterior border of the ripe segments being broader than the anterior giving the worm a serrated appearance.

The small head has four suckers and a rostellum of 34–48 large and small hooks in a double row but no neck.

The adult worms occur in the dog, cat, fox, lynx, coyote and several other wild carnivores. It is especially common in farm and suburban dogs having access to rabbit and hare viscera.

The intermediate hosts are rabbits, hares and rarely squirrels and other rodents.

**Life cycle** Similar to that of *T. hydatigena* and *T. ovis* except for different intermediate hosts and eventual sites of cysts in them.

Young stages of developing onchospheres after 2–4 weeks in the liver penetrate the liver capsule, a few developing into a bladderworm (*Cysticercus pisiformis*) in the peritoneal cavity attached to an organ. The cyst is elliptical in shape and is about the size of a pea. The migrating larvae in the liver produce tortuous tracts and sometimes hepatitis. The cysticerci may occur free in the peritoneal cavity but are usually found within the layers of the omentum or mesentery or beneath the serous capsule of the liver or kidneys. Usually only a few cysts are present but occasionally they are numerous resembling a bunch of grapes.

**R.** See **IA**.

**MT.** As for *T. ovis, T. hydatigena, T. multiceps*.

**CF.** Normally light infections of the adult worms in the definitive hosts produce no symptoms but severe infestations can cause diarrhoea and unthriftiness. The intermediate hosts can suffer digestive disturbances and even serious loss of condition where there is liver damage.

**P.** See *Life cycle*.

**D.** As for *T. hydatigena* and *T. ovis*.

**J.** Carcase and viscera: A and D or T, depending on number of cysts and carcase condition.

### *Taenia serialis*

**O.** *T. serialis* is distributed throughout the world. It is regarded by some authorities as not being distinct from *T. multiceps*.

**IA.** The adult worm is 20–72 cm long and 3–5 mm wide and possesses a prominent rostellum with one row of large and another of small hooks.

The *definitive hosts* are the dog, fox and other wild canids and the *intermediate hosts* are lagomorphs (rabbits, hares, squirrels, etc.) and rarely man, in which a coenurus (*Coenurus serialis*) is formed in the subcutaneous and intermuscular tissues (Plate 3, Fig. 15).

**R.** See **IA**.

**MT.** As for *T. multiceps* and *T. ovis*.

**CF.** In general there are no clinical signs in the definitive host, although severe infestations may cause unthriftiness and diarrhoea.

Subcutaneous cysts are palpable in the intermediate host and are more common in wild rabbits than in domestic ones. If numerous, they result in emaciation and death.

**P.** The cystic stage, which usually contains clear or turbid fluid, is termed *Coenurus serialis* and may be found almost anywhere in the body but most commonly in the intermuscular and subcutaneous tissues of the back, loins, and hind limbs. On occasions they involve the external muscles of mastication, forming a prominent swelling at the angle of the jaw. Cysts may even be found in the CNS. In 45 days post-infection the cysts are about the size of a cherry, but they can grow to 4 cm or more. Older cysts may contain pus.

Examination of unskinned rabbits should be made by firmly drawing the hand over the body from head to tail, when cystic elevations will be noted. If cysts have been punctured a depression in the muscle will be present.

**D.** As for *T. hydatigena* and other *Taenia* spp.

**J.** Carcase and viscera: A – with removal of a few cysts and if condition is good. T – if cysts are numerous and/or condition is poor.

## TAENIASIS DUE TO *TAENIA SAGINATA* (BEEF TAPEWORM) AND BOVINE CYSTICERCOSIS

**I.** *Taeniasis* due to *T. saginata* is an infection of the small intestine of *man* with the adult stage of the large beef tapeworm and *cysticercosis* is the tissue infection in *cattle* with its larval or cystic stage (*Cysticercus bovis*).

Many cases of taeniasis in man are asymptomatic, except for some anal pruritus due to emerging tapeworm segments but with severe infections human beings may experience loss of weight, anorexia, abdominal discomfort and digestive upset.

**O.** Taeniasis and cysticercosis are common where beef is eaten raw or imperfectly cooked. (many people prefer to eat rare beef and some consume raw sausages – a very dangerous practice since they contain head meat). Where cattle have access to human faeces due to poor personal hygiene habits the conditions often occur.

The incidence of *C. bovis* varies greatly between and within countries, and even between meat plants, a possible reflection of the competence and diligence of meat inspectors.

The diseases in man and cattle are common in Africa, especially in Zaire (high occurrence), with enzootic levels in Angola, Botswana, Burkina Faso, Mozambique, Namibia (*C. bovis* – 1.2% in slaughter cattle), Somalia, Sudan and Uganda. In the Matabeleland Province of Zimbabwe, *C. bovis* was detected in 2.16% of 100 000 bovine carcases during a period of 11 months. Lightly-infested carcases accounted for 95% of all positive cases, with live cysts occurring most commonly in older cattle and dead cysts in young stock, a reversal of the European situation (Pugh and Chambers, 1989).

Cuba and Guatemala also have enzootic levels but the diseases have been eradicated in Honduras (1986), Haiti and Colombia (1989), Peru (1988) and Haiti and Colombia (1989). In Uruguay the incidence of *C. bovis* is 0.25%.

Apart from Yemen and Lebanon, where *T. saginata* infection is enzootic, Asia does not appear to be seriously affected and the Philippines (1988), Kuwait (1986), Israel and Sri Lanka (1991) are free.

In Oceania, the diseases are constantly present in Fiji and New Zealand but have been eradicated from Samoa.

*T. saginata* infection has been eradicated from Germany and Greece (1988) and from Czechoslovakia in 1990.

Canada has a *C. bovis* incidence of 0.0018% in 2½ million cattle slaughtered annually.

At Belfast Meat Plant (N. Ireland) in 1989, the incidence of *C. bovis* was 0.4%, viable cysts accounting for 15% of the total. Degenerated and viable cysts usually occur singly or in very small numbers at this particular centre and generalised cases are rare, a situation which obtains throughout the British Isles. In 1989 in Northern Ireland, out of a total kill of 475 987 cattle there were 3 cases of generalised *C. bovis*, a percentage of 0.0006 or 0.39% of all bovine carcases condemned.

*T. saginata* in *man* is more common than *T. solium*. In Europe the human infection rate is probably less than 1%, but in Africa there are an estimated 12 million carriers with a 30% incidence in some African stockmen. In the USSR there are an estimated 49 million carriers.

A survey in Northern Ireland in 1967–68 revealed that 30 human cases of *T. saginata* taeniasis were treated in hospitals and 90 at home. In addition, a small number were found coincidentally, especially in maternity wards. The overall incidence in Northern Ireland is 8.16 per 100 000 of the population, although this does not include those individuals who do not seek treatment or in whom previous treatment was unsuccessful. Females were found to be more often affected than males in a ratio of at least 2:1.

In England, 82 cases of *T. saginata* infection were reported in 1976, 98 in 1977 and 58 in the first 32 weeks of 1978. All reported cases, however, only represent a very small proportion of the actual incidence.

In Britain, human infection due to *T. saginata* and bovine cysticercosis were virtually unknown before the Second World War, but the parasite appears to have become more prevalent since then. Some of this is undoubtedly due to the existence of antiquated sewage systems, the absence in many localities of sewage treatment, the increase in population movement and camping activities as well as the unhygienic habits of certain human beings.

**IA.** *Taenia saginata* lives exclusively in the small intestine of man. It averages 3.5–6 m in length but can reach lengths of 30 m or more. It possesses a scolex with four elliptical suckers but no rostellum or hooks (Plate 4, Fig. 20). The proglottids number up to 2000 and the uterus in each gravid segment possesses 15–35 delicate lateral branches and contains about 100 000 eggs.

The *intermediate cystic stage (C. bovis)* is found mainly in cattle, although other ruminants such as deer, reindeer, llama, buffalo, giraffe and antelope may harbour cysts.

**Life cycle** This is similar to that of *T. solium* except that the cysticercus stage of *T. saginata* occurs in cattle and some wild ruminants while the chief intermediate hosts of *T. solium* are pigs, wild boars and less commonly man (Fig. 18.4).

A small number of proglottids are passed out daily in the faeces of affected humans. Eggs are released in the process and are very resistant, remaining viable for months in grassland, rivers and sewage plants. The ova from a relatively few human carriers can be widely distributed in a wide variety of ways. Indiscriminate defaecation by humans can distribute gravid segments or ova and the latter can be disseminated via rivers and sewage sludge.

Most of the conventional *sewage treatment procedures* have not proved effective in eliminating tapeworm ova. Cattle grazing on land fertilised with either sewage sludge or farmyard manure may become infected, especially if no steps are taken to keep stock off such treated ground for at least 3 months, if left unploughed. The sensible practice of the deep injection of sewage sludge and slurry directly into the ground serves to reduce the risk of infecting cattle. The flood water of polluted streams may also disseminate ova onto pasture.

The resistant ova can remain infective on grassland for at least 8 weeks and in liquid manure for 71 days. It has been shown in Australia that *T. saginata* eggs can remain viable on dry pastures for 14 weeks, even up to 6 months if conditions are favourable.

It is also known that dissemination of ova takes place through the agency of insects and birds, especially seagulls, starlings and feral pigeons, which regularly feed at sewage plants, sewage outfalls on foreshores and refuse tips. As many as 150 eggs have been recovered from the intestine of a naturally infected seagull. *T. saginata* eggs have regularly been demonstrated in gull and starling droppings at such sites. These particular species of birds (which have increased greatly in numbers in recent years) have now developed a habit of roosting inland, making them a menace in the dissemination of *Taenia* eggs as well as other pathogens such as

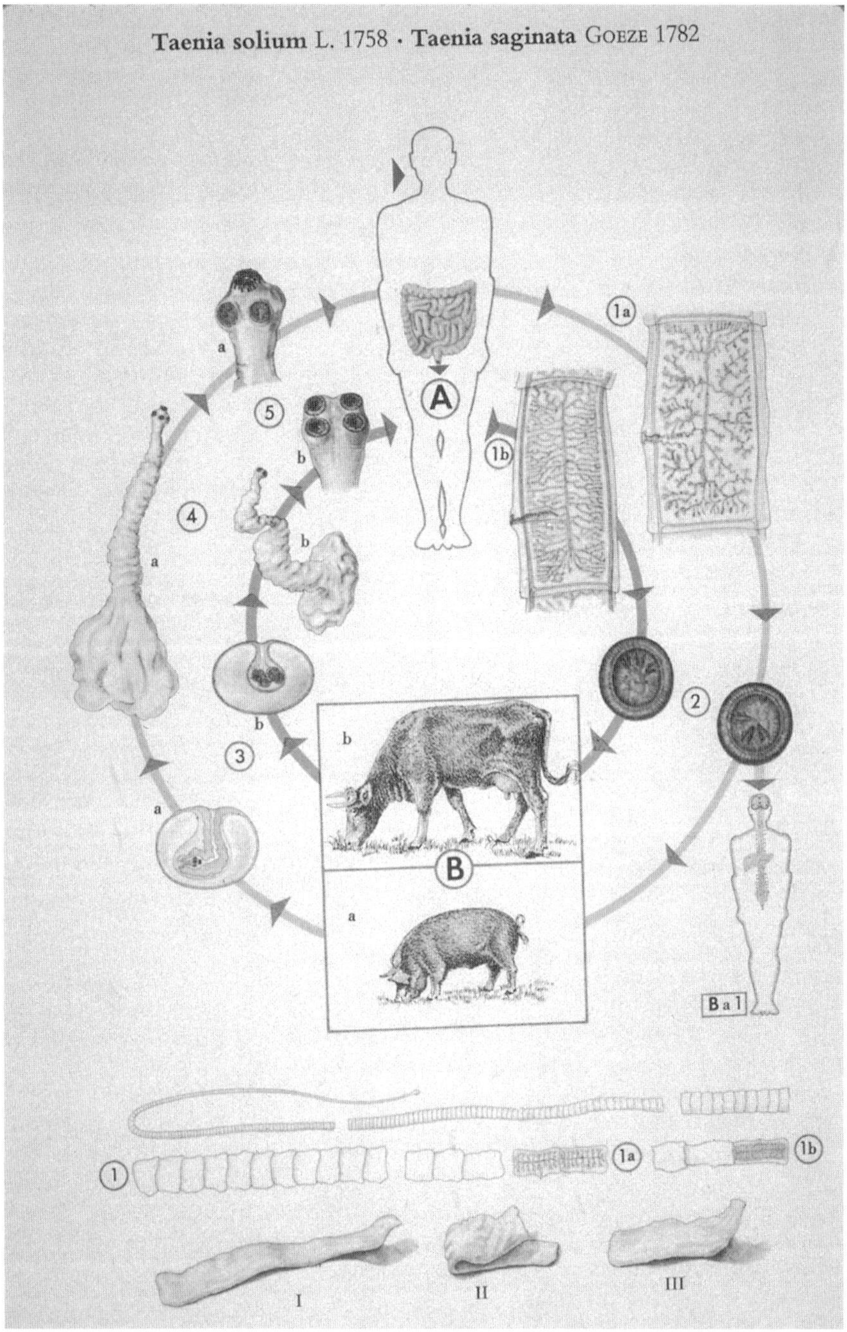


**Fig. 18.4** Life cycle of *Taenia saginata/Taenia solium*. (Courtesy of Prof. A. J. Trees.)

salmonella, campylobacter, ornithosis virus, etc.

These various agencies are responsible for diluting the initial infection, thus producing only a few cysts in cattle. However, if cattle, especially calves, ingest a large number of ova, generalised cases may ensue.

**Cystic stage** On ingestion by cattle and other ruminants such as llama, buffalo, gazelle, antelope and giraffe, the ova hatch in the intestine and the onchospheres penetrate the intestinal mucosa to reach the portal system and are then disseminated by the arterial system to develop into *cysticerci* (*C. bovis*) in skeletal and cardiac muscles. The main predilection sites are the masseter muscles, heart, diaphragm and tongue, but other sites may be involved.

The cystic stage is infective in about 10 weeks post-infection and can remain viable for up to 9 months. However, many begin to degenerate under the influence of tissue fluids and become caseous and eventually calcified.

*C. bovis*, the *beef measle*, is round or oval in shape and when fully developed consists of a scolex invaginated into a small fluid-filled vesicle (tail bladder). Surrounding this is an adventitious connective-tissue capsule formed by the reaction of the tissues of the host. The cysticerci present the following macroscopic appearance, according to their stage of development:

1 Very small cysts, about the size of a pinhead, with no scolex visible and surrounded by a delicate connective-tissue capsule.
2 Pinkish, oval cysts up to 1 cm × 0.5 cm in size, surrounded by a delicate, translucent capsule through which the scolex can be seen as a white spot.
3 At a later stage the capsule of the cyst becomes thickened, opaque and greyish-white in colour, the typical cysticercus being enclosed within. *C. bovis* is fully developed at about 18 weeks after infection but can be readily diagnosed at 6 weeks.

*Degenerative changes* often occur and cysts in the first stages of degeneration have been recorded as early as 6 weeks after infection, though such changes may not take place until 7 months. The onset of degeneration appears to be directly influenced by the supply of arterial blood to the muscle in which the cyst is lodged. For example, cysts in cardiac muscle are usually the earliest to undergo caseation and calcification. In endemic areas, degenerative changes may be considerably delayed and in an animal that becomes infected during the first 3 weeks of life cysts may remain viable for 30 months or even the entire life of the host.

However, in Australia experiments have shown that 9 months is the maximum longevity for *C. bovis* in cases of adult infection.

Cysts in varying stages of degeneration from caseation to calcification are frequently seen. Thus it is not uncommon to find the following:

**(a)** Oval cysts with a thick connective-tissue capsule which is formed by the host, is difficult to separate from the surrounding tissue and contains a yellowish-green caseous material. A dead cysticercus, usually with scolex evaginated, may be found in this material.
**(b)** Completely calcified cysts in which the cyst structure has been replaced by mortar-like concretions in the intermuscular connective tissue.

Cysts in bovine muscle may remain viable for up to 14 days after the death of the host.

The relatively large size of cysts in *calves* has in the past suggested prenatal infection but it is now known that calves are only infected after birth and that the metacestodes grow rapidly in the young animal. Infection in calves can occur by the ingestion of food contaminated with human faeces and by the licking of faecally soiled hands.

**Location of cysts** In general, *C. bovis* cysts are usually encountered singly, or in small numbers at meat inspection. Most are degenerated forms, viable cysts accounting for some 15% of the total. Generalised cases are relatively rare.

*C. bovis* cysts are most commonly found in the muscles of mastication, especially the masseter muscles, the heart, tongue, diaphragm, oesophagus, shoulder and occasionally in fatty tissues, lungs, liver and lymph nodes.

In cattle throughout Africa, important predilection sites are the muscles of the shoulder (musculus triceps brachii), a reason advanced for the frequent involvement of these muscles being the increased blood supply due to the long journeys undertaken by these animals.

In Zimbabwe, a survey of 100 000 bovine carcases showed that the head was the only organ affected in 58.4% of the positive cases, the shoulder in 20.1% and the heart in 7.9%. In the more heavily infested (condemned) cases, 81.1% had at least three sites involved (Pugh and Chambers, 1989).

**R.** The *definitive host* for *T. saginata* is man and the *intermediate hosts* are cattle, buffalo, deer, reindeer and wild ruminants such as wildebeest, giraffe and antelope.

**MT.** Infection in man follows the ingestion of raw or undercooked beef (*'measly beef'*) containing the cysticerci, while cattle and other ruminants are infected by consuming the eggs of *T. saginata*.

Only fresh, viable *C. bovis* cysts are infective for man.

**CF.** In *cattle and other animals*, cases of taeniasis are usually asymptomatic except when severe infestations occur when there may be diarrhoea and some loss of condition.

Most cases of bovine cysticercosis are acquired in early calfhood, particularly from birth to 28 days. In most European countries there is a seasonal incidence of cysticercosis, cysts being found most often at meat inspection during the late summer and autumn months, cattle having picked up the infection when put out to grass in the spring, the occurrence of the cysts coinciding with the 4–5 months required for development.

In *man*, there are usually no clinical disturbances except for pruritus ani, the patient being aware of discomfort in the perianal region. However, in more serious infestations loss of weight, gastrointestinal effects, nausea and nervousness may be evident.

**P.** See *Life cycle*.

**D.** In *cattle*, demonstration of viable *C. bovis* cysts in predilection sites at post-mortem is relatively easy but care has to be taken to differentiate minute forms from other entities such as fat globules and lesions of actinobacillosis (especially in the tongue).

The viability of cysts can be ascertained by placing them in normal saline solution with 30% ox bile or 5% sodium taurocholate and incubating at 37°C. Evagination of the unarmed scolex in viable cysts normally takes place within 1–2 h. Microscopic examination of the viable cyst will show the thin bladder wall and the scolex with four suckers but no rostellum or hooks.

Caseous and calcified degenerated cysts are more difficult to diagnose with accuracy.

In *man*, infection with the adult tapeworm is diagnosed by the demonstration of proglottids or eggs in the faeces or faecal swabs. The eggs of *T. saginata* and *T. solium*, however, cannot be differentiated morphologically and so reliance must be placed on the structure of the scolex (unarmed in the former and armed in the latter) and on certain other anatomical differences. Subcutaneous cysticerci in man are often palpable and can also be recognised by ultrasound, computerised axial tomography (CAT) or X-rays. Palpable cysts can be excised and examined microscopically. Serodiagnosis can be used to confirm the diagnosis.

### Efficiency of post-mortem inspection and treatment procedures

There is a practical limit to the number of incisions permissible because gross mutilation lowers the marketability of the carcase and also introduces contamination. As a result, many light infestations go undetected.

This has been confirmed by comparing detailed dissection of carcases with routine inspection procedures (Walther and Koske, 1980). In this experiment, 79 calves from a known *T. saginata* endemic area were slaughtered and the carcases were subjected to routine meat inspection procedures and subsequently to detailed dissection. While only 38.3% of infected carcases were detected at meat inspection, this figure was almost doubled on dissection, to 75.9%. Of these, 21.7% had cysts in the *triceps brachii* muscle only. During dissection, 34 (56.7%) of the animals were negative for *C. bovis* in the so-called predilection sites – masseter muscles, tongue, heart, oesophagus and diaphragm. Since the triceps incision is not used universally, this finding may be an indication for its adoption. However, this would probably meet with trade resistance, at least in the British Isles.

Although routine meat inspection measures may not be an absolute control for *T. saginata* infection in man, generalised infestations and many light ones will be detected.

The occurrence of a single degenerated cyst presents a problem. It is now considered that since live and dead cysts may co-exist in the same carcase, there is justification in subjecting such a carcase to freezing. A survey in Prague on lightly infested carcases showed co-existing live and dead cysts in 9.7% of positive cases.

The value of additional cuts in assessing the degree of infestation is questionable. Although these incisions may outdo the initial ones in the number of cysts found, the primary cut remains the most important for the detection of light infestations. It is certain that the shoulder cut should be insisted on in any of the African countries where *C. bovis* is prevalent. In Kenya, a modification of the shoulder cut is advocated – three incisions are made into the *triceps brachii* along with a further cut into the gracilis muscle parallel to the pubic symphysis.

Recent work on the efficiency of cold storage in killing *C. bovis* has thrown doubt on current techniques. Cartons (30 kg) of affected meat were exposed in a blast freezing tunnel with a conveyor cycle of 24 h and an average temperature of –30.9°C. A single cycle did not cause scolex death even if followed by 24 h cold storage. A double cycle caused scolex death if followed by 72 h cold storage. It was concluded that such a tunnel at a maximum temperature of –30°C would effectively kill cysticerci in boxed beef after a 48 h cycle followed by 72 h cold storage at –23.3°C.

Good eyesight is required for the efficient detection of *C. bovis*. The vast differences in detection rates, even among inspectors in the same meat plant, can only be explained by differences in vision, expertise and diligence.

*The development of an efficient, rapid ELISA test or other serodiagnostic test in the live animal would obviate much unnecessary mutilation and contamination and transform current meat inspection procedures.*

### Losses due to *C. bovis*

Losses of meat due to bovine cysticercosis are occasioned by the total condemnation of carcases with generalised infestation, the reduced value of carcases subjected to refrigeration, the cost of refrigeration, extra handling, transport, etc. It is reckoned that in Great Britain these losses amount to £100 per carcase or £4.0 million annually.

### Routine inspection procedures and judgements for bovine cysticercosis

Throughout the world the inspection techniques adopted and the final judgements exercised vary greatly. Only a small sample is given here.

#### MEMBER COUNTRIES OF THE EUROPEAN UNION

In Great Britain the relevant inspection procedures are contained in The Fresh Meat (Hygiene and Inspection) Regs. 1995 (Schedule 10, Part 1). These Regulations give effect to Council Directive 91/497/EEC, which amended and updated Directive 64/433/EEC on health problems affecting intra-Community trade in fresh meat; Council Directive 91/495/EEC on public health and animal health problems affecting the production and placing on the market of farmed game meat; Council Directive 92/45/EEC on public health and animal health problems relating to the killing of wild game and the placing on the market of wild game meat.

*Inspection procedure* (for bovines not less than 6 weeks old)

The procedure includes:

Visual inspection of the slaughtered animal and the organs belonging to it.

The external (masseter) muscles, in which two incisions must be made parallel to the mandible, and the internal masseters (internal pterygoid muscles) which must be incised along one plane, must be examined.

The tongue, having been freed to permit a detailed visual inspection of the mouth and fauces, must be visually inspected and palpated.

Visual inspection of the pericardium and the heart, the latter being incised lengthwise so as to open the ventricles and to cut through the interventricular septum;

Visual inspection of the diaphragm.

The cut muscles of the split carcase and the oesophagus should also be examined.

**Judgement**

Generalised *C.bovis*: Whole carcase, offal and blood unfit for human consumption.

Localised *C. bovis*: (a) Infected parts of carcase and offal removed – unfit for human consumption.

Remainder of carcase and offal to be kept in cold storage at a temperature not exceeding –7°C for a period of not less than 3 weeks or at a temperature of not less than –10°C for a period of not less than 2 weeks.

(Generalised and localised *C. bovis* are not defined.)

#### CANADA

*Inspection procedure*

1 Inspection of carcass, cut surfaces and organs.

2 Incisions shall be made through the centre of the internal pterygoid and external masseter muscles. Such incisions should be made

parallel to the mandible and extend right through the muscles.

3 Hearts shall be prepared for inspection by one of the following methods:

(i) Following visual examination of the exterior surface, the heart is incised by a longitudinal incision extending from its base to the apex through the wall of the left ventricle and the interventricular septum. The inner surfaces of the heart, including valves, shall be examined and the septum and left ventricular wall are incised by at least four deep incisions. All cut surfaces are examined for parasitic lesions.

(ii) A visual examination is made of the oesophagus. Whenever lesions suspicious of *cysticercus* infestation are found elsewhere in the carcase, the oesophagus shall be subjected to a thorough examination.

## Judgement

**(a) Index case** If on routine examination, one or more carcases are found to be affected with lesions suggestive of *C. bovis*, all affected carcases and their offal shall be held pending laboratory confirmation. As bovine cysticercosis is a *reportable disease* under the Animal Disease and Protection Act, the identity of the owner and the origin of the cattle must be established. To assist in this endeavour, as soon as a probable lesion is detected, the inspector should record all pertinent information which would assist in identifying the origin of the carcase(s), e.g. ear tags, brands, etc.

The Regional Office shall be informed that a suspect *C. bovis* lesion was detected and submitted for laboratory examination.

**(b) Laboratory confirmation** Appropriate lesions from affected carcases shall be excised with surrounding tissues, preserved in formalin, and forwarded to the Health of Animals Laboratory, Sackville, N.B., St. Hyacinthe, Quebec or Saskatoon, Saskatchewan or to ADRI/Nepean or ADRI/Lethbridge, for confirmation of the diagnosis. (Indicate on the laboratory submission form that the sample originates from an index case and therefore the carcase is being held pending laboratory confirmation. Also provide the phone number of the Regional Office for laboratory personnel to report their findings.)

Laboratory reports will reflect the results of histological examination of the submitted lesions and will consist of one of three possible options:

(i) The lesion was not caused by *C. bovis*. The pathologist will describe the lesion observed, adding the statement that the aetiology of the lesion was not *C. bovis*.

In this case, the carcase(s) from which the lesion originated may be considered not to be infested and should therefore be released without further treatment.

(ii) The lesion was caused by *C. bovis*. The pathologist will describe the lesion adding a statement which indicates that the aetiology of the lesion was *C. bovis*.

(iii) *C. bovis* cannot be ruled out as a possible cause of the lesion. In this case, the pathologist will describe the lesion observed, adding a statement which indicates that the lesion is consistent with that caused by *C. bovis*.

In the case of (ii) and (iii) above, the carcase(s) shall be considered infested and disposed of accordingly.

The laboratory will telephone the results of the examination directly to the Regional Office. The Regional Office will be responsible for transmitting this information to the Veterinarian-in-Charge.

When at least one carcase from a lot of cattle is considered to be infested, all carcases which originate from that lot and which exhibit gross lesions suggestive of *C. bovis* shall also be considered to be infested.

**(c) Disposition** *Infestation* shall be considered *extensive* where cysts are found in at least two of the following sites during routine primary inspection (heart, tongue, muscles of mastication, diaphragm and its pillars, oesophagus and musculature that is exposed during dressing operations) and in at least two of the sites exposed by incision into the rounds and forelimbs.

If on examination an inspector finds one or more lesions of *C. bovis* but the infestation is found to be of a lesser degree than that described above, the carcase shall be considered *slightly infested*. Carcases considered to be *slightly infested* shall be treated as follows:

(i) the cysts and surrounding tissues shall be removed and condemned; and

(ii) the carcase or the meat derived therefrom shall be held in a freezer under inspectional control at a temperature not exceeding −10°C for not less than 10 days; or

(iii) the meat is heated throughout, under inspectional control, to a temperature of at least 60°C.

**(d) Subsequent lots from the same premises** Subsequent lots of cattle which originate from *infected premises* and which are sent to slaughter under licence shall be subjected to a more detailed examination, including thorough slicing of the heart, the external and internal muscles of mastication, the muscular portion of the diaphragm, the tongue and the oesophagus and musculature exposed during the dressing operations of the carcase. All carcases exhibiting gross lesions suggestive of *C. bovis* shall be considered infested and disposed of accordingly. Laboratory confirmation is not required for this action.

**(e) Compensation** Under the Animal Disease and Protection Act, compensation is paid for carcases which are licenced to slaughter and subsequently condemned or treated due to cysticercosis.

### UNITED STATES OF AMERICA

*Inspection procedure*

1 Incise and observe lateral and medial masticatory muscles (cheeks) after tongue dropping.
2 Observe and palpate tongue.
3 Incise heart from base to apex or vice versa through interventricular septum and observe cut and inner surfaces.
4 As an alternative, at plant management's request, the heart may also be inspected as follows: After the inspector examines the heart's outer surface, a plant employee must completely evert it, after cutting through the interventricular septum and other tissues. The inspector then examines the inner surfaces and makes not more than four deep, lengthwise incisions into the septum and ventricular wall. If cysticercosis is suspected, more incisions shall be made. Cutting through the heart's walls should be avoided. If necessary, carcases and hearts shall be identified with consecutively numbered tags.
5 Observe the oesophagus and cut surfaces of muscles and pillars of diaphragm.

*When C. bovis is detected during the routine examination*, the *final inspection* is as follows:

1 The external and internal muscles of mastication, the heart and the muscular portion of the diaphragm, including its pillars, are thoroughly incised and examined, the peritoneum having first been removed from the diaphragm.
2 The tongue is thoroughly incised and examined.
3 The muscles of the oesophagus and all the cut muscular surfaces of the split carcase are examined.
4 When cysts are found in two or more of the above sites, one transverse cut is made into each shoulder 5–7.5 cm above the olecranon process and down to the humerus and an incision is made into each round so that the muscles are exposed in cross-section.

*When one beef carcase in a lot contains a tapeworm cyst*, the following procedure is required for all carcases in that lot:

1 Multiple incising of the interventricular septum and internal muscles of mastication. The oesophagus and cut surfaces of muscles exposed during the dressing operation are closely observed.
2 If available, and identified as part of the affected lot, hearts and cheeks from carcases which had passed inspection prior to finding the infected carcases are incised as above.

Inspectors are required to collect all live cysts from the heart and masticatory muscles, place them in formalin and send them to the Veterinary Services Laboratory in Ames, Iowa accompanied by full details of the carcases, tag numbers and owner's name and address.

The inspection for *C. bovis* may be omitted in the case of calves under 6 weeks of age.

## Judgement

1 Carcases of cattle displaying lesions of *C. bovis* shall be condemned if the *infestation is extensive* or if *the musculature is edematous or discoloured*. Carcases should be considered *extensively infested* if in addition to finding lesions in at least two of the usual inspection sites, namely the heart, diaphragm and its pillars, muscles of mastication, oesophagus, tongue and musculature exposed during normal dressing operations, they are found in at least two of the sites exposed by (i) an

incision made into each round exposing the musculature in cross-section, and (ii) a transverse incision into each forelimb commencing 2 or 3 inches above the point of the olecranon process and extending to the humerus.

2 Carcases of cattle showing *one or more tapeworm lesions of C. bovis but not so extensive as in (1) above*, may be passed for human food after removal and condemnation of the lesions with surrounding tissues. Provided that the carcases, appropriately identified by retained tags, are held in *cold storage* under positive control of a Program Inspector at a temperature not higher than 15°F (–9.4°C) continuously for a period of not less than 10 days, or in the case of boned meat derived from such carcases, the meat, when in boxes, tierces or other containers, is held under positive control at a temperature of not higher than 15°F (–9.4°C) continuously for a period of not less than 20 days. As an alternative to cold storage, such carcases and meat may be *heated throughout* to a temperature of at least 140°F (60°C).

Edible viscera and offal shall be disposed of in the same manner as the rest of the carcase from which they were derived, unless any lesion of *C. bovis* is found in these by-products, in which case they shall be condemned.

SOUTH AFRICA

*Inspection procedure*

Visual examination of the following tissues of all bovine animals is carried out for evidence of *C. bovis*:

1 Tongue (surface and substance palpated).
2 Masseter muscle, after making two deep linear incisions.
3 *Pterygoideus medialis* muscle, after making a linear incision parallel to the lower jaw.
4 The viscera, lungs and oesophagus.
5 The heart, after making a single incision through the LV and further incisions into the muscle if necessary.
6 The muscular diaphragm after removal of the peritoneum and making two incisions.
7 The cut surfaces of the carcase after splitting and incised if necessary.
8 *Triceps brachii muscle*, after making a deep transverse incision 5–7.5 cm above the point of the elbow. If *C. bovis* is found in this muscle, two further incisions parallel to the original ones are made.

**Judgement**

When one or two cysts are found on the majority of the cut surfaces, the carcase, meat and viscera are condemned. Otherwise, the carcase, meat and viscera are passed after treatment by: freezing at –10°C for 10 days; pickling in salt solution for 21 days at 8–12°C; steaming under moderate pressure (0.49 kg/cm$^2$) in an autoclave for 1 h; boiling at 95–100°C for 2½ h; or heating to a temperature of 95–100°C for 30 min.

AUSTRALIA

*Inspection procedure*

Under the Export Meat Regulations the following tissues of cattle over 32 kg of dressed weight are examined visually:

1 Tongue (also examined by palpation).
2 External and internal masseter muscles, after making two incisions into each masseter parallel to the plane of the lower jaw.
3 Heart, after making an incision through the interventricular septum and further incisions into the wall of the LV.
4 Diaphragm, after removal of the peritoneum.

When cysticercosis is found during the routine examination, further incisions are made into the predilection sites and the carcase musculature to determine the extent of infestation.

**Judgement**

Carcases showing one or more cysts in most of the incised muscles and oedematous or discoloured carcases are condemned. Carcases showing lesser infestation may be passed for food after removal of the affected parts and treatment of the carcase and its edible offal. Treatment involves refrigeration at –9.5°C for 10 days or, in the case of boned meat at –9.5°C for a period of not less than 20 days.

No carcase, including the head or viscera, may be exported if *C. bovis* is found in any organ or part.

NEW ZEALAND

*Inspection procedure*

The following tissues are examined visually:

1 Masseter muscles, after making several incisions into each masseter muscle.
2 Tongue, after making an incision into the base of the organ.
3 Oesophagus (also examined by palpation).
4 Heart, after making an incision through the LV and the ventricular septum from the base to the apex and making four further incisions into the muscle from the inside of the heart.

## Judgement

A carcase with more than two cysts in the muscles, excluding the heart, is condemned. When no more than two cysts are found in the carcase musculature, the cysts are removed and the carcase is passed for treatment by refrigeration at –10°C for 10 days. If freezing facilities are not available, the carcase, heart and the tongue are condemned.

No carcases in which *C. bovis* is found can be exported except in canned form.

## TAENIASIS DUE TO *TAENIA SOLIUM* (PORK TAPEWORM) AND SWINE CYSTICERCOSIS

**I.** *Taeniasis* due to *T. solium* is an infection of the small intestine of *man* with the adult stage of the pork tapeworm and *cysticercosis* the tissue reaction with its larval or cystic stage (*Cysticercus cellulosae*) which occurs most commonly in the musculature of the *pig* but also less commonly in other intermediate hosts such as man, dogs, rats and other mammals.

Zoonosis.

*T. solium* taeniasis and cysticercosis are of great public health and economic importance, the latter occasioned by the condemnation of pig carcases.

**O.** Although of only sporadic occurrence in Europe (Spain, Sweden, former Yugoslavia and Slovenia), *T. solium* has a high prevalence in many African countries (Tanzania, Angola, Burkina Faso, Chad, Gambia, Guinea Bissau, Mauritius and Mozambique), in Mexico and in South America (Ecuador, Guatemala, Honduras and Peru). Oceania is free except for East Timor, which has a high prevalence. Except for Cambodia and Lebanon, Asia is relatively free. The tapeworm has been eradicated from many countries – Czechoslovakia (1990), Finland (1947), Greece (1989), Lithuania (1991), Australia (1988), Philippines (1988), Canada (1985), Mauritius (1986), Namibia (1989), Cuba (1985), Haiti (1989) and Uruguay (1987).

In Mexico City, some 10% of street dogs harbour cysts, while in Madras about 1% of dogs are affected.

**IA.** The adult worm (*'armed tapeworm'*) is 1.8–4.8 m in length and possesses 800–900 segments which are distinguished from those of *T. saginata* by the gravid uterus, which has only 7–12 tree-like lateral branches while that of *T. solium* has 15–35. Each gravid proglottid contains some 40 000 eggs which are spherical in shape, those of *T. saginata* being oval.

The scolex is globular in shape and less than 1 mm in diameter. The rostellum possesses a double crown of 26–28 hooks. The neck is long and slender.

It usually occurs singly in man's intestine but in endemic areas, there may be several (as many as 25) tapeworms present.

The *life cycle* is similar to that of *T. solium* except that the *pig* usually acts as the *intermediate host*, although the cystic stage (*Cysticercus cellulosae*) may also occur less commonly in rats, cats, monkeys, sheep, cattle, deer, dogs and human beings.

Intermediate hosts are infected through the consumption of eggs in contaminated food or water. The onchospheres hatch in the intestine under the influence of gastric and intestinal juices, penetrate the intestinal wall into blood vessels or lymphatics, and are disseminated throughout the body to predilection muscle sites.

Intestinal infection in man (taeniasis due to *T. solium*) follows the ingestion of raw or undercooked infected (*'measly'*) pork, the adult worm developing in the small intestine. However, cysticercosis in man can also be acquired by the direct transfer of *T. solium* ova from the faeces of an individual harbouring an adult worm. Auto-infection due to reverse peristalsis of the intestine, once considered possible, is now known not to occur.

The fully developed *cysticercus* (*C. cellulosae*) is infective some 9–10 weeks after infection and

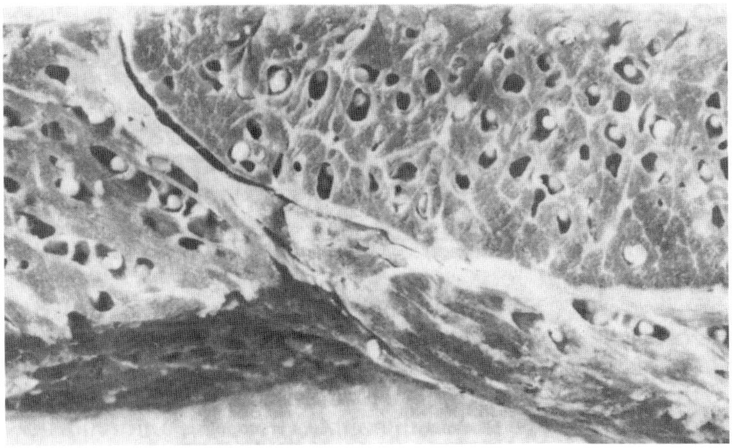

**Fig. 18.5** Measles of pork showing extensive invasion of muscle by *Cysticercus cellulosae*.

is about 20 × 10 mm in size, a delicate translucent structure with an invaginated head appearing as a small white spot. The size of *C. cellulosae* varies with its stage of development – at 20 days the cyst is the size of a pinhead, at 60 days the size of a pea with the head visible, while at 110 days all cysts are of equal size, elliptical in shape, with the scolex developed and invaginated.

*Predilection sites* are the heart, diaphragm and internal masseters, tongue, neck, shoulder, intercostal and abdominal muscles. The liver, lungs, kidney, eye and brain are less often affected, although 150 cysticerci have been found in the brain cortex. The deep muscles of the thigh are often involved, so that freedom from infection of the usual sites does not necessarily indicate the absence of cysts in the carcase musculature. The cysts in pig muscle (*'measly pork'*) may be scattered and few in number but one case is recorded in which some 3000 cysts were present in 453 g of muscle. *C. cellulosae* cysts can remain alive for several years but caseated and calcified cysts are non-viable (Fig. 18.5).

**R.** *Man* is the *definitive host* for *T. solium* and *pigs* the *main intermediate hosts* with rats, cats, dogs, sheep, cattle, deer, monkeys and man acting as lesser intermediate hosts.

Humans infected with *T. solium* excrete eggs into the environment as long as the worm is active in the intestine, a period which can last as long as 30 years. The eggs can remain viable outside the body for several months.

In countries where pork measles is endemic, the majority of infected pigs have a heavy infestation. This is explained by the fact that a person harbouring *T. solium* excretes 7–10 ripe segments daily, each segment containing some 30 000 ova which can be ingested by scavenging pigs. As with *T. saginata*, the unhygienic habits of some members of the human race perpetuate a serious disease.

**CF.** Cysticercosis in *pigs* is usually asymptomatic but heavy infestations can produce muscular stiffness and possible loss of condition.

In *man, clinical symptoms associated with the adult worm* in the small intestine can include abdominal pain, digestive disturbances, diarrhoea /constipation, nervousness and loss of weight but most cases are asymptomatic except for the irritation associated segments emerging from the anus. Eggs appear in the faeces 8–12 weeks after infection with the adult tapeworm.

In cases of *cysticercosis in man*, symptoms may appear days or years after infection. Cysticerci are formed in the subcutaneous tissues, striated muscles such as those of the shoulder, thigh or calf and other vital organs such as the brain, heart, liver, lungs and eye. While routine inspection of pig carcases and the adoption of other control measures have done much to reduce the incidence of *T. solium*, serious infections still occur in endemic areas. Suspect brain tumours often turn out to be *C. cellulosae* cysts, and epileptiform convulsions and death are frequently associated with neurocysticercosis. The prognosis is grave when cysticerci localise in the brain, heart and eye in particular.

**P.** See *Life cycle.*

**Carcase inspection** Suspect carcases should be split and exposed muscular surfaces examined, especially those of the diaphragm, abdomen, thigh and shoulder. The heart, tongue and larynx should also be included. In Africa the shoulder muscles are often infected and regulations in many African countries require that the *triceps brachii* muscle be incised by a cut about 2.5 cm above the elbow joint. This is claimed to detect infection in some 13% of carcases which would otherwise be missed.

*Diagnosis of adult tapeworm infection in man* is based on the morphology of gravid proglottids and the scolex in the faeces or on anal swabs. The scolex of each tapeworm has four suckers, but only *T. solium* is armed with hooks. (The ova of *T. solium* and *T. saginata* cannot be differentiated morphologically.) Recovery of the scolex after treatment ensures elimination of the worm.

*Subcutaneous cysticerci in man* may be visible or palpable. Microscopic examination of an excised cysticercus confirms the diagnosis. Cysticerci in visceral organs or the brain and spinal cord can be detected by X-rays, computerised axial tomography (CAT) or ultrasound.

The detection of products of *T. solium* in the serum of infected pigs can be made using a double homologous monoclonal antibody-based enzyme immunoassay (Rodriguez-del-Rosal *et al.*, 1989). These authors suggest that the ante-mortem diagnosis of swine cysticercosis is possible and useful in potentially preventing carcase condemnation losses, since as many as 80% of cysticercotic pigs could be detected and treated (praziquantel at 50 mg/kg per day for 15 days) before despatch for slaughter.

**J.** EC Council Directive 64/433/EEC (as amended) requires that meat from animals in which *generalised cysticercosis* has been diagnosed must be declared unfit for human consumption.

The Great Britain Fresh Meat (Hygiene and Inspection) Regulations 1995 prescribe that the whole carcase and all the offal and blood shall be condemned if found to be affected with *Cysticercus cellulosae.* No distinction is made between light and heavy infestations, nor is freezing advocated for localised infestations.

Codex Alimentarius (Alinorm 93/16A) prescribes that carcases and viscera affected with 'heavy infestations' be totally condemned, the designation of 'heavy infestation' to be prescribed by the controlling authority. Cases of 'moderate or light infestation or small numbers of dead/degenerated cysticerci' are to be subjected to freezing or heat treatment (q.v.).

United States regulations state that lightly affected pig carcases may be passed for cooking but those heavily infested must be condemned.

In Germany, lightly infested carcases may be cooked or pickled, though not frozen; such meat is classified as conditionally fit and may only be sold on the Freibank.

In South Africa, lightly infested carcases may be frozen.

### Methods of prevention and control (*T. saginata* and *T. solium*)

1 Education of public in personal hygiene – handwashing after defaecation and before eating; prevention of contamination of soil, water and food by use of proper toilet facilities; adoption of strict sanitation measures.
2 Prohibition of use of sewage effluent for soil irrigation or fertilisation. Alternatively, immediate ploughing in or direct deep injection of sewage into soil. (See also Control of Salmonellosis.)
 Prevention of access of livestock to human faeces, latrines, etc.
3 Effective pet and pest control.
4 Identification and immediate treatment of infected persons with effective taenicides such as praziquantel, niclosamide, etc.
 Encouragement of persons with suspect infection to seek proper medical treatment.
5 Effective meat inspection, condemnation and rendering procedures.
6 Efficient freezing and heating of meat (q.v.).
7 Thorough home cooking of beef and pork.
8 Investigation of contacts and source of infection.

## TREMATODES OR FLUKES

These are flattened, leaf-like, unsegmented parasites of which there are some 6000 species worldwide. They range in size from about 5 mm to several centimetres and can parasitise most vertebrates. They are found most commonly in fish, frogs and turtles but can also cause serious disease in ungulates, birds and sometimes man (especially the schistosomes or blood flukes). Some occur in invertebrates such as molluscs and crustaceans.

Most are endoparasites, but some are found externally. The majority of trematodes are hermaphroditic, but in some the reproductive organs are separate.

## Fascioliasis (distomatosis) or liver fluke disease

**I.** Liver fluke disease is an acute, subacute or chronic disease of the bile ducts and liver of mammals, especially ungulates (cattle, sheep, goats, buffaloes, deer, elk, moose and equidae) and sometimes man, caused by members of the genera *Fasciola, Fascioloides* and *Dicrocoelium*.

**O.** Worldwide, where cattle and sheep in particular are husbanded. *Fasciola hepatica* is common in the British Isles and Europe, while *F. gigantica* occurs in Africa, Middle East and Asia and *Fascioloides magna* in North America and Europe.

The disease is of great economic importance in many countries. In England and Wales about one million sheep livers are condemned annually. Chronic fascioliasis is the most common form of the disease in cattle, accounting for a 29% condemnation rate costing over £2 million in liver losses and a further £5 million in reduced liveweight gain and carcase quality.

In *Northern Ireland* the situation is relatively worse, the total weight of cattle and sheep livers condemned being greater than all the condemnations of carcase meat of cattle, sheep and pigs combined. Most recent figures show an incidence of 51% in cattle and 10% in sheep slaughtered. The annual loss of some 1000 tonnes of cattle and sheep liver amounts to £750 000, the overall losses due to fascioliasis in Northern Ireland being estimated at £4.5 million annually (Taylor, 1975).

German authorities have estimated that the parasite may reduce beef production by up to 10 per cent, milk production by 16% and be reponsible for loss of flesh in affected sheep by 25 per cent.

**IA.** *Fasciola hepatica (Distomum hepaticum)*, the common liver fluke, is approximately 30 mm long and 12 mm wide. It is pale brown in colour, flattened and oval in shape, being broadest anteriorly where it terminates in an oral sucker which surrounds the mouth and a ventral sucker situated about 2.5 mm behind the mouth. The cuticle is studded with numerous backwardly-directed spines which play an important part in the production of liver cirrhosis.

Like all flukes, *F. hepatica* is bilaterally symmetrical, both sides being similar. The *digestive system* consists of a pharynx, oesophagus, branched intestinal caeca and cloaca. The *nervous system* is composed of a pair of anterior ganglia and usually three pairs of nerve cords.

The parasite is hermaphrodite, the *female organs* comprising an ovary, oviduct, paired vitelline or yolk glands and uterus, while the *male organs* consist of two branched testes, vas deferens, seminal vesicle and armed cirrus. The eggs are brown in colour, oval and provided with an operculum or lid.

Excretion of waste products is achieved by a bladder and flame cells.

***Fasciola gigantica* (Giant liver fluke)** This trematode resembles *F. hepatica* in shape but is larger, being up to 75 mm long and 12 mm broad. Its morphology is similar to that of *F. hepatica* except that the anterior end possesses less defined shoulders. The life cycle involves different intermediate snail hosts, the most important of which are *Lymnaea auricularia, L. rufescens* and *L. acuminata*. *F. gigantica* occurs in cattle, sheep and buffaloes in Africa and Asia, causing acute and chronic disease in sheep but only chronic fascioliasis in cattle and buffaloes.

***Fascioloides magna* (Large American liver fluke)** This fluke measures up to 100 mm in length and is thick and oval in shape. It infests cattle, sheep, horses and pigs in North America and cattle, sheep and deer in Europe. Wild ruminants are affected in both continents. Deer are believed to be the normal hosts. A wide variety of snails, different from those of *F. hepatica* and *F. gigantica* act as intermediate hosts.

**Life cycle of *Fasciola hepatica*** Eggs laid by the adult worms in the bile ducts are excreted via the bile into the duodenum and passed out in the faeces. A single worm may lay over one million eggs during its lifetime. The rate of hatching depends mainly on temperature but this usually occurs in about 10 days when an embryo or *miracidium* is produced.

For further development and multiplication, the miracidium requires an *intermediate host* in the form of an amphibious mud snail, of which the most common is *Lymnaea truncatula*. Other intermediate snail hosts are *L. bulimoides* and *L. humilis* (N. America), *L. tomentosa* (Australia) and *L. viator* and *L. diaphena* (S. America). The actively motile miracidium must enter the mud snail within a few hours, otherwise it dies.

The optimum temperature for the miracidium to enter the snail is 15–24°C. It reaches the respiratory cavity of the mud snail and develops into a 1 mm long *sporocyst* which completes the final penetration into the snail. In the next 4–8 weeks the sporocyst gives rise to 6–8 *rediae*, each of which is 1–3 mm in length. In a further 4–6 weeks each redia becomes actively motile, migrates to the liver of the snail and produces 15–20 *cercariae*, each of which has a body 0.25–0.35 mm in length with a long tail, ventral and oral sucker and a bifurcated intestine. Development in the snail takes about 6–10 weeks.

The cercariae eventually escape from the rediae, leave the snail, lose their tails and either float in water or become encysted on grass stalks or aquatic plants on which they resemble grains of sand. The period of development from egg to encysted and infective cercariae takes 2–4 months. Cercariae may remain alive on pasture for up to 12 months and in dry hay for several weeks. A heavily waterlogged pasture enables cercariae to encyst farther up the blades of grass where they are more likely to be ingested by herbivores. Cercariae can, however, live in water and be swallowed by the final host.

In the final definitive host, the cercariae excyst in the small intestine owing to the action of the intestinal juices and in few days after infection penetrate the small intestine to reach the peritoneal cavity from which they bore through the liver capsule to migrate in the liver parenchyma.

In 7 weeks after infection, the immature flukes enter the bile ducts to reach sexual maturity and commence egg-laying.

Infection of mud snails occurs on two occasions during the year – summer and winter, the former being the more important, probably owing to the fact that many snails die during the winter months. *L. truncatula* begins to be active in March or April and lays eggs which give rise to a generation of snails, these producing more eggs 3–4 months later. Several generations of snails are produced between March and October. Summer infection results in disease in livestock from October onwards. Development of infection in snails is inhibited during the winter but recommences in the spring, with infection on herbage appearing in late spring and early summer and disease in animals occurring in July to October.

**Ecology of *L. truncatula*** The mud snail occurs most commonly on wet, badly drained land which has a slightly acid pH. This is especially true of *L. truncatula* and *L. bulimoides*, but others such as *L. tomentosa* are well adapted to an aquatic life and can drift long distances. Land which is frequently irrigated and where small springs and streams exist is also suitable for snail life.

**R.** See *Life cycle*. Fascioliasis is maintained in nature in a cycle between various vertebrate and snails of the genus *Lymnaea*.

**MT.** See *Life cycle*.

**CF.** Liver fluke disease occurs as an acute, subacute or chronic infection, the acute and subacute forms being evident mostly in sheep, while the chronic form in cattle is often asymptomatic.

In *sheep* the *acute* form occurs seasonally in the late summer and autumn, its timing being determined by the invasion of the liver by numerous young flukes in particular districts. Experimentally, it has been shown that if 5000 or more cercariae invade the liver parenchyma, sudden death due to extensive hepatic haemorrhage may occur without any premonitory symptoms. It takes place within 3 weeks of infection, mostly in younger animals.

Usually, however, there is weakness, dullness, anorexia, anaemia with oedema of the conjunctivae and abdominal pain. Death normally takes place within a few days of the onset of symptoms, which may be accompanied by dysentery and bloody epistaxis.

The *subacute* form differs from the acute type in that symptoms are more protracted, cercariae being ingested over a longer period. Loss of weight and anaemia are evident and sometimes submandibular oedema.

The *chronic* form of the disease, however, is the type most commonly encountered in sheep and cattle and is consistent with the ingestion of small numbers of cercariae over a long period of time. Infection occurs much later than in the previous two forms and symptoms, if they become evident, develop over a longer period. Should resistance be low, affected animals lose weight and develop anaemia with pallor of the mucosae. Animals on a high plane of nutrition can tolerate a higher fluke burden than those on a low plane.

In sheep there is submandibular oedema (*'bottle jaw'*), with oedematous swellings of the eyelids, throat, brisket and sometimes a pendulous appearance of the abdomen with diarrhoea. Loss of wool is marked, a feature which is especially evident in pregnant ewes. Some animals may die after 2–3 months, but survivors are emaciated for long periods and rarely recover weight. It is remarkable that some sheep survive despite the fact that virtually all liver tissue is destroyed and replaced by cirrhosis.

Susceptible cattle, after a slight initial weight gain, show loss of condition and milk yield and develop anaemia and chronic diarrhoea, especially if there is a superimposed pregnancy. Death, however, is relatively rare in the bovine, unless there is an associated disease. In contrast to the disease in sheep, most cattle show little impairment of health and well-nourished animals at slaughter are often encountered with markedly cirrhotic livers. It has been shown that while 50 adult flukes can cause clinical disease in sheep, some 250 are necessary in cattle.

Infection with *F. gigantica* produces much the same symptoms as those due to *F. hepatica*, while *Fascioloides magna* is of low pathogenicity in cattle, losses being due to liver condemnations as a result of extensive liver damage from thick-walled encapsulations. In sheep and goats, however, *F. magna*, even in light infestations, can cause acute symptoms and death due to hepatic haemorrhage caused by massive invasion of the liver with immature flukes.

**P.** The main lesions in fascioliasis occur in the liver parenchyma and bile ducts.

In the *acute* disease, in sheep large numbers of immature flukes invade the liver to produce acute swelling and congestion of the liver (acute parenchymatous hepatitis) in which the liver capsule is usually covered with fine fibrinous strands which may also occur in the peritoneal cavity. The liver itself assumes a paler colour than normal and is friable. Its parenchyma is extensively damaged with haemorrhagic tracts on the surface and in the substance. Immature flukes (1–2 mm) can be seen in the haemorrhagic tracts.

Rupture of the liver capsule occurs in very heavy infestations, with haemorrhage into the peritoneal cavity. The carcase presents a fevered appearance.

The acute type of the disease in sheep is sometimes associated with Black disease (q.v.) in which *Clostridium oedematiens (Cl. novyi)* proliferates in necrotic lesions caused by the immature flukes.

The *subacute* form of fascioliasis in sheep shows some degree of fibrosis as well as migratory tracts on the surface and in the parenchyma.

*Chronic fascioliasis* is by far the most common form of the disease in all animals, including man. The presence of adult flukes in the bile ducts gives rise to mechanical irritation of these passages and results in a chronic, pericanalicular atrophying cirrhosis with the formation of fibrous tissue in the walls of the bile ducts and surrounding liver tissue, including the portal canals. The fibrinous deposit on the liver capsule becomes organised and gives rise to a chronic perihepatitis which is often manifested in cattle and sheep by adhesion of the diaphragm to the anterior surface of the liver or by adhesion of the liver to the omentum. Fibrosis is usually greatest where immature fluke migration is most marked in the left lobe (ventral in position), but can occur elsewhere, e.g. in the portal canals and hepatic arteries, which become thickened. The walls of the bile ducts become very thickened owing to fibrosis and partial or complete occlusion is a frequent sequel. Flukes which fail to reach a bile duct become encapsulated in the liver parenchyma, especially in the left lobe, and form large rounded nodules with brown, greasy contents.

In *cattle* the thickened bile ducts eventually become calcified or *'pipey'* (*'pipe-stem liver'*) and casts of calcium are sometimes encountered blocking the bile ducts, making them difficult to cut with a knife. Such calcification does not occur in sheep and goats. The progress of fibrosis and scar tissue eventually results in the destruction of liver tissue with gross distortion of the organ, which becomes thickened and shortened, this being most apparent in sheep.

In cattle, flukes migrating through the liver may penetrate a radicle of the hepatic vein and be transported to the lung via the posterior vena cava, heart and pulmonary vein. In the base of the lungs they produce round cyst-like nodules varying in size from a hazel nut to a tennis ball. These initially contain coagulated blood and immature parasites and later become encapsulated with calcium and contain a thick, dark brown slime. In Britain some 20% of cattle with affected livers have accompanying lung lesions, but lung lesions rarely occur in sheep. Immature flukes may also be found in the mesenteric lymph nodes of cattle and sheep, appearing as millet seed to pea-sized nodules, at first yellow and pus-like but later greenish in colour and firm in consistency, with calcification in some cases. More rarely, encapsulated immature liver flukes may be found in the spleen, kidney, myocardium, subcutaneous tissues, under the parietal peritoneum and in the diaphragm.

The pathology of *F. gigantica* is essentially the same as that of *F. hepatica* but is less marked.

*Fascioloides magna* produces a severe reaction in *bovine* livers resulting in thick-walled encapsulations which do not communicate with the bile ducts. These, however, do not occur in *sheep*. In both species' infected livers there are black, tortuous tracts formed by migrating flukes.

*Fasciolopsis buski* is found in the small intestine of pigs, dogs and man in eastern Asia, especially China, Thailand and parts of India. It is a large trematode, measuring up to 7 cm in length and 10–20 mm wide. *Intermediate hosts* are pond snails of the genera *Planorbis* and *Segmentina* into which the miracidia penetrate with the eventual liberation of infective cercariae. These encyst on aquatic plants such as the water chestnut (grown in enclosed ponds) and cause infection when eaten raw. Infections in pigs are restricted to the small intestine, where there is enteritis, and on occasion, ulceration. Most cases, however, are asymptomatic.

Fascioliasis due to *F. hepatica* may occur in *pigs* at pasture without apparent symptoms. The difference in susceptibility is explained by the relatively large amount of fibrous tissue in the pig's liver, which acts as a barrier to fluke migration and high levels of precipitating antibodies to *F. hepatica*.

### *Human fascioliasis*

This has occasionally been described, man being an accidental host for *F. hepatica* and *F. gigantica*. Cases have been reported in Europe (especially France), Middle East, Australia, USA, South America and the Caribbean. Infection is acquired by the ingestion of uncooked aquatic plants, especially watercress, contaminated with free-swimming cercariae.

In most instances only a few flukes are present in the livers of infected persons, sufficient, however, to produce liver damage and enlargement along with abdominal pain, liver dysfunction with loss of weight, dullness and sometimes obstructive jaundice. On occasions, migrant larvae cause inflammation of the skin on the body and legs.

Infection in man with *Fasciolopsis buski*, when present in large numbers in the small intestine (but not the liver), produces symptoms associated with intestinal ulceration and toxaemia – anorexia, vomiting, diarrhoea or constipation, oedema of the face, abdominal wall and legs and sometimes ascites. Light infections, however, are frequently asymptomatic. In malnourished individuals, symptoms are more severe.

Humans in the Far East may also be infected with the flukes *Clonorchis sinensis* (also occurs in pigs), *Opisthorcis tenuicollis (O. felineus)* and *O. viverrini*, which have two intermediate hosts – snails and cyprinid fish (carp, tench, bream, chub, goldfish, etc.). Infection is acquired by eating raw infected fish.

## *Dicrocoelium dendriticum (D. lanceolatum)*

A member of the family *Dicrocoelidae*, this trematode is found in North and South America, North Africa, Asia and Europe (especially Yugoslavia, Spain, Switzerland) and certain parts of the British Isles – west coast of Scotland, Hebrides, north of England and western Ireland.

It occurs in a wide variety of animals – sheep, goats, cattle, deer, pigs, donkeys, elk, hares, rabbits and, occasionally, man.

It is 5–10 mm × 1.5 to 2.5 mm in size and lance-shaped, the body being widest at its middle. There are no cuticular spines.

**Life cycle** Two *intermediate hosts* – a *snail* and an *ant* – are required to complete its life history. The main snails are *Zebrina detrita* in Europe and *Cionella lubrica* in North America but the fluke can utilise a host of other species.

A feature of the life cycle is the formation of slime balls of cercariae in the snail. When expelled, these adhere to aquatic plants and are eaten by ants, mainly of the genus *Formica*, in which metacercariae are produced. The definitive hosts are infected by ingesting these metacercariae.

Infection with *D. dendriticum* is generally less severe than with *F. hepatica* but marked liver cirrhosis can occur with anaemia, oedema and emaciation.

### Eurytrema pancreaticum (pancreatic fluke)

This worm also belongs to the family Dicrocoelidae and is found in the pancreatic ducts and duodenum of sheep, goats, cattle, buffalo and man in Eastern Asia and parts of South America, especially Brazil.

It measures up to 19 mm × 9 mm and possesses the extensive, brown posterior uterus characteristic of the Dicrocoelidae.

Two *intermediate hosts* are required to complete the life cycle – *land snails* and *grasshoppers* or *tree crickets*.

Lesions include catarrhal inflammation of the pancreatic ducts and occasionally fibrosis resulting in duct blockage, atrophy of the pancreas and poor condition of the animal.

The infection is usually diagnosed post-mortem but can also be confirmed by demonstration of the small, brown eggs in the faeces.

### Diagnosis of fascioliasis

Fascioliasis should always be considered as a possible cause of ill-thrift in sheep and cattle, especially the former. It is frequently associated with parasitic gastroenteritis and verminous bronchitis.

Post-mortem examination will show the characteristic acute and chronic hepatic lesions. In the live animal the presence of the oval, operculated, brownish eggs of *F. hepatica* in faecal samples confirms the diagnosis but they must be distinguished from those of *Paramphistomum* (stomach flukes), which are larger and transparent. Serological tests, especially the ELISA, may be used.

*Differential diagnoses* include the above-mentioned parasitic entities, Jöhne's disease, deficiencies of copper and cobalt and infectious necrotic hepatitis (Black disease), eperythrozoonosis and anthrax in acute cases.

### Judgement

Cases of *acute fascioliasis* are rarely encountered at meat inspection. They must be condemned as fevered carcases.

*Chronic fascioliasis.* Markedly cirrhotic livers warrant condemnation but lightly affected organs can be trimmed provided lesions are well circumscribed.

Even in severely affected cases, the carcases are generally in good condition. But oedematous and emaciated carcases demand total condemnation.

Condemned livers may be consigned as inedible by-products or for petfood or pharmaceutical purposes.

### Control of fascioliasis

Control measures are directed at disrupting the life cycle of the fluke by land drainage, snail control using molluscicides on pasture and animal treatment with flukicides. Molluscicides include 0.5% copper sulphate solution (applied at a rate of 22.5 kg/ha), copper pentachlorphenate (11.2 kg/ha as a high volume spray of 4500 1itres/ha) and *N*-tritylmorpholene. Care must be taken with copper sulphate because chronic copper poisoning in sheep has resulted from its use.

Many modern anthelmintics – triclabendazole, rafoxanide, clorsulon, netobimin, ricobendazole, closantel, etc. – are effective against *F. hepatica*, some of them against immature flukes.

*Biological control* of fascioliasis has been mooted following the discovery of developing forms of *Echinostomatidae* (flukes similar to *F. hepatica*) in which no developing forms of *F. hepatica* were detected, suggesting some form of antagonism between the two species (Gordon and Boray, 1970). Further work along these lines has shown the presence of other forms of trematodes – *Xiphidiocercariae* in mud snails (*Lymnaea truncatula*) and adult lung flukes (*Haplometra cylindracea*) in the lungs of frogs –

but as yet no antagonistic mechanisms have been proved (Whitelaw and Fawcett, 1982).

In some regions, notably Northern Ireland, *climatic data are utilised to forecast* the emergence of cercariae and the severity of the following year's incidence of fascioliasis, enabling the strategic use of flukicides. These are usually administered to cattle and sheep towards the end of winter (to remove egg-laying flukes and reduce ground contamination), with another treatment in the spring (to kill overwintering cercariae) and a further autumn treatment to remove flukes from stock to prevent contamination.

To prevent *human infection*, education is necessary to persuade people to abstain from eating suspect watercress and other aquatic plants of unknown origin.

Treatment of *infected persons* with dihydroemetine and bithionol, along with investigation of contacts and source of infection is necessary.

### Schistosomiasis (bilharziasis, blood fluke infestation, snail fever)

**I.** An infection of blood vessels, especially the mesenteric and portal veins, kidneys and other organs of a wide variety of animals and man by adult male and female worms of the family *Schistosomatidae*, often associated with severe systemic symptoms.

**O.** The disease is widely distributed in Africa (including Madagascar and Mauritius), the Middle East, the Arabian Peninsula, China, Japan, Laos, Cambodia, Thailand, Malaysia, Brazil, Venezuela, Surinam, the Caribbean, the Great Lakes area and California, USA.

**IA.** The schistosomes are thin, elongated (up to 30 mm long), unisexual flukes existing as separate male and female forms. The female is very slender and longer than the male and lies, especially during copulation, in a longitudinal groove on the ventral surface of the male.

**Life cycle** In their predilection sites the females lay spined eggs which pass through the intestinal wall, etc., and leave the host in the faeces or urine. An aberrant predilection site is the nasal mucosa of ruminants and horses, in which *Schistosoma nasale* is found. Various *water snails* of the genera *Bulinus, Oncomelania, Planorbis* and *Lymnaea* act as *intermediate hosts* and are invaded by miracidia hatched from the eggs in water. In the snail the miracidia are followed by two generations of sporocysts to become cercariae. When mature, the cercariae leave the snail and invade the final host through the skin or mucous membranes. During penetration, the cercaria develop into immature schistosomula which are transported via the systemic circulation to the lungs in 1 week, and then to the portal and mesenteric vessels where pairing and egg-laying take place (Fig. 18.6).

**R.** Cattle, sheep, goats, water buffalo, horses, pigs and wild rodents are the principal

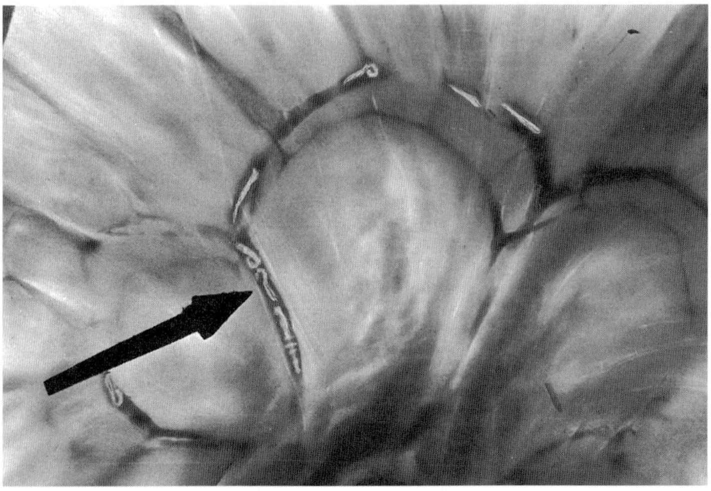

**Fig. 18.6** Adult male and female *Schistosoma matheei* in the mesenteric veins of an ox. In the newly slaughtered animal the parasites display active movement.

reservoirs for *S. mattheei, S. bovis, S. spindale, S. turkestanicum, S. japonicum* and *S. nasale*, while man is the main reservoir for *S. intercalatum, S. haematobium* and *S. japonicum*.

The various snail intermediate hosts are also reservoirs of schistosoma infection.

**MT.** Infection is acquired from water containing free-living cercariae which have developed in the snails. Animals become infected when standing in water containing the infective cercariae. Occasionally, oral infection may take place. These cercariae penetrate the skin of the final host and are transported to their predilection sites via the blood and lymph.

**CF.** The main symptoms, which are associated with the intestinal and hepatic forms of schistomiasis, consist of a haemorrhagic enteritis with blood and mucus in the faeces, anaemia, ascites and emaciation. Severe infections result in death within a few weeks, especially in sheep, goats and calves. More chronic cases develop egg granulomas with fibrous thickening of the intestinal wall and hepatic cirrhosis, while *S. nasale* cause a mucopurulent coryza and dyspnoea due to granulomatous lesions in the nasal cavities.

While acute and chronic forms occur, the disease in mild cases is often asymptomatic.

**P.** Infection with *S. mattheei* produces characteristic greyish-white granulomas or '*pseudotubercles*' in the intestinal mucosa, especially the small intestine. These form around the eggs and vary in size from 1 mm in diameter to elongated lesions as long as 200 mm and are accompanied by petechiae and ecchymoses. The intestinal lumen may contain large amounts of discoloured blood. There is fibrous thickening of the portal vessels and a grey, almost black discoloration of the liver in which granulomas, 1 mm in size, are scattered in the parenchyma. Similar granulomas are usually present in the bladder and in the nasal cavities (in *S. nasale* infection).

In both forms of schistosomiasis, adult flukes are found in the mesenteric, portal and intestinal veins, which are often dilated and tortuous. Similar lesions may also occur in the lungs, bladder and pancreas in severely infected animals.

**D.** Clinical signs, history and prevalence of the disease are suggestive of schistosomiasis but may be insufficient to confirm a diagnosis. At post-mortem examination the adult flukes may be seen in the mesenteric veins if these are stretched and the blood is not clotted.

Identification of the specific schistosome is based on the shape and size of the eggs and the presence/absence of spines and their location on the eggs.

In man, serological tests (circumoval precipitin, indirect immunofluorescent antibody, ELISA, radioimmunoassay) are used and are now being applied in animals.

**J.** As for *F. hepatica*.

### Paramphistomiasis

**I.** An infection of ruminants (cattle, sheep, goats and buffalo) with *paramphistomes* (amphistomes, conical flukes, rumen flukes) which cause rumenitis, reticulitis and abomasitis, diarrhoea, emaciation and death in severe cases over several weeks.

**O.** Worldwide, especially *Paramphistomum cervi*, while *P. hiberniae* occurs in cattle in Ireland, Scotland and The Netherlands; *P. scotiae* in cattle in Scotland and Ireland; *P. microbothrium* in Africa and Europe; *P. gotoi* in India.

*Gastrodiscoides aegyptiacus* has a conical anterior and a discoid posterior and is up to 18 mm long. It occurs in the large, and sometimes the small, intestine of equidae and pigs in Asia and Africa, causing a mild enteritis but on occasion, an acute, even, fatal colitis in horses due to the immature parasites.

Other genera such as *Calicophoron* (East Asia and Australia), *Cotylophoron* (Africa and other tropical and subtropical regions) and *Carmyerius* (Africa, Middle East and Pakistan) act like the paramphistomes.

**IA.** The adult worms are reddish in colour, pear-shaped and up to 15 mm long and 2–5 mm wide.

**Life cycle** The operculated eggs, laid by the adult worms in the 'stomachs', are passed in the faeces, hatch in water and infect snails similar to those which host schistosomes. Development in the snail is similar to that of *F. hepatica* (miracidium, sporocyst, rediae, cercariae). Cercariae encyst on herbage, are ingested by the final host, and excyst in the intestine where they remain for 3–5 weeks before migrating forward through the reticulum to the rumen. Eggs are laid by the adult worms 7–14 weeks after infection.

**R.** The definitive and intermediate hosts.

**MT.** Infection is acquired by the ingestion of infective cercariae on herbage or in water.

**CF.** Acute symptoms include severe diarrhoea, anorexia, anaemia, oedema, weakness, loss of condition with recumbency and death in a few days to several weeks. Mortality can be very heavy, especially in young cattle and sheep, older animals being more resistant. These symptoms are associated with the action of the immature worms in the small intestine (mainly duodenum and ileum) where their adhesion to the mucosa causes haemorrhage and necrosis.

In contrast, the adult worms in the rumen and reticulum are non-pathogenic except for *Carmyerius dollfusi*, which is a bloodsucker and causes anaemia. Less severe infestations result in some loss of condition with eventual recovery.

**P.** The adult flukes attached to the lining of the rumen and reticulum do not cause significant clinical disease, even when present in large numbers, but the immature forms embedded in the mucosa of the duodenum and ileum are responsible for severe enteritis, haemorrhage and necrosis.

**D.** Diagnosis is commonly made at post-mortem which reveals an intense necrotic enteritis with numerous parasites in the intestinal mucous membrane. Diagnosis can also be made by demonstrating the large, clear operculated eggs in the faeces which may also contain immature and adult worms.

**J.** As for *F. hepatica*.

## ARTHROPOD PARASITES

The *Arthropoda*, so-called because of their jointed limbs, constitute the largest phylum in the animal world and include the insects, crustaceans, centipedes, millipedes, scorpions, spiders and mites.

Other distinguishing features are the protective outer cuticle (which is shed at a moult or ecdysis), a segmented body and head, specialised sense organs, a blood vascular system containing spaces (haemocoeles), bilateral symmetry and separate sexes.

Arthropods are of great economic importance worldwide, being responsible for transmitting pathogens, e.g. protozoa and viruses, to man and animals – African horse sickness, Rift Valley fever, bluetongue, lumpy skin disease, malaria, plague, trypanosomiasis, filariasis, yellow fever, etc.

The adult flies cause harm by their stings and bites, while the larvae of certain members act as scavengers causing '*strike*' in sheep and contamination of meat (blow fly larvae). Ticks are involved in causing babesiosis, theileriasis, tick paralysis, etc., and mites, the smallest of the members of the phylum (0.25 mm), cause mange and sheep scab.

### *Gasterophilus* spp. infestation (bot fly)

**I.** An infestation of the stomach and subcutaneous tissues of equidae, and less commonly, pigs, dogs, birds and man, by the larvae (bots) of the bot flies.

**O.** Worldwide.

**IA.** The adult flies (*Gasterophilus intestinalis, G. haemorrhoidalis, G. inermis* and *G. pecorum*) resemble bees, are active in late summer, especially August, and lay their yellow eggs on the hairs of the forelegs, shoulders and breast. The eggs hatch in 5–10 days and the larvae, after being ingested, bore through the buccal mucosa and wander in the tongue (*G. intestinalis* and *G. haemorrhoidalis*) and submucosa, eventually reaching the stomach after several months. The bots are thick, segmented, pink or red in colour and 15–25 mm long.

They attach themselves mainly to the cardiac area of the stomach, although some may be found in the pharynx, duodenum, upper portion of the oesophagus and rectum. Two ecdyses are made and in 10–12 months the bots leave the host in the spring to pupate on the ground for 3–5 weeks, when adult flies emerge.

**R.** Infected equidae.

**MT.** See **IA**.

**CF.** The adult flies act like warble flies, frightening animals when ovipositing by their hovering and darting flight. Infestation results in unthriftiness, colic and anorexia in cases of heavy infestations.

**P.** Lesions are most severe with *G. intestinalis*. Inflammation, thickening, abscessation and ulceration of the gastric mucosa are evident where the larvae adhere. The attachment points are pitted. In some cases perforation may occur. Other lesions include stomatitis and pleurisy. Death may ensue in very heavy infestations. Up to 500 bots have been recorded in the stomach, but the usual number is about 30.

**D.** The activity of the flies, the presence of botfly eggs on the coat and stomatitis, ill thrift, etc., may suggest a tentative diagnosis. Pharyngeal larvae can be detected. Stomach bots are often encountered at post-mortem.

**J.** Carcase and viscera: A and D (stomach and other affected organs), provided carcase condition satisfactory.

### Lice infestation (pediculosis)

**I.** Infestation of the skin of all domestic animals, poultry and man with adult lice, larvae and eggs.

**O.** Worldwide.

**IA.** Lice are small, flattened, wingless insects varying in size from 0.3 mm to 11 mm. They are white, brown, yellow or black in colour and possess a *head* with modified parts for chewing or sucking and segmented antennae, a *thorax* which may be segmented or unsegmented, a large segmented *body* and three pairs of well developed *legs*.

There are two main groups – *Mallophaga* (chewing or biting lice) and *Siphonculata* (sucking lice).

**Life cycle** Most spend their whole life cycle on the host. *Eggs* are laid on hairs or feathers and hatch to produce *nymphs*. These undergo three moults to become *adults*, the whole process lasting 2–4 weeks. Breeding commences in the autumn, the greatest numbers being attained in the spring.

Important tick species in animals and poultry are the following

Cattle – *Damalinia bovis* (biting louse); *Haematopinus eurysternus* (short-nosed sucking louse), *H. quadripertusus* (tail louse) (N. America and Oceania), *H. tuberculatus* (buffalo louse) (Asia, Australia and Oceania); *Solenopotes capillatus* (long-nosed sucking louse)

Sheep – *Damalinia ovis* (biting louse); *Linognathus africanus* (also affects goats), *L. ovillus* (sucking face louse) (Australia, NZ, Scotland); *L. pedalis* (sucking foot louse), *L. stenopsis* (sucking goat louse)

Goats – *Damalinia caprae* (biting louse), *D. crassiceps, D. limbata; Bovicola painei*

Pigs – *Haematopinus suis* (sucking louse)

Horses – *Damalinia equi* (biting louse); *Haematopinus asini* (sucking louse)

Poultry – *Chelopistes meleagridis* (large turkey louse); *Cuclotogaster heterographus* (head louse); *Goniocotes gallinae* (fluff louse); *Lipeurus caponis* (wing louse); *Menacanthus stramineus* (body louse); *Holomenopon leucoxanthum* ('wet feather' in ducks)

Man – *Pediculus humanus capitis* (head); *P. humanus corporis* (body); *Phthirus pubis* (genital area)

**R.** Affected livestock and people. Outbreaks of head lice are common in school children and institutions.

**MT.** Direct contact with infested animals and indirect contact with contaminated blankets, harness, grooming equipment, etc. In man, the body louse *Pediculus humanus corporis* is the vector of epidemic typhus, trench fever and louse-borne relapsing fever

**CF.** Lice are most prevalent on livestock during the winter months. The irritant effects of these ectoparasites produce scratching, rubbing, licking and restlessness. The coat becomes rough and matted. In sheep the wool is damaged, assumes a yellowish colour and is soiled by lice faeces. Lameness accompanies the activity of the foot louse (*L. pedalis*). Milk and egg production may be reduced. In pigs the constant scratching produces an allergic dermatitis.

All lice are host-specific, but people handling infested stock, especially poultry, frequently acquire lice from them and suffer temporary irritation.

**P.** See **CF**.

**D.** Examination of body coat and feathers readily reveals lice or eggs ('nits').

**J.** Carcase and viscera: Usually A, provided carcase condition is satisfactory and no other lesions are present.

## Mites (order Acarina)

The *mites* are close relatives of the ticks, scorpions and spiders.

They are tiny parasites and range in size from less than 0.5 mm to about 6 mm in length. Their shape varies from round to elongated, with bodies which may be soft or hard like the ticks' and flattened or bulbous. They possess a *head, thorax* and *body* which may be covered partly or wholly with spines. *Nymphs* and *adults* generally have four pairs of legs, while larvae have three pairs.

They occur throughout the world in different habitats. While most are free-living, others are of considerable economic importance, living usually as ectoparasites on, but sometimes in, animals, birds, plants and insects. Some act as intermediate hosts of diseases transmissible to man, animals and crops while others are pests of stored grain and food products, even cheese.

An important cause of house-dust allergy in man are the mites *Dermatophagoides pteronyssinus* in Europe and *D. farinae* in the USA.

The importance of mites in meat inspection is associated with the damage to hides and fleeces, possible loss of condition in hosts, and their nuisance value to the handlers of animals, especially poultry.

Mites are host-specific but on occasions they may temporarily infest other host species.

The sexes are separate and the *life cycle* (completed in 2–3 weeks) is similar to that of ticks – egg, larval, nymphal (one or two) and adult stages, the latter three stages staying on the host and feeding on epidermis, serum, etc., and in some cases burrowing into the skins, e.g. *Cnemidocoptes mutans* which causes *'scaly leg'* in poultry and *Sarcoptes scabiei* causing sarcoptic mange in sheep, goats, cattle, equidae and other animals.

Important mites in farm livestock are as follows:

- *Chorioptes* spp. – Chorioptic mange in horses, sheep, goats, cattle and rabbits.
- *Demodex* spp. – Follicular mange in cattle, sheep, goats, pigs, horses and dogs.
- *Notoedres* spp. – Notoedric mange in rabbits and cats.
- *Psoroptes* spp. – Psoroptic mange in sheep (sheep scab), goats and horses.
- *Sarcoptes* spp. – Sarcoptic mange in sheep, goats, cattle, horses, rabbits and man (scabies).
- *Trombicula* spp. (Harvest mites) – Pests of grain and dermatitis in horses, cattle and pigs.

Important mites in poultry (see Disease of Poultry) include:

- *Cnemidocoptes gallinae* (depluming itch mite).
- *Cnemidocoptes mutans* (*'scaly leg'* mite).
- *Dermanyssus gallinae* (red mite).
- *Laminosioptes cysticola* (subcutaneous mite).
- *Magninia cubitalis* (depluming mite).
- *Ornithonyssus (Liponyssus) sylvarium* (northern mite).
- *Ornithonyssus bursa* (tropical mite).

## Mange (acariasis)

**I.** A contagious disease caused by *mites* in which there is skin irritation, loss of hair and wool, pruritus and sometimes debility leading to death.

**O.** Mange occurs worldwide.

**IA.** Mites of the genera *Chorioptes, Demodex, Notoedres, Psoroptes* and *Sarcoptes*.

**R.** Larvae, nymphs and adult mites and infested animals.

**MT.** Transfer of parasites by direct contact and indirectly through contaminated inert materials. Mange can co-exist with ringworm and lice infestation.

**CF** and **P.** *Chorioptic mange* – severe skin irritation with stamping of the feet, biting and rubbing of pasterns ('itchy leg') and tail in horses and cattle ('leg mange', 'barn itch'), loss of hair and allergic dermatitis in sheep. Cattle often unaffected. Lesions takes the form of an exudative dermatitis with formation of papules and scabs. Scrotum of rams may be affected.

**Demodectic mange (follicular mange)** This rarely produces clinical signs in animals despite the formation of microscopic nodules and papules on the neck, face, shoulder, brisket and sometimes the whole body of animals, especially cattle. These lesions are so small as to be overlooked. These are usually white in colour and contain a thick, whitish material containing numerous mites. On rare occasions, larger abscesses may develop from the papules with thickening of the skin into folds.

**Notoedric mange** Cats are most often affected with notoedric mange and rabbits less often. The mites are burrowers and create a thickening of the skin with a yellowish crust, especially on the ears, face and neck.

**Psoroptic mange (*sheep scab, body mange, ear mange*)** This occurs mainly in *sheep (Psoroptes ovis)* but also affects *cattle* (*P. natalensis* and *P. bovis*), *P. caprae* and *rabbits (P. cuniculi)*.

Psoroptic mange is a disease of great economic importance throughout the world and, along with sarcoptic mange, is a notifiable disease in many countries. It has been largely brought under control in many regions, although pockets of infestation still persist in many areas, probably owing to inefficient dipping/treatment measures. Losses are associated with damaged fleeces, loss of wool and condition in sheep, weight loss in other species due to intense skin irritation and itchiness, and even death in goats and rabbits (from septic meningitis) in severe cases.

The mites, unlike *Sarcoptes*, are host-specific and in all species puncture the skin to cause a dermatitis with serum formation. The animals scratch and bite at the affected areas, which may cover the whole body. In sheep the areas most commonly affected are the woolly parts of the body – shoulders, back, breast and base of tail – while the ears, face and neck of other species are predilection sites. The lesions commence as small papules which increase in size as bare crusty patches.

Psoroptic mange in cattle (*'barn itch'*) in the USA assumes a chronic form and is a notifiable disease which must be treated by government officials.

**Sarcoptic mange** Sarcoptic mange is caused by variants of *Sarcoptes scabiei*, the cause of scabies in man, e.g. *S. scabiei* var. *bovis, S. scabiei* var. *suis*.

Sarcoptic mange is most common in pigs, horses, dogs and rabbits but is less common in sheep, goats and cattle.

The mites pierce the skin and create burrows to produce an intense exudative dermatitis, the serum coagulating to form crusts. The skin becomes rough, thickened and wrinkled owing to connective-tissue formation and wool and hair are lost. Pruritus is evident with loss of condition in the more severe cases.

Hypersensitivity to the mites develops in some cases and is probably responsible for the pruritus which occurs after 3 weeks.

**D.** *Differential diagnoses* include parakeratosis, infectious dermatitis, pityriasis rosea, ringworm and infestation with lice and *Tyroglyphus* mites.

Diagnosis is confirmed by the examination of skin scrapings taken from areas with crusting/erythematous papules, i.e. active areas, clearing the sample with 10% NaOH or KOH and examining under low power (×40) microscope. The use of a small amount of mineral oil on the scalpel blade facilitates the collection of scrapings.

**J.** Judgement in mange depends on the severity of the infestation, condition of carcase, absence/presence of pesticide residues, etc.

## Screwworm infestation

This condition is a myiasis, an invasion of the animal body with larvae of the blow-flies (screwflies) *Callitroga hominivorax* and *Chrysomia bezziana*.

**O.** *C. hominivorax* (New World screwworm) is found in North and South America and *Chrysomia bezziana* (Old World screwworm) in Africa, southern Asia and Papua New Guinea.

Screwworm infestation occurs in all species of farm livestock, birds and wildlife as well as man. So serious has been the situation in North Africa that FAO introduced an eradication programme in 1989 using the sterile insect technique. This involves the artificial breeding of millions of adult flies which are sterilised as pupae by gamma rays and released as sterile males (40 million a week) to mate with normal females to produce sterile eggs. The final result is the eradication of screwworm flies, which has been achieved in Libya (1991) and Mexico (1991) and most of the USA (1976).

**IA.** The adult flies are bluish-green in colour, 10–15 mm long, slightly larger than the house fly, *Musca domestica*, and are similar in appearance to other blow flies.

The females lay 200–400 eggs in rows on wounds, cuts, bites (e.g. tick bites), navels and other parts of the body. In 10–18 h the larvae (which resemble wood screws) hatch and burrow into the flesh, feeding on fluids and tissues. In 7 days the larvae emerge, fall to the ground and pupate in the soil and after 1–8 weeks (depending on temperature) adult flies emerge to breed in 1 week.

**R.** Infested livestock, birds and man.

**MT.** See **IA**.

**CF.** and **P.** Infested wounds show cavitation, haemorrhage, necrosis and liquefaction with a fetid reddish-brown liquid staining the hair or wool in the vicinity. Unattended wounds become very large owing to multiple infestation and may result in the death of the animal due to septicaemia. There is intense irritation and restlessness.

**D.** The nature of the wound and the presence of the characteristic larvae (screwworms) confirm the diagnosis.

**J.** As for mange cases.

### Sheep blowfly strike (Cutaneous myiasis)

**I.** An invasion of the skin of sheep with larvae of the following blow flies:

*Lucilia sericata* (Britain, New Zealand, USA, Canada)

*Lucilia cuprina* (Australia, New Zealand, South Africa)

*Lucilia illustris, Phormia regina, Protophormia terraenovae, Cochliomyia macellari* (USA, Canada)

These blow flies, like the screwworms and *Sarcophaga* spp. have larvae which are sarcophagous, i.e. they eat flesh. Eggs are laid below the fleece tip, especially in the breech and tail, to which the flies are attracted by faeces and urine. The *eggs* hatch in 1–to 3 days, depending on temperature, to produce *first-* and *second-stage larvae* or *maggots*. The latter, some species of which bear mouth hooks and body spines, burrow into and devour the flesh to produce large wounds. Any part of the body may suffer *'fly strike'*.

The animal is irritated and restless, loses condition and may die owing to toxaemia/septicaemia.

Losses due to deaths, loss of body weight, fleece damage, cost of treatment/control, etc. can be considerable.

*Control measures* include dipping of sheep with appropriate insecticides, selective breeding to produce narrow breeches, 'mules' operation to remove breech wrinkles, docking of tails at fourth coccygeal joint, crutching or dagging (removal of wool round tail and breech).

### Sheep ked (*Melophagus ovinus*)

An ubiquitous wingless fly, about 7 mm long, and brownish in colour. The female fly lives on the sheep for several months and produces 10 or so larvae over this period. These adhere to the wool, pierce the skin with their mouth parts and suck blood causing irritation, permanent staining of wool, rubbing and scratching by the sheep and loss of condition.

*Control* is as for 'fly strike'.

### Sheep nostril or nasal fly (*Oestrus ovis*)

While *Oestrus ovis* appears to have decreased in Europe, it is still an important parasite in South Africa, Mediterranean region and Brazil.

In addition to infesting sheep, it is sometimes found in camels, dogs, and man.

The adult fly is hairy, greyish-brown in colour and about 12 mm long. It lays its whitish larvae around the nostrils without alighting. These migrate into the nasal cavities and paranasal sinuses, e.g. frontal sinus, where they cause a mucoid, and later a mucopurulent and sometimes haemorrhagic, catarrh with nasal discharge.

Larvae in sinuses may die and calcify, but occasionally erosion of bone may ensue with septic sinusitis and symptoms resembling infection with *Coenurus cerebralis* (*'false gid'*). Such cases usually die.

Affected animals display dyspnoea, sneezing and loss of condition.

*Judgement of fly strike, ked and nostril fly* infestation cases is as for mange.

## TICKS

*Ticks*, of which there are some 850 species occur worldwide, are ectoparasites which act as reservoirs and vectors in the transmission of major diseases (viral, rickettsial and protozoal) in animals and man such as African tick typhus, anaplasmosis, babesiosis, cowdriosis, ehrlichiosis, louping ill, Lyme disease, Nairobi sheep disease, Q fever, Rocky Mountain spotted fever, theileriasis, tick-borne encephalitis, tick paralysis, tick pyaemia and tularaemia.

In addition to farm livestock and man, ticks also parasitise birds and wildlife such as small carnivores, bats, beetles and lizards.

**Classification** Ticks belong to the class *Arachnida*, order *Acarina*, sub-order *Ixodoidea* (hard and soft ticks), family *Argasidae* (soft ticks – fowl ticks and tampans) and family *Ixodidae* (hard or true ticks), which is the most important group.

**Structure** Most ticks are 15 mm or less in size but some reach 30 mm. Adult ticks consist of a round or oval *body* with *four pairs* of *legs*. The ventral aspect of the body bears mouth parts and on its dorsal surface a hard plate or *scutum* (complete in the male ixodid but only an anterior half in females, nymphs and larvae) is present in hard but not in soft ticks. Adult ticks possess distinct *genital* and *anal pores* on their ventral surface and possess four pairs of legs (three pairs in nymphs). A unique sensory organ, *Haller's organ*, is present on the foreleg tarsi of all ticks.

**Life cycles** This is fairly straightforward with four developmental stages: egg, larva, nymph, adult male and female. With a few exceptions all feed on blood, the number of hosts utilised varying with individual species. There are two main genera of veterinary importance: *Argasidae* (soft ticks) and *Ixodidae* (hard ticks).

**Argasidae** These occur most frequently in arid tropical and subtropical areas, but recently *Argas persicus*, an important tick in poultry, has become established in more temperate regions. Its larvae feed for 7–10 days while nymphs feed and moult twice and adult ticks as often as 5 or 6 times, laying eggs between each meal, the life cycle taking some 4 months to complete using multiple hosts. *Argas persicus*, which causes death through blood loss, also transmits the spirochaete *Borrelia anserina*, the cause of avian spirochaetosis, and the rickettsial parasite *Aegyptianella pullorum*, which is responsible for *aegyptianellosis* (anaemia and diarrhoea) in all the domestic fowls.

Several species of *Argas* (and *ixodid*) ticks are involved in transmitting the neurotoxin of *tick paralysis* in calves, lambs, goats, dogs, cats and man.

Some species of *Ornithodoros* ticks act as vectors of the *African swine fever* virus, of the *Borrelia* spirochaetes of *relapsing fever* (tick or recurrent fever) in *man*.

**Ixodidae** This more important genus of ticks parasitises many animals and human beings. Their life cycles involve one-host, two-host or three-host cycles, the females extracting more blood than males and dying after ovipositing. Most ixodids have a three-host cycle in which larvae, nymphs and adults feed on three different hosts. Two-host ticks have larvae and nymphs feeding on one host and adults on another while in one-host ticks all three stages feed on the same host.

***Amblyomma* spp.** are involved in transmitting heartwater, tularaemia, Rocky Mountain spotted fever, Q fever, Lyme disease and tick typhus in man besides creating serious wounds which may become infected with screwworms.

***Boophilus* spp**. All five members are one-host ticks and act as vectors in anaplasmosis, babesiosis (piroplasmosis, Texas fever) and theileriasis. *B. annulatus* (North American tick) has been eradicated (along with *B. microplus*) from the USA but is active in central America and Africa and causes great losses due to Texas fever. *B. decoloratus* (blue tick) transmits anaplasmosis and babesiosis in Central Africa, while *B. microplus* (tropical cattle tick) occurs in tropical and subtropical Asia, Australia, Central America and Mexico.

***Dermacentor* spp.** are mainly three-host ticks, except for *D. nitens* and *D. albipictus*, which are one-host forms. They are mostly confined to N. America, Europe and Asia and transmit numerous viruses in addition to rickettsiae, *Francisella tularensis, Anaplasma marginale, Babesia, Coxiella burnetii* and *Theileria ovis*.

***Haemaphysalis* spp.** All have a three-host cycle and are involved in tick paralysis besides acting as transmitting the agents of Q fever, tularaemia, anaplasmosis, babesiosis, tick-borne encephalitis, theileriasis and brucellosis.

***Hyalomma* spp.** Most are three-host but some are two-host and one-host ticks. Involved as vectors in theileriasis, babesiosis, anaplasmosis, Q fever, tick typhus, tick paralysis, Crimean-Congo haemorrhagic fever (CCHF) in man and animals and bovine sweating sickness.

***Ixodes* spp.** Largest genus of the family Ixodidae. All are three-host ticks and inhabit temperate and tropical forest and grassland regions parasitising animals, birds and man. *I. ricinus* (castor bean tick, sheep tick) occurs in Europe, British Isles, N. Africa and parts of Asia and transmits babesiosis, louping ill, tick-borne fever, tick pyaemia, Q fever, Lyme disease, anaplasmosis, Rocky Mountain spotted fever and Russian spring-summer encephalitis in various parts of the world.

***Rhipicephalus* spp.** occur in Europe, Asia and Africa and parasitise domestic and wild animals. Most are three-host ticks but *R. bursa, R. evertsi* and *R. glabroscutatum* have two-host cycles.

Like many other ticks rhipicephalids act as vectors for babesia, anaplasma, theileria, ehrlichia, rickettsia and leishmania and Crimean-Congo haemorrhagic fever (Congo virus disease) in man.

### Economic losses due to ticks

These are mainly occasioned by deaths from anaemia due to blood loss, secondary bacterial infection and toxaemia. In other instances there is reduced performance and damage to hides and fleeces caused by bites, the damage taking the form of small rounded areas of necrosis which is often followed by secondary fly attack resulting in serious skin infection.

All species of ticks act as severe skin irritants and some can cause febrile illness in animals and man through the injection of salivary toxins and arboviruses.

## *HYPODERMA* SPP. (WARBLE FLIES, HYPODERMOSIS, CATTLE GRUBS)

There are two main genera – *Dermatobia* and *Hypoderma*.

### *Dermatobia hominis*

This is the *tropical warble fly* or *torsalo* and occurs in central America from Mexico to Argentina. It is an important parasite of cattle, sheep, goats, pigs, buffaloes, dogs, cats, rabbits, man and many wild animals.

The adult fly is about the same size as *Hypoderma* – 12–15 mm long with a life span of 4 days.

**Life cycle** Eggs are laid on numerous insects (mainly mosquitoes and bloodsucking flies) and then carried to the various hosts. The larvae penetrate the skin and remain in the subcutaneous tissue for 5–10 weeks. Painful swellings are produced by the larvae, which breathe through a pore. Infection often ensues through the activity of muscid flies and screwworms.

The larvae eventually escape, fall to the ground and pupate for up to 10 weeks when the adult fly emerges. The complete cycle takes 80–120 days.

**Losses due to Dermatobia** These resemble those due to *Hypoderma* – damage to hides and skins, skin irritation and reduced performance.

### *Hypoderma* spp.

**Distribution** The four main species, *H. bovis, H. lineatum, H. diana* and *H. aeratum* are distributed over Europe, Asia, Africa (mainly Morocco and Tunisia) and the Americas (mainly USA, Brazil, Ecuador and Guyana).

Warble fly infestation has been eradicated from Cyprus (1952), Denmark (1966), Isle of Man (1964), N. Ireland (1990), Channel Isles (1987), Czechoslovakia (1971), Malaysia (1986), Oman (1991), Namibia (1974), Chile (1962) and Colombia (1988). In Great Britain no clinical cases were reported in 1996.

In the *United Kingdom*, Warble Fly is a *Notifiable Disease* under the Warble Fly Order of 1982. A testing service (based on the ELISA test) is now available whereby farmers who have cattle that may have been exposed to infestation can have blood samples taken for examination. In addition, the State Veterinary Service and Meat Hygiene Service have mounted a market and abattoir surveillance scheme to identify affected animals. Treatment of herds in which positive cases are found is mandatory and movement restrictions are imposed except for cattle destined for slaughter and calves under 12 weeks of age. Farmers are urged to be on the look-out for signs of warbles and encouraged to treat their cattle in the autumn as a precautionary measure. Imported animals must be treated on arrival, while infested animals are sent back to the country of origin.

Preliminary results from the GB 1994/95 blood serum survey involving some 300 000 samples show that warbles are present in indigenous cattle, albeit in small numbers.

### *Hypoderma bovis (common European warble fly, northern cattle grub)*

The adult flies are hairy (greenish-yellow and black in colour) and measure 15 mm in length. They are an important parasite of cattle and bison and less commonly horses and man.

**Life cycle** The adult flies are active from the beginning of summer until autumn (mainly June to August). Warm weather favours their activity, but cattle may be attacked during low temperatures. The flight of flies is limited, rarely exceeding 5 km. Individual flies live only 2–7 days, during which time the female attaches as many as 370 eggs to the roots of the hairs of the host, mostly on the outer aspect of the lower limbs and on the belly. The eggs are laid singly. *H. bovis* does not suck blood.

In 3–7 days the 1 mm long larva hatches, enters the skin through a hair follicle by means of its cutting mouth hooks and wanders in the subcutaneous tissue. Muscle is not invaded, but larvae utilise its intermuscular connective tissue. Movement is facilitated by means of proteolytic enzymes which dissolve tissue. Migration to the back is made by way of the crura of the diaphragm, the intercostal muscles at about the ninth rib or the spinal canal. First-stage larvae (5–13 mm in size) are often found in *'winter resting sites'* in the epidural fat of the spinal canal between December and March. First-stage larvae may also be found in other parts of the body, including the surface of organs.

From the spinal canal the larvae migrate towards the skin of the back through the intervertebral foramina. On the back they form swellings (2–3 cm in diameter) from just behind the shoulders to the angle of the haunch and extending some 18–20 cm on either side of the vertebral column. Small holes in the skin are produced by a dermatolytic toxin, enabling the larvae to breathe the oxygen necessary for further development. Larvae (which may number 1 to 200 or more) are visible on the back from around mid-February until May (warble stage). At this stage the mature third-stage larvae are about 28 mm long and segmented with spines, yellowish in colour at first and brownish later.

After a second resting period of 28–35 days, the larvae emerge from the back and fall to the ground to pupate. In about 1 month the adult fly escapes from the black pupal case through the operculum.

The entire life cycle of *H. bovis* takes about 1 year. Infested animals may show no evidence of grubs.

### *Hypoderma lineatum (heel fly, common cattle grub)*

The adult fly is smaller than *H. bovis*, measuring about 13 mm. *H. lineatum* appears about one month earlier than *H. bovis*.

**Life cycle** Eggs are laid chiefly on those parts of the body in contact with the ground when the animal is lying. The favourite location is the heel. The eggs are about 1 mm long and are laid in rows of 6–14 on a single hair.

The life cycle resembles that of *H. bovis* except that the first-stage larvae find their way to the oesophagus, where they are found in the submucous tissue and oriented along the long axis of the gullet. The pale, translucent larvae are easily demonstrated if the external connective tissue is removed and the oesophagus is inflated and finally dried. These oesophageal larvae are 5–13 mm in length and are found in this location from December to mid-February (period of peak incidence) after which they migrate towards the skin of the back.

The presence of larvae in the oesophageal wall is sometimes manifested by an inflammatory exudate which extends to the mediastinum and gives rise to a yellow gelatinous condition of the mediastinal fat.

*H. lineatum* is never found in the spinal canal but its general pathological effects are similar to those of *H. bovis*.

### *Hypoderma diana*

This species is found in Scotland and Europe infesting *red* and *roe deer* and sometimes *sheep* (Dempsey, 1983). Its life cycle and effects are similar to those of *H. lineatum*, deaths in deer often occurring in severe infestations.

*Hypoderma aeratum* affects goats and sheep in the Middle East and India.

### Clinical signs

*Warbles* affect young animals more often than adults. The activity of the adult female flies is associated with the condition known as *'gadding'* in which the animal rushes about violently with the tail held high. On occasions, kicking at the belly is evident. This nervousness is believed to be caused by the ovipositing female fly and her unusual flight sound. There is a variable loss of condition and milk yield consistent with the degree of infestation. Injuries may ensue from the uncontrolled rushing around.

The swellings on the back are soft and painful to the touch. There may be as many as 300 present. Should the spinal canal be involved, posterior paralysis may ensue, a condition which can occur in horses as well as cattle.

In *H. lineatum* infestation where the oesophagus contains larvae, bloat may occur because of the inability to orally eject gas from the rumen.

### Pathological changes and losses due to warbles

The incidence of warbles in cattle varies from year to year. If flies are active in a particular summer, the incidence of warbled hides will be high in the following year. Fly activity results in lowered milk production in dairy cows and occasional injuries from gadding.

A survey carried out by the UK Meat and Livestock Commission in May 1985 showed a hide infestation rate of 0.01%, the incidence in 1978 when the eradication programme began being 38.0%, a remarkable reduction in incidence. An eradication scheme commenced in Northern Ireland in 1967 reduced the prevalence from 50% to 0.01% in 10 years.

*H. bovis* larvae in the epidural fat cause fat necrosis, connective-tissue autolysis, oedema and inflammatory changes which may extend to bone, producing a periostitis and osteomyelitis. Such changes can result in nervous symptoms and even paralysis. *H. lineatum* larvae in the oesophagus produce inflammation and oedema which may interfere with swallowing and eructation. The oesophagus itself is rendered unfit as a constituent for sausage. In the USA, 'grubby gullets' are commonly encountered in packing houses in autumn and winter.

Larvae under the skin of the back cause soft, painful swellings about 3 cm in diameter. They damage the subcutaneous and muscular tissues, especially the sirloin. This condition is known as *'licked beef'* or *'butcher's jelly'* and is revealed when the hide is removed as a diffuse, haemorrhagic oedema.

Various estimates have been made of the losses of meat from condemnations, weights of up to 1.8 kg being quoted in Britain in the past. An investigation in Canada in 1970 showed that 1–5 larvae resulted in a trimming of 0.4 kg of meat, 6–10 larvae 0.7 kg and 11 or more a loss of 1.2 kg of meat. Trimming of carcases reduces their overall value.

It is customary to grade hides according to the number of warble holes present. In the USA, hides with 5 or more holes are Grade 2, but a hide with numerous holes is rejected for tanning and converted into inedible by-products. In the USA in 1960 it was estimated that one-third of all cattle hides showed warble damage, the percentage in Germany in 1969 being 2.6%.

Where countries have undertaken eradication schemes, losses due to meat condemnation and hide damage are non-existent.

While the assessment of losses due to hide damage is relatively easy, those associated with reduced weight gain and milk yield are difficult to estimate with accuracy. A cost–benefit analysis of warble fly eradication was carried out by the UK Ministry of Agriculture in 1975/6. This showed that the benefits of eradication nationally would be $12 million, taking into account losses in value caused by direct damage to meat ($4.6 million) and hides ($5.8 million). Slower growth rate, loss of milk yield and injuries were not included in the study.

### Judgement of warble cases

Usually only trimming of meat is necessary, at the most.

## REFERENCES

Borland, E. D., Keymer, I. F. and Counter D. (1980) *Vet. Rec.* **106**, 265.

Brown, D., Hinton, M. H. and Wright, A. I. (1984) *Vet. Rec.* **115**, 300.
Clarkson, M. J. (1978) *Vet. Rec.* **102**, 259.
Chambers, P. G. (1991) *Vet. Rec.* **129**, 431–432.
Collobert, *et al.* (1995) *Vet. Rec.* **136**, 463–465.
Crooks, J. L. (1980) *Vet. Rec.* **106**, 466.
Dempsey, J. (1983) *Meat Hygienist* (May/June), 15.
Edwards, G. T. (1982) *Vet. Rec.* **110**, 511.
Fogarty, U. M. G. (1994) *Vet. Rec.* **134**, 515–518.
Gibson, McM. and Lanning, D. G. (1981) *Vet. Rec.* **107**, 165.
Gordon, H. McL. and Boray, J. C. (1970) *Vet. Rec.* **86**, 288.
Livesey, C. T., Herbert, I. V., Willis, J. M. and Evans, W. T. (1981) *Vet. Rec.* **109**, 217.
Meat and Livestock Commission (1985) Report.
Mellor, P. S. (1973) *J. Helminth.* **47**, 97.
Mitchell, G. B. B. and Linklater, K. A. (1980) *Vet. Rec.* **106**, 466.
Palmer, S. R. and Biffin, H. B. (1987) *Epidemiol. Infect.* **99**, 693.
Pattison, H. D., Thomas, R. J. and Smith, W. C. (1980) *Vet. Rec.* **107**, 415.
Pugh, K. E. and Chambers, P. G. (1989) *Vet. Rec.* **125**, 480–484.
Rodriguez-del-Rosal, E., Correa, D. and Flisser, A. (1989) *Vet. Rec.* **124**, 488.
Taylor, S. M. (1975) *Agriculture in Northern Ireland*, Vol. 49, No. 8.
Torgerson, P. R. (1992) *Vet. Rec.* **131**, 218–219.
Walther, M. and Koske, J. K. (1980) *Vet. Rec.* **106**, 401.
Whitelaw, A. and Fawcett, A. R. (1982) *Vet. Rec.* **110**, 500–501.

## FURTHER READING

Soulsby, E. J. L. (1982) *Helminths, Arthropods and Protozoa of Domesticated Animals*, 7th edn. London: Ballière-Tindall.

# Chapter 19
# Metabolic Diseases and Nutritional Deficiencies

## METABOLIC DISORDERS

While in general most of these conditions will be treated on the farm, those not responding to therapy will inevitably find their way to the meat plant as casualties. A special category is the so-called *'downer cow syndrome'* (q.v.) which is most commonly a sequel to parturient paresis (milk fever) in cows but may be associated with metritis, dystocia, septic mastitis, ketosis, arthritis, hypomagnesaemic tetany, hindquarter injury or similar conditions.

It is not uncommon for cases of hypomagnesaemic tetany in cows to occur in the meat plant lairage – cases of sudden death in high-yielding cows suddenly deprived of feed under cold conditions and necessitating differentiation from anthrax.

Metabolic diseases (hypocalcaemia, hypomagnesaemia, hypophosphataemia, hypoglycaemia, etc.) represent the *'diseases of production'* and are associated with an imbalance or deficiency in uptake of nutrients (including major minerals and trace elements) and the requirements of the animals for maintenance, production of milk and meat and reproduction.

A few of the metabolic diseases are *inherited*, e.g. mannosidosis in Aberdeen-Angus, Galloway and Murray Grey cattle in which there is a deficiency of the enzyme mannosidase resulting in nervous symptoms, ataxia, abortion and neonatal death. Other examples are ceroid lipofuscinosis of sheep (q.v.), porcine syndrome in pigs (q.v.), photosensitisation in sheep (q.v.) and osteogenesis imperfecta (brittle bone) in cattle.

Most, however, are *acquired* and result from the influence of defective systems of breeding, feeding and management for optimum results in terms of milk, meat, fertility and prolificacy. All too often these entail ill health and deaths, the overall cost of which is reckoned by many to be greater than that due to specific infective diseases. The quest for increased production has created a situation in which the animal is unable to sustain normal physiological concentrations of specific nutrients. This situation is exemplified in particular by milk fever in cows in which the secretion of calcium is greater than that supplied by the diet or bones. In other forms of metabolic disease, e.g. pregnancy toxaemia in ewes and beef cows, fat cow syndrome, the onset of disease, and often death, is occasioned by a sudden reduction of intake of a nutrient or nutrients.

Associated with the prevalence of some of the metabolic diseases has been the development of intensive systems of grassland management, with an emphasis being placed on the use of simple seed mixtures and heavy applications of fertiliser, especially nitrogen. The philosophy of Stapleton (1949) that 'the technique of grassland improvement consists first of establishing wild white clover and then the better grasses, and always arranging matters that edible herbs are within reach of the grazing animal' is not always adhered to, often with dire results. The essential homeostasis of the animal, because of the high demands placed upon it, frequently exacerbated by pregnancy, lactation, adverse environmental conditions and other forms of stress, is upset and the mineral and energy balances of the body are thrown out of gear.

The principal *acquired metabolic disorders* in the food animals are as follows:

Hypomagnesaemic tetany (grass tetany, grass staggers, lactation tetany, Hereford disease) – cattle and sheep.

Pregnancy toxaemia – ewes and cows (fat cow syndrome).

Parturient paresis (milk fever) – cows and ewes.

Ketosis (acetonaemia, ketonaemia) – cattle.
Porcine stress syndrome (malignant hyperthermia, PSE, back muscle necrosis, transport myopathy) – pigs (q.v.).
Dark, firm, dry meat (DFD) (q.v.) – cattle and pigs.
Post-parturient haemoglobinuria – cows.
Azoturia (paralytic myoglobinuria) – horses.
Transit tetany (recumbency) of cows, ewes and mares.
Equine hyperlipaemia.
Congenital porphyria of cattle and pigs (q.v.).
Downer cow syndrome (q.v.).

## Hypomagnesaemic tetany

This is probably the major metabolic disorder and occurs in cows and ewes, being responsible for great losses in many parts of the world where it is also the most common cause of sudden death in bovines.

High-producing dairy cows (the condition sometimes occurs in pregnant beef cows) and ewes grazing lush pastures, those that are undernourished and animals in good condition subjected to a check in feeding, are especially liable. Stress and concurrent low levels of calcium may also act to trigger off the disease. Magnesium levels may be satisfactory in grass, forage and feedingstuff but the uptake by the animal is inadequate, the exact reason being unknown, and when serum magnesium levels fall below 1.8 mg/dl hypomagnesaemic tetany is liable to occur.

The condition is characterised by low serum levels of magnesium and sometimes of calcium.

**Clinical signs** in the *acute form* comprise convulsions, twitching of muscles and ears, bellowing, incoordination, galloping, salivation, retraction of eyelids in between periods of quiescence. Affected animals are hyperaesthetic, i.e. abnormally sensitive to stimuli. Death usually occurs within 2 hours. The *subacute form* may last up to 4–5 days, after which recovery may take place, with or without treatment. Such cases display similar symptoms along with opisthotonus of the head, trismus (lockjaw), frequent urination and defaecation and straddling gait. The *chronic form* of hypomagnesaemic tetany includes dullness, inappetence, ataxia, reduced milk yield and vague nervous symptoms. Sudden death may also occur in the chronic form.

**Post-mortem lesions** Apart from extravasations of blood in the pericardial sac, subendocardial, pleural, peritoneal and intestinal mucosal haemorrhages, there are few significant findings. Bruising of prominent parts caused by the animal's erratic behaviour is usually evident.

*Differential diagnoses* include BSE, anthrax, listeriosis, lead poisoning, nervous form of ketosis in ewes, rabies and virtually all conditions in which nervous symptoms are displayed.

## Pregnancy toxaemia of ewes/acetonaemia in cows

Both these conditions represent disorders of energy metabolism at a time when the demand for increased carbohydrate intake is greatest, in which fatty acids are incompletely metabolised with the production in the blood and urine of *ketones* along with hypoglycaemia (low blood sugar). Both conditions are essentially the same except that twin-lamb disease occurs in the latter third of pregnancy in ewes carrying twins or triplets while acetonaemia in cows affects those in early post-calving lactation. The increased need for glucose is for the two or more fetuses in the ewe and for milk in the cow.

**Pregnancy toxaemia of ewes** is usually a highly fatal disease and is associated with nervous symptoms (twitching of ears, periorbital muscles, head and leg muscles), stargazing, apparent blindness, ataxia, teeth grinding, coma and death. If the ewes lamb or abort, many will recover. Any factor which causes a sudden reduction in feed intake during the last third of pregnancy in ewes carrying multiple lambs is liable to precipitate the disease.

**Lesions of pregnancy toxaemia** Fatty degeneration of the liver, which is pale yellow or greyish in colour. Two or more dead lambs which may show decomposition.

**Acetonaemia of cows** has causes and biochemical changes similar to those of twin-lamb disease but the disease is not as serious. The demand for glucose in early heavy lactation is great and, if there is insufficient glycogen in the liver, fat stores become involved with the eventual production of volatile fatty acids and ketones. Two types of the disease are evident – *wasting form* in which there is anorexia, reduced milk yield, rapid loss of condition, lethargy, disinclination to move and the odour of ketones in the breath and milk, and *nervous form* which involves incoordination, circling, hyperaesthesia, bellowing, chewing and licking.

Acetonaemia may be an accompaniment with other diseases such as metritis, acute mastitis and traumatic pericarditis.

**Post-mortem changes** in bovine acetonaemia are similar to those of twin-lamb disease in relation to liver changes. Marked loss of condition attends the wasting form, while bruising of parts of the body may be evident in the nervous type.

In *fat cow syndrome* (fatty infiltration of the liver) which occurs in high-producing cows just before and after calving, the liver is grossly enlarged, yellowish in colour, friable and greasy to the touch. Such hepatic changes may also accompany peracute mastitis and metritis.

### Parturient paresis (milk fever)

This non-febrile metabolic condition is characterised by acute hypocalcaemia occurring at or soon after parturition in mature dairy cows and in pregnant and lactating ewes, goats and mares.

In all species the onset is sudden with the development of excitability, ataxia, paralysis and frequently coma and death. Although the exact aetiology is not clear, there appears to be an inability to mobilise calcium, especially in older animals. Like other metabolic diseases, milk fever is often associated with certain precipitating factors such as excitement, fatigue and reduction in food intake and, as with hypomagnesaemic tetany, there may be an inherited predisposition to the disease.

**Symptoms** include ataxia, recumbency, head turned to one side, inappetence, constipation, coma and death without treatment or unsuccessful treatment.

**Post-mortem findings** Nil, except for the presence of coincident disease. In some cases changes associated with the 'downer cow syndrome' (q.v.) are evident.

The aetiology, epidemiology, symptoms and PM findings, etc., are similar in ewes, goats and mares.

### Transit tetany (transport tetany, railroad disease, staggers)

Prolonged transport, especially during hot weather, is sometimes responsible for a highly fatal condition of nervousness, muscular tremors, posterior paresis and recumbency in well-fed cows and ewes in advanced pregnancy and also in non-pregnant ruminants.

While long journeys are usually involved, other predisposing factors include overcrowding and inadequate ventilation during transit, heavy pre-transport feeding, deprivation of food during shipment, free access to water and exercise after transport. There appears to be no consistent serum mineral deficiency with hypocalcaemia, hypophosphataemia, hypoglycaemia and hypomagnesaemia being recorded in different cases.

**Lesions** As for 'downer cow syndrome'.

### Post-parturient haemoglobinuria

A condition of low incidence and high mortality in high-yielding dairy cows in which there is anaemia and haemoglobinuria occurring 2–4 weeks after parturition. The exact cause is unknown, but the condition may be associated with a hypophosphataemia since feeding on low-phosphorus diets can precipitate the disease. On the other hand, feeds low in copper and selenium have been incriminated as well as haemolytic agents in certain plants such as rape, turnips and kale. Predisposing factors include prolonged housing and cold weather.

**Symptoms** of anaemia are evidenced by the pallor of the conjunctivae and other mucous membranes at the outset of the disease. Later stages display jaundice, inappetence, reduced milk yield and weakness.

**Lesions** Icterus, anaemia, fatty infiltration of liver, dark reddish coloured urine.

### Azoturia (paralytic myoglobinuria, exertional rhabdomyolysis)

This disease of equidae occurs during forced exercise, usually after a period of inactivity on full feed. It is associated with the rapid formation of large amounts of lactic acid from muscle glycogen and results in degenerative changes in muscles, especially of the hindquarters.

Excessive feeding on grain predisposes to the condition as does poor management with regard to exercise.

**Symptoms** Stiff gait, posterior paralysis, recumbency, haemglobinuria.

**Lesions** The muscles of the hindquarters (gluteal, quadriceps) are dark and moist with pale areas indicative of Zenker's coagulative necrosis. The myocardium, larynx and diaphragm may be similarly affected. The kidneys are swollen and show brownish-red streaks in the medulla with dark brown urine in the bladder.

## Equine hyperlipaemia

A metabolic disease of high mortality in pony mares in late pregnancy or early lactation in which fatty changes occur in most viscera and associated with undernutrition and fatty acid mobilisation and esterification (esters are compounds formed by combination of acid with an alcohol with loss of water).

**Symptoms** Depression, twitching of muscles, inappetence, loss of weight, ventral oedema, coma and death in most cases.

**Lesions** The liver is very enlarged, yellow or orange in colour, and may be ruptured with extensive haemorrhage. Similar changes occur in the kidneys, adrenal gland and skeletal muscle.

**Judgement of metabolic diseases. Each case requires careful assessment** A, T or D, depending on overall condition.

## Photosensitisation

In this condition photodynamic agents – hypericin, fagopyrin, saponin, psoralen, phylloerythrin, etc. – in the blood causes the skin of animals to be hypersensitive to light, especially sunlight, resulting in dermatitis and oedema. Such substances are mainly derived from plants, but certain chemicals, e.g. phenothiazine, tetracyclines, corticosteroids and carbon tetrachloride, can act as direct photodynamic substances.

The disease is encountered most often in sheep and cattle, although it can affect any species. Poultry have been severely affected by the ingestion of species of the plants *Ammi*. It is worldwide in distribution.

The *lesions* are confined to the white unpigmented areas of the skin of the face and ears in the large farm animals. These areas become reddened and oedematous with serum exudation. There is a tendency for necrosis to develop. In many instances, especially in the *secondary* form, there are associated jaundice, gastroenteritis and other clinical signs.

**Congenital photosensitisation** This is due to a simple recessive gene and occurs in mutant Southdown and Corriedale lambs in New Zealand and the USA. Excess phylloerythrin and bilirubin are present in the blood owing to hepatic insufficiency and may lead to progressive skin damage and death. There is an accompanying kidney dysfunction. The condition is similar to *congenital porphyria (pink tooth)* in certain breeds of cattle (Ayrshire, Holstein, Shorthorn, Danish) and pigs (q.v.) in which defective haemoglobin metabolism results in large amounts of porphyrins being present in the blood, with deposits of these pigments in the bones and teeth, which are stained amber or reddish-brown.

Photosensitisation may be primary or secondary, the latter being the more common form in animals. In *primary photosensitisation* the photodynamic agent is absorbed directly through the skin or the gastrointestinal mucosa and reaches the skin in an unchanged form. Fairly large amounts of the plant have to be eaten in order to cause a reaction.

Substances and plants associated with primary photosensitisation include:

Hypericin (*Hypericum*, St John's Wort)
Fagopyrin (*Fagopyrum esculentum*, Buckwheat)
8-Methoxypsoralen (furocoumarin) (*Ammi majus, Ammi visnaga, Cymopterus watsonii*)
Perloline (*Lolium perenne*, perennial ryegrass), in combination with the mould *Pithomyces chartarum* causes facial eczema in sheep
Saponin *Medicago sativa,* alfalfa, lucerne
? *Trifolium hybridum* (Alsike clover)

*Secondary* or *hepatogenous photosensitisation* occurs when liver cells are damaged by ingested hepatoxins and phylloerythrin (a porphyrin and end-product of chlorophyll metabolism) is liberated into the bloodstream. These hepatoxins include sporidesmin, phomopsin and saponin in plants while others are found in fungi, e.g. *Pithomyces chartarum* and *Periconia* spp. on Bermuda grass, and in certain bacteria, e.g. cyanobacteria on blue-green algae (q.v.).

*Phylloerythrin* is a photosensitising agent that is normally excreted in the bile, but when liver damage is present it accumulates in the tissues and skin, where it absorbs light energy to produce the typical lesions of photosensitisation. The liver damage is essentially associated with an inability to excrete bile and may be due to bile duct obstruction or some other interference with bile excretion, e.g. in fascioliasis.

**Judgement of photosensitisation** A, T, D, K, I, L depending on severity of body condition.

## NUTRITIONAL DEFICIENCIES

In many parts of the world, even in advanced agricultural areas, livestock are often faced with an inadequate intake of various nutrients. The most frequent nutritional deficiency is that of *energy and protein starvation*, which occurs mainly during winter and times of drought, especially where supplementary feeding is not carried out. In addition to a lack of feed intake, the provision of food of poor quality can result in *malnutrition*, especially in calves given inferior milk replacers. Sudden deficiencies in energy supply can lead to starvation ketosis and pregnancy toxaemia in fat cattle and pregnant ewes. Adverse weather conditions may also play a part in precipitating nutritional deficiencies.

In addition to energy and protein, the major minerals calcium, phosphorus, sodium/chlorine and potassium, and the microminerals (trace elements) cobalt, copper/molybdenum, iodine, iron, magnesium, manganese, selenium, sulphur and zinc are required for optimum metabolism of most species. Deficiencies of many of these elements occur throughout the world, some in specific geographical regions, and result in poor condition, severe parasitic infestations, mainly parasitic gastroenteritis and bronchitis, and huge losses from reduced body weight, lowered reproductive performance and deaths. Susceptibility to various types of disease is also enhanced. Vitamin deficiency, chiefly of A, D, E and K, invariably accompanies malnutrition.

An inventory of scientific papers on the frequency and financial impact of non-infectious and production diseases carried out by FAO/OIE/WHO (1995) in 1970–1989 showed the following rankings based on literature citations:

| | |
|---|---|
| Multifactorial causes of production loss: | 37% |
| Inorganic and organic agents: | 17% |
| Nutritional deficiencies: | 15% |
| Physical agents: | 12% |
| Genetic diseases: | 8% |

Metabolic diseases, diseases of unknown aetiology and neoplasias made up the balance of citations. Female reproductive disorders (50%) and neonatal mortality (37%) were the two largest subcategories under the multifactorial causes of production loss. Nutritional deficiencies and metabolic diseases obviously assume major importance throughout the world.

They pose problems for the meat inspector in relation to carcase condition and judgement, especially where there is a concurrent oedematous condition in the carcase. In general, however, they are not serious public health entities.

*Emaciation with generalised oedema – cachexia –* indicative of starvation, is usually accompanied by a heavy worm burden in the alimentary and respiratory tracts and is a principal reason for total carcase condemnation in most meat inspection protocols – a reasonably straightforward procedure. But where subclinical disease conditions complicate the situation, the task of judgement is made more difficult, especially in those countries where the category of 'conditional approval' does not exist and carcase and offal judgement is an 'all or nothing' affair. Where heat treatment is available, carcase judgement is less of a problem.

While true deficiencies of some minerals and trace elements exist in certain parts of the world, certain fertiliser treatments may make particular elements unavailable for the grazing animal. For example, the level of selenium is low in new clover pasture, but is rendered even lower by the undue application of superphosphate. Excessive application of nitrogen has on occasion led to outbreaks of nitrite and nitrate poisoning, especially in cattle and sheep.

While deficiencies of these essential elements can occur, excesses result in poisoning.

### Calcium (Ca)

*Calcium* is essential for the proper formation of bones and teeth, for satisfactory nerve, heart and muscle function and the clotting of blood. Vitamin D is essential for the adequate uptake and utilisation of calcium.

An inadequate supply in the diet results in poor growth and ossification of bone, which becomes brittle and liable to spontaneous fracture, general growth and development being retarded. Rickets in the young animal in conjunction with phosphorus deficiency and osteomalacia in the mature animal may result from a calcium deficiency. The need for calcium is greatest in high-yielding dairy cows in early lactation.

### Sodium chloride (NaCl)

This essential compound is required for the acid–base mechanisms of the body and for the proper functioning of osmosis. Diets low in salt, especially those based on cereal grains, in regions where pasture is naturally deficient and where soils are heavily treated with potash, eventually cause *pica* with loss of body weight and milk yield. Affected animals tend to chew various solid objects (wood, metal, dirt, etc.) and show incoordination and cardiac insufficiency with frequent high death rates.

Salt deficiency is more liable to affect young growing animals, females in heavy lactation and animals suffering loss in sweat through exercise. Hot environmental conditions are also prone to cause a deficiency.

The deficiency can be corrected by providing salt licks or loose salt containing trace elements.

### Cobalt (Co)

*Cobalt* is a component of *vitamin* $B_{12}$ (*cyanocobalamin*), which is essential for the formation of red blood cells and for the maturation of the nuclei and division of all body cells. In ruminants, $B_{12}$ is synthesised in the rumen by microorganisms.

Cobalt deficiency occurs in regions where the soils are deficient in cobalt, leading to an unavailability in forages. Those containing less than 0.07 ppm of cobalt are considered cobalt-deficient and are found in parts of North America, South Africa, Australia, New Zealand and Scotland.

Lack of dietary cobalt results in inappetence, emaciation, reduced reproductive performance, reduction of milk yield and retarded growth.

**Post-mortem changes** Extreme emaciation with brown deposits of the pigment haemosiderin in the liver and spleen. It is also responsible for *'white liver disease'* in sheep in New Zealand, Australia, Norway and the United Kingdom in which liver cells are damaged, the liver assuming a greyish-white appearance.

### Copper (Cu)/molybdenum (Mo)/sulphur (S)

*Copper* is required for the mobilisation of iron in the synthesis of haemoglobin. Besides being a constituent of many body enzymes, copper is essential for the maintenance of bone osteoblasts and the synthesis of melanin and keratin.

*Molybdenum* is an essential component of the enzymes xanthine oxidase, aldehyde oxidase and nitrate reductase, while *sulphur* is a constituent of the amino acids methionine, cystine and cysteine, the anticoagulant heparin, the hormone insulin, vitamin $B_1$ (thiamin), keratin and several enzymes.

A *deficiency of copper* per se results in retarded growth, diarrhoea, anaemia, loss of hair and wool pigmentation, bone fragility, myocardial fibrosis, infertility and, in many cases, incoordination in cattle. The coat becomes rough and changed in colour – from black and red to rusty red and – in some cases, coat licking, ataxia and paresis occur.

*Shortage of copper* in soils and forage is a serious problem in many parts of the world, especially Australia, New Zealand, USA and Europe. It is responsible for *'swayback'* (*enzootic ataxia*) in sheep and goats (q.v.), falling disease of cattle in Australia, licking disease in cattle in Holland and anaemia in sucking pigs. Falling and licking diseases are associated with various nervous symptoms, pivoting on forelegs, bellowing, coat licking, etc., and often sudden death.

Combined with a *deficiency of cobalt*, it is involved in *coast sickness* in Australia and *salt sickness* in the USA, both of which display the typical symptoms of copper deficiency.

Where copper deficiency is associated with an *excess of molybdenum and sulphate* (secondary copper deficiency), the typical syndromes of unthriftiness and/or diarrhoea occur and are referred to as *Teart* or *peat scours* in cattle and sheep and *pine* in calves (Britain, New Zealand and Canada).

**Post-mortem lesions** in *copper deficiency* include anaemia, emaciation and bone fragility (osteoporosis), sometimes with enlarged joints. In swayback there is hydrocephalus with an increase in cerebrospinal fluid and occasionally cerebral oedema.

## Iodine (I)

Small traces of *iodine* are required for the proper functioning of the thyroid gland in growth and metabolism, iodine being a component of thyroxine and triiodothyronine. These hormones act along with calcitonin, which is concerned with plasma calcium homeostasis.

*Deficiency of iodine* results in thyroid gland enlargement (*goitre*) (Plate 2, Fig. 10), which occurs in certain regions worldwide where iodine is lacking in the soil and water supplies, e.g. around the Great Lakes in North America. Certain plants – e.g. kale, cabbage, Brussels sprouts, turnips, soybeans – and linamarin in linseed meal contain *goitrogens* which inhibit the action of thyroxin, thus producing goitre. Along with a deficient secretion of thyroxine, cretinism (dwarfism) and myxoedema (mucinous thickening of the skin) may result, the former mainly in foals but possibly in all species, and the latter in neonate piglets.

**Post-mortem lesions** include enlargement of the thyroid gland, myxoedema, alopecia and deficient bone formation.

## Iron (Fe)

*Iron* is the main constituent of the haem molecule of haemoglobin, the colouring matter of red blood cells, and is thus vital for the transport of oxygen in the body. It also occurs in other respiratory enzyme systems.

A *deficiency* produces *anaemia* in newborn piglets and sometimes calves and lambs without access to iron.

**Lesions** Anaemia, pallor of mucosae, subcutaneous oedema of carcase, thin watery blood, hypertrophy of heart and of the liver, which shows fatty changes.

## Magnesium (Mg)

*Magnesium* is essential for all mammals, being involved in many different enzyme systems, especially those concerned with energy exchange. It is necessary for normal nerve function. It is present in small amounts in all tissues, mostly in bone in combination with phosphate and bicarbonate.

A deficiency in the diet leads to low blood magnesium which, however, does not always result in hypomagnesaemic tetany (q.v.), a highly fatal disease of recently calved cows and lambed ewes. Although cases treated early respond to magnesium therapy, the deficiency is not a straightforward one of magnesium, since many other factors complicate its absorption and metabolism.

**Post-mortem lesions** There may be pericardial, endocardial, peritoneal, and subcutaneous haemorrhages in some cases.

## Manganese (Mn)

*Manganese* is found in all cell mitochondria and in melanin besides being an important element in many enzyme systems, e.g. liver arginase. It is involved in glucose utilisation and in the formation of cartilage and bone matrix and the rigidity of connective tissue.

A *deficiency* leads to bone deformities, enlarged joints, fetlock knuckling in neonates and retarded growth and infertility in cows and ewes.

## Phosphorus (P)

*Phosphorus* is an essential body element, being involved in almost all metabolic processes; its action is controlled by calcium and vitamin D. (Vitamin D is necessary for the absorption and utilisation of phosphorus and calcium.) It is essential for cell metabolism, being a constituent of nucleic acids and phosphatides, and as phosphate forms some 70% of bone and teeth. It also provides the energy for muscles in the form of adenosine triphosphate and creatine phosphate.

In many parts of the world, e.g. South Africa, Australia and North America, soils and forages are deficient in phosphorus.

A *deficiency* in the diet culminates in retarded growth, pica, infertility and osteodystrophy – failure of bones to develop in calves (rickets) or distortion of bones with enlargement of joints, fragility and associated incoordination of posture and gait in adult cattle (osteomalacia). Post-parturient haemoglobinuria may be a sequel to phosphorus deficiency in cows.

### Potassium (K)

*Potassium* is an essential chemical element in the maintenance of acid–base and water balance in the body and, with sodium and calcium, in the proper functioning of the heart.

*Deficiency* is rare since most diets have adequate supplies of the chemical. However, P-deficient soils may be responsible for low dietary levels which can cause inappetence, poor growth, anaemia and diarrhoea.

### Selenium (Se) and vitamin E

*Selenium* is an essential mineral nutrient which protects body tissues, especially the heart, liver and skeletal muscle. It is a component of glutathione peroxidase (GSH-Px), an enzyme which acts in conjunction with vitamin E to protect cellular membranes and lipid cells from attack by endogenous peroxides, which cause degeneration and necrosis. Selenium is also a constituent of several proteins and enzymes and plays an important part in detoxifying metals like arsenic, copper, cadmium, lead, mercury and silver.

Several diseases of livestock are associated with *selenium and vitamin E deficiency* and include the following:

- Enzootic (nutritional) muscular dystrophy – all species
- Susceptibility to infectious and parasitic diseases – all species
- Exudative diathesis
- Iron hypersensitivity } pigs
- Hepatosis dietetica } pigs
- Mulberry heart disease } pigs
- Weakly neonates
- Retained fetal membranes – cattle
- Bone marrow defects and anaemia – all species
- Ill thrift – all species
- Infertility – sheep, cattle, pigs
- Exudative diathesis } poultry
- Nutritional muscular dystrophy } poultry
- Encephalomalacia } poultry

Although an indispensable element at a level of 0.30 ppm in the diet, an excess (3 ppm and above) of selenium can cause serious disease and death, as indeed can any mineral or vitamin.

### Nutritional muscular dystrophy (NMD) (nutritional myopathy, white muscle disease, stiff lamb disease)

This myopathy (degeneration of muscle) occurs most often in calves but may affect lambs, goat kids, foals, poultry and pigs (in which it usually accompanies other diseases such as mulberry heart disease and hepatosis dietetica).

It is encountered in areas where soils and associated forage and grain crops contain inadequate amounts of *selenium*, e.g. USA, Canada, Australia, New Zealand and Europe, especially the United Kingdom and Scandinavia. Marginal deficiencies probably occur throughout the world in specified regions. Along with a lack of *vitamin E* there may also be an interference with the uptake of selenium due to an excess of sulphur. Diets high in unsaturated fatty acids may produce NMD, hepatosis dietetica and exudative diathesis.

A congenital form of NMD in which the heart is affected usually results in death in very young animals a few days after birth.

Young growing animals affected with NMD show stiffness of gait, diarrhoea, dyspnoea and often an inability to feed because of muscular rigidity.

**Lesions** Groups of muscles, bilaterally affected, are paler in colour than normal and may show longitudinal whitish or greyish striations of degeneration or even a pronounced general whiteness. Damaged areas are oedematous and friable. Similar lesions may be present in the diaphragm, and heart (especially under the endocardium).

### Mulberry heart disease (MHD)

This highly fatal condition usually affects young rapidly growing pigs, 6–16 weeks of age, but can occur in older pigs. The diets fed are mainly soybean, barley and other grains deficient in selenium and vitamin E but high in unsaturated fatty acids.

**Symptoms** may be absent because of the rapidity of death, but in animals seen alive there is anorexia, muscular stiffness, apathy and depression with vague nervous symptoms because of CNS involvement.

**Lesions** Multiple linear epicardial and endocardial haemorrhages and necrosis with hydropericardium, the fluid being straw-coloured, gelatinous and containing fibrin. Lesions of muscular dystrophy are also present, although sometimes overlooked. Carcases are in good condition.

The enlarged liver has a nutmeg appearance due to acute haemorrhagic necrosis and there is evidence of interlobular oedema in the lungs and marked gastric mucosal congestion. Older pigs may show oedema of the subcutaneous tissues and spiral colon resembling that in oedema disease. Advanced cases may show areas of focal necrosis in the brain.

The basic lesion common to the haemorrhagic changes is a microangiopathy in the form of hyalinisation of the walls of arterioles.

(Mulberry heart disease, hepatosis dietetica, exudative diathesis and NMD in pigs are sometimes referred to as the VESD (vitamin E and selenium deficiency) syndrome because of a common aetiology.)

### Hepatosis dietetica

This is a degenerative disease of the liver associated with sudden death in which there is extensive hepatic necrosis. It is similar to MHD except for some variations in symptoms and post-mortem findings.

**Lesions** Extensive subcutaneous oedema and mottling of the liver with attached fibrinous strands, the mottling being related to foci of necrosis and haemorrhage which may also be present in the heart and skeletal muscles. The body cavities often contain straw-coloured fluid.

### Exudative diathesis

As with MHD and hepatosis dietetica, this condition is seen in young growing pigs but also occurs in chicks and broilers.

It is an extensive oedema of the subcutaneous tissues and body cavities. In poultry the accumulation of fluid occurs over the breast and thighs, under the wings, in the pericardial sac and intermuscular tissues.

### Vitamin deficiencies

The requirements for vitamins vary greatly in the different species. For example, vitamins B, C and K are synthesised by ruminants and so are not required in the diet except where a thiaminase is active in the feed which destroys thiamin. This can occur in certain maize silages or wet maize gluten feed which contain sulphate or sulphite.

Apart from vitamin E (and selenium) and vitamin D deficiency (Plate 2, Fig. 12), which are only encountered occasionally, vitamin deficiencies are rarely met with in meat inspection, even as casualties. They do, of course, accompany cases of malnutrition.

Vitamin A is required by all species to maintain the integrity of all epithelial tissues. A deficiency in cattle and sheep may be manifested by lachrymation, conjunctivitis and diarrhoea, which may be accompanied by respiratory involvement including coughing and nasal discharge. Night blindness, associated with opacity of the cornea, and xerophthalmia may occur in cattle and sheep, and sterility in young bulls is occasionally connected with aspermatogenesis. Vitamin A deficiency may be due to an inadequate intake of carotene (provitamin A), which is converted into vitamin A in the small intestine or to a lack of preformed vitamin A. An extremely rare condition in young finishing cattle is subcutaneous oedema or anasarca, believed to be caused by vitamin A deficiency, which can also be associated with stillbirths in cattle, sheep and pigs.

### Judgement of nutritional deficiencies

Many of the conditions described will not be presented at meat inspection because they occur in neonates or are associated with sudden death.

**Total condemnation** (T) Cases associated with emaciation and with generalised oedema.

**Approved as fit** (A) Less severe cases with satisfactory body condition. Or D, K, I, L.

## REFERENCES

FAO/OIE/WHO (1995) *Animal Health Yearbook 1995.* Rome: Animal Production and Health Division, FAO.

Stapleton, R. G. (1949) *The Land Now and Tomorrow.* London: Faber and Faber.

# Chapter 20
# Diseases Caused by Environmental Pollutants

(See also Chapter 13.)

Man and animals are increasingly being exposed to pollutants in the environment, some of which pose direct threats to life while others find their way into the food chain and thence into the tissues of both man and beast (Fig. 20.1). Man's greed in the exploitation of the earth's resources; the worst features of urbanisation; oil spillages at sea; the problems associated with industrial and mining operations; chemical waste discharges into rivers and the atmosphere; the increasingly sophisticated, and often negative and productional, practices in agriculture and the food industry; the litter problem; the problems of human and animal sewage and now of radioactivity – all are harmful and demand immediate and rational control measures.

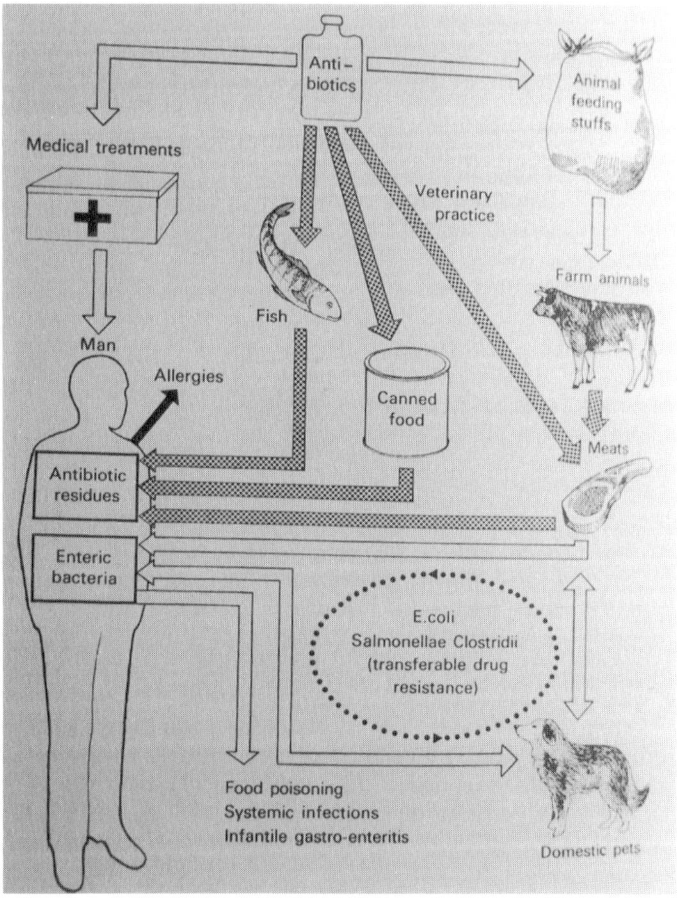


**Fig. 20.1** Chemical and bacterial residues in animals and man. (From J. Lucas, *Our Polluted Food*, 1975, by courtesy of Charles Knight & Co., London)

Happily, and not before time, the seriousness and complexity of the situation is being realised and measures are afoot to deal with at least the major pollutants.

The changes produced by bacteria, viruses, protozoa, rickettsiae, etc.) are mainly occasioned by specific *toxins*, the organisms entering the body via the digestive, respiratory and urogenital tracts and by the skin and conjunctivae. In the case of staphylococcal food poisoning and botulism, however, toxin is ingested with the food in which it is formed, except in infant botulism, in which toxin is formed by *Cl. botulinum* in the intestinal tract. The exact mode of action of the so-called rogue '*prion*' of BSE in the CNS is as yet unknown.

The resulting *lesions* in the animal body may be well- or ill-defined depending on the causal organism, a situation which also applies to the chemical and plant poisons.

While it is unlikely that *acute cases of poisoning* in livestock will be encountered at the meat plant where an adequate system of casualty certification is in force, although the extreme possibility always exists, it may be that some cases may be presented in which there are elevated levels of chemicals – e.g. fluorine, antimicrobials, pesticides and bacterial toxins – in their tissues.

*Poisoning* should always be suspected where a number of animals, previously in good health, suddenly develop clinical signs. This is especially so if the symptoms appear after mass treatment, e.g. spraying or dipping for ectoparasites, dressing for warbles using systemic organophosphorus compounds, the laying down of rodenticides or molluscicides containing copper; the careless disposal of tins of paint and other lead-containing items; and the grazing of certain pastures containing poisonous plants.

While most cases of poisoning are accidental, some are malicious, often perpetrated by grudge-holding individuals.

Again, poisoning and deaths in animals may take place as a result of proximity to a factory explosion, such as occurred at Seveso in Italy in 1974 and at Bhopal in India in December 1984, when almost 2000 people died and 200 000 were rendered ill from the toxic effects of *dioxin*, deaths and sickness also occurring in animals.

Traces of *dioxin* have been detected in milk from cows grazing near a chemical waste disposal plant in Scotland (December 1984) but the exact cause of the losses (200 cows and calves) is uncertain.

The proximity of a factory to grazing livestock has been a hazard in several parts of the world, with elevated levels of poison, e.g. sodium fluoride dusts and gases, falling on grass and forage crops. *Fluorosis*, or chronic fluorine poisoning, has occurred in cattle grazing adjacent to factories producing acid phosphate from rock phosphate, or engaged in the production of aluminium and the manufacture of bricks from fluorine-bearing clays.

## POISONING (INORGANIC AND ORGANIC)

*Toxic substances* ingested directly or in a feedingstuff may cause damage depending on a variety of factors – initial dose of poison, solubility in water, quantity and quality of food ingested, rate of elimination from body, metabolic pathway, concentration in tissues, sensitivity of tissues to poison, etc.

Should the substance be insoluble, it will normally be unabsorbed and will pass through the gastrointestinal tract and be eliminated in the faeces, usually without ill-effect. Soluble substances are absorbed from the small or large intestine. Some then reach the liver via the portal vein, where they are detoxified (if of low toxicity), and thence the bloodstream and body tissues or kidneys, with elimination in the urine. Some may leave the liver by the bile duct to be excreted in the faeces. Poisons of simple chemical structure are more easily and directly absorbed from the intestine into the blood and lymphatic systems and tissues. Another route of absorption from the gastrointestinal tract is via the lymphatics and bloodstream.

The *gastrointestinal tract* is the organ most frequently damaged directly by toxic chemicals and plant poisons. Ingested radioactive elements like strontium-90 and caesium-137 produce changes in the gut similar to those produced by external radiation – haemorrhagic and/or ulcerative gastroenteritis.

In the tissues, poisons may interfere directly with enzyme action or indirectly through action on DNA and RNA. Pathological changes ensue if adequate amounts are ingested, these including necrosis and various other degenerative effects. More seriously, there may be alterations in nucleic acids resulting in teratogenicity or tumour formation. Certain substances ingested over a long period of time may cause teratogenicity.

Severe restrictions were imposed on the Dutch dairy industry in mid-1989 following the finding of dioxin in milk samples. The source was believed to be two of the large incinerators for burning Holland's industrial waste, there being failure to reach the required temperature of 1200°F.

### *Factors influencing the action of poisons*

Such factors include the dose, physical and chemical form of the poison and the species, age, size and condition of the animal. The dose of the poison, its amount, duration and frequency of exposure are important factors in determining the severity of the poisoning, as is the solubility of the poison – the more soluble the greater the amount absorbed. Poisons contained in vegetable oils are more dangerous than those in aqueous solutions. Cattle, because of their inquisitive nature, appear in general to be more prone to poisoning than other species, although the large size of the rumen with its microfloral synthesising ability tends to have a protective effect. Young animals are more often affected, probably because their detoxifying efficiency is underdeveloped and also because they are less discerning. The amount of the poison ingested in relation to the body weight of an animal largely determines detoxifying ability, while hungry animals in poor condition are more liable to ingest harmful substances.

Variations in susceptiblity occur, sheep, for example, being especially prone to copper poisoning, although the same species is resistant to poisoning by ragwort (*Senecio jacobaea*).

### *Diagnosis of poisoning*

A particular problem for the veterinarian at ante-mortem inspection is that of differential diagnosis. Some cases of poisoning, e.g. lead toxicity, produce nervous symptoms which may be confused with those in some infective diseases such as listeriosis.

A full record of the history of the animal(s) presented for slaughter, clinical signs and lesions are essential in addition to a complete veterinary certificate.

A particular concern for the practising veterinarian is the animal injured shortly after treatment with chlorinated hydrocarbons and carbamates, etc., for warble fly infestation or any other treatment where a withdrawal period is necessary before slaughter. *Animals in which chemical residues are believed to exist must not be certified for slaughter for human food*.

### *Collection of samples*

As with all cases in which a microbiological examination is warranted, *specimens of several organs* in addition to intestinal contents, should be carefully collected for *forensic tests*, even if the lesions dictate total condemnation of the carcase and offal. Specimens should be packed individually, preferably in plastic containers, and properly labelled. If the specimens have to travel some distance, they should be packed in ice or solid carbon dioxide, ensuring that each container is tightly sealed.

The principal organs to be tested are the *liver* (in all cases) and *kidney* (where arsenic, lead, copper, mercury and phosphorus are suspected). In the case of *fluorine*, samples of *bone*, *teeth* and *urine* are collected; bone and blood samples are also required if lead poisoning is suspected. *Blood* is also useful for examination where copper and strychnine are under suspicion.

### *Poisons involved*

These comprise organic and inorganic substances, poisonous plants, mycotoxins and radioactive materials. Only a few of the more common substances are discussed here, the reader being referred to specialist texts such as that by Humphreys (1988).

## Lead

### *Sources*

*Lead* is an important constituent of the earth's crust, from which it is mined for industrial purposes, being used as an alloy in solders, bearing metals, as white lead and chrome yellow in paints, as red lead in anti-rust agents, as lead glazes for earthenware and as an additive in petrol. Some of its previous uses are now discontinued or are being abandoned, e.g. in water pipes, petrol, paints and lead arsenate in insecticidal sprays.

However, many potential sources of lead for livestock still remain – old lead-containing paints on woodwork and other structures, and in putty, linoleum, tarpaulins, roofing felt, batteries, lead weights for angling, grease and lubricating oils.

Lead poisoning is generally regarded as the most common form of poisoning in the United Kingdom and probably in the world, occurring especially in young cattle. The inquisitive nature of cattle and their licking and chewing habits cause them to ingest lead and other noxious substances.

Besides these sources, lead may also be found in feedingstuffs. A novel and serious outbreak of lead poisoning in cattle (dairy cows, beef cattle and calves) occurred in south-west England and Wales in 1989 through the consumption of feed contaminated with maize gluten imported from Holland. Some 1700 farms had been supplied with the noxious feed, which caused illness in numerous animals and a total of 35 deaths. In order to safeguard public health, strict controls were placed on the movement and slaughter of animals and a testing programme covering milk, dairy products, beef and beef offals was instituted under the Food Protection (Emergency Prohibitions) (Contamination of Feedingstuffs) Order 1989. Derestriction of controls was subject to negative results of blood samples.

### *Clinical signs*

There may be sudden death without premonitory symptoms. Nervous symptoms predominate, with bellowing, head pressing and other forms of abnormal behaviour. Dullness, apparent blindness and excitability may occur in addition to diarrhoea, constipation, muscular spasms, etc.

### *Lesions*

Only some 2% of the lead ingested is absorbed – always in an inorganic form – the remainder being excreted in the faeces. It binds with proteins in the same way as mercury, cadmium and zinc and is thus easily transported to various parts of the body, where it exerts special effects on the kidneys, liver, RBCs and the CNS. *Acute poisoning:* gastroenteritis, epicardial and endocardial haemorrhages, pulmonary congestion, liver and kidney degeneration. *Chronic poisoning:* softening and cavitation of the CNS with yellowish discoloration and normocytic anaemia. The author (J.F.G.) has noted very fine petechiation of the thymus gland as a very constant finding in chronic lead poisoning in calves.

### *Differential diagnosis*

*Listeria* meningoencephalitis, BSE, Aujeszky's disease, brain abscess, hypomagnesaemic tetany, polioencephalomalacia, *Cl. perfringens* Type D enterotoxaemia, sporadic bovine encephalitis, mercury poisoning, *Haemophilus* meningoencephalitis, rabies, hypovitaminosis A and all conditions with acute onset of nervous symptoms without previous history.

## Acids and alkalis

Strong *acids* (e.g. sulphuric, hydrochloric, nitric, phenolic) and alkalis (e.g. sodium, potassium and calcium hydroxides) are corrosive substances that are very destructive to tissues.

The phenols and cresols are used extensively as disinfectants (e.g. at 2.5%), hydrochloric and sulphuric acids (e.g. 5%) less so. Various forms of alkalis, e.g. caustic soda (sodium hydroxide) and calcium hydroxide (hydrated lime) are used as 2% dilutions, while sodium carbonate (washing soda) is frequently used as a cleansing agent as a 4% w/v solution for washing vehicles prior to disinfection. On occasions, grain and roughage are treated with caustic to improve digestibility.

### *Lesions*

Corrosive action on all mucous membranes – stomatitis, oesophagitis, gastroenteritis with hyperaemia, oedema and thickening of the mucosae.

## Ammonia ($NH_3$) compounds and urea

*Ammonium compounds*, e.g. ammonium sulphate and nitrate, are used as fertilisers, urea on occasion being added to feed for cattle. Ammonia gas is frequently generated in badly ventilated animal houses and can be harmful in concentrations above 100 ppm.

### *Lesions*

Pulmonary congestion and oedema with petechial haemorrhages, catarrhal bronchitis and gastroenteritis.

### Arsenic (As)

*Arsenic* is still available in many different situations, although less commonly today – dips for controlling ectoparasites, rodenticides, wood preservatives, weed killers, defoliants, etc.

*Lesions*

Haemorrhagic gastroenteritis, degenerative changes in liver, kidney, heart and adrenal glands. Endocardial haemorrhages. Chronic cases may show fatty degeneration of liver and kidneys.

### Cadmium (Cd)

*Cadmium* occurs as a contaminant in zinc mining and sewage sludge but is no longer a constituent in anthelmintics for pigs, being considered too toxic. It is used in fungicides and is currently of interest as an environmental pollutant.

A measure of its widespread occurrence is shown by the fact that the National Surveillance Scheme for Residues in meat (NSS) detected *cadmium* in one sheep sample and in 28 out of 29 samples of horse kidneys during 1985. Horses are more often affected, being older than other species at slaughter. In the UK voluntary agreement exists with horse slaughterhouses whereby all offals are discarded from animals destined for human consumption.

Poisoning is rare, most cases occurring from aerial pollution of pastures near mining operations and by accidental ingestion of farm chemicals.

*Lesions*

Many of the adverse effects of cadmium have been determined in experimental animals. Cadmium accumulates in the liver, kidney, bone and pancreas. Its appearance in muscle appears to vary with the different species, but it can cause nutritional myopathy in herbivores and pigs, especially where dietary calcium and phosphorus are deficient. The metal is a potent kidney toxin causing acute tubular necrosis and renal failure, mainly in pigs and horses. In poultry, cadmium poisoning leads to nephritis, enteritis, myocardial haemorrhages and hydropericardium.

### Chemical pesticides

These chemicals include the herbicides, fungicides and insecticides.

**The *herbicides*** are used to destroy noxious weeds as general weedkillers in particular areas or as selective herbicides, large volumes of which are used for the protection of crops. The wide variety includes the organic carbamate and thiocarbamate compounds (see insecticides below), amides (diphenamide, propanil, bensulide), chlorophenoxy compounds (2,4,5-T, 2,4-D, dalapon, MCPA, silvex, etc.), dinitro compounds (dinoseb, dinitrocresol, dinitrophenol, etc.), dipyridyl compounds (paraquat, diquat), glyphosphate, triazine compounds (propazine, atrazine, simazine, etc.) as well as the inorganic arsenicals, sodium chlorate and borax.

Most cases of poisoning are due to the accidental ingestion of fairly large amounts of the herbicides or access to contaminated grazing. Spray drift from booms used for applying herbicides can cause problems for grazing animals. The palatability as well as the toxicity of some poisonous plants are increased with the use of certain hormone weedkillers.

Depending on the compound the *clinical signs* of toxicity include salivation, ataxia, depression, dyspnoea, bloat, muscular spasms hyperaesthesia and the *necropsy findings* include gastroenteritis, liver, kidney and lung congestion. In the case of the very toxic diquat and paraquat, there is severe stomatitis, colic, enteritis, pulmonary oedema and haemorrhage.

**The *fungicides*** consist of inorganic compounds of copper, arsenic, mercury and sulphur as well as organic compounds (dinitrocresol, pentachlorphenol (PCP), dithiocarbamate and derivatives). *Post-mortem findings* include generalised congestion, anaemia, enlargement of the liver, nephritis and cystitis.

The *insecticides* include the carbamates (carbaryl, propoxur), chlorinated hydrocarbons (aldrin, benzene hexachloride (BHC), chlordane, DDT (dichlorodiphenyltrichloroethane), DDD, dieldrin, endrin, heptachlor, organophosphates (dichlorvos, chlorpyrifos, malathion, diazinon, phosmet, coumaphos, fenthion, etc.), benzyl benzoate, pyrethrin, rotenone and the insect growth regulators – methoprene, phenoxycarb and pyriproxyfen.

The *carbamates* are moderately toxic and act in a similar way to the *organophosphates* (OP) by inactivation of acetylcholinesterase (AChE). With both compounds there is salivation, vomiting, hypermobility of the gastrointestinal tract, diarrhoea, urination, bronchial constriction, muscle twitching and paralysis. The organophosphates have multiple use as animal and plant insecticides, fungicides, defoliants, rodenticides and insect repellents.

Poisoning by *organophosphates* may occur through consumption of contaminated feeds and feed crops, overdosing, or swallowing of OP dip or contaminated water. OP compounds vary greatly in toxicity, which can be enhanced by isomerisation during storage and by higher temperatures (e.g. malathion, fenthion, diazinon). Toxicity also varies in different species, cattle being more sensitive than sheep to phosmet, ronnel, dimethoate and crufomate, more sensitive than pigs to phorate, but more resistant than other species to fenthion.

Inhibition of AChE results in the accumulation of acetylcholine (ACh) at neuromuscular junctions, death in severe cases being due to neurotoxicity – asphyxia from respiratory depression, paralysis of respiratory muscles, bronchoconstriction, bradycardia and cyanosis.

Poisoning by these insecticides has been recorded in all species of animals, although less commonly today.

In man, nausea, vomiting, colic, salivation, blurred vision, mental confusion, dyspnoea and coma have been recorded. Reported adverse effects following sheep dipping operations using OPs is currently being investigated in the UK.

**Lesions of incecticide toxicity** These insecticides are general CNS stimulants causing congestion and oedema of the brain and spinal cord. There is congestion of most organs, with epicardial haemorrhages, pulmonary oedema with blood-tinged froth in the trachea and larynx. Chronic cases may show focal centrilobular necrosis of the liver. Chlordane causes vascular damage with subcutaneous petechiae and intestinal and myocardial ecchymoses.

## Copper

*Copper poisoning* (acute and chronic) is one of the more common forms of farm animal poisoning, especially in sheep, probably because of the wide use of the metal in agriculture – in fungicides, seed dressings, parasiticides, mineral mixtures (used where molybdenum and sulphate are lacking in the diet), and feed additives for growth promotion. Copper is often used to prevent copper deficiency in cattle and sheep.

Poisoning by copper results in a haemolytic crisis and is influenced by many different stress factors as well as by the ingestion of certain hepatotoxic plants. The alkaloids of subterranean clover (*Trifolium subterraneum*), Heliotrope (*H. europaeum*) and Ragwort (*Senecio* spp.) ingested over a long period cause retention of copper in the liver.

### *Lesions*

*Acute* poisoning: haemorrhagic gastroenteritis with ulceration and rupture of the abomasum in some cases.

*Chronic* poisoning: Enlarged yellowish liver, icterus, haemoglobinuria, enlarged gunmetal-coloured kidneys.

## Dioxins (tetrachlorodibenzodioxin, TCDD)

*Dioxins* are extremely toxic teratogens which can occur as contaminants during the manufacture of certain auxin herbicides (chlorophenoxy acids), the so-called 'hormone' weedkillers, e.g. 2,4-D and 2,4,5-T, and the fungicides trichlorophenol, pentachlorophenol and their derivatives. TCDD is one of the most poisonous substances known.

These compounds are widely used in agriculture – the chlorophenols as fungicides, mainly in the preservation of timber, and the auxin herbicides for the destruction of weeds in grain crops. Formulations of the latter were used extensively in the early 1960s by the American forces in Vietnam to defoliate jungle areas, the local diets being seriously contaminated at the same time.

The presence of dioxins as contaminants in herbicides and fungicides can have serious consequences for grazing livestock. They may also be present in by-products from plants manufacturing the chlorophenols and the auxin herbicides. They are also sometimes present as contaminants in chlorinated biphenyl products.

*Lesions*

Dioxin is fairly rapidly absorbed and produces centrilobular changes in the liver and kidneys. In poultry the lesions are similar to those of chick oedema disease – accumulation of clear yellowish fluid in subcutaneous tissues and body cavities.

## Feed additives

A wide variety of pharmaceutical or nutritional substances (antimicrobials, fungicides, anthelmintics, arsenicals, oestrogens, coccidiostats, urea, animal and poultry wastes, copper, etc.) are added to livestock feeds to improve growth and feed utilisation. Improperly used they can cause illness and death.

*Oestrogens*

Administered *oestrogenic* substances (oestradiol, oestriol, oestrone, diethylstilboestrol, zearalanol, etc.) are banned in some countries and strictly controlled in others. They can lead to excessive sexual activity in cattle – mounting, head butting, roaring and pawing of the ground by steers – while larger doses can produce preputial, vaginal and rectal prolapse, raising of the tail head, nymphomaniac behaviour in females, with injuries in both sexes. Infertility in males and females is common, with abortion, swelling of the vulva and vagina, relaxation of pelvic ligaments, and endometritis also occurring. Sheep may also be similarly affected, an added symptom being urethral obstruction due to calculi.

Oestrogenic substances are also found naturally in certain plants – subterranean clover (*Trifolium subterraneum*), perennial ryegrass (*Lolium perenne*), lucerne (*Medicago sativa*), red clover (*Trifolium pratense*), white clover (*Trifolium repens*).

**Lesions caused by oestrogens** In addition to the clinical signs, chronic cervicitis, enlarged clitoris and cystic endometritis are observed in cattle and sheep. In pigs rectal inflammation, necrosis and prolapse, nephritis and ureteritis, prostatitis and enlargement of the seminal vesicles occur.

*Antimicrobials*

Although most are of low toxicity, improper use of antimicrobials can cause changes varying from diarrhoea, thinning of intestinal wall and gastrointestinal haemorrhage to neuromuscular damage and aspergillosis, depending on the particular antimicrobial used.

*Urea*

Urea and other forms of organic (e.g. biuret) and inorganic (e.g. ammonium phosphate) sources of nitrogen are sometimes added to feeds for ruminants. Toxic amounts can result in sudden death and in less severe cases, severe colic, bloat, aspiration of rumen contents and convulsions.

*Animal and poultry wastes*

The ever-constant tendency to utilise low-cost materials for feeding to livestock often has adverse results. While making a contribution to the reduction of pollution, the practice of feeding hydrolysed poultry feathers, poultry by-product meal, boiler litter, dehydrated paunch products, meat meal tankage, blood meal, etc., has to be related to their possible content of antibiotics, arsenicals, bacteria, coccidiostats, heavy metals, hormones, mycotoxins, sulphonamides and so on.

Serious bacterial disease in the form of *botulism* (q.v.) following the feeding of waste materials has occurred in addition to poisoning in sheep from the use of poultry litter containing high levels of *copper sulphate*. Although cattle and other species are less susceptible to copper toxicity, there remains the serious question of copper residues in meat and milk. Chicken litter containing *dinoestrol diacetate* has been responsible for abortions in a beef herd.

Because of the possible sequelae of toxicity and undue tissues levels in livestock fed recycled animal wastes, a withdrawal period of 30 days is necessary before slaughter of the fed animals. The use of sewage sludge is dangerous because of the possible bacterial, viral and parasitic (e.g. *T. saginata* eggs) content.

## Fluorine (F)

*Fluorine* is present in many natural minerals such as fluorite (fluorspar), cryolite and fluorapatite and in many soils and water sources.

Poisoning (fluorosis) is rare and though it has occurred in the acute form owing to the accidental ingestion of sodium fluoride, it occurs more as a chronic entity from the grazing of pastures and forages and the inhalation of air contaminated with fluorine dusts and hydrofluoric acid from factories engaged in aluminium and calcine ironstone mining, phosphate fertiliser and feed manufacture, brick manufacture from fluorine-containing clays, etc.

*Lesions*

*Acute poisoning*: Haemorrhagic gastroenteritis, liver and kidney congestion have been reported in pigs.

*Chronic poisoning*: Mottling, staining and excessive wear of teeth, softening and thickening of bones, which become whitish in colour with the appearance of exostoses.

### Hydrocyanic (prussic) acid (HCN) and cyanides.

The most common source of the extremely toxic HCN is cyanogenetic glucosides in certain plants, e.g. *Acacia, Eucalyptus, Lotus, Panicum, Prunus, Sorghum* spp., but poisoning can also occur from the ingestion of contaminated effluent from mining operations (gold mining) and the plating of chrome and nickel and from the careless use of HCN-containing rodenticides.

*Lesions*

The quick-acting HCN causes rapid death due to CNS anoxia. There is widespread carcase and organ congestion with bright red, unclotted blood, haemorrhage in the lungs and trachea and petechiation in the abomasum and small intestine. Subepicardial and subendocardial haemorrhages are evident, along with the smell of bitter almonds on opening the abdomen.

### Mercury (Hg)

*Mercury* occurs in both inorganic and organic forms and has been used variously as an antiseptic, e.g. mercuric chloride (corrosive sublimate), in counter-irritant ointments (yellow mercuric oxide, red mercuric iodide, mercuric nitrate) and as a parasiticide, diuretic and purgative. Beside its pharmaceutical use, mercury is utilised as an agricultural and industrial fungicide and in dental fillings.

Mercury poisoning is rare but can occur through the ingestion of soluble compounds (e.g. by the licking of skin dressings and ointments or the eating of mercurial seed dressings and contaminated feeds), via the skin or by inhalation of vapour.

*Lesions*

*Acute cases*: Gastroenteritis with petechiation of mucosae.

*Chronic cases*: Enlargement and congestion of liver and kidneys. Pulmonary congestion with haemorrhages. Petechiation of kidneys, liver and nasal mucosa.

### Molybdenum (Mo)

An essential trace element in plants, *molybdenum*, can, however, occur in soil in sufficient amounts to cause chronic molybdenum poisoning (molybdenosis) or *'teart'* (q.v.) through the ingestion of herbage containing 20–100 ppm of molybdenum. Other sources of poisoning include the contamination of pasture from industrial operations (molybdenum is used as an alloying agent in the production of various alloys and in the hardening of steel) and the treatment of grassland for growth.

*Lesions*

*Acute*: Marked gastroenteritis with ulceration. Icterus.

*Chronic*: Yellowish enlarged liver. Icterus. Enlarged kidneys and spleen.

### Nitrate (NO3)/nitrite ($NO_2$)

Both salts are used in curing brines, machine oils, fertilisers and explosives, nitrite being the more poisonous entity. Certain plants (*Brassica* spp. (rape, turnips, etc), *Lolium* spp. (ryegrasses), Amaranthus spp. (redroot), *Beta vulgaris* (sugar beet), *Avena sativa* (oats)) contain high amounts of nitrates and can be toxic, as can high levels of nitrates in water (ponds, wells, etc.) affected by fertiliser and feedlot run-off.

*Lesions*

Gastroenteritis. Chocolate-coloured blood due to methaemoglobinaemia. General congestion of carcase. Cardiac, tracheal and serous membrane petechiation. Poor clotting of blood.

## Phosphorus (P)

White or yellow *phosphorus* is rarely used today as a rodenticide, making phosphorus poisoning relatively uncommon. Pigs and poultry are especially susceptible to the accidental ingestion of rat/rabbit baits or the poisoned pests. In some instances poisoning by malicious intent occurs.

*Lesions*

Severe haemorrhagic gastroenteritis. Enlarged, yellowish liver with evidence of haemorrhages and necrosis.

## Other rodenticides

*Antu* (α-naphthylthiourea) causes pulmonary oedema, hydrothorax, congestion of trachea and kidneys.

*Bromethalin* is a neurotoxin which produces muscle tremors, hyperaesthesia, paraplegia and depression with CNS oedema.

*Cholecalciferol* causes hypercalcaemia and hyperphosphataemia, kidney failure with mottling of the kidneys, diffuse haemorrhagic gastroenteritis and plaques on the large abdominal vessels and viscera.

*Red squill (Urginea maritima)* is a plant containing a glycoside rarely used today. Poisoning is rare because of its unpalatability and the fact that large doses are required. Haemorrhagic gastroenteritis is a prominent post-mortem lesion.

*Sodium fluoroacetate/fluoroacetamide* is very toxic, inducing cardiac depression and CNS stimulation with convulsions. Post-mortem lesions include generalised carcase congestion, cyanosis, subepicardial haemorrhages and dilated heart.

*Strychnine* is the alkaloid in the trees *Strychnos nux-vomica* and *Strychnos ignatii* and was once used in rodenticides as a tonic, in feral animal bait and for the malicious poisoning of dogs and cats.

Strychnine stimulates the spinal cord and medullary centres by blocking the action of the inhibitory neurotransmitter amino acid glycine. Clinical signs of toxicity show initial muscle stiffness and tremor followed by tetanic convulsions with marked extensor muscle rigidity and extension with opisthotonus. These signs can be activated by sudden sounds, light or touch and last for 1–4 minutes, after which there is a period of relaxation which gradually lessens as the condition worsens. Post-mortem lesions are consistent with asphyxia – venous congestion of lungs and meninges.

*Thallium sulphate* and *acetate* are cellular poisons which have been banned as rodenticides. Poisoning results in gastroenteritis, which may be haemorrhagic, ulcerated and necrotic extending to the mouth and gums, dermatitis, alopecia and hyperkeratosis in chronic cases.

*Warfarin* is an anticoagulant derived from coumarin, the substance responsible for the smell of new-mown hay, which is converted to dicoumarol, the active principle produced when sweet clover (*Melilotus alba* and *M. officinalis*) spoils. Warfarin has been responsible for numerous poisonings in domestic animals as well as causing fetal death and abortion by depressing plasma prothrombin and other coagulation factors, mainly VII, IX and X.

Sweet clover (dicoumarol) poisoning is caused by the ingestion of large quantities of spoiled sweet clover hay or silage. The normal constituents of coumarin and melilotin are converted into dicoumarol by the action of moulds.

*Post-mortem findings*

These include extensive internal haemorrhage and extravasations of blood in the subcutaneous and connective tissues.

## Selenium (Se)

Selenium is an essential trace element necessary to prevent nutritional myopathy in cattle and sheep, hepatosis dietetica in pigs and exudative diathesis in chicks. Excess amounts, however, result in acute, subacute or chronic selenosis in areas where soils contain significant amounts of organic and inorganic selenium. Soluble forms of these compounds are taken up by certain plants, e.g. *Acacia, Aster* spp., *Astragalus* spp.,

*Gutierrezia* spp, *Pentstemon* spp., which are consumed by cattle and sheep.

Acute selenosis results in fairly rapid death and causes *post-mortem changes* in the form of generalised haemorrhages and ascites. Subacute and chronic selenosis ('alkali disease' or 'blind staggers') results in general necrotic and cirrhotic changes, especially in the liver and spleen, ascites, congestion, haemorrhage and cerebral oedema.

## Sodium chloride (NaCl)

Deaths from the consumption of excessive quantities of salt have occurred in all species, including poultry, where there has been an accompanying deprivation of water. Poisoning may be associated with salt hunger in cattle and contaminated feed and drinking water in all species. The toxic dose for ruminants is very high, but poultry are susceptible to relatively small amounts.

### *Lesions*

Gastroenteritis with blood-stained fluid faeces, watery blood and cerebral oedema in ruminants and pigs. Poultry show anasarca and ascites, nephritis, myocardial haemorrhages, cardiac hypertrophy and hydropericardium.

## Zinc (Zn)

The pharmaceutical sources of *zinc* include the sulphate (emetic and ophthalmic astringent), acetate and benzoate (internal astringents), oxide, stearate and gelatin (protectants) and undecylenate (fungicide). Zinc phosphide is used as a rodenticide, while compounds of zinc have various uses in industry – galvanising of metal, plumbing and paints.

*Poisoning* with zinc is rare but has occurred from the careless use of zinc-containing products and from the contamination of pasture in the vicinity of mines and factories utilising zinc.

### *Lesions*

*Acute cases*: pulmonary emphysema; kidney haemorrhages; hepatic degeneration; pale flabby myocardium.

*Chronic cases:* Catarrhal gastritis and enteritis, internal haemorrhages especially in axillary spaces.

## Poisonous plants

The flora responsible for poisoning in livestock in different parts of the world are extremely numerous and only a few are mentioned here. Some of these – *Brassica* spp., *Trifolium* spp., *Hypericum* spp., and *perennial ryegrass* – are treated elsewhere.

Common *poisonous plants* in the UK include the blue-green algae; bracken fern (*Pteridium aquilina*); *Brassica* spp. (rape, kale, turnips, charlock); buttercup (*Ranunculus* spp.); clovers – alsike, ladino, red, strawberry, subterranean (*Trifolium* spp.); (deadly nightshade (*Atropa belladonna*); horse tail (*Equisetaceae* spp.); *Hypericum* spp. (St John's Wort, etc.); laburnum (*Cystissus laburnum*); larkspur (*Delphinium* spp.); oak (*Quercus* spp.); perennial ryegrass (*Lolium perenne*); ragwort (*Senecio jacobea*); rhododendron (*Ericaceae* spp.); *Solanum* spp. (woody and garden nightshade, Japanese cherry, potato); and yew (*Taxus baccata*).

## Poisonous fungi

(See Fungi and Mycotoxicosis.)

## Poisonous algae

*Algae* are primitive plant-like organisms living in water and varying in size from microscopic cells to large seaweeds several metres in length. Although they are normally responsible for providing food for aquatic life (and may eventually be used for feeding livestock), there are some species which are extremely toxic for animals, birds, fish and man.

Strains of the genera *Anabena, Aphanizomenon, Chlorella, Microcystis, Nodularia, Oscillatoria* and others have caused poisoning and deaths in stock drinking water from stagnant ponds, lakes, etc. Such events have occurred during periods of heavy growth (algal bloom) of these blue-green algae at times of high temperature, drought, shallow water with high organic content, etc., and have been most common in North America, South Africa and Australia, but also in the UK.

The three most common species of blue-green algae known to produce potent toxins in fresh water are *Anabena flos-aqua* (exogenous neurotoxin), *Aphanizomenon flos-aqua* (endogenous saxitoxin) and *Microcystis aeruginosa* (β-peptide toxin). *Blue-green algae* can also produce polysaccharides which cause severe skin irritation and oral blisters, while some elaborate a photodynamic pigment, phyocyan, which is responsible for photosensitisation.

*Exotoxins* are secreted by the algae into the water; endotoxins remain within the organisms, and either the algae have to be consumed by the animal or the toxin has to be released into the water on the death of the algae. The optimum temperature for toxin production is about 25°C.

*Anabena flos-aqua* is believed to be the cause of the most serious incidents of algal poisoning, causing death by paralysis of the CNS and respiratory arrest. Ruminants, especially sheep, have been most often affected but cases have occurred in dogs.

*Chlorellosis* is an infection of mammals due to the ingestion of chlorophyll-containing algae of the genus *Chlorella* and has been recorded in cattle, sheep, beaver and man. It has been encountered in sheep during meat inspection in the Sudan (Zakia, 1989).

### *Lesions*

These vary according to the species involved, the severity of the condition and the toxins ingested. While some cases are peracute with sudden death, others are more chronic in character. Lesions range from congestion of the CNS with pulmonary oedema and hydrothorax in peracute cases to hepatic necrosis, haemorrhagic gastroenteritis, widespread petechiation, visceral congestion, ascites, jaundice and photosensitisation.

Done and Bain (1993) describe an outbreak in which 20 sheep and 15 dogs were affected in Rutland, England in 1989. Post-mortem lesions in the *sheep* revealed dark, congested livers with coagulative necrosis and haemorrhage. In the dogs there were widespread petechial haemorrhages, dark congestion of the liver and haemorrhagic lesions in the liver, kidney, stomach and small intestine.

The *post-mortem findings* in *chlorellosis* include a grossly enlarged liver and hepatic lymph nodes with delineation of the hepatic lobules, with a bright green pigment giving it a honeycomb appearance.

## JUDGEMENT OF INORGANIC AND ORGANIC (INC. PLANT AND ALGAL) POISONING

Total condemnation.

## RADIOACTIVE CONTAMINATION

Radioactive contamination arises from both natural and artificial sources, the latter having assumed greater importance since the Second War World. *Natural* sources of radioactive materials include the presence of radium, uranium, polonium, rubidium, thorium, potassium, radio carbon and the gas radon (a daughter product of radium) in soil, rocks and waters and the constant interactions of cosmic rays, infrared, light (visible and ultraviolet), radio and X-rays in the atmosphere. As a result there have always been tiny amounts of these radioactive substances in the food of man (Fig. 20.2).

*Artificial* forms in varying amounts originate from many different sources. While harmful forms of ionising radiation were once limited to high-energy X-rays for diagnosis and therapy, hazards now include nuclear reactors, cyclotrons, linear accelerators, chemical industries, laboratories, etc. The testing of atomic weapons and the waste discharges from nuclear power stations and other sources have further added to the problem of safety from radioisotopes. Discharges of radioactive wastes from industry, hospitals and laboratories, however, are not generally regarded as sources of contamination of food.

In recent times, *accidental escapes of radiation* from nuclear reactors have occurred, the most notable being the Three Mile Island reactor in Pennsylvania, USA in March 1979 where, happily, major radiation exposure did not occur because of the lower doses of radiation. However, the explosion at the *Chernobyl power complex* in the Ukraine in April 1986 resulted in extremely high radiation doses, with 20 deaths and numerous injuries as well as extensive radiation fallout throughout western Europe, Asia and the USA (Fig. 20.3).

### *Radiation damage*

Ionising radiation consists of X-rays, neutrons, protons, alpha, beta and gamma rays emitted

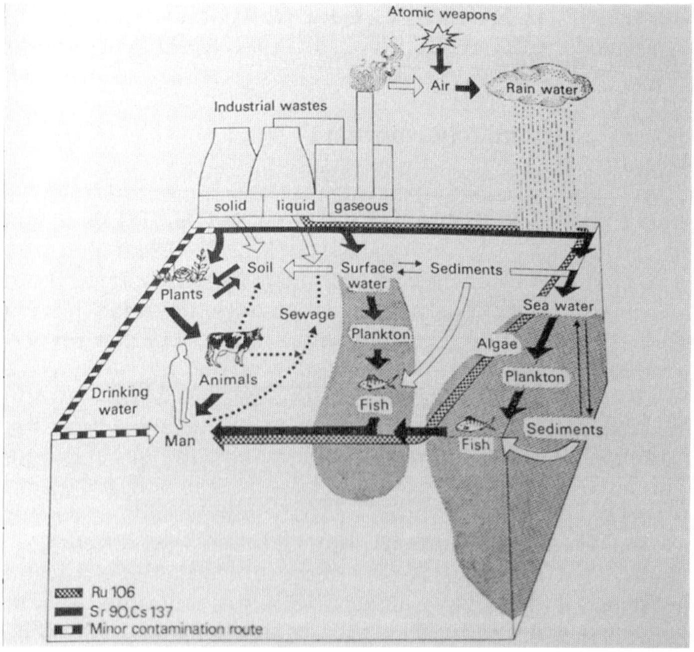


**Fig. 20.2** Radioactive food chains. (From J. Lucas, *Our Polluted Food*, 1975, by courtesy of Charles Knight & Co., London)

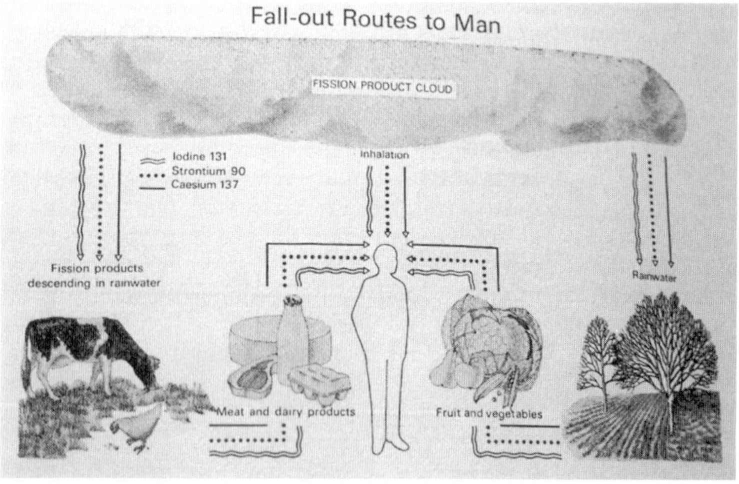


**Fig. 20.3** Fall-out routes to man and animals. (From J. Lucas, *Our Polluted Food*, 1975, by courtesy of Charles Knight & Co., London)

by certain radioactive substances (see above). Radioactive nuclei emit two forms of radiation – electromagnetic radiation (gamma rays) and particulate radiation, e.g. beta particles. All can cause damage to the living tissues of animals and man either directly as somatic effects which occur within days, or indirectly by creating changes in the DNA of proliferating cells (genetic effects) – changes which may not become evident until years later. Somatic and genetic effects are determined by the *total dose* and the *dose rate* of radiation. Immediate somatic lesions are produced by large doses, while low doses can cause delayed somatic and genetic effects.

Other factors involved include the body area exposed, the distribution of the dose and the target tissues, the more active cells being most sensitive. The lymphoid cells are damaged first, followed by the testes and ovaries, bone marrow cells, epithelial cells of the alimentary tract, skin, liver, lungs, biliary tract, kidneys, pleura and peritoneum, nerve cells, bone, muscle and connective tissue. High doses produce cell necrosis while sublethal doses cause disturbances in cell metabolism –

decreased mitosis and DNA synthesis, etc. – resulting in organ hypoplasia, atrophy and eventual fibrosis with a wide variety of conditions such as decreased fertility, anaemia, leukopenia, skin ulceration, cataracts, squamous cell carcinoma, leukaemia and genetic defects.

Such effects can be produced by direct action on the animal body or by the ingestion of herbage contaminated by fallout, which introduces beta and gamma radiation to the alimentary tract.

### UK Chernobyl mark and release scheme

Although the Chernobyl reactor plant explosion caused serious radioactivity fall-out, no apparent abnormality was noted in any grazing livestock. However, concern was expressed about possible levels of contamination in the environment and the food chain following the passage of the plume across Britain in May 1986.

A survey carried out by the Ministry of Agriculture, Fisheries and Food (MAFF) found high levels of *radiocaesium* in upland areas in England (Cumbria), north Wales and Scotland where rainfall had coincided with the passage of the radioactive plume. Monitoring of the sheep grazing these areas showed serious contamination, many being above the limit recommended by the European Commission of 1000 becquerels of caesium per kilogram (Bq/kg).

The only other type of radioactivity encountered was *iodine* but this decayed quickly owing to its short-lived property.

A system of *live monitoring* (*'Mark and Release'*) was devised by the UK Ministry of Agriculture which placed movement and slaughter restrictions on those areas where sheep showed levels of caesium above 1000 Bq/kg while allowing the marketing of sheep below this figure. Individual monitoring using a portable hand-held instrument was carried out before any animal was allowed to leave the farm. Sheep with levels above 1000 Bq/kg were marked with a special paint (changed every 3 months), enabling them to be moved under licence but not slaughtered. Sheep moved to clean pasture reduced their caesium levels in a few weeks, the caesium being excreted naturally. Close collaboration with meat plants established which marked animals were eligible for slaughter and which were ineligible. Random sampling of sheep meat at selected meat plants showed the highest level in 1991 to be 533 Bq/kg compared with 335 Bq/kg in 1995. Mean figures in 1995 of all samples were 30–50 Bq/kg.

The total number of animals failing the test has been very small – the failure rate in 28 000 sheep monitored in Cumbria in 1986 being 12%, with no failures in 1995 in 43 000 sheep tested. Similar results were obtained in Wales and Scotland. Consistent with these results has been a gradual reduction of caesium contamination in vegetation in these areas, making it possible to gradually reduce the areas under restriction.

Final removal of restrictions on the movement and slaughter in parts of Cumbria took place on 12 January 1996, but restrictions still continue in upland areas of Wales, southern Scotland and Northern Ireland. Acid, peaty soils allow radioactivity to remain soluble and thus available for uptake into the vegetation.

The overall effect of the 'Mark and Release' monitoring programme in the United Kingdom has been the effective protection of the public, no appreciable reduction in the consumption of sheepmeat and no interference with the sheep farming industry as a result of the Chernobyl reactor plant explosion.

### UK Terrestrial Radioactivity Monitoring Programme (TRAMP); UK Food and Agriculture Monitoring Programme (FARM)

The UK Ministry of Agriculture has been monitoring radionuclides in foodstuffs and in agricultural and marine materials since the 1950s. Since 1986 its Science Division has undertaken a comprehensive monitoring programme for radioactivity in terrestrial foodstuffs to confirm the effectiveness of the controls for the routine release of low-level radioactive waste from 23 licensed nuclear sites in England and Wales. Similar arrangements apply in Scotland. The programmes are also designed to check on possible accidental releases of radioactivity from nuclear sites. In mid-1996 cracks were detected in pipe welds in the nuclear reactors at Hinkley Point B in Somerset and Hunsterton B in Ayrshire, but without any leakage of radioactivity. Immediate shut-down was ordered, this taking place in all such instances.

Releases of low-level wastes can only be made with the authority of the Chief Inspector of HM Inspectorate of Pollution (HMIP) and the Minister of Agriculture under the Radioactive Substances Act of 1993.

Strict regulations also apply to the standards of construction and operation of nuclear power generators and other establishments where radioactivity is generated, the protection of the public and the food chain being of paramount importance.

Results of the TRAMP and FARM programmes for 1997 showed that public exposure from anthropogenic radioactivity due to consumption of milk and foodstuffs grown around licensed nuclear sites was well within acceptable UK and EU limits, which confirmed the adequacy of regulatory controls applied to radioactive emissions from licensed nuclear sites. Sampling of milk, crops and animals was carried out for the nuclides of tritium, carbon-14, sulphur-35, strontium-90, caesium-137, plutonium-238, plutonium-239+240, plutonium-241 and americium-241.

## Nordic model on food safety after nuclear accidents

In 1988 a group of officials from the five Nordic countries (Sweden, Norway, Finland, Denmark and Iceland) designed a model for response to nuclear accidents which included recommendations on intervention levels in food, their final report being made in April 1991.

The Nordic Model was concerned with the protection of the individual and society at large by the management of food supplies and food safety after nuclear accidents through the production, distribution, sale and consumption of food and drink. The overriding aim was to keep the radiation dose for the population as low as reasonably possible by the institution of appropriate countermeasures.

### *Recommendations*

1. Radiation doses to the population should be kept as low as reasonably possible. The introduction of countermeasures should be optimised to ensure that the net result is beneficial to individuals and society.
2. The dose from all radionuclides in all foodstuffs in the diet to which individual members of the population are exposed should not, except in extreme accident situations, exceed the following:
   - *Primary Intervention Level I*: 5 mSv (millisieverts) as a result of dietary intake during the first 30 days following a radioactive fall-out.
   - *Primary Intervention Level II*: 5 mSv as a result of dietary intake during the remaining part of the first year following a radioactive fall-out.
   - *Primary Intervention Level III*: 1 mSv per year as a result of dietary intake during the second and subsequent years following a radioactive fall-out, calculated as an average over several years.
3. There should be a set of common Nordic *Permanent DILs* (Derived Intervention Levels) for radionuclides in food, valid for normal, i.e. non-accident situations and identical to the Guideline levels laid down by the Codex Alimentarius Commission for foods in international trade as follows:
   - 1 Bq/kg for the sum of plutonium-239, americium-241 and corresponding radionuclides (actinides) in milk and infant foods.
   - 10 Bq/kg for the sum of plutonium-239, americium-241 and corresponding radionuclides (actinides) in all other foods.
   - 100 Bq/kg for the sum of strontium-90, iodine-131 and corresponding radionuclides in milk and infant foods.
   - 100 Bq/kg for the sum of strontium-90 and corresponding radionuclides *in all other foods.*
   - 1000 Bq/kg for the sum of caesium-134, caesium-137 and corresponding radionuclides in milk and infant foods.
   - 1000 Bq/kg for the sum of iodine-131, caesium-134, caesium-137 and corresponding radionuclides *in all other foods.*

A set of Nordic *Emergency DILs* for radionuclides should be set to come into effect when a country experiences a nuclear accident. These should apply for 30 days and replaced within a maximum of 30 days by appropriate Intervention Levels.

*Primary Intervention Levels* (PIL): Maximum upper levels of radiation doses which should not be exceeded. A reasonable maximum dose level resulting from intake of food over a one-year period would be 1 mSv, the starting point of the Nordic Model.

The Primary Intervention Level for the first 30 days immediately following a nuclear accident is set at 5 mSv, for the remainder of the first year after an accident the level is 5 mSv and in subsequent years 1 mSv as an average over several years.

PILs provide a reasonable margin of safety.

*Derived Intervention Levels (DILs)*: Maximum levels of radioactive substances in foodstuffs, expressed in Bq/kg. Conversion of mSv per year to Bq/kg involves factors such as the composition of the diet, the degree and distribution of radioactive contamination in the various types of foodstuffs.

## Glossary

*Anthropogenic*: Man-made.

*Absorbed dose*: Amount of energy given off by ionising radiation to unit mass of material, e.g. tissue. SI unit is gray (Gy).

*Activity*: Amount or quantity of a radionuclide. Describes the rate at which radioactive decay takes place.

*Cosmic rays*: Ionising radiation from outer space acting on the earth.

*Dose*: Amount of radiation received by materials and tissues.

*Dose equivalent*: Quantity obtained by multiplying the absorbed dose by a factor to allow for the different effectiveness of the various ionising radiations in causing harm to living tissue. SI unit is sievert.

*Fall-out*: The radioactive fission products settling on earth after the testing of nuclear weapons or explosion at a nuclear plant.

*Isotope*: Nuclide having the same number of protons but a different number of neutrons, that is, a different atomic mass.

*Nuclide*: A species of atom defined by the charge, mass, number and quantum state of its nucleus.

*Radiation*: Energy emitted by radionuclides as waves or streams of particles through space or materials.

*Radionuclide*: Unstable nuclide emitting ionising radiation.

### *Units for the measure of radiation*

Bq (*becquerel*): SI unit of radioactivity – the quantity of a radionuclide that undergoes one decay or transformation per second.

C (*coulomb*): SI unit of exposure to radiation. 1 coulomb per kilogram (C/kg) = 3876 roentgen.

Gy (*gray*): SI unit of energy absorbed by a tissue or substance, equal to the transfer of a joule of energy per kg (1 J/kg) of absorbing material.

R (*roentgen*): Quantity of X or gamma ionising radiation in air. Superseded by coulomb.

Sv (*sievert*): SI unit of radiation absorbed dose equivalent, equal to the same biological effect as 1 gray of high energy X and gamma radiation.

## REFERENCES

Done, S. H. and Bain, M. (1993) *Vet. Rec.* **133**, 600.

Humphries, D. J. (1988) *Veterinary Toxicology*, 3rd edn. London: Baillière-Tindall.

Zakia, A. M., Osheik, A. A. and Halima, M. O. (1989) *Vet. Rec.* **125**, 625–626.

## FURTHER READING

Lucas, J. (1975) *Our Polluted Food*. London: Charles Knight.

# Chapter 21
# Disease Data Retrieval and Feedback

The slaughter and inspection of large numbers of food animals and poultry, besides providing wholesome meat and offal for human consumption, can, through *accurate diagnosis and recording*, also contribute to the following desiderata:

1. Reduction of losses due to disease and injury through feedback to livestock producers and practising veterinary surgeons.
2. Demonstration of trends and variations in animal disease incidence due to husbandry methods, season, geographical location, etc.
3. Tracing of affected herds as part of national disease control programmes.
4. Extent, cost and reasons for condemnations due to disease and injury.
5. Use of information regarding animal housing and husbandry, including breeding data, to improve standards on the farm, including those of animal hygiene.
6. Demonstration of certain subclinical conditions.
7. Forecasting of disease outbreaks in conjunction with meteorological data.
8. Enhancement of the clinical competence of the practising veterinary surgeon regarding data on client's slaughtered stock, especially casualty animals.
9. Provision for research investigations.
10. Quality control check on inspection standards.

The meat plant has, therefore, an important role to play in epidemiology and preventive veterinary medicine, not only in relation to post-mortem findings but also following examination of the live animal prior to slaughter.

Except for a few countries with efficient meat inspection services such as Sweden, Denmark, Holland, Australia, New Zealand, USA and Northern Ireland, this valuable source of information is, regrettably, not being fully exploited worldwide. Among the reasons for this deficiency are lack of coordination between those in charge of meat inspection, the traditional 'iron curtain' which exists between the livestock production and slaughter/meat inspection in many countries, practical difficulties in slaughter line recording (e.g. fast rail speeds, inadequate inspector manning levels), traditional marketing systems and the absence of a foolproof, efficient animal identification system – a major stumbling block.

## MEAT INSPECTION RECORDING SYSTEMS

Many variations are in existence. Those countries which possess cooperative livestock/meat systems, e.g. the Scandinavian countries, are better placed to organise an efficient recording and feedback of information to producers.

Skovgaard (1990) has provided the ideal arrangement for an integrated meat hygiene service in which data collection is an important function (Fig. 21.1).

Information from the farm which would be of value to the meat inspectorate would include disease incidences; mortality and morbidity rates in livestock; use of antibiotics, hormones, etc.; details of feed consumption; and results of laboratory investigations (microbiological, serological, chemical for residues).

*Proper use of the data emanating from ante-mortem inspection at the farms of origin combined with the feedback of disease data from the meat plant to the farms is an essential part of a modern meat inspection service and the safety assurance of the final product.* Systems devoid of these essentials are basing carcase and offal judgements on

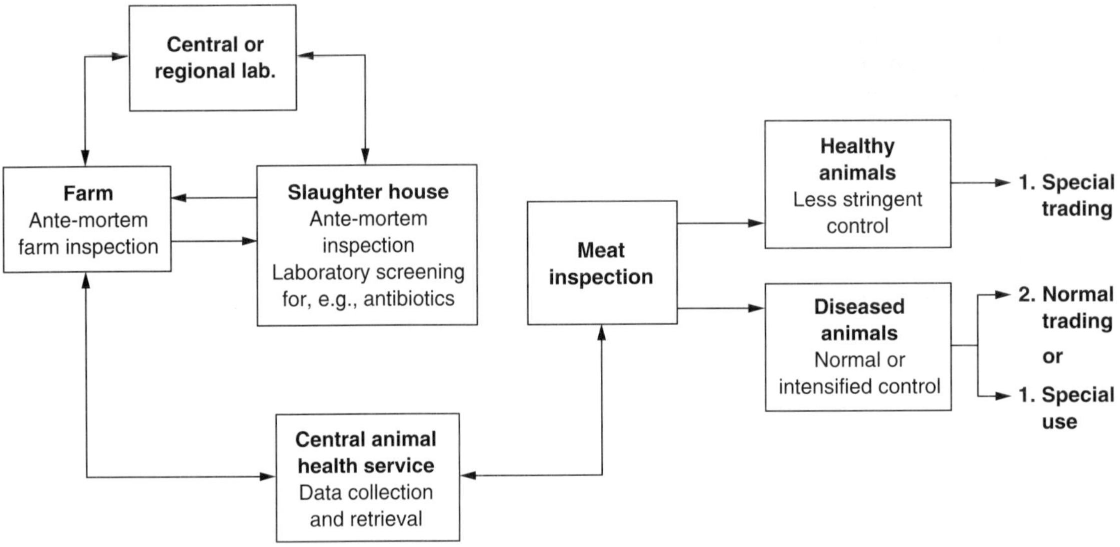


**Fig. 21.1** Flowsheet for an integrated 'meat hygiene' service. Investigations on, e.g. (1) death and disease rate during rearing; (2) use of antibiotics, hormones, etc.; (3) feed consumption; (4) laboratory findings – serological (bacteria, parasites), microbiological (pathogenic bacteria), chemical (residues). (After Skovgaard, 1990)

flimsy evidence and, by concentrating solely on visual procedures, are missing diseases of zoonotic importance, e.g. salmonellosis, campylobacteriosis, yersiniosis, giardiasis, listeriosis.

Inherent in any scheme for the utilisation of abattoir data is the need for precise diagnoses, standard nomenclature for the diseases encountered, and recognised forms of presentation of the disease data. There is no point in referring back vague or inaccurate information to livestock producers. Equally important is efficient identification of live animals as well as of their carcases and offal, which must be correlated. The system in the abattoir must include full details of the carcase and species, disease condition, part of carcase affected, weight of meat and offal condemned and, if necessary, be supplemented by the results of laboratory examinations. The disease conditions to be recorded should be of a type that are readily identified, of economic importance in the animal health and/or public health sphere and easily controllable. It is essential for the meat inspectorate to cooperate fully in such a scheme.

If the occurrence of abnormalities on post-mortem examination and the reference back to producers were combined with subsequent visits by practising veterinary surgeons (who should also be informed of the disease findings), it is likely that preventive measures would be much more effective.

## New Zealand

In 1974 the *New Zealand* Ministry of Agriculture and Fisheries (NZMAF) commenced a computerised system of meat inspection data recording as a quality control check on meat inspection procedures and to monitor 18 conditions in cattle, sheep, pigs and goats (Christiansen and Hellstrom, 1979). This programme ('Diseases and Defects' system) records the incidence of actinoform lesions, arthritis, bruises and wounds, caseous lymphadenitis, contamination, *C. bovis, C. ovis*, emaciation, pleurisy, facial eczema, faulty castration, neoplasms, pyogenic lesions, sarcocysts, septicaemic-like lesions, skin lesions, tuberculosis and xanthoses.

Coloured tickets with the disease/defect in abbreviated form in consecutive numbers are attached to the carcase from a dispenser. Condemned tickets are used for condemned whole carcases along with the disease/defect ticket. The total number of tickets in each class is then recorded by a clerk.

Monthly returns of the number of cases and condemnations in each disease category are made by each plant to the NZMAF together with the weekly kill figures. The disease/defect data are then punched on cards and the data are afterwards transferred to a master magnetic tape for storage.

Monthly reports are produced giving the number of animals, by species and geographical location, affected with each condition, in addition to the number of total condemnations.

### Sweden

The Swedish Meat Hygiene Service has an extremely close liaison between meat inspection, regional laboratories, livestock production and field veterinarians. Meat inspection is divided into primary and secondary sections, the former dealing with control for human consumption and the latter with the diagnosis of animal disease, its feedback to the farmer and its utilisation in disease prevention. The findings in meat inspection do not always involve condemnation of the carcase or parts of it; some serve to identify herds infected with respiratory diseases, mastitis, *Salmonella*, etc., so that eradication programmes can be initiated. In this way, healthier stock can be raised and the public can be protected from food poisoning. It has been found that very small lesions in certain organs, e.g. kidney and liver, may indicate that toxins or other substances are present on the farm without the knowledge of the farmer or the practising veterinary surgeon.

The Swedish Meat Inspection Service cooperates very closely with the organised Animal Health Service, which is established under the supervision of the Swedish Board of Agriculture and the National Food Administration. All diagnoses and information from meat inspection are reported to the Animal Health Service and to the farmers. Veterinary pathologists have been employed since 1977 to work exclusively in the meat inspection sphere and 37 of the official microbiological control laboratories are headed by veterinarians, these laboratories being distinct from the meat plant laboratories. During the last 10 years a special group of 11 laboratories has been established (the Swedish Laboratory Service Ltd) which provides facilities for veterinary, food and water investigations.

### Canada

In the Food Production and Inspection Branch of Agriculture Canada, all parts of carcases condemned are recorded (with reason for rejection) by direct computer data entry on the kill floor. *All carcase condemnations, with the reason for seizure, are reported to the livestock producer concerned* (Clarke 1989, personal communication).

Some 73 disease conditions are currently being reported. Each meat plant submits monthly reports to headquarters in Ottowa for entry into a data bank, summary sheets of condemnation statistics being sent back to each plant along with information for the region and Canada as a whole in order to detect differences in condemnation rates (which could be ascribed to regional variations and/or suspect inspection standards). The data bank is also used to answer queries from producer groups, research organisations, universities, etc. Several forms in English and French are utilised to provide extensive information on disease entities. These include a Certificate of Condemnation (whole and part carcases), a copy of which is sent to the owner of the animal, one being retained on file; an Ante-mortem Screening Record (to record lots of animals examined live); an Ante-mortem Veterinary Inspection Report (to transfer information gained on ante-mortem inspection to the meat inspection staff); and an Ante-mortem and Post-mortem Disposition Report (to record pathological changes encountered at AM and PM).

Codes are assigned to 130 disease conditions, 48 carcase sites, 11 provinces and 24 species of livestock which, in addition to cattle, sheep, pigs, poultry and horses, include buffalo, deer, elk, moose, wild Russian boars, yaks, reindeer, musk oxen and caribou.

Specific instructions to meat inspection staff are provided for form completion to ensure uniformity of recording and to detect any major differences in condemnation rates as well as to assess trends in disease incidence and to establish any necessary disease control measures.

An overall picture of disease incidence as revealed by meat inspection is obtained by

Canada's centralised service, which inspects some 97% of all meat products produced in Canada, the remainder being the responsibility of the Provincial Meat Inspection Service. All meat plants registered under the Federal Meat Inspection Act have a full-time veterinarian on site during operations.

### Denmark

Data banks containing meat inspection findings have been in operation in Denmark since 1964 and in Sweden since 1970, similar arrangements applying in both countries.

The Danish Swine Slaughter Inspection System's aim is to create a method for the surveillance of health and disease in bacon pigs and to establish disease-control programmes. The system is facilitated by a direct form of marketing through national farmers' cooperative associations and uses slap marks coded for individual farms on the pigs. A centralised computer-based recording scheme for bacon factories utilises a uniform code of diagnoses to identify lesions causing partial and total condemnation. These diagnoses are in the form of two-digit numbers which can be grouped into 20–25 disease categories made by veterinarians.

Data from almost all the 12 million bacon pigs slaughtered annually are stored and processed on the central computer, which summarises the weekly data by herd at each factory, monthly and yearly disease statistics by bacon factory being provided by the Danish Meat Research Institute at Roskilde.

Analysis of the disease data with the institution of control measures (herd health programmes, genetic selection, clinical trials, etc.) have proved very successful. It is accepted that in all abattoir disease data collection, the nature of the lesions detected is that of gross pathology resulting in partial or total condemnation. Since diseases responsible for high mortality are obviously not included, this limits this form of disease survey, making concurrent *farm surveys* essential for an overall estimation of national disease incidence to be gained.

All the information from the Danish Swine Slaughter Inspection Data System is made available to the producers involved. They have benefited from control programmes in several ways, for example, although lung and pleura lesions comprise about two-thirds of all diagnoses and were increasing from 1964 to 1972, there has since been a steady fall in their incidence and in the overall disease rate at slaughter.

Zachrau (1992) has given details of three ID systems (barcodes, 'vision' system using slaughter numbers, and radiofrequency (RF) tags) successfully used in Danish bacon factories, all being based on pig ear marks. Computer-based on-line data capture systems have been used on slaughterlines since 1977 in almost all Danish bacon factories, the final data being conveyed to the Danish Agriculture EDP centre for statistical production control and payment to the producer. The information collected comprises meat inspection findings, skatole content of entire male pigs, carcase classification and weights.

**Barcode system** Instead of marking individual pigs (applies also to vision system and RF tags), each gambrel on which the pig is hung is permanently marked with an easily read barcode label (2 to 5) printed on an aluminium foil in a two-coloured serigraphy or made as a laser-engraved aluminium plate in two colours, both types protected by a heat-, cold- and chemical-resistant enamel.

The barcodes are read as they pass helium/neon laser scanners with a scanning frequency of 400 scans/second and with a built-in fast microprocessor and specially developed software. These scanners are located at eight specific points – inspection, weighing, sampling from entire pigs, classification, sorting, dispatch, cutting/bacon. Should reading quality of the codes fall below a certain limit, an alarm is activated. Gambrels after use are washed in an automatic washing machine and those with codes of poor reading quality are replaced. This system has the lowest overall cost but highest maintenance cost.

**'Vision' system** Earlier trials with reading stamp or brand marks on the actual carcases were unsatisfactory because bite and scrape marks interfered with readings, so a stainless steel plate with a laser-cut ID number is welded on to the lower side of each gambrel. This number is illuminated by a special light and recorded by a vision camera at each reading station. An associated multiplexer control unit converts the numbers into data signals for transmission to the external computer system. The overall cost is high, but maintenance cost is low.

**RF-tags** RF-tags or microchips (small radiotransmitters) are fitted in a hole in each gambrel and protected so as to withstand the 150°C of the singeing machine and the –40°C of refrigeration. This system has medium overall cost and low maintenance cost.

All three systems are suitable for meat plant use, although some differences exist between them (Table 21.1)

Using these systems, Danish bacon factories are able to compile detailed statistics on carcase classification and meat inspection and relay this information back to the producers. For cattle, a database has been established from which data for individual animals from birth up to and including slaughter can be obtained.

*Quality control and traceability with certification of meat plants and livestock producers will undoubtedly become essential requirements for the future as a result of supermarket and consumer demands.*

## Australia

A major part of the National Animal Disease Information Service is associated with the collection of abattoir data, information also being obtained from 18 veterinary diagnostic laboratories, each of which has a minicomputer. Records are maintained on floppy disks at each laboratory for all farms served by the laboratory, with a central computer being located at the Australian Bureau of Animal Health. This latter maintains consolidated records on magnetic tape for all regions, analysing the database and providing printouts of herd histories and disease eradication activities.

It is recognised in Australia that, although meat plants and laboratories cannot provide a true picture of national animal disease incidence, they are of value in disease conditions not materially affected by sample bias and as indicators of certain emerging, disease trends (Roe, 1979).

## Northern Ireland

The collection of meat inspection data was instituted in 1969 following a survey in 1954–55 of mortality and morbidity on 623 farms and of condemnations in 18 abattoirs (Gracey, 1960).

It is generally recognised that many specific diseases are responsible for much economic loss in livestock and that accurate recording in the meat plant is an inexpensive method of monitoring these. A computerised retrieval system has been devised which links abattoir, meteorological and economic data relating to specific disease conditions since 1969 and enables an ongoing assessment of important production diseases to be made. For example, since 1976 there has been an overall increase in pig liver condemnations due to hepatic cirrhosis mainly caused by migrating *Ascaris suum* larvae, despite the fact that this disease was thought to be adequately controlled by management and the fairly widespread use of anthelmintics.

**Table 21.1** Comparison of three ID systems according to Zachrau.

| | Barcode | Vision | RF tag |
|---|---|---|---|
| Resistance to dirt | Low | Medium | High |
| Reading distance | <1 m | <4 m | <15 mm |
| Temperature stability | Good | Very good | Good |
| Speed/reading | Medium | Low | Low–medium |
| Alphanumerical info. | | | |
| Code 2 of 5 No. | No | Yes | Yes |
| Resistance to chemicals | Good | Very good | Good |
| Resistance to rime | Fair | Good | Very good |
| Visually readable | Yes | Yes | No |

Use of abattoir data has been made in relating disease incidence to weather conditions and in the forecasting of outbreaks. For example, the incidence of pneumonia and pleurisy in sheep has been shown to have statistically significant correlations with several lagged weather variables, the most important being wind chill with a lag of 2 months ($P$ <0.001) (McIlroy *et al.*, 1989). Fascioliasis, a serious parasitic disease of great economic importance in many parts of the world, including Northern Ireland, has been made the subject of accurate forecasts, enabling the effective operation of control measures, by integrating liver condemnations due to liver fluke with a concurrent meteorological database (McIlroy, 1990).

McIlroy and colleagues (1988) have also reported the development of an integrated computerised data analysis system for the evaluation of diseases in food animals. This system combines databases containing abattoir pathology, meteorological and economic data and allows the monitoring of economically important diseases in cattle, sheep and pigs in Northern Ireland. Data have been held since January 1969 and reports are available in both tabular and graphical formats. Figures are available on some 20 diseases and contamination in relation to partial and total carcase seizures as well as all types of offal. These authors indicate that accurate abattoir pathology data can provide an effective and inexpensive method of disease surveillance in livestock.

A national meat inspection recording system has been devised utilising forms for each abattoir from which weekly return is made, all the resulting data being analysed at the Department of Agriculture's headquarters in Belfast. Detailed disease data are available on the incidence of several major diseases and the main reasons for condemnations of carcases and offal in the various species of livestock in nine abattoirs (slaughtering cattle and sheep), five bacon factories and nine poultry plants.

## Meat plant statistics

In 1951 the Oake Interdepartmental Committee on Meat Inspection in Great Britain reported that 'abattoirs can and should play a part in disseminating knowledge about animal disease and also provide assistance to those responsible for combatting animal disease and improving animal health'. This Committee also stated that information resulting from meat inspection records could provide valuable evidence of the incidence of disease in particular herds, in particular areas, or in the country as a whole. Standardisation and increased accuracy of records would enable comparisons to be made with individual abattoirs.

In a report to the UK Humane Slaughter Association and Council of Justice to Animals, Rimmer (1989) found numerous anomalies in the recording of disease data in British abattoirs. The paucity, inaccuracy and incompleteness of information was ascribed to inadequate meat inspector manning levels, fast slaughter rates and substandard inspector training. In addition to the economic effects, it was concluded that accurate meat inspection records, properly applied at producer level, could also improve the welfare of food animals. It was found, however, that livestock owners rarely utilised these records, believing them not to be cost-effective. This was considered to be associated with the provision of doubtful diagnoses. Rimmer also reported on the causes of condemnations at a poultry plant and found that half the birds were rejected for 'oedematous oviduct', a condition of rare occurrence and a doubtful cause of total condemnation.

It has to be recognised that, in the United Kingdom, the feedback of disease data from meat plants to farms of origin is as yet a rare occurrence, but it is beginning to be applied in the poultry sector in which ante-mortem farm inspection is now taking place.

In Great Britain no national meat inspection records are as yet available. Only limited information is on hand from the annual records of Community Health Officers on the weight of meat and offal rejected as unfit for human consumption and the percentage of carcases totally or partially condemned for various diseases. With the setting up of the Meat Hygiene Service on 1 April 1995, this situation will undoubtedly change.

A valuable review of some animal diseases, encountered at meat inspection in England and Wales during 1969–78 was provided by Blamire *et al.* (1980). During this period there was a significant decrease in condemnations due to fascioliasis, an increase in losses caused by bruising, with abscesses in livers responsible for considerable losses in cattle and sheep.

Ascariasis and hydatidosis continued to be important reasons for lung and liver rejection, while pneumonia and pleurisy had a high incidence in pigs and adult cattle. In a previous paper, Blamire *et al.* (1970) suggested that an efficient meat inspection service had an important contribution to make in the monitoring of animal disease, especially of chronic and ill-defined conditions which are not apparent to the farmer but are of considerable economic and public health importance.

Loss of liver in lambs due to the presence of liver fluke and taeniasis (mainly *C. tenuicollis*) have been reported to be costing a meat plant at Cullompton in Devon, England, in the region of £1000 a week (11 pence a lamb). The average annual throughput of this plant is 450 000 lambs and the incidence of tapeworm cysts is about 8%. This particular company took action by informing its suppliers of these findings. Advice offered on the control of tapeworms in dogs has shown good results (*Farmer's Weekly* 1984).

In Scotland, Cuthbertson (1983) carried out a sheep disease surveillance based on condemnations at three abattoirs over a period of 3 years. Carcase condemnations were mainly due to arthritis, abscesses and emaciation, with percentages (of the total kill) of 0.7%, 0.2% and 0.1%, respectively, as averages for the whole period. Viscera condemned were predominantly livers (5.5%) because of abscesses, liver fluke and 'other parasitism' (mainly *C. tenuicollis*) and lungs (2.2%) due to pneumonia, pleurisy and parasitism. *Muellerius capillaris* was the main cause of lung parasitism.

In Norway, Flesja and Ulvesaeter (1980) analysed the post-mortem data from 254 342 bacon pigs. The following conditions were found to be of importance:

1 Pyaemia and abscesses with tail lesions, severe pneumonia and anaemia.
2 Pyaemia with polyarthritis and claw lesions.
3 Atrophic rhinitis with all recorded chest lesions and perihepatitis.
4 Severe pneumonia accompanied by pleurisy, pericarditis and numerous 'whitish spots' in the liver.
5 Marked pneumonia with polyarthritis and other liver lesions.
6 Pleurisy with pericarditis, peritonitis and other liver lesions.
7 Lesions of the tail with anaemia, marked pneumonia, polyarthritis and arthritis.

Tuberculosis was not correlated with any other disease condition, but scabies was positively correlated with white spot liver.

Examples of diseases currently being monitored on selected farms supplying livestock to several abattoirs in England and Scotland by the Meat and Livestock Commission include (for sheep) liver fluke, abscess (liver, lung, thoracic cavity), bruising, *C. tenuicollis*, hydatid cysts and yellow discoloration; (for cattle) liver fluke, abscess (carcase and offal), *C. bovis*, bruising and warble fly; (for pigs) ascariasis, abscess (carcase), arthritis, bruising and pneumonia (Pratt, 1979).

Accurate diagnoses, standardisation of disease nomenclature, adequate inspection manning levels, suitable methods of on-line recording, proper meat inspector training and a centralised veterinary meat inspection service are essential components of an efficient disease data retrieval and feedback system.

Hill (1988) detected major differences in condemnation rates and causes of rejection in different parts of the United Kingdom, many of these being occasioned by a lack of these requisites. This author examined pig abattoir records from four regions in the UK and found them inadequate for the following reasons:

1 Lack of standardised reasons for carcase condemnations.
2 Weight of condemned meat and offal not included.
3 Comparison between abattoirs impossible.
4 Ante-mortem data not available.
5 Unnecessary restriction of availability of records for interested parties.

It was concluded that the whole system of meat inspection recording and transmission of information required urgent attention if it was to contribute to pig production, abattoir operations and animal welfare. Not only could such information form the basis of animal health/zoonoses preventive schemes, it would also enable research to be directed along practical lines and thereby reduce the huge losses incurred in animal disease and injury.

## Northern Ireland

The main reasons (in order of importance) for condemnations in cattle, sheep and pigs are given in Tables 21.2, 21.3 and 21.4.

**Table 21.2** CATTLE. Reasons for carcase condemnations, N. Ireland, 1995.

Bovine kill: 451780.
Condemnations: Total: 4205 (0.93% of kill)
Carcases: 873 (20.8% of total condemnations; 0.19% of kill)
Parts: 3332 (79.2% of total condemnations; 0.74% of kill)

| Reason | Carcases | % of total | Parts | % of total |
|---|---|---|---|---|
| 1 Oedema | 199 | 4.7 | 32 | 0.8 |
| 2 Fever/septicaemia | 169 | 4.0 | | |
| 3 Abscesses/pyaemia | 112 | 2.7 | 483 | 11.5 |
| 4 Gastritis/peritonitis | 58 | 1.4 | 19 | 0.5 |
| 5 Pneumonia/pleurisy | 36 | 0.9 | 2 | 0.05 |
| 6 Tumours | 35 | 0.8 | 10 | 0.2 |
| 7 Tuberculosis | 32 | 0.8 | 42 | 1.0 |
| 8 Emaciation | 30 | 0.7 | | |
| 9 Imperfect bleeding | 18 | 0.4 | | |
| 10 Arthritis | 17 | 0.4 | 478 | 11.4 |
| 11 Bruising | 12 | 0.3 | 1316 | 31.3 |
| 12 Nephritis/nephrosis | 12 | 0.3 | | |
| 13 Uraemia | 10 | 0.2 | | |
| 14 Actinobacillosis | 2 | 0.05 | 3 | 0.07 |
| 15 Parasitic diseases | 2 | 0.05 | | |
| 16 Pericarditis | 2 | 0.05 | | |
| 17 Miscellaneous | 127 | 30.20 | | |
| **Totals** | **873** | **20.8** | **(3332)** | **(79.2)** |
| Per cent of total kill | 0.19 | | 0.7 | |

**Table 21.3** SHEEP. Reasons for carcase condemnations, N. Ireland, 1995.

Sheep kill: 637356
Condemnations: Total: 4107 (0.64% of kill)
Carcases: 813 (19.8% of total condemnations; 0.13% of kill)
Parts: 3294 (80.2% of total condemnations; 0.52% of kill)

| Reason | Carcases | % of total | Parts | % of total |
|---|---|---|---|---|
| 1 Oedema | 118 | 2.9 | 11 | 0.3 |
| Pneumonia/pleurisy | 118 | 2.9 | 11 | 0.3 |
| 2 Emaciation | 114 | 2.8 | | |
| 3 Arthritis | 113 | 2.8 | 2086 | 50.8 |
| 4 Fever/septicaemia | 111 | 2.7 | | |
| 5 Abscesses/pyaemia | 66 | 1.6 | 605 | 14.7 |
| 6 Imperfect bleeding | 21 | 0.5 | 157 | 3.8 |
| 7 Peritonitis | 19 | 0.5 | | |
| Contamination | 19 | 0.5 | 48 | 1.2 |
| 8 Nephritis/nephrosis | 12 | 0.3 | | |
| Uraemia | 12 | 0.3 | | |
| 10 Bruising | 9 | 0.2 | 273 | 6.6 |
| 11 Parasitic diseases | 6 | 0.15 | | |
| Tumours | 6 | 0.15 | | |
| 12 Decomposition | 6 | 0.15 | 5 | 0.1 |
| 13 Miscellaneous | 63 | 15.3 | 38 | 0.9 |
| **Totals:** | **813** | **19.80** | **(3294)** | **80.2** |
| Per cent of total kill | 0.13 | | 0.52 | |

**Table 21.4** PIGS. Reasons for carcase condemnations, N. Ireland, 1995.

| | | |
|---|---|---|
| Total kill | | 1 040 888 |
| Condemnations: | Total: | 15 288 (1.50% of kill) |
| | Carcases: | 6766 (44.3% of total condemnations; 0.7% of kill) |
| | Parts: | 8522 (55.7% of total condemnations; 0.8% of kill) |

| Reason | Carcases | % of total | Parts | % of total |
|---|---|---|---|---|
| 1 Abscesses/pyaemia | 2485 | 16.3 | 2259 | 14.8 |
| 2 Arthritis | 1086 | 7.1 | 5115 | 3.50 |
| 3 Pneumonia/pleurisy | 617 | 4.0 | | |
| 4 Fever/septicaemia | 514 | 3.4 | | |
| 5 Peritonitis | 390 | 2.6 | | |
| 6 Imperfect bleeding | 122 | 0.8 | | |
| 7 Bruising | 42 | 0.3 | 894 | 5.8 |
| 8 Oedema | 38 | 0.2 | | |
| 9 Emaciation | 37 | 0.2 | | |
| 10 Contamination | 26 | 0.2 | 60 | 0.4 |
| 11 Pericarditis | 21 | 0.1 | | |
| 12 Nephritis/nephrosis | 15 | 0.1 | | |
| 13 Uraemia | 15 | 0.1 | | |
| 14 Tumours | 13 | 0.09 | | |
| 15 Miscellaneous | 1345 | 8.80 | 213 | 1.4 |
| **Totals** | **6766** | **44.30** | **(8522)** | **55.7** |
| Per cent of total kill | 0.65 | | 0.82 | |

### Cattle

*Generalised oedema, fever/septicaemia* and *abscesses/pyaemia* continued to be a major cause of total carcase condemnations with *bruising* the main reason for seizure of parts of carcases.

*Contamination* did not result in total carcase condemnations but was a significant cause of partial condemnation and even more so of offal, an indication that the standard of cleanliness of livestock presented for slaughter leaves a lot to be desired.

*Fascioliasis*, affecting 31.6% of the total kill, is still a serious source of loss of edible liver, as well as of loss of condition, deaths and abortions in cattle. If the liver condemnations classed as 'cirrhosis' are added, the incidence of liver fluke becomes 34.2%.

*Neoplasia*, mainly as enzootic bovine leukosis, was responsible for the seizure of 35 carcases and numerous organs, revealing an incidence of 0.04 of the total animals slaughtered.

*Tuberculosis* was responsible for the seizure of 36 carcases and 76 parts besides being encountered in many organs – an indication of the difficulty experienced in its total eradication.

### Sheep

Oedema, pneumonia/pleurisy, emaciation, arthritis, fever/septicaemia and abscesses/pyaemia caused most condemnation.

### Pigs

In terms of whole-carcase condemnations, oedema, pneumonia/pleurisy, emaciation, arthritis and fever/septicaemia are the major causes of pigmeat loss. But when partial condemnations are taken into account, the most serious condition is undoubtedly arthritis. Abscesses and pyaemia, resulting from wounds of various types with resulting infection, are an indication that attention should be paid to proper handling and sterile injection methods.

*When compared with the condemnations recorded in Northern Ireland in 1954–55 (Gracey, 1960), the causes, apart from tuberculosis – an important disease in cattle and pigs at that time – are virtually the same today.*

Faecal contamination was responsible for considerable loss of offal, resulting from transference of dirt from hides/fleeces/skins and the possible rupture of stomachs and intestines during evisceration.

It is interesting to note that the highest rate of carcase meat condemnation takes place in pigs, with the least in sheep, and cattle assuming an intermediate position, surely a reflection of respective husbandry methods.

## Poultry disease statistics

Yogaratnam (1995) analysed the causes of carcase rejection at a poultry processing plant in England receiving approximately 3,365 million birds from 87 broiler units in 1992. Carcase rejection rates of 3% or more were recorded in birds from 13.2% of the rearing houses distributed among 48% of the growing units. Higher rejection rates occurred in the units with an average flock size of over 100 000 birds and from rearing houses of more than 30 000 birds.

The main causes of condemnation were dead on arrival, disease and miscellaneous conditions, the most common disease being *coli septicaemia* (Tables 21.5, 21.6).

**Table 21.5** Reasons for rejection of broiler carcases (Yogaratnam, 1995).

| Cause | % of total slaughter |
|---|---|
| Dead on arrival | 0.24 |
| Disease conditions | 1.57 |
| Miscellaneous conditions | 0.28 |
| **Total** | **2.09** |

**Table 21.6** Reasons for rejection of broiler carcases from farms with high rejection rates. (Yogaratnam, 1995).

| Disease | % of total rejects |
|---|---|
| Pericarditis/perihepatitis/air sacculitis | 42.80 |
| Septicaemia/toxaemia | 29.63 |
| Emaciation | 19.45 |
| Ascites | 5.91 |
| Hydropericardium/pericarditis | 1.01 |
| Skin lesions | 0.62 |
| Joint lesions | 0.31 |
| Jaundice | 0.16 |
| Tumours | 0.11 |
| **Total** | **100.00** |

The high rate of birds found dead on arrival was ascribed to severe stress occasioned by rough methods of catching and transportation. The use of mechanical harvesters for catching and modular systems for transport have been shown to reduce this high rate and subsequent downgrading of carcases. Mechanical harvesters, however, are only suitable for use in relatively large poultry houses.

Coli septicaemia, which includes pericarditis, perihepatitis and air sacculitis, the most common cause of condemnation, accounted for almost 43%.

Diseases of the musculoskeletal system are an important economic and welfare problem in broilers, as evidenced by the percentage of joint lesions (0.31%) and emaciation (19.45%) due to inability to feed. Leg weakness probably also contributes to the development of hock burn and breast blisters.

Fluid pericarditis (1.01%) is a septicaemia which may be caused by a variety of microorganisms, including *S. enteritidis*.

Yogaratnam estimates, based on these findings, that the British broiler industry is currently losing £16.5 million annually because of disease.

## Use of abattoir data in epidemiology

The use of pathological data from meat plants can be used to evaluate the epidemiological aspects of certain diseases (see above).

In Northern Ireland, a recent study (Goodall *et al.*, 1993) examined the monthly percentage condemnations in slaughter pigs due to pneumonia and pleurisy for each of the 21 years since 1969. Combining the data with a meteorological database, it was shown that while there was no consistent seasonal pattern in the percentage of lung condemnations, in general maximum levels occurred in midsummer and minimum levels in midwinter. Predictable seasonal patterns were found for all the major weather variables. The average monthly air temperature correlated in most of the 21 years with the percentage of lung condemnations, this being possibly due to the increased levels of ammonia and dust in pig houses. A decrease in lung condemnations between 1979 and 1984 may have been due to the introduction of new antibiotics. Between 1985 and 1989, however, there was a significant increase in lung condemnations which corresponded with the increased identifications of *Actinobacillus (Haemophilus) pleuropneumoniae* in Northern Ireland, a situation which also obtained elsewhere in the United Kingdom.

## IDENTIFICATION AND REGISTRATION OF ANIMALS

In the European Union, the minimum requirements for the identification and registration of animals are contained in Council Directive 92/102/EEC of 27 November 1992 for the purposes of:

1. Veterinary and zootechnical checks in intra-Community trade in certain live animals and products.
2. Veterinary checks on animals entering the Community from Third Countries.
3. Management of certain Community Aid agriculture schemes.
4. Rapid and efficient exchange of information between Member States.
5. Keeping of records of animals on holdings and records of dealings.
6. *Rapid and accurate tracing of animals.*

The Directive refers primarily to *cattle*, the marking of sheep, pigs, goats and buffalo being left to a later date.

(The relevant legislation for Great Britain is the Bovine Animals (Records, Identification and Movement) Order 1995.)

### Registration and identification requirements

**ARTICLE 3** Up-to-date list of all holdings with details of species of animals, keepers and marks. Exceptions: Holdings with only 3 sheep or 3 goats or 1 pig kept for own use or consumption.

*Holdings* include farms, markets, slaughterhouses, showgrounds, zoos and city farms.

**ARTICLE 4** Register of all cattle and pigs with records of all births, deaths (except for pigs) and movements.

Register of all sheep and goats and their movements.

**ARTICLE 5** *Identification marks*:

- To be applied before animals leave holding.
- Must not be removed or replaced without competent authority permission.
- Illegible or lost marks must be replaced with new approved marks and so recorded in register.
- Ear tags to be approved, tamper-proof, easy to read, incapable of re-use and animal-welfare-friendly.

**Cattle** All cattle born after 1 October 1994 must have a tag in the right ear within 36 hours of birth for dairy calves and 30 days for other calves or when the calf is moved off the holding of origin if earlier.

The code consists of a country code, e.g. UK for United Kingdom, herd mark and a five-digit individual number for each animal. The total number of characters must not exceed 14.

**Cattle records** Information required: date of birth, death, movement or ear tag loss, ear tag number, breed, age, sex, dam's official identification. Replacement ear tag number (if necessary). Premises from which moved with name and address of person from whom delivery was taken. Premises to which moved with name and address of person taking delivery.

Records to be kept for 10 years and made available to authorised inspectors on request.

For movements to a market or slaughterhouse, a movement document (to travel with the animals) must be completed containing the farmer's name and address, address of destination, date of movement and each animal's ear tag number.

**Pigs** Pigs require some form of identification, e.g. a paint mark, a tattoo (including slapmark tattoos) or an ear tag for every movement. This mark must be recorded in the on-farm movement record and on the movement document. Pigs for export require an ear tag or tattoo bearing the country code and the herd mark as well as an individual number.

**Pig Records** All off-farm movements require a movement document which in the UK will act as a licence under the Movement and Sale of Pigs Order. Details of the health status of the pigs is required along with the number to be moved, their description, ID marks and addresses of premises from which and to which moved.

**Sheep and goats** All holdings with sheep and goats are now registered on a central record. They must be marked in such a way that holding of origin can be traced. On export they must be marked with a tag or tattoo indicating country of origin and flock of origin.

Although EC Directive 92/102 requires all sheep and goats to be permanently marked with an ear tag or tattoo for movements within Great Britain, a national system of identification is allowed as an alternative to permanent marking.

**Information required** Total number of sheep and goats on holding to be recorded annually, the number of female sheep and goats over 12 months of age or which have given birth and all movements of sheep or goats, stating the holding of origin, destination, identifying mark and date of movement.

**Marking of sheep and goats** It is not necessary to mark sheep and goats until they leave the holding of origin, except for export when ear tags or tattoos are necessary. These require the country code, e.g. UK for United Kingdom, and the flock mark allocated by the local Animal Health Office, e.g. UK AH 1234. For tags and individual numbers, a P must be inserted between the flock mark and the individual number to avoid confusion with cattle which carry a similar code.

For a national system of identification for movements within GB, it is proposed that sheep and goats be marked with an ear tag, tattoo, horn brand, paint mark or combination. A movement document giving details of date of movement, address from and to which the animals are moving, number of animals and identifying marks has been proposed subject to approval by the European Commission.

**Sheep and goat records** Information required: Annual stock take, e.g. at tupping, dipping or shearing. Number of sheep eligible for premium payments. Records must be kept for 3 years, and following permanent movement off the holding, for a further 3 years.

#### ARTICLE 10

The possibility of introducing *electronic identification* to be decided by the European Commission not later than 31 December 1996 in the light of progress achieved by the ISO.

### Purposes of identification

1. *Disease control*

The present system of ID of cattle was introduced for this specific purpose, mainly in relation to the eradication of bovine tuberculosis and brucellosis.

An essential element in the control of any animal disease is the need to quickly identify the origin of the animal(s), in-contacts and any premises through which it (they) may have passed. Foot-and-mouth disease and classical swine fever are two conditions of importance in this connection.

Efficient animal identification allows tracing forwards and backwards in establishing the origin of disease outbreaks and their dissemination. Systematic screening using laboratory tests is made possible.

Animals which have been vaccinated in national programmes can quickly be identified.

Animal identification is necessary where import controls operate to prevent the introduction of exotic diseases. This becomes even more important with the advent of the European Single Market and the abolition of border controls, the latter being regarded by many experts as an unduly hasty decision. A measure of the amazing spread of certain exotic diseases is the current presence in Europe of rabies, contagious bovine pleuropneumonia, African horse sickness and African swine fever – diseases which were previously confined to Africa or Asia.

2. *Individual herd health and performance*

A reliable system of recording histories of animals and groups of animals is essential for a successful herd health programme.

At present most breeding programmes in all species are carried out in a haphazard manner. Selection of sires is mainly based on production performance, e.g. 2000 gallons (10 000 litres) in first lactations of dams and daughters for dairy bulls. In all species there is an emphasis on phenotype rather than genotype. Yet many animal diseases are known to be hereditary in origin and it is likely that more will be added to the list in the future.

Animal health and production data considered necessary to assess herd performance can be collected with an efficient

ID system linked to a computer-based recording system.

A proper tamper-proof system of identification which would overcome current defects was recommended by the Wilson Committee in 1990, set up to review existing systems of cattle identification, milk recording and genetic evaluation in the United Kingdom. They reported as follows:

> The unique identification of every (bovine) animal in the United Kingdom is fundamental to livestock improvement. The identity of the animal is the primary source of information for all subsequent records. At the farm level, this unique identification is vital for management and disease control purposes, but at the genetic level animal identification is required to enable the data from all related cattle to be assembled and collated so that breeding values can be ascribed to cows and bulls alike.
>
> The ability to identify every animal uniquely in the country would have enormous benefits for the cattle industry. It would enable a 'log book' to be maintained for every animal so that each time an event occurred (such as sale to another farmer) the database could be updated. Such a procedure would enable the protection of the industry from adverse criticism to disease outbreak or potential human health risk. Such a methodology would provide the industry with an unprecedented tool for animal management, animal health and animal movement control. In the wider EEC context it would reduce fraud. For this reason, we consider it probable that a harmonised system of animal identification and animal travel documentation will become mandatory by EEC regulations.
>
> For the reasons stated above, a *database* containing all information on all UK cattle would be a national asset and would perform many functions 'for the public good'; it would contain information of value not only for individual farmers but also for the whole of the cattle industry and the consuming public.
>
> (See Wilson Committee Report 1991, below.)

### 3. *Public health*

EC Council Directive 86/469 concerning the examination of animals and fresh meat for the presence of residues and EC Directive 85/358 which deals with substances having a hormonal and thyrostatic action provide for sampling at the farm and the abattoir.

The need for efficient identification is obvious in this area and in others such as zoonoses, meat inspection findings, etc., otherwise any subsequent legal action could be jeopardised.

### 4. *Meat inspection*

An important source for the promotion of public health and animal health is the meat plant where accurate diagnoses are made.

Disease and injury in the food animals cause huge economic losses throughout the world besides being responsible for serious food-poisoning outbreaks in man.

Information on the extent of many of these losses is provided in many countries, e.g. Australia, Canada, Denmark, Holland, New Zealand, Northern Ireland, Sweden and the USA.

As yet, however, full use is not being made of disease data retrieval and feedback to producers to control animal disease and prevent zoonoses. Still less information is available from the farm to assist the meat inspectorate in the diagnosis of disease and carcase judgement.

### 5. *Animal welfare*

Animal welfare violations of whatever form would be more conclusively dealt with were efficient animal ID available.

### 6. *Trade, consumer confidence and fraud*

Efficient animal identification can be considered as the key to unlocking all the information required for a successful and profitable producer–retailer–consumer relationship.

It can be utilised by the producer to improve his efficiency, by the marketeer to enhance his business, by the retailer as part of his quality assurance and by the statutory bodies that oversee the whole marketing cycle.

Fraud, which is rife in certain parts of the animal and food industry, not least in the European Union, should be reduced, along with the trade in unfit meat, with the introduction of tamper-proof ID linked to bar coding and trace-back systems.

## Current systems of identification and limitations

These vary to some extent in the different species and include metal and plastic ear tags, plastic leg and tail bands, freeze marks and hoof brands, sketch cards and passports (cattle), marking aerosols and paints, horn branding and ear notching (sheep), ear tags, slap imprints and tattoos (pigs).

All these methods are considered unsatisfactory for the following reasons:

1. Liability to damage.
2. Ease of removal, either accidental or malicious.
3. Difficulty of reading, especially when damaged or dirty.
4. Limitation to a single number, or number plus letter.
5. Confusion liable between digits, e.g. 3 and 8, 4 and 6.
6. Exclusive use on the farm – of limited value when animal leaves the farm.
7. Liability to infection, especially with metal ear tags.
8. Possible welfare problem with insertion of tag into sensitive appendage, with or without subsequent infection.
9. Use of ear contraindicated because of resistance by animal.
10. Being currently under producer control, liable to misuse.

## Electronic identification of livestock

The development of an efficient, tamper-proof *electronic system of animal identification* (envisaged in Directive 92/102/EEC) providing positive identification with name of owner and address, and (for cattle) number of animal, HB number, date of birth, sex, breed, name of dam and sire is considered essential for disease control and genetic improvement purposes as well as the prevention of fraud.

Such a system must be combined with a record of animal movements.

Automatic identification technology has made great strides in less than 20 years and is utilised in many different industries, e.g. retailing, warehousing and distribution. The bar code used for the pricing of individual retail items is the main technology, but many other techniques are available such as magnetic stripe, radiofrequency (RF) tagging, machine vision, smart cards and voice recognition. All these systems are capable of feeding information from a microchip into a computer.

The essential components of an electronic ID system are a means of encoding the required information on a *microchip* and applying it (in this case to an animal), and a *reader/scanner* and *software* to feed the data to a *computer*. In the case of live identification, it is envisaged for practical purposes that with an implanted microchip or transponder, a hand-held reader/scanner with a visual display unit (VDU) will be adequate, except where specialised information is required.

The reader/scanner is applied to, or reasonably close to, the encoded microchip, which is usually implanted subcutaneously in the animal. Where a greater distance from the animal is necessary, a RF tag is used. In this case the tag contains a transponder as a tiny transmitter/receiver which sends out signals automatically when the correct interrogation is received. These RF tags have many applications in industry, healthcare and farming, for example, for automatic feeding of cattle, poultry and pigs.

The injectable *microchip* (semiconductor transponder) consists of a tiny transmitter and antenna. When the scanner or read-out unit is brought close to the transponder, the latter is charged with energy and transmits its ID number on the scanner's display unit. For the implanted chip to function properly it must be hermetically-sealed and cause no reaction in the tissues or discomfort to the animal. It is vital that the transponder does not migrate or break in the tissues. It is also essential that all microchips are retrieved from the carcases on completion of recording.

## Cattle databases and passports

Several countries, notably Denmark and Northern Ireland, already possess systems of bovine identification with details of movements (passports) recorded on a central government computerised database. Any deficiency lies in the actual identification of the individual animal.

In the UK, the Wilson Committee advocated in 1991 that a central Cattle Data Centre (CDC) be established in the United Kingdom with the purpose of linking together and coordinating:

**(a)** All existing cattle databases.

**(b)** Cattle identification on a unique number basis.

**(c)** Cattle ancestry and its validation.

**(d)** All milk recording to the International Committee for Animal Recording (ICAR) standards, including DIY recording.

**(e)** Beef recording.

**(f)** Genetic evaluation of cattle.

**(g)** Linear assessment of cattle.

## REFERENCES

Blamire, R. V. *et al.* (1970) *Vet. Rec.* **97**, 243.
Blamire, R. V. *et al.* (1980) *Vet. Rec.* **106**, 195.
Christiansen, K. H. and Hellstrom, J. S. (1979). *Proc. 2nd Int. Symp. Veterinary Epidemiology and Economics*, p. 47.
Cuthbertson, J. C. (1983) *Vet. Rec.* **112**, 219.
*Farmer's Weekly* (1984) 3 August, p. 46.
Flesja, K. I. and Ulvesaeter, H. O. (1980) *Acta Vet. Scand.* **74** (Suppl. 74).
Goodall, E. *et al.* (1993) *Vet. Rec.* **132**, 11–14.
Gracey, J. F. (1960) *Survey of Livestock Diseases in Northern Ireland*. Belfast: HMSO.
Hill, J. R. (1988) *Meat Inspection Records and Their Use. A Need for Change?* Potters Bar, Herts: Humane Slaughter Association.
McIlroy, S. G. *et al.* (1988) *Computers and Electronics in Agriculture*, Vol. 3, p. 147. Amsterdam: Elsevier Science.
McIlroy, S.G. *et al.* (1989) *Vet. Rec.* **125**, 79.
McIlroy, S. G. *et al.* (1990). *Prevent. Vet. Med.* **9**, 27.
Pratt, J. H. (1979) *Meat Hygienist* **16**, 25.
Rimmer, H. (1989) *Meat Inspection Records. Their Use in Promoting Animal Welfare*. Potters Bar: Humane Slaughter Association.
Roe, R. T. (1979) *Proc. 2nd Int. Symp. Veterinary Epidemiology and Economics*, pp. 26–34.
Skovgaard, N. (1990) *Proc. Round Table Conf., World Association for Veterinary Food Hygiene. The Scientific Basis for Harmonising Trade in Red Meat* (Hannan, J. and Collins, J. D., eds), Dublin.
The Wilson Committee Report (1990) Submitted January 1991. Professor P.N. Wilson, Chairman.
Yogaratnam, V. (1995) *Vet. Rec.* **137**, 215–217.
Zachrau, R. (1992) Danish Meat Research Institute Manuscript no. 1016E.

# Appendix I
# By-products of the UK Meat Industry

| Raw by-products | Processed by-products | Use |
|---|---|---|
| Edible raw blood | Plasma and red cells | Adhesive for sausages, etc., blood sausages or pudding |
| Inedible raw blood | Blood meal | Adhesive for livestock and poultry feed, petfood, fertiliser, glues, foam fire extinguishers |
| | Blood albumen | Leather preparation, mordant |
| Edible raw fat | Edible fat | Frying purposes (suet, lard) |
| | Oleo oil | Shortening |
| | Oleostearin | Candy, chewing gum |
| | Cracklings | Petfood, meat meal |
| Inedible raw fat | Inedible fat | Adhesives for livestock and poultry feed, lubricants, soap candles, glycerin, biodegradable oils, liquid detergents |
| Inedible raw material, mixed | Inedible fat | *See above* |
| Condemned material and whole condemned carcases | Meat and bone meal | Livestock and poultry feed |
| Raw bone classified as edible | Edible fat | Shortening |
| | Bone pieces | Bone gelatin, bone meal, tallow, petfood |
| Raw bone classified as inedible | Inedible fat | *See above* |
| | Bone pieces | Bone glue, bone meal, buttons, handles |
| Cattle feet | Neatsfoot oil | Fine lubricants |
| | Feet and meal | Bone meal, tallow, glues, gelatin, 'dog chews', buttons, cow-heel jelly |
| Sheep feet | Meal | Tallow |
| | Feet | Possible edible use |
| Pig feet | Feet | Edible use |
| | Meal | Fertilisers, glues, gelatin |
| Horns and hooves | Extracted protein | Foam fire extinguishers |
| | Meal | Mixed with livestock feed, fertilisers |
| | Horns, hooves | Buttons, handles, etc. |
| Stomach (cattle) | | |
| Rumen | Edible tripe | Edible use |
| | (Rendered) | Petfood, meat meal |
| Reticulum | Edible tripe | Edible use |
| | | Petfood, meat meal |
| Omasum | | Petfood, meat meal |
| Abomasum | | Petfood, meat meal, rennet (from suckling calves) |

| Raw by-products | Processed by-products | Use |
|---|---|---|
| Stomach (sheep) | | |
| Rumen | Edible tripe | Edible use, haggis casings |
| Reticulum, omasum, abomasum | | Petfood, meat meal |
| Stomach (pig) | | Processing and manufacture, petfood, pepsin, haggis casings, chitterlings |
| Hide (cattle) | Prewashed hide | Leather goods, collagen casings |
| | Hair | Felt, upholstery |
| | Trimmings (inedible) | Fertilisers |
| Hide (sheep) | Pelt | Woolskins, rugs, clothing, chamois leathers |
| | Wool | Textiles, upholstery |
| Hide (pig) | Tanned skin | Leather goods |
| | Gelatin | Jellied food products |
| Large intestines (cattle and sheep) | Rendered | Meat meal |
| Colon, caecum, rectum (pig) | Edible use | Chitterlings |
| | Rendered | Meat meal |
| Small intestines (cattle) | | Casings, surgical sutures, heparin |
| Small intestines (sheep) | | Meat meal, casings, surgical sutures, tennis racket strings |
| | Rendered | Meat meal |
| Small intestines (pig) | | Casings, heparin |
| Oesophagus | | Casings, meat meal |
| Trachea | | Meat meal |
| Mammary gland (cattle) | | Meat meal, petfood, pharmaceuticals |
| Mammary gland (pig) | | Meat meal |
| Cheek and head trimmings (cattle and pigs) | | Meat products, sausages |
| Lungs | | Petfood, heparin |
| Tongue | | As tongue, processing |
| Brains | | Edible |
| Heart | | Edible |
| Liver | | Edible, pharmaceuticals |
| Diaphragm (cattle) (thick and thin skirt) | | Edible, processing |
| Spleen | | As spleen, petfood, processing |
| Tail | | As tail |
| Kidney (cattle) | | As kidney, processing |
| Kidney (sheep) | | As kidney |
| Kidney (pig) | | As kidney |
| Bladder | | Meat meal, tallow (not pig) |
| Gall | | Cleaning agent in leather manufacture, paints, dyes, pharmaceuticals |
| Gallstones | | Pharmaceuticals |
| Spinal cord (cattle) | | Meat meal, pharmaceuticals |
| Genital organs | | Meat meal, pharmaceuticals |
| Pancreas (cattle and pigs) | | Insulin |
| Pituitary, thymus, thyroid (cattle) | | Pharmaceuticals |

# Index

**Note:** Page numbers in **bold type** refer to main references.


abamectin, 315
abattoir, 5, 166
  admission of diseased or injured animals, 192–3
  animals arriving dead, 195
  data, epidemiology, 734–5
  emergency slaughter, 194
  fever, 416, 608–9
  management, 181–2
  small units, 82–3
abdomen nodes, 38–9
abomasal ulcer disease, 466
abomasum, 24, 465
abortion, 461, 489, 532, 600, 609
abrasions, 409
abscess, 278, 453–5, 499, 500
  formation, 427
  judgement, 455
  pigs, 253
acariasis, 690–1
acceleration concussion, 202
acceptable daily intake (ADI), 300, 302, 303
accidents, 410
  BSE, 575–6
acetonaemia in cows, 700–1
acetone, 66
acetylcholinesterase (AChE), 714
*Achromobacter*, 346
acid treatments, 237
acids, 712
*Acinetobacter*, 106, 346
*Acinetobacteria*, 104
acne, 428
actinobacillosis *see* actinomycosis
*Actinobacillus*, 389
*Actinobacillus (Haemophilus) pleuropneumoniae*, 735
*Actinomyces* pyogenes, 253, 254, 454
*Actinomyces* spp., 389
actinomycosis, 493, 506–7
activated sludge process, 141
actomyosin, 61
additives, 300
adenosine triphosphate (ATP), 61, 110, 115, 159, 160, 186, 377
  bioluminescence, 377–8
  detection system, 379
  monitoring, 377
adhesive tape, 342
adrenal cortex, 47
adrenal (suprarenal) bodies, 47–8
adrenaline, 7, 47
adrenocorticotrophic hormone (ACTH), 185
*Aedes camptorhynchus*, 606
*Aedes lineatopennis*, 596
aerobic digestion, 141
aerobic mesophilic count (AMC), 357
aerobic plate count (APC), 357
aflatoxicosis, 351
aflatoxins, 318
African horse sickness (AHS), 554–5
African pig disease, 555–6
African swine fever (ASF), 555–6
African trypanosomiasis, 633
agar contact or impression, 360
agar plate
  methods, 357
  streaking with spores, 403
agar plate counts (APCs), 357
agar sausage, 342
agar slope or slant cultures, 364
age determination by dentition, 51–3
age guide, 22
ageing of meat, 126
Agriculture Act 1970, 263
Agriculture (Miscellaneous Provisions) Act 1968, 16, 171
agrochemicals, 313
air chillers, 272
air circulation rates, 110
air emboli, 443
air sampling, 362
alarm reaction, 185
*Alcaligenes*, 346
algae, 633–4, 718–19
alimentary tract, **464–70**
  tuberculosis, 547
alkalis, 712
alkaptonuria, 438
alkyl phenol ethoxylates (APEOs), 161
allergies, 410–11
allotriophagia, 459
Alpine, 14
*Alternaria*, 106
aluminium, 145
*Amblyomma* spp., 693
American trypanosomiasis, 633–4
*Amidostomum anseris*, 284
ammonia, 109, 140, 712
amoebiasis, 616–17
ampicillin, 306
amyloidosis, 439–40
anabena flos-aqua, 719
anabolic, 309
anaemia, 440–1, 479
anaerobic digestion, 141
anaesthesia, 205–6
  electric shock, 208
  electrical, 209
  gas concentration, 208
anaphylaxis, 422
anaplasia, 444
anaplasmosis, 604–5
anatipestifer infection, 279
anatomy, **19–55**
  descriptive terms, 19–20
androgen, 7, 309
androstenone, 67
aneurysm, 441
animal-based proteins, 58
animal behaviour, 84
Animal Disease and Protection Act, 676
Animal Health Act 1981, 173, 195
animal identification, 191, 245, **735–9**
Animal Products (Examination for Residues and Maximum Residue Limits) Regulations 1997, 379
animal registration, **735–9**
animal waste *see* waste; waste disposal
animal welfare, 171–2, 737
animal welfarists, 4
Animals (Scientific Procedures) Act 1986, 195
Animals (Sea Transport) Order 1930, 177
anorexia, 459
ante-mortem inspection, 84, **189–92**, 243–4
  poultry, 272–3
  records, 192
anterior mediastinal nodes, 38
anterior nodes, 40
anthelmintics, 314–16
  maximum residue levels, 315
anthrax, 195, 249, 411, 507–9
  in man, 509
  procedure, 509
anthrax blood/transudate smears, 372–3
antibacterials, 309
  residues, 402
antibiotics, 305, 306, 308
  residues, 402
  resistance, 331
antibodies, 310, 423
antigens, 423
antimicrobials, 299, 305–8, 715
  statutory survey results, 308
  tests, 307–8
antioxidants, 125
ANTU, 717
aphagia, 459
aphthous fever, **583–7**
aplasia, 444
apoptosis, 432
appendicular skeleton, 21
apramycin, 306
apron of chain-mail, 410
arachnoid mater, 45
Argasidae, 693
argon, 212–13
  anaesthesia, 205
arizonosis, turkeys, 281
arsenic, 316, 713
arteriosclerosis, 441–2
arteritis, 441
arthology, 20–3
arthritis, 254, 493–4
arthropod parasites, **688–92**
Arthus reaction, 410
ascarid worms, 247
*Ascaris suum*, 94, 643
*Ascarops strongylina*, 642
ascites, 285
aseptic canning, 116
ASPCA restrainer pen, 218
aspergillosis, 283, 610
*Aspergillus*, 94, 106
*Aspergillus flavus*, 318, 351, 610
*Aspergillus fumigatus*, 283, 610
*Aspergillus niger*, 610
*Aspergillus parasiticus*, 318
ass, tapeworms, 659
asthma, 410
atherosclerosis, 442
atomic absorption spectrometry, 316
atrophic rhinitis, 509–10

atrophy, 444
Aujeszky's disease, 556–7
Australia
  *Cysticercus bovis* inspection procedure, 677
  meat inspection records, 729
autoimmune disease, 423
autolysis, 344
automatic pelt removal, 92
automatic stunning devices, 212
autonomic nervous system, 45–6
avermectins, 314
avian epidemic tremor, 15
avian influenza, 277
axial skeleton, 21
axillary node, 38
axon, 44
azoturia, 701–2

B lymphocytes, 423
*Babesia*, 397, 618, 625
babesiosis, 617–18
bacillary haemoglobinuria, 514–15
bacillary white diarrhoea (BWD), 279
*Bacillus*, 106, 328, 345
*Bacillus anthracis*, 389, 411, 508
*Bacillus cereus*, 335–6, 381
*Bacillus subtilis*, 307
back bleeding, 214
back-up stunner, 211
bacon
  fat, 348
  new dry cure, 106
  production, **104–6**
  smoking, 106
  traditional dry cure, 105–6
bacteraemia, 194, 451
bacteria, 140, 340, 421, 462, 464
  cured product, 106
  in canned foods, 121–2
bacterial diseases, 465, 467
bacterial poultry diseases, **277–83**
bacterial residues, 709
bacterial resistance, 422
bacteriological examination, 247, **339–44**, 373–4
bacteriological monitoring, 256
bacteriological standards, 343–4
bacteriological test, 353
balancing tanks, 141
balantidial dysentery, 618–19
balantidiosis, 618–19
*Balantidium coli*, 94
Balkan grippe, 416
Balkan influenza, 416
banned substances, 303
barbone, 537
barcode system, 728
barking, 286
bedding, 166
beef
  cleansing, 237
  measle, 672
  production systems, 6–7
  ripening, 71
  sides, tenderstretch method of hanging, 72
  slaughter, cutting and packing, 91
  tapeworm, **669–74**
Belgian Blue, 5
benign theileriosis of cattle, 627
benzylpenicillin, 306
Berkshire, 12
*Besnoitia* spp., 397
besnoitiosis, 619
best before date, 353–4
beta-adrenergic blocking agents, 7
beta-agonists, 7, 300, 311–12
  testing, 312
bighead in rams, 515
bilateral severance, 215
bile acids, 435
bile pigments, 434
bilharziasis, 686–7
bilirubin, 435
  test, 498
biochemical oxygen demand (BOD), 139–40, 161
biochemical tests, 366
biocidal active components, 149
biocide, 150, 168
biological tests, 56–7
biological treatment systems, 141
biosecurity, 15
birds, muscles, 50
bison, 6
bite marks, 188
black disease, 517
black pith, 433
black spot, 351
blackhead, 284
blackleg, 515
bladder, 41, 486–7
blastomycosis, 611–12
bleb, 428
bleeding, 199, 209, 212, 213
  area, 88
  cattle, 214–15
  efficiency, 216–17
  hygienic, 88
  imperfect, 456–7
  insufficient, 287
  trough, 88
blepharitis, 502
blight, 530
blister, 428
Blonde d'Aquitaine, 5
blood, 32–3, 362, 363, 479–80
  agar, 364
  by-products treatment, 133–4
  collection, 216
  diseases, **440–4**
  edible, 133–4
  inedible, 134
blood fluke, 485, 686–7
blood meal, drying, 134
blood platelets, 33
blood smears, 360, 400
blood vessels, 478–9
bloody scours, 542–3
bloom, 102
blue-eared pig disease, 557
blue tongue, 557–8
bluish-green moulds, 352
boar
  carcase, 54
  definition, 13
  odour, 67
  taint, 13
body temperature, 456
boiling test, 66
bolt velocity check, 204
bones, 20–3, 491–3
  by-products treatment, 135
  carcase, 22
  classification, 21
  marrow, 444
  protein, 58
  taint, 349
  tuberculosis, 548
*Boophilus*, 617
*Boophilus annulatus*, 617
*Boophilus* spp., 693
bootwash/apronwash facilities, 92
bootwashing equipment, 87
Border-Leicester, 9
*Bordetella*, 389
*Bordetella bronchiseptica*, 510
Borna disease, 580
*Borrelia burgdorferi*, 415
*Bos indicus*, 6
*Bos taurindicus*, 6
*Bos taurus*, 6
bot fly, 688–9
botulism, 518, 715
bovine
  congenital erythropoietic protoporphyria (BCEP), 436
  cysticercosis, **669–74**
  inspection procedures, 674
  farcy, 523–4
  foetus, 44
  herpesvirus 1 (BHV-1), 586
  hides, 135
  leukaemia virus (BLV), 579
  lymphosarcoma, 578–80
  malignant catarrh (BMC), 558
  nocardiosis, 523–4
  Offals (Prohibition) Regulations 1989, 564
  papular stomatitis, 558–9
  petechial fever, 605–6
  pleuropneumonia, 521–3
  viral diarrhoea (BVD), 576–7
  viral leukosis, 578–80
bovine spongiform encephalopathy (BSE), 75, 214, 244, 246, 247, 410, **559–76**
  accidents, 575–6
  advisory notes for farmers, 575–6
  breeding, 576
  calving, 576
  checks, 564
  chronology, **565–74**
  handling of suspect animals, 576
  hygiene, 576
  initial examination of suspect cases, 564
  number of cases, 560
  post-mortem examinations, 564–75
  precautions to be taken by meat plant personnel, 575
  precautions to be taken by persons handling known or suspected cases, 564–75
  research, 576
  treatments, 576
bowel oedema, 520
brachial node, 38
bradsot, 515–16
Brahman, 6
brain, 45, 500
braxy, 515–16
breast blisters, 285
breeding strategy, 189
British Hampshire, 12
British Meat Survey (BMS), 304
British Saddleback, 12
*Brochothrix thermosphactum*, 348
broiler, 264, 265, 266, 268, 285
  carcase, 274
    rejection, 734
  definition, 15
  industry, 261
bromelin, 72
bromethalin, 717
bronchial nodes, 37, 41
bronchiolitis, 471
bronchitis, 471
bronchopneumonia, 179, 472
brown fat disease, 65
Brown Swiss, 5
browning, 106
*Brucella*, 389, 489
*Brucella abortus*, 411–12
*Brucella melitensis*, 412
*Brucella suis*, 412
brucellosis, 411–12, 510–11
  in man, 511
bruising, **187–9**, 254, 497–8
  and mixing of animals, 188
  incentives and education, 189
  internal ham, 216
  poultry, 284–5
  rabbits, 290
BSE *see* bovine spongiform encephalopathy (BSE)
*Bubalus bubalis*, 2, 5
bubonic plague, 554
buffalo, 2, 6
Building Regulations 1991, 78
bukoses, 479–80
bull, 6, 7
  beef, 7
  carcase, 53
  definition, 8
  viscera, 25

bulla, 428
bullock, 6
  carcase, 35, 53
  definition, 8
bunging
  cattle, 233
  technique, 254–5
*Bunostomum phlebotomum*, 638
*Bunostomum trigonocephalum*, 638
bursitis, 494
button ulcers, 542, 600
by-products treatment, **129–41**
  blood, 133–4
  bones, 135
  edible, 129
  fats, 130–1
  hides, 135–6
  inedible, 129
  intestines, 131–3, 133
  preliminary treatment, 140–1
  premises, 130
  processing, 130
  secondary treatment, 141
  skins, 135–6
  stomach, 131–3
byssinosis, 411

cadmium, 317, 713
Caisson disease, 443
calcification, 433
calcium, 703–4
calcium chloride-infused bovine muscle, 73
Calcofluor white/Fungifluor kit, 372
calf, 7
  age estimation, 459
  carcase, 54
  diphtheria, 535
  lymphosarcoma, 580
  omphalophlebitis, 254
  post-mortem examination, 250
  stomach, 24
  thymus, 47
*Callitroga hominivorax*, 691
CAMP (Christie, Atkins, Munch-Petersen) test, 369
*Campylobacter*, 104, 232, 252, 281–2, 324, 326, 328, 330–2, 383–4, 512
*Campylobacter jejuni*, 282, 332
campylobacteriosis, 281–2, 512
Canada
  *Cysticercus bovis* inspection procedure, 674–6
  meat inspection recording, 727–8
cancer, 3, 7
  *see also* tumour
candidamycosis, 612–13
candidiasis, 283, 612–13
candidosis, 612–13
Canicola fever, 413, 530–1
cannibalism, 286
canning, 72
  bacteria in, 121–2
  can manufacture, 118
  ham, 121
  meat, 120–1
  microbiological examination, 125
  operations, 119
  public health aspect, 124–5
  quality of containers, 125
  rust or damage, 124
  spoilage, 122–4
  traditional methodology, 117–18
  treatment of food, 118–19
Canpak system, 90
caprine pleuropneumonia, 521–3
Captive Birds Order 1976, 415
captive bolt pistol, 202, 203, 205, 211
car park, 98
carbamates, 714
carbohydrate, 60, 145, 147
carbon dioxide anaesthesia, 200, 205, 208, 212
carboxylic acids, 317
carcase
  bacteriological examination, **339–44**, 373–4
  boar, 54
  bones, 22
  broiler, 274, 734
  bull, 53
  bullock, 35, 53
  calf, 54
  cattle, 53, 250
  condemned, 191, 449
  contamination, 223, 255
  cow, 54
  deer, 17
  ewe, 54
  fevered, 287
  freezing, 108
  gilt, 55
  gimmer, 54
  goat, 55
  heifer, 53–4
  hog, 54–5
  horse, 55
  identification, 245–8
  immature, 458
  lamb, 10
  line dressing, 89
  neoplasms, 449
  ox, 55
  pig, 13, 54, 131
  ram, 54
  samples, 341
  sheep, 54, 55
  stamping, 247
  storage, 108
  testing, 310
  wether, 54
cardiac arrest, 199
cardiovascular system, 450, **475–80**
*Carica papaya*, 73
carotene, 64
caseous lymphadenitis, 512–14
caseous necrosis, 430
Cash instruments, 202
Cash penetrative stunners, 204
cast ewe, definition, 10
castrates, 6
castration, 7, 67
casualty animal, **192–4**
  decision on-farm, 193
  meat plant, 193–4
casualty slaughter, 192, 195
catarrhal fever, 558
catarrhal inflammation, 425
catch basins, 80
catecholamines, 47
cattle, **4–8**
  abscess formation, 454
  benign theileriosis of, 627
  bleeding, 214–15
  breeds, 5–6
  bunging, 233
  carcase, 53
  carcase condemnations, 732
  contamination, 733
  databases, 738–9
  dehairing, 226
  dressing, 230
  foot rot of, 534–5
  growth promoters, 7
  horns, 50
  identification, 245, 735
  lairage, 84–5
  meningoencephalitis of, 537–8
  mycoplasmal arthritis in, 521–2
  nematodes in, 638–40
  neural tissue embolism in, 204
  parasitic gastroenteritis of, 638–40
  passports, 738–9
  pneumonic pasteurellosis of, 538–9
  polyarthritis, 528
  post-mortem inspection, 248
  records, 735
  rectum, 233
  red dysentery in, 620–1
  registration, 735
  slaughter, 226
  stunning, 214–15
  tapeworms, 659
  tuberculosis, 545, 546, 548
Cattle Data Centre (CDC), 738
cattle grubs, 694–6
cattle lungworm, 657
cattle plague, 596–8
cattle tick fever, 617–18
CBPP *see* contagious bovine pleuropneumonia (CBPP)
CCPP *see* contagious caprine pleuropneumonia (CCPP)
cefquinone, 306
cell, 19
  injury and death, **429–32**
central nervous system (CNS), 44, 45, 501, 599
  tuberculosis, 548
cereal, 58
cerebellum, 45
cerebrum, 45
cervical abscess, 454
*Cervus canadensis*, 17
*Cervus elaphus*, 17
cestodes, 636, 637, 658–60
chabertiasis, 656
Chagas' disease, 632–4
Charolais, 5
cheese, 8, 14
chelation, 147–8
chemical agents, 422
chemical energy, 146
chemical oxygen demand (COD), 140, 161
chemical residues, **299–319**, 709, 711
  detection limit, 303
  legislation, 300–1
  maximum residue levels (MRLs), 302–3
  regulations, 301
  sample collection, 303–4
  sample handling, 305
  statutory surveillance programmes, 304–5
chemical spoilage, 123–4
chemical tests, 56, 352–3
chemical treatments, 237–8
chemiluminescence, 353
Chernobyl mark and release scheme, 721
Chernobyl power complex, 719
Cheviot, 8–9
chicken, 16
chicken anaemia agent (CAA), 276
chill rooms, 110
chilled meat, 406–7
chilling, 106, 108, 109, 111
  poultry, 271–2
*Chlamydia psittaci*, 414, 415
*Chlamydia* spp., 389–90
chlamydiae, 465, 467
chlamydiosis, 282, 414–15
chlorellosis, 719
chloride, 140
chlorinated hydrocarbons, 312
chlorine, 237, 272
chlorpromazine, 7
cholangiohepatitis, 285
cholangitis, 468
cholecalciferol, 717
cholecystitis, 468
cholera in turkeys, 278
chronic wasting disease (CWD), 559
*Chrysomia bezziana*, 691
Cincinnati-Boss (CB) pen, 218
circling disease, 531–3
circulatory system, 31–4
citrate utilisation test, 375
CJD Surveillance Unit (CJDSU), 563
classical histoplasmosis, 612
classical swine fever (CSF), 599–600
clean/healthy livestock production, **163–72**
cleaning
  chemical reactions, 147–8
  chemistry, 144–8
  energies, 146
  EU directives, 144

cleaning—*continued*
foam, 150–2
food plants, 143–4
gel, 152
manual, 150
monitoring, 158
physical reactions, 146–7
procedures, **156–8**
safety, 160–1
sequence, 156
spray, 152
time, 146
training, 160
Cleaning Schedule, 156
cleanliness testing, 159–60
cleansing-in-place (CIP), 147, 152–4
clearance rates for drugs, 299
clenbuterol, 7
clipping, 166
Cloisonné kidney, 434
closantel, 314, 315
clostridial cellulitis, 418
clostridial diseases, 514–19
*Clostridium*, 328, 330, 345, 390
*Clostridium botulinum*, 117, 124, 335, 381, 518, 710
*Clostridium nigrificans*, 124
*Clostridium novyi*, 517
*Clostridium oedematiens*, 683
*Clostridium perfringens*, 138, 278, 285, 326, 334, 381–2, 451, 516, 517
*Clostridium pufrefaciens*, 349–50
*Clostridium putrificum*, 350
*Clostridium septicum*, 278, 516
*Clostridium sporogenes*, 349
*Clostridium tetani*, 518
cloudy swelling, 430
cloxacillin, 306
coagulase test, 368
coagulative necrosis, 430
cobalt, 704
coccidia, 620
coccidioidal granuloma, 610–11
*Coccidioides immitis*, 610
coccidioidomycosis, 610–11
in man, 611
coccidiosis, 283, 289, 291, 620–1
Codex Alimentarius Commission, 108, 109, 125
cold shortening, 110
colibacillosis, 519–20
coliform
gastroenteritis, 520–1
infections, 279
colisepticaemia, 275
carcase rejection, 274
collagen, 50, 427
colony counts of mesophilic aerobes, 357
colony-forming unit (CFU), 357
colony morphology, 373
colour, 70, 71, 106, 124
comminuted meats, 68
Committee on the Medical Aspects of Food and Nutrition Policy (COMA), 2, 3
common cattle grub, 695
Communicable Disease Surveillance Centre (CDSC), 326
communication system, 98
Compact $CO_2$ Immobiliser, 206
complement fixation, 56, 415
compound light microscope, 380
concrete, 145
condemnation, 130, 136, 191, 253, 255, 449, 461, 480, 487, 491, 494, 499, 501, 502, 731–4, 736
condemned meat room, 96
condensation, 101
conditionally approved for human consumption, 255
conditioning (tenderising), **71–4**
congenital abnormalities, 422
congenital cysts, 429
congenital defects, 314, 471, 500
congenital malformations, 450
congenital photosensitisation, 702
Congo virus disease, 578
conjunctivitis, 502
connective tissue, 19, 50
proteins, 59
consciousness, assessment, 199
contagious agalactia, 490
of goats, 522–3
of sheep, 522–3
contagious bovine pleuropneumonia (CBPP), 421, 472, 521–3
contagious bovine pyelonephritis, 524
contagious caprine pleuropneumonia (CCPP), 521–3
contagious ecthyma, 412, 577–8
contagious equine metritis (CEM), 488
contagious opthalmia of cattle, sheep and goats, 606
contagious pustular dermatitis (CPD), 412–13, 577–8
contagious vulvo-vaginitis, 523
contamination, 155–6, **223–38**
carcase, 223, 255
chemical, 225, 321
chemical treatments, 237–8
deer, 295
dirty animal, 225–6
documentation, 240–1
equipment, 224
faecal, 163, 254–5
gastrointestinal tract, 233–5
methods of reducing, 225–35
monitoring faecal, 252
operatives, 224
poultry, 270, 286
prevention, 247
rabbits, 292
radioactive, **719–23**
slaughterline, 229
sources, 223
trimming, 237
utensils, 224
water, 225, 236
continuous powered system, 90
Control of Substances Hazardous to Health Regulations 1991 (COSHH), 245
convenience foods, 4
converters, 1
copper, 317, 704–5, 714
copper sulphate, 715
corned beef, 121
Cornish game, 262
corrective action, 240
corridor disease, 626
corrosion inhibition, 148
*Corynebacterium*, 345
*Corynebacterium equi*, 251, 395
*Corynebacterium pseudotuberculosis*, 454, 513, 612
*Corynebacterium renale*, 524, 525
costocervical nodes, 36
cow
acetonaemia in, 700–1
carcase, 54
definition, 8
horns, 50
ossification, 22
udder, 44
uterus, 42–3
*Cowdria ruminantium*, 399, 607–8
cowdriosis, 607–8
cowpox, 591
*Coxiella burnetii*, 399, 416, 608
creatine phosphokinase (CPK), 498
cretinism, 46
Creutzfeld–Jakob Disease (CJD), 559, 563
Crimea-Congo haemorrhagic fever (CCHF), 578
criteria, specification, 240
critical control points (CCPs), 158, 239, 244
crossbreeding, 2
croupous inflammation, 425
crushed bone and waste, 58
cryogenic freezing, 112, 115
cryptococcosis, 611–12
*Cryptococcus neoformans*, 611
cryptosporidiosis, 621–2
*Cryptosporidium*, 397, 621, 622
*Culex annulirostris*, 606
culture
evaluation, 365–6
failures, 405
for *Salmonella* organisms, 281
incubation of, 365
membrane slide, 361
methods, 364
culture media, 363–4
anaerobic, 364
inoculation of, 364
curing, **103–4**
common defects, 106
hide, 136
ingredients, 103
salts and additives, 103
cutaneous cysts, 439
cutaneous myiasis, 692
cutaneous streptothrichosis, 524–5, 613–14
cuts, 409
cutting
bacon and ham, 104
meat, **69–75**
cutting rooms, 97, 274
cyanides, 716
*Cyathostoma bronchialis*, 284
cyst, 428–9, 439, 484, 646–7, 672, 673
*see also* hydatid cyst
cysticerci, 249
*Cysticercus bovis*, 57, 116, 246, 248, 249, 250, **669–74**
cysts, 672, 673
index case, 675
laboratory confirmation, 675
*Cysticercus cellulosae*, 1, 116, 251, 680
*Cysticercus pisiformis*, 291
*Cysticercus tenuicollis*, 295, 517
cystitis, 524
*Cystoisospora*, 620
*Cytoecetes (Ehrlichia) phagocytophila*, 609
*Cytoectes phagocytophila*, 543

dairy worker fever, 413
Dandy–Walker syndrome, 500
dark, firm and dry (DFD) meat, 6–7, 62–3, 186
dark ground (dark field) microscopy, 380
data retrieval and feedback, **725–39**
DDT, 312
dead-on-arrivals (DOAs), 273
decomposition, **344–53**
assessment, 352–3
danger to man, 352
fat, 348–9
decontamination, post-slaughter, 235–8
deep inguinal nodes, 39
deep samples, 342
deer, **16–17**, **293–6**, 347
calves, 17
contamination, 295
culling, 295
epizootic haemorrhagic disease of, 582
farmed, 292
handling, 17, 293
hill, 17
husbandry, 17
inspection, 294
lairage, 86–7
lowland, 17
meat, 17
park, 294–5
rutting, 17
slaughter, 294
stunning, 294
wild, 294
deerfly fever, 419, 553–4
deficiency diseases, 422
dehairing, pig, 93
demodectic mange, 690–1
dendrites, 44
Denmark, meat inspection data banks, 728–9

dentition, age determination by, 51–3
*Dermacentor*, 617, 693
dermamycosis, 614–15
dermaphytosis, 614–15
dermatitis, 411
*Dermatobia hominis*, 694
dermatomycosis, 416–17
dermatophilosis, 524–5, 613–14
*Dermatophilus congolensis*, 525, 613
dermatophytes, 396
dermatophytosis, 416–17
dermoid cysts, 429
desert fever, 610–11
detained meat room, 96
detergents, 150
  application, 157–8
  design and choice, **148–9**
  safety, 160–1
development, abnormalities, 444–6
diarrhoea, 281, 519–20
*Dicrocoelium dendriticum* (*D. lanceolatum*), 684–5
*Dictyocaulus viviparus*, 657
dietary factors, **2–4**
diethylstilboestrol, 7, 303, 309, 310
digestive system, **23–9**, 450
dinoestrol diacetate, 715
*Dioctophyma renale*, 485
dioxins, 714–15
dip lift, 206
dip slide, 361
diphtheritic inflammation, 425
*Diphyllobthrium latum*, 660
dirty animal, contamination, 225–6
dirty livestock, 166
discoloration, 106, 124
disease
  acquired, 421
  causes, 421
  data recording, 244
  genetically determined, 422–3
  infective, 421
  nature of, 421
disinfectants, 150
  design and choice, 150
  non-oxidising, 149
  oxidising, 149
  safety, 160–1
disinfection, 158
  EU directives, 144
  food plants, 143–4
  monitoring, 158
  principles, 149
dispersion, 147
dissolved air flotation, 141
distomatosis, **681–6**
DNA, 19, 57, 710
  probes, 343
DNase (deoxyribonuclease) test, 368
documentation, contamination, 240–1
dog, tapeworms, 659
doramectin, 315
dorsal, 20
Dorset-Down-cross, 10
Dorset Horn, 9
dorso-costal node, 37
dourine, 631
Downer syndrome, 497
drainage, meat plant, 80
drains, collection of material from, 361
drenching guns, 168
dressing techniques, 230
dried blood and plasma, 58
drip (weeping), 115
dripping, 131
drive races, 84
driving disease, 592–3
drop plate method, 357
dropsy, 443–4
Droughtmaster, 6
drugs
  clearance rates for, 299
  *see also* chemical residues
dry matter, 140
drying, 102
  blood meal, 134
Dubin–Johnson syndrome, 437
duck, 15–16
  wax stripping, 269
duck virus enteritis, 275
ductus arteriosus, 32
ductus venosus, 32
Due Diligence defence, 156
dura mater, 45
durability, processed foods, 353
Duroc, 12
dysplasia, 444

ear, 502
East Coast Fever (ECF), 625–6
EC Directive, 7, 12, 79
EC Directive 64/433, 95, 107, 110, 224, 227, 252, 300, 674, 680
EC Directive 69/349, 107
EC Directive 70/524, 300
EC Directive 71/118, 107
EC Directive 77/99, 75
EC Directive 79/112, 353
EC Directive 79/373, 300
EC Directive 80/778, 361
EC Directive 81/476, 110
EC Directive 81/602, 300, 301, 309
EC Directive 81/851, 300
EC Directive 81/852, 300
EC Directive 85/358, 301
EC Directive 85/649, 300
EC Directive 86/469, 300, 301, 310, 737
EC Directive 88/146, 301
EC Directive 88/657, 358, 359
EC Directive 89/153, 301
EC Directive 89/187, 301
EC Directive 89/395, 353
EC Directive 89/610, 301
EC Directive 90/153, 301
EC Directive 90/515, 301
EC Directive 91/497, 458, 189, 244, 246, 252, 256, 674
EC Directive 91/628, 174
EC Directive 91/664, 301
EC Directive 92/23, 301
EC Directive 92/45, 294
EC Directive 92/102, 191, 244, 738
EC Directive 92/117, 272
EC Directive 93/119, 198, 199, 205, 208, 214
EC Directive 93/43, 224
EC Directive 94/59, 649
EC Directive 94/495, 86
EC Directive 95/23, 232
EC Directive 95/29, 174
EC Directive 96/22, 300, 301
EC Directive 96/23, 300, 304, 379
EC Directive 96/239, 49
EC Directive 96/362, 49
EC Fresh Meat Directive, 227
EC Regulation 1538/91, 262
EC Regulation 1906/90, 354
ecchymoses, 452
*Echinococcus granulosus*, 660–2
*Echinococcus multilocularis*, 662
*Echinococcus vogeli*, 662–3
ectoparasites, 284
edible fat, 51
edible fat room, 97
effluent
  control, 159
  discharge, 140
  treatment, 139
egg drop syndrome, 15
egg peritonitis, 286
*Ehrlichia ondiri*, 605
*Eimeria*, 397, 620
*Eimeria steidae*, 289
*Eimeria tenella*, 283
elaeophoriasis, 656
electric goads, 198
electrical stimulation (ES), 72–3
electricity, 80
electrocorticogram (ECoG), 200
electroencephalogram (EEG), 200
electromagnetic radiation, 126
electronic identification of livestock, 738
electroplectic fit, 212, 267
electroplectic shock, 208
ELISA (enzyme-linked immunoabsorbent assay) test, 56
emaciation, 287, 459
embolism, 442–3
embryo transfer, 2
embryonic cysts, 429
emergency reaction, 185
emergency slaughter, 192, 193–4
  abattoir, 194
  on-farm, 194
empyema, 426
emulsification, 146
encephalitis, 500, 532, 600
encephalomalacia, 500
endocarditis, 254, 441, 477
endocardium, 31, 476–7
endocrine system, 46–50
end-of-lay hens, definition, 15
endosteum, 21
endotoxins, 455
energy deficiency, 703
*Entamoeba histolytica*, 616
enteric colibacillosis, 520–1
enteric infections, 323–5
enteritis, 466, 532, 541–2, 600
  rabbits, 290
*Enterobacteriaceae*, 138, 270
enterotoxaemia, 516–18
*Enterotoxigenic colibacillosis*, 520
Environmental Assessment (EA), 78
environmental pollutants, **709–23**
Environmental Statement (ES), 78
enzootic balanoposthitis, 525
enzootic bovine leukosis (EBL), 449, 578–80
enzootic staphylococcosis, 543
enzyme, 73, 344
enzyme-linked immunoassays, 310
enzymolysis, 148
eosinophilic myositis, 495, 625
*Eperythrozoon*, 399
eperythrozoonosis, 606
*Eperythrozoonosis suis*, 606
ephemeral fever, 581–2
epicardium, 31, 476
epidermal inclusion cysts, 429
epidermophytosis, 416–17
epididymitis, 490
epinephrine, 7
epineurium, 45
epithelial tissues, 19
epithelioma of the eye, 449–50
epizootic cellulitis, 583
epizootic haemorrhagic disease of deer, 582
epizootic lymphangitis (EL), 612
eprinomectin, 315
equidae
  septicaemia of, 538
  strongylosis (strongylidosis) of, 654–5
equine
  ehrlichial colitis, 607
  ehrlichiosis, 607
  encephalomyelitis, 580–1
  hyperlipaemia, 702
  infectious anaemia (EIA), 581
  influenza, 582–3
  monocytic ehrlichiosis, 607
  post-mortem inspection, 251
  sarcoid, 463
  typhoid, 583
  viral arteritis (EVA), 583
  viral rhinopneumonitis, 583
equipment
  contamination, 224
  design, 82
  wash, 97
erysipelas, 278, 413, 526–8
erysipeloid, 413
*Erysipelothrix insidiosa*, 278
*Erysipelothrix rhusiopathiae*, 249, 252, 254, 390–1, 413, 526

erythromycin, 306
erythropoietic factor, 41
*Escherichia*, 346
*Escherichia coli*, 104, 170, 232, 235, 237, 252, 279, 324, 328, 332–3, 384
*Escherichia coli* enterotoxaemia, 520
EU directives *see* EC Directives
European Union, *Cysticercus bovis* inspection procedure, 674
*Eurytrema pancreaticum*, 685
evaporation, 101
evisceration, poultry, 269–71
ewe
  carcase, 54
  cast, definition, 10
  definition, 10
  pregnancy toxaemia of, 700
  udder, 44
  uterus, 43
excess fat, 51
exertional rhabdomyolysis, 701–2
exotic meat production, **289–98**
exotoxins, 455, 719
exsanguination, 200
exudate, 363
exudation cysts, 429
exudative diathesis, 707
exudative epidermitis in pigs, 543
eye, 501–2, 530
eyeworm disease, 657

Factories Act 1961, 410
factory-blindness, 144
faecal coliforms, 362
faecal contamination, 163
faeces, 363, 399–400
  collection, 361
fallopian tubes, 487
FAO, 108
farcy, 528–9
  *see also* glanders
Farm Animal Welfare Co-ordinating Executive, 212
Farm Animal Welfare Council (FAWC), 86, 217
Farmer's lung, 410
*Fasciola gigantica*, 681
*Fasciola hepatica*, 314, 681–2
fascioliasis, **681–6**
  human, 684
*Fascioloides magna*, 681, 684
*Fasciolopsis buski*, 684
fast antimicrobial screen test (FAST), 402–5
fasting, prior to slaughter, 183
fat, 51
  by-products treatment, 130–1
  decomposition, 348–9
  differentiation, 55
  edible fat rendering, 131
  emboli, 443
  necrosis, 431, 469, 470
  rancidity, 348, 407
  sources, 3
fats, oils and greases, 140, 144
  saponification of, 147
fatty change, 438–9, 452
fatty liver, 468
  haemorrhagic syndrome (FLHS), 285
feather pecking or pulling, 286
febantel, 315
Federal Meat Inspection Act, 190
feed additives, 715
feeding
  effect on odour, 65–6
  influence on animal tissue, 64–5
fenbendazole, 315
ferkelgrippe *see* swine influenza
fermentation of sugars, 375
Ferris wheel, 198
fetal blood, 33
fetal circulation, 32
fetuses, 457
fever, 452, 456
fibrinous inflammation, 425
fibrinous pericarditis, 476
fibroma, 287
fibrosis, 427
fiery red areas, 106
fight and flight, 47
fight or flight syndrome, 185
Finnish Agreement, 167
Firearms Act 1968, 205
first-aid, 410
first-aid room, 98
fish, 1
fissure, 428
flamed glass slides, 360
flat-souring, 123
flatworms, 636
*Flavobacterium*, 346, 391
fleece, 223, 230
flight zones, 182
flora, 366
florenicol, 306
fluids, 362
fluke, 247, 636, 637, **680–8**
flukecides, 314
fluorine, 317, 715–16
  poisoning, 710
*Fluorosis*, 710
foam, cleaning, 150–2
focal necrosis of liver, 535
focal symmetrical encephalomalacia, 517
fogging, 152
follicular mange, 690–1
folliculitis, 428
food
  adulteration, 57
  animals, 1–18
  consumption, 3
  debasement, 57
  ingredients, 58–9
  substitution, 57
  tampering, 68–9
Food Act 1984, 57, 58
Food Animal Residue Avoidance Databank (FARAD), 299
food poisoning, **321–36**
  bacterial, 328
  food vehicles in, 326–7
  location of general outbreaks, 327
  management, 336–8
  notification, 323
  organisms, 251
  outbreak control group (OCG), 336
  outbreak surveillance, 325–8
  risk factors in, 327
  surveillance, 322–3
  types, 321–2
food poisoning organisms, 247
Food Processing Engineering Ltd (FPE) plant, 82–3
food safety, 258
  after nuclear accidents, 722–3
Food Safety Act 1990, 336
Food Safety Inspection Service (FSIS), 236
food vehicles in food poisoning, 326–7
foodborne disease, 328
foodborne pathogens, 328
foot-and-mouth disease (FMD), **583–7**
foot rot
  of cattle, 534–5
  of goats, 534
  of pigs, 534
  of sheep, 534
footwear, 410
foramen magnum, 45
foramen ovale, 32
foreign bodies, 68
foreleg, 21
four-plate test (FPT), 307, 308
fowl
  cholera, 278
  heart, 31
  intestines, 26
  kidneys, 42
  liver, 27
  ovaries, 44
  pancreas, 29
  respiratory system, 30
  spleen, 34
  testes, 44
  typhoid, 280
fractures, 493
  poultry, 284–5
Francis disease, 553–4
*Francisella (Pasteurella) tularensis*, 553
*Francisella tularensis*, 391, 419
free bullet pistol, 204–5
free fatty acid (FFA), 131
  hydrolytic rancidity, 407
freeze drying, 113
freezer burn, 115
freezing, 96, 106, 107, 111–12, 114
  carcases, 108
  effect on pathogenic microorganisms and parasites, 115–16
  horse meat, 651–2
  of meat, 650–1
fresh meat dispatch area, 97
Fresh Meat (Hygiene and Inspection) Regulations 1995, 189, 192, 458, 680
Friesian, 5
frozen meat, **114–16**
fungal diseases, 471, 472
fungal poultry diseases, 283
fungi, 396–7, 462, 464, 467, 610
fungicides, 300, 713
*Fusarium*, 106
*Fusarium necrophorus*, 468
*Fusobacterium necrophorum*, 425, 535

gall bladder, 468
gall sickness, 604–5
galvanic corrosion, 145
game, 72, 347
gamma-irradiator, 127
gangliosidosis, 440
gangrene, 431–2
gangrenous dermatitis, 277
gas emboli, 443
*Gasterophilus* spp., 688–9
gastric nodes, 39, 41
gastroenteritis, 519–20
gastrointestinal campylobacteriosis, 512
gastrointestinal parasites of ruminants, **638–42**
gastrointestinal tract, 223, 710
  contamination, 233–5
geese, 15–16
gel cleaning, 151
gelatin, 135
gelatin strips, 246
general adaptation syndrome, 185
General Agreement on Tariffs and Trade (GATT), 238, 263
General Food Hygiene Regulations, 224
genetic abnormalities, 487
genetic defects, 462, 464
genetic engineering, 2, 189
genetically determined disease, 422–3
genitalia, 41
  tuberculosis, 548
germ tube test, 396
Gerstmann–Straussler–Scheinker syndrome, 559, 560
gestagen, 309
giant liver fluke, 681
*Giardia*, 252, 397, 622
giardiasis, 622
Giemsa stain, 372
gilt
  carcase, 55
  definition, 13
  uterus, 43
gimmer
  carcase, 54
  definition, 10
glanders, 528–9
glands, collection and yield, 49–50

glass containers, 121
glass-packed foods, 121
*Globocephalus longemucronatus*, 644
glomerulonephritis, 483
Gloucester Old Spot, 12
gloves, 226–7, 410
glucocorticoids, 47
glutamic-oxaloacetic transaminase (GOT), 498
glycogen storage disease, 439
gnathostomiasis, 656
goat, **13–14**
  breeds, 14
  carcase, 55
  contagious agalactia of, 522–3
  foot rot of, 534
  identification and registration, 736
  kidneys, 42
  meat, 14
  Nairobi sheep disease (NSD), 587–8
  nematodes in, 640
  parasitic gastroenteritis of, 640–2
  plague, 590
  pneumonic pasteurellosis of, 539
  post-mortem examination, 250
  records, 736
  skins, 135
  stomach, 25
  tapeworms, 659
  teeth, 53
  tongue, 23
  tuberculosis, 546
  udder, 44
goatpox, 591
goatpox virus (SGPV), 591
*Gonglyonema pulchrum*, 642
Good Manufacturing Practices (GMP), 238
Graff–Reinert disease, 588–9
Gram-negative bacteria, 367
Gram-negative cocci and bacilli, 371
Gram-negative organisms, 346–8
Gram-positive cocci and bacilli, 371
Gram-positive non-sporing rods, 367
Gram-positive organisms, 345–6
Gram's stain, 370–1
granulation tissue, 427–8
granulomatous inflammation, 427
gravity rail system, 90
greases *see* fats, oils and greases
greasy pig disease, 543
green offal, 130
green struck, 347
greening, 106
gross clean/preparation, 156–7
growth hormone (GH), 7
growth promoters, 7, 309
  testing, 310–11
guards, 410
guinea fowl, 16
gullet worm, 642
Gumboro disease, 274
gut and tripe room, 96–7
gut oedema, 520
gut sweetbread, 29

HACCP (hazard analysis critical control points), 158, 160, 238, 244, 263, 344
haemal lymph nodes, 35–6
haemangioma, 286
*Haemaphysalis*, 617, 693
haematin, 434
haematogenous pigments, 434
haematoma, 249, 429, 440
*Haematopinus suis*, 592
haematuria, 486
haemoglobin, 61, 434
haemoglobinaemia, 480
haemoglobinuria, 486
haemolysis, 365
haemolysis test, 369
haemolytic jaundice, 435
haemopericardium, 476
haemophilosis, 529–30
*Haemophilus*, 474
*Haemophilus somnus*, 529
haemorrhage, 209, 213, 440, 452, 466, 475–7, 487, 496–7
haemorrhagic
  dysentery, 542–3
  inflammation, 425
  jaundice, 413, 530–1
  septicaemia, 537
haemosiderin, 434, 498
hair, 223, 230
hairballs, 466
Half-Bred, 9
*Halobacterium*, 346
halogenated hydrocarbons, 314
ham
  canning, 121
  cooked, 105
  internal bruising, 216
  production, **104–6**
  taint in, 349–50
hamartoma, 468
hand-stunning devices, 211
handwashing facilities, 87
hares, 347
Hazard Analysis Critical Control Points. *See* HACCP
head
  cattle, 248
  restraints, 198
head-to-brisket system, 209
headgear, 226
healing efficiency, 428
health and safety, 245
  legislation, 409–10
  *see also* safety
Health and Safety at Work Act 1974, 409
Health and Safety Executive (HSE), 409, 410
health foods, 4
health risks, 240
heart, 31, 475–8
  cattle, 249
  congenital conditions, 478
heartwater, 607–8
heat-thermal processing, **116–25**
heated beef, 347
heavy metals, 300, 316–17
heel fly, 695
heifer
  carcase, 53–4
  definition, 8
helminth parasites, 284, **636–8**
hepatosis dietetica, 707
herbicides, 300, 313, 713
Herd Health Surveillance, 257, 258
hereditary malformations, 450
Hereford, 6
heritable hypomyoglobinaemia, 441
*Heterakis gallinarum*, 284
*Hexamita meleagridis*, 284, 398
hexamitiasis, 284
hexoestrol, 310
hide, 96, 130, 166, 223
  by-products treatment, 135–6
  curing, 136
  manurial pollution, 163
high-performance liquid chromatography (HPLC), 308
high pressure techniques, 127–8
high-risk material, 136
high-voltage electrophoresis (HVE) bioautography, 308
Highland cattle, 5
hindleg, 21
hindquarter nodes, 38–9
hip joint, 494
hippurate hydrolysis test, 368
*Histomonas meleagridis*, 284, 398
histomoniasis, 283
*Histoplasma capsulatum*, 612
hock burn, 285
hog
  carcase, 54–5
  cholera, 599–600
  flu *see* swine influenza
hogg, definition, 10
hormones, 46, 48, 300, 309
  testing, 310–11
horns, 50
  bruising due to, 188
horse, 1
  carcase, 55
  fat, 56
  heart, 31
  kidneys, 42
  liver, 27
  lungs, 30
  nematode infections in, 655–6
  spleen, 34
  stomach, 26
  tapeworms, 659
  tongue, 23
  tuberculosis, 545
horse meat
  examination, 649
  freezing, 651–2
  inspection, 651
horsepox, 592
Horses (Sea Transport) Order 1952, 177
hot boning, 69–70
housing
  density, 166
  structure and layout, 166
human consumption, conditionally approved for, 255
humane slaughter, **197–222**
Humane Slaughter Association (HSA), 213, 267
hyaline degeneration, 439
*Hyalomma*, 617, 693–4
*Hyalomma rufipes*, 39
hydatid cyst, 249, 429, 493, 549–50, 662
hydatid disease, **660–9**
  in man, 664–5
hydrant points, 85
hydrocarbons, 109
hydrocyanic (prussic) acid, 716
hydrofluorocarbons (HFs), 109
hydrogen ion concentration, 406
hydrogen sulphide, 124
hydrogen sulphide test, 369
hydrogen swell, 123
hydrolysis, 147
hydropericardium, 274, 476
hydrophobia, **593–5**
hydrophobic surfaces, 146
hydropic degeneration, 439
hydrops allantois, 489
hydrops amnii, 489
hydrosalpinx, 488
hygiene, **223–41**
  assessing operational, **238–41**
  assessment systems (HAS), 241
  basic techniques, 227–9
  equipment and application methods, 150–5
  integrated approach, 191
  monitoring, **158–60**, 378–9
  requirements for waste processing plants, 137–8
  service flowsheet, 726
hygroma, 494
*Hyostrongylus rubidus*, 642–3
hyperaemia, 442
hyperbilirubinaemia, 434
hyperplasia, 444
hyperthermia, 456
hypertrophy, 444
*Hypoderma*, 694–6
*Hypoderma aeratum*, 696
*Hypoderma diana*, 295, 695
*Hypoderma lineatum*, 695, 696
hypodermic syringe, 167
hypodermosis, 694–6
hypomagnesaemic tetany, 700
hypoplasia, 444
hypostasis, 443
hypothrichosis cystica, 463

icterus, 434–6
identification of organisms, 366–9
iliacs, 39
immaturity, 457–8
immune responses, 423
immune system, 422, 423
immunoassay, 308, 310, 318
immunological factors, 422
impact damage, 81
imperfect bleeding, 456–7
implants, 311
Imported Meat Monitoring Programme (IMMP), 304
Imported Meats Point of Destination Sampling (IMPoDS) survey, 304
impression plates, 342
inclusion body hepatitis, 275
incubation
  of cultures, 365
  period, 451
India ink film, 381
indole test, 369
industrial nurse, 98
inedible area, 97
inedible rendering plants, **138–41**
infarct, 249, 429, 432, 484
infection, **409–19**, 421
  generalized systemic, **450–62**
  mode of spread, 450–1
infectious bovine rhinotracheitis (IBR), 586
infectious bulbar paralysis, 556–7
infectious bursal disease (IBD), 15, 274
infectious diseases, **505–634**
  judgement, 505–6
infectious enzootic hepatitis of cattle and sheep *see* Rift Valley fever (RVF)
infectious keratoconjunctivitis, 530, 606
infectious laryngotracheitis, 276
infectious necrotic hepatitis, 517
infectious ophthalmia, 530
infective microorganisms, 421
inflammation, **424–8**, 466
  acute, 424–7
  chronic, 427–8
influenza, equine, 582–3
infrared radiation, 126
ingesta, 469
inherited conditions, 422–3
injection abscesses, 454, 498
injuries, 187
  occupational, 409–10
inoculation of culture media, 364
insecticides, 312, 713–14
inspection
  ante-mortem, **189–92**, 243–4
  deer, 294
  meat, 68, 91, 305, 737
    recording systems, **725–35**
    traditional versus entirely visual, 251
  post-mortem, 194, **244–58**
  rabbit, 290
intercostal node, 37
interdigital dermatitis (scald) in sheep, 535
interdigital necrobacillosis, 534–5
intermittent powered system, 90
internal parasitism of pigs, **642–8**
internal retropharyngeal nodes, 36
International Commission on the Microbiological Specification of Foods (ICMSF), 343–4, 358
International Organisation for Standardisation (ISO), 191
interstitial nephritis, 484
interstitial pneumonia, 473
intestines, 26, 130, 223, 465
  by-products treatment, 131–3
  cattle, 249
intracellular accumulations, **432–40**
intracellular blood parasites, 360
inverted dressing, 232
iodine, 705, 721
iodine value, 56
ionizing radiation, 126
iron, 705
irradiation, 126
ischaemia, 442
ischaemic heart disease (IHD), 2
ischiatic node, 39
ISO11784, 191
ISO11785, 191
isolation block, 95
isolation media, 364–5
*Isospora*, 620
ivermectin, 315
*Ixodes*, 617, 694
*Ixodes ricinus*, 415, 543, 609
Ixodidae, 693

Jaagsiekte, 592
Japanese encephalitis (JE), 580, 586–7
jaundice, 434, 502
jelly pockets, 106
Jewish slaughter, 217–20
Jöhne's disease, 536, 580
joints, 493–5
  tuberculosis, 548
jowl abscess, 454

kangaroo meat, 57
kata, 590
keratinisation, 439
keratitis, 502
kidney, 41–2, 248, 254, 483–6
  cattle, 249
  fat and channel (pelvic) fat (KKCF), 69
  residues, 402
  stones, 485
  tuberculosis, 547
  worm of pigs, 645
*Klebsiella*, 346, 391
knives, 410
  hygienic use of, 227–9
  multiple knife technique, 229
  sterilising, 227–8
Kosher slaughter restraining systems, 218
Kreis test, 349
Kuru, 559

labelling, 57, 353–4
la bouhite, 588–9
laboratory
  analyses, 300
  equipment, 355–6
  examination, 246, 247, **363–407**
  facilities, **355–407**
  methods, trichinae, 648–9
  procedures, quality control, 647–8
  records, 366
  reports, 323–5
  surveillance, 325
lacerations, 409
*Lactobacillus*, 106, 345
Laikipia lung disease, 588–9
lairage, 83–7, 166
  animal husbandry, **181–4**
  cattle, 84–5
  construction, **180–1**
  deer, 86–7
  design, 198
  flight zones, 182
  handling facility, 197–9
  moving animals within, 181–2
  ostriches, 296
  pig, 85–6
  poultry, 265
  sheep, 85, 182
  watering, 182
lamb, 10
  definition, 10
  lymphadenitis of, 538
  slaughter, 225
  washing, 225
*Lamblia*, 622
lambliasis, 622
lamziekte, 518
Landrace, 12
large American liver fluke, 681
Large Black, 12
Large White, 12
laryngeal necrobacillosis, 535
laryngitis, 471
lateral retropharyngeal nodes, 36
laundry, 98, 226
lead, 316, 711–12
leanness, 459
*Legionella*, 391–2
legislation
  ante-mortem inspection, **189–92**
  chemical residues, 300–1
  health and safety, 409–10
  poultry, 266
  processed foods, 353
  slaughter, 213–15
  transport, 173–4
Leishman stain, 372
*Leishmania* spp., 398
Lelystad agent, 557
leptomeningitis, 500
*Leptospira*, 392
*Leptospira biflexa*, 413
*Leptospira interrogans*, 413
*Leptospira interrogans complex*, 530
leptospirosis, 413, 530–1
lesions, regional distribution, 462
leucocytes, 33
*Leucocytozoon*, 284
leucocytozoonosis, 284
*Leuconostoc*, 345
leukaemia, 479–80, 578–80
leukosis, 276
levamisole, 315
lice infestation, 689–9
ligamentum nuchae, 50
lighting, 96
  meat plant, 80–1
limberneck, 518
limbs, 20
limits of quantification (LOQ), 310
Limousin, 5
line dressing, 89–92
  advantages, 90
  disadvantages, 90–2
linguatulae, 249
lipids, 59–60
lipofuscin, 437
liquefaction (colliquative) necrosis, 431
liquid batch cultures, 364
liquid nitrogen, 112
listerellosis, 413–14, 531–3
*Listeria*, 252, 328
*Listeria monocytogenes*, 292, 333–4, 343, 382–3, 413–14, 421, 532, 533
listeriosis, 292, 413–14, 500, 531–3
  human, 533
liver, 26–8, 254, 466–7
  abscesses, 454, 535
  cattle, 249
  disease, 467–8
  enlarged, 285
  focal necrosis of, 535
  functions, 26
  hyperlasia, 468
  rupture, 468
  tuberculosis, 547
liver fluke disease, **681–6**
livestock
  dirty, 166
  electronic identification of, 738
  healthy, 167–9
  mortality during transport, 178–9
  production, **163–72**
  reception area, 83
  research, 461–2
  transport, 172–80
    loading/unloading, 172–3, 175
  washing, 87
  weather safety index chart, 179
  world production, 4
lobar pneumonia, 472–3
lockjaw *see* tetanus

louping ill, 414, 588
Lovibond comparator, 406
low-risk material, 136
Luing, 5
lumbar nodes, 38
lumpy jaw *see* actinomycosis
lumpy skin disease (LSD), 587
lumpy wool, 524–5
lumpy wool disease, 613–14
lungs, 29–30, 472
  cattle, 249
  tuberculosis, 546
lungworm, 295
luteal cysts, 429
luteinising hormone releasing hormone (LHRH), 67
Lyme disease, borreliosis, 415–16
*Lymnaea bulimoides*, 682
*Lymnaea diaphena*, 682
*Lymnaea tomentosa*, 682
*Lymnaea truncatula*, 682
*Lymnaea viator*, 682
lymph nodes, 34–5, 36–41, 254, 460, 481
  carcase, 250, 251
  cattle, 248
  haemal, 35–6
  head and neck, 36–8, 40
  pig, 40–1
  submaxillary, 250
lymphadenitis, 452, 481
  of lambs, 538
lymphangitis, 441, 481
lymphatic system, 34–6
lymphatic vessels, 34, 481–2
lymphatics, 441
lymphoblastoma, 287
lymphocytes, 34
lymphocytic inflammation, 425
lymphocytoma, 578–80
lymphomatosis, 578–80
lymphoproliferative disease, turkeys, 276–7
lymphoreticular system, **480–3**
lyophilisation, 113
lyssa, **593–5**

MacConkey agar, 374
*Macracanthorhynchus hirudinaceus*, 486, 644
mad cow disease *see* bovine spongiform encephalopathy (BSE)
mad itch, 556–7
maedi, 588–9
maedi-visna, 588–9
magnesium, 705
malformations, 450
malignant aedema, 517–18
malignant carcinomas, 287
malignant catarrhal fever, 558
malignant head catarrh, 558
malignant hyperthermia, 64
malignant lymphoma, 578–80
malignant theileriosis, 627
malleus, 528–9
malnutrition, 459, 703
  *see also* nutrition
mammary glands, 50, 489–90
manganese, 705
mange, 690–1
manure, disposal, 87
manure bay, 97–8
marbled lung, 521
marbling, 51
Marek's disease, 15, 276
marker organism, 378–9
marking dyes, 245
marking of meat, 649–50
marrow, 21
mastitis, 489–90
  rabbits, 290
materials of construction, 145
maximum recovery diluent (MRD), 359
maximum residue level (MRL), 302–3
meat
  ageing, 126
  annual consumption, 3
  by-products, 741–2
  canning *see* canning
  chemical and biological differentiation, **56–9**
  composition, **59–61**
  condemned *see* condemnation
  curing *see* curing
  cutting, **69–75**
  drainage, 80
  exotic production, **289–98**
  frozen, **114–16**
  hygiene, **223–41**
    integrated approach, 191
    service flowsheet, 726
  identification, 245
  inferior, 255
  inspection, 68, 91, 305, 737
    recording systems, **725–35**
    traditional versus entirely visual, 251
  integrated inspection/hygiene, 257
  marking of, 649–50
  microbiology *see* microbiology
  plant
    and throughputs, 4
    area size, 79
    construction and equipment, **77–99**
    doors, 81–2
    drainage, 79
    electricity, 80
    environment, 78
    facilities, 79–82
    floor and wall finishes, 81
    floor plan, 78
    hygiene, monitoring, 378–9
    lighting, 80–1
    plans submission, 78
    plumbing plan, 78
    sanitation, **143–62**
    site, 77–8
    site plan, 78
    statistics, 730–1
    ventilation, 81
    water, 79–80
  preservation, **101–28**
    *see also* chilling; freezing; heat-thermal processing; refrigeration
  quality, **61–9**
    and stress, 185–6
    effect of stunning, 211
    effects of breeding and pre-slaughter stress, 62–4
    physical and chemical changes, 61
    poultry, 213
  re-inspection, 246
  species differentiation, 407
  stored, 101–2
Meat and Livestock Commission, 246
mechanical energy, 146
mechanical handling systems, 82
mechanically-recovered meat (MRM), 58, 74–5
*Mecistocirrus digitatus*, 638
median plane, 20
medical certification, 227
medical examinations, 227
medicines
  administration, 302
  record keeping, 302
  safe use, 301–2
  statutory surveillance programmes, 304–5
  withdrawal times, 302
  *see also* chemical residues
Medicines Act Veterinary Information Service (MAVIS), 304
Mediterranean Coast Fever, 626–7
medulla oblongata, 45
melanin, 433–4
melioidosis, 533–4
  human, 534
*Melophagus ovinus*, 692
membrane filters, 362
membrane slide cultures, 361
meningitis, 500
meningoencephalitis of cattle, 537–8
mercury, 316–17, 716
mesenteric emphysema, 470
mesenteric nodes, 38
mesophilic aerobes, colony counts of, 357
metabolic disorders, 699–703
  acquired, 699
  inherited, 699
metacestodes, 637, 658
metallic foreign bodies, 68
metaplasia, 444
metastasis, 443
*Metastrongylus elongatus*, 652
*Metastrongylus pudendotectus*, 652
*Metastrongylus salmi*, 652
metazoan parasites, 422
methyl red test, 375
metritis, 488
  in rabbits, 290
*Microbacterium*, 345
microbial contamination, 155
microbial counts, 344
microbial specifications, 358
microbial spoilage, 122–3
microbiological analysis, 342–3
microbiological assessment, 159
microbiological criteria, 248
microbiological examination
  of fresh meat, 401
  of processed meat, 401
microbiological guidelines, 343
microbiological limits, 358, 359
microbiological specifications, 343, 358
microbiological standards, 343, 358
microbiological techniques, 344
microbiological testing, 357
microbiology, 158, **339–54**
*Micrococcus*, 106, 345
*Micrococcus luteus*, 307
microorganisms, 169, 170
  infective, 421
*Micropolysporum faeni*, 410
microscopy, 369–73, 380–1
microsporosis, 416–17, 614–15
*Microsporum*, 614
middle cervical nodes, 36
Middle White, 12
mild steel, 145
milk, 8, 14
milk fever, 701
milker's nodule, 592
Minced Meat Preparations (Hygiene) Regulations 1995, 75
mineralocorticoids, 47
minerals, 60
mites, 690
modified-atmosphere packaging (MAP), 70–1, 116
moistened membrane filters, 360
molybdenum, 704, 716
moniliasis, 283, 612–13
monitoring
  bacteriological, 256
  faecal contamination, 252
  hygiene, **158–60**
  implementation, 240
  plant hygiene, 378–9
mononucleosis, 413–14, 531–3
*Moraxellae*, 104, 346, 392
mortality, transport, 178–9
motility test, 375
moulds, 342, 350–1, 396
  growth, 113
moxidectin, 315
mucoid degeneration, 440
mucolipidosis, 440
*Mucor*, 94, 106, 352
mucormycosis, 613
mucosal disease complex (MD), 576–7
mucous inflammation, 425
mucous membranes, 24
mud fever, 413, 530–1
*Muellerius capillaris*, 657
mulberry heart disease (MHD), 706–7
mule, 9
  tapeworms, 659

*Multiceps multiceps. See Taenia multiceps*
*Multiceps serialis*, 291
multiple knife technique, 229
Murray-Grey, 5
muscle, 254, 362, 495, 496, 499
  differentiation, 55
  tissue, 19, 248
  tuberculosis, 548
muscular system, 50, **495–9**
Muslim slaughter, 220–1
musty taint, 67
mycobacteria, 550
*Mycobacterium*, 392–3
*Mycobacterium avium*, 544
*Mycobacterium bovis*, 248, 544
*Mycobacterium farcinogenes*, 612
*Mycobacterium kansasii*, 550
*Mycobacterium paratuberculosis (jöhnei)*, 536
*Mycobacterium tuberculosis*, 544
*Mycoplasma*, 393, 512
*Mycoplasma agalactiae* var. *bovis*, 522
*Mycoplasma hyopneumoniae*, 522
*Mycoplasma hyorhinis*, 522
*Mycoplasma hyosynoviae*, 522
*Mycoplasma mycoides* var. *Mycoides SC*, 521
mycoplasmal arthritis
  in cattle, 521–2
  in pigs, 522
mycoplasmal (enzootic) pneumonia in pigs, 522
mycoses, 610
mycota, 396–7
mycotic dermatitis, 613–14
mycotic lymphangitis, 523–4
mycotoxins, 318, 351
myelomalacia, 500
myocarditis, 441, 477
myocardium, 31, 477
myodegeneration, 496
myofibrillar protein, 59
myoglobin, 61
myoglobinuria, 486
myositis, 495–6
myxomatosis, 291

N5 disc, 403
NADP, 468
nagana, 631–2
Nairobi sheep disease (NSD), 587–8
nasal passages, 470–1
National Sampling and Surveillance Scheme (NSS), 303, 379
neck-cutting, poultry, 267–8
necrobacillosis, 534
necrosis, 429–32
necrotic enteritis, 277
necrotic rhinitis, 535
necrotic stomatitis, 535
*Neisseria*, 393
*Neisseria meningitidis*, 422, 451
nematodes, 636
  in cattle, 638–40
  in goats, 640
  in sheep, 640
  infections, **653–60**
    in horses, 655–6
neoplasia, **446–50**
neoplasms, 462, 464, 465, 467, 470–2
  poultry, 286
*Neospora*, 623
neosporosis, 622–3
nephritis, 483
nephrosis, 485
nerve cells, 44
nervous system, 44–6, 450, **499–501**
nervous tissue, 19
netobimin, 315
neural tissue embolism in cattle, 204
neurofilariasis, 656
neurons, 44
new variant-CJD (nv-CJD), 563–4
New York Dressed (NYD) birds, 271
New Zealand, 9, 10
  *Cysticercus bovis* inspection procedure, 678
  meat inspection data, 726–7
Newcastle disease, 15, 277
nitrate, 103, 716–17
nitric oxide, 103
nitrite, 103, 716–17
nitrogen, 140
nitrosomyoglobin, 103
nitrous oxide anaesthesia, 205
nitroxynil, 314
no observable effect (NOEL), 302
*Nocardia*, 393–4
noise, 182
non-meat proteins, 58
non-protein nitrogen, 60
noradrenaline, 7, 47
norepinephrine, 7
nortestosterone, 310
Northern Ireland
  condemnations data, 731–4
  meat inspection data, 729–30
notoedric mange, 691
NSAIDs, 317–18
Nubian, 14
nuclear accidents, food safety after, 722–3
nutrition, 464
  *see also* malnutrition
nutritional deficiencies, 462, 467, 471, 703–7
nutritional muscular dystrophy (NMD), 706
nutritional myopathy, 706

obesity, 438
obturator foramen, 72
occupational disease, prevention of, 419
occupational injuries, 409–10
ochratoxins, 318
ochronosis, 438
odour, 65–9, 365
  abnormal, 68
  absorption, 66
  control, 161
  due to abnormal metabolism, 66
  sexual, 67–8
oedema, 443–4
oedema disease, 520
*Oesophagostomum brevicaudum*, 652–3
*Oesophagostomum dentatum*, 652–3
*Oesophagostomum georgianum*, 652–3
*Oesophagostomum quadrispinulatum*, 652–3
*Oesophagostomum radiatum*, 249
*Oesophagostomum* spp., 644
oesophagus, 23, 223, 233
  cattle, 249
oestradiol, 309, 310, 311
oestrogen, 7, 309, 715
oestrus, 461
*Oestrus ovis*, 692
off-flavour, 67
offal, 97, 130, 136
  edible, 238
  storage, 108
  washing, 238
Ohara's disease, 419, 553–4
oils *see* fats, oils and greases
omasum, 24, 465
omphalophlebitis, calves, 254
on-the-rail dressing, 88–92
*Onchocerca armillata*, 654
*Onchocerca gibsoni*, 654
*Onchocerca* spp., 653–4
*Onchocerciasis*, 653
ondiri disease, 605–6
operatives
  contamination, 224
  hand washing, 226
ophthalmia, 502
oral necrobacillosis, 535
Oregon disease, 287
orf, 412, 577–8
organisms, identification of, 366–9
organoleptic changes, 127
organophosphates, 312, 313, 714
organs, 19
ornithosis, 283, 414–15
ossification, 22–3
  cows, 22
osteitis, 492
osteoarthritis, 492
osteochondrosis, 492
osteodystrophia fibrosa, 493
osteogenesis imperfecta, 493
osteology, 20–3
osteomalacia, 492
osteomyelitis, 278, 492
osteopetrosis, 493
osteoporosis, 493
ostrich, **295–8**
  dressing, 297
  lairage, 296
  restraint, 297
  slaughter, 298
  stunning, 297
outer integument, 223
oval tunnel, 206
ovarian (follicular) cysts, 429
ovaries, 48, 487
  fowl, 44
overscald, 287
oversticking, 214
ovine encephalomyelitis, 588
ovine progressive pneumonia, maedi, maedi-visna, 588–9
ovine pulmonary carcinoma, 592–3
ox
  adrenal glands, 47
  carcase, 55
  heart, 31
  kidneys, 41
  liver, 26
  lungs, 29–30
  lymph nodes, 36–9
  pancreas, 29
  skeleton, 20
  spleen, 33–4
  stomach, 23–4
  teeth, 52
  thyroid, 46
  tongue, 23
oxfendazole, 315
oxidase (cytochrome *c* oxidase) test, 368
oxidase-positive bacteria, 367
oxidation of coloured materials, 148
oxyclosanide, 314

paints, 145
pale, soft, exudative (PSE) muscle tissue, 11, 63–4, 86, 186
pancreas, 29, 468–9
pancreatic fluke, 685
pancreatitis, 468–9
papain, 72
paper labels, 245
papilla, 428
papillomatosis (warts), 589–10
papule, 428
paralytic myoglobinuria, 701–2
paramphistomiasis, 687–8
paranasal sinuses, 470–1
parasites, 462, 464, 465, 467, 469, 477, 485, **635–97**
  specimen collection, 399–400
parasitic cysts, 429
parasitic diseases, 471, 472, 495, 501
parasitic gastroenteritis, 638
  of cattle, 638–40
  of goats, 640–2
  of sheep, 640–2
parasitic infections, 116, 493, 502, 549–50
parasitic infestations, 473
parasitic poultry diseases, 283–4
parasitism, internal, 166
parasympathetic system, 46
parathyroids, 46–7
paratuberculosis, 536
paratyphoid, 539–42

paravaccinia, 592
parotid nodes, 36, 40
parrot fever, 414–15
partitions, 174
parturient paresis, 701
parturition, 461
passageways, curved, 84
*Pasteurella*, 394
*Pasteurella* (*Moraxella*) *anatipestifer*, 279, 537
*Pasteurella haemolytica*, 179, 537, 538, 539
pasteurella haemolytica, 539
*Pasteurella multocida*, 278, 291, 510, 537, 538
pasteurellosis, 278–9, 291, 537
pathogenic bacteria, 140
pathogens, **381–99**
  food-borne bacterial, **381–8**
  identification, 374–8
  non-food-borne bacterial, **389–96**
pathological lesions, 428–32
pathological ossification, 433
pathology, **421–503**
pawpaw, 73
pediculosis, 689–9
pelts, 130
penetrative type of percussive stunner, 202
penicillin, 106
*Penicillium*, 318
*Penicillium notatum*, 351
penis, 491
pens, 84
pericarditis, 274, 441, 476
pericardium, 475–6
  tuberculosis, 547
perineurium, 45
periodontal disease, 464
periosteum, 21
periostitis, 278
peripheral nervous system, 44, 45
peritoneum, 469–70
  tuberculosis, 547
peritonitis, 469, 470
permitted substances, 303
peroxide value (PV), 407
personnel
  contamination risk, 155–6
  facilities, 98
pest control, 82
pest of small ruminants (PPR), 590
pesticides, 300, 312–16, 713
  testing, 313–14
pet food industry, 129
pH effects, 62–3, 72, 140, 307–8, 345
pH estimation, 353
pH measurement, 406
pH value, 406, 453
  fresh slurry, 170
pharmaceutical products, 130
pharmacokinetics, 299
pharyngeal necrobacillosis, 535
phenols, 313
phenylbutazone, 317–18
phlebitis, 441
phosphorescence, 350
phosphorus, 705, 717
photosensitisation, 437, 702–3
phylloerythrin, 703
*Physocephalus sexalatus*, 642
pia mater, 45
pica, 459
pickle application, 104–5
Piedmontese, 5
pig, **10–13**
  abscesses, 253, 454
  breeds, 11–12
  carcase, 54, 131
    condemnations, 733–4
  definition, 13
  dehairing, 93
  dressing, 232–3
  exudative epidermitis in, 543
  fat, rancidity, 348
  flu *see* swine influenza
  foot rot in, 534
  grading, 13
  heart, 31
  hides, 135
  identification, 245, 735
  inspection, 257
  internal parasitism, **642–8**
  kidney worm of, 645
  lairage, 85–6
  liver, 27
  lungs, 30
  lymph nodes, 40–1
  meat examination, 648–9
  meat production, 12–13
  mycoplasmal arthritis in, 522
  mycoplasmal (enzootic) pneumonia in, 522
  pneumonic pasteurellosis of, 538
  post-mortem examination, 250–1
  pre-slaughter stress, 198
  production, 12
  records, 735
  rectum, 235
  registration, 735
  scalding, 93
  slaughter, 215–16
  slaughter hall, 92–4
  spleen, 34
  stomach, 25
  stunning, 198
  teeth, 53
  thorny-headed worm of, 644
  thyroid, 46
  toe nails, 233
  tongue, 23
  tuberculosis, 545
  vertical scalding, 94, 232
  viral encephalomyelitis of, 603
piglet, definition, 13
pigmentation, 433, 473, 485, 501
pigments, 61
pineal gland, 48–9
pink eye, 530, 583, 606
piroplasmosis, 617–18
pithing, 88, 214
pituitary gland, 48
pizzle rot, 525
placenta, 46
planning application, 78
plant sanitation, **143–62**
plants, poisonous, 718
plastic tag, 245
plastics, 145
plate count, 343, 357
pleurae, 472
  tuberculosis, 547
pleurisy, 254, 474–5
pluck, 30–1
pneumonia, 254, 472–3
  of ruminants, 657–8
pneumonic pasteurellosis, 539
  of cattle, 538–9
  of goats, 539
  of pigs, 538
  of sheep, 539
pneumorickettsiosis, 416, 609–9
poached egg eye, 605
pododermatitis, 534–5
poisoning, 710
  diagnosis, 711
  inorganic and organic, **710–19**
poisonous plants, 718
poisons, 463, 465, 467
pollution parameters, 139–40
polyarthritis
  of cattle, 528
  of sheep, 528
polychlorinated biphenyls (PCBs), 314
polychlorinated naphthalenes (PCNs), 314
polymerase chain reaction (PCR) analysis, 57
polyphosphates, 105
popliteal nodes, 39, 41
porcine poliomyelitis, 603
porcine reproductive and respiratory syndrome (PRRS), 557
porcine stress syndrome (PSS), 64, 499
pork
  pale, soft, exudative (PSE), 86
  tapeworm, 678–80
porphyrin, 436–7
portal circulation, 31–2
portal nodes, 38, 41
posterior mediastinal nodes, 38
post-mortem
  examination, 311
    BSE, 564–75
    current regime, 255
    decision-making, **252–5**
    improvement proposals, 255–8
    poultry, 269
  findings, 179
  inspection, 194, **244–58**
    EC procedure, 246–8
    poultry, 273
    rabbits, 290
  specimens, 362
post-parturient haemoglobinuria, 701
post-rinsing, 158
post-slaughter decontamination, 235–8
post-weaning diarrhoea, 520–1
potable water samples, 79, 361–2
potassium, 706
potassium peroxide (3%) test, 366–7
Potomac horse fever, 607
poultry, **14–16**
  ante-mortem inspection, 272–3
  bacterial diseases, **277–83**
  bruising, 284–5
  catching and crating, 264–5
  chilling, 271–2
  contamination, 270, 286
  dead-on-arrival, 284
  defeathering, 269
  disease, 274
    statistics, 734
  diseases of the female reproductive system, 286
  effects of stunning on meat quality, 213
  evisceration, 269–71
  feedingstuffs, 263
  flock health, 263
  fractures, 284–5
  frozen, 344
  fungal diseases, 283
  harvesting procedures, 264
  lairage, 265
  legislation, 266
  modular system, 265
  neck-cutting, 267–8
  neoplasms, 286
  parasitic diseases, 283–4
  pelleting of feed, 263
  post-mortem examination, 251, 269
  post-mortem inspection, 273
  preslaughter inspection, 266
  production, **261–87**, 272
  reception and unloading, 265–6
  scalding, 268–9
  shackling, 266
  skeleton, 23
  slaughter, 211–13, 262, 264, 266–8
    on-farm, 213
  spray-washing, 271
  stunning, 266–8
  tuberculosis, 282
  unfit for human consumption, 273–4
  viral diseases, **274–7**
Poultry Breeding Flocks and Hatchery Scheme Order 1994, 281
pour plates, 364
poussin, 262
  definition, 15
pox diseases, 590–1
practical storage life (PSL), 112
pre-packed foodstuffs, 353
pre-rinsing, 157
pre-slaughter
  check, 247
  feeding of sugars, 186
  handling and meat quality, **184–6**

pre-slaughter—*continued*
  handling/restraint, 197–9
  inspection, poultry, 266
  stress, 184–5
precipitin test, 56
precrural nodes, 39, 40
pregnancy, 461
  toxaemia of ewes, 700
prepectoral nodes, 36
prepuce, 491
prescapular nodes, 37, 40
preservatives, 125–7, 313
presternal calcification, 493
primal cuts, 116
primary photosensitisation, 702
prion disease *see* bovine spongiform encephalopathy (BSE)
probiotics, 7
Processed Animal Protein Order 1989, 263
processed foods
  durability, 353
  legislation, 353
progesterone, 309–11
prone sticking, 216
propanolol, 7
protective clothing, 224, 226
protein, 4, 59, 144–5, 147
  starvation, 703
Pro Ten Process, 73
proteoglycan, 71
*Proteus*, 106, 394
*Protostrongylus rufescens*, 295, 657
protozoa, 397–9, **616–34**
pseudo-cowpox, 592
pseudo-glanders, 533–4, 612
pseudomembranous inflammation, 425
*Pseudomonas*, 104, 106, 346, 394–5
*Pseudomonas* (*Malleomyces*) *mallei*, 528, 612
*Pseudomonas* (*Malleomyces*) *pseudomallei*, 533
pseudorabies, 556–7
pseudotuberculosis, 279, 554
  of rabbits, 292
psittacosis, 283, 414–15
psoroptic mange, 691
public health, 737
Public Health Act 1966, 411
Public Health (Control of Diseases) Act 1984, 321, 336
pullorum disease, 280
pulmonary abscesses, 473–4
pulmonary adenomatosis, 592–3
pulmonary circulation, 31
punctures, 409
purified-protein-derivative (PPD) tuberculin, 549
purple staining, 124
purulent inflammation, 425–6
purulent pericarditis, 476
pus, 362, 363
putty brisket, 493
pyaemia, 453
pyelonephritis, 484, 524
pyoderma, 428
pyometra, 488
pyosalpinx, 488
pyothorax, 426
pyrexia, 456

Q fever, 416, 608–9
  in man, 609
quail disease, 277
qualitative criteria, 240
quality assurance, 158, 244, 340–1
quality control, 238
  waste processing plants, 138
  *see also* HACCP; meat
quantitative criteria, 240
Query fever, 416, 608–9
quick chilling, 110

rabbit, **16**, **289–92**
  contamination, 292
  death before slaughter, 290
  fever, 419, 553–4
  inspection, 290
  meat, 16
  post-mortem inspection, 290
  processing plants, 16
  production, 289
  pseudotuberculosis, 292
  salmonellosis, 292
  slaughter, 289–90
  trimming, 292
  tuberculosis, 292
  tumours, 291
rabies, **593–5**
  control, 595
  tests, 595
radiation damage, 719–21
radioactive contamination, **719–23**
radioactivity monitoring, 721–2
rafoxanide, 314
ragwort, 711
rail vehicles, 174
ram
  bighead in, 515
  carcase, 54
  definition, 10
ramp angles, 173
rancidity, 106, 348
  fat, 407
  oxidative, 407
rapid methodologies, 343
reagents, storage, 403
rearing, definition, 13
receptaculum chyli, 34
recontamination, 155–6
records, ante-mortem, 192
rectum, 223
  cattle, 233
  pigs, 235
  sheep, 235
red blood cells, 33
red deer, 16–17
red dysentery in cattle, 620–1
red meat, inspection, **243–59**
red nose, 586
red offal room, 97
red squill, 717
red stomach worm, 642–3
reducing bodies, 61
redwater, 617–18
redworm infestation, 654–5
refractive index, 56
refrigerants, 112
refrigerated meat
  storage of, 113–14
  transport of, 113–14
refrigerated road vehicle, 113
refrigeration, **106–14**
  accommodation, 95
  EU regulations, 107–9
  instrumentation, 112
  mechanical, 109
regional ileitis, 466
reindeer, slaughter, 213
relative humidity, 179
  meters, 112
renal disease, 483
renal node, 38
rendering plants, inedible, **138–41**
renin, 41
reoviruses, 275
repetitive strain injury (RSI), 409
reproductive system, 42–4, 450, **487–91**
research, livestock, 461–2
residues
  antibacterial, 402
  antibiotic, 402
  kidney, 402
  sampling, 379–80
  sulfonamide, 402
  *see also* chemical residues
respiratory system, 29–31, **470–5**
Retail Animal Products Survey (RAPS), 304
retention cysts, 429
reticuloendotheliosis, 276
reticulum, 24, 465
  cell sarcoma, 578–80
retroperitoneum, 469–70
retropharyngeal nodes, 36
RF-tags, 729
rhabditiasis, 656
rhinitis, 410
rhinosporidiosis, 614
rhinotracheitis, turkeys, 275
*Rhipicephalus*, 617, 694
*Rhizopus*, 106
*Rhodococcus equi*, 395
ribs, 22
Richmond Committee, 167
rickets, 492
*Rickettsia*, 399
*Rickettsia phagocytophila*, 609
*Rickettsiae*, 465, 603–4
rida, 598
Rift Valley fever (RVF), 596
rigor mortis, 61–2, 115, 186
rind, 58
rinderpest, 596–8
ringworm, 292, 416–17, 614–15
rinse systems, 154–5, 341, 361
  high-pressure, 154
  low-pressure, 154
  medium-pressure, 154
ripening, 71
risk assessment, 252
  principles, 241
risk factors in food poisoning, 327
RNA, 19, 710
road vehicles, 174, 176
rodding, 235, 255
rodent glanders, 533–4
rodenticides, 717
roller strips, 245
Romagnola, 5
Romney Marsh, 9
rough handling, 187
roundworms, 636
rubbers, 145
rumen, 24, 465
ruminants
  gastrointestinal parasites of, **638–42**
  pneumonia of, 657–8

sacral nodes, 39
sacroplasmic proteins, 59
sacrum, 22
safety
  cleaning, 159
  helmets, 410
  *see also* health and safety
Salers, 5
*Salmonella*, 104, 115, 138, 170, 180, 251, 252, 263, 264, 325, 326, 328, 329–31, 344, 384–6, 540
  organisms, culture for, 280
*Salmonella cholerae suis*, 425
*Salmonella dublin*, 194, 329
*Salmonella enteritidis*, 271, 325, 329, 330, 452
  vaccination, 281
*Salmonella gallinarum*, 280
*Salmonella paratyphi*, 93
*Salmonella pullorum*, 279, 329, 330
*Salmonella typhi*, 329
*Salmonella typhimurium*, 93, 102, 325, 330, 331
*Salmonella* v. *arizona*, 281
*Salmonella virchow*, 330
salmonellosis, 180, 279–81, 466, 539–42
  rabbits, 292
salpingitis, 279, 488
salt, 103
samples, 356–7
  carcase, 341
  chemical residues, 305
  collection, 303–4, 403, 711
  despatch to approved laboratories, 649
  storage, 363
  transport, 363

sampling, **356–63**
  air, 362
  plans, 358, 359
  residue, 379–80
  techniques, **359–63**
San Miguel sea lion virus disease, 602
sanitation, plant, **143–62**
saponification of fats, oils and greases, 147
*Sarcocystis*, 495, 623
sarcocystosis, 623–5
sarcoma, 276, 287
sarcoptic mange, 691
sarcosporidiosis, 623–5
sausage, 347–8
  casings, 130
sawdust livers, 535
scabbard, hygienic use, 229
scalding, pig, 93
*Schistosoma mattheei*, 485
schistosomiasis, 686–7
Schwann cells, 44
scientific experiments, 195
scotoma, 144
scours, 519–20
scrapie, 598–9
scrapie-associated fibrils (SAF), 599
screening, 140–1
  tests, 310
screwworm infestation, 691–2
secondary photosensitisation, 702
security arrangements, 98
selenium, 317, 706, 717–18
self-adhesive cellophane tapes or labels, 360
semi-solid cultures, 364
*Senecio jacobaea*, 711
septic pericarditis, 476
septic shock, 455
septicaemia, 254, 274, 287, 451–3, 532, 541
  clinical signs and lesions, 452
  diagnosis, 452
  judgement of, 452
  neonatorum, 519–20
  of equidae, 538
septicaemic colibacillosis, 520
septicaemic pasteurellosis, 539
serous fluids, 363
serous inflammation, 426
*Setaria* spp., 485
sewage sludge, 171
sex determination, 53–5
sex hormones, 48
sexual odour, 67–8
shackle washer, 269
shake cultures, 364
sharp freezers, 111
sheath rot, 525
sheep, **8–10**
  adrenals, 47
  age, 22
  blowfly strike, 692
  breeds, 8–10
  carcase, 54, 55
  condemnation, 732, 733
  contagious agalactia, 522–3
  Downland, 9
  dressing, 230–2
  fat, 131
  foot rot of, 534
  heart, 31
  hill breeds, 8–9
  identification and registration, 736
  interdigital dermatitis (scald) in, 535
  internal parasitism, 166
  kidneys, 42
  lairage, 85, 182
  liver, 27
  lowland breeds, 9
  lungs, 30
  Nairobi sheep disease (NSD), 587–8
  nematodes in, 640
  parasitic gastroenteritis of, 640–2
  pneumonic pasteurellosis of, 539
  polyarthritis, 528
  post-mortem examination, 250
  production, 9–10
  records, 736
  rectum, 235
  slaughter, 166, 215
  slaughter hall, 92
  spleen, 34
  stomach, 25
  tapeworms, 659
  teeth, 52
  thyroid, 46
  tongue, 23
  tuberculosis, 546
  viscera, 25
sheep dips, 313
sheep ked, 692
sheep nostril or nasal fly, 692
sheeppox, 591
sheeppox virus (SPV), 591
shellfish toxin, 318
*Shigella*, 386
shipping fever, 179, 538–9
Shorthorn, 5, 6
shrinkage, 101, 111
Simmental, 5
*Simondsia paradoxa*, 643
skeletal disorders, 493
skeletal system, **491–5**
skeleton, 21
  ox, 20
  poultry, 23
skin, 50, 96, 166, 223, 450, **462–4**
  by-products treatment, 135–6
  diseases, 411, 462
    diagnosis, 463
  lesions, 250, 463
  leukosis, 580
  rashes, 410
  sepsis, 417–18
  tuberculosis, 550
slaughter, **163–96**
  assessment of unconsciousness, 199–200
  casualty, 192
  deer, 293
  emergency, 192–4
  fasting prior to, 183
  hall, **87–99**
    bleeding area, 88
    condemned meat room, 96
    cutting rooms, 97
    detained meat room, 96
    edible fat room, 97
    emergency unit, 95
    environment, 224–5
    equipment wash, 97
    fresh meat dispatch area, 97
    gut and tripe room, 96–7
    hide and skin store, 96
    inedible area, 97
    isolation block, 95
    layout and flowlines, 229–30
    manure bay, 97–8
    on-the-rail dressing, 89–92
    personnel facilities, 98
    pig, 92–4
    red offal room, 97
    refrigeration accommodation, 95
    sheep, 92
    stunning area, 87–8
    vehicle washing, 98
    veterinary laboratory, 99
    veterinary office, 98–9
  humane, **197–222**
  Jewish, 217–20
  lambs, 225
  legislation, 213–15
  licence, 199
  miscellaneous methods, 213–14
  mobile facility, 83
  Muslim, 220–1
  ostriches, 298
  pigs, 215–16
  poultry, 211–13, 262, 264, 266–8
    on-farm, 213
  process, 199
  programme, 245
  rabbits, 289–90
  religious, 217
  resting of animal prior to, 183–4
  sheep, 166, 215
  transport to, 173
  *see also* pre-slaughter
sleeping sickness, 633
slide catalase test, 367
slides, 369–73
slit samplers, 362
slurry, 169–70
smears, 369–73
snail fever, 686–7
snow moulds, 351
social stress, 182
sodium ascorbate, 105
sodium chloride, 103, 704, 718
sodium fluoroacetate/fluoroacetamide, 717
soils, 144–5
solid carbon dioxide, 113
solubilisation, 147
sore mouth, 577–8
sour side, 347
souring, 349
South Africa, *Cysticercus bovis* inspection procedure, 677
sow
  definition, 13
  udder, 44
  uterus, 43
species identification tests, **55–9**
specified bovine material (SBM), 130, 563
Specified Risk Material, 248
specified risk material (SRM), 131
specimens
  identification, 363
  parasite collection, 399–400
*Sphaerophorus necrophorus*, 454, 578
spinal cord, 45, 500
spine, 21
spiramycin, 306
spirochaetales, 399
spirochaetosis, 291
*Spirometra mansoni*, 660
*Spirometra mansonoides*, 660
spleen, 33, 248, 254, 482–3
  cattle, 249
  tuberculosis, 547
splenic lymph nodes, 38
spoilage, 106, **344–53**, 407
  canning, 122–4
sponges, 341
Spongiform Encephalopathy Advisory Committee (SEAC), 563
spores, 403
  staining of, 370
sporocyst, 638
*Sporothrix schenckii*, 615
sporotrichosis, 615–16
spray chillers, 272
spray cleaning, 152
spray-washing, poultry, 271
squab, production, 298
squamous cell carcinoma, 287, 449
stab cultures, 364
staff, self-declaration form, 228
stag, 53
  definition, 8
staining, 369–73
  of spores, 370
  techniques, 370
stainless hollow knife, 88
stainless steel, 145
stains, 396
  types, 370
standard plate count (SPC), 357
*Staphylococcus*, 125, 328, 345, 386–7
*Staphylococcus aureus*, 102, 252, 254, 278, 326, 328, 334, 422, 451, 543
*Staphylococcus hyicus*, 543
starches, 145
starvation, 459
static water chillers, 272
steam extraction, 79
steam hoses, 154
steam pasteurisation, 236

steam sterilisation, 237
steam vacuum sterilisation process, 237
steel, hygienic use, 229
steer, 6, 53
  definition, 8
*Stephanurus dentatus*, 485, 645
sterilisation, 92, 236
  knives, 227–8
sternum, 22
steroids, 309
sticking point, 224
stiff lamb disease, 706
stilbene, 309
stockmanship, 166
stomach, 23–6, 130, 223
  by-products treatment, 131–3
  cattle, 249
storage
  fresh meat, 116
  refrigerated meat, 113–14
  temperatures, 112
strawberry foot rot, 524–5, 613–14
streak for colony isolation, 374
streak plates, 364
streptococcosis, 418
*Streptococcus*, 125, 345, 395
*Streptococcus faecalis*, 249
*Streptococcus liquefaciens*, 123
*Streptococcus pneumoniae*, 451
*Streptococcus pyogenes*, 451
*Streptococcus suis* type 2, 418
*Streptococcus zooepidemicus*, 418
*Streptomyces avermitilis*, 314
streptomycin, 306
stress, 457
  and meat quality, 185–6
  pre-slaughter, 184–5
*Strongyloides ransomi*, 644–5
strongylosis (strongylidosis) of equidae, 654–5
*Strongylus edentatus*, 655
*Strongylus equinus*, 655
*Strongylus vulgaris*, 654–5
structured surveys, 303
*Struthio camelus*, 296
strychnine, 717
stunning, 198, 199
  and meat quality, 211
  area, 87–8
  box, 198
    design and bruising, 188
  cattle, 214–15
  deer, 294
  effectiveness, 200
  electrical, 200, 208–12, 266–7, 290
    high-voltage, 210
    low-voltage, 210, 212
  gas, 267
  head to back/leg, 210–11
  mechanical, 201, 268
  methods, **200–11**
  non-penetrative percussion, 202
  ostriches, 297
  pen, 88
  percussive, 200–5
    head sites, 202–5
  pigs, 198
  pneumatic, 202
  poultry, 266–8
  water-bath, 267
  water-jet, 205
subcutis diseases, 463–4
subdorsal node, 37
submaxillary nodes, 36, 40
subprimal cuts, 116
substrates, 145
Suffolk-cross, 10
sugars
  fermentation, 375
  pre-slaughter feeding, 186
sulfonamide residues, 402
sulphiding, 118
sulphonamides, 303, 306
sulphur, 704
superficial inguinal (male) nodes, 39
superficial samples, 341
supramammary (female) nodes, 39
suprasternal node, 37
surface contact or impression plate, 361
surface materials, 145
surface plate method, 357
surface slices, 341
surfaces, contamination, 156
surra, 631–3
suspended solids, 140
swabs, 341, 359–60, 403
swamp fever, 581
sweating, 101
Sweden, meat inspection recording, 727
sweep plate technique, 361
swine
  cysticercosis, 678–80
  dysentery, 542–3
  erysipelas, 249, 526–8
  fever (SF), 599–600
  herd disease, 413
  herd fever, 530–1
  influenza, 600–1
  vesicular disease (SVD), 601
  vesicular exanthema of, 602
swinepox, 592
swollen head syndrome (SHS), 275
sympathetic system, 46
*Syngamus trachea*, 284
syringomyelia, 500
systemic circulation, 31
systemic disturbance, 191
systems, 19

T *lymphocytes*, 423
*Taenia hydatigena*, 295, 665–6
*Taenia marginata*, 665–6
*Taenia multiceps*, 666–7
*Taenia ovis*, 667–8
*Taenia pisiformis*, 291, 668
*Taenia saginata*, 248, **669–74**, 678–80
*Taenia serialis*, 291, 669
*Taenia solium*, 678–80
*Taenia taeniaeformis*, 291
taeniasis, **669–74**, 678–80
taint, 65–9
  in fat, 349
  in hams, 349–50
Talfan disease, 603
Tamworth, 12
tanning, 136
tapeworms, 284, 636, 658–60
  asses, 659
  cattle, 659
  dog, 659
  goats, 659
  horses, 659
  mules, 659
  sheep, 659
TCDD, 714–15
teeth, 52–3
telangiectasis, 467–8
temperament and bruising, 188
temperature, 191
  control, 179
  indicator-recorders, 110
  indicators, 112
  recording facilities, 95
  water, 155
tendercut process, 72
tenderising, **71–4**
  by electrical stimulation, 72–3
  by infusion of calcium chloride, 73
  pre-slaughter, 73–4
tenderness of meat, 71
tenderstretch method of hanging beef sides, 72
tenosynovitis, 275
terminal ileitis, 466
terminal rinsing, 158
terrazzo, 145
Teschen disease, 603
testes, 48, 250, 490–1
  fowl, 44
testosterone, 309, 310, 311
tetanus (lockjaw), 418–19, 518–19
tetanus toxoid, 409
tetrachlorodibenzodioxin, 714–15
tetracyclines, 306
Texas fever, 617–18
thallium sulphate, 717
*Thamnidium*, 352
thawed frozen meat, 406–7
*Theileria*, 398, 625, 627–8
*Theileria parva*, 625, 626
theileriosis, 625
thelaziasis, 657
therapeutic products, 299
thermal energy, 146
thermal processing *see* heat-thermal processing
thiabendazole, 314, 315
thin ewe syndrome, 514
thin-layer chromatography, 308
thiobarbituric acid (TBA), 349
thoracic duct, 34
thorny-headed worm of pigs, 644
three-day sickness, 581–2
thrombocytes, 33
thrombosis, 442
thrush, 283, 612–13
*Thuga accidentalis*, 412
thymic leukosis, 580
thymus, 47, 483
thyroid, 46
tibia sours, 350
tick pyaemia, 543
tick-borne diseases, 617
tick-borne fever (TBF), 609
tick-borne meningopolyneuritis, 415–16
ticks, 692–4
tilmicosin, 306
tinea, 416–17, 614–15
tissue factor, 442
tissues, 19
Toggenburg, 14
toilet facilities, 87
toilet rooms, 98
tongue, 23
torulosis, 611–12
total count agar (TCA), 342–3
total viable count (TVC), 344, 357
toxaemia, 274, 455
toxic goitre, 46
toxic shock, 455
toxic substances, 710
toxins, 318, 421, 463, 465, 467, 710
*Toxoplasma*, 398
*Toxoplasma gondii*, 629–30
toxoplasmosis, 628–9
tracheitis, 471
training, cleaning, 159
tranquillisers, 300
transit erythema, 463
transit fever, 179, 538–9
Transit of Animals Order 1927, 177
Transit of Animals (Road and Rail) Order 1975 (amended 1988; 1992), 173–5
transit tetany, 179
transmissible gastroenteritis (TGE), 601–2
transmissible mink encephalopathy (TME), 559
transmissible spongiform encephalopathies (TSEs), 559
transponders, 245
transport, 166
  air-conditioned vehicles, 176
  conditions induced by, 179
  fresh meat, 107
  journey plan, 174
  legislation, 173–4
  livestock, 172–80
    loading/unloading, 172–3, 175
  loading/unloading, 188
  loss of weight during, 177–8
  mortality, 178–9
  refrigerated meat, 113–14
  separation of animals, 175
  unfit animal, 174

Transport of Animals (General) Order 1973 (amended 1988; 1992), 175–7
traps, 80
traumatic injury, **187–9**
traumatic reticuloperitonitis, 469
travel oedema, 63
trematodes, 636, 637, **680–8**
tremblante du mouton *see* scrapie
trenbolone, 309, 310
*Treponema*, 395–6
*Treponema hyodysenteriae*, 542–3
*Treponema pallidum*, 415
trichinae, laboratory methods, 648–9
*Trichinella*, 116
*Trichinella* cysts, 646–7
*Trichinella spiralis*, 645
trichinellosis, **645–8**
  control, 652
trichiniasis, **645–8**
trichinoscope, 648–9
trichinosis, **645–8**
*Trichomonas*, 628
*Trichomonas foetus*, 398, 627
trichomoniasis, 627–8
*Trichophyton*, 614
*Trichophyton mentagrophytes* var. *granulare*, 292
trichophytosis, 416–17, 614–15
*Trichuris suis*, 653
*Trichuris trichiura*, 94
triclabendazole, 315
trimethoprim, 306
trimming
  contamination, 237
  rabbits, 292
tripe, 132–3
trisodium phosphate, 237, 272
tropical theileriosis, 626–7
true sweetbread, 47
*Trypanosoma gambiense*, 634
*Trypanosoma rhodesiense*, 634
*Trypanosoma (Schizotrypanum) cruzi*, 633
trypanosomes, 630–4
trypanosomiasis, 629–4
tsetse fly-transmitted African trypanosomiasis, 630–2
tube coagulase test, 368
tuberculin test, 549
tuberculosis, 249, 250, 460, 476, 490, 543–53
  affections of specific organs, 546–9
  alimentary tract, 547
  bones, 548
  cattle, 545, 546, 548
  central nervous system, 548
  deer, 295
  differential diagnosis, 549–51, 550
  genitalia, 548
  goats, 546
  horses, 545
  joints, 548
  judgement, 551–3
  kidneys, 547
  lesions, 545
  liver, 547
  muscle, 548
  pathogenesis, 545
  pericardium, 547
  peritoneum, 547
  pigs, 545
  pleura, 547
  poultry, 282
  rabbits, 292
  reactions in different species, 546
  sheep, 546
  skin, 550–1
  spleen, 547
  udder, 548
tuberculous enteritis, 545
tuberculous meningitis, 500, 545
tuberculous meningoencephalitis, 548
tularaemia, 419, 553–4
tumour, **446–50**, 474, 475, 478, 482, 486–90, 493, 494, 499, 500, 502, 579
  rabbits, 291
tup, definition, 10
turbinate atrophy of pigs, 509–10
turkey, 15, 266, 272
  arizonosis, 281
  cholera, 278
  egg kidney, 600
  lymphoproliferative disease, 276–7
  rhinotracheitis, 275
turkey haemorrhagic enteritis (THE), 275–6
twinning, 2
tylosin, 306
*Tyzzeria* spp., 399
Tyzzer's disease, 291

udder, 44, 249–50
  tuberculosis, 548
UK Fresh Meat Directive 1995, 226
ulcer, 428
ulcerative enteritis, 277
ultraviolet radiation, 126
umbilical cord, 32
unconsciousness, assessment, 199
undulant fever, 511
unfit for human consumption, poultry, 273–4
United States of America, *Cysticercus bovis* inspection procedure, 676–7
upper cervical nodes, 40
uraemia, 486
urea, 58, 712, 715
urease test, 369, 375
ureter, 41, 486–7
urethra, 41, 486–7
*Urginea maritima*, 717
urinary calculi, 485
urinary organs, 41
urinary system, **483–7**
urine, 363, 486
urogenital system, 41–2
USDA regulations, 191–2
use by date, 354
utensils, contamination, 224
uterus, 42–4, 488–9
  cattle, 249

vaccination, *Salmonella enteriditis*, 281
vaccinia, 591
vacuolar degeneration, 439
vacuum packing, 70, 113
vagina, 489
variolae, 590–1
variolovaccinia, 591
vasculitis, 441
veal calves, 7
vegetable protein products, 4
vegetarians, 4
vehicle
  design, 188
  washing, 98
veins, 441
venepuncture, 564
venison, 72
ventilation, 79
  meat plant, 81
ventral, 20
vents, 80
verification checks, 240
vermin, 225
verminous bronchitis, 657–8
verotoxin-producing *Escherichia coli* (VTEC), 332–3
vertebral column, 21
vesicle, 428
vesicular exanthema of swine (VES), 602
vesicular stomatitis, 602–3
veterinary laboratory, 99
Veterinary Medicines Directorate, 304–5
veterinary office, 98–9
*Vibrio*, 387–8
*Vibrio parahaemolyticus*, 335
vibrionic dysentery, 542–3
vices, 285
viraemia, 451
viral diseases, 471
viral encephalomyelitis of pigs, 603
viral papular dermatitis, 603
viral papular stomatitis, 603
viral poultry diseases, **274–7**
viruses, 328, 421, 463, 465, 467
viscera
  bull, 25
  inspection table, 88
  missing, 292
  sheep, 25
vision system, 728
vitamin, 60
  deficiencies, 707
vitamin A, 707
vitamin B, 707
vitamin C, 707
vitamin D, 707
vitamin E, 706
vitamin K, 707
Voges–Proskauer test, 375–6
volatile fatty acids (VFA), 141
vulva, 489

wapita, 17
warble fly, 295, 694–6
warfarin, 717
warthog disease, 555–6
washes, 341, 361
washing
  lambs, 225
  livestock, 87
  machine, 152
  offals, 238
  pre-slaughter, 168
waste, high- and low-risk, 136
waste disposal, 168, 715
waste processing plants
  hygiene requirements for, 137–8
  quality control, 138
waste water disposal system, 80
water, 58–9, 321
  activity, 102
  availability, 102
  contaminated, 155, 225, 236
  content of meat and offal, 345
  lairage, 84
  meat plant, 80
  non-potable, 79
  potable, 79, 361–2
  temperatures, 155
water buffalo, 5
watering, lairage, 182
watery pork, 63–4
wax stripping, ducks, 269
weaner, definition, 13
weeping, 115
Weil's disease, 413, 530–1
Welfare of Animals during Transport Order 1994, 192
Welfare of Animals during Transport Order 1994 (with amendments), 174
Welfare of Animals (Northern Ireland) Act 1972, 171
Welfare of Poultry (Transport) Order 1988 (amended 1989; 1992), 175
Welsh, 12
western duck disease *see* botulism
wet carcase syndrome, 499
wet preparation (hanging drop), 380–1
wether
  carcase, 54
  definition, 10
wetting, 146
whipworm, 94
whiskers, 352
white blood cells, 33
white liver disease, 468
white muscle disease (WMD), 496, 706
white spot, 351–2
Whitmore's disease, 533–4
wholesome food, 57
Wholesome Meat Act, 190
wild animals, 1

wild boar, 2, 11
wind chill chart, 179
wings, 23
withdrawal periods, 168
wooden tongue *see* actinomycosis
Wood's lamp, 396
wool, 8, 9
work-station, layout, 230
World Health Organisation (WHO), 108, 227
worm nodule disease, 653
wound repair, 428
Wright–Giemsa stain, 372

xanthosis, 437
xiphoid (ventral mediastinal) node, 38

yeasts, 342, 396
yellow fat, 65, 438
*Yersinia*, 388
*Yersinia enterocolitica*, 252, 333, 388, 554
*Yersinia pestis*, 554
*Yersinia pseudotuberculosis*, 279, 554
yersiniosis, 554
yoghurt, 14

Zebu, 5, 6
Zenker's necrosis, 431
zeranol, 309, 310
Ziehl–Neelsen stain, 371–2
zinc, 145, 718
zone of maximum ice formation, 114
zoonoses, 292, 411
*Zoonosis*, 608
zygomycosis, 613